Neuropathologic Evaluation

From Pathologic Features to Diagnosis

Neuropathologic Evaluation

From Pathologic Features to Diagnosis

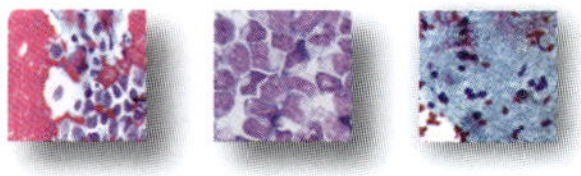

MURAT GOKDEN, M.D.
Professor of Pathology
Director of Neuropathology
Department of Pathology
University of Arkansas for Medical Sciences
Little Rock, Arkansas

Wolters Kluwer | Lippincott Williams & Wilkins
Health
Philadelphia • Baltimore • New York • London
Buenos Aires • Hong Kong • Sydney • Tokyo

Acquisitions Editor: Ryan Shaw
Senior Product Manager: Julia Seto
Vendor Manager: Bridgett Dougherty
Senior Manufacturing Manager: Benjamin Rivera
Senior Marketing Manager: Caroline Foote
Senior Designer: Stephen Druding
Production Service: SPi Global

Two Commerce Square
2001 Market Street
Philadelphia, PA 19103 USA
LWW.com

Printed in China

Library of Congress Cataloging-in-Publication Data
Gokden, Murat.
Neuropathologic evaluation: from pathologic features to diagnosis / Murat Gokden.
p. ; cm.
Includes bibliographical references and index.
ISBN 978-1-4511-1655-7
I. Title.
[DNLM: 1. Nervous System Diseases—diagnosis. 2. Nervous System Diseases—pathology. WL 141]
616.8'0475—dc23
2012020849

---

10 9 8 7 6 5 4 3 2 1

CCS1012

In memory of my late father, Abdurrahman Gokden, M.D.

Preface

"What do you see and what does it mean?"
H.T. Karsner, M.D.[1]

When a patient presents to a clinic, our clinical colleagues evaluate that patient's signs and symptoms through a systematic history taking and physical examination, sort through pertinent differential diagnoses, and formulate a working diagnosis for further investigation utilizing additional resources, including clinical laboratory, radiology, and biopsy, to make a diagnosis. If a tissue sample is obtained and sent to pathology, an analogous process takes place. The patient presents with particular tissue changes to the pathologist, who evaluates these changes grossly and microscopically to identify particular findings, leading to a list of differential diagnostic possibilities that need to be further investigated and sorted out by utilizing special techniques such as special stains, molecular diagnostic techniques, and electron microscopy, to make a diagnosis. No patient presents to the clinic with a diagnosis of cerebral infarct, but likely with hemiplegia or mental status changes; no tissue presents to the pathologist with a diagnosis of oligodendroglioma, but with a cellular lesion with round nuclei and clear cytoplasms, both of which can be seen in several other pathologic processes. Each simple alteration in a cell represents a complex underlying biologic process. The more accurately we, as diagnosticians, can recognize such changes, the closer we can bring the advances in basic science to our patients and the more positively we can influence their management. Identification of morphologic changes remains the mainstay in this quest and will likely continue to do so for many years to come in spite of all the progress made in many other areas.[2,3] It was with these ideas that my personal attempts to systematically organize gross and microscopic findings and put in writing the diagnostic thinking process eventually transformed into this text.

There are many great and comprehensive books covering all components of neuropathology, both neoplastic and nonneoplastic, with emphasis on diagnostic and basic science aspects, organized in a way to cover various entities in great detail. The purpose of this book is not to provide yet another neuropathology book or to compete with well-established texts, but to complement the available knowledge by focusing on its practical diagnostic application as it occurs in routine neuropathologic evaluation. This way, *Neuropathologic Evaluation from Pathologic Features to Diagnosis* is expected to provide a guide for further reading and investigation based on the findings identified in the tissue. Though the contents of this book are second nature to many experienced neuropathologists, not every neuropathologist practices all aspects of neuropathology at all times, and therefore they too may benefit from the availability of a quick reference in unusual situations. Neuropathology, with its broad coverage of neoplastic, nonneoplastic, forensic, autopsy, neuromuscular, and pediatric fields, studying a system with complex anatomic features and cell populations quite different than the usual epithelial and mesenchymal cells common to other body sites, and with frequent involvement by systemic processes, may be intimidating

[1]Vogel FS. Satisfactions and uncertainties that frequent an extended life. *J Neuropathol Exp Neurol*. 2010;69:207–213.

[2]Rosai J. The continuing role of morphology in the molecular age. *Mod Pathol*. 2001;14:258–260.

[3]Rosai J. Why microscopy will remain a cornerstone of surgical pathology. *Lab Invest*. 2007;87:403–408.

to those who are not specifically trained in or have not developed some experience by practicing it. I believe that the approach taken in this book will prove useful for the nonneuropathologists in their diagnostic practice, for the neuropathology and pathology trainees to make sense out of various tissue changes, and for any others who need a source for quick practical reference and review. With these thoughts in mind, it is organized according to gross and microscopic findings the tissues present to us and discusses the differential diagnoses for these findings and some details of specific entities when relevant. Since it is intended primarily to be a quick reference source, to provide the information as concisely as possible for any given finding and related entity, some repetition and overlap among various explanations were allowed. When possible, references were selected from broad review papers to provide further reading on the specific entities.

Approximately 70% of this book was written on personal time, that is, after hours, weekends, and "vacations," without taking extra time from routine work responsibilities, but by taking that time away from my family, my wife, Neriman Gokden, M.D., and my son, Alper Gokden, loved ones, friends... I would like to thank all of them for sharing the fun times and frustrations and for their support, patience, and understanding throughout my virtual absence for over 1.5 years. I have been very fortunate to have come in contact with too many influential individuals to thank in this limited space, making me strongly believe in retrospect that the best thing one individual can do for another is to simply provide an opportunity for the better. First and foremost, I would like to express my gratitude to my parents: my mother, Nebahat Gokden, and my father, Abdurrahman Gokden, M.D., my first teachers in life. I am grateful to M. Serefettin Canda, M.D., and Tulay Canda, M.D., my first teachers in pathology at Dokuz Eylul Medical School, Izmir, Turkey, who somehow managed to inspire me to the specialty of pathology and to academia. I am indebted to my mentors, Robert E. Schmidt, M.D., Ph.D., Kevin A. Roth, M.D., Ph.D., and Steven L. Carroll, M.D., Ph.D., in the Division of Neuropathology, Washington University School of Medicine, St. Louis, Missouri, for the opportunity to become a part of this great subspecialty through their effective training by example and humility. Taking pictures of specimens was part of the culture and a joy I was introduced to there. Many are used in this book. Thank you, Bob, also for asking me if I still wanted to start neuropathology in my 3rd year of residency. That was certainly encouraging. I have received invaluable support as a neuropathologist from my senior neuropathology colleagues, Robert E. Mrak, M.D., Ph.D., and Muhammad M. Husain, M.D., at the University of Arkansas for Medical Sciences, Little Rock, Arkansas, as well as all neuropathologists I have met, and continued to learn from them. Thank you! I would like to thank Donald E. Sandlin and Sara L. Thompson, M.Ed., for their administrative assistance with formatting of the text and pictures. Last but not the least, many thanks to the editors and other professionals at Lippincott Williams & Wilkins for their expertise and for making the realization of this work possible.

Never does a work attain the heights of our desires.[4] I hope that it is useful to all those who study and practice neuropathology.

Murat Gokden

---

[4] Marinoni A. *España*. New York: The Macmillan Company; 1926.

Contents

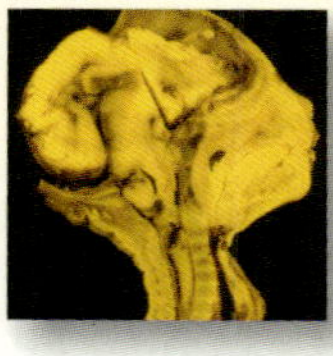 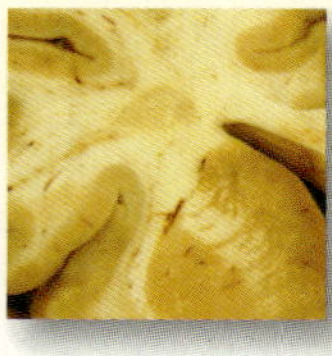 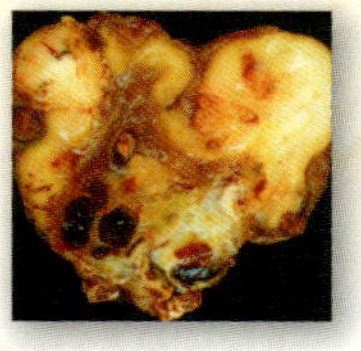

CHAPTER 1

Gross Features

Introduction

This chapter focuses on a variety of gross features. For all practical intents and purposes, gross neuropathology has become more and more limited to autopsy neuropathology, paralleling the progress made in premortem diagnostic and surgical techniques. The progress in research and diagnostic neuropathology has allowed the neuropathologist to be able to diagnose more complex diseases more accurately and with even smaller amount of tissue, taking the advantage of many special stains and molecular diagnostic techniques. Additional complex social, financial, and legal issues have also played a role in the dramatic decrease in autopsy numbers. All these factors combined, the volume of autopsy, and therefore gross neuropathology, has diminished significantly, even though its role in medical practice and education has become all the more important. As a reflection of these changes, pathology and even neuropathology training have been affected, some graduates potentially not feeling as comfortable with nonneoplastic/autopsy neuropathology as they do with surgical neuropathology. This section aims to provide a general understanding of gross findings and what they mean. As such, they are discussed mainly in the context of autopsy material. Knowledge of the general gross features of the disease processes is certainly very helpful in correlations with radiologic findings, approaching the surgical specimens (see "Surgical Specimens" below) and even in the interpretation of microscopic findings, the latter being especially important in the context of intraoperative consultation (IOC). An attempt is shown to organize the content in a somewhat real-life pattern, starting from the skin, as one would do at autopsy, and avoid repetitions among sections as much as possible. As a result, some findings that are expected to be discussed in one section may be found in a more specific section; for example, basal ganglionic hemorrhage in "parenchymal hemorrhage" instead of "cut surfaces." This chapter and Chapter 4 "Radiologic Features" complement each other.

Even though the component organs of the central nervous system (CNS) are referred to as individual organs, they are actually composed of substructures that are grouped together to form subsystems organized functionally and anatomically. Based on the principle of selective vulnerability, in most situations, a disease process involves one or more of these subsystems, rather than the entire brain, resulting in quite specific and highly predictable changes, both morphologically and clinically. Therefore, there is an amazing logical clinicopathologic correlation that can be demonstrated in many of these pathologic conditions. As a result, gross examination of the CNS structures is more involved than just the traditionally so-called brain cutting, which is essentially "gross neuropathologic examination," and is more than just simply "serial sectioning" and submitting "representative sections" for microscopic examination. In a given scenario, one may have to be prepared with the details of the clinical and radiologic findings and equipped with adequate neuroanatomic knowledge to modify the gross examination approach to identify and examine certain structures. For any deviation from normal and especially subtle abnormalities to be identified, one has to be familiar with the normal appearances and variations of normal.

Skin and External Findings

Changes in the skin may provide clues for further examination. These typically have already been identified and can be found in clinical notes; however, it is important to search for them for documentation and to guide the neuropathologic evaluation. It has to be remembered that the time of autopsy is the only chance for the pathologist to examine the skin.

Ecchymoses, abrasions, lacerations, and *avulsions* are typically associated with *blunt force* impact, while stab wounds and gunshot wounds are *penetrating injuries*. They point to potential areas of pathologic findings in the underlying structures. These findings need to be evaluated altogether to provide useful information to reconstruct the premortem events, especially in medicolegal and forensic cases. They can help interpret brain contusions for coup versus contrecoup injury, whether the head was in motion and whether the individual was conscious, even though forensic case construction is a complicated process that is dependent on many factors, including the scene information. Nonetheless, an external sign of trauma should be an indication to specifically look for internal injury, including hemorrhages in various compartments, fractures, and evaluation of the opposite side of the brain for injury as part of a contrecoup injury. In general, several practical rules should be kept in mind. *Coup injury* occurs on the same side of the brain as the impact, and the head is still at the time of the impact, for example, when hit while sitting. *Contrecoup injury* occurs on the side of the brain opposite to the impact, and the head is in motion at the time of the impact, for example, when falling on the ground.[1,2] An individual tends to fall backward while conscious, making occipital head injury more

List of Findings/Checklist for Skin and External Findings

• AT A GLANCE

- *Trauma*
  - Ecchymosis
  - Abrasion
  - Laceration
  - Avulsion
  - Blunt force trauma
  - Penetrating trauma
  - Coup injury
  - Contrecoup injury
  - Scar
  - Caput succedaneum
- *Vascular lesions*
  - Deep-seated hematoma
  - Periorbital hematoma
  - Hemangioma
  - Vascular malformation
- *Skin lesions*
  - Hypomelanotic macules
  - Hypomelanosis of Ito
  - Livedo reticularis
  - Basal cell carcinoma and other skin cancers
  - Dyskeratotic pits
  - Café-au-lait spots
  - Epidermoid cyst
  - Sebaceous tumor
  - Trichilemmoma
  - Nodules
  - Freckles
  - Nevi
  - Nevus of Ota
  - Hyperpigmentation
  - Skin tag/dimple
  - Pilonidal sinus/cyst
  - Hairy patch
- *Mass lesions*
  - Peripheral nerve sheath tumor
  - Myxoma
  - Meningioma
  - Meningocele
  - Meningoencephalocele
  - Meningomyelocele
  - Lipoma
- *Others*
  - Dysmorphic features
  - Cyclopia
  - Proboscis
  - Anencephaly
  - Rachischisis
  - Head size/circumference
  - General appearance
  - Eyes, iris, lens
  - Cerebrospinal fluid leak

likely, and forward when unconscious, making frontal/facial injury more likely. The location, size, shape, number, and pattern of the skin lesion and the characteristics of its edges should be documented by diagrams and pictures. This may require shaving the hair for better examination and documentation. In the case of gunshot wounds, it is also important to identify entry and exit wounds, where applicable. Dating of *contusions* based on their color, as color is variable based on the depth, skin pigmentation, and size of the lesion, may not be accurate. Microscopic examination may provide better means of determining the age of the lesion. The great majority of these cases are forensic and are handled by forensic pathologists at the medical examiner's office or crime laboratory. In some institutions, autopsy pathologists, as well as neuropathologists, also handle forensic autopsies. In addition, in situations where the victim died after being admitted to and received care at a hospital, autopsy examination may rest on the shoulders of the pathologist in that institution. Therefore, a basic conceptual knowledge of how to handle these situations is necessary for the neuropathologist, even though its details are beyond the scope of this text. In medical autopsies, previous surgical *scars* can also serve as indicators of underlying pathology or history thereof. Old or recent scars, their location and extent, whether they are infected or bleeding are points that may potentially help with subsequent steps such as looking for infection/sepsis, submitting wound cultures, or raising the possibility of bleeding/clotting disorders. In the context of surgical procedures, the presence of shunts and catheters should be noted. *Caput succedaneum* is a self-limited hemorrhagic edematous accumulation in the subcutaneous tissues of the scalp due to birth trauma.

Aside from contusions, *discolorations in skin* may indicate *deep-seated hematomas*. Especially hemorrhage that occurs in the tight scalp may track along the tissue planes and accumulate in areas of the face and neck, where skin and soft tissues are loose. Therefore, they may indicate a more serious pathology in the underlying tissues elsewhere, including the brain. *Periorbital hematoma* (raccoon eyes, black eyes, spectacle ecchymoses) is a sign of skull base fracture, especially those involving orbits. *Vascular lesions* in the skin may be associated with syndromes that have nervous system components,[3] that is, neurocutaneous syndromes or phakomatoses **(Table 1.1)**. Sturge-Weber syndrome (encephalofacial angiomatosis) consists of *capillary hemangioma* in the skin of the trigeminal nerve distribution, ocular angioma, and meningeal angiomatosis. It is reported that the brain is not involved if the vascular nevus does not involve the ophthalmic branch distribution of the trigeminal nerve.[4] Ataxia telangiectasia[5] is characterized by *telangiectasias* of the skin and conjunctiva, immune system impairment, and predisposition to develop various malignancies, including hematolymphoid malignancies, melanoma, carcinomas, and primary brain neoplasms. Telangiectasia in skin and sclera appears by the end of the first decade, usually earlier, but ataxia is typically present from the beginning of walking. *Cutaneous arteriovenous malformation (AVM)* may be associated with Wyburn-Mason syndrome,[6] which also includes retinal, cerebral, mandibular, or maxillary AVMs. AVMs can also be a component of Osler-Rendu-Weber syndrome (hereditary hemorrhagic telangiectasia), along with mucous membrane involvement.[7]

Other notable examples of such syndromes have different skin lesions. Tuberous sclerosis (Bourneville's disease) is characterized by skin lesions, most commonly *hypomelanotic macules*, among many others, cortical tubers, subependymal nodules, and subependymal giant cell astrocytomas (SEGAs), as well as other organ components, such as renal angiomyolipomas, and lymphangiomyomatosis.[8,9] *Hypomelanosis* of Ito has hypopigmented skin lesions in the form of streaks and whorls associated with brain abnormalities such as megalencephaly, loss of cortical layering, neuronal heterotopias, and lesions resembling cortical tubers.[10,11] Sneddon syndrome consists of *livedo reticularis* (a web-like purple mottling of skin), ischemic strokes, and a variety of neurologic features.[12] Nevoid basal cell carcinoma syndrome (Gorlin syndrome) includes *basal cell carcinomas* of the skin, *dyskeratotic pits* of palms and soles, odontogenic keratocysts, macrocephaly, and medulloblastoma, especially the nodular/desmoplastic variant.[13] Skin lesions are also seen as part of brain tumor polyposis syndrome (BTPS, Turcot syndrome), along with astrocytomas/glioblastomas, medulloblastomas, adenomatous polyposis coli, and colorectal cancers. They may be of various types, such as *café-au-lait spots*, *epidermoid cysts*, or *sebaceous tumors*, and the

TABLE 1.1 Summary of associations of skin lesions with syndromes that involve the nervous system

Skin Lesion	Condition	Main CNS Features	Other Prominent Features
Capillary hemangioma	Sturge-Weber syndrome	Meningeal capillary hemangiomas Ischemic cortical changes Parenchymal vascular mineralization	Internal organ and choroidal hemangiomas
Telangiectasia	Ataxia-telangiectasia	Telangiectasias Cerebellar atrophy	Immune system impairment Hematolymphoid malignancies Melanoma and carcinomas
AVM	Wyburn-Mason syndrome Osler-Rendu-Weber syndrome	AVM Vascular malformations	Retinal AVM Vascular malformations of mucous membranes Pulmonary arteriovenous fistulae
Hypomelanotic maculae Facial angiofibroma Ungual fibromas	Tuberous sclerosis	Cortical dysplasias SEGA Subependymal nodules Radial band heterotopia	Renal or other organ angiomyolipoma Retinal hamartomas LAM Cardiac rhabdomyoma
Livedo reticularis	Sneddon syndrome	Ischemic strokes	Antiphospholipid antibody syndrome SLE
Basal cell carcinoma Dyskeratotic pits	Gorlin syndrome	Medulloblastoma	Odontogenic keratocyst
Café-au-lait spots Epidermoid cyst Sebaceous tumor	BTPS (Turcot syndrome)	Glioblastoma Medulloblastoma	Adenomatous polyposis coli and colorectal cancers
Café-au-lait spots Axillary–inguinal freckles	NF1	Optic nerve glioma Infiltrating astrocytoma PNST	Sphenoid wing dysplasia
Café-au-lait spots	NF2	Schwannoma Meningioma Glioma Glial hamartia Meningioangiomatosis Schwannosis PNST	Subcapsular lens opacity
Trichilemmoma	Cowden syndrome	Dysplastic gangliocytoma of the cerebellum	Multiple internal organ malignancies and hamartomas
Various skin cancers	Li-Fraumeni syndrome	Astrocytomas Medulloblastoma and PNET Choroid plexus carcinoma	Other organ malignancies
Spotty pigmentation Blue nevus Myxoma	Carney's complex	Psammomatous melanotic schwannoma Pituitary adenoma	Myxoma

CNS, central nervous system; AVM, arteriovenous malformation; SEGA, subependymal giant cell astrocytoma; LAM, lymphangiomyomatosis; SLE, systemic lupus erythematosus; BTPS, brain tumor polyposis syndrome; NF, neurofibromatosis; PNST, peripheral nerve sheath tumor; PNET, primitive neuroectodermal tumor.

type of CNS neoplasms vary depending whether the syndrome is type 1 or type 2.[14] The typical skin lesion of Cowden syndrome is a *trichilemmoma* in association with dysplastic gangliocytoma of the cerebellum (Lhermitte-Duclos disease); breast, thyroid, and endometrial cancers, and multiple hamartomas of multiple tissue types.[15] Especially adult-onset Lhermitte-Duclos disease is diagnostic of Cowden syndrome. A variety of *skin cancers* and CNS neoplasms, along with malignancies of many other organs, may be seen in the context of Li-Fraumeni syndrome.[16] The most common CNS neoplasms in this syndrome are infiltrating astrocytomas of various grades as well as medulloblastoma/primitive neuroectodermal tumor (PNET) and choroid plexus carcinomas. *Café-au-lait spots* **(Fig. 1-1)** are most famous in neurofibromatosis type 1 (NF1; von Recklinghausen disease). Neurofibromas can be noted as *cutaneous nodules* and *pedunculated lesions*. Other skin lesion in this syndrome is *axillary and groin freckles*. Many other dysplastic lesions and peripheral nervous system (PNS) and CNS neoplasms, such as malignant peripheral nerve sheath tumor, pilocytic astrocytoma, as well as many other organ neoplasms can be seen. Café-au-lait spots are also seen in a large subpopulation of patients with neurofibromatosis type 2 (NF2). NF2 also may have cutaneous nodules representing schwannomas, along with meningiomas, gliomas, and schwannomas in the CNS.[17] Glial hamartia and meningioangiomatosis can be seen, among others. Alternatively, multiple skin nodules representing multiple schwannomas may indicate schwannomatosis.

Carney complex is associated with *spotty pigmentation, skin or mucosal myxomas,* and epithelioid *blue nevi*, among other features, but the CNS components are psammomatous melanotic schwannoma or somatotroph pituitary adenoma.[18] *Congenital nevi* can be seen in association with intracranial melanoma or a diffuse proliferation of melanocytes throughout the subarachnoid space.

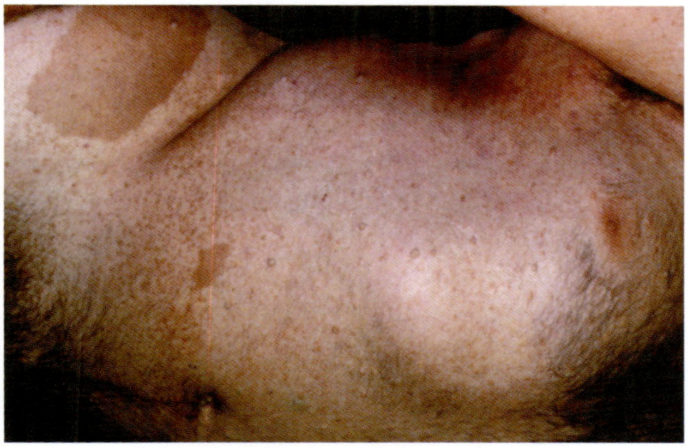

Figure 1-1. Café-au-lait spots are tan-brown macular pigmentations of variable sizes and irregular borders. Multiple nodular lesions representing cutaneous neurofibromas are also present in this NF1 case.

Large or multiple congenital nevi, especially in head and neck skin, may represent neurocutaneous melanosis, in which a diffuse proliferation of leptomeningeal melanocytes is present, with a risk of developing skin and primary CNS melanomas.[19] Some of these patients may also have other malformations,[20] such as Dandy-Walker malformation, Sturge-Weber syndrome, and cerebellar abnormalities. *Nevus of Ota* can also be associated with meningeal melanocytic lesions, along with congenital *hyperpigmentation* of skin, ocular, and orbital soft tissues.[21]

Aside from primary lesions of skin and subcutaneous soft tissues, and those lesions that may represent indirect findings associated with nervous system pathology, some CNS disorders can be identified directly during external examination. For instance, what may appear to be a *subcutaneous mass lesion* may actually represent a meningioma that has invaded through the bone, or an ectopic meningioma.[22] Some such subcutaneous masses, especially softer ones in midline locations such as occipital region, may also represent meningoceles or meningoencephaloceles. Occipital region is a common location for encephalocele, although they can rarely occur laterally in the parietal region. Anterior encephaloceles can be visible at the nose ridge in many cases; in others, they may extend into paranasal sinuses, orbit, or nasal cavity. It is not surprising to find disorganized neuroglial tissue in a surgical specimen removed as a nasal polyp. They are traditionally termed "nasal glioma," a misnomer.[23,24] Especially in the lumbosacral region in children, meningomyelocele sacs are common and may not always be ulcerated and obvious. In this region, a skin tag, lipoma, skin dimple, sinus tract (pilonidal sinus or tract), or a pigmented or hairy area may indicate an underlying spina bifida occulta.[25] "Fawn's tail" is a lipoma with an overlying skin tag that looks like a tail **(Fig. 1-2)**.

Spina bifida and *meningoceles and encephaloceles* may be part of other syndromes. It is beyond the scope of this text to delve into the specific features of numerous syndromes, in which CNS is involved.[26,27] One notable example of such an association is Chiari type I malformation, which can be associated with occipital encephalocele as well as lumbosacral meningomyelocele. The latter is also a part of Chiari type II (Arnold-Chiari) malformation. Cervical and occipital encephalocele, including cerebellum in its contents, can be seen in Chiari

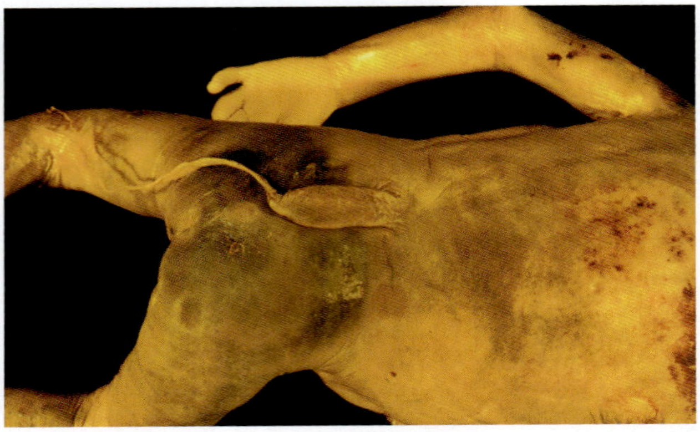

Figure 1-2. Fawn's tail, as with any other skin lesion, can be present in the lumbosacral region as an indication of an underlying neural tube defect, such as meningomyelocele.

III malformation.[28–30] Meckel-Gruber syndrome is also associated with an occipital encephalocele.[31] It should be kept in mind that when a malformation is identified, it is usually accompanied by other malformations in other parts of the nervous system as well as in many other organs. Especially in neonatal and fetal autopsies, knowledge of clinical concerns and head ultrasonographic findings will greatly increase the yield of neuropathologic evaluation. If untreated, especially lumbosacral meningo(myelo)celes **(Fig. 1-3)** commonly become eroded and infected, resulting in local and widespread CNS infections and death. Therefore, spinal and intracranial infection should be searched for in these cases.

As mentioned above for spina bifida, meningocele, meningomyelocele, and encephalocele, especially in fetal and neonatal autopsies, many *dysmorphic features identified by external evaluation* can turn out to be part of a more complex syndrome. There are numerous syndromes in which CNS is a part, and it is beyond the scope of this text to discuss the details of each and every one of them. However, being aware of the clinical concerns and findings, and especially knowledge of head ultrasonography findings, will increase the yield of neuropathologic evaluation. Some examples are as follows: Anencephaly is the *absence of the skull vault* with disorganized neurovascular (area cerebrovasculosa) tissue over a flat skull base, and protruding eyes **(Fig. 1-4)**. It can be associated with variable degrees of *rachischisis*. Dysmorphic

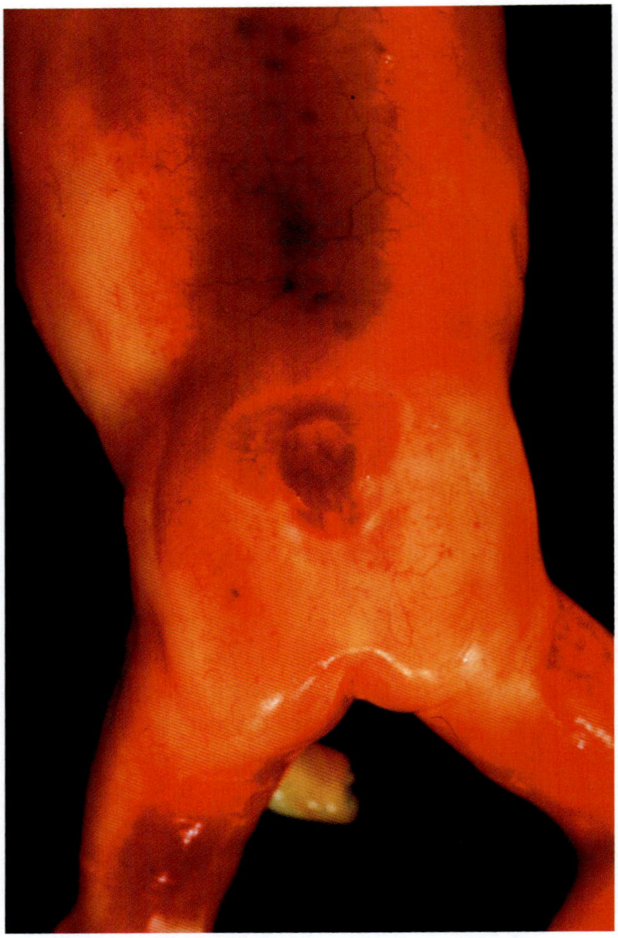

Figure 1-3. Lumbosacral meningomyelocele in a stillborn fetus.

features such as proboscis, cyclopia **(Fig. 1-5)**, nasal pit, hypo-, or hypertelorism may be an indication of more serious, usually midline, nervous system malformations, for example, holoprosencephaly, olfactory aplasia, or corpus callosum agenesis. Microcephaly, macrocephaly, and hydrocephaly can alert one to the presence of additional pathology and provide clues to the nature of it. In addition, other abnormalities such as craniosynostosis can be the cause of these dysmorphic features and should be noted at the time of autopsy (see also discussions on "Bones" and "Brain Weight" below).

General appearance of the body also provides clues to any endocrine abnormalities, in this case, in regard to pituitary gland disorders. Gigantism, acromegaly, and cushingoid habitus should alert one to direct more attention to sella turcica and pituitary gland, an organ that is prone to be

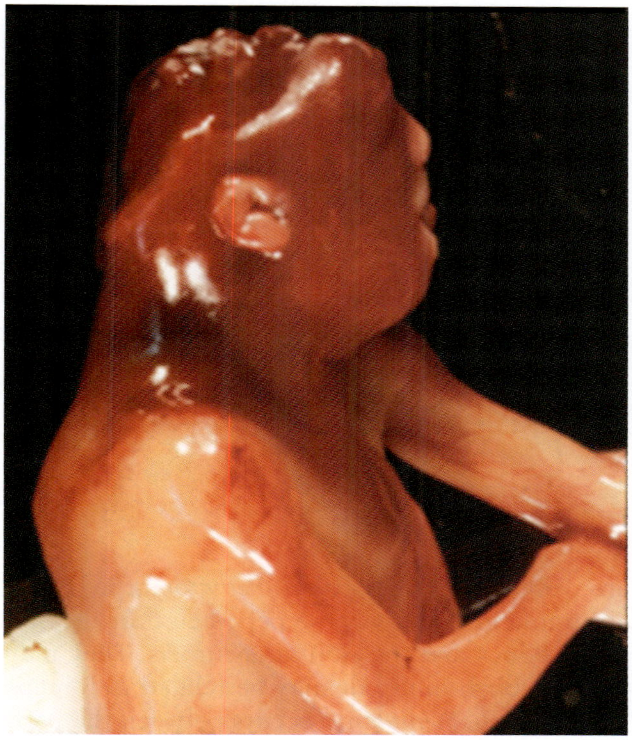

Figure 1-4. Anencephaly: Calvarial bones are not formed, resulting in protruding appearance of the eyes, and an irregular aggregate of tissue, area cerebrovasculosa, is present instead of a well-formed brain.

ignored and sometimes even forgotten at the time of autopsy. Muscle wasting, especially in a particular distribution, such as proximal, distal, around large joints, or in association with erythematous skin lesions, may prompt sampling of skeletal muscle and peripheral nerve for evaluation for neuromuscular diseases, which is not routinely done at autopsy. They may also indicate systemic disease that can involve CNS.

Just like examination of the skin, inspection of the *eyes* may also provide an insight to the underlying or associated processes. Lisch nodules are hamartomas of *iris* and are seen in NF1. *Lens* opacities can be seen in NF2, although this is difficult to evaluate with any degree of certainty postmortem. Hypopigmented iris spots can be associated with tuberous sclerosis. Ocular surfaces can be involved by nevus of Ota, which in turn can be associated with meningeal melanocytomas or melanomas.

Hemorrhage or cerebrospinal fluid (CSF) leak from the nose or ear indicates a skull base fracture.[32]

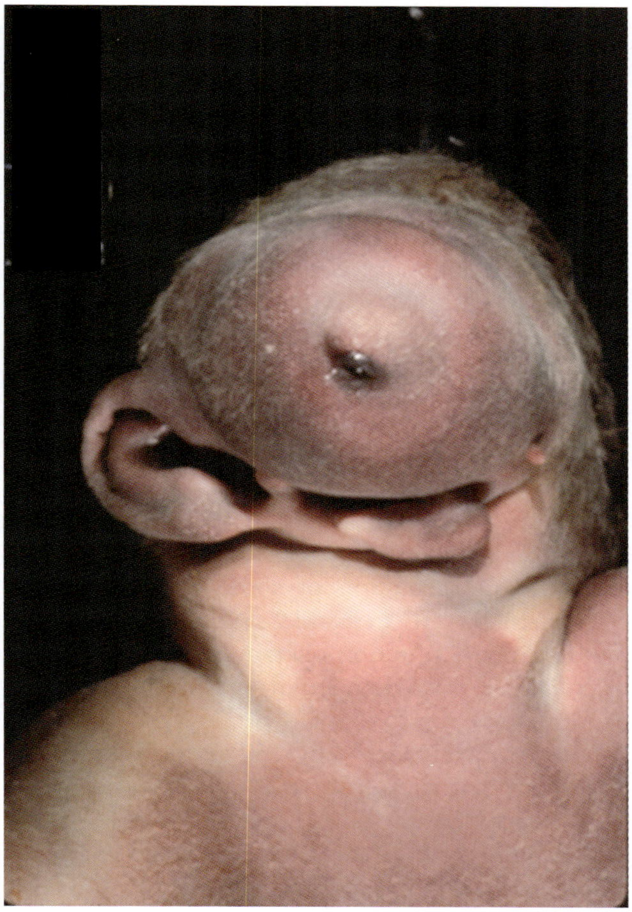

Figure 1-5. Severe dysmorphic features, consisting of a central single eye (cyclopia) and a round protuberance (proboscis). Ears are fused under the proboscis.

Unless they are large and very obvious, they need to be sought for. Such a leak also indicates a communication between intracranial cavity and outside environment, raising the possibility of intracranial infection. Sometimes, CSF leaks can simply occur in association with encephaloceles, for example, anterior/ethmoidofrontal encephalocele.

Bones

The importance of identification and documentation of the status of the bones and related lesions come from the fact that they may prove crucial for accurate interpretation of many findings in the CNS. If one is not careful or documentation is not done appropriately during autopsy,

List of Findings/Checklist for Bones

• AT A GLANCE

- Surgery site
- Subcutaneous hematoma
- Subgaleal hematoma
- Cephalhematoma
- Periorbital hematoma
- Cerebrospinal fluid leak
- Status of fontanelles
- *Fractures*
  - Linear
  - Depressed
  - Bursting
  - Diastatic
  - Open
  - Closed
  - Skull base
- *Thickening–thinning*
  - Neoplasms
  - Cysts
  - Hyperostosis
  - Dysplasia/agenesis
  - Malformations
- *Others*
  - Penetrating injury
  - Parenchymal injury
  - Thermal injury

accurate interpretation of some lesions may be compromised. If available, radiologic findings facilitate the evaluation of bones, especially vertebral lesions, since detailed evaluation of vertebrae is not readily possible.

External surfaces of calvarial bones are exposed when the scalp is peeled. *Subcutaneous hemorrhages* can be seen, indicating sites of injury. *Surgical intervention sites*, the type and extent of the surgical approach, are also better appreciated. At this point, presence of shunts, reservoirs, burr holes **(Fig. 1-6)**, craniectomy, metal plate to cover craniectomy site, dural graft, skeletal muscle, and adipose tissue packing of surgical sites are revealed.[33–35] *Subgaleal hematoma* is blood accumulation between the periosteum of the calvarial bones and the skin aponeurosis. They may indicate birth injury or may be related to forceps use.[36,37] *Cephalhematoma* occurs between the periosteum and bone.

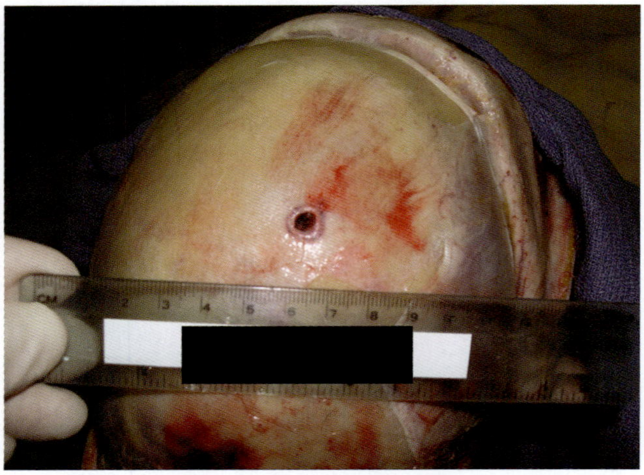

Figure 1-6. A burr hole is seen indicating in this autopsy case a previous stereotactic biopsy site.

Skull fractures[38] should be sought, in some cases by removing large hematomas under the periosteum as necessary. They can be linear, depressed (when fragments are displaced at least equal to the thickness of skull bone), bending (if the displacement does not qualify as depressed, although not a common term), bursting (outward displacement of fragments), diastatic (if sutures are separated, resulting in sawtooth appearance of its edges), or a combination of these. Diastatic fractures are more likely to occur in younger individuals in whom the sutures are not completely ossified. The fractures can also be open (compound) or closed, depending on whether they are exposed due to injuries in the overlying scalp and soft tissues. Skull fractures are common in child abuse cases, and this possibility should be kept in mind in the evaluation of pediatric cases.[39,40] In cases of multiple linear fractures, it is possible to identify which fracture occurred first, as the subsequent linear fracture lines do not extend beyond the previous fracture lines.[41] *Penetrating injuries* can be evaluated at this point. Bullet or other penetrating objects can be evaluated based on the shape of the entry site. Entry sites of the bullets can be identified by the inward spreading of the bone fragments, which can be carried into the brain parenchyma along with the bullet.

Fractures are usually but not necessarily associated with underlying *parenchymal injury*. Likewise, there does not necessarily have to be a skull fracture for a parenchymal injury to be suspected traumatic. In burn victims exposed to extreme thermal injury, boiling of brain in the intracranial water may result in pressure fractures due to increased intracranial pressure. They in turn may be associated with artifactual epidural hematomas, due to oozing of the bone marrow through the pressure fracture sites. Such hemorrhages can also be seen without the skull fractures, however. They should not be confused with true epidural hematoma and true fracture. There is external discoloration of parenchyma in thermal injury as a result of baking of the tissues, essentially representing coagulation of tissue.[38] *Skull base fractures*[42–44] should be sought after the removal of cranial contents and may not be readily apparent. Peeling the skull base dura may be needed to find them. They should be searched for especially if there is CSF or blood discharge from the ears or nose.[45] Hinge fractures are fractures, typically diastatic, that run across the skull base at the anterior aspects of petrous ridges to usually involve the sella. They result in the separation of anterior and posterior portions of the skull base and are the result of the skull being crushed. Bilateral petrous bone fractures may indicate a blow to the chin. Ring fractures around the foramen magnum indicate a fall with spine impacting on the skull base. Fractures involving the orbital bones may occur away from the actual trauma site and may result in periorbital hematoma (black eyes, raccoon eyes, spectacle ecchymosis). Red-purple hemorrhages under the dura of the orbital skull base strongly suggest an underlying orbital roof fracture. Growing fractures occur when leptomeninges protrude through the dura and a fracture site to gradually form an enlarging cyst and result in enlargement of the fracture. This is seen almost always in the first few years of life. Fractures in general pose a high risk for intracranial infections by providing a passage for the microorganisms into the cranial contents. This is true even for the closed fractures if they involve the paranasal sinuses and upper aerodigestive tract.[35]

In children, the status of the *fontanelles* should be checked and evaluated relative to age. Whether they are depressed or distended provide an idea about the intracranial pressure as well as hydration status. Fontanelles and sutures that fuse early (craniosynostosis) is one of the causes of secondary microcephaly.[46] Likewise, expansion of the suture lines and enlargement of the head circumference is associated with hydrocephalus or other conditions with increased intracranial volume.

Irregular *thickening or thinning of bones* and *mass lesions* may indicate sites of pathologic processes within the bone or in the adjacent intracranial structures. This applies to calvarium as well as skull base and spine. The knowledge of radiologic findings is very helpful with specifically searching for bone lesions that do not form obvious mass lesions or other changes. Diffuse changes and some focal lesions can be evaluated on the cut surfaces. Paget's disease causes irregular diffuse thickening of bones that is seen on cut surfaces as spongy in the earlier stages and dense and compact in the later stages. Fibrous dysplasia presents as an expansile lesion with solid, compact cut surfaces. Osteoma, osteoid osteoma, Langerhans cell histiocytosis, giant cell tumor, hemangioma **(Fig. 1-7)**, and essentially any bone lesion in the context of bone pathology can be seen.[47] Rarely, truly intraosseous meningiomas can be seen, but a bone invasive meningioma should be ruled out in those cases.[48] Of particular importance are areas of hyperostosis, presenting as irregular thick areas with compact cut surfaces associated with underlying

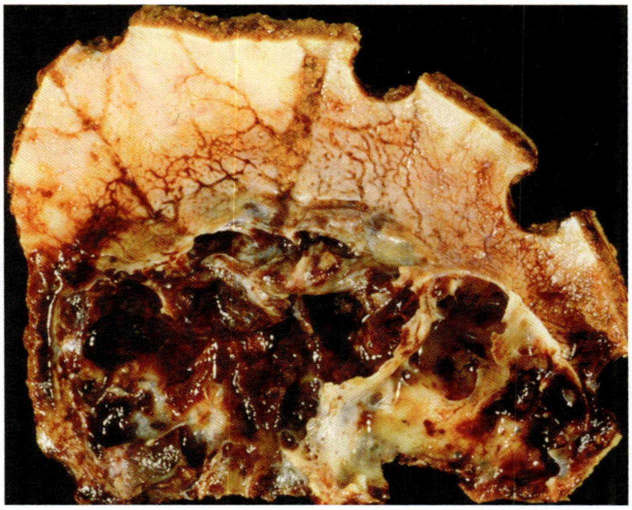

Figure 1-7. Cavernous hemangioma of the frontal bone in a resection specimen. The hemangioma has hemorrhagic spongy surfaces.

meningiomas, which can frequently invade into and through the bone.[49] The presence of such a meningioma should be apparent when the bone is removed (or when the brain is removed in the case of skull base lesions). Some superficial hamartomatous lesions, and low-grade, long-standing lesions such as dysembryoplastic neuroepithelial tumor, can cause erosion of the inner surface of the skull bones and thinning of the bone. Epidermoid and dermoid cysts are other developmental lesions that can be seen in association with bone and cause variable degrees of erosions. Dermoid cysts are essentially limited to midline, while epidermoid cysts can be seen in essentially any skull bone.[50] Metastatic carcinoma, involvement by myeloma **(Fig. 1-8)**, or Langerhans cell histiocytosis are other common lesions that can be encountered in the bones.[47,51] Thickening of skull bones can also be seen in Batten's disease (neuronal ceroid lipofuscinosis). Hyperostosis frontalis interna is the irregular thickening of inner surface of frontal skull by irregular bony proliferation[52,53] **(Fig. 1-9)**. It has no known clinical significance but may result in frontal brain atrophy. Aside from this peculiar condition, hyperostosis of the cranial bones is associated with meningiomas and likely is the result of reaction of the bone to invasion by meningioma.

In lumbosacral spine, the absence of vertebral arches indicates *spina bifida* occulta. Being the mildest form of the dysraphic defects, the only external suggestion for it might be an overlying skin lesion. *Dysplasias or agenesis* of sphenoid bone is one of the features that may be seen in NF1, with other bone abnormality in this syndrome being dysplasias or thinning of the long bone cortices.[17] Chiari I malformation can be associated with skeletal abnormalities involving the skull base, such as platybasia, basilar invagination (basilar impression),[54] or Klippel-Feil syndrome.[55] Foramen

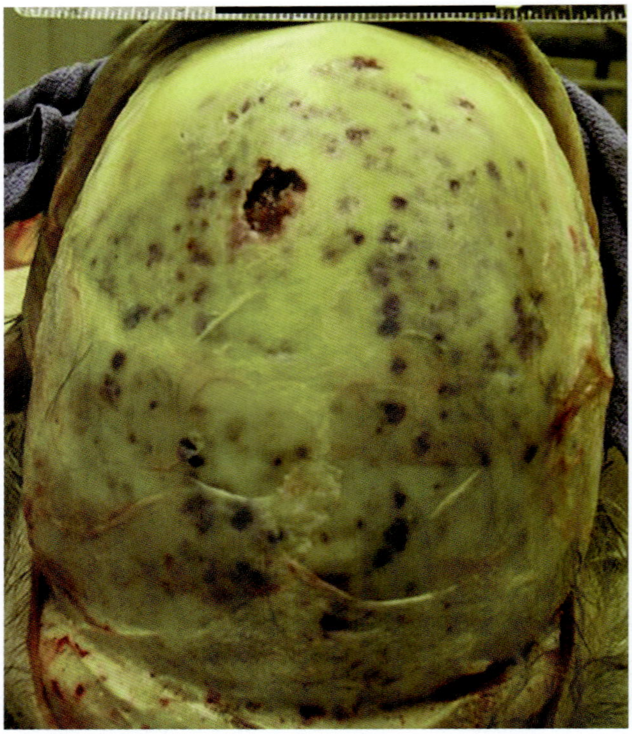

Figure 1-8. Numerous lytic lesions of variable sizes widely distributed over the bones in a multiple myeloma patient.

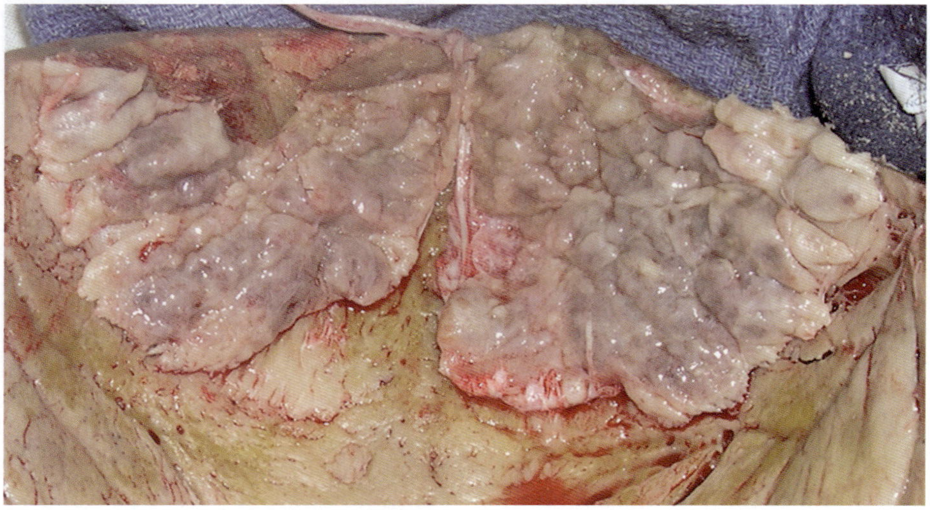

Figure 1-9. Hyperostosis frontalis interna identified as an incidental findings during an autopsy for Creutzfeldt-Jacob disease (CJD).

magnum is enlarged in Chiari II malformation, resulting in cerebellar herniation and downward displacement of brainstem. Cranial dysplasias may result in hydrocephalus by exerting pressure on venous return and CSF reabsorption. Vertebrae need to be examined for abnormalities that can cause nontraumatic cord injury, such as atlantoaxial subluxation; dural thickening; kyphotic and/or scoliotic deformities; dysplastic, neoplastic, infectious diseases of bone and connective tissue; and intervertebral disc and joint diseases, in addition to epidural, dural, subdural, and subarachnoid processes.[56–59] Atlantoaxial dislocation is a serious life-threatening complication seen especially with the rheumatoid arthritis and ankylosing spondylitis involving the atlantoaxial joint.[60] Occipitalization of the atlas (i.e., fusion of the atlas and the occipital bone) is another serious condition that can give rise to neurologic symptoms by compromising the cervical spinal cord.[61]

Epidural Space

Epidural hemorrhage occurs typically due to middle meningeal artery injury as a result of skull fracture and is therefore an arterial hemorrhage, although a group of hematomas can be of venous origin.[62] As soon as the hemorrhage is identified, it should be documented by photographs. Being arterial in origin, it develops rapidly and is almost always fresh. Therefore, it will disintegrate and will be lost since it has no significant clot formation or organization. An idea about its volume should be provided by three-dimensional (3-D) measurements as much as possible, as direct volume measurement is not practical and will likely not be accurate. It is usually temporoparietal, corresponding to the trajectory of the middle meningeal artery, and is unilateral. It is rare in the spinal cord. A skull fracture in this area or a history of lucid interval should alert one to the potential presence of an underlying epidural hematoma.[63] Blood dyscrasias and metastatic malignancies are relatively rare causes of epidural hematoma. In burn victims, a diffuse epidural hemorrhage is also seen as a thin layer of clotted blood and is attributed to intense heat (see “Bones” above).[64] Whenever possible, hematoma should be sectioned in search for solid tissue areas that may represent a metastatic malignancy or organization. The latter is usually in the form of shiny, gray-white membranes surrounding the hematoma. Microscopic examination should be performed to assess the age of the hematoma and for other potential findings. Other evidence for traumatic injury as well as secondary changes in the brain, such as swelling and herniations, should be sought. In the spinal cord, they may provide clues to bone injury and underlying cord injury.

Epidural pus[65] can accumulate as a result of direct extension of infections from neighboring bones (osteomyelitis) or paranasal sinuses (sinusitis). Especially infections originating from frontal sinuses and mastoid air cells result in epidural abscesses in the anterior and posterior fossae, respectively, where the dura mater is loosely attached to the bone. Since this is not possible in other areas where dura mater is tightly attached to the bone, the infections from other sinuses tend to penetrate the dura to result in subdural spread. When widespread, it is called epidural empyema and is life threatening due to both its mass effect and to infection. Pus tends to be most prominent near the originating focus. In cases of venous spread, it can be associated with venous thrombosis. In chronic cases, the infection can be walled-off and turn into an abscess. In spinal cord,[38,66] epidural abscess or empyema develops from osteomyelitis or Pott's disease.

Epidural infections are particularly associated with osteomyelitis in the spine.[67] Abscess formation is commonly seen in the thoracic levels, with typical well circumscription and granulation

List of Findings/Checklist for Epidural Space

AT A GLANCE

- Hemorrhage
- Pus
- Fracture
- Bone infections
- Abscess/empyema
- Metastatic neoplasms
- Primary bone/soft tissue neoplasms
- Herniated nucleus pulposus
- Dorsal root ganglia

tissue wall. Intravascular drug abuse, as well as any other source of bacteremia, is a risk factor.[68] Retroperitoneal and posterior mediastinal infections can spread through the intervertebral foramina into the spinal canal. Likewise, infectious agents can be inoculated by penetrating trauma.[69] Infections should be cultured, intraoperatively or at autopsy.

Epidural space is a common site in the spine for *metastatic malignancies*. Many *bone and soft tissue neoplasms*, benign or malignant, can extend into this space and present with cord compression. Therefore, knowledge of clinical history and clinical and radiologic findings should help direct attention to the appropriate location. Especially in the spinal cord, the extradural (in contrast to intradural extramedullary or intramedullary) location of a lesion helps narrow down the differential diagnostic possibilities to metastatic neoplasms, primary bone and soft tissue neoplasms, and neoplastic or reactive hematolymphoid lesions, as well as infections. Herniated intervertebral discs resulting in various neurologic conditions may become an issue during pathologic evaluation, especially at autopsy.[70] The latter can break off to migrate in the spinal canal to result in confusing conditions.[71] A few dorsal root ganglia are usually seen attached to the epidural surface of the spinal dura mater after removal at autopsy. They are irregular tan-brown nodular structures of several millimeters up to about a centimeter on the posterolateral epidural aspects of the spinal dura mater. When they are of particular interest for the case, as in degenerative diseases involving them or evaluation for sensory neuropathies as in diabetes mellitus, careful removal of the spinal cord along with its dura mater will help identify many dorsal root ganglia a lot easier.

Dura Mater and Subdural Space

In cases of epidural or subdural hematoma, if the fresh blood clot has washed away and not been documented during autopsy, a vague *blood-tinged appearance* **(Fig. 1-10)** on dura surface may be the only sign of it. The terms "intradural" and "subdural" may occasionally be used interchangeably, especially in the spinal cord. However, "intradural" sometimes means truly within the fibrous tissue of the dura mater. Very focal and subtle *intradural hemorrhages*[72] can occur as the earliest sign of anoxic/ischemic injury or other stress in the prenatal period and infancy. In the case of describing location of lesions in the spinal canal, such as intradural extramedullary, intradural is used to mean subdural location. What is being said should be clear from the context in which the term is used. Dural grafts, surgical sites, and shunt insertion sites are identified by examining the dura mater.

Mass lesions of variable sizes and consistencies may be identified especially on the inner surface of the dura mater. Many of these are incidental findings at autopsy. Irregular, plaque-like *calcifications*

List of Findings/Checklist for Dura Mater and Subdural Space

• AT A GLANCE

- Intradural hemorrhage
- Subdural hemorrhage
- Empyema
- Calcification–ossification
- Diffuse thickening
- Mass lesions/meningiomas
- Soft tissue, hematolymphoid, metastatic neoplasms
- Skull base/vertebral canal
- Dural sinuses
- Traumatic dural tears

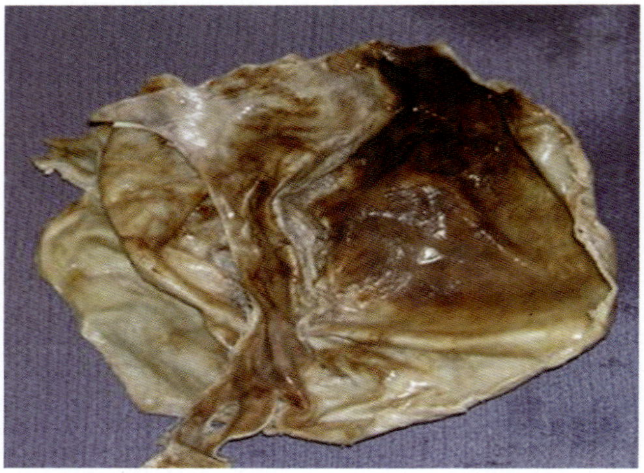

Figure 1-10. Blood-tinged appearance of the inner surface of dura mater after an acute subdural hematoma was washed away.

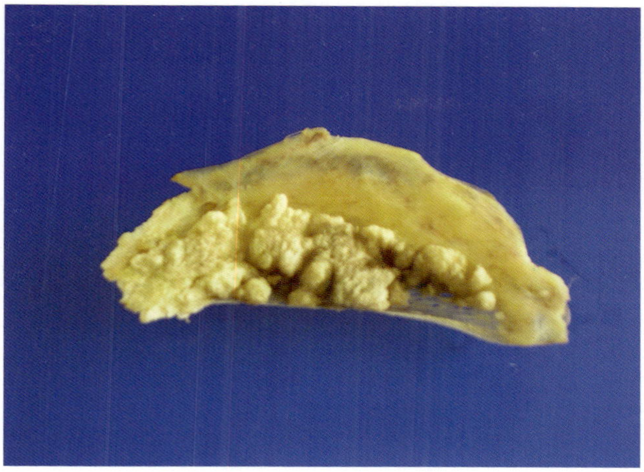

Figure 1-11. Extensive irregular nodular calcifications on falx cerebri commonly seen as a normal finding. Some such lesions may represent extensively calcified meningiomas, typically psammomatous meningiomas.

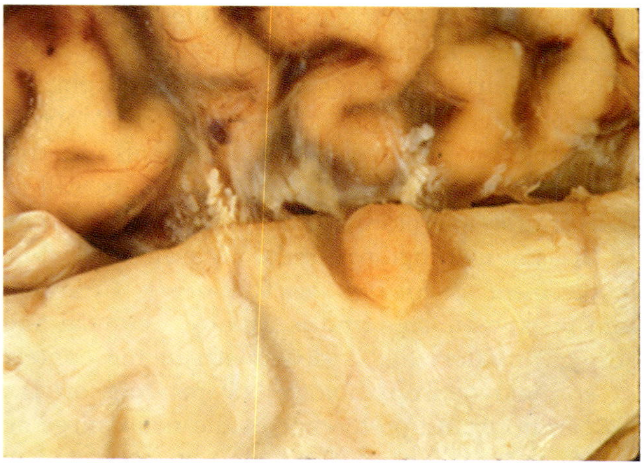

Figure 1-12. Incidental nodule remaining attached to the inner surface of the reflected dura mater, representing a meningioma.

or ossifications can be seen commonly in the falx cerebri, in the parasagittal region or tentorium, are usually age-related changes, and are of no known significance **(Fig. 1-11)**. Meningiomas are nodular lesions of up to several centimeters. Some of these are extremely calcified and need decalcification. Microscopic examination commonly shows them to be psammomatous meningiomas. More diffuse and widespread *plaque-like thickening* or growth involving the dura and meninges can be seen in diffuse growth pattern of meningioma, that is, meningioma en plaque.[73] This type of growth pattern may also be seen in metastatic malignancies, in benign or malignant hematolymphoid proliferations, and in the rare condition of pachymeningitis.[74] In the case of meningiomas, lymphoplasmacyte-rich meningioma especially can present with a plaque-like growth pattern.[75] Rarely, a calcifying pseudoneoplasm of the neuraxis is identified.[76] Meningiomas are neoplasms arising from the arachnoid cap cells that are intimately associated with dura mater, and therefore, they present as dura-based mass lesions that can be identified incidentally attached to the dura mater **(Figs. 1-12 and 1-13)**. Skull base should also be inspected after the removal of the brain, as skull base meningiomas in olfactory groove, sphenoid wing, clinoid process, petroclival, foramen magnum and cavernous sinus, and occasionally other lesions can be present. *Multiple* dura-based mass lesions likely represent multiple meningiomas. This can be a sporadic occurrence, may be associated with NF2,[77] or may represent a postradiation meningioma development.[78]

When possible, an effort should be shown to examine *dural sinuses*. These are essentially venous channels and may harbor metastatic malignancies and thromboses.[79,80] Superior sagittal *sinus thrombosis* is a dramatic event resulting in extensive bilateral congestion and subsequent hemorrhagic infarction of the parasagittal brain tissue due to blockage of venous return. Thrombus should be distinguished from *postmortem clot*. The former is firmly attached to the sinus wall, is hard instead of

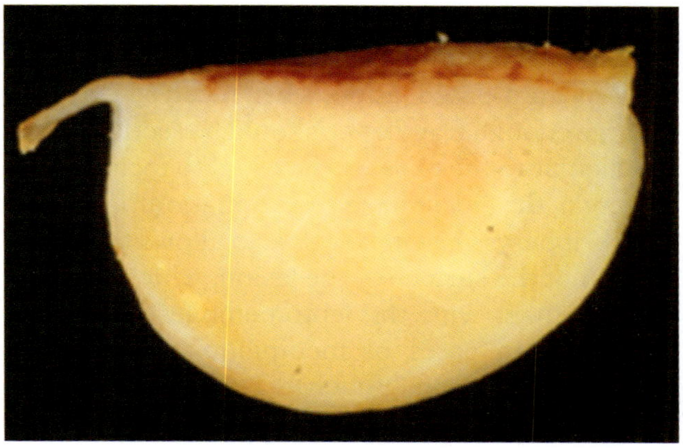

Figure 1-13. Section of the nodule shows the dura-based well-circumscribed nodular mass with solid tan-white cut surface.

friable, and tends to expand the lumen. If in doubt, microscopic examination should clarify the issue, although early thromboses tend to be friable and may dislodge during sectioning. The thrombosis should be investigated, is that it may also be due to neoplastic involvement of the sinus as well as dehydration and clotting disorders, among others. In cases of meningioma in the parasagittal region, *involvement of superior sagittal sinus* is an important prognostic sign and is usually a clinical and surgical matter that is dealt with in the context of surgical neuropathology.[81] Depending on the observations and preference of the neurosurgeon, intraoperative consultations may be requested to evaluate the involvement of dural sinus by meningioma, similar to *"dural margin"* evaluations that are sometimes requested during meningioma resections. Usually distorted by the thermal artifact, these small fragments of dura mater invariably contain at least a few clusters of meningothelial cells, raising the question of normally prominent arachnoid cap cell population, hyperplastic groups reacting to the neoplasm, or actual involvement by meningioma. The decision may be straightforward but usually becomes a somewhat subjective one depending on the experience of the neuropathologist and definitely requires incorporation of the intraoperative observations and the histologic similarity to the meningioma at hand if there is a previous sample for diagnosis. An occasional source of error is when the hyperplastic meningothelial tissue is received for intraoperative consultation from a "brain tumor" and shows many meningothelial cells, which may result in a diagnosis of meningioma, when the actual lesion is something else, such as a schwannoma, hematoma, or glioma.

Any dura-based lesion, when received in toto or in large enough fragments, should be sectioned perpendicular to the dural surface and to include dura mater in the microscopic examination, including the periphery. This approach also allows the examination of the surface of the lesion, which is facing or in contact with the leptomeninges and brain. Especially in cases of meningioma, this allows identification of any attached brain tissue and its examination for invasion by meningioma. Many mesenchymal and hematopoietic lesions, benign or malignant, as well as metastatic carcinomas occur in association with the dural and leptomeningeal soft tissues.[82] **(Fig. 1-14)**. Infectious granulomas

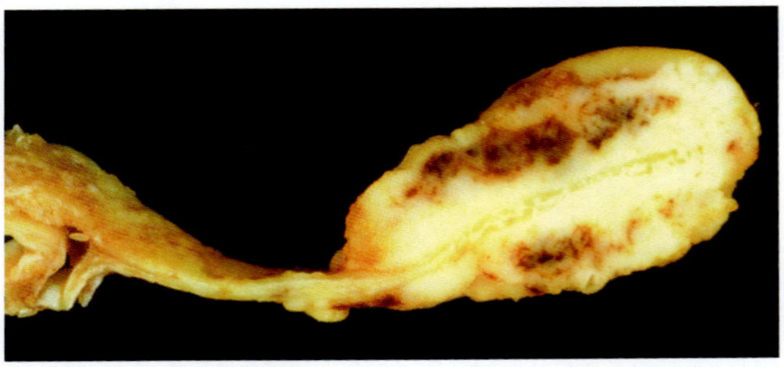

Figure 1-14. Metastatic carcinoma attached to falx cerebri. Cross section of collapsed superior sagittal sinus is seen on the left.

may reach significant sizes to present as a mass lesion and, when in dura mater, may mimic meningiomas. Subdural mass lesions in the spinal cord are described as being intradural extramedullary.[83] In this context, it is possible to see essentially every type of mesenchymal neoplasm, primary or metastatic, including drop metastases. As in other locations, *lipoma* is a yellow, soft, lobular mass that commonly occurs attached to falx cerebri and may be associated with partial or complete agenesis of corpus callosum, with or without other abnormalities and facial dysmorphic features.[84] It can also be seen in cerebellopontine angle, suprasellar region, sylvian cistern, and in the lumbosacral spinal cord. Many of these, especially of the spinal cord lesions, are not true neoplasms but represent prominent adipose tissue resulting in a mass. It is not uncommon to see such irregular adipose tissue attached to the posterior surface of the spinal dura mater or in other locations[85] **(Fig. 1-15)**.

While *subdural space* has traditionally and historically been referred to as a "space," the space actually forms by separation of the dural border cells when there is an accumulation.[86] *Subdural hemorrhage* occurs typically due to bridging vein **(Fig. 1-16)** injury as a result of trauma and is therefore a venous hemorrhage in the great majority of the cases. However, in a significant subpopulation of cases, there seems to be no history of trauma[87] **(Table 1.2)**. Parasagittal frontoparietal region is a common location, with many cases, and more commonly in children, being bilateral. It is rare in the spinal cord. Older age and brain atrophy increase the risk of subdural hemorrhage by increasing the distance the bridging veins travel and make them more vulnerable to injury, even

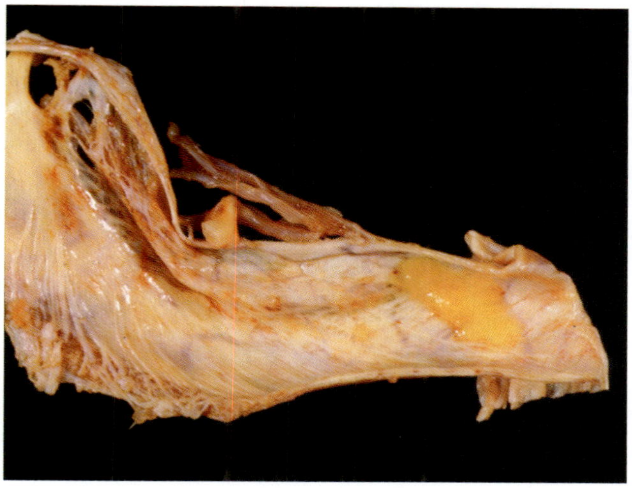

Figure 1-15. A piece of mature adipose tissue attached to falx cerebri, identified as an incidental finding at autopsy, with no associated abnormalities.

with no apparent trauma. A small percentage may occur at the margins of old traumatic scars.[88] Other rare occurrences are as a risk factor in ventricular decompression of hydrocephalus or as a complication of pneumoencephalography. A history of alcoholism also increases the risk of subdural hemorrhage. Blood dyscrasias and metastatic malignancies are other rare causes of subdural hemorrhage.[89] As with epidural hematoma, in situ

TABLE 1.2 Common causes of subdural hemorrhage

Bridging vein injury/trauma
Brain atrophy
Traumatic scars
Hydrocephalus decompression
Pneumoencephalography
Alcoholism
Bleeding diathesis
Metastatic malignancies
Dural tears
Prematurity

pictures should be taken for documentation, and 3-D measurement should be recorded to provide an idea about the size of the hematoma, which is crucial especially if there is no previous radiologic documentation. Whenever possible, hematoma should be sectioned in search for solid tissue areas that may represent a metastatic malignancy or organization. The latter is usually in the form of shiny, gray-white *membranous structures* surrounding the hematoma **(Fig. 1-17)**. Microscopic examination should be performed to assess the age of the hematoma[90] and for other potential findings. The so-called pseudomembranes are composed of granulation tissue with neovascularization and

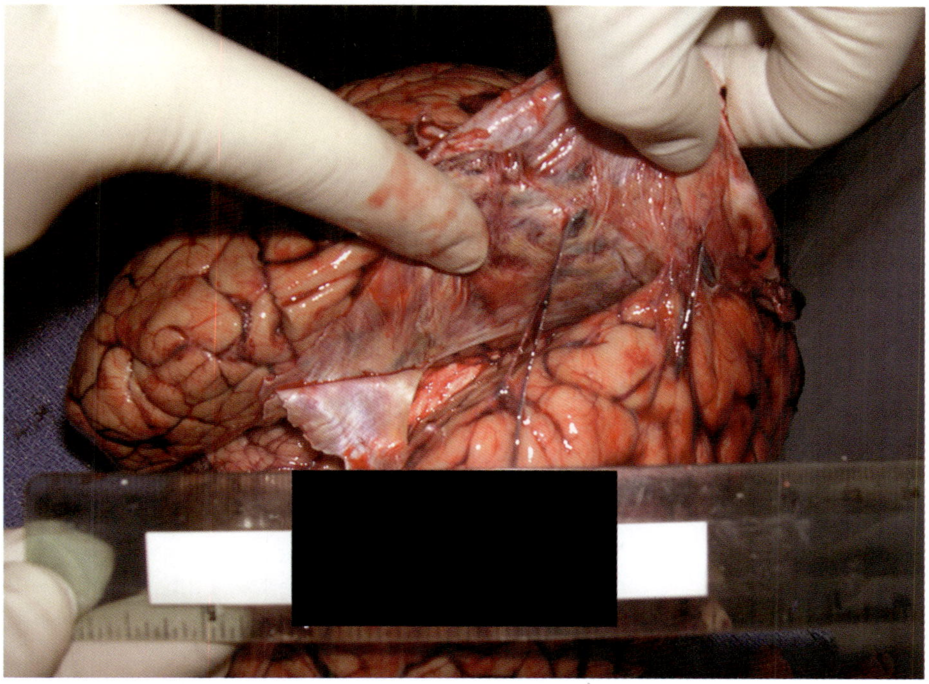

Figure 1-16. Delicate bridging veins traversing the distance between the brain and dura mater, stretched here for better demonstration.

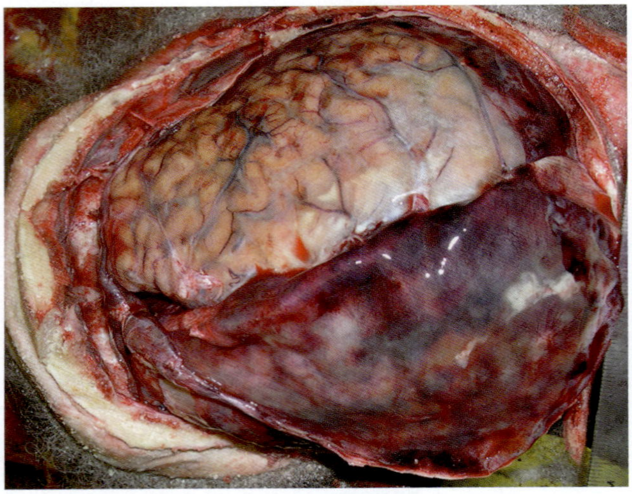

Figure 1-17. Chronic subdural hematoma remaining attached to the reflected dura mater. Organization with formation of granulation tissue membranes covering the hematoma, resulting in a shiny surface. Organization also creates a jelly-like clear appearance.

are prone to rebleeding in chronic, organizing hematomas. They are commonly removed and submitted to pathology as part of subdural hematoma evacuation specimens. Other evidence for traumatic injury, for example, diffuse axonal injury (DAI) and skull fractures, as well as secondary changes in the brain, such as swelling and herniations, should be sought. Depending on the amount of material, generous sampling for microscopic examination should be done, especially in surgical cases with a history of malignancy and especially hematolymphoid malignancy. In the spinal cord, associated contusions and epidural hemorrhages may be present in traumatic cases. In pediatric population, subdural hemorrhages are typically perinatal lesions or may be a result of child abuse, such as shaken baby syndrome.[91] They may be associated with *dural tears*, indicating distortion of the head. *Subdural empyema* can be identified as a diffuse pus accumulation, either as part of a generalized process in the CNS or due to direct extension of infection from vertebral osteomyelitis **(Fig. 1-18)**, which may become walled-off and localized in chronic cases. It is a common complication of upper aerodigestive tract and middle ear infections[92] **(Fig. 1-19)**.

Some of the other rare conditions to be mentioned are subdural hematoma associated with Menkes (kinky hair) disease,[93] coagulation problems, sinus thrombosis and subdural hemorrhages with L-asparaginase use in cancer treatment,[94] and complications related to shunts placed for management of hydrocephalus especially in the elderly.[95]

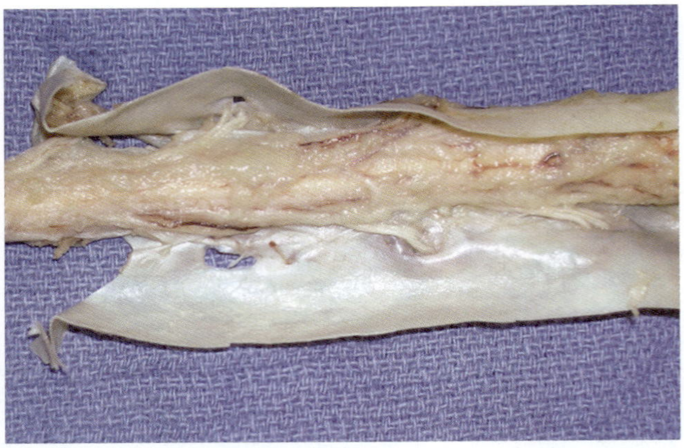

Figure 1-18. Prominent thick yellow pus under the spinal dura mater covering the spinal cord surface.

Leptomeninges and Subarachnoid Space

The usual smooth and glistening appearance of the leptomeninges can change by a variety of

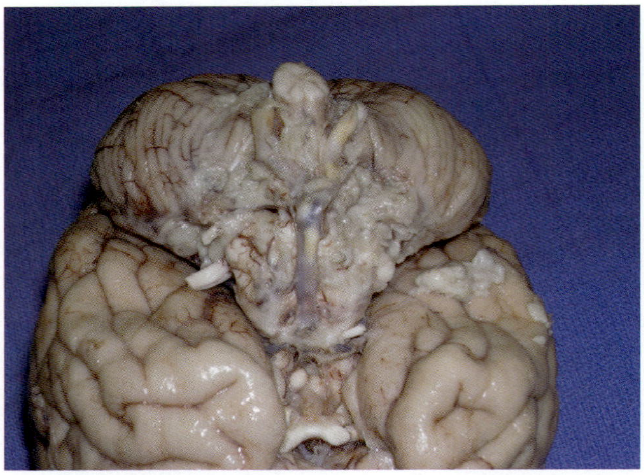

Figure 1-19. Thick yellow subdural pus is covering the basal surface of the brain. There was a subdural empyema in this case, secondary to extension of the process from a chronic and advanced middle ear infection.

List of Findings/Checklist for Leptomeninges and Subarachnoid Space

AT A GLANCE

- Subarachnoid hemorrhage
- Blood-tinged arachnoid surface
- Aneurysm
- Arterial dissection
- Traumatic injury
- Pus
- Mucinous appearance
- Fibrosis/thickening/granular appearance
- Cysts
- Underlying parenchymal injury/infarct
- Brown discoloration
- Fibrohyaline plaques

processes that involve the subarachnoid space. *Subarachnoid hemorrhage*[96,97] creates a red–brown dusky appearance when focal and mild **(Fig. 1-20)**. It is common to see if there is prominent *congestion*. Blood-tinged leptomeningeal surfaces can be due to *contamination of blood* during the autopsy or from a fresh and washed away *subdural hemorrhage*. True subarachnoid processes cannot be wiped away, as they are under the leptomeninges. A larger amount of blood is readily obvious. Most common scenario in autopsy setting is the rupture of a *saccular (berry) aneurysm* of the basal arteries[98] **(Fig. 1-21)**. It is important to identify the source of this hemorrhage and evaluate the aneurysm for the presence of *thrombosis* in the lumen and *rupture* site and, if a procedure such as coil placement has been performed **(Fig. 1-22)**, whether it is in place or damaged the aneurysm wall **(Table 1.3)**. These cases should be evaluated fresh to avoid hardening of blood clot after fixation. After documentation by pictures, the clot should be gently washed after dissecting the overlying leptomeninges if they have not been already ruptured, before the brain is transferred into formalin. Knowledge of the radiology and operative notes is important to help identify the aneurysm even if it is readily obvious, as they can be multiple aneurysms previously identified, and the pathologist is expected to confirm premortem findings. Since the majority of the aneurysms are located in the major basal vessels of anterior and posterior circulations, careful removal of these vascular systems in toto before or after fixation and subsequent dissection of any attached soft tissues or residual blood clots under a dissection microscope is a good approach, which may take some time in return for peace of mind **(Fig. 1-23)**. Again, the aneurysm should be documented by pictures, any foreign material removed gently, and the aneurysm is then cut perpendicular to the original artery **(Fig. 1-24)** to allow for microscopic examination of the aneurysm neck and the potential rupture site, which is usually toward the tip. In small lesions, obtaining multiple levels upfront is helpful to enable a thorough

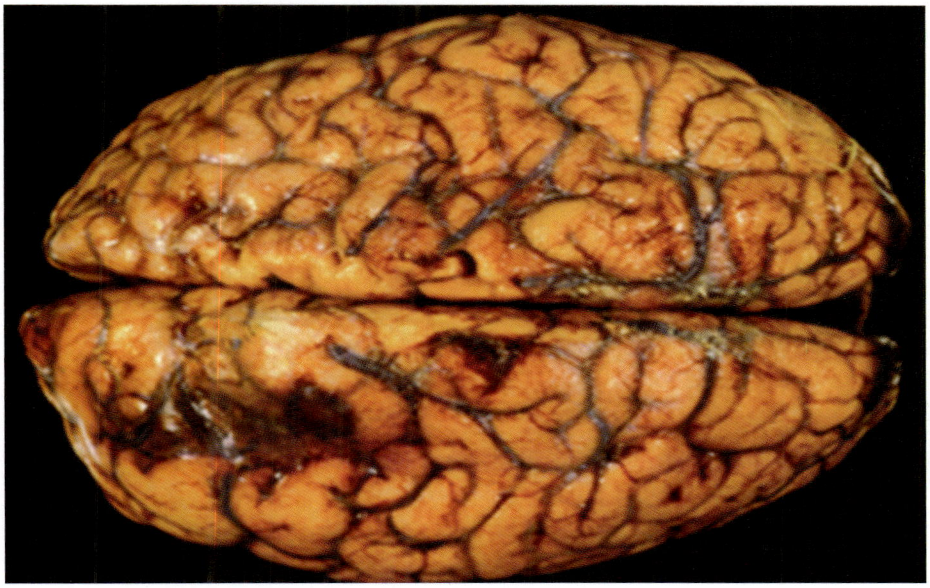

Figure 1-20. Subarachnoid hemorrhage over the left frontal lobe.

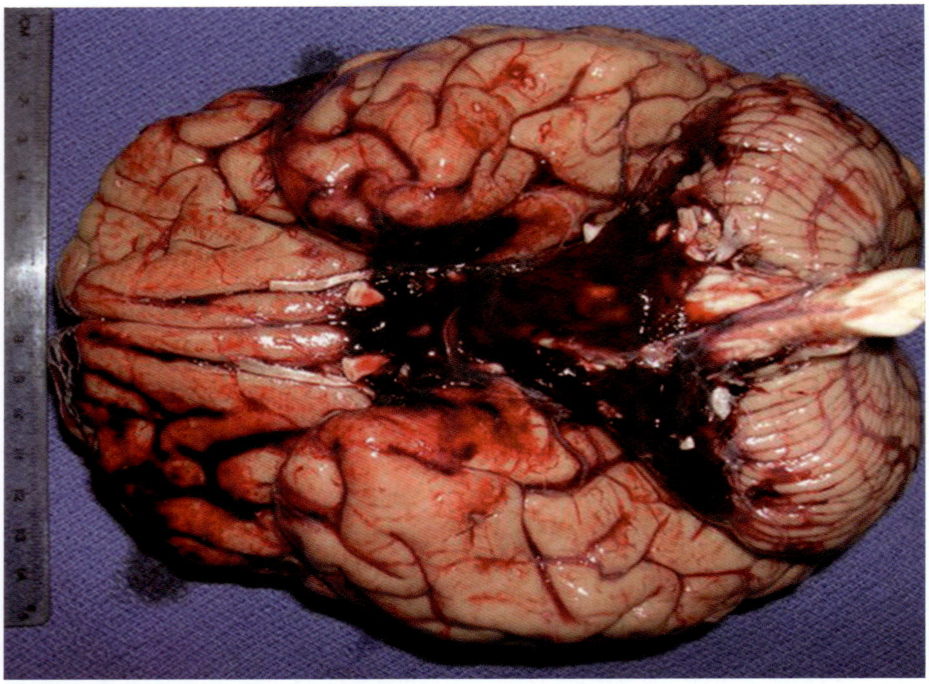

Figure 1-21. Basal subarachnoid hemorrhage due to a saccular aneurysm rupture. The hemorrhage is covered by the shiny, delicate arachnoid membrane and cannot be wiped away, although in some cases with abundant hemorrhage, arachnoid membrane can be breached and the hematoma becomes subdural.

examination without losing tissue to trimming of the block for subsequent requests. An elastic tissue stain such as Verhoeff-Van Gieson and a Masson's trichrome to highlight fibrin accumulation in and around potential subtle rupture site are useful. Subarachnoid hemorrhage can be associated with *traumatic aneurysms*[99] **(Table 1.4)**. These are usually associated with a history and other evidence of traumatic injury. Therefore, vessels within the hemorrhage should be examined for such changes

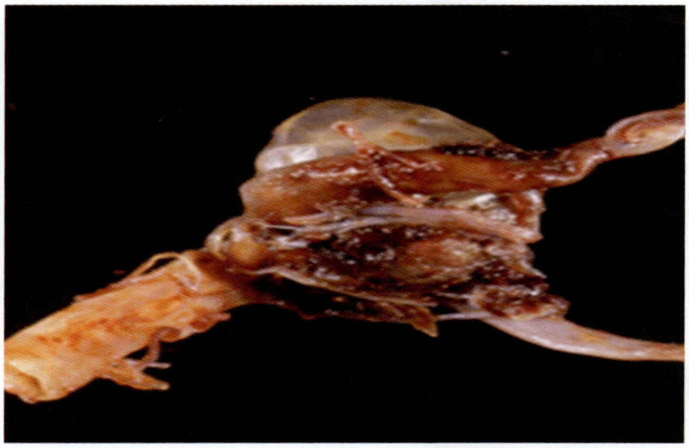

Figure 1-22. Blood clot has been dissected out to show the coiled saccular aneurysm.

TABLE 1.3 Approach to aneurysms at autopsy (typically for basal vessels but is applicable to other areas)

1. Inspect in situ
2. Take pictures
3. Remove brain
4. Take pictures of fresh brain
5. Wash blood clot gently as much as possible
6. Dissect and remove blood clot as much as possible, paying attention not to tear any aneurysm or vessels
7. Identify aneurysm (or other suspected hemorrhage site), note any rupture site, perforation by coils, etc.
8. Fix in formalin
9. Dissect out basal vessels (anterior and posterior circulation) gently (may be done prefixation; however, vessels are more likely to be torn). Preferably use stereotactic microscope
9. Note any clips, coils, etc.; take pictures; and remove any metal objects gently
10. Section the aneurysm perpendicular to the parent vessel to demonstrate its neck
11. Submit sections, order elastic and trichrome stains and levels upfront in small aneurysms to avoid unnecessary tissue loss due to subsequent trimming of the block

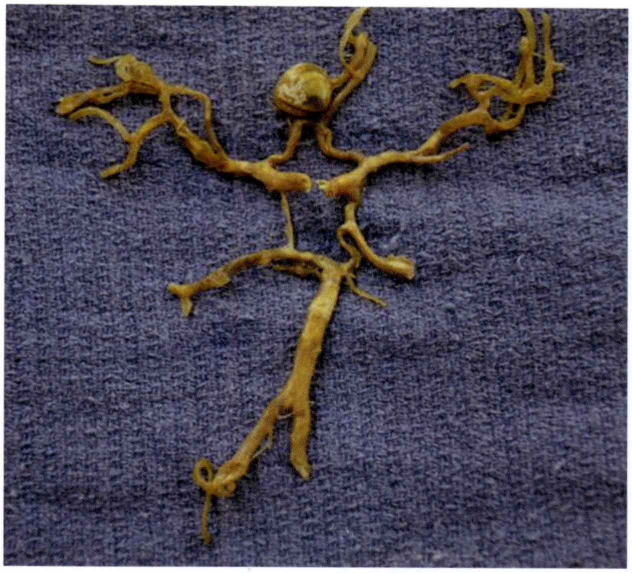

Figure 1-23. A saccular aneurysm is present at the bifurcation of the anterior communicating artery and right anterior cerebral artery.

for documentation. Likewise, trauma directly can cause leptomeningeal, vascular, and parenchymal injury, such as contusion, which can be seen on the leptomeningeal surfaces as subarachnoid hemorrhage. Basilar and vertebral artery tears, as well as internal carotid artery tears, dissections, and dissecting aneurysms can result from hyperextension of the neck.[100] Subarachnoid blood, as well as inflammation, can cause vascular spasm and result in *infarcts* in the brain tissue.[101,102] These are usually one or more superficial small infarcts. Larger ones can be felt as cortical softening and seen as dusky areas. In addition, bacterial meningitis, especially those due to *Neisseria meningitidis*, can result in patchy subarachnoid hemorrhages due to vascular injury.[103] *Angiostrongyliasis*, caused by Angiostrongylus cantonensis, can result in subarachnoid hemorrhage due to meningitis and vascular necrosis, which can further cause thrombosis and infarcts.[104] *Hyperthermia*, including malignant hyperthermia, may be associated with parenchymal and meningeal hemorrhages.[105,106] The syndrome of meningocerebral angiodysplasia and renal agenesis has very vascular leptomeninges, sometimes associated with subarachnoid hemorrhage. Angiodysplasia is in the form of ectatic capillaries and veins and can be seen in leptomeninges as well as in the brain, cerebellum, and brainstem.[107] In the leptomeninges, subarachnoid hemorrhages are seen. Cyclosporine A also results in subarachnoid hemorrhages, although this is a rare occurrence.[108] Amphetamines, methamphetamine, methylenedioxymethamphetamine (ecstasy), and cocaine are other drugs that can result in subarachnoid hemorrhages, along with parenchymal hemorrhage.[109,110]

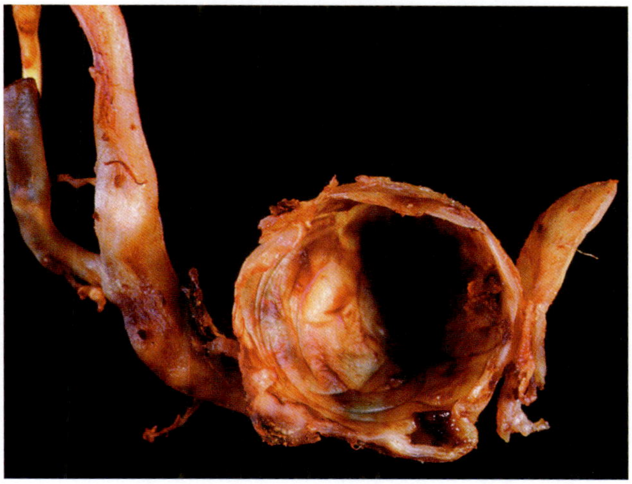

Figure 1-24. The aneurysm has been sectioned and the contents removed. Cross section of the artery it is originating from is seen at the bottom of the aneurysm.

TABLE 1.4 Common causes of subarachnoid hemorrhage

Saccular (berry) aneurysm
Other aneurysms
Coagulation disorders, anticoagulants
Extension of parenchymal hemorrhage
Bacterial meningitis
Medications and illegal drugs
Angiostrongyliasis
Hyperthermia
Meningocerebral angiodysplasia
Metastatic neoplasms
Hematolymphoid neoplasms
Rule out melanocytic lesions

Yellow–green *pus* accumulation in the subarachnoid space **(Fig. 1-25)**, usually throughout the brain surface or preferentially over the convexities, is typical for acute bacterial meningitis but may also be seen in fungal infections. It is also associated with prominent vascular congestion and brain edema. The exudate may not always be prominent, and all

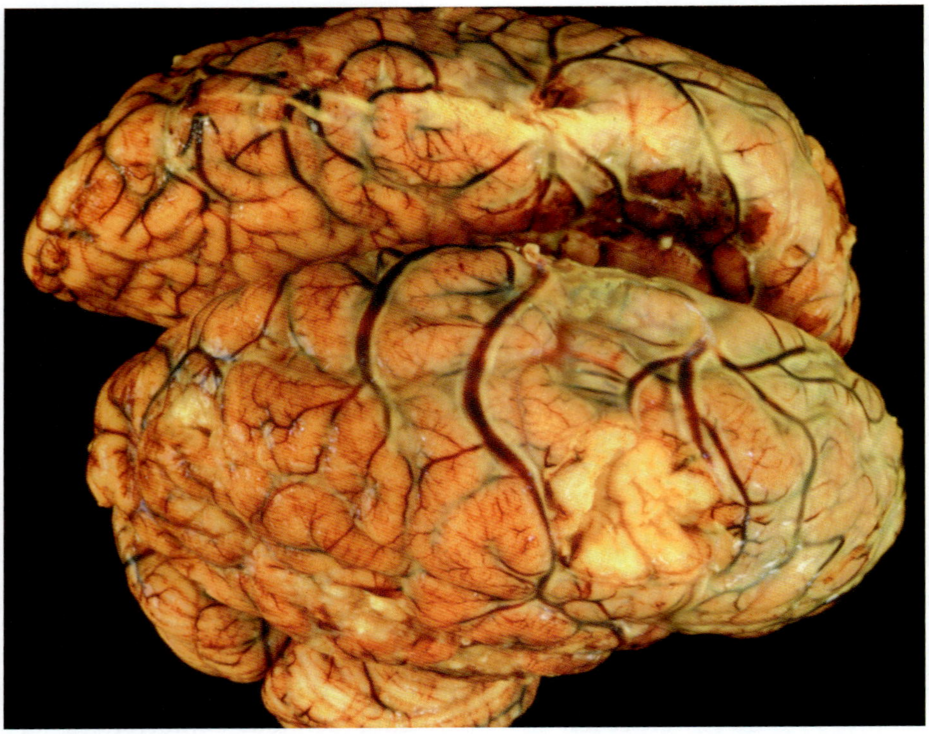

Figure 1-25. Bacterial meningitis with diffuse subarachnoid yellow pus, more prominent on the frontal lobes in this case, along with congested vessels.

there may be seen is a mild cloudy fluid collection rather than obvious pus. This is especially true in newborns, where the only obvious finding may be brain edema, especially if the course is rapidly fatal due to brain edema, leaving not much time for inflammatory response to develop. In these cases, *viral (aseptic) meningitis* is another consideration. The causative microorganism has usually been identified by CSF cultures and, in the case of autopsies, by premortem studies; however, in many cases, further work-up by special stains for *microorganisms*, depending on the clinical situation, may be required to cover the bacterial and fungal microorganisms by Gram-Twort and Grocott's/Gomori's methenamine silver (GMS) stains, respectively. The bacteria may be very difficult to find, but a diligent search usually is rewarding. It may be impossible to find bacteria in autopsy cases where the patient has received treatment. In autopsies, *postmortem growth* and *contamination* of the material are two major pitfalls. In such cases, there is usually no significant inflammatory component or a clinical history of meningitis is not present. Therefore, every finding should be interpreted in the given context. One exception to the *absence of inflammatory infiltrate* is immunocompromised patients. Fungal infiltration of the leptomeninges creates a grayish, more solid appearance. Especially cryptococcal meningitis has a thick, *mucinous appearance* **(Fig. 1-26)**. Histoplasmosis creates a yellow-gray exudate in the meninges.

In cases of *sepsis*, bacteria may be identified in the blood vessels and in the cytoplasm of

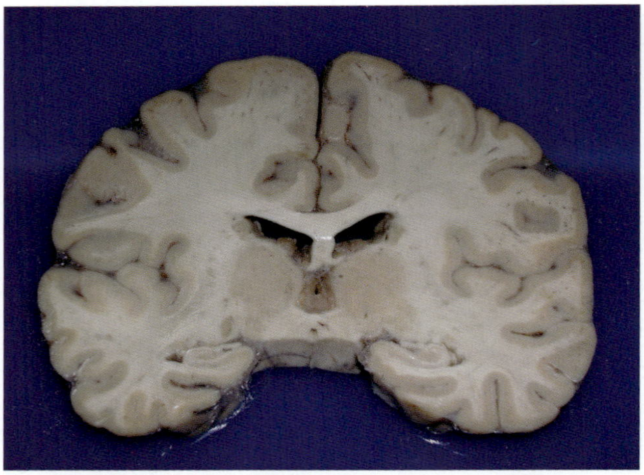

Figure 1-26. Diffuse involvement of subarachnoid space by a gray, mucinous material in this case of cryptococcal meningitis, best seen in the sulci. There is also ventricular involvement with similar features.

polymorphonuclear (PMN) leukocytes within the blood vessels, but this requires a long search and lots of luck. Fortunately, there are premortem blood cultures in most cases. A postmortem artifact, corresponding to the gross appearance of Swiss-cheese artifact, is a *multicystic parenchymal change*.[38] The cysts are the result of gas-forming bacteria, which can be demonstrated in the cysts in many situations, which made their way to the CNS as a result of sepsis or putrefaction of intestinal tissues in decomposing bodies. Although rare in the CNS, Fusarium infections can cause meningitis and abscesses.[111] North American blastomycosis, caused by Blastomyces dermatitidis, results in meningitis and sometimes abscess or granulomas, with a fibrous patchy thickening of meninges, exudates, and fibrosis.[112]

A *fibrotic thickening* of the leptomeninges **(Table 1.5)** with a *granular texture* suggests a chronic and likely granulomatous inflammatory process, such as tuberculous meningitis[113] or sarcoidosis.[114] These usually have a predilection to involve the basal surfaces of the brain. Meningovascular syphilis and general paresis (chronic meningoencephalitis) result in fibrous thickening of meninges,[115] with an appearance similar to that of tuberculosis. Fungal meningitis also has a tendency to involve basal surfaces. Leptomeninges are thickened with a gelatinous appearance in Batten's disease (neuronal ceroid lipofuscinosis) and in mucopolysaccharidoses.[116] HTLV-1-associated myelopathy (HAM), a.k.a. tropical spastic paraparesis, results in spinal cord atrophy and leptomeningeal and parenchymal vascular fibrosis that involves especially the lower thoracic region. Cysticercosis may be numerous, mainly involving the meninges, cortex, and ventricles. It can degenerate to become a firm white nodule, which eventually calcifies. In the ventricles and meninges, it may float around in the form of *clear cysts*. When the organism is dead, intense granulomatous reaction may result in fibrous thickening of the meninges.[117] Coenurosis,[118] caused by Coenurus cerebralis, a rare parasitic disease that can involve the ventricles, especially the fourth ventricle, and subarachnoid space, also has cysts that can measure up to several centimeters.

A firm and diffuse thickening may also be due to the rare idiopathic hypertrophic pachymeningitis,[119] which mainly affects dura mater, but may also involve leptomeninges. Fibrosis of the parasagittal leptomeninges can also be normally seen as an age-related change. Leptomeningeal glial heterotopias, depending on their prominence and extent, can be seen as focal patchy opacities of leptomeninges. Cerebro-ocular dysplasia has, among other findings, glial and mesenchymal proliferation in the subarachnoid space resulting in thickened leptomeninges obscuring sulcal–gyral pattern.[120] Another cause for large areas of diffuse plaque-like thickening and opacity is meningioma en plaque, a diffusely growing meningioma without the formation of a dominant mass.[17] Metastatic carcinomas can result in a similar appearance, that is, leptomeningeal carcinomatosis,[121] sometimes erroneously but habitually referred to as carcinomatous meningitis. It is also common for leptomeninges to be involved by hematolymphoid processes, especially leukemic infiltrates, which are very similar to subarachnoid hemorrhage in gross appearance. Some primary CNS neoplasms have a tendency to infiltrate the subarachnoid space and spread through cerebrospinal fluid (CSF). Pineal region neoplasms, including germ cell tumor (GCT) and medulloblastoma, are well-known for this. Especially medulloblastoma can widely infiltrate the leptomeninges to appear as an icing, simulating fibrosis **(Fig. 1-27)**. Another example of craniospinal spread of primary CNS neoplasm is in the form of multiple drop metastases and is commonly seen as multiple nodules typically on the spinal cord and spinal nerve surfaces. Aside from the pineal region neoplasms, ventricular, cerebellar,

TABLE 1.5 Causes of leptomeningeal thickening and opacification

Chronic inflammation
Granulomatous inflammation (tuberculosis, fungal infections, sarcoidosis)
Syphilis
Neuronal ceroid lipofuscinosis
Mucopolysaccharidosis
HTLV-1-associated myelopathy (HAM)
Parasitic infestation (cysticercosis, coenurosis)
Idiopathic hypertrophic pachymeningitis
Aging
Glial heterotopias
Cerebro-ocular dysplasia
Meningioma en plaque
Meningeal carcinomatosis
Fibrohyaline plaques (spinal cord, multifocal)

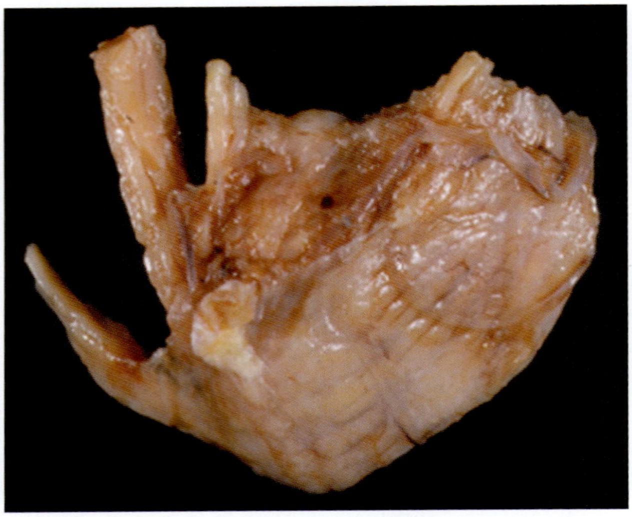

Figure 1-27. Diffuse infiltration of the leptomeninges by medulloblastoma, creating a gray-white, opaque layer, simulating fibrosis.

and fourth ventricle neoplasms; ependymomas; meningiomas; gliomas; and literally any type of neoplasm can show this type of spread **(Fig. 1-28)**.

A *dark brown discoloration* of the leptomeninges, usually on the brainstem surfaces, anterior surface of cervical spinal cord, and base of the brain, is due to melanocytes that are normally present and are more prominent in black race. It may superficially resemble subarachnoid hemorrhage but is not as homogenous or diffuse. In cases of melanosis and melanomatosis, the diffuse proliferation of benign and malignant melanocytes, respectively, the pigmentation is more prominent and widespread. It may mimic subarachnoid hemorrhage, although it is darker and brown, rather than dark red. Melanocytoma and melanoma tend to occur as localized lesions in the distribution of

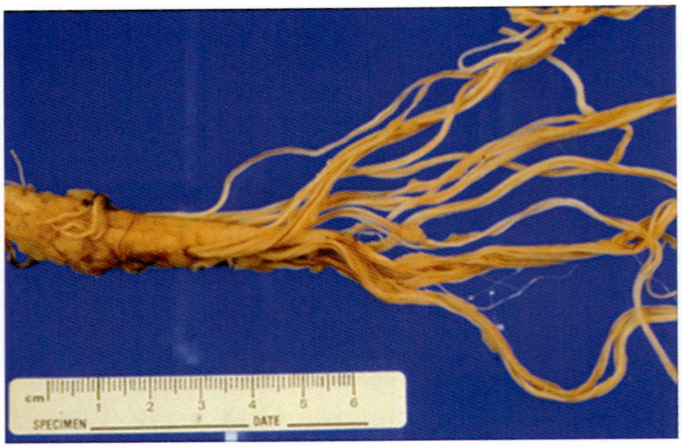

Figure 1-28. Multiple nodules are present on the spinal cord and the spinal nerves in the cauda equina, representing drop metastases from an ependymoma, that is, ependymomatosis.

melanocytes, most commonly in association with the cervical and thoracic spinal cord leptomeninges, as extramedullary, intradural mass lesions. In cases where nerve roots are involved, they may mimic other neoplasms such as schwannoma and meningioma, although pigmentation is helpful in considering a melanotic lesion. The identification of pigmentation may be difficult as it may appear as hemorrhage. Melanotic schwannomas should also be considered in such pigmented mass lesions. In melanocytoma, melanoma, and melanomatosis, metastasis should be ruled out.[122]

Fibrohyaline plaques are thin, irregular, firm, multiple, and gray-white plaque-like structures attached to the posterior leptomeninges of the lower spinal cord that represent a common finding with no known significance **(Fig. 1-29)**. They are more common with increasing age, can get calcified and ossified, and can be identified radiologically.

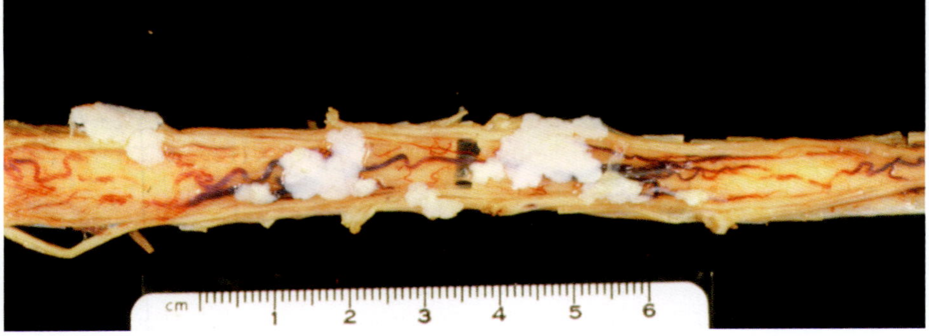

Figure 1-29. Multiple thin fibrohyaline plaques on the posterior surface of the spinal cord, associated with the leptomeninges.

Blood Vessels

Atherosclerotic changes are frequently prominent in older age in the basal vessels as *yellow plaques*. They can be focal or can involve long segments of an artery, making it feel like a firm tube rather than its usual collapsible soft consistency with clear walls. When calcified, they may be difficult to cut without crushing, which should be avoided especially if the vessel wall needs microscopic examination for subtle changes, such as early arterial dissection. Mild decalcification is useful in such cases. Basilar artery can be extremely dilated and can become *tortuous, forming an "S" shape*, called dolichoectasia.[123] This is due to the deformation of the artery wall due to hypertensive and atherosclerotic changes. Close examination of basal arteries can reveal dramatic findings, such as complete occlusion of internal carotid artery by *thrombus*, or milder versions of this theme. Therefore, vasculature may be dissected diligently in search for embolic/thrombotic processes. Such an attempt is especially recommended in cases with large infarcts. Thrombosis in the vessels should be distinguished from *postmortem clot*, which is loosely attached, if any, to the vessel wall; can easily be removed; and is friable. Thrombi are firm, tend to be tightly attached to the vessel wall, and distend the lumen **(Fig. 1-30)**. They may show red and white areas (lines of Zahn) due to settling and separation of red and white blood cells. Early thrombi may be difficult to tell apart from postmortem clot. Microscopic examination clarifies this issue, although the vessel should be sectioned carefully to avoid breaking and dislodging the thrombus. Thrombi result from a wide variety of disorders. *Thromboemboli*,[124] most notably of cardiac origin due to atrial fibrillation, local thrombus formation due to disorders of the vessels, such as complicated atherosclerosis, aneurysms, and vascular inflammatory disorders, or systemic problems with coagulation, thrombophilia, antiphospholipid antibodies, polycythemia, dehydration, oral contraceptive use, smoking, and paraneoplastic thrombotic conditions, among many others, can be involved **(Table 1.6)**. Therefore, microscopic examination of the thrombosed vessel wall and review of clinical and other laboratory findings can be very useful in further explaining the thrombotic event **(Fig. 1-31)**. Venous sinus thrombosis is discussed in "Dura Mater and Subdural Space" above. *Emboli* other than thromboemboli, such as adipose tissue, can also be identified, though they are more common to see microscopically. Pediatric population

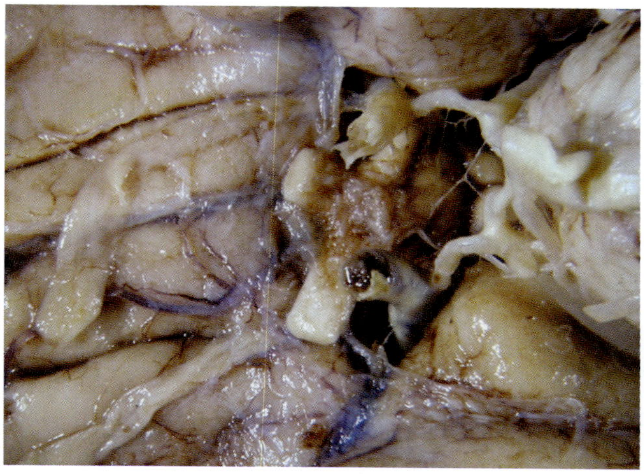

Figure 1-30. Right internal carotid artery is distended by a thrombus completely occluding the lumen in this patient who was found unresponsive in his house.

List of Findings/Checklist for Blood Vessels

• AT A GLANCE

- Atherosclerosis
- Dolichoectasia
- Thrombus/postmortem clot
- Emboli/thromboemboli
- Arterial dissection/dissecting aneurysm
- Saccular and other aneurysms
- Vascular nodularity/thickening
- Malformations

TABLE 1.6 Common causes of thrombi
Thromboembolus (atrial fibrillation)
Complex atherosclerosis
Aneurysms, other vascular disorders
Systemic coagulation disorders
Thrombophilia
Antiphospholipid antibody syndrome
Polycythemia
Dehydration
Oral contraceptive use
Smoking
Paraneoplastic thrombotic disorders

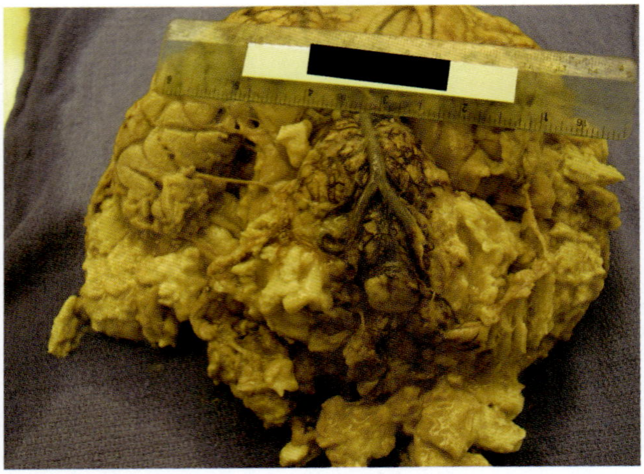

Figure 1-31. Diffuse thrombosis of the entire anterior and posterior circulation, more prominently of both vertebral arteries and basilar artery, resulting in extensive infarction predominantly of the brainstem, cerebellum, and occipital lobes. Vertebral and basilar arteries are diffusely distended by thrombosis. The patient was a 40-year-old woman, who was found dead in her apartment. No clinical history was available; however, autopsy showed lobar pneumonia and polarizable crystals in the lungs, consistent with intravenous drug use.

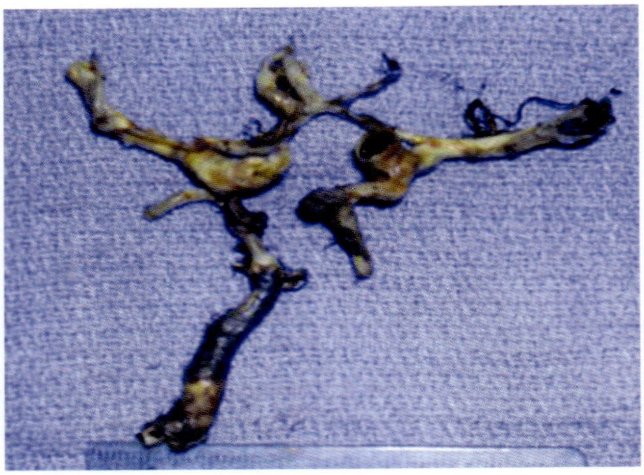

Figure 1-32. Basilar artery is expanded and its adventitia is hemorrhagic due to the dissecting aneurysm seen in Figure 1-33.

is not immune to thrombotic events,[125] and vessels should be examined in detail in pediatric cases as well.

Arterial dissection and *dissecting aneurysm*[126,127] commonly occur in the supraclinoid segment of the internal carotid arteries and in the vertebral arteries **(Figs. 1-32 and 1-33)**. Sometimes, it may be necessary to take the sphenoid bone as a block together with the sella turcica. It can then be cut on both sides following the internal carotid artery trajectories to expose the cavernous sinuses and the cavernous segments of the internal carotid arteries to further examine for dissection or cavernous sinus thrombosis. They are also seen in vertebral arteries and less commonly as isolated basilar artery aneurysm. The aneurismal artery may show a fusiform expansion, and there may be evidence of hemorrhage in and around its adventitia. The term *fusiform aneurysm* is sometimes used interchangeably with dissecting aneurysm [128]; however, fusiform aneurysm refers to an elongated sausage-like expansion of the artery due to any damage to the artery wall resulting in this type of deformity, although dissecting aneurysms can assume this appearance, also. Basilar and vertebral artery tears can also occur as a result of hyperextension injury. *Saccular (berry) aneurysms* are also seen in the basal arterial system, sometimes as an incidental findings They are discussed in more detail together with subarachnoid hemorrhage, since that is the main context they are seen in neuropathology (see "Leptomeninges and Subarachnoid Space" above). Multifocal *irregularities of vascular contours* and *nodular thickenings* may indicate a generalized involvement of vascular system by vasculitis, granulomatous inflammation, or primary angiitis of the CNS.[129] Moyamoya disease also causes irregular thickenings of the basal arterial system[130] **(Fig. 1-34)**. Ecchordosis physaliphora is an incidental finding seen anterior to the basilar artery and represents an ectopic notochord rest **(Fig. 1-35)**.

Vascular malformations are seen as irregular conglomerations of vascular structures of variable sizes and shapes, usually forming a localized mass lesion. AVM and cavernous angioma (cavernoma) are the most commonly seen vascular malformations on the meningeal surfaces. AVMs can be superficial and identified on the leptomeningeal surfaces. On the posterior surface of the lumbar spinal cord, prominence of tortuous vasculature may be an indication of Foix-Alajouanine syndrome, which is an arteriovenous fistula, rather than an AVM.[131] On the anterior surface of the lumbosacral spinal cord, AVM can be present. Both of

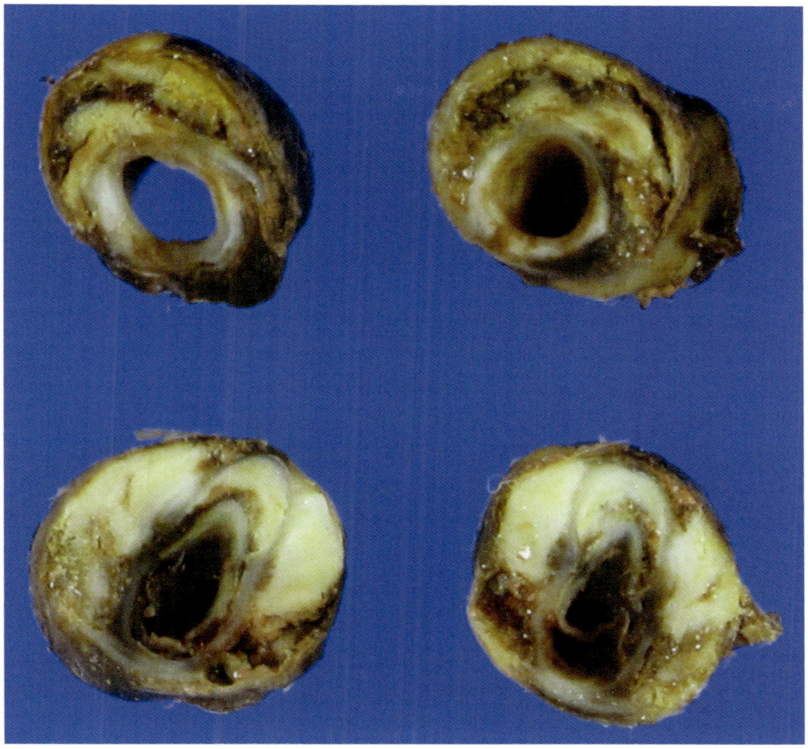

Figure 1-33. Cross sections of the dissecting aneurysm of the basilar artery seen in Figure 1-32. Extensive atherosclerotic changes are seen as *yellow-white* thickening, while dissection is seen as hemorrhagic intramural lines, together severely obliterating the lumen. Hemorrhage reaches the adventitia in some areas.

these lesions result in venous congestive myelopathy, and depending on the stage of the disorder, the underlying spinal cord may be variably gliotic, firm, and shrunken.[132] Intramedullary AVMs can also be found in the spinal cord, resulting in more acute changes. Cavernous hemangiomas are frequent in the skull bones. Vascular malformations may be associated with some syndromes, for example, PHACE, that is associated with posterior fossa malformations, arterial abnormalities, coarctation of aorta, and eye abnormalities.[133] AVMs may be seen as part of other malformations or syndromes (see "Skin and External Findings" above), such as Sturge-Weber syndrome, NF1, hereditary

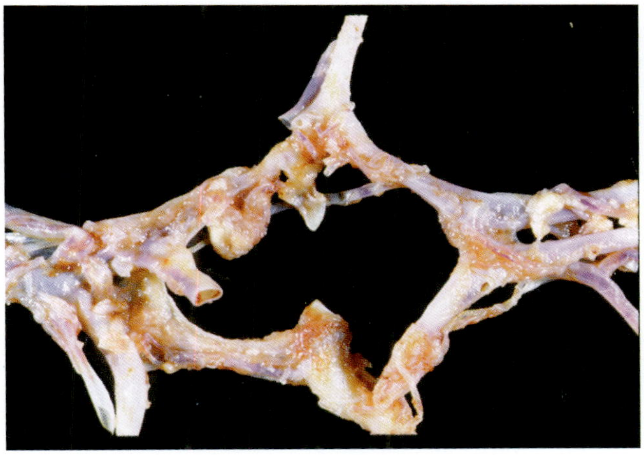

Figure 1-34. Moyamoya disease: Distorted, irregular nodular, and thick basal vasculature.

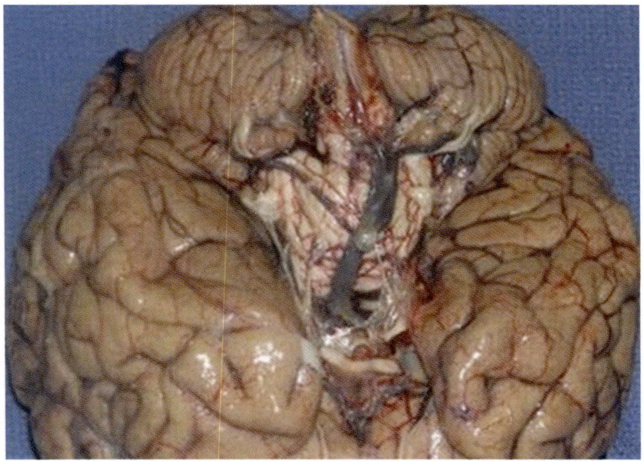

Figure 1-35. Ecchordosis physaliphora: A glistening nodule of tissue is seen attached to the basilar artery as an incidental finding.

hemorrhagic telangiectasia, Marfan syndrome, and Wyburn-Mason syndrome. Cavernomas are typically multiple in hereditary forms.[134]

Brain Weight

Healthy human *adult brain weight* is 1,300 to 1,400 g in the male and 1,275 to 1,375 g in the female, or about 2% of body weight, although these figures are highly variable, ranging from 1,100 to 1,700 g in the male and 1,050 to 1,550 g in the female. The *gender difference* is due to general body size difference and not to any significant structural variations. Racial differences in each gender are also minimal.[135–139] Brain reaches adult weight around 12 years of age, with a gradual decline becoming prominent especially after about seventh decade, where up to about 10% of the original weight may be lost. It is possible to find brain weights outside these given ranges with no functional or morphologic pathology. Brain weight is more crucial with more practical accuracy in prenatal and postnatal life. Detailed charts correlating brain weight with gestational weeks and subsequent stages of life up to 12 years of age are available. Similar charts are also available to compare brain weight with body weight and various measurements of the body.[140] The *weight of the cerebellum*, excluding brainstem, and its comparison with brain weight can provide additional insight.[141] The normal *cerebrum-to-cerebellum ratio* is about 10% to 11% in both genders. The weights of the cerebellum and brainstem together account for approximately 12% of the total brain weight.[142] Changes in this ratio may be used as an indicator of more prominent atrophy of either component. This ratio is decreased in posterior fossa abnormalities, especially in cerebellar malformations. Typically, a small cerebellum or other obvious malformation is grossly identified, such as in pontocerebellar hypoplasia. However, this method has not been commonly used in practice. Instead, visual evaluation and subsequent systematical examination of relevant tissues constitute the usual approach. Brain weight differs in *fresh and fixed brains*. There is about 5% to 10% increase in brain weight after fixation. The difference seems to be greater in pediatric than in adult brains.[142] Given the wide ranges of normal weight and no definitive criteria associated with it, the difference does not appear to be critical for practical purposes. However, it has become customary to qualify the brain weight as fixed or unfixed weight. When possible, the weight should be measured fresh.

Brain weight outside the normal range for age and gender indicates significant pathology in pediatric population, such as a malformation or growth retardation. It is also *decreased* in conditions with significant tissue loss, such as periventricular leukomalacia. The significance of brain weight and the limits of normal are more flexible in adults. In the older population, decreased brain weight may indicate a neurodegenerative disease, such as Alzheimer's disease (AD), where tissue is lost due to the degenerative process, although it is not unusual to see discrepancies between brain weight and the degree of histopathology. In general, *increases* in brain weight can also be due to generalized edema, as seen in hemodynamic disturbances or in infections due to associated edema, as in encephalitis or meningitis.

One area where brain weight is crucial is the assessment for microcephaly (microencephaly) or macrocephaly (megalencephaly).[143] *Microcephaly* refers to a small head, and *microencephaly* refers specifically to small brain; however, they are frequently used interchangeably in daily practice **(Table 1.7)**. Microcephaly can result from *bone disorders*, such as craniosynostosis, interfering with the development of the brain and growth of the head.[144,145] *Primary microencephaly* is when the brain weight is more than 3 standard deviations

List of Findings/Checklist for Brain Weight

• AT A GLANCE

- Brain weight
- Cerebrum-to-cerebellum ratio
- Increased brain weight
- Decreased brain weight
- Head circumference
- Microcephaly/microencephaly (primary or secondary)
- Macrocephaly/megalocephaly/megalencephaly (primary or secondary)
- Hemimegalencephaly

below the mean for age and sex.[146] There should not be any other reason, such as prenatal injury, radiation exposure, or craniosynostosis, to cause the microencephaly. If no gross abnormalities are identified in the small brain and the gyral pattern is normal, then it is termed *microencephaly vera*. If the gyral pattern is simplified or abnormal (also may be termed oligogyric microencephaly or microlissencephaly), it is termed *microencephaly with simplified gyral pattern*.[147] Whether the gyral pattern is normal or abnormal implies different pathogenetic mechanisms, and it is therefore important to accurately identify these cases. Periventricular heterotopias should be sought in cases with abnormal gyral pattern. Microencephaly can be associated with *chromosomal and single gene defects* such as trisomy 21 (Down syndrome),[148] trisomy 18 (Edwards syndrome),[149] criduchat syndrome (5p syndrome),[150] Wolf-Hirschhorn syndrome (4p syndrome),[151] and fragile X syndrome. Microencephaly can also be seen in cases of X-linked mental retardation.[152] There are, of course, many other syndromes with a microencephaly component, and these should be evaluated on a case by case basis with the help of the resources dedicated to genetic disorders, syndromes, and malformations. In some genetic disorders, there is *progressive postnatal microencephaly*, although these children may be normal at birth. Many represent metabolic diseases. Alpers disease, Rett syndrome, and infantile neuronal ceroid lipofuscinosis are some examples, which demonstrate postnatal and progressive microencephaly. Cases of *secondary microencephaly* typically are of nongenetic nature. *Environmental factors* such as conditions resulting in intrauterine growth retardation, for example, placental problems and intrauterine infections, children of uncontrolled phenylketonuric mothers, fetal alcohol syndrome, teratogenic agents, and radiation exposure are some of the notable causes.

Macrocephaly or megalocephaly refers to a larger than normal head, and *megalencephaly* refers to a brain that weighs 2.5 or more standard deviations over the normal weight for age and sex, although various definitions including intracranial volume measurements are also used[153] **(Table 1.8)**. Many associations have been described.[154] It is also divided into *primary and secondary* groups based on etiologic factors. Some are *isolated cases* with no other explanation; however, many others are associated with mental retardation and some kind of gross or microscopic structural abnormalities, such as polymicrogyria. Others may be familial or associated with other abnormalities, such as achondroplasia or endocrine abnormalities. *Secondary megalencephaly* is usually seen in inborn errors of metabolism or leukodystrophies, such as Alexander's disease, where a substance accumulation causes enlargement of the brain, or neurocutaneous syndromes. Megalencephaly can also be associated with NF1, due to increases in cerebral volume. Cases with Cowden syndrome/Lhermitte-Duclos disease may have macrocephaly/megalencephaly, which is considered a major criterion for this syndrome.[155] *Hemimegalencephaly or unilateral megalencephaly* is a rare malformation that can be isolated or syndromic.[156] The surface of the involved side may show agyria or pachygyria and may be firm.

TABLE 1.7 Selected causes of microcephaly

Bone disorders
Microcephaly vera
Microcephaly with simplified gyral pattern
Trisomy 21
Trisomy 18
Cri-du-chat syndrome
Wolf-Hirschhorn syndrome
Fragile X syndrome
X-linked mental retardation
Progressive postnatal microcephaly (e.g., leukodystrophies)
Intrauterine infections
Phenylketonuria
Fetal alcohol syndrome
Teratogenic agents
Radiation

TABLE 1.8 Selected causes of macrocephaly

Idiopathic
Familial
Endocrine abnormalities
Achondroplasia
Storage diseases
Syndromic (e.g., NF1, Cowden syndrome)
Hemimegalencephaly

Head circumference is used as a measure of brain development in pediatrics.[157] One major cause of megalocephaly, in its strict meaning referring to a large head, is *hydrocephalus*. Paradoxically, with the pressure of the accumulated CSF, there is actually reduction in the size and weight of the brain in time, in spite of the enlarged head. Intrauterine or perinatal *infections* resulting in destructive lesions in the brain are associated with microencephaly/microcephaly typical for varicella, CMV, rubella, and congenital toxoplasma infections involving the brain.[158]

External Surfaces

The external surfaces of brain and spinal cord provide critical guidance for further sectioning and examination. *Pattern of atrophy* of various distribution and degree gives an idea about neurodegenerative diseases, especially dementing conditions. Atrophy, as it applies to this discussion, indicates neuron loss and associated gliosis and is associated with decreased brain weight (see "Brain Weight" above). Cortical atrophy causes *thinning of gyri* and *widening of sulci* **(Table 1.9)**. AD results in a *generalized cortical atrophy* **(Fig. 1-36)**, although occipital lobes and motor cortex tend to be somewhat spared in AD, with the most prominent atrophy in the medial temporal lobes. Dementia with Lewy bodies (DLB) also shows generalized atrophy, though not as prominent as in AD, and also tends to spare the occipital lobes. Huntington's disease results in a mild, generalized cortical atrophy, in addition to its involvement of basal ganglia, especially caudate nucleus and putamen. Generalized atrophy is also a component of Guam parkinsonism–dementia complex,[159] general paresis (syphilitic chronic meningoencephalitis),[160] and prion diseases. In prion diseases, atrophy is primarily in the cerebral cortex, and in some cases, it may also involve cerebellum and brainstem. In the later stages of subacute sclerosing panencephalitis (SSPE),[161] prominent cortical atrophy can be seen, along with white matter changes due to demyelination. Neuroaxonal dystrophies constitute a rare group of conditions associated with generalized atrophy of the brain and cerebellum.[162] Atrophy can be a result of systemic processes such as uremic encephalopathy[163] and inborn errors of metabolism **(Fig. 1-37)**. Ifosfamide, an alkylating agent,

List of Findings/Checklist for External Surfaces

AT A GLANCE

- Atrophy
- Pattern of atrophy
- Brain atrophy
- Cerebellar atrophy
- Brainstem atrophy
- Spinal cord atrophy
- Softening
- Depression
- Discoloration
- Expansion of the gyri, cerebellar folia, brainstem, and spinal cord
- Flattening of surfaces (generalized or focal)
- Cerebral malformations
  - Agyria/pachygyria/lissencephaly
  - Holoprosencephaly
  - Polymicrogyria
  - Polygyria
  - Brachycephaly
  - Atelencephaly
  - Anencephaly
  - Hydranencephaly
  - Basket brain
  - Porencephaly
  - Schizencephaly
  - Agenesis of corpus callosum
  - Encephalocele
- Cerebellar malformations
  - Cerebellar agenesis
  - Agenesis of vermis
  - Midline cyst
  - Rhombencephalosynapsis
- Spinal cord
  - Diplo- and diastematomyelia
- Exophytic growth
- Herniations
  - Cingulate (subfalcine)
  - Uncal (transtentorial)
  - Cerebellar tonsillar
  - Upward cerebellar transtentorial
  - Fungating (transcalvarial)
  - Frontal-to-middle cranial fossa
  - Spinal cord

TABLE 1.9 Diseases that result in brain atrophy and its distribution on external examination

Disease or Agent	Typical Pattern of Atrophy
AD	Generalized Relative sparing of motor and occipital cortices
DLB	Generalized, less prominent than AD Relative sparing of occipital cortex
FTLD	Frontal and temporal lobes Sparing of posterior superior temporal gyrus
Huntington's disease	Generalized, mild
CBD	Preferentially parietal, posterior frontal, perirolandic, asymmetric
ALS	Motor cortex
Inborn errors of metabolism	Generalized
Prion diseases	Generalized May also involve cerebellum and brainstem
SSPE	Generalized, in later stages
Syphilitic chronic meningoencephalitis	Generalized
GPDC	Generalized
Neuroaxonal dystrophies	Generalized Cerebellum is also involved
Uremic encephalopathy	Generalized
Ifosfomide	Generalized, in children
Mercury poisoning	Calcarine cortex, cerebellum

AD, alzheimer's disease; DLB, dementia with Lewy bodies; FTLD, frontotemporal lobar degeneration; CBD, corticobasal degeneration; ALS, amyotrophic lateral sclerosis; SSPE, subacute sclerosing panencephalitis; GPDC, Guam parkinsonism–dementia complex.

can result in brain atrophy in children.[164] Atrophy may have a more *selective pattern*. Frontotemporal lobar degeneration (FTLD) has a predominantly frontotemporal atrophy pattern **(Fig. 1-38)** with sparing of the posterior part superior temporal gyrus, especially in Pick's disease **(Fig. 1-39)**. Corticobasal degeneration also has a selective atrophy pattern involving parietal, posterior

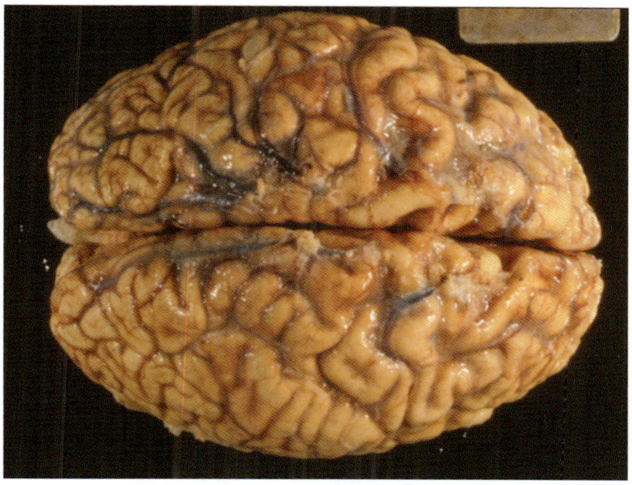

Figure 1-36. Diffuse cortical atrophy that is characterized by thinning of gyri and widening of sulci. Occipital lobes on the left side of the picture are relatively spared as they appear more compact.

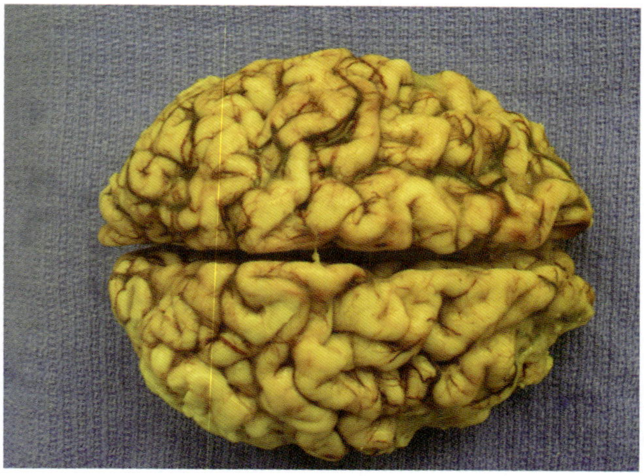

Figure 1-37. Diffuse atrophy is seen in this brain from a child who died of leukodystrophic process. The entire brain appears small and shrunken.

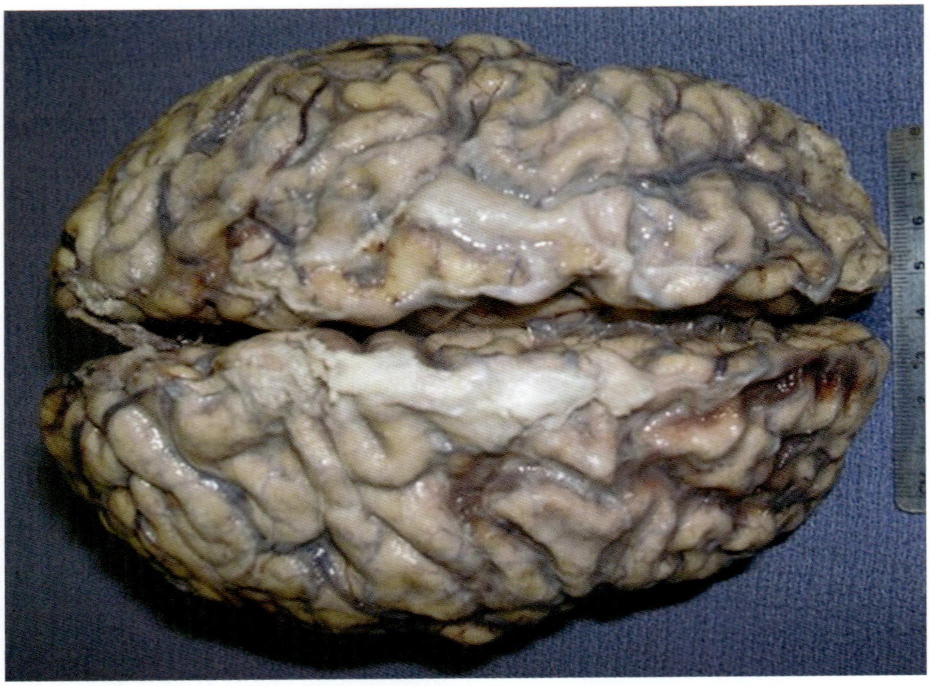

Figure 1-38. Prominent cortical atrophy involving mainly the frontal lobes in this brain with FTLD.

frontal, and perirolandic areas. Mercury poisoning (Minamata disease) can selectively result in degeneration of the calcarine cortex, along with cerebellar degeneration.[165] Selective precentral (motor) cortex atrophy is seen in amyotrophic lateral sclerosis (ALS). Such selective atrophy patterns are difficult to appreciate in mild cases and unless conscious attention is paid. *Spinal cord* should also be carefully evaluated for the atrophic appearance of anterior spinal nerve roots relative to posterior spinal nerve roots in motor neuron disease (MND). On cross sections of the spinal cord, shrinkage and tan discoloration of the anterior horns are identified in such cases. Taking a microscopic section of the motor cortex together with the adjacent gyri before the brain is cut is more practical to show the relative neuron loss and gliosis in the former, as orientation may become difficult after the brain is sectioned. Sampling of skeletal muscle is also helpful to evaluate for neurogenic atrophy. Similar spinal cord and skeletal muscle findings are also applicable to spinal muscular atrophies (SMA). Atrophy of the dorsal columns of the spinal cord and the posterior spinal nerve roots are features seen in Friedreich's ataxia. In general, however, atrophy of spinal cord structures by external examination can be extremely difficult in most cases but can be seen better on cross sections. Several patterns of *tract degeneration* can be seen better this way and provide important information (see Chapter 2, "Tract Degeneration"). In advanced cases of generalized degeneration of spinal cord components for any reason, the associated gliosis will result in a firmer and a string-like feel to palpation of the spinal cord. In Pelizaeus-Merzbacher disease, the sparing of peripheral nerves can be seen in spinal cord exam

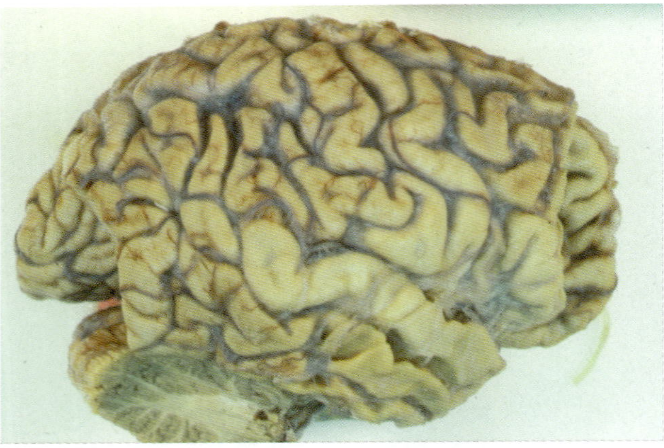

Figure 1-39. Frontotemporal atrophy with relative preservation of superior temporal gyrus, especially its posterior part, is typical for Pick's disease. Tissue has been removed from the right frontal and occipital poles, and cerebellum for research.

grossly, with white, normally myelinated spinal nerves contrasting with dusky shrunken atrophic spinal cord.[166] Cerebellar degeneration is common. HAM, a.k.a. tropical spastic paraparesis, results in spinal cord atrophy as a result of involvement of multiple tracts and leptomeningeal and parenchymal vascular fibrosis that is especially prominent in the lower thoracic region.[167] *Brainstem components and cerebellum* may be entirely or selectively atrophic **(Table 1.10)** in various neurodegenerative diseases. In cases where this type of atrophy is prominent, the posterior fossa contents appear smaller than the brain when seen from the basal aspect of the brain. In cases of *cerebellar atrophy*, such as cerebellar cortical degeneration, the *occipital poles can be seen protruding beyond the cerebellar boundaries*. The cerebellar folia are thin and widely separated, akin to the cortical atrophy in the brain with thin gyri and widened sulci. In cases where the midbrain is particularly atrophic, the *interpeduncular fossa becomes wider and deeper* between the thin cerebral peduncles. Paraneoplastic cerebellar degeneration is usually not prominent on gross examination, although it may be quite severe, typically in association with ovarian and breast carcinomas. In *pontine atrophy*, the fullness of basis pontis is diminished with a shrunken appearance. Atrophy of the midbrain and tegmentum pontis can be seen in progressive supranuclear palsy (PSP). In multiple system atrophy (MSA) **(Fig. 1-40)**, which encompasses olivopontocerebellar atrophy (OPCA), Shy-Drager syndrome, and striatonigral degeneration, various patterns of atrophy are seen in the cerebellum and brainstem depending on the pattern of involvement. Autosomal dominant cerebellar ataxias (ADCAs)[168,169] mainly consist of spinocerebellar ataxia (SCA) **(Fig. 1-41)** and its many subtypes based on genetic features,

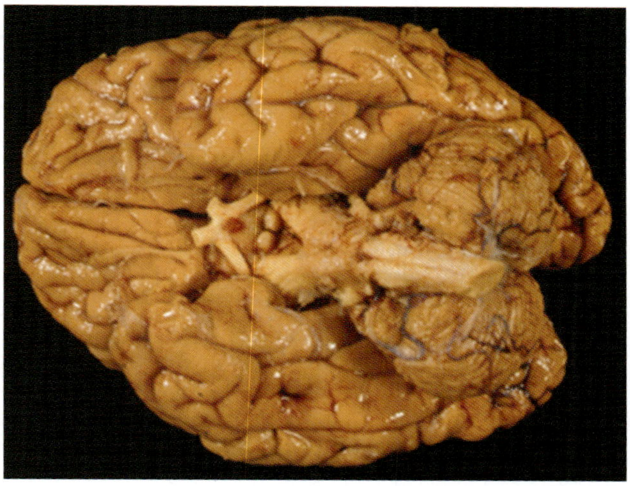

Figure 1-40. Multiple system atrophy: Cerebellum and brainstem are extremely atrophic, and occipital poles are seen protruding well beyond the cerebellar hemispheres. Especially the pons and midbrain show prominent atrophy, resulting in widened interpeduncular fossa.

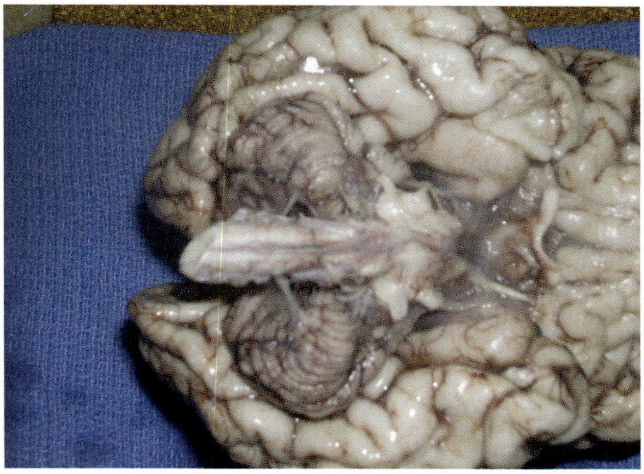

Figure 1-41. Findings similar to those seen in Figure 1-40, that is, extremely atrophic cerebellum and brainstem, especially pons, and occipital lobes protruding beyond the cerebellum due to cerebellar atrophy, are seen in this child's brain with SCA. Evaluation of cut surfaces and identification of specific structures by microscopic examination that show neurodegeneration, as well as genetic testing and clinical correlation, are needed to further characterize and subtype these complex processes.

TABLE 1.10 Diseases that result in cerebellar and/or brainstem atrophy
Cerebellar cortical degeneration
Spinocerebellar ataxia (SCA)
Dentatorubropallidoluysian atrophy (DRPLA)
Progressive supranuclear palsy (PSP)
Olicopontocerebellar atrophy (OPCA)
Shy-Drager syndrome
Striatonigral degeneration
Idiopathic late-onset cerebellar atrophy
Celiac disease
Intoxications (toluene, mercury)
Medications (phenytoin, lithium)

dentatorubropallidoluysian atrophy (DRPLA), and episodic ataxias. The more prominent of these, SCA1 (atrophy of cerebellum, pons, inferior olives, neuron loss in spinal cord), SCA2 (OPCA, neuron loss in substantia nigra, striatum, globus pallidus), SCA3 (Machado-Joseph disease; cerebello-olivary sparing, but neuron loss in dentate nucleus, superior cerebellar peduncle, and spinocerebellar tract degeneration), SCA6 (cerebellar cortex degeneration that is most prominent in vermis), SCA7 (cerebellar cortical atrophy, spinocerebellar and olivocerebellar tract degeneration), as well as DRPLA, result in various atrophic patterns depending on the type and severity of the disease. In idiopathic late-onset cerebellar ataxia, cerebellar atrophy is most prominent in the superior part of cerebellum, especially vermis.

Various structures and tracts can be smaller than usual as a result of agenesis or atrophy, usually in the brainstem and cerebellum; however, these small structures and subtle changes are better identified on microscopic evaluation. Asymmetric unilateral cerebellar hemispheric atrophy may indicate contralateral extensive cerebral destructive lesions. Cerebellar degeneration can be associated with systemic diseases, such as celiac disease,[170] toluene,[171] and mercury[165] intoxications. Medications such as phenytoin[172] and lithium[173] can cause cerebellar degeneration and atrophy.

Softening can be identified by visual examination if it results in shrinkage or depression of the tissue, but it can look unremarkable and best felt by palpation. *Fetal autopsy brains* are invariably entirely soft and tend to fall apart even after fixation and when handled gently, if not during removal. Especially in premature babies and intrauterine fetal demise cases, the intracranial contents may literally be liquid, which is a hopeless situation for appropriate evaluation. In other cases, this fragmentation due to soft nature of the tissues can be avoided to some degree by fixing the brain in Bouin's solution, which makes the tissues harder. It results in bright yellow discoloration of the tissues but does not interfere with interpretation. If the body can be kept for a few days after the autopsy, it is preferable to open the cranium and fix the brain in situ together with the body to minimize handling and tissue damage. If this is not possible, the brain can be removed under water and then fixed in Bouin's solution. Since many times the question of some kind of malformation or syndromic association is the question, in situ examination and keeping the brain intact as much as possible for adequate gross examination are crucial. Any help from premortem head ultrasound and other clinical, imaging, and laboratory findings should be sought for. In an otherwise intact *adult brain*, even if the fixation is suboptimal, the external surfaces are usually fixed uniformly and better than the deep tissues, and focal soft areas may still represent a lesion. Areas that remain soft due to inadequate fixation are the deep areas. They appear pink and are diffuse without any relation to anatomical structures on cut surfaces and do not interfere with external examination. Softening is frequently due to an infarct, which may be at any stage of development. Underlying hemorrhage or a cystic lesion, such as an abscess, can also cause a focal softening. In these cases, due to the accumulation of additional material, the brain surface appears distended and flattened, whereas in infarcts, due to tissue loss, the lesion also appears somewhat depressed. In addition, the conditions that result from mass lesions are prone to cause midline shift and herniations. This type of reaction can sometimes be seen in infarcts of subacute stage, when edema can be severe and results in a mass effect. It is not always easy to identify cerebellar tonsillar or transtentorial herniation due to the variably present usual indentations on the parenchymal surfaces in these regions. In true herniations, among other findings, a softening of the herniated portion of the parenchyma is identified. This is due to the relative ischemia of the herniated portion and can be associated with congestion and punctuate hemorrhages. In *spinal cord*, infarcts create soft segments of variable lengths. Midthoracic level is the preferred location for the watershed spinal cord infarcts due to the vascular supply of the cord. Necrotizing myelopathy results in a long continuous segment of spinal cord necrosis. It predominantly involves lumbosacral region and advances cranially, sometimes involving the entire spinal cord, which can be felt like a fluid-filled tube **(Fig. 1-42)**. Demyelinating lesions of acute stage can be felt as soft areas in the spinal cord upon external evaluation, because of the cord's naturally thin parenchyma. If the removal of the cord is not carried out gently, there is usually some distortion and crush artifact at the point where forceps is

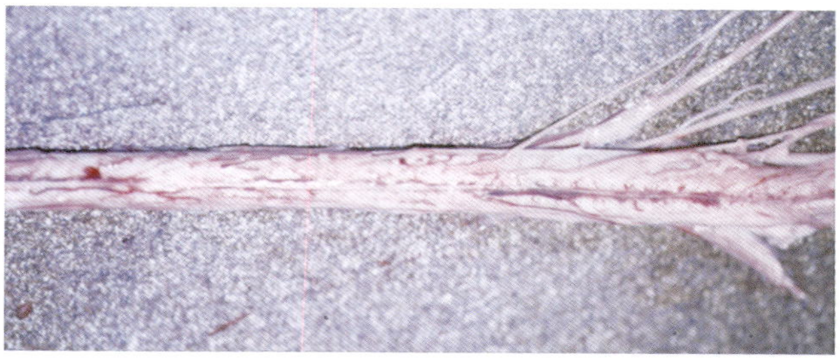

Figure 1-42. This spinal cord appears unremarkable on inspection; however, it was extremely soft throughout its length due to necrotizing myelopathy. The white specs on it represent necrotic parenchyma oozing through its surface while handling the specimen. The patient was undergoing intrathechal chemotherapy for craniospinal involvement by acute lymphoblastic leukemia.

applied and the cord is pulled. This area will not fix as good as the intact tissue and will remain soft. Variable length segments, usually focal, can feel soft due to hydromyelia or syringomyelia.

Depression of the brain surface may be due to an underlying tissue loss or an external pressure. Infarcts are soft and cause some degree of depression of that area due to underlying tissue loss. A meningioma focally compressing the brain will leave its impression on the brain surface, which fits perfectly to the meningioma like a puzzle. Due to long-standing pressure by a large mass lesion, the gyral–sulcal pattern of the lining surfaces of the depressed area is flattened. These features suggest the presence of a mass lesion, even if the dura and the actual mass are not available for examination. Other neoplastic and nonneoplastic lesions of soft tissue and hematopoietic nature are other common causes that may present in a similar manner. Sometimes, a large surface area is depressed with ill-defined borders. The gyral–sulcal pattern is also flattened and the brain appears asymmetric. This pattern is common with long-standing subdural hematomas **(Fig. 1-43)**. It is also possible with epidural hematomas but is seen only occasionally, since epidural hematomas are unlikely to remain for long enough time to cause this type of disfiguring changes on the brain surface. Epidural and subdural empyema and metastatic deposits are other potential accumulations to cause similar changes. Random artifactual regional flattening of brain surface is also very common if the brain is not suspended in formalin during fixation and is left to rest at the bottom of the container. Its surfaces are otherwise unremarkable, unless there are other lesions coincidentally. Very small pitting type depressions of the brain surface can be identified upon very careful and close examination of the brain surface in cases of cortical microinfarcts. When many and prominent, they can create a granular surface focally or covering large areas and may be

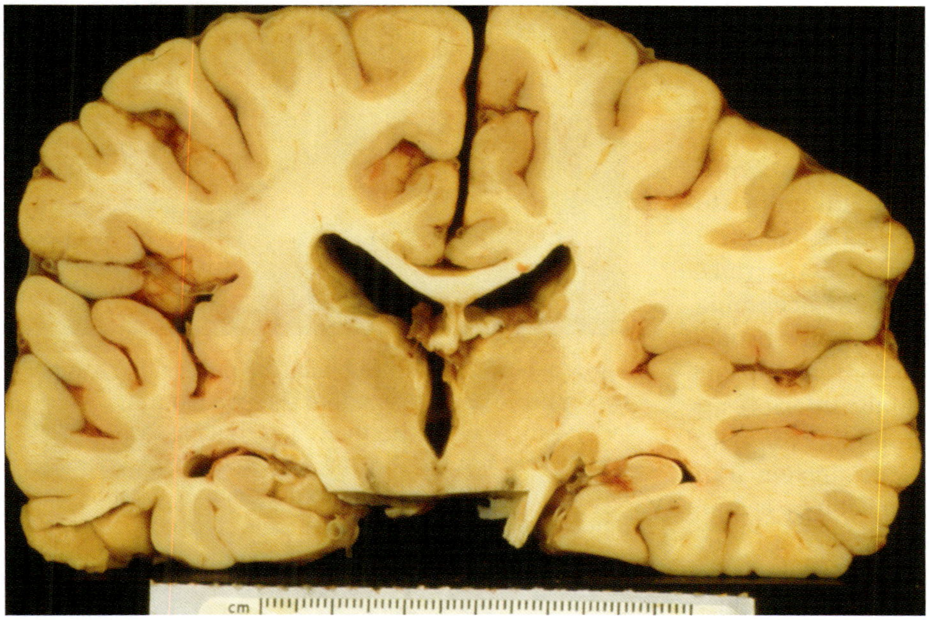

Figure 1-43. On the right side of the picture, the convexity of the cerebral hemisphere is flattened due to the presence of a subdural hematoma (removed). Similar appearance can be caused by the brain resting on the bottom of the container during fixation, if it is not suspended in the fixative.

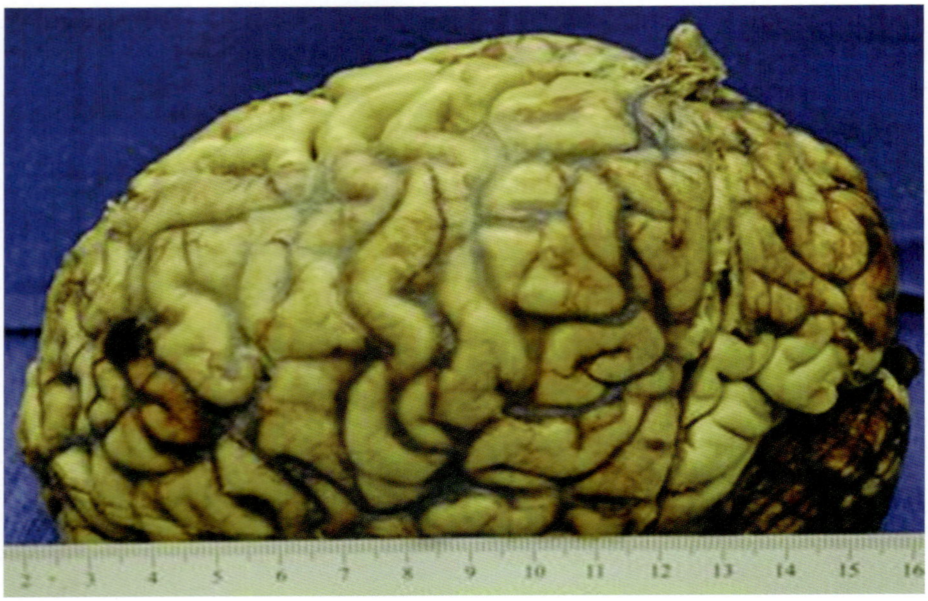

Figure 1-44. While leptomeninges are smooth and transparent, the parenchymal surface has a granular, pitted appearance due to numerous microinfarcts. The patient had severe systemic and coronary arteriosclerosis, atrial fibrillation resulting in numerous thromboemboli and cerebral small vessel disease.

a component of a widespread circulatory disorder, such as multi-infarct dementia or other embolic phenomena **(Fig. 1-44)**. In the spinal cord, demyelinating or hypoxic/ischemic lesions can result in surface depressions due to the gliosis and shrinkage of the plaques in chronic stage. When multiple, they result in irregular contours of the spinal cord.

Many *discolorations* actually represent the changes in the leptomeninges, such as subarachnoid hemorrhage and meningitis (see "Leptomeninges and Subarachnoid Space" above), leaving only a few changes that alter the usual color of neuroglial parenchyma proper to be mentioned here. An overall dusky tan-brown discoloration is seen in the so-called respirator brain or in cases of global hypoxic/ischemic injury, which is also friable in spite of extended fixation attempts **(Fig. 1-45)**.Focal orange-brown discoloration, usually associated with depression of the tissue, is seen in contusions, which go along with hemorrhage and subsequent hemosiderin pigment accumulation and tissue loss **(Fig. 1-46)**. They are usually multiple small foci located on the contusion-prone basal surfaces of the brain, mainly inferior surfaces of frontal and temporal lobes, temporal poles, and anterior surfaces of the brainstem. Tan-brown discoloration of parenchyma can be seen in thermal injury as a result of baking of the tissue, that is, coagulation of the tissue. Soot and gunpowder residue can be seen focally on the parenchymal surface in gunshot wounds as a dark brown to black discoloration, depending on the range of the shooting. Neoplasms and hemorrhages that are superficial enough to be observed by inspection may cause focal discolorations associated with

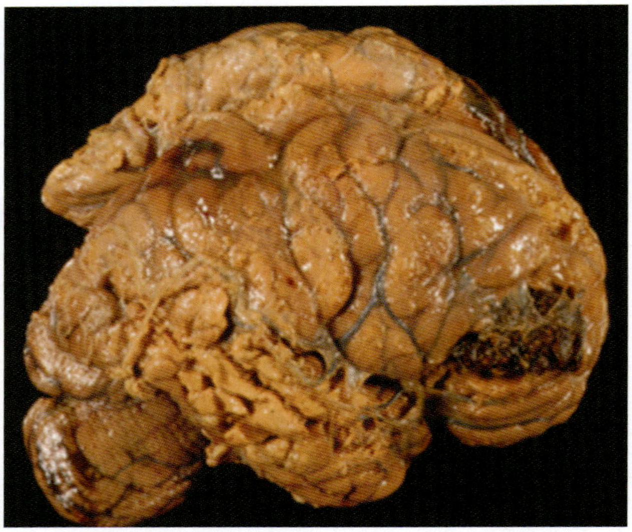

Figure 1-45. Respirator brain: The patient had a large hypertensive hemorrhage that extended into the ventricular system, as well as to the subarachnoid space as seen on the right frontal lobe, resulting in extensive edema. He became unconscious and was placed on respirator. The intracranial pressure overcame the systemic blood pressure, stopping perfusion and oxygenation of the brain, resulting in this global anoxic state and brain death. The entire brain is necrotic with dusky and friable appearance.

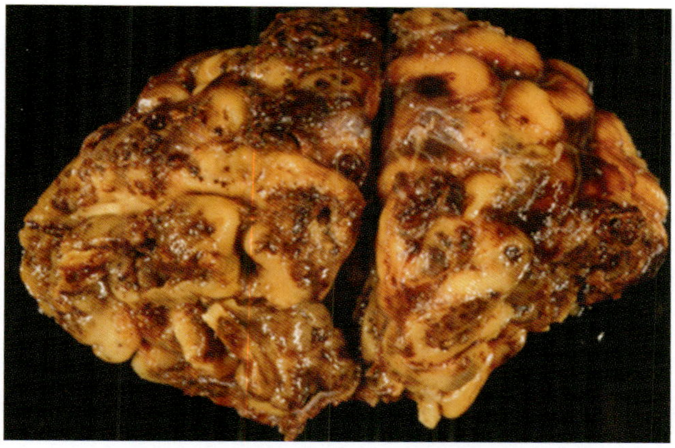

Figure 1-46. Numerous contusions seen on the parenchymal surface as hemorrhagic and slightly depressed lesions of variable sizes and shapes. Some can be soft due to tissue necrosis. If the patient lived long enough, the blood would be resorbed, leaving orange-yellow shrunken lesions behind, as a result of hemosiderin pigment and gliosis.

hemorrhage, necrosis, or any pigments. A localized white appearance with a firm quality to the brain surface may be seen in meningioangiomatosis, owing to the extensive collagenization.

Expansion of gyri, cerebellar folia, brainstem, and spinal cord indicates an accumulation of cells and/or other material within the parenchyma. A generalized expansion of gyri, which is accompanied by and is not as dramatic as the flattening of their surfaces, is typical for conditions associated with brain edema **(Table 1.11)**, either isolated or in association with conditions such as encephalitis **(Fig. 1-47)** or Reye syndrome. While there are many reasons for brain swelling, a few prominent other reasons may be hyponatremia,[174] hypoglycemia,[175] hepatic encephalopathy,[174] acute lead encephalopathy,[176] and carbon tetrachloride,[177] ethylene glycol,[178] methanol,[179] carbon monoxide,[180] ethanol,[181] heroin,[182] and cyanide[183] intoxications. Due to the increase in the intracranial pressure, herniations follow, usually bilateral tonsillar and transtentorial, as associated findings. More localized swelling of similar nature can be seen in the areas of the brain overlying mass lesions, such as abscess, hemorrhage, subacute infarct, or metastatic carcinoma. While metastatic malignancies result in gyral expansion by the edema they cause, as much as the mass effect, infiltrating gliomas result in gyral expansion due to the infiltrating neoplastic cells. Any of the infiltrating glial neoplasms is capable of this effect, although it is more commonly seen with oligodendroglioma, which has a tendency to infiltrate the cortex and later the leptomeninges **(Fig. 1-48)**. Malformations of cortical development, especially focal cortical dysplasia as seen in the tubers of tuberous sclerosis or as a sporadic lesion, result in a focal expansion of one or more gyri focally **(Fig. 1-49)**. They are also felt, especially

TABLE 1.11 Conditions associated with brain edema

Generalized
Infectious
Encephalitis
Metabolic
Reye syndrome
Hyponatremia
Hypoglycemia
Hepatic encephalopathy
Toxic
Acute lead encephalopathy
Carbon tetrachloride
Ethylene glycol
Methanol
Ethanol
Carbon monoxide
Heroin
Cyanide
Localized
Hemorrhage
Infarct
Metastasis
Abscess

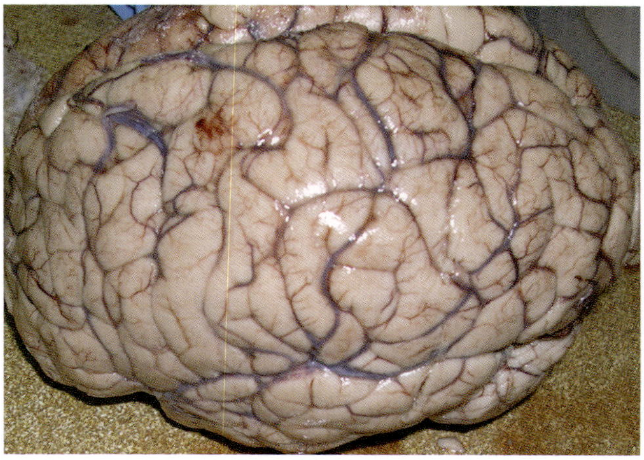

Figure 1-47. Diffuse brain edema resulting in swelling and flattening of its surfaces due to compression against the calvarium.

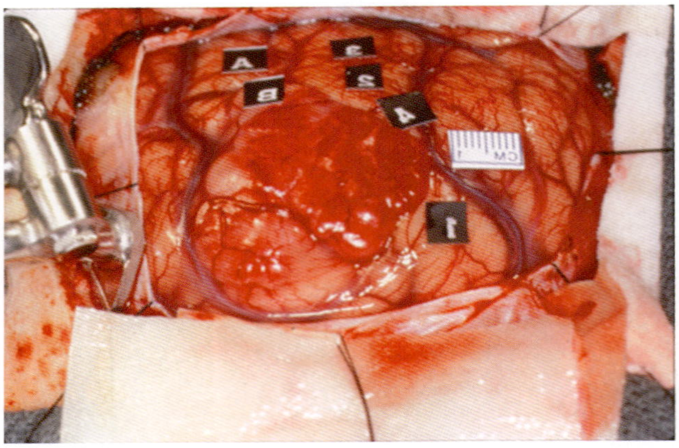

Figure 1-48. Intraoperative appearance of a focal area (seen as a hyperemic area) of a few expanded gyri due to infiltration by an underlying oligodendroglioma.

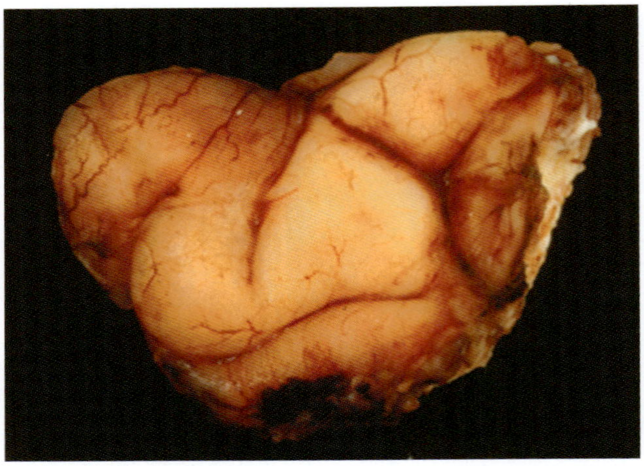

Figure 1-50. Surgical excision specimen of a sporadic focal cortical dysplasia with expanded gyral pattern, although this may be difficult to appreciate when in isolation in such small specimens.

in fresh brains, as distinct nodules that are firmer than the brain tissue. This type of expansions due to primary neoplastic or malformative disorders can also be appreciated in surgical resection specimens **(Fig. 1-50)**, although it may be difficult to appreciate the gyral expansion in small specimens, without the luxury of comparison with normal gyri. In *cerebellum*, focally or as widespread and prominent as to occupy one entire hemisphere, prominent expansion of the folia sometimes nearly to the size of the cerebral gyri is seen in dysplastic gangliocytoma of the cerebellum (Lhermitte-Duclos disease) **(Fig. 1-51)**, which can be associated with Cowden syndrome,[15] especially in adult cases. Therefore, in full autopsies, other organs that may harbor malignancies as part of this syndrome should be carefully investigated. Focal nodular expansion of a group of folia, similar to focal cortical dysplasia in the brain, may represent cerebellar cortical dysplasia. It may also be widespread to involve the entire cerebellum, creating a multinodular surface. Dysplastic cerebellar cortex can be focally seen

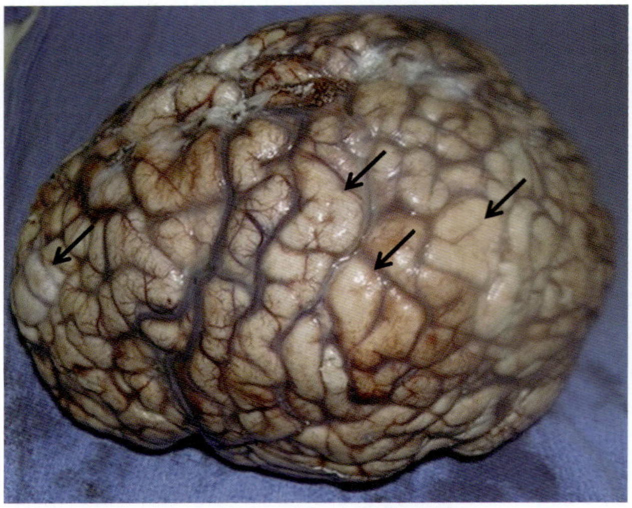

Figure 1-49. The appearance of "tubers" representing focal cortical dysplasias in this case of tuberous sclerosis. They appear as focal expansions of gyri (*arrows*).

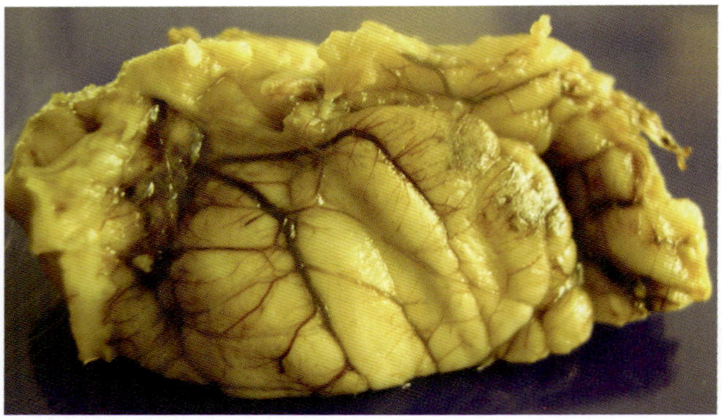

Figure 1-51. Dysplastic gangliocytoma of the cerebellum (Lhermitte-Duclos disease). The cerebellar folia are extremely expanded, almost resembling cerebral gyri. Although the patient was 29 years of age, which made it more likely to have a syndromic association with Cowden syndrome, he did not present for follow-up and further investigation.

commonly especially in flocculonodular lobes as an incidental finding. In *spinal cord*, a nodular or fusiform expansion of the parenchyma indicates a parenchymal accumulation resulting in mass effect. These are commonly primary neoplasms, such as ependymoma and astrocytoma. In addition, hydromyelia and syringomyelia can cause similar appearance. Schistosomiasis, among other findings, can involve the cord and result in segmental swelling. It usually involves lumbosacral spinal cord segments and only rarely the thoracic and cervical.[184] Diffuse swelling is associated with more generalized processes such as myelitis.

Other abnormalities of external pattern essentially refer to the numerous *malformations*. Fetal brain has various normal surface appearances depending on the sulcal–gyral development according to the week of gestation. *Agyria* refers to the smooth brain surface without the gyri **(Fig. 1-52)**. It is also sometimes used synonymously with lissencephaly type I. Lissencephaly type II refers to a still smooth surface but with a cobblestone appearance and is different than pachygyria. Agyria can be associated with Miller-Dieker syndrome,[185] together with olivary nucleus dysplasia. Neu-Laxova syndrome[186] also has agyria along with microcephaly, agenesis of corpus callosum, and cerebellar hypoplasia. If there is some degree of gyral development but in the form of less than expected numbers and broad gyri, it is then called *pachygyria*, which is sometimes known as macrogyria. *Holoprosencephaly* is the continuation of cerebral cortex from one hemisphere to the other. In the alobar form, the interhemispheric fissure is not formed and the brain is in the shape of one "sphere" rather than two hemispheres **(Fig. 1-53)**. Semilobar variant is the partial formation of the interhemispheric fissure and is somewhere in the spectrum between alobar and lobar holoprosencephaly. In partial or lobar holoprosencephaly, when the observer looks down between the cerebral hemispheres, corpus callosum is not seen. Instead, a continuous cerebral cortex is seen. It is better seen on coronal cut surfaces **(Fig. 1-54)**. This should not be confused with subfalcine herniation of cingulate gyrus. Small and crowded gyri, that is, *polymicrogyria*, can be a very small focus or may occupy the entire brain surface **(Fig. 1-55)**. Polymicrogyria may be the result of multiple different etiologies, such as metabolic diseases, hypoxic/ischemic injury, as part of various syndromes, peroxisomal, mitochondrial, or infectious. A combination of pachygyria and polymicrogyria is seen in Zellweger syndrome.[187] Temporal lobe has broad gyria with polymicrogyria in thanatophoric dwarfism. A polymicrogyria-like irregular surface can be present in *atelencephaly*, which is the absence of cerebral hemispheres and lateral ventricles, but diencephalic structures or their remains are present. *Polygyria* is an increase in the number of otherwise

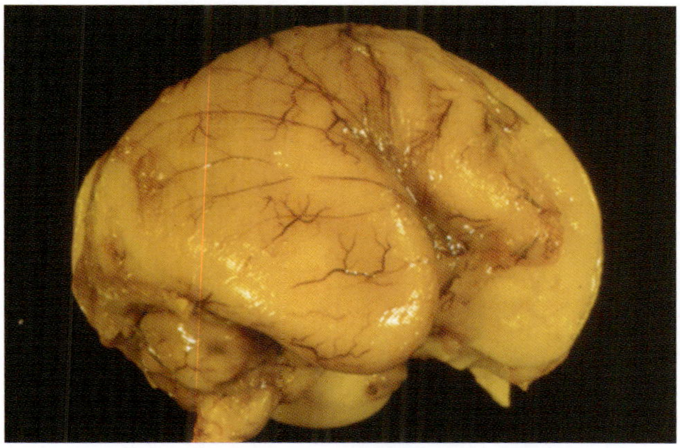

Figure 1-52. Agyria: This brain is from a 30-week gestational age fetus with intrauterine demise. The external appearance is consistent with approximately 21 week of development. The yellow color is the result of fixation in Bouin's solution.

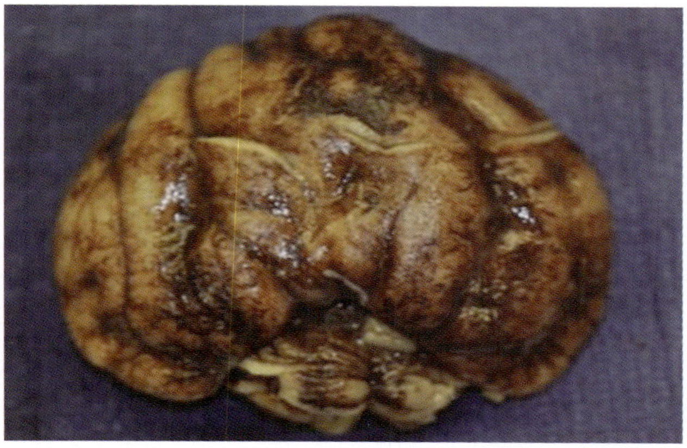

Figure 1-53. Alobar holoprosencephaly, posterior view. Interhemispheric fissure is not present, and the entire cerebral cortex of right and left hemispheres is continuous over the midline. There is also pachygyria. There is an attempt for gyrus formation, but they are broad, resulting in a somewhat flat surface. (Compare with agyria in Figure 1-52.)

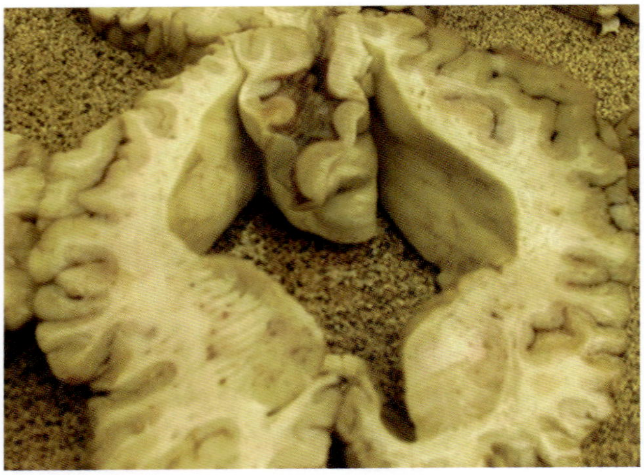

Figure 1-54. Cut surface of lobar holoprosencephaly. The interhemispheric fissure is present, resulting in the division of right and left cerebral hemispheres, but the cortical ribbon, though very thin, continues without interruption across the midline to the other side in the depth of the interhemispheric fissure.

normal gryi and is therefore different than polymicrogyria. It can be seen as part of X-linked hydrocephalus. Polygyria is typically associated with hydrocephalus that develops early in life. *Brachycephaly* is the anteroposteriorly short brain, especially in the frontal lobes, with flattened occipital lobes, resulting in a somewhat rounded appearance, and is seen in Down syndrome. Superior temporal gyrus is thin. In *spinal cord, diplomyelia* and *diastematomyelia* refer to the duplication and splitting of the spinal cord, respectively. In the latter, the spinal cord appears to have been divided longitudinally, resulting in two hemicords, and is seen as a cleft running along the spinal cord in the sagittal plane for variable distances. *Triplomyelia* is a rare condition where there are three spinal cords.

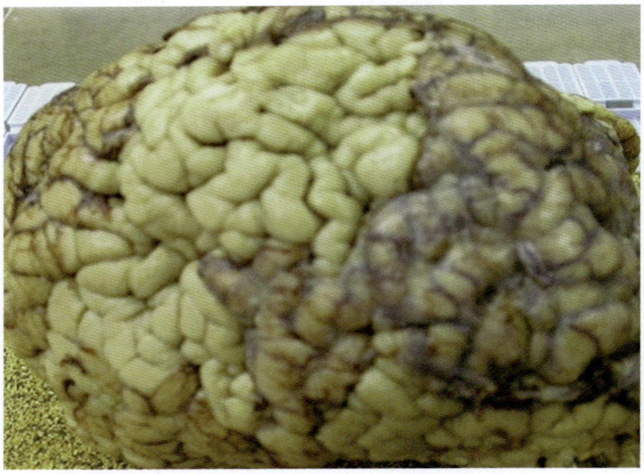

Figure 1-55. The cerebral cortex has a crowded, busy appearance in polymicrogyria. The leptomeninges have been partially peeled to better demonstrate the even smaller nodulations on the surfaces of the gyri, corresponding to the areas of incomplete sulcus formation.

Tissue defect is used here to imply a missing component, either as a result of destruction or malformation. The most dramatic of these is *anencephaly*. Anencephaly refers to the absence of brain with a remaining conglomerate of irregular, disorganized neurovascular tissue (area cerebrovasculosa). Skull bones are not formed. Pituitary gland can be protected by diaphragma sellae. Due to the absence of bony structures of the forehead, the eyes become more prominent and protrude outward, creating a characteristic facial appearance (Fig. 1-4). Extreme cases of hydranencephaly can create a confusion regarding the terminology and accurate identification. In *aprosencephaly*, in addition to atelencephaly, eyes, optic nerves, mamillary bodies, hypothalamus, and pituitary gland are also absent but brainstem is preserved **(Fig. 1-56)**. The cranial

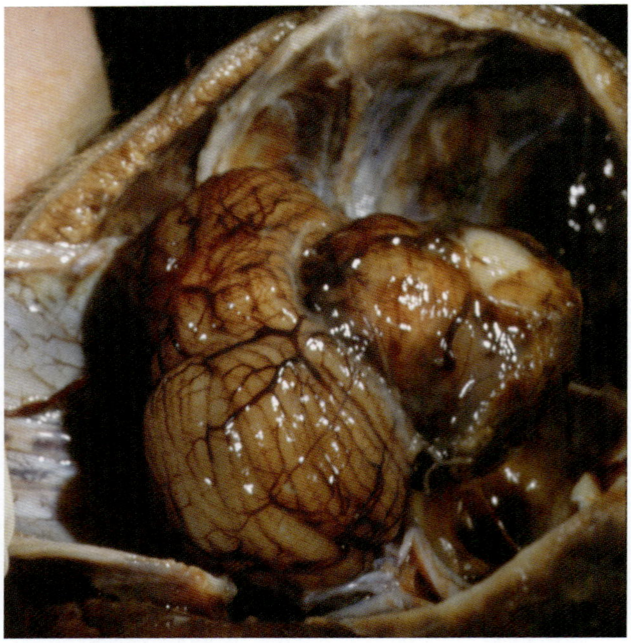

Figure 1-56. Aprosencephaly. The intact calvarium is opened and shows absence of brain. Only the cerebellum and a few nodules representing brainstem structures are seen.

vault has formed and is intact. In *hydranencephaly*, the calvarium is intact, and the brain substance has been destroyed after it has developed, resulting in a cyst that literally occupies the entire cranial cavity with only the extremely thin residual subpial neuroglial tissue forming the membranous "cyst lining" (see "Cystic Lesions" below). It is debated whether the hydranencephaly in Fowler's syndrome (proliferative vasculopathy and hydranencephaly)[188] is of developmental or destructive (encephaloclastic) in nature. *Basket brain* results from extensive destruction of brain parenchyma bilaterally, leaving intact only the paramedian portions and cingulate gyri as the handle of a basket **(Fig. 1-57)**. A more limited and focal destruction but still severe enough to create a hole in the brain parenchyma is *porencephaly*, which may be unilateral or bilateral and symmetrical **(Fig. 1-58)**. There may be confusion between the terms porencephaly and schizencephaly, and they may even be used interchangeably. While they are similar lesions and both are thought to be due to tissue destruction, porencephaly is preferred when the destruction extends deep enough to reach and connect with the ventricular system, whereas *schizencephaly* implies a variable degree of a slit-like or larger tissue loss with no connection to the ventricular system. Schizencephaly may sometimes be used for bilateral large porencephalic defects creating a slit-like symmetrical damage. Whether such a lesion is the result of an insult during developmental stage or after the development is completed can be evaluated by paying attention to the edges of the pore. If the lesion occurred before the development has been completed, the surrounding gyri will be malformed and create a radial arrangement around the lesion, which is covered only by leptomeninges. Hydranencephaly, basket brain, and porencephaly are typically the result of destructive lesions that occur in the second trimester. In adults, a large cystic, *remote infarct* may result in a similar cystic structure; however, it is covered by leptomeninges and a thin layer of subpial tissue that remained intact by obtaining its nutrition from the surface leptomeninges, and the original gyral pattern is preserved. In cases of trauma, if a large contusion is resorbed, the surface will also be damaged, and this thin subpial layer may not survive due to the physical insult coming from outside the brain. *Corpus callosum* is evaluated by gently separating the hemispheres and looking down to see the smooth white matter substance of corpus callosum. In fetal brains, it is easily disrupted while removing and handling the brain, imitating agenesis, allowing one to see directly the ventricles. True agenesis can

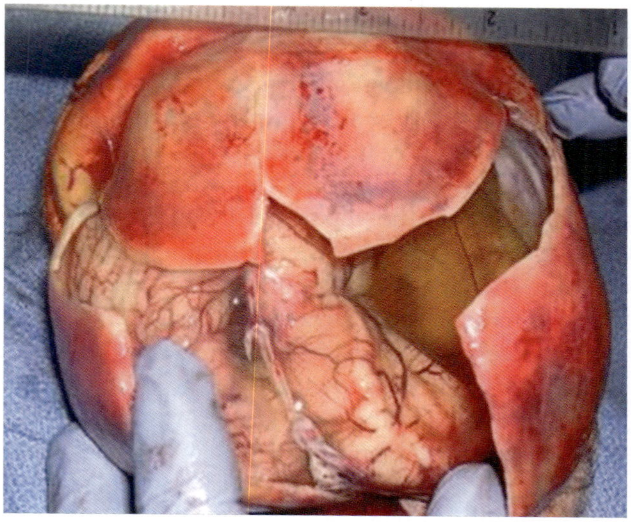

Figure 1-58. A large right-sided porencephaly seen in situ at autopsy. The *tan-brown* area represents the defect filled with CSF and the overlying distended arachnoid membrane. The defect was in continuity with the ventricular system.

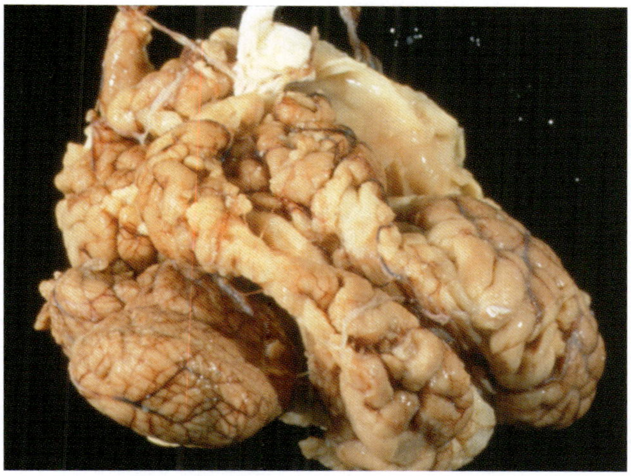

Figure 1-57. Viewed from the top, this brain shows extensive bilateral cerebral destruction mainly in the middle cerebral artery territories, resulting in large defects on both sides. The cerebellum is artifactually displaced to the right as a result of extremely soft and fragmented nature of the specimen. Mainly the parasagittal regions remain intact in the brain, creating an appearance reminiscent of a basket handle, though a milder form.

still be identified on cut surfaces and by microscopic examination (see "Cut Surfaces" below). In some cases of corpus callosum agenesis, a lipoma, cyst, or a meningioma can be seen in place of corpus callosum and apparently in the way of its development. In cases of suspected corpus callosum agenesis, the hemispheres can be separated by making a midsagittal cut through the interhemispheric fissure to evaluate the cingulate gyri on medial view. In true agenesis, cingulate gyrus does not form as a regular anteroposterior straight gyrus but is irregular and convoluted above the remnants of the corpus callosum. To perform this evaluation, it is not always necessary to cut the brain in this fashion. The hemispheres can be separated gently to observe the status of the cingulate gyrus, and the brain cutting can continue in the frontal plane as usual. Agenesis of corpus callosum can be associated with Aicardi syndrome,[189] Andermann syndrome,[190] Apert syndrome,[191] acrocallosal syndrome,[192] and Meckel-Gruber syndrome[193] and is a component of many others.[190,191] In the *cerebellum*[194,195] **(Table 1.12)**, *Dandy-Walker malformation* creates an appearance that is similar to porencephaly in the brain, in the sense that there is agenesis of the vermis and a tissue defect, together with dilated fourth ventricle, creating a cystic cavity through the cerebellum, which is covered by leptomeninges posteriorly, connecting to the fourth ventricle **(Fig. 1-59)**. Dandy-Walker malformation can be associated with many other malformations, both in the CNS and systemically. Spina bifida, occipital meningocele, polymicrogyria, pachygyria, corpus callosum agenesis, microcephaly, and cerebellar hypoplasia can be identified upon external evaluation in association with it. There are other syndromes that should be kept in mind and investigated in the absence of cerebellar vermis. *Joubert syndrome* also includes midbrain abnormalities and malformations of the medulla oblongata and typically lacks the cystic changes of Dandy-Walker malformation, although rare cases can have them. Cerebellar vermis is absent. Together with a deep interpeduncular fossa, "molar tooth sign" is created in the midbrain in this syndrome, although it also is not specific. Further differentiation can be performed by careful and systematic microscopic examination of cerebellar and brainstem structures to identify a variety of

TABLE 1.12 External features of common cerebellar malformations and disorders

Syndrome/Malformation	Cerebellar Features	Other Features
Dandy-Walker	Agenesis of vermis Dilated fourth ventricle Posterior midline cyst	Spina bifida, occipital meningocele, polymicrogyria, pachygyria, corpus callosum agenesis, microcephaly, cerebellar hypoplasia
Joubert syndrome	Agenesis of vermis Posterior midline cyst is not typical but rarely present	Deep interpeduncular fossa, malformations of medulla oblongata, occipital meningocele
Cerebello-oculo-renal syndrome (CORS; Joubert syndrome type B)	Agenesis of vermis	Similar to Joubert syndrome, also retinal and renal dysplasia
Walker-Warburg syndrome (cerebro-ocular dysplasia)	Hypoplastic vermis	Hydrocephalus, agyria, retinal dysplasia, and encephalocele (HARD+E)
Tectocerebellar dysraphia	Agenesis of vermis	Occipital encephalocele, tectum deformation
Rhombencephalosynapsis	Agenesis of vermis Fused cerebellar hemispheres Hypoplastic cerebellum	
Cerebellar agenesis	Partial or complete absence of cerebellum May be unilateral	Occipital encephalocele
Pontocerebellar hypoplasia	Atrophic cerebellum Vermis relatively spared	Atrophic pons
Werdnig-Hoffmann disease (acute infantile spinal muscular atrophy)	Uniform cerebellar hypoplasia	Anterior horn degeneration, motor nerve and skeletal muscle atrophy
Granule cell aplasia	Atrophic cerebellum	
Fetal alcohol syndrome	Cerebellar dysplasia or hypoplasia	Microcephaly, agenesis of corpus callosum, migration disorders

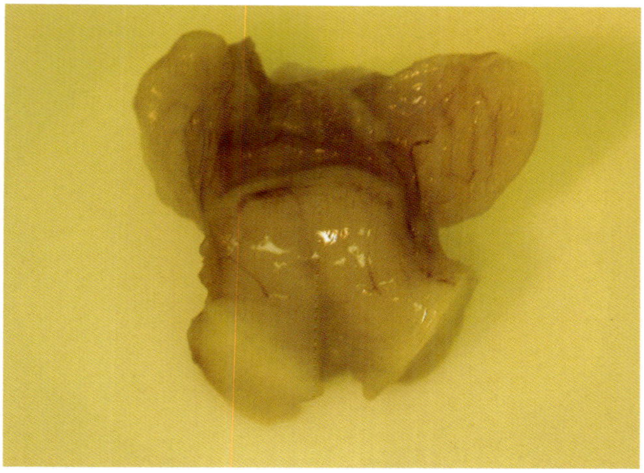

Figure 1-59. Dandy-Walker malformation. Cross section of the midbrain is seen from the top view in the center. The two wing-like structures toward the upper right and upper left corners of the picture represent cerebellar hemispheres. They are not connected in the middle, where vermis is absent. Instead, there was a midline cyst that was connected to the fourth ventricle. The CSF-filled cyst collapsed when the brain was removed, leaving behind the midline cavity between the cerebellar hemispheres and the crumbled arachnoid membrane.

dysplastic lesions. It can be associated with occipital meningocele. Clinical features are also very different and helpful in this differential diagnosis. *Cerebello-oculo-renal syndrome* (CORS) has the additional components of retinal and renal dysplasias and is considered a variation of Joubert syndrome, or Joubert syndrome type B. *Walker-Warburg syndrome* (cerebro-ocular dysplasia), in addition to cerebellar vermal hypoplasia, also has hydrocephalus, agyria, retinal dysplasia, and encephalocele (HARD+E). In *tectocerebellar dysraphia*, there is variable degree of cerebellar vermis agenesis along with occipital encephalocele, in which cerebellum may participate, as well as deformation of tectum. In contrast, when the two cerebellar hemispheres are fused in the presence of vermis agenesis, it represents a form of cerebellar hypoplasia termed *rhombencephalosynapsis*. *Cerebellar agenesis* is usually partial, and residual parts of the cerebellum can be seen. It can be unilateral and may be associated with occipital encephaloceles or in utero vascular problems. Pontocerebellar hypoplasia is another cause of atrophic cerebellum and pons that is seen in pediatric population. Cerebellum may assume a flattened appearance. Vermis is relatively spared compared to hemispheres. A uniform homogeneous cerebellar hypoplasia may be seen together with some cases of Werdnig-Hoffmann disease. Granule cell aplasia results in an atrophic cerebellum. Various cerebellar dysplasias and hypoplasias may be seen as part of fetal alcohol syndrome. As in the cranial nerves and pituitary stalk, *traumatic tears* commonly seen at the pontomedullary region require careful in situ examination and removal of the brain to avoid confusion with artifactual tears. Distinguishing them from true tears may become impossible as axonal swelling cannot be seen if the injury was rapidly fatal and petechial hemorrhages may not develop in cases of such instantaneous death.

Exophytic growth of a lesion on the surface of the CNS parenchyma can be identified easily and is typical of a few neoplasms. Pilocytic astrocytomas, especially in brainstem and hypothalamus, may have an exophytic growth pattern. They are firm, lobulated masses with irregular surface. Another relatively rare neoplasm is liponeurocytoma that typically arises in the cerebellum but sometimes can present as an exophytic mass in the cerebellopontine angle. Schwannoma, arising in this region from the cranial nerves, is also another exophytic mass (see "Cranial and Spinal Nerves" below). *Nodular cortical dysplasia* (a.k.a. brain wart due to wart-like protrusion of cortex on brain surface) forms lesions of a few millimeters on the brain surface.[196] In the conus medullaris of the *spinal cord*, a sausage-like expansion of the parenchyma with a gelatinous consistency is typical for myxopapillary ependymoma **(Fig. 1-60)**. Likewise, paraganglioma also presents as a similar filum terminale mass **(Fig. 1-61)**. The drop metastases and other metastatic malignancies that may be seen on the external surfaces of the brain and spinal cord parenchyma are actually leptomeningeal lesions, which are discussed in "Leptomeninges and Subarachnoid Space" above. Exophytic or not, external examination, both palpation and inspection, can reveal other obvious mass lesions that are superficial enough to be identified before cutting the brain **(Figs. 1-62 and 1-63)**. Encephalocele forms a mass lesion covered by skin, although its malformative nature is readily obvious **(Figs. 1-64 and 1-65)**.

Herniations should be searched for during external evaluation. When one looks down through the interhemispheric fissure by gently separating

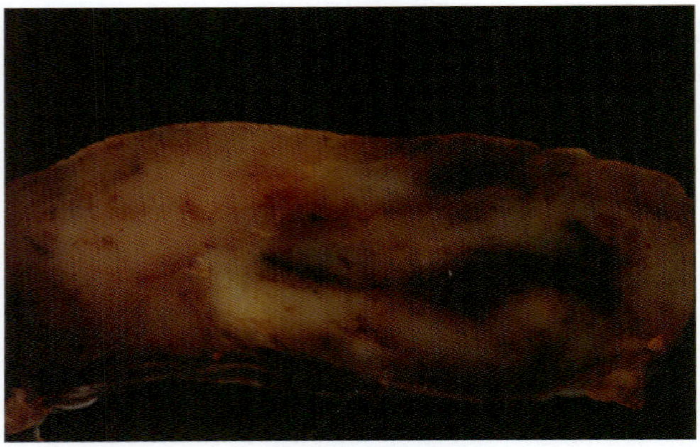

Figure 1-60. Myxopapillary ependymoma. A sausage-like round, elongated, tan-brown, gelatinous neoplasm is attached to the filum terminale that is seen as a longitudinal fibrous band of tissue at the bottom of the neoplasm. Conus medullaris is seen attached to it as a white nodular structure in the left bottom corner of the picture. The neoplasm is covered by glistening arachnoid membrane.

the cerebral hemispheres apart, corpus callosum should be seen as a white, homogeneous structure with its flat surface. In cases of *cingulate gyrus herniation (subfalcine herniation)*, the herniated cingulate gyrus will be seen blocking the view of corpus callosum **(Fig. 1-66)**. In *transtentorial herniation (uncus herniation)*, when the base of the brain is inspected, medial temporal lobes will be seen to extend toward the midline, typically with a linear indentation on its surface, corresponding to the edge of the tentorium. *Kernohan's notch* is the linear impression of the contralateral tentorium on that side of the midbrain due to brainstem being pushed to the contralateral side by the herniating uncus **(Fig. 1-67)**. Due to this pressure on the brainstem, an anteroposterior elongation of the

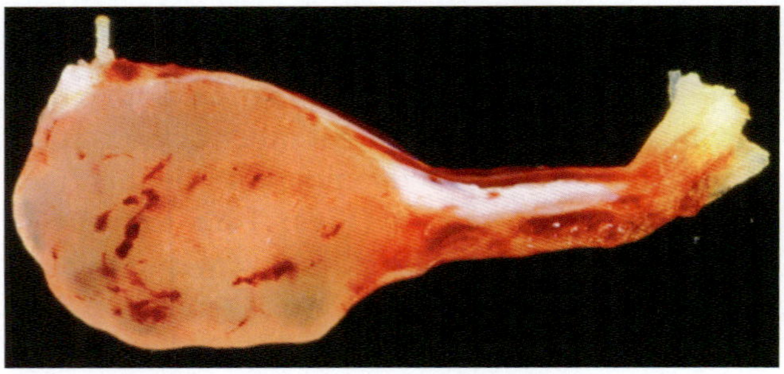

Figure 1-61. This nodular structure resected from the filum terminale showed a paraganglioma.

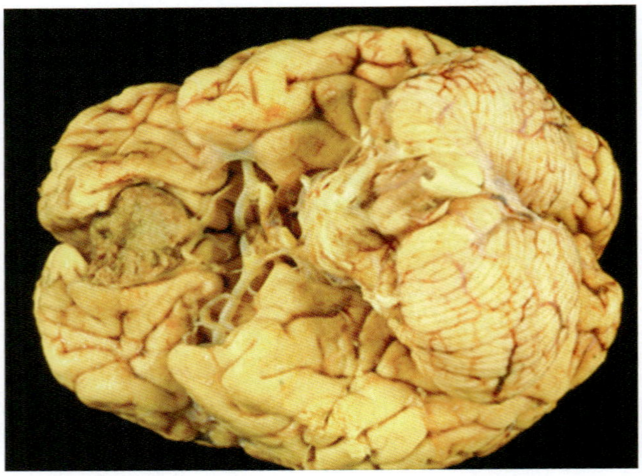

Figure 1-62. A tan-brown well-circumscribed mass is present protruding between the frontal lobes. This was a meningioma attached the anterior part of the falx cerebri.

brainstem can be seen as an additional supportive finding for the herniation **(Fig. 1-68)**. *Cerebellar tonsillar herniation* may be difficult to tell apart from normal variations of indentation of the cerebellar parenchyma due to the irregularity of the skull base. It is not unusual to normally see a wide semicircular groove over the cerebellar tonsil. True herniation into the foramen magnum creates a narrow, tongue-like downward extension of the cerebellar tonsil, closely wrapping around the medulla and cervical spinal cord **(Fig. 1-69)**. This

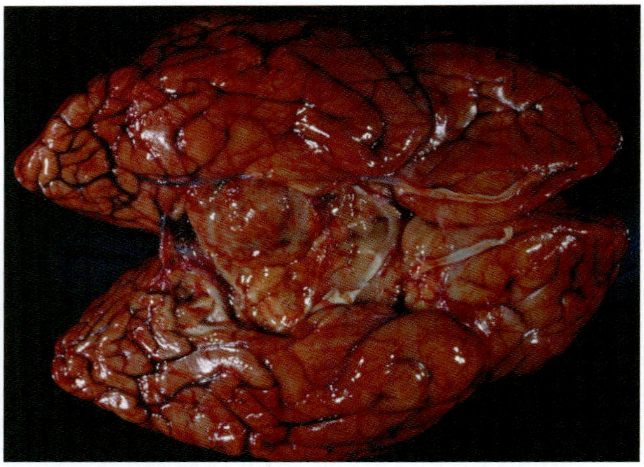

Figure 1-63. There is a large, bosselated mass between the cerebral hemispheres, destroying the midbrain and the midline structures. This was a lymphoma in the center of the brain, crossing the midline and creating extensive mass effect.

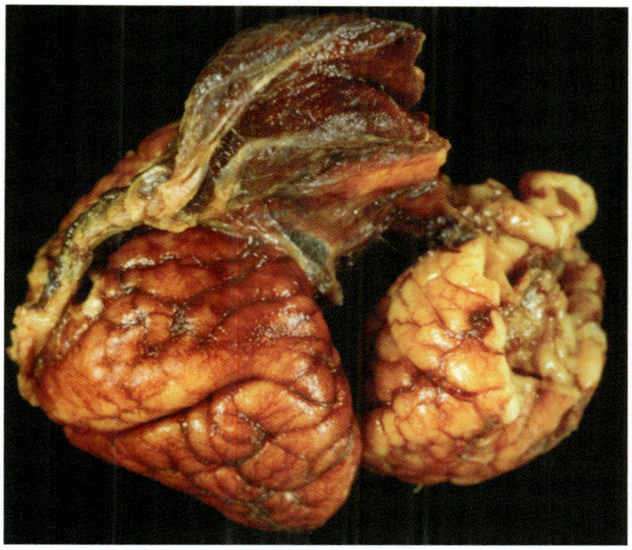

Figure 1-64. Occipital encephalocele contents, consisting of bilateral occipital poles. The gyral pattern is disorganized. The skin covering is seen on top of the contents.

may interfere with the CSF circulation, resulting in hydrocephalus. A relatively rare herniation is the *upward transtentorial herniation* of the cerebellum as a result of mass lesions in the posterior fossa, typically of the cerebellum. The linear impressions of the tentorium cerebelli are then seen on the superior surface of the cerebellum, usually in a roughly circular shape. Midbrain and pons are compressed by the herniating cerebellum posteriorly. Aqueduct may be compressed, resulting in hydrocephalus. Another relatively rare herniation is the *herniation of the frontal lobe into the middle cranial fossa*. This typically involves the inferior posterior portion of the frontal lobe and occurs in space-occupying

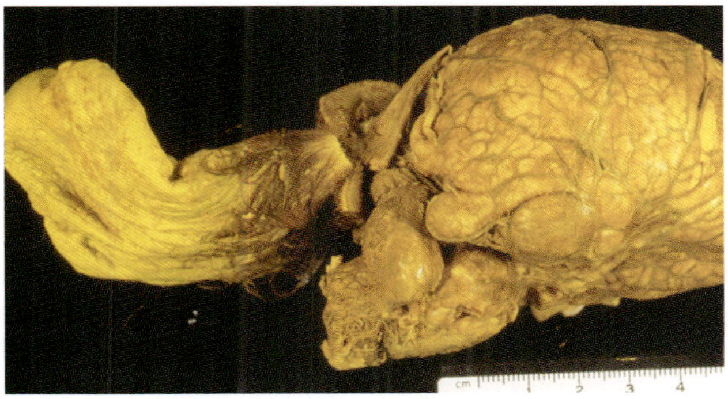

Figure 1-65. Brain and an attached encephalocele covered by skin (**left side**), removed intact at autopsy.

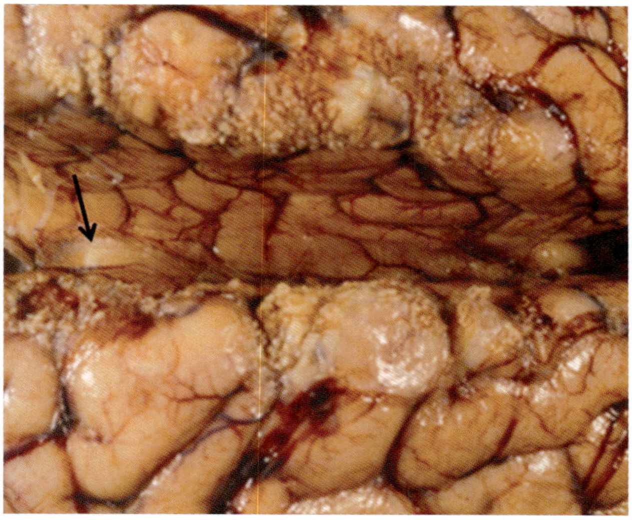

Figure 1-66. Subfalcine herniation. When the interhemispheric fissure is separated and one looks down from the top, corpus callosum should be seen throughout its entire length. In this case, only a small part of corpus callosum can be seen (*arrow*), as most of the view is blocked by the herniating cingulated gyrus.

lesions of the frontal lobe. In these cases, the linear impression of the sphenoid ridge can be seen over the basal surface of the frontal lobe. A *fungating herniation* of the brain convexity occurs outward through calvarial defects, such as after cranial fractures or craniectomy. This type of herniation may especially occur after evacuation of a hematoma or resection of mass lesions due to reactive brain swelling **(Fig. 1-70)**. In general, herniated portions of the neuroglial parenchyma show changes ranging from softening, punctate hemorrhages (herniation contusions), and dusky discoloration to frank infarcts depending on the severity and duration of the herniation as a result of hypoxic/ischemic damage due to compression of the tissues in their herniated state. Herniations are accompanied by a generalized brain swelling or focal mass lesions in areas that may result in the particular herniation. Paying attention to these features should help distinguish variations of normal from true herniations and avoid overdiagnosis. The term *spinal cord herniation* refers to the displacement of the spinal cord parenchyma under the pressure of a mass lesion or shifting of tissues after lumbar puncture and therefore is conceptually different than the brain herniations. The term spinal cord herniation

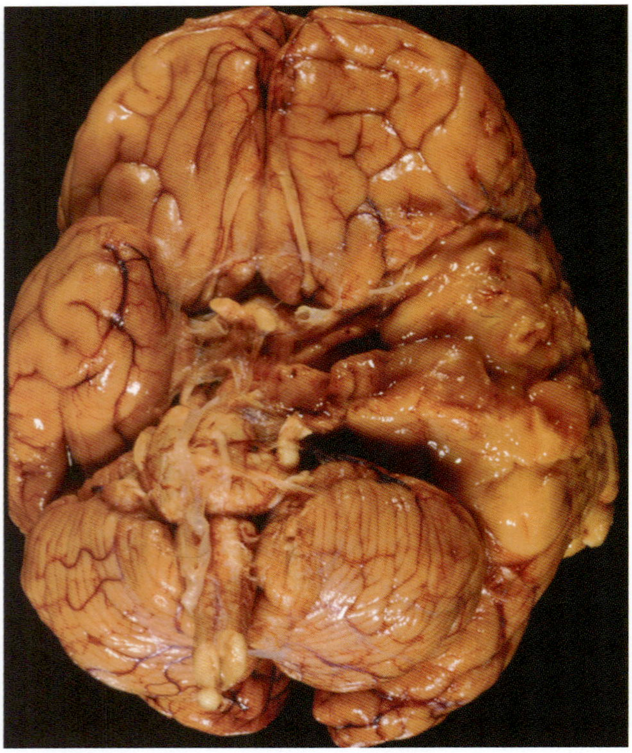

Figure 1-67. Left transtentorial herniation. The left medial temporal lobe has been displaced toward the midline compared to the right side, pushing the brainstem and cerebellum toward the other side. The herniating tissue is swollen, appears soft and friable due to ischemic changes.

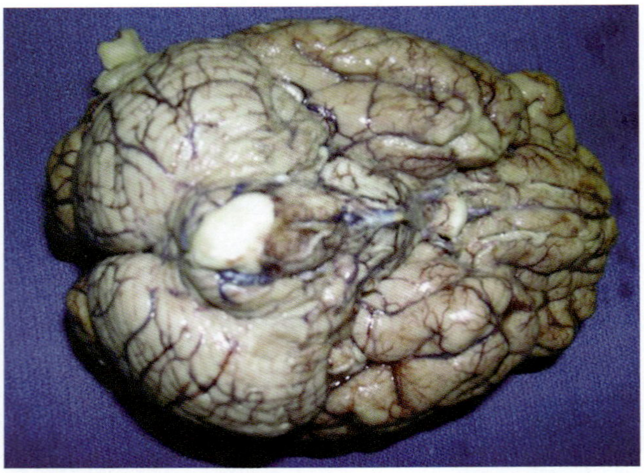

Figure 1-69. Bilateral cerebellar tonsillar herniation. Both cerebellar tonsils extended down into the foramen magnum. Here, they are seen tightly wrapping around the medulla oblongata and superior cervical spinal cord, with a prominent circular groove around them, representing the impression of the edges of foramen magnum. The brain is diffusely swollen with flattened gyri and narrowed sulci.

may sometimes be used to refer to the actual herniation of spinal cord parenchyma from a spinal dural defect, a very rare condition. Cerebellar tonsillar herniation can be associated with Chiari I and Chiari II (Arnold-Chiari) malformation. The latter also shows beaking of tectum and kinking of cervicomedullary junction **(Fig. 1-71)**. Due to the downward displacement of the spinal cord, the spinal nerve roots tend to exit the spinal cord and proceed in an upward direction.

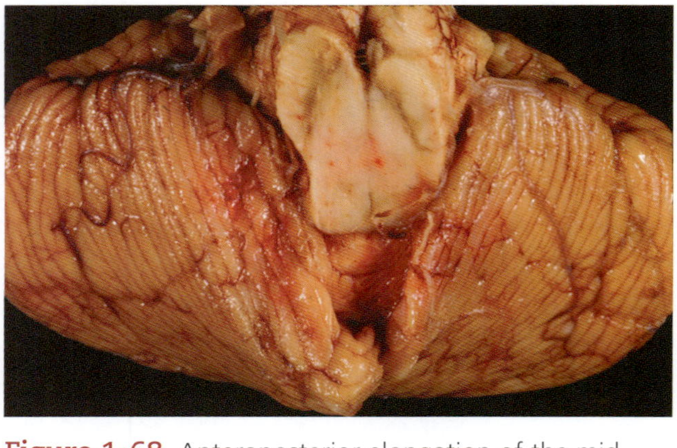

Figure 1-68. Anteroposterior elongation of the midbrain as a result of compression by the medial temporal lobe in transtentorial herniation, which can be bilateral or unilateral, usually severe.

Cranial and Spinal Nerves

Preferably during the removal of the brain and spinal cord, but if that is not possible, definitely during gross examination, *nerve roots* should be inspected. Whether they are present, symmetrical, and intact should be evaluated. A subtle form of midline defect, for instance, is simply the *absence of olfactory bulbs and tracts*, historically referred to as arrhinencephaly,[197] which can be identified by paying attention to the basal surfaces of the frontal lobes. They are commonly torn if one is not careful during the removal of the brain; therefore, the nerve roots should ideally be inspected at the time of autopsy, also by inspecting the skull base. This is usually more of a problem with fragile brains in the

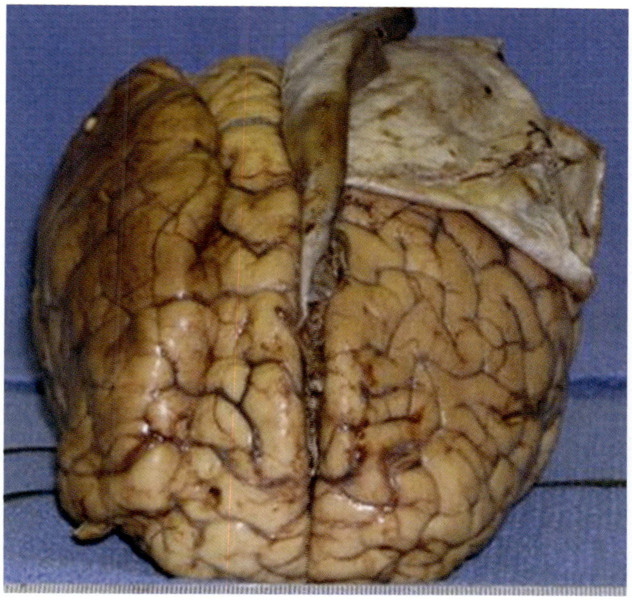

Figure 1-70. Transcalvarial herniation. Another severely and diffusely swollen brain (seen from the front) that shows a large fungating herniation of the brain parenchyma on the right hemisphere. The herniating parenchyma is elevated from the surface and is surrounded by a groove, representing the edges of the calvarial defect. The brain swelling occurred as a result of head trauma, and a craniectomy was performed to alleviate the rapidly increasing intracranial pressure due to uncontrollable swelling. Instead, the brain continued to swell and herniated through the surgery site.

pediatric population, where malformations constitute a bigger concern. However, if this examination is not possible at the time of autopsy, for instance, as in the brains received for consultation, other features can help with accurate interpretation. If the tract appears incomplete bilaterally or unilaterally, it likely developed appropriately but was torn during removal. In true agenesis, they will be entirely absent, bilaterally or rarely unilaterally, in which case, the gyri recti will be disorganized and the olfactory grooves will not have formed **(Fig. 1-72)**. Cribriform plate may not have formed. Olfactory aplasia may be incidental, or may be associated with holoprosencephaly, Meckel-Gruber syndrome, corpus callosum agenesis, septo-optic dysplasia, and Kallmann syndrome. In *aprosencephaly*, there is atelencephaly and in addition, eyes, optic nerves, mamillary bodies, hypothalamus, and pituitary gland are not developed. Cranial nerve

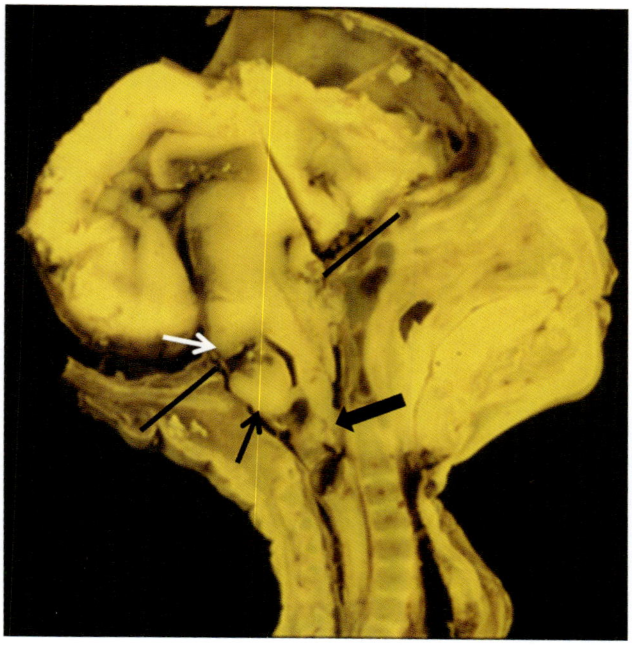

Figure 1-71. Arnold-Chiari malformation. An approximately midsagittal section through the fetus that was a product of terminated pregnancy due to multiple malformations identified in utero. Essentially the entire posterior fossa contents (cerebellum: *black arrow*; brainstem is seen anterior to cerebellum) are displaced caudally through the foramen magnum into the cervical spinal canal (*black lines* indicate the level of skull base and the distance between them is the widened foramen magnum). There is beaking of the tectum (*white arrow*) and kinking of the spinal cord (*block arrow*) approximately at the level of cervicomedullary junction. The yellow color of the specimen is due to previous fixation in Bouin's solution for hardening the specimen during fixation.

List of Findings/Checklist for Cranial and Spinal Nerves

AT A GLANCE

- Artifactual tear
- Agenesis
- Olfactory aplasia (incidental or syndromic)
- Optic nerve agenesis (aprosencephaly)
- Avulsion
- Contusion
- Entrapment neuropathy
- Atrophy/degeneration
- Motor neuron disease
- Discoloration/irregularities/demyelination
- Mass lesions
- Diffuse expansion

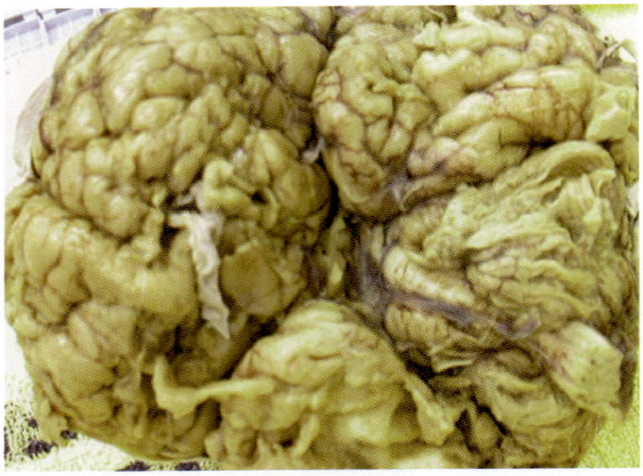

Figure 1-72. Agenesis of olfactory nerves: The true agenesis is identified by the absence of orderly gyri recti and the presence of irregular convoluted gyration on the basal surfaces of the frontal lobes. Widespread polymicrogyria is also present, especially over the frontal lobe surfaces bilaterally.

avulsions may occur as a result of traumatic injury.[198] Olfactory, auditory, facial, and optic nerves are commonly involved. They may be difficult or even impossible to distinguish from artifactual tears during the removal of brain. Traumatic tears are typically associated with hemorrhage, and microscopic examination likely reveals additional damage, such as axonal spheroids. Again, evaluating the nerves in situ at the time of the autopsy should be extremely helpful. In cases where death occurs instantaneously, however, no changes, including hemorrhage, may be present. Cranial nerve damage can also be due to *contusions*, especially in the olfactory bulbs, which are compressed by the weight of the brain against the skull base, resulting in anosmia.[199]

Trigeminal neuralgia and other similar compression syndromes are the result of pressure to a nerve root usually by an artery.[200] These are frequently corrected surgically and do not constitute an issue during postmortem evaluation nor do they generate surgical specimens. Cranial and/or spinal nerve roots can be entrapped in processes involving the meninges, particularly those of the dura mater, resulting in *entrapment neuropathy*. These processes can be inflammatory, neoplastic, or idiopathic conditions, resulting in increase in volume of the dura mater, usually in the form of fibrosis, to compress the nerve roots. Granulomatous diseases such as tuberculosis, sarcoidosis, fungal infections, or idiopathic conditions such as idiopathic hypertrophic pachymeningitis, or the similar condition associated with systemic autoimmune/connective tissue disorders can result in such entrapment.[201] Also, focal mass lesions arising from the adjacent tissues can secondarily infiltrate or compress the nerve roots. Systemic diseases affecting the bone, including skull base, and bone dysplasias resulting in the distortions of the foramina in the skull base can cause cranial or spinal neuropathies.[202,203]

Peripheral nerve sheath tumors can be seen as *mass lesions* associated with the nerve roots. Schwannomas are in the form of a well-defined mass eccentrically growing off of a nerve root, although the latter can be difficult to identify when the neoplasm is large enough to compress and obscure the nerve. Schwannomas may be sporadic neoplasms in the cranial nerves **(Fig. 1-73)**. Neurofibromas result in a *diffuse enlargement*, sausage-like, somewhat irregular nodular thickening and tortuosity of the nerve. They have a smooth, glistening external surface because of the overlying leptomeninges covering the nerve root. In a patient with a first-degree relative, however, a vestibular schwannoma or two nonvestibular schwannomas or two or more neurofibromas are diagnostic of NF2. A similar diffuse expansion of the optic nerves, uni- or bilaterally, with or without involvement of the chiasm, may also be due to pilocytic astrocytoma of the optic nerve/tract, commonly referred to as optic glioma, a term that should

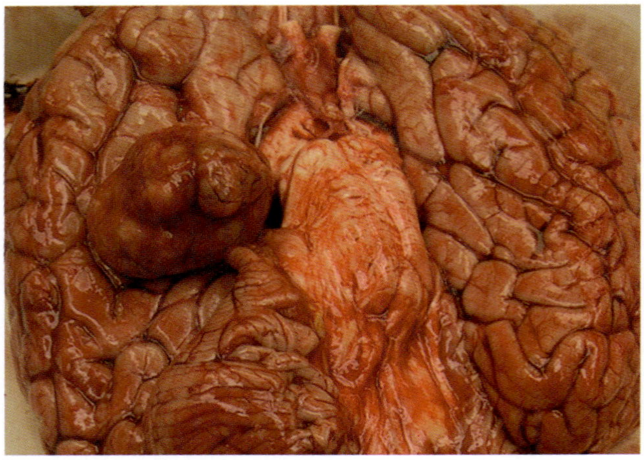

Figure 1-73. Vestibular schwannoma with a lobular appearance.

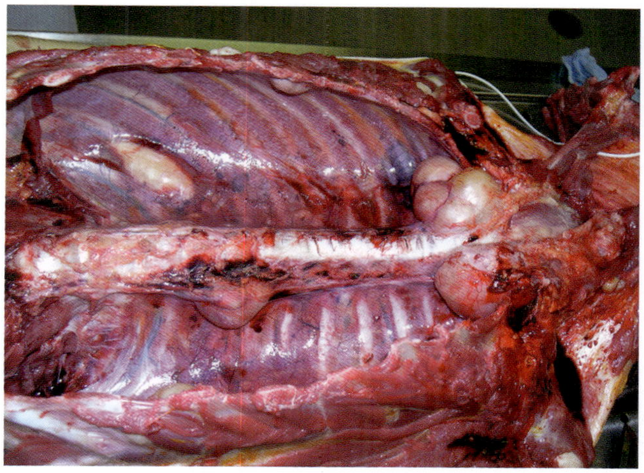

Figure 1-74. Multiple lobulated masses of peripheral nerve sheath tumors are present mainly in paraspinal locations, as well as in the intercostal nerves in this NF2 patient. Some of these neop asms showed malignant component together with neurofibromas.

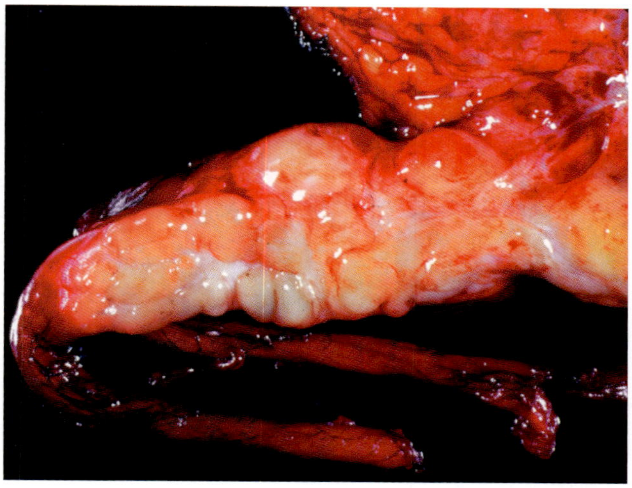

Figure 1-75. Plexiform neurofibroma consisting of a diffuse enlargement of peripheral nerves and a convoluted, multinodular appearance described as "bag of worms."

be avoided since occasionally diffuse astrocytomas can involve the optic nerves, also. Pilocytic astrocytoma of the optic nerve is one of the manifestations of NF1.[17,204] Multiple neurofibromas in paraspinal location, associated with spinal nerve roots, can be seen in NF1 **(Fig. 1-74)**. Plexiform neurofibromas, which may be grossly recognized by their multinodular "bag of worms" appearance **(Fig. 1-75)**, as well as MPNST can be seen in these locations, also in association with NF1. Multiple nodules or diffuse sheet-like accumulations on the spinal cord and spinal nerve surfaces may represent drop metastases from CNS neoplasms, such as ependymoma or medulloblastoma. Optic nerve meningiomas ensheath the nerve and may also appear as diffuse expansion of the nerve.[205] However, meningioma forms a firm, coarse, and gray-white encasing, obscuring the glistening external surface of the nerve. Neural neoplasms also arise in the peripheral ganglia, such as adrenal medulla, and mainly include paraganglioma and neuroblastoma with or without variable degree of differentiation, for example, ganglioneuroblastoma **(Fig. 1-76)**. *Cerebellar cortical degeneration* shows degeneration of cerebellar cortex, olivary nuclei, and visual system, including *optic nerves*, superior colliculi, lateral geniculate bodies, and visual cortex, sparing pons.[206,207] Various degenerative diseases that involve the *brainstem* motor nuclei may show degeneration of *cranial nerves,* and some also involve anterior horn neurons in spinal cord to result in spinal nerve atrophy, for example, hereditary bulbar palsies of types I and II, van Laere syndrome, and Fazio-Londe disease, respectively.[208] Type I also shows involvement of sensory *vestibulocochlear nerves* and ventral cochlear nuclei.

In the spinal cord, if special attention is paid to removal in an attempt to preserve the nerve roots

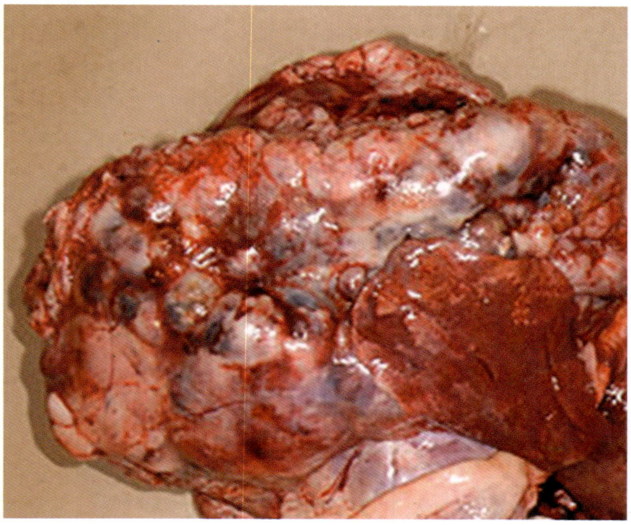

Figure 1-76. Multilobular retroperitoneal ganglioneuroblastoma originating from adrenal medulla.

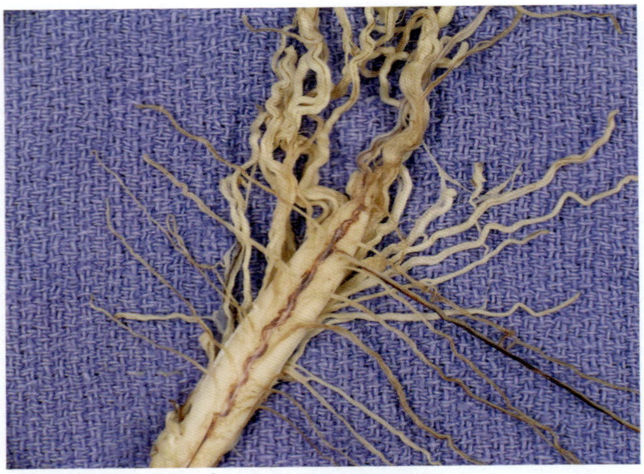

Figure 1-77. Atrophic anterior (motor) spinal nerves (spread perpendicular to the spinal cord) compared to unremarkable posterior (sensory) nerve roots (spread diagonally to the spinal cord) in a patient with acute infantile spinal muscular atrophy (Werdnig-Hoffmann disease).

and to the detailed examination, it is possible to examine individual nerve roots by spreading them apart. This way, thin anterior spinal nerves relative to the posterior nerves can be documented in diseases involving the motor system, such as ALS and SMA (acute infantile form, i.e.,Werdnig-Hoffmann disease **(Fig. 1-77)**; intermediate form; chronic form, i.e., Kugelberg-Welander syndrome). Anterior nerve roots and nerves are atrophic due to anterior horn neuron loss. They may involve brainstem cranial nerve nuclei and dorsal root ganglia. Some variants may be associated with cerebellar atrophy or hypoplasia.

Optic nerve is frequently involved in multiple sclerosis (MS) and neuromyelitis optica (Devic's disease)[209,210] **(Table 1.13)**. The involved nerve appears tan and shrunken, distorting its usual full and bright white-tan appearance. In chronic and extensive lesions, entire optic nerves and chiasm may appear shrunken and feel like a firm thin cord. Optic atrophy can be seen in association with some medications, such as chloramphenicol[211] and ethambutol.[212] Optic nerves are also thin in cerebro-ocular dysplasia.

TABLE 1.13 Disorders affecting the optic nerves

Optic nerve meningiomas
Optic nerve glioma
PNST and MPNST
NF1
MS
Neuromyelitis optica
Trauma
Cerebellar cortical degeneration
Cerebro-ocular dysplasia
Chloramphenicol
Ethambutol

Cut Surfaces

Traditionally, the brain is cut in the frontal plane unless a specific situation dictates otherwise to better demonstrate a lesion or better examine a structure. While standard sectioning is adequate in the great majority of cases, sometimes the plane of sectioning may need to be adjusted so that it can pass through a particular area of interest or a suspected lesion identified during external examination. A systematical approach to evaluate every component is necessary to identify subtle lesions. Some *artifacts* can mimic true lesions. Poorly fixed brains can have pink and soft areas that can mimic an early infarct. These areas are typically in the deep parenchyma, where the fixative needs more time to reach. They are not limited to a particular anatomical structure but rather a circular area involving the basal ganglia, thalamus, and periventricular white matter. Sometimes, the bases of the gryi and sulci are also included **(Fig. 1-78)**. One of the confusing situations occurs with the tangential sections of cortical gray matter, seen as well-circumscribed islands of tan tissue surrounded by white matter. These are usually in the superficial white matter and can mimic chronic demyelination plaques. In addition, if the section passes close enough to an underlying sulcus, they feel softer than the surrounding tissue, further raising the suspicion for a true lesion. Another potentially confusing artifact is a focal tissue loss due to a dull knife catching and dislodging a piece of brain tissue, resulting in a cavitary or friable area of several millimeters, mimicking a microinfarct or demyelination. This can be resolved by evaluating the corresponding area on the opposite slice. Artifacts are typically one-sided, while the true lesions are typically present on the slices on both sides of the cut. Nonetheless, some defects can be difficult to sort

List of Findings/Checklist for Cut Surfaces

AT A GLANCE

- Artifacts
- Cortical ribbon
  - Thickness
  - Color
  - Consistency
  - Watershed zones
- Atrophy and its distribution (also see "External Surfaces")
  - Cerebral cortex
  - Hippocampus
  - Mamillary bodies
  - Basal ganglia and thalami
  - White matter
  - Cerebellum
  - Brainstem
  - Spinal cord
- Thickening and irregularity of cerebral cortex
- Firm nodules
- Gray-white matter junction
- Double cortex
- Heterotopias
- Expansion of gyri
- White matter
  - Demyelination (focal, diffuse)
  - Destructive lesion (infarct, hypoxic–ischemic changes, cavitary lesions)
  - Volume loss
  - Discoloration
  - Status of U-fibers
- Basal ganglia and thalami
  - Atrophy
  - Lacunae
  - Cavitary lesions (bilateral, symmetrical, random)
  - Discoloration
- Cerebellum
  - Atrophy
  - Thickening
  - Artifact
- Brainstem
- Softening
- Calcification
- Hemorrhage (see "Parenchymal Hemorrhage")
- Ventricular system (see "Ventricular System")
- Cystic change (see "Cystic Lesions")
- Mass lesions
  - Solid
  - Cystic
  - Consistency
  - Borders
  - Multiplicity
  - Involvement of corpus callosum/crossing the midline
- Midline shift
- Herniations

out, and a microscopic section should be submitted when in doubt. The *leptomeningeal lesions* can easily be lost after sectioning if particular attention is not paid to their localization. Minimal subarachnoid hemorrhages and fibrotic, granulomatous, and nodular areas may become difficult to identify on cut surfaces. In addition, especially when cutting tissue sections for microscopic examination and not so much during serial sectioning of the brain, leptomeninges can easily be stripped off of the surface and not represented on the slide, potentially resulting in loss of diagnostic clues. This is particularly a problem in surgical specimens and fetal brains. In the latter, the "slimy" nature of the tissue results in such separation even when handling the brain. In such cases, the displaced leptomeninges can be lumped together and submitted separately for microscopic examination. In some situations, leptomeninges can be intentionally and partially stripped in an attempt to better demonstrate certain characteristics of the parenchymal surface, for example, atrophy, polymicrogyria, and pitted surface in microinfarcts; however, this is not a preferred method for diagnostic work.

Cortical ribbon should have a uniform thickness, with the exception of focal, tangentially cut areas. It has a homogeneous texture and color with a sharp gray-white matter junction. Any deviation from this usual appearance may indicate a pathologic process and needs to be sampled. It may be *blurred* with mild swelling as an early change in an infarct. Subtle *collapsed* appearance or its obvious disappearance over an unremarkable white matter indicates a laminar infarct **(Fig. 1-79)**. Especially the watershed zone location of such changes is associated with a global drop in perfusion, such

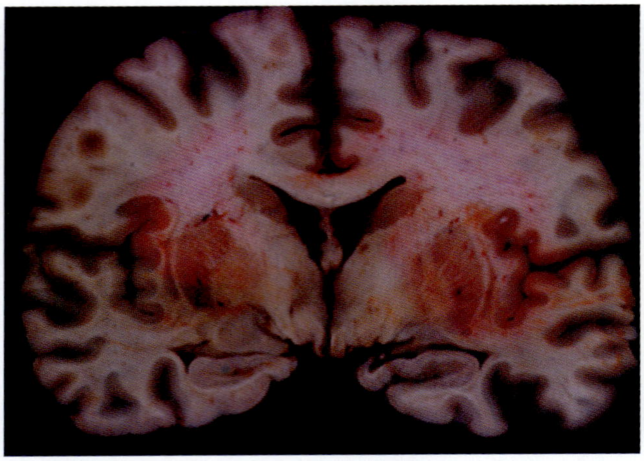

Figure 1-78. Poor fixation resulting in the deeper areas of the brain to remain soft and pink. Coincidentally, this particular brain also shows multiple dusky cortical areas representing hypoxic/ischemic injury. Although basal ganglia and insular cortices appear to be affected more prominently, the poorly fixed pink region also involves the centrum semiovale, creating a circular outline.

as a hypotensive episode; however, they may be more extensive in hypoperfusion states. In its acute stages, especially in the first few days, it is soft and granular, friable. In cases with reperfusion, a *hyperemic appearance* and petechial hemorrhages may be seen **(Fig. 1-80)**. In some cases, such hemorrhages may be the predominant feature, that is, hemorrhagic infarct. In subacute stage, infarct has a collapsed appearance **(Fig. 1-81)**. In chronic stage, it can barely be seen as a thin line due to astrocytosis and shrinkage. If a hemorrhagic component is present, an orange-yellow discoloration is also seen. Focal, *dusky red-brown discoloration* indicates the early hypoxic/ischemic injury. Microinfarcts secondary to small vessel disease or embolic showers create an irregular cortex with variable thickness. These represent the cut surfaces of the granular leptomeningeal surface appearance. Focal groupings of *hemorrhages* in the cortex, associated with

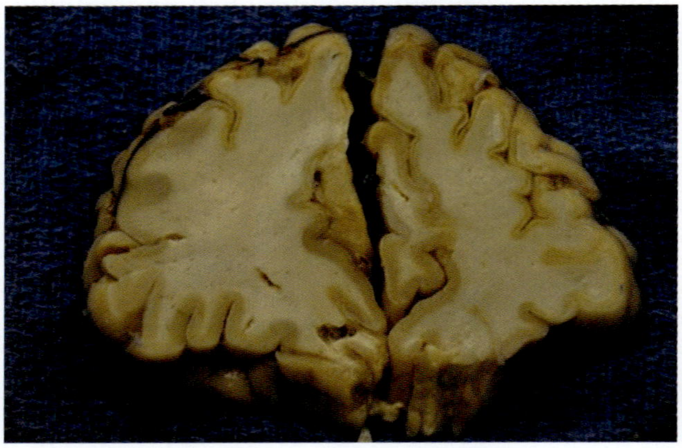

Figure 1-79. Cortical infarcts. Long stretches of cortical gray matter appears thin, collapsed, and pale, more prominently in the parasagittal regions. The changes stand out especially when compared to the relatively uninvolved cortex in other areas.

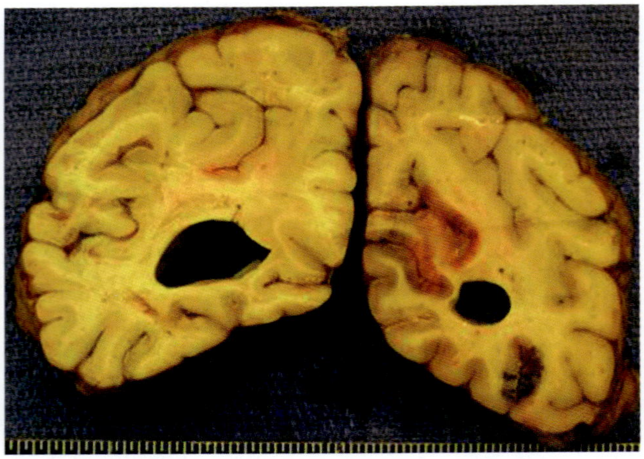

Figure 1-80. Acute infarcts in the right occipital lobe. In addition to tan-brown discoloration in areas of the cortical ribbon, there are punctuate hemorrhagic foci. They tend to involve the depths of the gyri and not the surface, consistent with their hypoxic/ischemic nature.

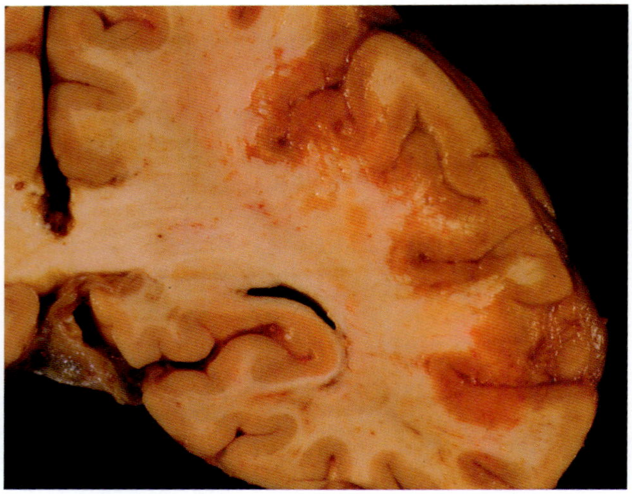

Figure 1-81. Subacute infarcts. The involved areas of the cortex and underlying white matter appear collapsed and soft. The changes are pronounced in the depths of the gyri, consistent with their hypoxic/ischemic nature.

subarachnoid hemorrhage, represent contusions (see "Parenchymal Hemorrhage" below).

The earliest changes associated with hypoxic/ischemic damage are very subtle. There may be a no changes in appearance or there may be a mild red-brown *discoloration*. Otherwise, especially in the white matter, the only indication may be *softening* of the tissue. This is best appreciated when a finger is run over the cut surface of fixed tissue as a depression felt due to soft consistency of the lesion compared to adjacent areas. As the infarct progresses through acute, subacute, and chronic stages, a gradual change from depressed, friable, gelatinous appearance to *collapsed*, **(Fig. 1-82)** and eventually *cystic* appearance can be seen **(Fig. 1-83)**. These changes are highly variable depending on the size of the lesion, metabolic rate, oxygenation and perfusion, collateral circulation, and restoration of circulation of the tissue. Infarcts can be very focal or can involve an entire hemisphere, for instance, in cases of embolic occlusion of internal carotid artery. Their appearance is altered by the presence of a *hemorrhagic component*, due to leaking of necrotic vessels as part of the initial event, or as reperfusion hemorrhage when the necrotic vessels cannot withstand the pressure of re-established blood flow.[213] Depending on the age of the hemorrhage, these hemorrhagic infarcts can be associated with different colors

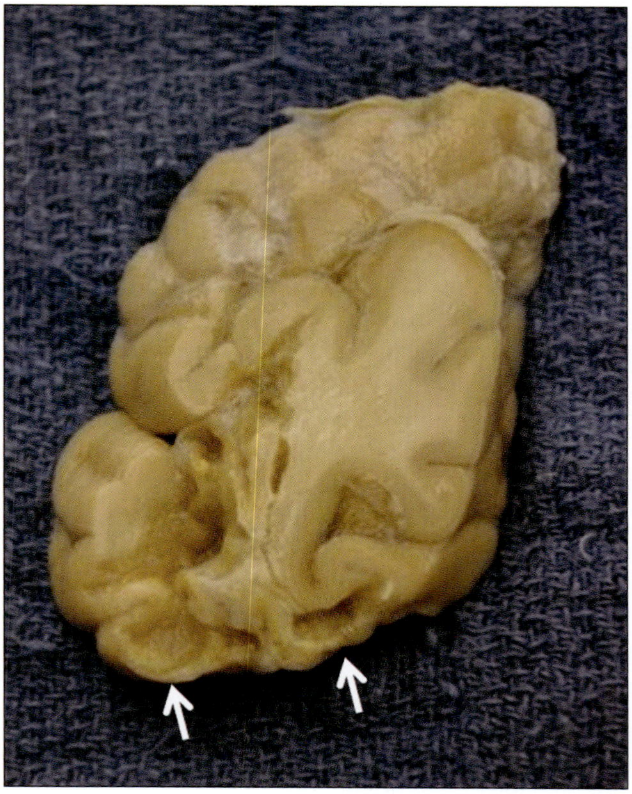

Figure 1-83. Remote infarct. The lesion has become largely cystic. A mild yellow-orange discoloration is present on its lining, suggesting a hemorrhagic component, now likely represented by hemosiderin pigment. Thin pial–subpial layer of tissue remains relatively intact as a membranous structure overlying the lesion (*arrows*), supporting its hypoxic/ischemic, rather than traumatic, nature.

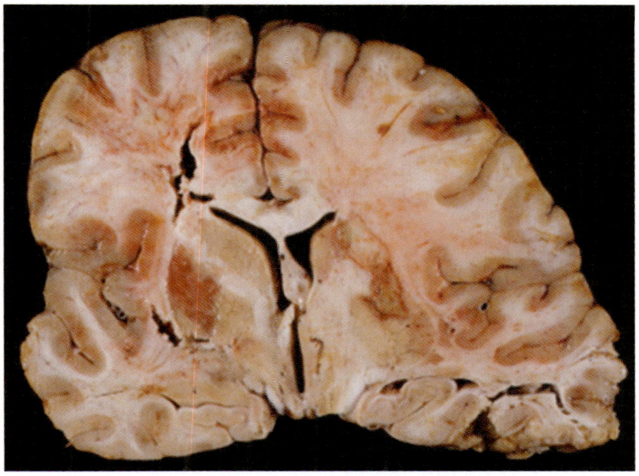

Figure 1-82. Multiple infarcts involving cortex, white matter, and basal ganglia. Especially the ones in the right striatum and left centrum semiovale are sharply demarcated, a feature that becomes more obvious grossly as the infarcts progresses into the subacute stage.

from bright red in fresh hemorrhage to orange-yellow in remote hemorrhage. These color changes usually parallel the evolution of the infarct through its stages. Differentiating a superficial hemorrhagic infarct from a contusion can be difficult. Infarcts tend to have a triangular outline with the base of the triangle toward the brain surface; however, this can only be appreciated in larger lesions. Hemorrhages and infarcts can be associated with porphyrias due to the hypertension seen in these cases. CNS involvement is seen in hepatic porphyrias.[214] Leptomeninges and the pial layer are not involved in the lesion if it is hypoxic/ischemic in nature. Upon close examination, a viable, gliotic, thin *membranous subpial layer* **(Fig. 1-83)** can be identified and sometimes can only be appreciated by microscopic examination. In traumatic injury, the leptomeninges and the subpial layer are also damaged and show hemorrhage and disruption. Therefore, in problematic cases, including the leptomeningeal surface in the section becomes important. In addition, contusions tend to be multiple and tend to involve the crests of the gyri, while hypoxic/ischemic lesions tend to involve the depths of the gyri. Drowning has no specific gross findings but a diffuse gray matter darkening due to hemoconcentration.[38] Because the neurodegenerative diseases are so diverse with involvement of different subsystems and components of the CNS, *patterns of atrophy* involving various combinations of these structures provide information regarding the nature of the disease. *Cortical atrophy* is seen, similar to its appearance on external examination, as thinning of the gyri and widening of sulci on cut surfaces. These features are especially prominent in the sylvian fissure. The fibrous tissue bands of the leptomeninges can be seen traversing the sulci with the vascular structures hanging in the subarachnoid space. Ventricles show compensatory dilatation (see "Ventricular System" below). A generalized atrophy is usually seen in advanced cases of dementing neurodegenerative diseases, such as AD **(Fig. 1-84)**. In FTLD, frontal and temporal lobes are preferentially affected. In addition, other structures are also involved depending on the type of FTLD.[215,216] In frontotemporal degeneration, parkinsonism linked to chromosome 17, atrophy preferentially involves the anterior–inferior parts of temporal lobes, frontal lobes, and anterior cingulate gyrus. Substantia nigra may be pale, and basal ganglia atrophy may be seen. FTLD-U (frontotemporal lobar degeneration with ubiquitin-only immunoreactive changes) also shows frontotemporal atrophy and basal ganglion atrophy; substantia nigra pallor may be seen as well. FTLD-MND and FTLD-NF (FTLD with neurofilament inclusions), in addition to frontotemporal atrophy, basal ganglia atrophy may also be seen. *Atrophy of the hippocampus* is a common finding in dementing diseases, such as AD and FTLD. It is also seen in hippocampal sclerosis, also referred to as mesial temporal sclerosis. Cornu ammonis is attenuated and the temporal horn of the lateral ventricle becomes enlarged due to volume loss in hippocampus **(Fig. 1-85)**. Unilateral atrophy of one hippocampus indicates a localized process, such as mesial temporal sclerosis in epilepsy patients, as seen in hippocampectomy specimens. These are mentioned in the respective discussions of regional pathology below. Areas involved by Rasmussen encephalitis appear atrophic.[217] Some cases may have coexisting neoplasms, cavernous angiomas, or

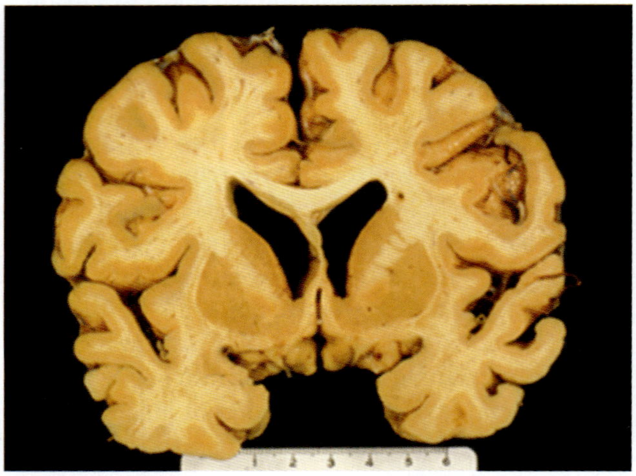

Figure 1-84. Generalized atrophy. The gyri appear shrunken and sulci widened. The changes are better seen in the sylvian fissure, where the vessels are seen freely in the widened subarachnoid space. Ventricular system is dilated as a result of parenchymal volume loss, that is, hydrocephalus ex vacuo, with blunting of the angles of the lateral ventricles.

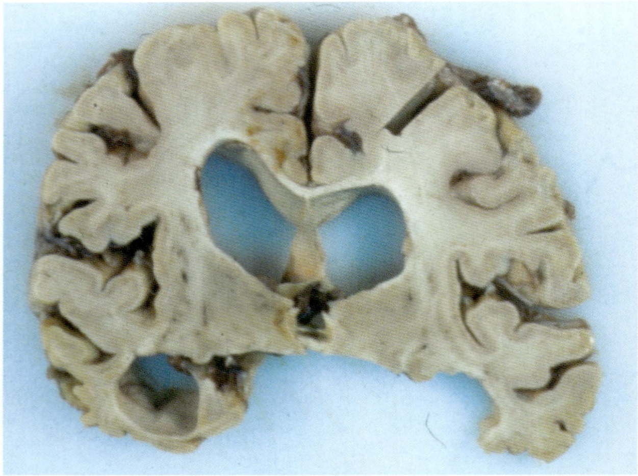

Figure 1-85. Prominent atrophy in a case of Pick's disease. Some tissue, including right hippocampus, has been removed for research. The left hippocampus is extremely atrophic, and there is prominent hydrocephalus ex vacuo, including the temporal horns of the lateral ventricles. The severe atrophy results in pointy tips of the gyri.

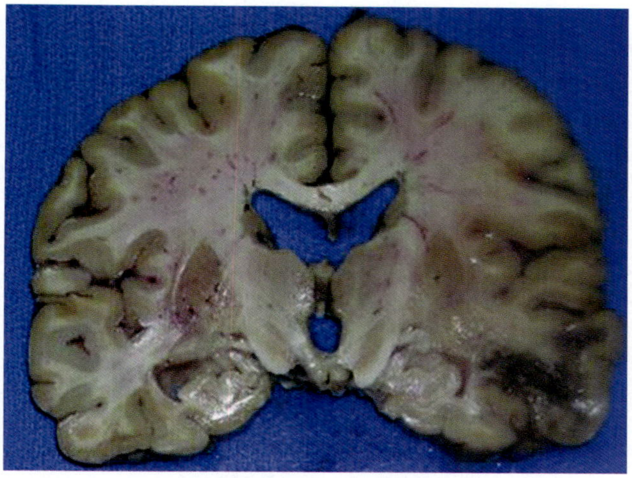

Figure 1-86. Cerebritis predominantly involving the right temporal lobe white matter. The lesion has irregular borders, and although there is liquefaction and early cavity formation, indicating progression to abscess formation, the process is more diffuse than it grossly appears. There is also a mild edema in the entire right hemisphere, which is slightly larger than the left.

malformation of cortical development. An irregular, somewhat dusky hemorrhagic and soft lesion of variable size and shape within the brain parenchyma may represent cerebritis **(Fig. 1-86)**. It has gross features similar to subacute infarct, including edema, although the edema is a lot more prominent in cerebritis, frequently with midline shift and potential for herniation. In addition, it is quite ill-defined compared to the well-circumscribed infarct. Alpers-Huttenlocher syndrome (progressive neuronal degeneration of childhood) results in thin, friable, dusky cortex, especially prominent in calcarine cortex, and may involve white matter.[218] It also has liver pathology, consisting of microvesicular steatosis and fibrosis. Multiple infarcts of variable sizes and stages, simultaneously or metacronously, may occur when there is a systemic process involving multiple vessels, such as an embolic shower. Fat emboli, multiple thromboemboli due to atrial fibrillation, hypercoagulable states, intravascular lymphoma **(Fig. 1-87)**, and erythrocyte sickling **(Fig. 1-88)** are some examples. There may or may not be a definitive clinical history to provide clues, and the brain lesions may be quite subtle, especially if seen earlier in their development. Ventricular shunt catheter tracts are easy to recognize if the shunt is in place, in which case

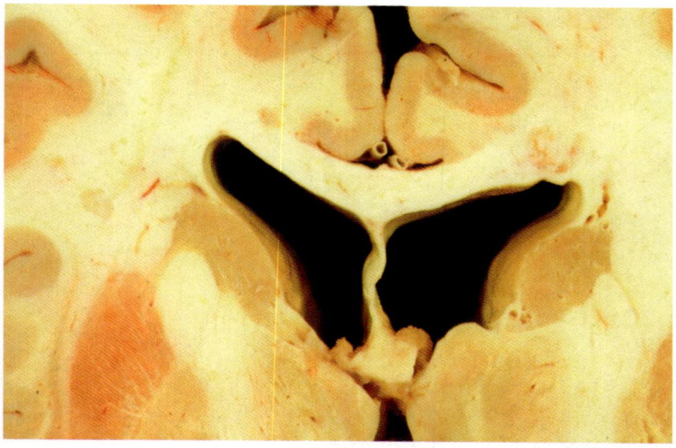

Figure 1-87. Intravascular lymphoma. Multiple small lesions in the periventricular white matter have slightly discolored and depressed appearance. The differential diagnosis includes demyelination. Microscopic examination showed them to be microinfarcts as a result of vascular occlusion by intravascular lymphoma in this patient with mental status changes.

its functionality and location should be noted. The usual tract is in the white matter next to the lateral ventricle angle and is perpendicular to the ventricle surface **(Fig. 1-89)**. Depending on the duration of its presence, the cavity may be gliotic in longstanding cases and may be hemorrhagic in recent cases. Rarely, due to a variety of factors, the shunt may be buried into the parenchyma in the ventricular wall and may cause a cavity that can be taken

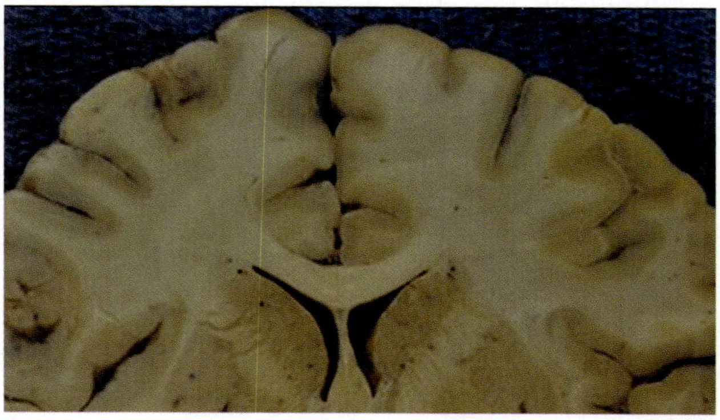

Figure 1-88. Multiple acute infarcts in a patient with sickle cell trait. Although the changes are very subtle grossly, white matter in both hemispheres had ill-defined soft areas that microscopically showed acute ischemic changes. They form mildly discolored areas with irregular borders. They were associated with prominent sickled erythrocytes within the vessels.

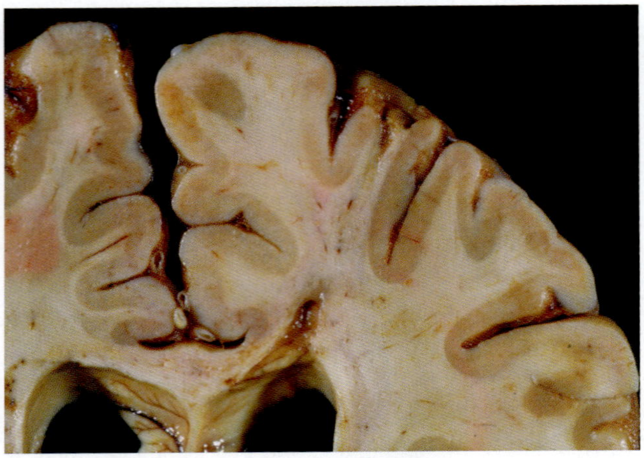

Figure 1-89. Shunt tract. A slit-like cavity is present in the right frontal lobe white matter and lies perpendicular to the lateral ventricle surface. If the shunt has been pulled out before the examination, these lesions can cause confusion with infarcts. It can also be traced all the way up to the surface in serial sections.

for a true pathologic process, such as an infarct. Therefore, it is appropriate to leave the shunts and any other surgical evidence in place until the time of brain cutting, so that they are documented in detail.

Irregular *thickening of cortical gray matter* may indicate a malformation of cortical development, such as focal cortical dysplasia. Usually, there is expansion of the cortex associated with an *expansion of the gyrus*, which can also be seen on external examination. Typically, the *gray-white matter junction is blurred* with the colors of gray and white matter gradually fading into each other **(Fig. 1-90)**, and the lesion has a *firmer consistency*. A white, firm quality to the cortical gray matter, essentially limited to the cortical ribbon in a band-like manner, may be due to meningioangiomatosis and the associated extensive collagenization. Prominent and large lesions can be felt as *firm nodules* especially during the handling of fresh whole brain **(Fig. 1-91)**. A similar appearance can be seen in neoplasms infiltrating the gray-white matter junction, such as oligodendroglioma **(Fig. 1-92)**, the cells of which have a tendency to infiltrate the gray matter and accumulate under the pia mater. If calcification and astrocytosis are also present, the lesion may have a *pale tan-yellow* appearance. Polymicrogyria is seen as irregular attempts at rudimentary gyration but with no separation into true gyri with intervening sulci or leptomeninges. Instead, they form a solid cortical ribbon but with *irregular up and down winding of gray matter* with intervening white matter streaks **(Fig. 1-93)**. It can be widespread or focal and, when focal, it has a predilection for perisylvian region. Cortical ribbon may appear extremely thick due to the presence of band heterotopias, which runs parallel to the pial surface to form a *double-cortex appearance*. Laminar/band heterotopias, in subcortical white matter, may engulf claustrum in it and is separated from cortex by a thin white matter layer. A cortical

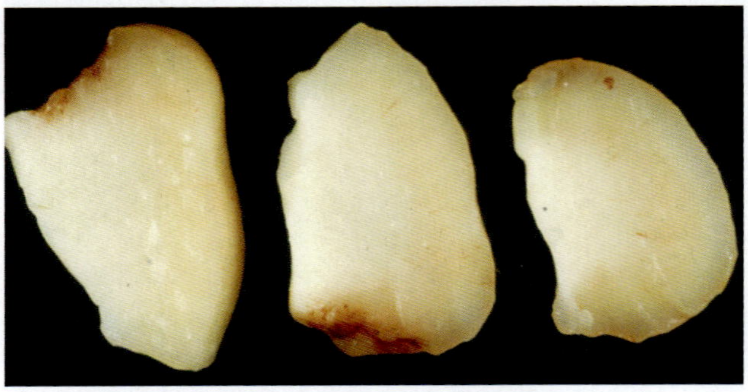

Figure 1-90. Focal cortical dysplasia. Serial sections of the surgical specimen of focal cortical dysplasia show mild pallor of cortical gray matter and blurring of the gray-white matter junction, especially prominent on the section on the left.

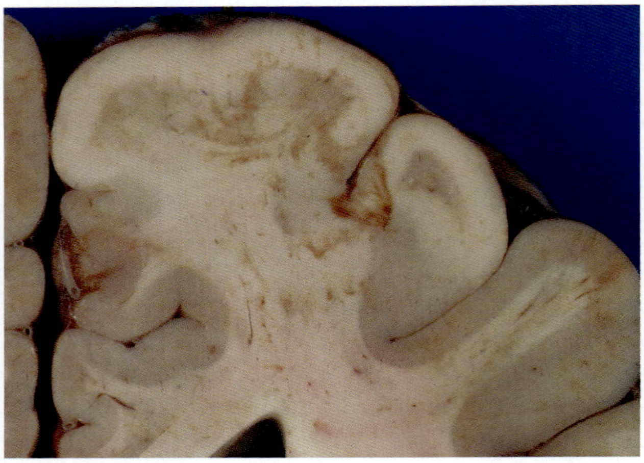

Figure 1-91. Tuber in a case of tuberous sclerosis. Pallor of cortical gray matter stretches over multiple gyri. The underlying white matter shows somewhat tan discoloration due to prominent gliosis, therefore creating a negative image of the gray-white matter junction. Especially such large and multiple cortical dysplasias can be felt grossly as firm nodules in the soft parenchyma before fixation.

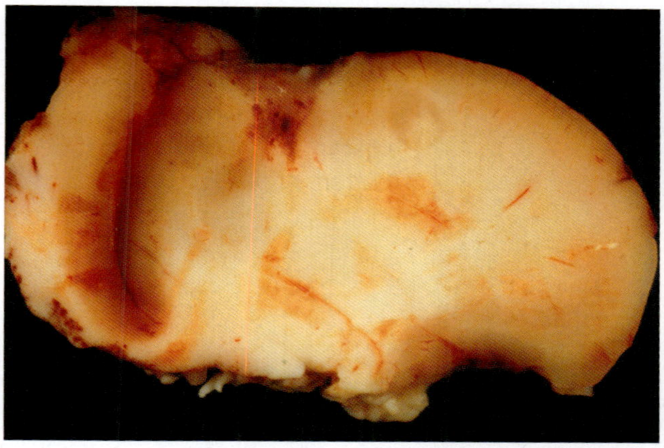

Figure 1-92. Oligodendroglioma. Cut surface of the surgical specimen of oligodendroglioma resection shows expansion of the gyrus with blurring of the gray-white matter junction due to infiltration of the gray matter by the underlying oligodendroglioma, which has a tendency to do so.

malformation with features of focal cortical dysplasia but in a diffuse manner is seen in unilateral cortical dysplasia with hemimegalencephaly. It may be isolated or in association with various syndromes. Dentate gyrus dysplasia and hypoplasia of hippocampus can be associated with trisomy 18.[219]

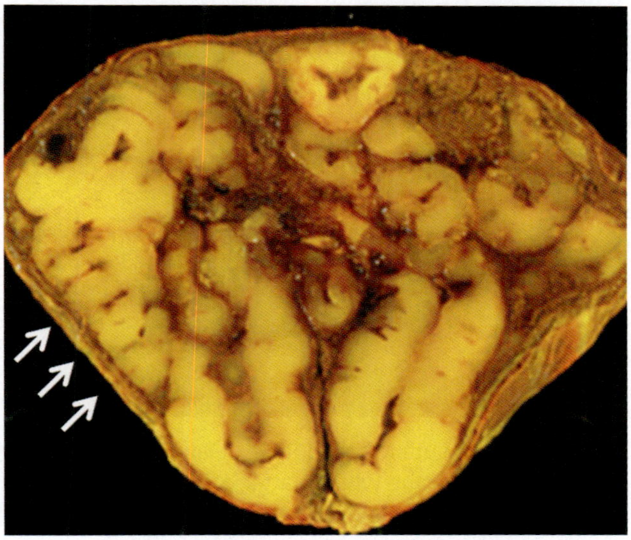

Figure 1-93. Polymicrogyria in encephalocele. Cut surface of distorted brain parenchyma in an encephalocele sac formed by the skin. The *arrows* indicate the polymicrogyria where there appears to be attempted gyrus–sulcus formation. Microscopically, the leptomeninges do not follow the attempted sulcus formation formed by the cortical layers.

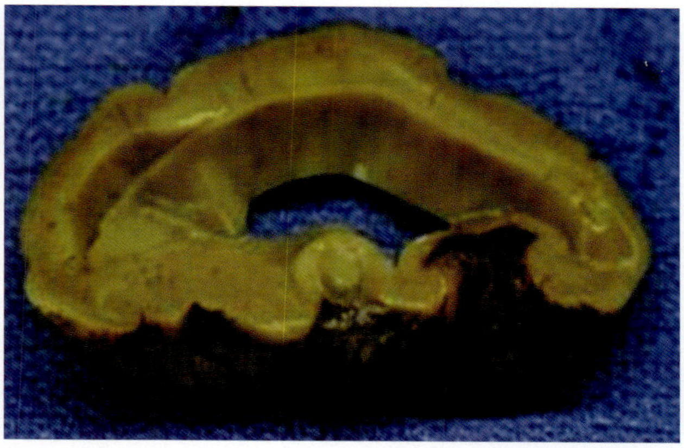

Figure 1-94. Alobar holoprosencephaly and thick cortical ribbon. Cortex is continuous and no interhemispheric fissure is present. The cortical gray matter is thick, forming essentially the entire parenchymal thickness, with minimal amount, if any, of white matter, which is also contributed by the prominent hydrocephalus and possible other damage to the periventricular white matter.

Cortex is *uniformly thick* in agyria/pachygyria. They are extensive lesions involving one or both hemispheres. In holoprosencephaly, cortex is continuous (cingulosynapsis) **(Fig. 1-94)**. Interhemispheric fissure has formed in the lobar form, in contrast to alobar form, which may be partial. Sagittal sinus and falx cerebri may be absent.

Gray matter foci in the white matter may represent a tangential section of the gray matter of an underlying gyrus, as discussed above. Heterotopic gray matter nodules can be of variable sizes and numbers but typically as an aggregate of a few nodules of a few millimeters, with irregular borders. They can be anywhere in the white matter, though with a predilection for periventricular areas **(Fig. 1-95)**. Demyelinating lesions, especially the chronic plaques of MS, can produce an appearance that looks like gray nodules in the white matter **(Fig. 1-96)**.They also have irregular borders and a firmer consistency relative to the surrounding tissue. Usually, wedge-shaped or *triangular-shaped* and somewhat linear ill-defined solid lesions in the white matter, especially noticed in association with cortical dysplasia nodules, subependymal nodules, and SEGA, likely represent radial glioneuronal heterotopias in tuberous sclerosis. The base of the lesion is typically toward the brain surface.[220] Heterotopias and cortical dysplasias in brain and cerebellum may be associated with fetal mercury exposure.[221] Focal lesions of variable sizes, shapes,

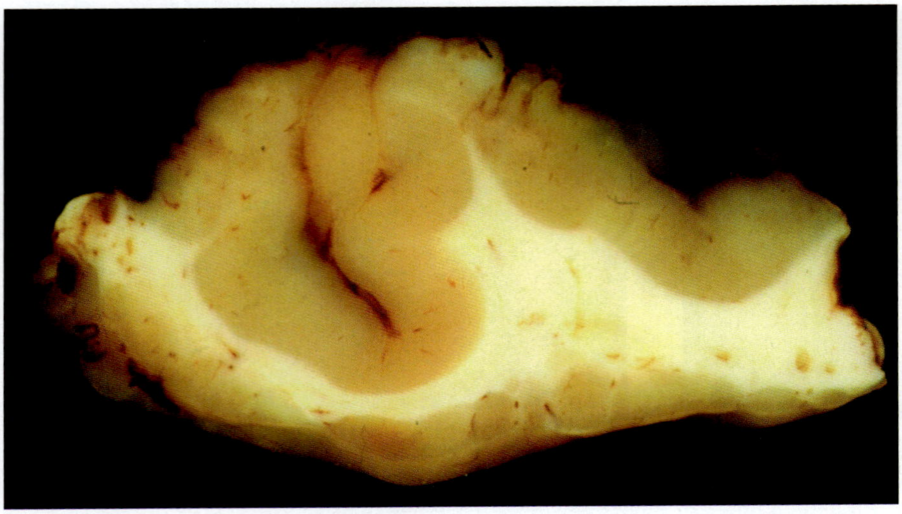

Figure 1-95. Nodular heterotopic gray matter. Cut surface of this surgical specimen shows multiple gray matter nodules present adjacent to the ventricular surface (bottom of the specimen).

and numbers in the white matter should also bring to mind the demyelinating processes. Their appearance changes according to the stage of development they are in. Acute plaques are soft and have a *gelatinous appearance* **(Fig. 1-97)**. It may be difficult to differentiate them from early infarcts based on gross features alone. In general, they tend to be located in a *periventricular location* in the deep white matter and have irregular geographic borders. However, white matter location is not the absolute rule, and involvement of gray matter is also seen. In other words, lesions in gray matter may not necessarily represent another pathologic process. Larger lesions may have a configuration as though they are closely associated with the ventricle walls. As the lesion becomes chronic, in concordance with decreasing inflammation and increasing astrocytosis, it starts to acquire a *tan-gray color and a firm consistency*. MS lesions are typically multiple and *polyphasic*, that is, lesions of different stages of development can be seen at the time of examination, and are randomly

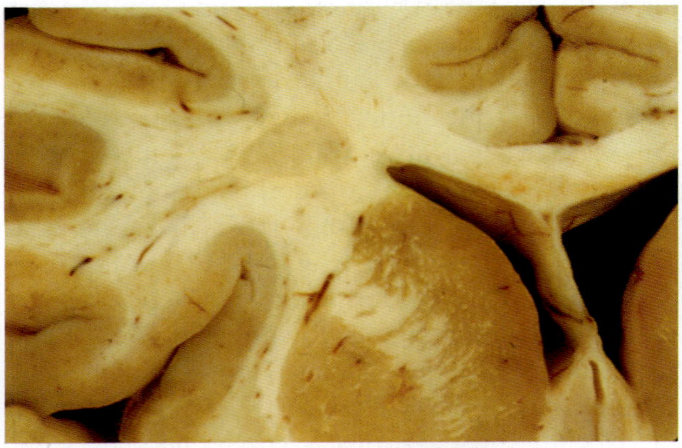

Figure 1-96. Chronic MS plaque. A tan, well-circumscribed lesion is seen in the left frontal lobe white matter. The color is due to gliosis, which is also responsible to the firm consistency of these lesions, in contrast to acute lesions.

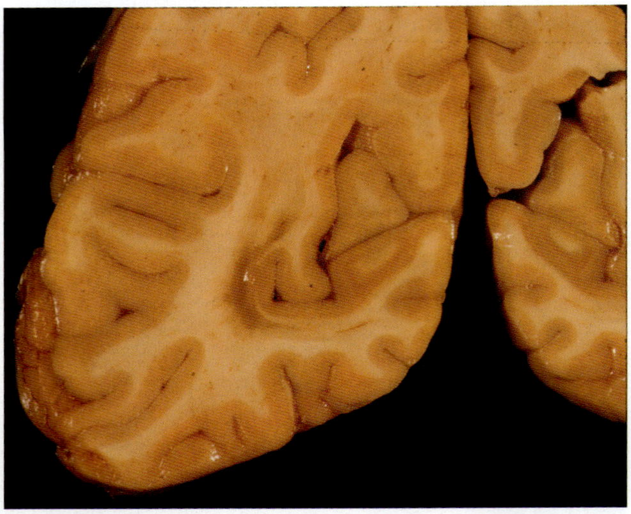

Figure 1-97. Acute MS plaque. A gelatinous depressed lesion is present in the white matter of the left occipital lobe. This appearance is due to high cellularity contributed by the inflammatory cells, edema and myelin loss in the absence of gliosis. There are other plaques in other areas of the white matter. Judging by their more solid and tan quality, they appear more advanced in their evolution, resulting in this polyphasia of the lesions, supportive of MS.

distributed without being limited to a particular anatomical–functional subsystem. Optic radiations have a somewhat tan color that makes them stand out in white matter as ill-defined areas. They are seen in the periventricular white matter next to the temporal and occipital horns of the lateral ventricles and can sometimes look like a demyelinating or discolored white matter pathology. Lesions with similar features that *involve corpus callosum, usually centrally*, are typical of Marchiafava-Bignami disease, which is associated with chronic alcoholism, with or without malnutrition. Although corpus callosum involvement is the hallmark, especially the genu and the body, there may be similar lesions in optic chiasm, anterior and posterior commissures, and middle cerebellar peduncles, as well as necrosis of striatum in some cases and white matter involvement.[222] The lesions, especially those in the corpus callosum, are surrounded by at least a thin rim of uninvolved tissue.

Corpus callosum agenesis (see also "External Surfaces" above and "Ventricular System" below) should be looked for and differentiated from artifactual tear, especially in pediatric cases. Corpus callosum agenesis can be seen on cut surfaces **(Fig. 1-98)** and also results in a typical *"bat-wing" appearance of the lateral ventricles*. Corpus callosum may become thin in a variety of conditions resulting in tissue loss. Corpus callosum, along with white matter tracts in centrum semiovale, cerebral peduncles, and brainstem, is also a common place to be involved by DAI,[223] where petechial hemorrhages are present **(Table 1.14)**. The presence of such petechial hemorrhages in a variable pattern can also be seen in AHL (see "Parenchymal Hemorrhage" below). Chronic changes of DAI in survivors consist of variable degrees of discolored and atrophic white matter, thin corpus callosum, dilated lateral and third ventricles, and atrophic brainstem, cerebral peduncles, and pyramids. Cerebral autosomal dominant arteriopathy with subcortical infarcts and leukoencephalopathy (CADASIL) and its recessive form cerebral autosomal recessive arteriopathy with subcortical infarcts and leukoencephalopathy (CARASIL)[224] involve the white matter *diffusely*, with the involvement of bilateral anterior temporal lobes, and external capsule being common and prominent. White matter becomes *discolored* dusky-tan, *collapsed and friable* in advanced cases **(Fig. 1-99)**. SSPE,[225] especially in later stages of the disease, can produce prominent white matter demyelination and destruction, resulting in a collapsed appearance with compensatory ventricular dilatation. Extensive and diffuse myelin loss with collapsed and friable appearance of white matter is typical for leukodystrophies.[226] White matter has lost its bright white color and has a dusky-tan appearance. *Sparing of U-fibers* is characteristic **(Fig. 1-100)**, but they are involved in Canavan's disease. In addition, in orthochromatic leukodystrophy, white matter can have a greenish hue. The involvement, while generally diffuse, may show some variation in some of the leukodystrophies. More *severe involvement of the occipital lobes* is typical for adrenoleukodystrophy, although somewhat similar pattern may also be seen in Krabbe's disease **(Fig. 1-101)**. In contrast, metachromatic leukodystrophy and Alexander's disease tend to involve *predominantly frontal lobes*. White matter pathology may be extremely pronounced, resulting in essentially complete loss of white matter with residual *cavitation* in vanishing white matter disease.[227] It is important to save fresh tissue from such cases, especially if premortem diagnosis has not been established, so that genetic and biochemical analyses can be performed for accurate identification of the process. Some cases of vanishing white matter disease have been associated

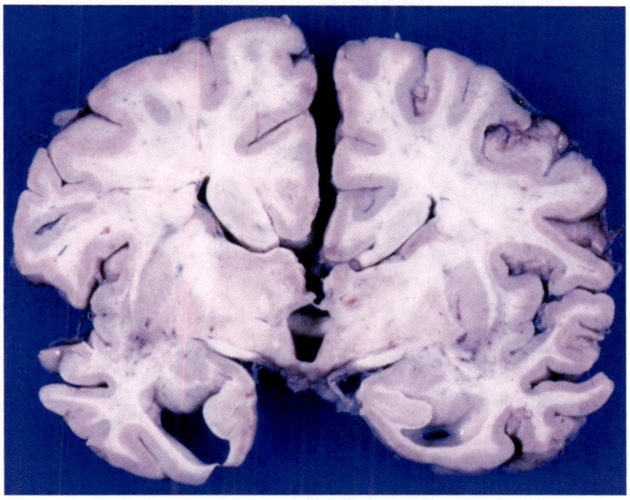

Figure 1-98. Agenesis of corpus callosum. Corpus callosum is not present as an incidental finding in this adult patient. The lateral ventricles have assumed a bat-wing appearance. Misdirected myelinated fibers running longitudinally on both sides underneath the cingulate gyri form the Probst bundles.

TABLE 1.14 Differential diagnosis of diffuse white matter involvement

Disorder/Agent	Predominant Location	Other Findings
DAI	Long tracts, corpus callosum, cerebral peduncles	Petechiae, other findings of trauma; discoloration and atrophy in chronic cases
AHL	Localized or diffuse	Petechiae
CADASIL	Anterior temporal lobes, external capsule common	Discoloration, collapse, cavitation
SSPE	Periventricular	Demyelination, destruction, especially late stages
Congenital rubella and toxoplasma infections	Periventricular	Destructive lesions, calcifications
Leukodystrophies (general)	Diffuse, U-fibers spared	Myelin loss, discoloration, collapse, cavitation
ALD	Occipital lobes more severe	—
Krabbe's disease (globoid cell leukodystrophy)	Occipital lobes more severe, though not as prominent as ALD	—
Canavan's disease (spongiform leukodystrophy)	U-fibers are not spared	—
Alexander's disease	Frontal lobes more severe	—
Vanishing white matter disease	Diffuse	Cavitation
Toxic-metabolic/medications		
Fucosidosis	Diffuse	White matter is firm, bright white
Nimorazole	Cerebral, cerebellar	White matter necrosis, brainstem, dentate nucleus involvement
Sulfonamides	Gray and white matter	Necrosis, with or without hemorrhage
Methotrexate	Variable, preferentially periventricular with intrathecal administration	MNL, hemorrhagic infarcts possible
Amphotericin B, BCNU, cisplatin, cytosine arabinoside, CHOP, radiation, AIDS	Variable	MNL
Fludarabine	More severe in occipital lobes, pyramids, and spinal cord posterior columns	MNL, may be perivascular, may involve cortex
Intoxication (CO, methanol)	Diffuse	U-fibers spared in CO poisoning
Mitochondrial disorders	Diffuse	
Leigh's disease (subacute necrotizing encephalomyelopathy)	Periventricular	Shrunken and discolored, older lesions may be cavitary, many other areas involved
Binswanger disease/small vessel disease	Usually deep white matter	Microinfarcts
Systemic embolic, thrombotic events	Diffuse or patchy	Many microinfarcts or multiple large infarcts
Perinatal telencephalic leukoencephalopathy/PVL	Focal or diffuse, preferentially periventricular	Collapse, discoloration, calcification, cyst formation
Hydrocephaly	Immediate periventricular	Softening
Giant axonal neuropathy	Deep white matter, brain, cerebellum, spinal cord	Softening, discoloration
Neuroaxonal dystrophies	Deep white matter, U-fibers spared	Softening, discoloration
Whipple's disease	Patchy, gray and white matter	Yellow-gray discoloration
Nasu-Hakola disease	White matter degeneration, U-fibers spared	Rusty brown discoloration of basal ganglia, thalamus involvement
HIV encephalitis	Diffuse	Softening, discoloration

DAI, diffuse axonal injury; AHL, acute hemorrhagic leukoencephalopathy; CADASIL, cerebral autosomal arteriopathy with subcortical infarcts and leukoencephalopathy; SSPE, subacute sclerosing panencephalitis; ALD, adrenoleukodystrophy; MNL, multifocal necrotizing leukoencephalopathy; BCNU, 1,3-bis-(2-chloroethyl)-1-nitrosourea; CHOP, cyclophosphamide, hydroxydaunorubicin, oncovin, prednisolone; AIDS, acquired immunodeficiency syndrome; CO, carbon monoxide; PVL, periventricular leukomalacia; HIV, human immunodeficiency virus.

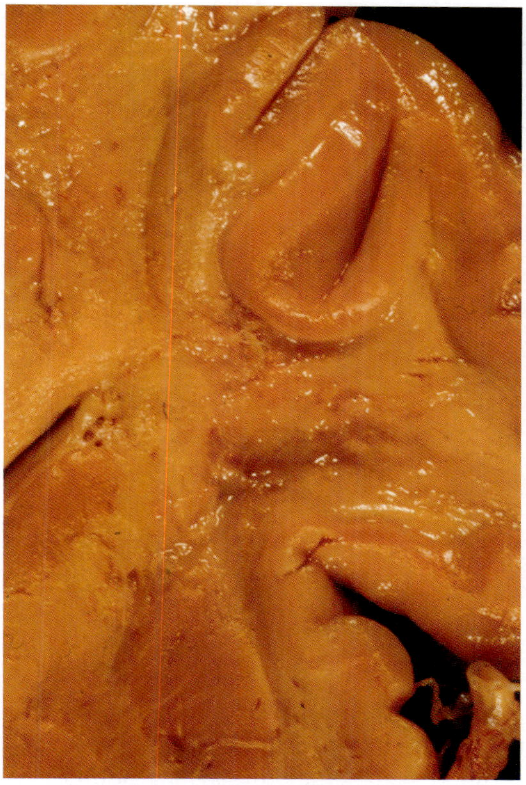

Figure 1-99. CADASIL. The white matter has a collapsed, friable, and discolored appearance in this advanced case.

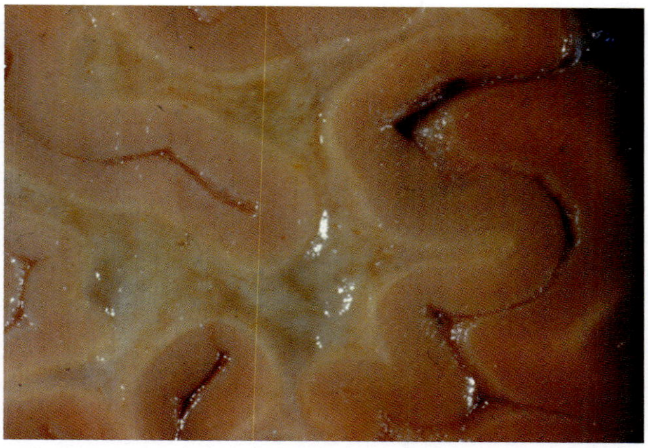

Figure 1-100. Adrenoleukodystrophy. Due to extensive myelin loss, the white matter is discolored and has a collapsed appearance. The subcortical U-fibers are preserved and can be seen as *white lines* underneath the cortical gray matter.

with ovarian failure and termed ovarioleukodystrophy, while adrenoleukodystrophy also has adrenal cortical and Leydig cell involvement. Many storage diseases, for example, gangliosidoses and mucopolysaccharidoses, result in cerebral atrophy due to neuron loss. Fucosidosis also results in firm and bright white matter. Mitochondrial diseases,[228] such as MELAS (mitochondrial myopathy lactic acidosis and stroke-like episodes), result in foci of necrosis and cavitation of different stages in cortex, involving more the crests of gyri. Occipital lobes are involved more severely. Basal ganglia, thalamus, and cerebellum involvement is less often. Another mitochondrial disorder, MERRF (myoclonal epilepsy with ragged red fibers) tends to involve dentate nuclei and olivary nuclei, resulting in their brown discoloration and shrinkage. The brain may be otherwise grossly normal. A variety of toxic causes may result in multifocal or diffuse damage that typically predominantly involves the white matter. Nimorazole causes cerebral and cerebellar white matter necrosis and Leigh's disease–like lesions in brainstem and dentate nuclei. Sulfonamides cause gray and white matter necrosis with or without hemorrhage. Methotrexate causes cerebral and spinal white matter necrosis described as multifocal necrotizing leukoencephalopathy that can occur with or without radiation treatment.[229,230] It can be preferentially periventricular if methotrexate is administered intrathecally. There may be hemorrhagic infarcts due to vascular damage. Multifocal necrotizing leukoencephalopathy is a descriptive term for this type of lesion that can also be seen as a result of amphotericin B, BCNU [1,3-bis-(2-chloroethyl)-1-nitrosourea], cisplatin, cytosine arabinoside, CHOP (cyclophosphamide, hydroxydaunorubicin, oncovin, prednisolone), radiation treatment, and AIDS.[214,231–234] Similar lesions, although in a relatively more diffuse pattern, can be seen in carbon monoxide, cyanide and methanol poisoning, global hypoxia, and mitochondrial disorders. Fludarabine[235] also may cause necrotizing leukoencephalopathy predominantly in occipital lobes, additionally involving pyramids and posterior columns of spinal cord. In addition to multifocal necrotizing leukoencephalopathy seen in AIDS, HIV encephalitis diffusely involves the white matter and results in a dusky discoloration **(Fig. 1-102)**. White matter lesions may be perivascular or more confluent and may involve overlying cortex. Cocaine, in addition to parenchymal hemorrhages, can result in infarcts

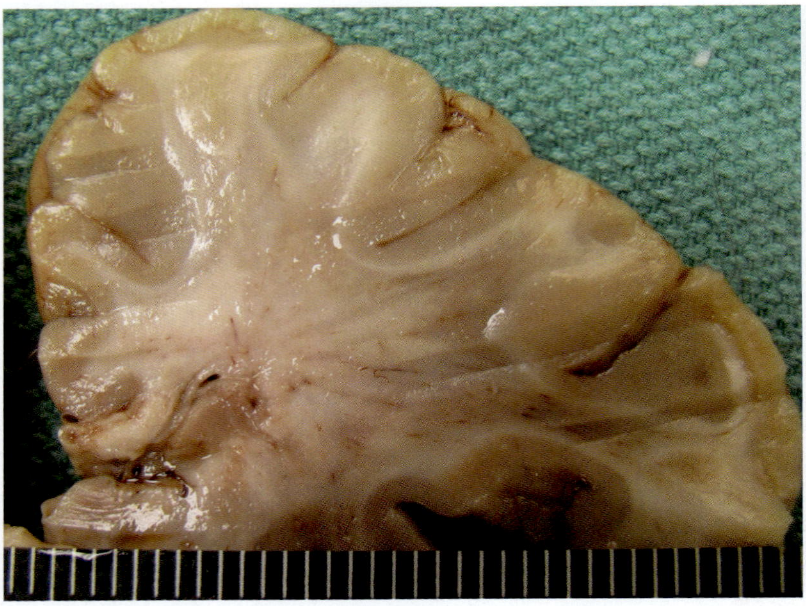

Figure 1-101. Krabbe's disease (globoid cell leukodystrophy). Common to the great majority of leukodystrophies, the white matter is diffusely involved and shows tan discoloration with preservation of the U-fibers.

due to thromboemboli that arise from the heart affected by the cardiomyopathy it may cause.[236] A similar etiology can cause infarcts in a neurodegenerative disease, Friedreich's ataxia, if there is associated cardiomyopathy.[237] While acute ethanol intoxication is associated with congestion, edema, and petechial hemorrhages, chronic alcoholism results in white matter volume loss and anterior superior vermis degeneration.[238] The crests of the folia tend to be more affected than their depths in contrast to hypoxic–ischemic damage, where the depths of the folia tend to be affected more. Vascular dementia cases may present with variable findings depending on the type of vascular pathology. Small vessel disease[239,240] is typically associated with white matter ischemia with collapsed and pitted appearance, ventricular dilatation, lacunar infarcts mostly in basal ganglia, pons, and thalamus. Since subcortical white matter is usually preserved, widespread sampling especially of deep white matter is needed to identify vascular changes. This condition is also termed Binswanger's disease (subcortical arteriosclerotic leukoencephalopathy). Virchow-Robin spaces are dilated (etat crible and etat lacunaire) and the cortical surface is granular and pitted due to multiple cortical microinfarcts (which may also be seen in other conditions associated with multiple emboli, thromboses, etc.). Large vessel disease is associated with frank infarcts of variable size, which may be in critical locations such as pons and basal ganglia, also involving the internal capsule. Global hypoperfusion results in hippocampal sclerosis and watershed infarcts, likely due to hypotensive episodes associated with atherosclerosis. Diffuse white matter involvement with softening and discoloration but with sparing of U-fibers, resulting in a generalized brain atrophy and ventricular dilatation, is also seen in neuroaxonal dystrophies.[241] Giant axonal neuropathy[242] shows deep white matter degeneration in brain, cerebellum, and spinal long tracts. In hydrocephalus, increased pressure within the ventricular system that is caused by the accumulation of CSF results in ventricular dilatation. The resultant pressure on the brain tissue

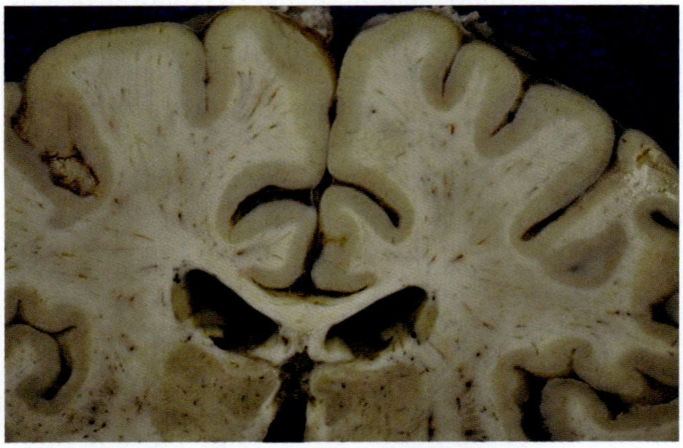

Figure 1-102. HIV encephalitis. There is a subtle diffuse dusky appearance to the white matter due to extensive myelin loss.

can result in subsequent degeneration and softening of the white matter due to fluid escaping into the tissues. Whipple's disease can involve the gray and white matter and may cause yellow-gray discolored foci in the parenchyma.[243] In *destructive lesions involving the white matter*, for example, periventricular leukomalacia, loss of white matter thickness, thinning of cortex, and dilatation of ventricles are residual lesions after the actual destruction is healed **(Fig. 1-103)**. Scattered white specks of calcification may be seen **(Fig. 1-104)**. The distance between the lateral ventricle and overlying cortex is diminished due to white matter loss. In active lesions, periventricular white matter is soft, discolored, and friable. In early hypoxic–ischemic conditions in childhood, white matter becomes dusky, making the relatively pale cortex to stand out as a distinct linear structure. This type of widespread hypoxic/ischemic injury results in the destruction of white matter and the depths of the gyri, while the crests of the gyri remain as mushroom-like broad structures. This appearance is called ulegyria **(Fig. 1-105)**.

On cut surfaces of the brain and especially in the basal ganglia, *cavitary areas of a few millimeters* can be found. These represent aging and/or hypertensive changes and are usually due to *dilated Virchow-Robin spaces* around thickened and tortuous blood vessels. The vessel can usually be seen within the cavity on close inspection **(Fig. 1-106)**. These cavities are different than cystic infarcts of less than 1.0 to 1.5 cm in maximum dimension called *lacunae*. The appearance that results from multiple perivascular cavities is called *etat lacunaire* **(Fig. 1-107)** in gray matter and *etat crible* in white matter **(Fig. 1-108)**. Sometimes, *etat*

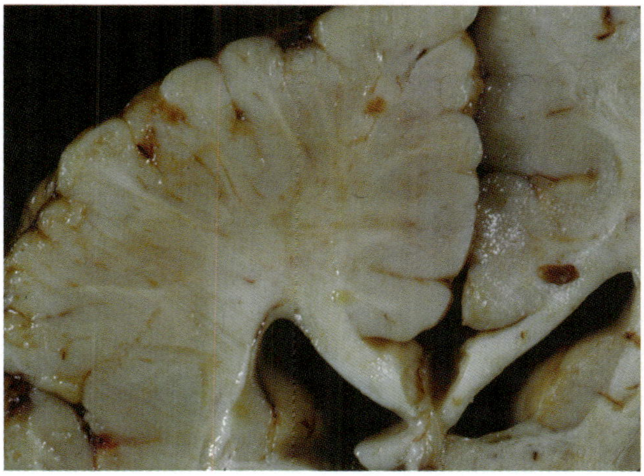

Figure 1-103. Prominent white matter loss due to previous destructive event, most likely periventricular leukomalacia. The distance between the cortex and ventricles is reduced, and the ventricles show compensatory dilatation.

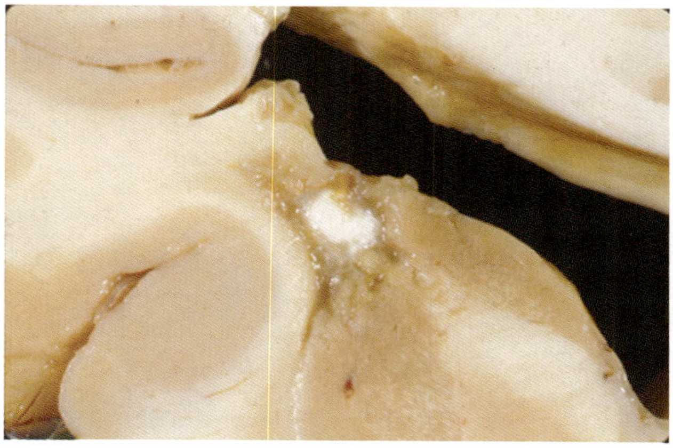

Figure 1-104. Periventricular leukomalacia with calcification. The periventricular destructive lesion is cavitary with a white calcified area. The white matter is diminished in amount.

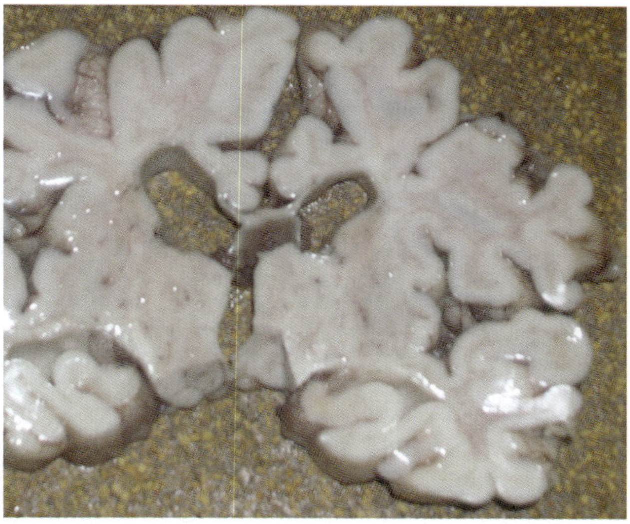

Figure 1-105. Ulegyria. The gyri have bases disproportionately narrower than their superficial portions, creating a somewhat mushroom-like appearance. There is also extensive white matter loss with thinning of corpus callosum and dilatation of ventricles. The cause is most likely a severe previous hypoxic/ischemic destruction involving the periventricular white matter and the depths of the gyri.

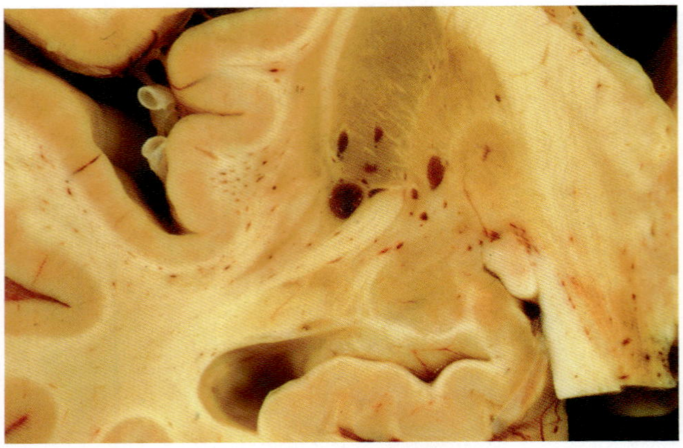

Figure 1-106. Dilated Virchow-Robin spaces. Multiple cavitary areas are seen in the basal ganglia. Blood vessels are present in them and can be seen within the largest one. These cavitary lesions represent dilated Virchow-Robin spaces around the distorted blood vessels affected by hypertensive and atherosclerotic changes.

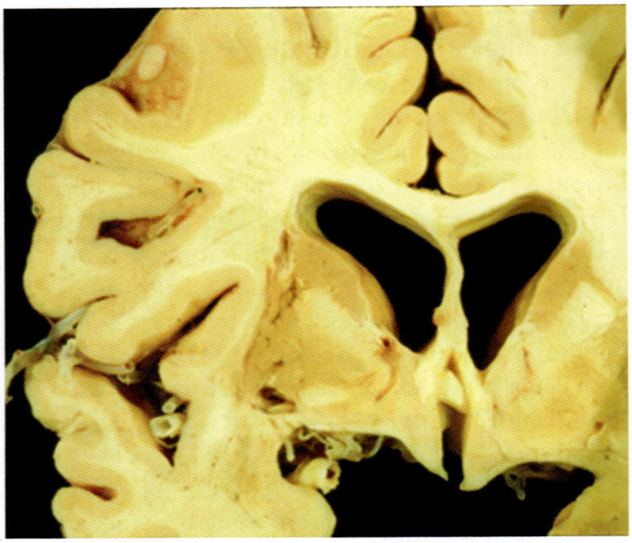

Figure 1-107. Etat lacunaire. Multiple irregular cavitary lesions, measuring less than 1.0 to 1.5 cm, are present in the left putamen. They are small cystic infarcts creating a lacunar appearance.

cavitaire is applied to a cavitary state that is simply the result of mixture of multiple cavities consisting of infarcts and dilated Virchow-Robin spaces. Telangiectasia is typically an incidental finding and can look as an obvious vascular lesion or may appear as an *ill-defined dusky area*, usually about 1.0 to 2.0 cm in maximum dimension, in the white matter, commonly in temporal lobe or brainstem **(Fig. 1-109)**. Dentate nucleus of the cerebellum normally has prominent vessels in the white matter in its hilum that may look like a telangiectasia, even microscopically. Of the other *vascular malformations*, venous malformation (venous angioma) is also usually an incidental finding at autopsy, as it rarely causes bleeding. It is seen as a focal aggregate of what appears to be congested vessels in the white matter. It can be associated with other vascular malformations. Cavernous angioma (cavernoma) appears as a round, well-circumscribed, firm vascular lesion with hemorrhagic cut surface.

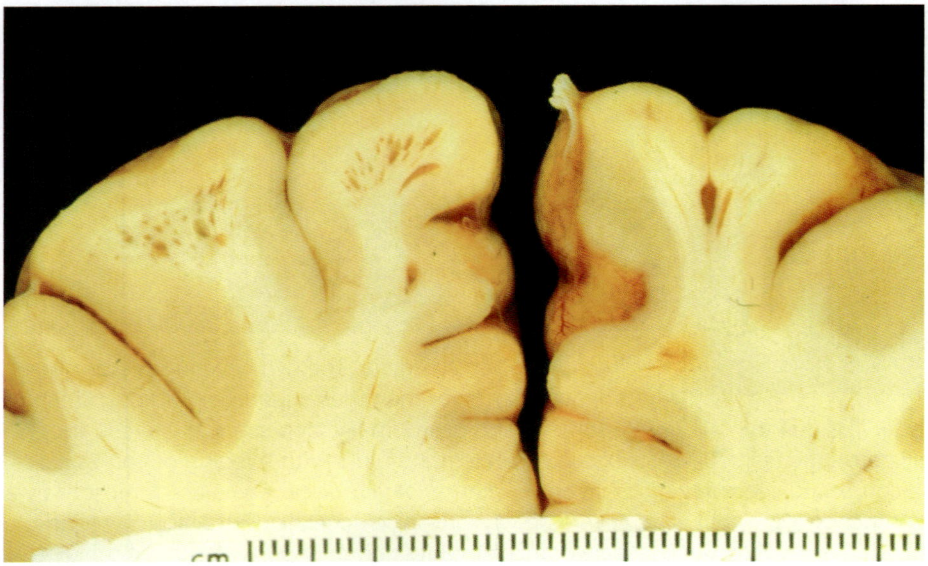

Figure 1-108. Etat crible. Multiple pinpoint vacuoles are seen in the superficial white matter of the left hemisphere, representing dilated Virchow-Robin spaces associated with the small vessel disease.

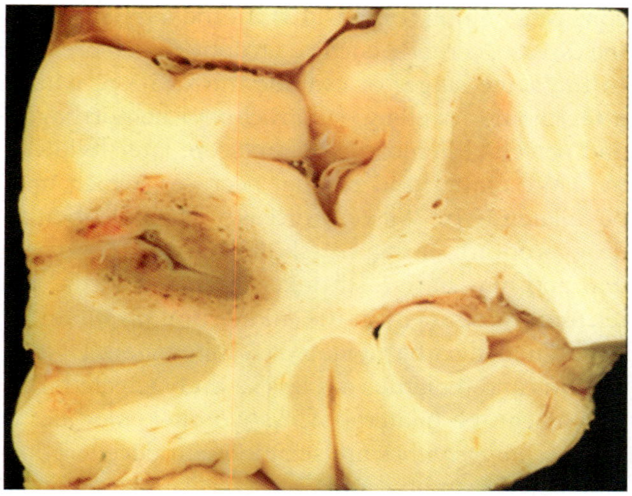

Figure 1-109. Telangiectasia. An incidental localized *tan-brown* area is seen in the temporal lobe, involving the superficial white matter and cortical gray matter. Larger ectatic vessels can be seen grossly.

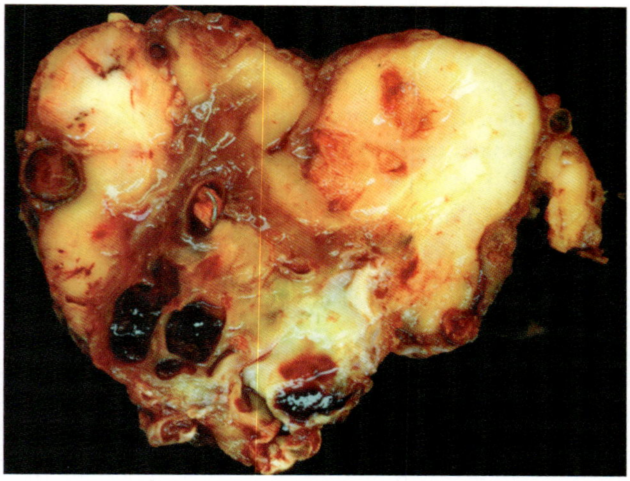

Figure 1-111. Arteriovenous malformation. Vascular channels are irregularly distributed in the brain parenchyma. The intervening parenchyma and the overlying cortical gray matter are discolored due to previous hemorrhages, as well as shrunken due to hypoxic/ischemic changes as a result of shunting of blood directly from arterial to venous system.

It is similar to AVM grossly; however, AVM is more irregular, has admixed brain tissue among its vessels on close inspection, and usually involves a leptomeningeal surface, or may even predominantly be superficial **(Fig. 1-110)**. Both cavernous angiomas and AVMs show evidence of previous old hemorrhages in the form of yellow-tan, dusky areas representing hemosiderin pigment at their periphery or admixed within the lesion **(Fig. 1-111)**. They are firm and may be gritty while cutting due to extensive fibrosis in the vessels and calcifications. Close inspection reveals the vascular nature of these lesions. Angioinvasive fungal microorganisms result in hemorrhagic necrotic, one or more lesions of variable sizes (see "Parenchymal Hemorrhage"). In chronic stages, some of these

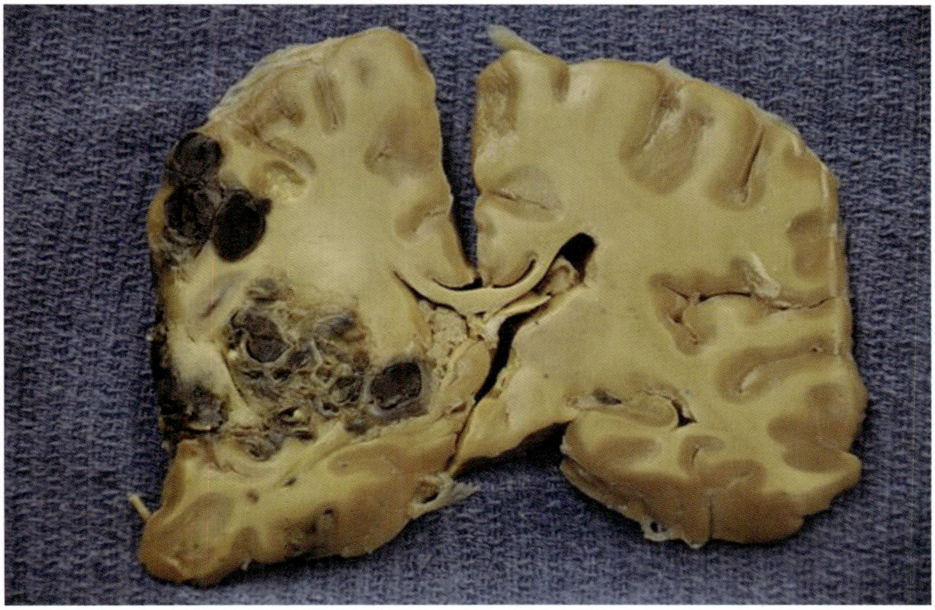

Figure 1-110. AVM. Many vascular channels of variable sizes are present in the left hemisphere. The malformation has irregular borders with brain parenchyma admixed with the vessels. It also involves the leptomeningeal surface.

may be walled-off to form cystic lesions with fibrotic walls. Chromoblastomycosis lesions are also necrotic but, in addition, have brown discoloration due to pigmented fungi and may appear like hemorrhage. Frontal lobe parenchyma is preferred, but they may extend to meninges and ventricles. In addition to the necrotic lesions, coccidioidomycosis can cause endarteritis, resulting in infarcts and leukomalacia.

Basal ganglia are involved in a variety of disorders with different ethiopathogenesis **(Table 1.15)**. Multiple, usually a few millimeters well-circumscribed collections of *mucinous, gelatinous material* likely represent Cryptococcus meningitis infiltrating the brain parenchyma following Virchow-Robin spaces. They may be abundant and may eventually form a *spongy appearance* in the parenchyma, preferentially involving the basal ganglia, or they may form abscesses **(Fig. 1-112)**. *Bilateral necrosis of the striatum* is seen in the condition descriptively termed bilateral striatal necrosis, which results in cavitary lesions bilaterally in the putamen and caudate nuclei. Internal capsule is also involved. There is a history of preceding febrile illness.[244] Holotopistic striatal necrosis (familial striatal degeneration)[245] can cause similar lesions, or may result in *atrophy* due to neuron loss and gliosis. It may be associated with cerebellar and cortical degeneration. Other unusual disorders that involve the striatum bilaterally to cause cavitary lesions are Leber's hereditary optic neuropathy, bilateral striatal necrosis, and MS-like mitochondrial disease. Neuroacanthocytosis results in striatal and cerebral cortical atrophy due to neuron loss and gliosis.[246] Cavitation of putamen may be associated with mitochondrial DNA depletion syndrome, with lesions similar to Leigh's disease.[247] Carbon monoxide poisoning,[248] in its acute stage, results in brain swelling, congestion, and cherry-red color (seen especially in fresh state). After 1 to 2 days, widespread white matter petechiae and larger hemorrhages are present in the globus pallidus, usually but not necessarily bilaterally and symmetrically. After several days, the pallidal lesions gradually become cavitary, and white matter foci of necrosis may be present, sparing the U-fibers. Huntington disease, depending on the severity, can result in extensive atrophy of the striatum and loss of the natural convexity of the caudate nucleus into the ventricular lumen. Instead, it becomes flat and may even assume a concave contour **(Fig. 1-113)**. In the later stages of the disease, cerebral cortical atrophy is also present. In the acute stages of cyanide intoxication, within a few hours, swelling, subarachnoid hemorrhages, and petechial hemorrhages are seen, later followed by white matter and pallidal necroses, which may be bilateral. In Wilson's disease (hepatolenticular degeneration), striatum shows *brown discoloration* and may have a shrunken appearance, the latter more prominent in the midportion of putamen, which may also be cavitated in this region. Globus pallidus and thalamus are less severely affected. The lesions can be bilateral. A *rusty brown color and a shrunken appearance* are seen in neurodegeneration with brain iron accumulation type 1 (a.k.a., pantothenate kinase–associated neurodegeneration formerly known as Hallervorden-Spatz disease),[249] in which substantia nigra is also involved in addition to basal ganglia. They are also present in the pars reticularis of substantia nigra. Severe basal ganglionic and internal capsule destruction may result in the degeneration and atrophy of cerebral peduncles. Nasu-Hakola disease (polycystic lipomembranous osteodysplasia with sclerosing leukoencephalopathy)[250] is a disease that is associated with adipocyte membrane abnormalities and cerebral white matter degeneration. U-fibers are spared. Basal ganglia have rusty brown discoloration. Thalamus may be involved. *Yellow discoloration* of particular areas is seen in kernicterus. Especially in hippocampus, subiculum, subthalamic nucleus, globus pallidus, lateral geniculate nucleus, substantia nigra, dentate nucleus, and various brainstem nuclei are variably affected. While the discoloration is quite obvious, the pigment may be microscopically very subtle. Leigh's disease (subacute necrotizing encephalomyelopathy)[228] has *symmetrical tan-brown discolorations* involving striatum, subthalamic nucleus, substantia nigra, inferior olives, and brainstem tegmentum. Cerebellar degeneration is commonly present. Older lesions may be cavitary. Different stages of lesions can be seen simultaneously. Periventricular white matter, optic nerves, spinal cord, and cerebellar white matter may have myelin loss and therefore can appear atrophic and discolored. Rubella infection, along with microcephaly, calcifications, and hydrocephalus, results in cystic destructive lesions in the parenchyma, especially in periventricular regions, basal ganglia, and thalamus. Similar lesions can be seen in congenital toxoplasma infection, which can also involve subpial

TABLE 1.15 Differential diagnosis of basal ganglia lesions

Disorder/Agent	Predominant Feature in Basal Ganglia	Other Features
Bilateral striatal necrosis	Cavitary lesions in putamen and caudate	Internal capsule involvement
Holotopistic striatal necrosis (familial striatal necrosis)	Cavitary lesions or atrophy in putamen and caudate	Degeneration of cerebral cortex and cerebellum
Marchiafava-Bignami disease	Necrosis and cavitary lesions in putamen and caudate in some cases	Demyelinating lesions in corpus callosum, anterior and posterior commissures, middle cerebellar peduncles, optic chiasm
Leber's hereditary optic neuropathy	Cavitary lesions in putamen and caudate	Optic atrophy, mitochondrial disease with cavitation
Mitochondrial DNA depletion syndrome	Cavitary lesions in putamen	Leigh's disease–like cavitary lesions
Leigh's disease (subacute necrotizing encephalomyelopathy)	Tan-brown discoloration and cavitary lesions of caudate and putamen	Involvement of many other areas, including white matter and spinal cord
CO intoxication	Globus pallidus cavitary lesions, bilateral (after several days in survivors)	Brain swelling, petechiae, cherry-red color, white matter necrosis, U-fibers spared
Cyanide intoxication	Globus pallidus necrosis, bilateral	Brain swelling, petechiae, white matter necrosis
Methanol intoxication	Putamen necrosis, cavitary lesions, bilateral	White matter, internal capsule, claustrum
Cryptococcosis	Multicystic appearance	Widespread cysts and abscesses, meningitis
Wilson's disease (hepatolenticular degeneration)	Atrophy and brown discoloration of caudate and putamen	May be more prominent and cavitary in the midportion of putamen; globus pallidus, and thalamus involvement mild
Neurodegeneration with brain iron accumulation type 1*	Rusty brown and atrophic basal ganglia	Substantia nigra, internal capsule involvement
Nasu-Hakola disease	Rusty brown discoloration of basal ganglia	Thalamus, white matter involvement
Kernicterus	Yellow discoloration of globus pallidus	Hippocampus, subthalamic nuclei, substantia nigra, dentate nucleus, lateral geniculate nucleus involvement
Vascular disorders affecting the basal vessels, great vein of Galen	Infarcts, hemorrhages, hemorrhagic infarcts	Other areas may be involved
Huntington disease	Atrophy of caudate and putamen	Cerebral cortical atrophy in later stages
Other neurodegenerative diseases Neuroaxonal dystrophies DRPL atrophy Multiple system atrophy ALS	Predominantly globus pallidus involvement	Other structures involved depending on the disease
Pallidal degenerations	Predominantly globus pallidus atrophy	Various other structures depending on the disease
Juvenile and acute pallidal degenerations	Globus pallidus atrophy	Pallidoluysian tract, subthalamic nucleus
Pallidoluysian degeneration	Globus pallidus atrophy	Subthalamic nucleus, substantia nigra, and ventrolateral thalamic nuclei
Pallidonigrospinal degeneration	Globus pallidus atrophy	Substantia nigra, subthalamic nucleus, pontine tegmentum, anterior horns of spinal cord

DNA, deoxyribonucleic acid; CO, carbon monoxide; DRPL, dentatorubropallidoluysian; ALS, amyotrophic lateral sclerosis.
*a.k.a., pantothenate kinase associated neurodegeneration; formerly known as Hallervorden-Spatz.

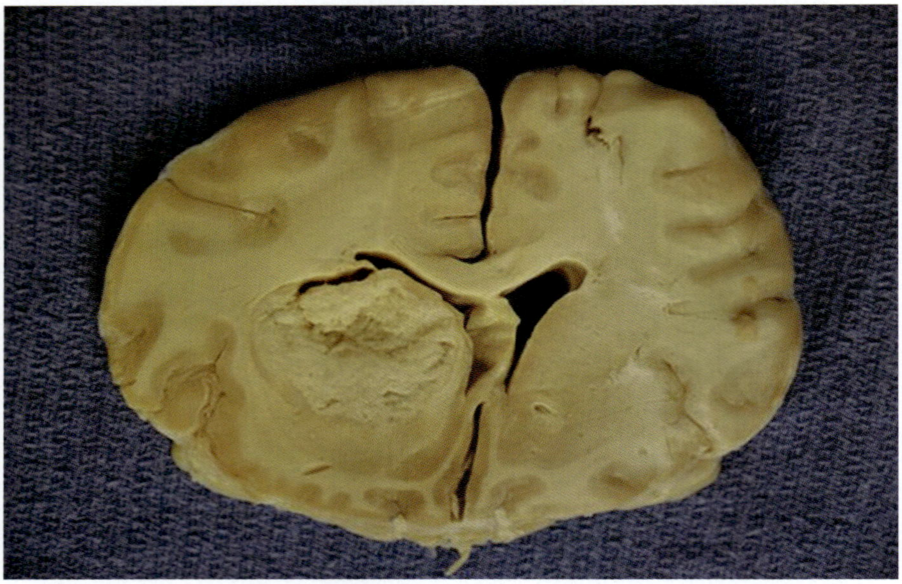

Figure 1-112. Cryptococcal abscesses. The larger one in the left basal ganglia also creates a mass effect with midline shift to the right. It is filled with gray-white gelatinous/mucinous material, which appears solid after fixation. Similar material is also present in the leptomeninges and in the sulci on the basal aspect of the brain.

regions. Basal ganglia infarcts can be caused by the infectious and inflammatory conditions, or aneurysmal subarachnoid hemorrhages involving the basal meninges and creating vascular necrosis or spasm. Globus pallidus can be involved in many other conditions, such as neuroaxonal dystrophy, DRPLA **(Fig. 1-114)**, MSA, ALS, and neurodegeneration with brain iron accumulation type 1. Pallidal degenerations[251] can have, in addition to involvement of globus pallidus, various patterns of involvement depending on their clinical forms and are commonly termed descriptively based on this involvement. Juvenile and acute pallidal degenerations tend to involve pallidoluysian tract and subthalamic nucleus. Pallidoluysian degeneration additionally involves subthalamic nucleus, substantia nigra, and

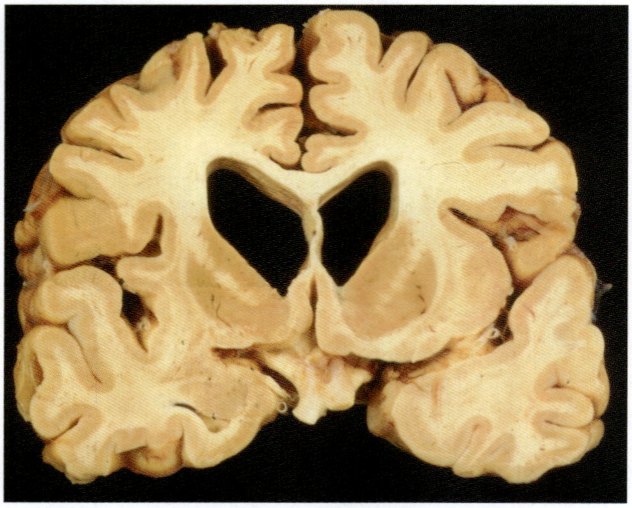

Figure 1-113. Huntington disease. The striatum on both sides shows prominent atrophy, resulting in the loss of the usual convexity of the caudate nuclei into the lateral ventricles. Instead, they have a flat surface. There is also cortical atrophy and compensatory hydrocephalus.

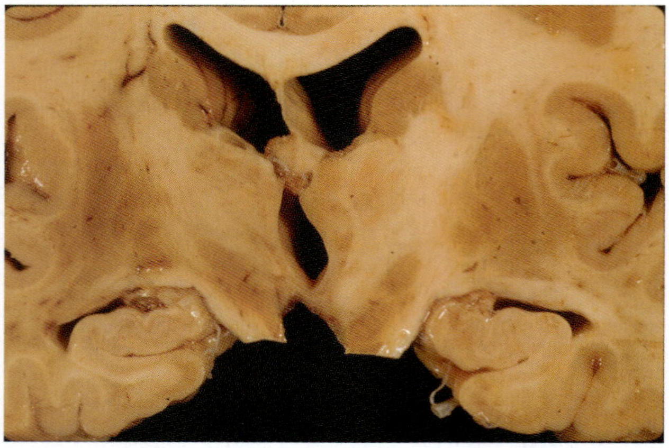

Figure 1-114. Dentatorubral-pallidoluysian atrophy. Although the section is asymmetrical, the globus pallidus seen better on the left side appears shrunken with a tan-orange discoloration. Substantia nigrae are pale. Subthalamic nuclei, seen on both sides immediately above the substantia nigrae as oval structures, also appear shrunken and discolored.

ventrolateral thalamic nuclei. Pallidonigrospinal degeneration additionally involves substantia nigra and anterior horns with variable involvement of subthalamic nucleus and pontine tegmentum.

Thalamus can be involved by a variety of processes, just like basal ganglia. Rarely, the involvement is isolated as a pure thalamic degeneration. However, many times, it is part of a more complex process. Thiamine deficiency, resulting in Wernicke's encephalopathy, typically involves mamillary bodies, hypothalamus, medial thalamic nuclei, periaqueductal region, and floor of fourth ventricle. While the most common scenario is in the context of chronic alcoholism, it is not limited to alcoholics and can be seen in other setting such as gastrointestinal disorders and total parenteral nutrition. In the acute stage, there is congestion and petechial hemorrhages. In chronic stage, gradual shrinkage, gliosis, and tan-brown discoloration are seen. Involvement of medial thalamic nuclei is also seen in cases of Korsakoff syndrome. X-linked hydrocephalus[252] can have several additional findings on cut surfaces, including polygyria (not microgyria), absence of pyramids, fusion of thalami, and corpus callosum agenesis. Some of the other conditions that may involve thalamus are multiple system atrophy, SCAs, Huntington disease, Nasu-Hakola disease, neuroaxonal dystrophy, fatal familial insomnia, and Creutzfeldt-Jakob disease (CJD). Thalamus and basal ganglia can have an irregular variegated gray and white appearance, creating a marble-like cut surface, called status marmoratus. It is due to aberrant myelination of these structures after a hypoxic/ischemic damage that occurs before the active myelination is completed.

Atrophy of the cerebellum, similar to that of the brain, is seen as thin folia and widened sulci instead of the usual compact appearance. It is seen in many neurodegenerative conditions that involve the cerebellum, as discussed in more detail in "External Surfaces" above **(Fig. 1-115)**. Various *malformations* involving the cerebellum can be associated with agenesis, hypoplasia, or structural abnormalities that can be identified on cut surfaces (see "External Surfaces" above). Some other disorders[253] that can include cerebellar degeneration among their constellation of grossly identifiable findings and that are not mentioned elsewhere are Menkes (kinky hair) disease, which can be associated with frequent subdural hematomas; ataxia-telangiectasia, which can have thalamic and spinal cord posterior column degeneration, telangiectasias of conjunctiva, and skin lesions in sun-exposed skin; carbohydrate-deficient glycoprotein syndrome type I, which is associated with small and flattened basis pontis; autosomal dominant cerebellar ataxia type II (ADCA II), which can show pontine atrophy; infantile neuroaxonal dystrophy; and idiopathic late-onset cerebellar ataxia, in which cerebellar atrophy is most prominent in the superior part of the cerebellum, especially in the vermis. *Thickened cerebellar folia* in a localized or diffuse manner is seen in dysplastic gangliocytoma of the cerebellum (Lhermitte-Duclos disease), due to the presence of many large ganglion cells instead of the small internal granule cells **(Fig. 1-116)**. An artifactual appearance creating a glassy white line throughout the cerebellar folia is called *etat glace* **(Fig. 1-117)** and is the result of autolysis of the internal granule cells.

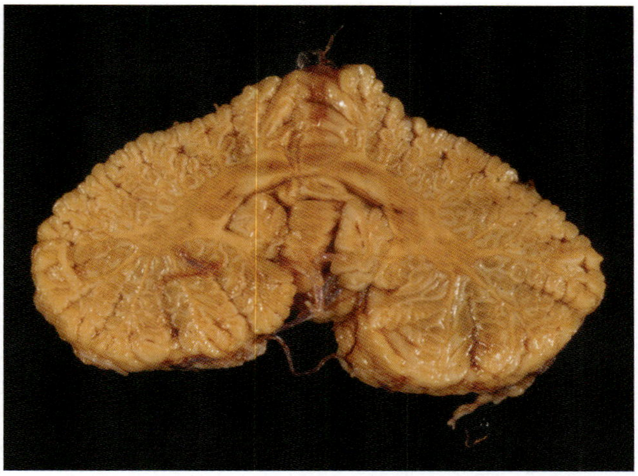

Figure 1-115. Cerebellar degeneration. The entire cerebellum appears small and shrunken. A tan discoloration of the residual white matter is also present. Both dentate nuclei are difficult to identify due to atrophy. (Compare with Figure 1.117.)

Osmotic demyelination syndrome (central pontine and extrapontine myelinolyses) is typically seen as a central tan, butterfly-shaped friable and *depressed lesion in basis pontis* **(Fig. 1-118)**. Even in dramatic lesions with near-complete involvement of pons, the epicenter of the lesion is *central*. In contrast, MS plaques involving brainstem tend to be multiple, randomly distributed and have

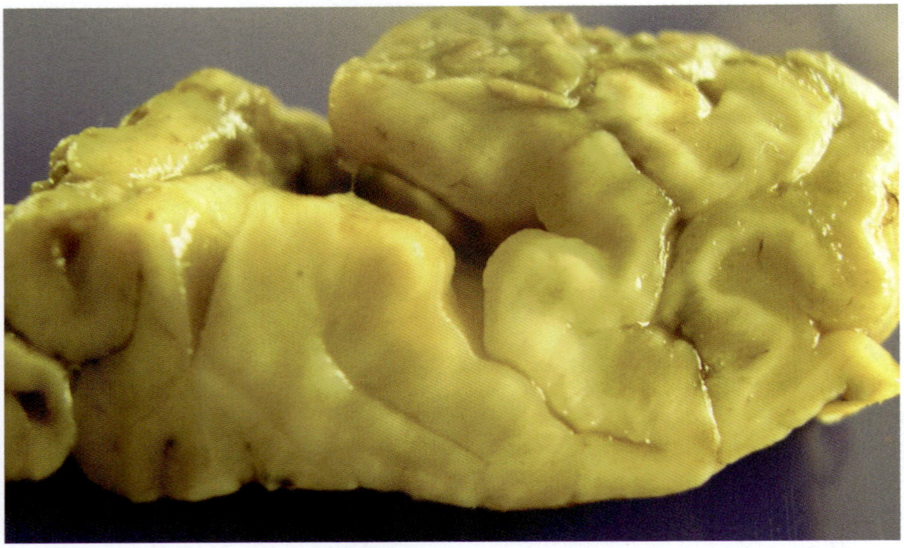

Figure 1-116. Dysplastic gangliocytoma of the cerebellum (Lhermitte-Duclos disease). The cerebellar folia resemble cerebral gyri due to thickening mainly as a result of the usual small neurons of the internal granule layer are replaced by larger ganglion cells.

a tendency toward *subpial* regions. Pigmented regions of the brainstem, substantia nigra, and locus ceruleus are pale due to neuron loss and may have tan discoloration due to gliosis in neurodegenerative diseases that involve these regions, the prototype of which is Parkinson's disease **(Fig. 1-119)**. The gross assessment of pigmentation does not always provide accurate information about the disease status of these structures. Neuromelanin pigment may remain for a long time in the neuropil until it is cleared, still creating a pigmented appearance even though there may be significant neuron loss **(Table 1.16)**. Since pigmentation is a result of dopaminergic metabolism, these structures have not yet been completely pigmented in the pediatric population and until about 20 years of age and are normally nonpigmented or pale.[254] PSP (Steele-Richardson-Olszewski syndrome) is also associated with pigment loss in substantia nigra and locus ceruleus. In addition, dentate nuclei **(Fig. 1-120)**, midbrain, pontine tegmentum, and globus pallidus may be atrophic. PSP may be associated with brainstem and/or basal ganglionic infarcts. Such cases are termed combined PSP. Postencephalitis parkinsonism can be seen in survivors of encephalitis

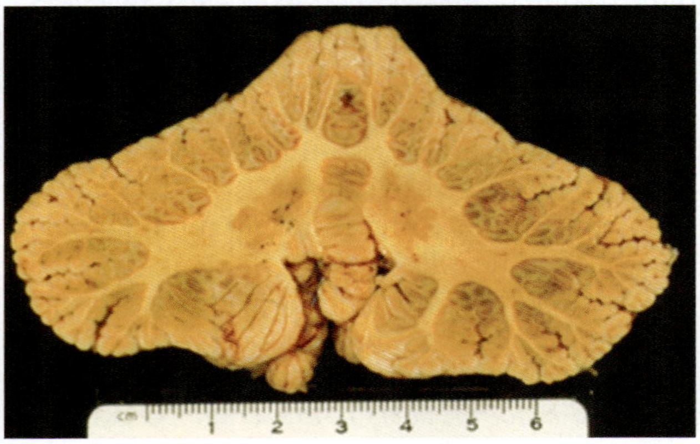

Figure 1-117. Etat glace. Autolysis of internal granule layer neurons results in this artifact characterized by cloudy white discoloration of the cerebellar folia.

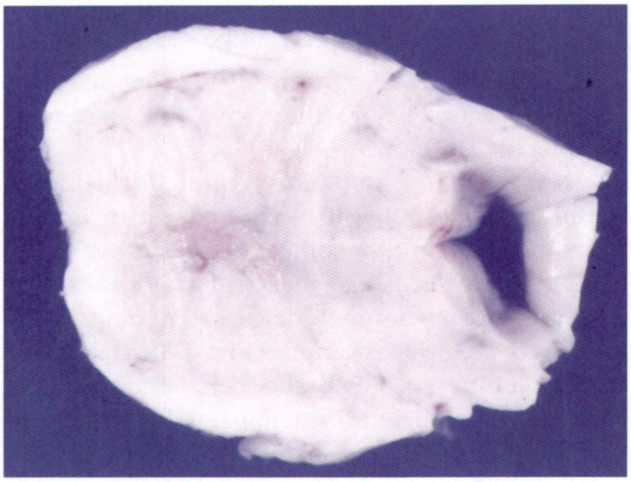

Figure 1-118. Osmotic demyelination syndrome (central pontine myelinolysis). The typical lesion characterized by myelin loss creates a soft, friable area in the center of the basis pontis.

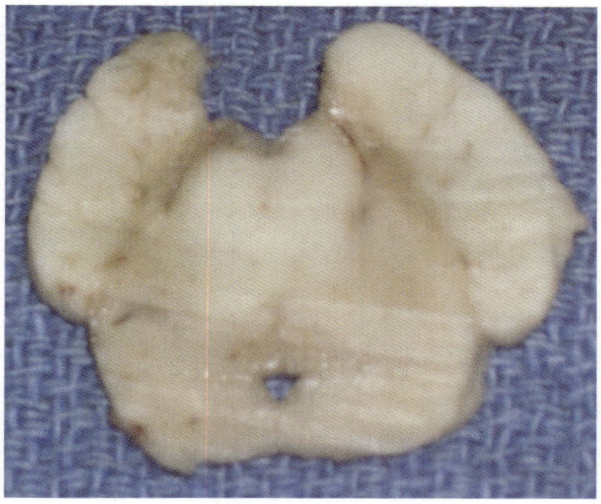

Figure 1-119. Parkinson's disease. The substantia nigrae are pale due to loss of pigmented neurons. They also appear collapsed as a result of volume loss and gliosis.

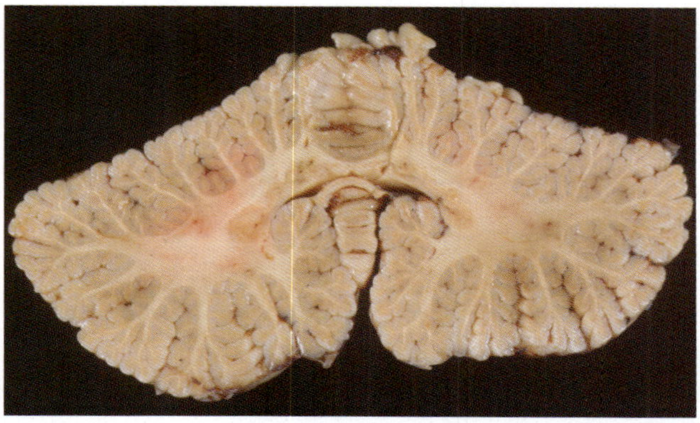

Figure 1-120. Progressive supranuclear palsy. While the cerebellum appears full without significant atrophy, both dentate nuclei appear discolored and shrunken as a result of degeneration of their neurons and associated gliosis.

lethargica (von Economo disease).[255] Substantia nigra and locus ceruleus may be pale due to the destruction of the neurons during the disease process, the nature of which is not entirely clear. Mild generalized atrophy may be seen. In corticobasal degeneration, substantia nigra and locus ceruleus are pale. In addition, there are posterior frontal, parietal, and perirolandic cortex atrophy but not necessarily symmetrically. Arteriosclerotic pseudoparkinsonism is a term that is used to refer to the destruction of the substantia nigra by cavitary infarcts. Ischemic lesions can also be present in basal ganglia, especially putamen, and frontal white matter. Guam parkinsonism–dementia complex,[256] in addition to a generalized cerebral atrophy, has pale substantia nigra and locus ceruleus. The presence of substantia nigra and locus ceruleus pallor and subsequent diagnosis of Parkinson's disease in a patient with dementia should prompt consideration of DLB, even if another dementing disease, such as AD has already been identified. Substantia nigrae are shrunken and show rusty brown discoloration in neurodegeneration with brain iron accumulation type 1, along with basal ganglionic involvement, especially globus pallidus. Brainstem components may be atrophic entirely or in various combinations in neurodegenerative diseases, depending on the

TABLE 1.16 Differential diagnosis of substantia nigra pallor and degeneration

Disease/Agent	Other Features
Pallor is normal in the first 2 decades of life[254]	—
Parkinson's disease	Pallor of loci cerulei
PSP	Pallor of loci cerulei, midbrain, pontine tegmentum, globus pallidus involvement
Corticobasal degeneration	Pallor of loci cerulei, basal ganglionic and cortical atrophy
DLB	Pallor of loci cerulei, cortical Lewy bodies, other cerebral cortical dementing neurodegenerative disease may be present
Postencephalitis parkinsonism (encephalitis lethargica)	Mild generalized cerebral atrophy in some cases
Arteriosclerotic pseudoparkinsonism	Infarcts in substantia nigra, basal ganglia, other regions
GPDC	Pallor of loci cerulei, generalized cerebral atrophy
Neurodegeneration with brain iron accumulation type 1	Rusty brown discoloration of substantia nigrae, basal ganglionic involvement

PSP, progressive supranuclear palsy; GPDC, Guam parkinsonism–dementia complex; DLB, dementia with Lewy bodies.

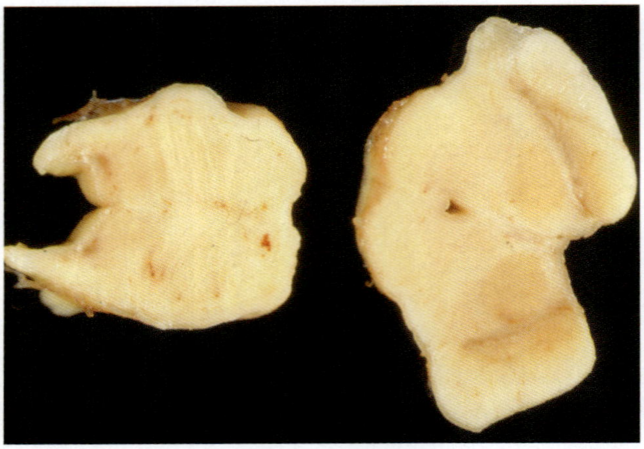

Figure 1-121. Multiple system atrophy. Brainstem, and mainly basis pontis, is atrophic. The interpeduncular fossa is widened due to midbrain volume loss. Basis pontis has shrunken almost to the size of its tegmentum.

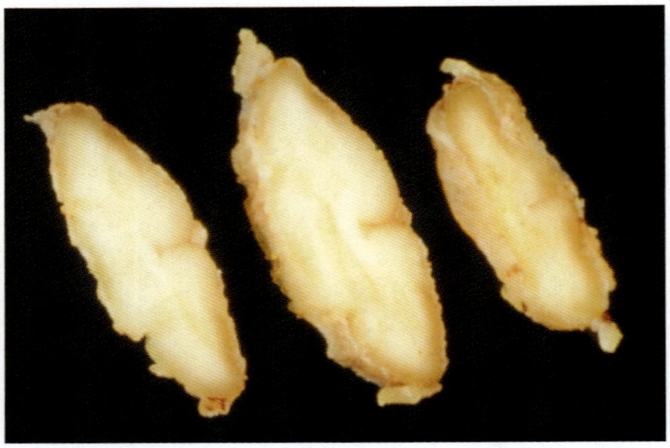

Figure 1-123. MS, spinal cord, chronic stage. Cut surfaces of spinal cord show volume loss, a collapsed appearance, and tan-yellow discoloration.

nature of the disease process involving the structures in the brainstem, such as MSA **(Figs. 1-121 and 1-122)**.

Spinal cord is commonly involved by demyelinating disease, especially MS and neuromyelitis optica (Devic's disease). Demyelinating lesions (plaques) render the spinal cord to have a *collapsed appearance* in the involved areas. The usual gray and white matter distinction and the butterfly-shaped anterior and posterior horns may not be as apparent due to loss of myelin, interfering with the usual contrast of these structures **(Fig. 1-123)**. As in the brain lesions, the plaques may be *soft and gelatinous* in acute stages and *shrunken, firm*, and tan in chronic stages. The demyelinating lesions in neuromyelitis optica are aligned longitudinally in the spinal cord and span long stretches, typically longer than three vertebrae. Syringomyelia is a longitudinal slit-like *cavity* of variable length in the spinal cord, posterior to the central canal, usually in the cervical and upper thoracic region. The majority of idiopathic cases are associated with Chiari I. Others form as a result of resorption of destructive lesions, such as contusions or infarcts. If it involves the medulla, then it is called syringobulbia. In brainstem, the slit lies behind the fourth ventricle, with which it may be communicating. It may also be isolated in the brainstem without syringomyelia. Hydromyelia and hydrobulbia refer to the dilatation of the central canal and are lined by ependyma.

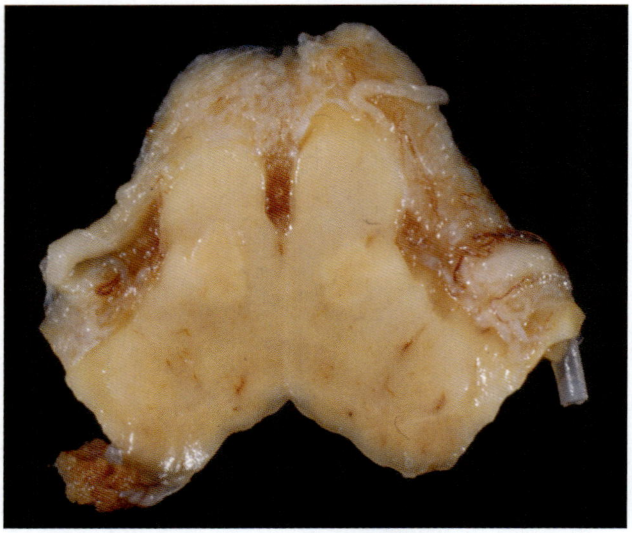

Figure 1-122. Multiple system atrophy. There is also involvement of medulla oblongata, with generalized volume loss and prominent atrophy of inferior olivary nuclei.

Mass lesions are occasionally seen as a whole and at autopsy as most have previously undergone surgical procedures for resection or to at least obtain a tissue diagnosis with subsequent treatment. When a mass lesion is identified, its borders with the surrounding tissues and cut surfaces provide important clues to its nature. *Cystic lesions* and cyst contents are discussed in "Cystic Lesions" below. As for *solid mass lesions*, in general, homogeneous cut surfaces without hemorrhage or necrosis tend to represent low-grade or benign neoplasms. Variegated cut surfaces with areas of hemorrhage and necrosis, possibly

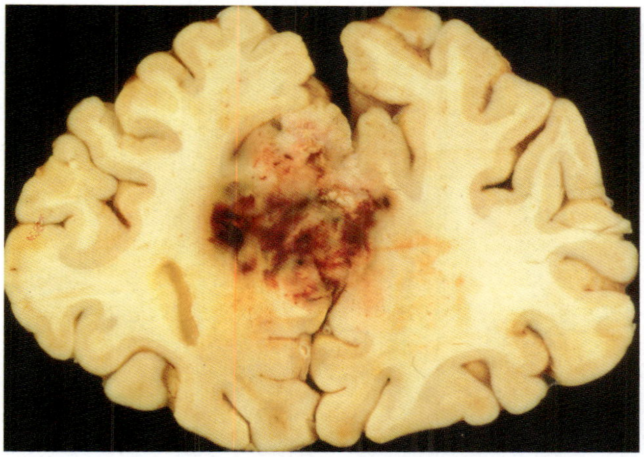

Figure 1-124. Glioblastoma multiforme. A mass lesion with variegated hemorrhagic, necrotic, and solid cut surface is seen. It has irregular and ill-defined borders. It infiltrates the genu of corpus callosum to cross to the opposite hemisphere, a feature associated with high-grade neoplasms.

with a combination of solid and cystic areas, likely represent a malignant neoplasm, which may be primary, such as glioblastoma multiforme (GBM) **(Fig. 1-124)**, or metastatic, such as metastatic carcinoma. There are exceptions, as should be expected. Schwannomas typically have cut surfaces that fit better to those of a malignant neoplasm **(Fig. 1-125)**. Medulloblastomas, on the other hand, have solid homogeneous cut surfaces. Metastatic neoplasms within the neuroglial parenchyma tend to be *well-circumscribed* due to their expansile growth with peripheral edema**(Fig. 1-126)**, while gliomas tend to have *ill-defined borders* due to their widely infiltrative nature **(Fig. 1-124)**, although some gliomas, for example, ependymomas, typically have grossly well-circumscribed borders. Extra-axial mass lesions

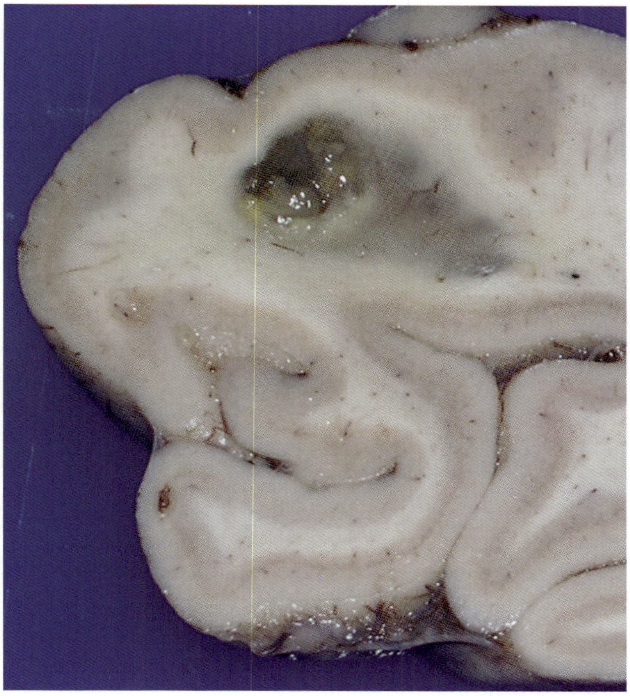

Figure 1-126. Metastatic adenocarcinoma. A well-circumscribed nodule with a gelatinous cut surface due to mucin content and *yellow-green* color representing necrosis is present in the white matter of occipital lobe. In spite of its small size, abundant peripheral edema that is typical for metastatic malignancies is present, seen as a discoloration of the adjacent white matter.

usually show expansile growth with borders that are well-delineated and can be easily separable from the brain parenchyma **(Fig. 1-127)**. The so-called well-circumscribed gliomas such as pilocytic astrocytoma, ganglioglioma, and pleomorphic xanthoastrocytoma (PXA) are prone to better gross total resection due to this feature. The *consistency* of the cut surfaces

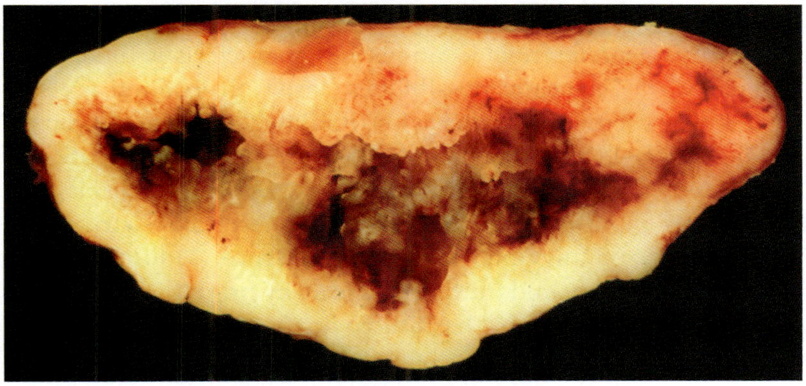

Figure 1-125. Schwannoma. The central regions of the neoplasm show hemorrhage and cyst formation as a degenerative change. These changes are not associated with malignancy, in spite of their worrisome appearance.

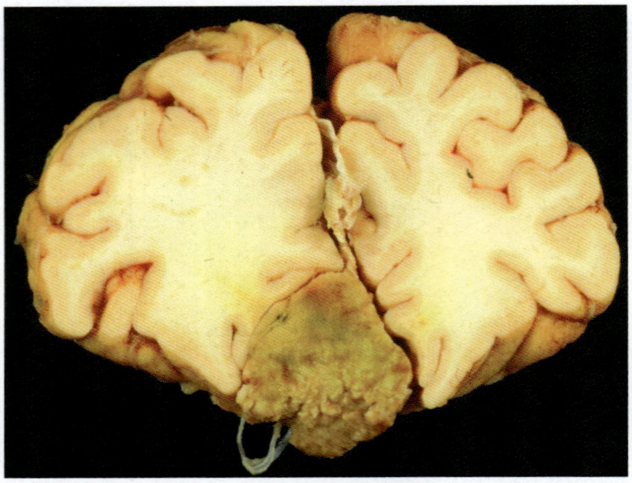

Figure 1-127. Meningioma. The extra-axial mass is attached to anterior falx cerebri, has solid cut surface, and grows in an expansile fashion to push the brain parenchyma. Otherwise, it appears easily detachable from the brain parenchyma, unless it shows brain invasion, as seen in some of the high-grade meningiomas, underscoring the importance of examining brain–meningioma interface for brain invasion in surgical specimens.

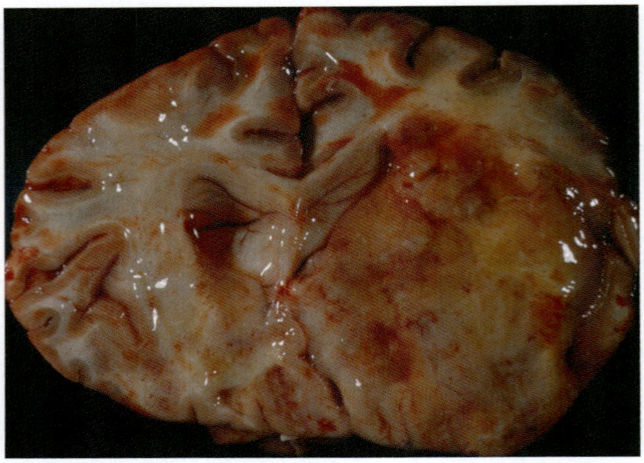

Figure 1-128. Lymphoma. A large mass occupies more than half of the right hemisphere on this section. It has an apparently soft, solid, tan-white cut surface, described as "fish-flesh."

may provide additional clues to narrow down the differential diagnostic possibilities. Fibrous, soft tissue lesions, such as solitary fibrous tumor, tend to have an elastic consistency, while high-grade neoplasms are soft due to necrosis. Small blue cell neoplasms such as medulloblastoma and lymphoma characteristically have fish-flesh, soft, homogenous white cut surfaces **(Fig. 1-128)**. Tumefactive infectious lesions usually represent large granulomas, which may coalesce and become necrotic. They tend to have irregular but well-defined borders. Tuberculosis and many fungal infections, such as coccidioidomycosis, paracoccidioidomycosis, and blastomycosis, may present this way. Mass lesions with necrotic, inflammatory component can be associated with parasitic infections, such as strongyloidiasis (Strongyloides stercoralis),[257] which can cause vascular pathology and secondary infections by bacteria.

Involvement of corpus callosum and crossing to the opposite side, creating a butterfly appearance, is associated with high-grade neoplasms **(Fig. 1-124)**. The neoplasms that are well-recognized with this type of pattern are most commonly GBM, metastatic carcinoma, and lymphoma. Multiplicity of mass lesions can also provide some clues to their nature, although there are no definitive rules and many exceptions. Disease processes that arrive in the CNS through the blood stream tend to cause multifocal lesions. They also tend to be preferentially located at the gray and white matter junction where the blood flow is slow. This is typical for bacterial and fungal abscesses, cysticercosis, and metastatic carcinomas. Rarely, sporadic primary neoplasms of the CNS can be multifocal. Some of those cases are debated to be prominent mass-forming foci in a more diffusely infiltrating glioma and are in fact connected. Those neoplasms associated with various syndromes tend to be multiple, for example, bilateral vestibular schwannomas in NF2, as well as other neoplasms in the setting of neurofibromatosis,[17] and multiple hemangioblastomas associated with von Hippel-Lindau syndrome.[258] Some examples for other lesions that can be multifocal are lymphoma, toxoplasmosis, progressive multifocal leukoencephalopathy (PML), germ cell neoplasms, vascular malformations, and postradiation meningiomas.[259] The preferential locations and characteristic differential diagnostic possibilities based on location are discussed together with "Radiologic Features" Chapter 4 to facilitate correlation and minimize repetition.

Midline shift is identified as the curving or shifting of midline formed by the midline structures, mainly interhemispheric fissure, septum pellucidum, and third ventricle away from the hemisphere involved by the pathologic process toward the other side. It is associated with space-occupying lesions, such as neoplasms, hemorrhage, edema, and cerebritis **(Fig. 1-129)**. In severe cases, there may be accompanying herniations, typically unilateral cingulate **(Fig. 1-130)** and uncal **(Fig. 1-129)**. The involved hemisphere can be seen as larger than the uninvolved hemisphere and as enlarged in all directions. Sometimes, it can be difficult to appreciate the presence of a lesion in the background of extensive swelling. These cases may represent diffuse glioma, cerebritis trauma, or postsurgical brain swelling as can be seen with subdural hematoma evacuation. If available, reviewing sequential radiologic studies and clinical findings for clues for focal lesions can be helpful with focusing in the area of the lesion.

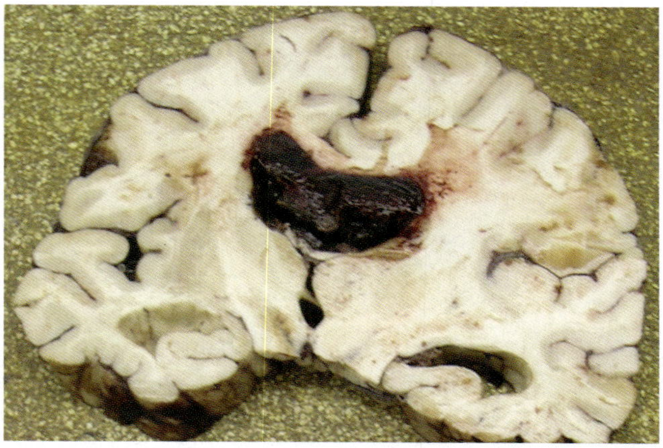

Figure 1-130. Subfalcine (cingulate gyrus) herniation. The right cingulate gyrus has herniated underneath the falx cerebri (removed), pushing against the opposite cingulate gyrus and blocking the superior view of the corpus callosum. There is also a mild right-to-left midline shift. The lateral ventricles are filled with hemorrhage, which originated from a hypertensive hemorrhage in the right basal ganglia (not shown).

Parenchymal Hemorrhage

Hemorrhage in the neuroglial parenchyma usually presents in a pattern based on multiplicity and location to allow for narrowing down the differential diagnostic possibilities to at least a few broad categories. When possible, 3-D measurements of the hematoma should be obtained to give an idea about its volume. This is especially important when there is no radiologic record. Measuring its volume directly is also possible but is not as practical. One of the most common scenarios is a large, single focus of *hemorrhage in the basal*

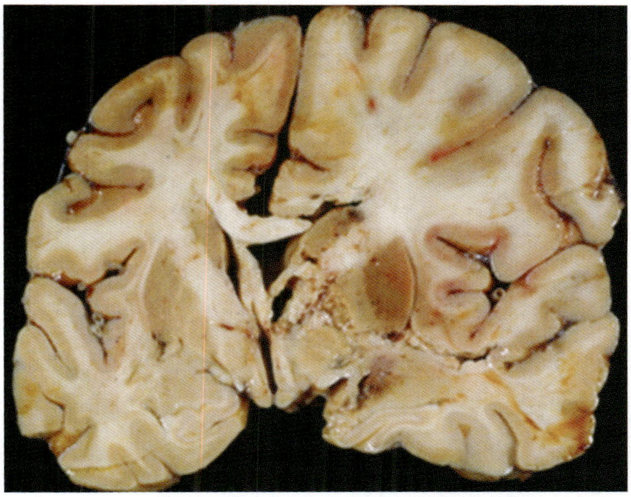

Figure 1-129. Midline shift. The right hemisphere is significantly larger than the left as a result of edema associated with a large infarct involving the basal ganglia and surrounding structures. It appears soft, partially depressed, and cystic, consistent with subacute stage. There is right-to-left midline shift, as well as right transtentorial herniation, seen as the protrusion of the right medial temporal lobe toward the midline.

List of Findings/Checklist for Parenchymal Hemorrhage

• AT A GLANCE

- Hemorrhage pattern (single, multiple, deep, superficial, petechial, dissecting into parenchyma from subarachnoid space, or vice versa)
- Ganglionic hemorrhage
- Lobar hemorrhage
- Brainstem hemorrhage
- Contusions
- Herniations
- Shunts
- Neoplasms (metastatic or primary)
- Vascular malformations
- Hematologic disorders
- Infectious diseases
- Toxic/metabolic disorders
- Hemorrhagic infarct
- Venous thrombosis
- Germinal matrix hemorrhage/hypoxic–ischemic injury

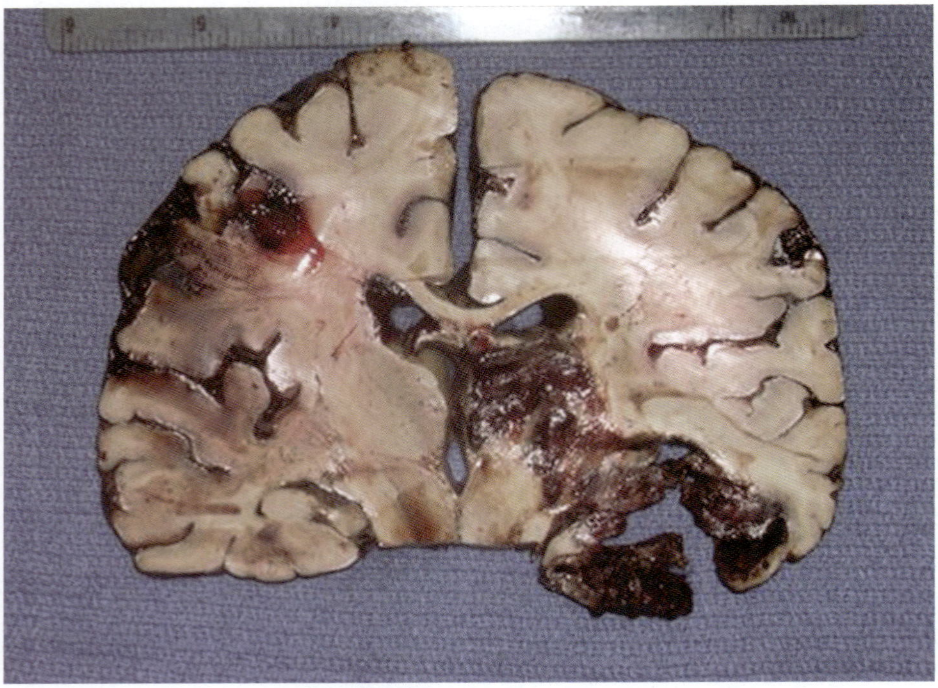

Figure 1-131. A thalamic hypertensive hemorrhage dissects the parenchyma to reach the subarachnoid space and covers the entire brain surface. It has not yet made its way into the ventricular system. The hemorrhagic foci in the left parietal cortex and in the angle of the left lateral ventricle are related to shunt. There is also global hypoxic/ischemic change seen as dusky discoloration of the parenchyma, likely due to extended vegetative state by being bound to respirator.

ganglia, usually dissecting the brain parenchyma to reach ventricular system or subarachnoid space **(Fig. 1-131)**. This is typical for *hypertensive hemorrhage*[260–262] **(Fig. 1-132)**. Hypertensive hemorrhage can also occur in *pons* as a large focus expanding the brainstem **(Fig. 1-133)** and may dissect into the midbrain, medulla oblongata, along the cerebellar peduncles, and into the fourth ventricle. This type of pontine hemorrhage should be distinguished from *Duret hemorrhage*, which results from stretching and tearing of vessels within the parenchyma in cases of transtentorial (uncal) herniation **(Fig. 1-134)**. Parenchymal hemorrhages especially close to the *base of the brain* may be the

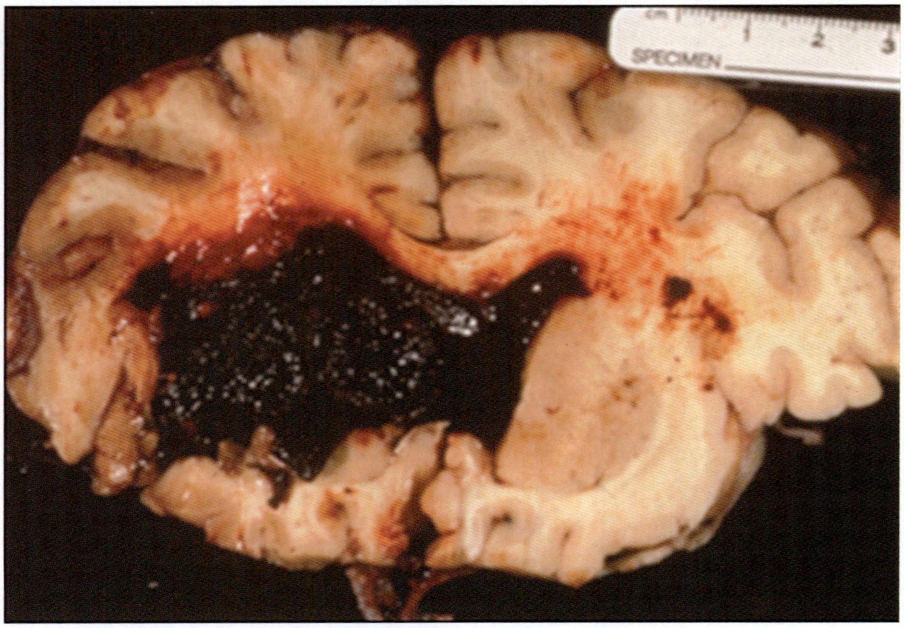

Figure 1-132. Hypertensive hemorrhage in the left striatum (ganglionic hemorrhage), filling the ventricular system and also dissecting into the subarachnoid space. There is left-to-right midline shift.

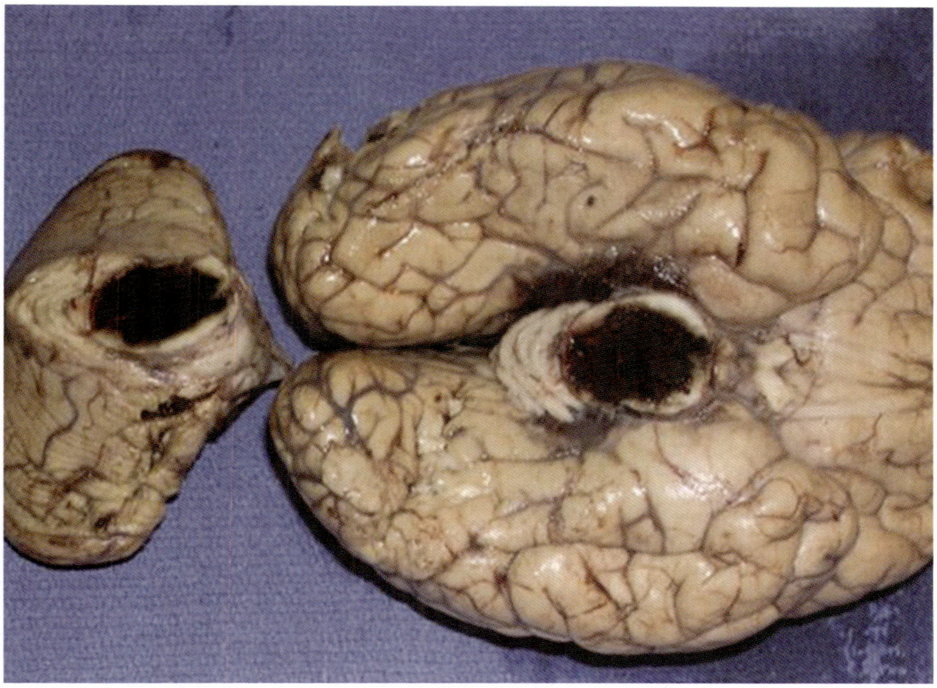

Figure 1-133. Large hypertensive brainstem hemorrhage, likely associated with large ganglionic and ventricular hemorrhage. There is prominent brain swelling, indicated by the flattening of the sulcal–gyral pattern. Bilateral transtentorial (uncal) herniations are present, resulting in the hemorrhagic appearance of both parahippocampal gyri, more prominent on the right side (herniation contusions).

result of *aneurysm rupture* in the basal arteries and the hemorrhage dissecting into the brain parenchyma. It may even extend into the ventricular system. When brain hemorrhage is *multifocal* and with a preferentially *superficial* epicenter, that is, the so-called lobar hemorrhage **(Fig. 1-135)**, *cerebral amyloid angiopathy* (congophilic angiopathy) should be considered[260,262,263] **(Table 1.17)**. It commonly involves the occipital lobe.[264] *Trauma* is another cause that is likely to produce superficial and multiple hemorrhagic foci.[223] These represent *contusions*, tend to be in the form of *multiple* small foci, which may coalesce to form larger lesions. The traumatic nature of these hemorrhages can be supported by the additional evidence of tissue injury in the leptomeninges, subdural and epidural compartments, bone, and skin, although these are neither necessary nor invariably present. In addition, they tend to occur in the basal portions of the brain and anterior aspect of the brainstem, where neuroglial tissue comes into close contact with the irregular bony surfaces of the skull base **(Fig. 1-136)**. *Ventriculostomy tract* should not to be confused with lacerations, especially if the shunt catheter has been removed. Some shunt tracts may bleed, mimicking contusions or other hematomas. Hemorrhage in association with catheter can rarely be spontaneous or may result secondarily from the coagulopathic state, such as anticoagulant use, severe burns, and tissue plasminogen activator administration. Groups of *punctate hemorrhages* localized to the *cerebellar tonsil* or *uncus* are seen in cases of cerebellar tonsillar or transtentorial

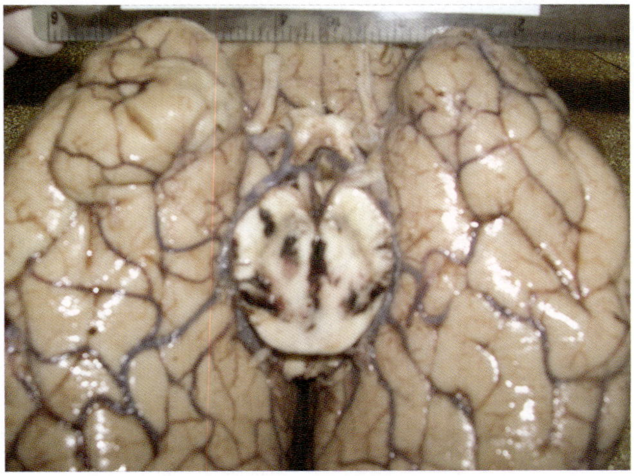

Figure 1-134. Multiple hemorrhages in the brainstem result from stretching of and damage to the penetrating vessels as the herniating uncus pushes the brainstem and are called Duret hemorrhages.

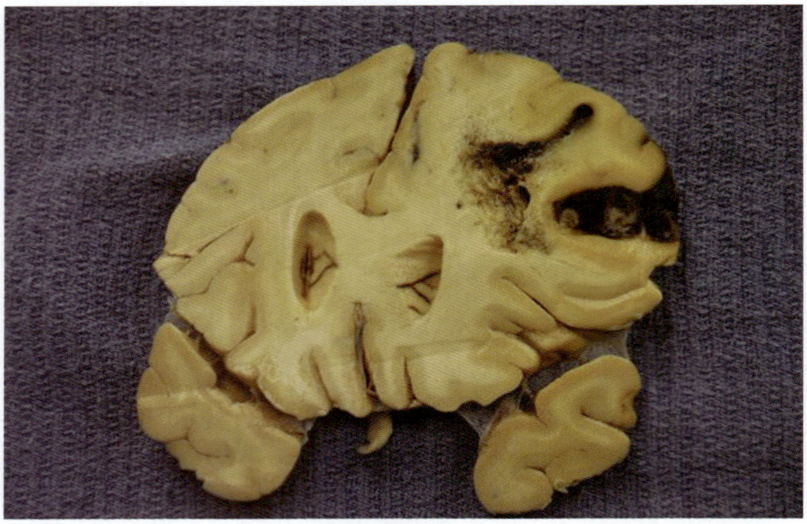

Figure 1-135. Cerebral amyloid angiopathy. In this case, a superficial frontal lobe hemorrhage is present and also involves the leptomeninges. If the patient survived previous hemorrhages, there may be evidence of remote events that may have possibly become cystic, with rusty brown discoloration due to hemosiderin pigment accumulation.

herniations, respectively, and are also associated with softening of these tissues due to ischemia **(Fig. 1-137)**.

Metastatic malignancies[89] with a tendency to bleed are another cause of one or more hemorrhagic foci in the brain, usually at the *gray-white matter junction*, although this is difficult to appreciate in most cases with large lesions and certainly is not the rule **(Table 1.18)**. Melanoma[265] and renal cell carcinoma[266] are two common causes of hemorrhage due to metastatic malignancy. In the case of melanoma, abundant *melanin pigment*, if present, may simulate hemorrhage in the absence of actual hemorrhage **(Fig. 1-138)**. Hematologic malignancies, such as leukemic involvement, can also present as hemorrhagic lesions.[267] *Primary neoplasms*,[268,269] notably, glioblastoma, oligodendroglioma, and pilocytic astrocytoma, or *vascular malformations* such as AVM, or vasculitides can be the cause of hemorrhage.[270] Choriocarcinomas are also well-known for their hemorrhagic/necrotic nature. All of these can present for the first time as hemorrhage. Therefore, whether it is an autopsy examination or a surgical specimen for hematoma evacuation, all hematomas, but especially intraparenchymal hematomas, should be sampled very carefully and generously in an attempt to identify any underlying cause, be it beta-amyloid accumulation in vessel walls or a neoplastic process. An attempt should be made during gross evaluation to pick preferentially any solid tissue fragments, which may represent admixed brain tissue or lesional tissue, which should be submitted

TABLE 1.17 Common causes of multifocal hemorrhage

Cerebral amyloid angiopathy
Metastatic neoplasms (see Table 1.18)
Contusions
Vasculopathies
Angioinvasive fungi
Parasites (Ameba, Trypanosoma, Trichinella)

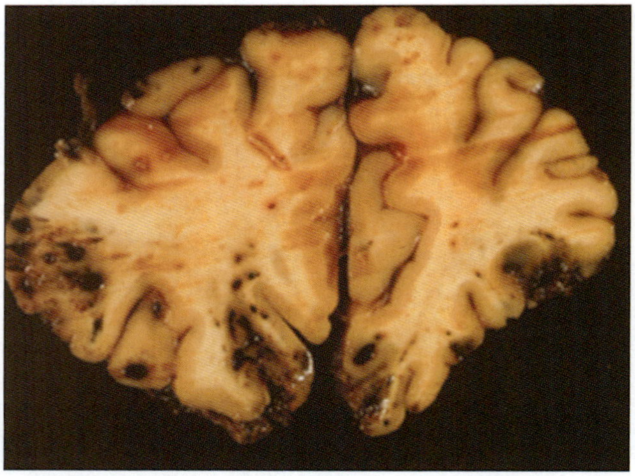

Figure 1-136. Multiple superficial contusions of variable sizes, mainly concentrated on the basal surfaces of the frontal lobes. Many of them, especially the medial ones, are in contact with the leptomeninges, without an intact pial membrane, supporting their traumatic origin, rather than hemorrhagic infarct.

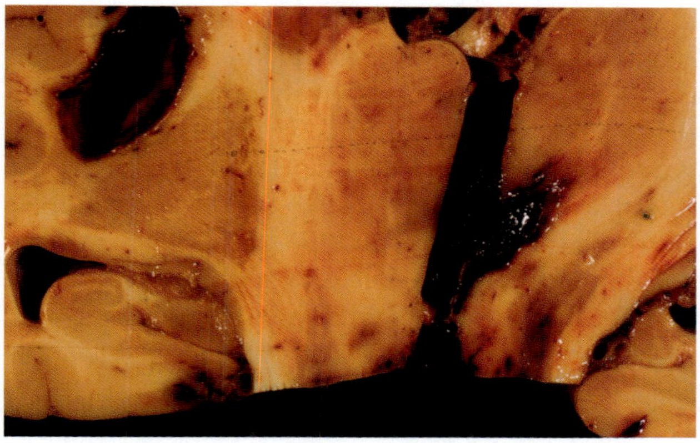

Figure 1-137. Transtentorial herniation of the left parahippocampal gyrus. Compared to the other side, it is in close contact with and pushing the midbrain and also has punctate hemorrhagic foci (herniation contusions). See also Figure 1-133.

TABLE 1.18 Neoplasms that can commonly present with hemorrhage

Metastatic
Melanoma
Renal cell carcinoma
Leukemia
Choriocarcinoma
Primary
Oligodendroglioma
GBM
Pilocytic astrocytoma

for microscopic evaluation. Even what appears to be obvious blood clot may contain admixed small fibrovascular component in the background to provide clues about any vascular problems.

Multiple white matter-centered microhemorrhages indicate a more widespread involvement of the cerebral vasculature **(Table 1.19)**. *Accelerated (malignant) hypertension* can result in *fibrinoid necrosis* of parenchymal arterioles and subsequent petechial hemorrhages in small clusters. Acute hemorrhagic leukoencephalopathy can be due to an autoimmune reaction to previous infections such as systemic viral infections or respiratory infections and also can be seen in association with inflammatory bowel disease, methanol poisoning, and arsenic-containing medication use. *Fat embolism*[271] and *DAI*[223] are other conditions where multiple petechial hemorrhages are seen in white matter. The brain in fat embolism can be grossly normal within the first 2 days. Petechial hemorrhages occur in 2 to 4 days. There may be perivascular gray discolorations, which indicate tissue damage and may progress to small perivascular infarcts if patients live longer **(Fig. 1-139)**. Although more prominent in the white matter, gray matter areas can also be involved. Hemorrhages in DAI are predominantly associated with well-organized long tracts, such as corpus callosum, cerebral peduncles, and brainstem. It may or may not be associated with other evidence of trauma. *Disorders of*

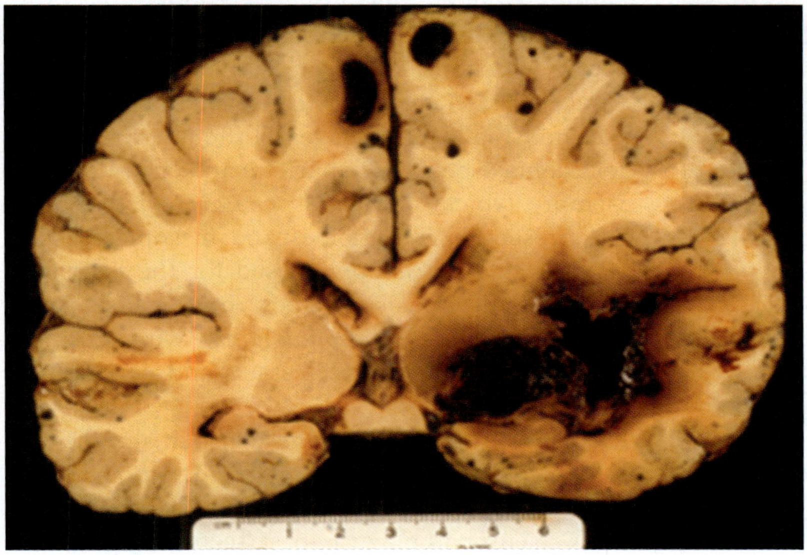

Figure 1-138. Multiple pigmented foci, many measuring a few millimeters and are mainly superficial, favoring gray-white matter junction. The patient had a history of melanoma of the skin but presented with a stroke due to the hemorrhage in the right temporal metastatic focus.

TABLE 1.19 Differential diagnosis of petechial hemorrhages

Diffuse axonal injury
Fat embolism
Malignant hypertension/small vessel disease
Acute hemorrhagic leukoencephalopathy
Hematologic disorders
Disseminated intravascular coagulation
Idiopathic thrombocytopenic purpura
Thrombotic thrombocytopenic purpura
Sickle cell disease
Metabolic
Wernicke's encephalopathy
Pancreatic encephalopathy
Toxic
Lead
Ethanol
Methanol
Methamphetamine
Cocaine
Medications
Amphetamine
Sulfonamide
Cyclosporine A
Melarsoprol
Infections
Rickettsia
Malaria

coagulation, such as disseminated intravascular coagulation, thrombotic thrombocytopenic purpura and idiopathic thrombocytopenic purpura, and especially anticoagulant medication use, can also result in widespread white matter petechial hemorrhages or larger multiple hemorrhages.[272,273] *Sickle cell disease* is a relatively rare cause of hemorrhage, especially in adults.[274] A rare cause of such white matter petechial hemorrhage pattern is the microvascular damage due to *malaria* infection,[275] resulting in ring-and-ball type hemorrhage and tissue damage. Brain is pale gray with petechial hemorrhages, especially in white matter.

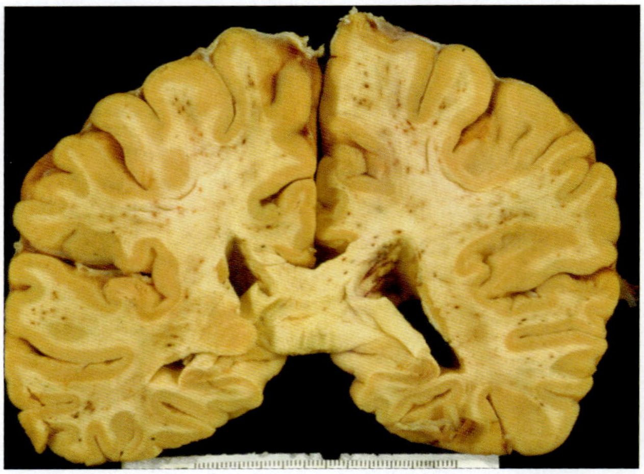

Figure 1-139. Numerous petechial hemorrhages diffusely involving the white matter in a patient with fat embolism. Many of these foci are also associated with a gray discoloration, consistent with early perivascular infarcts.

Petechial hemorrhage in *mamillary bodies* is seen in acute stages of *Wernicke's encephalopathy*.[276] Parenchymal hemorrhage, mainly in the form of multiple petechial hemorrhages, can be one of the findings associated with a number of *toxic conditions. Acute lead encephalopathy* is characterized by swelling, congestion, and petechial hemorrhages due to endothelial swelling and vascular necrosis.[277] *Ethylene glycol*[278] and acute *ethanol*[279] intoxications can result in congestion, edema, and petechial or larger hemorrhages. *Methanol* poisoning[179] is characterized by edema and global hypoxic–ischemic injury, as well as petechial hemorrhages and hemorrhagic infarctions that are most typical in putamen and claustrum bilaterally. *Amphetamine, methamphetamine,* and *methylenedioxymethamphetamine (ecstasy)* can sometimes result in a necrotizing vasculitis involving various types of vessels and subarachnoid and parenchymal hemorrhages, as well as arterial and venous infarcts.[260,280] *Cocaine* can cause subarachnoid and parenchymal hemorrhages. Rupture of a saccular aneurysm, if there is one, can be seen as a result of sudden increase in blood pressure. Among *medications, sulfonamides*, due to endothelial swelling and necrosis, can result in gray and white matter necrosis, with or without hemorrhage. *Cyclosporine A* can rarely cause subarachnoid and parenchymal hemorrhages, although white matter edema especially in parietal and occipital lobes is more typical.[281] *Organic pentavalent arsenicals* are present in insecticides and in some medications such as *melarsoprol* used for the treatment of trypanosomiasis.[282] They may cause *acute hemorrhagic leukoencephalopathy* with fibrinoid necrosis of white matter vessels and perivascular hemorrhages.

Several *infectious agents* can damage the vessels to cause hemorrhagic lesions. Brain is swollen and has petechial hemorrhages in *rickettsial infections*. Neuropathology is best seen in typhus and Rocky Mountain spotted fever. Opportunistic fungal

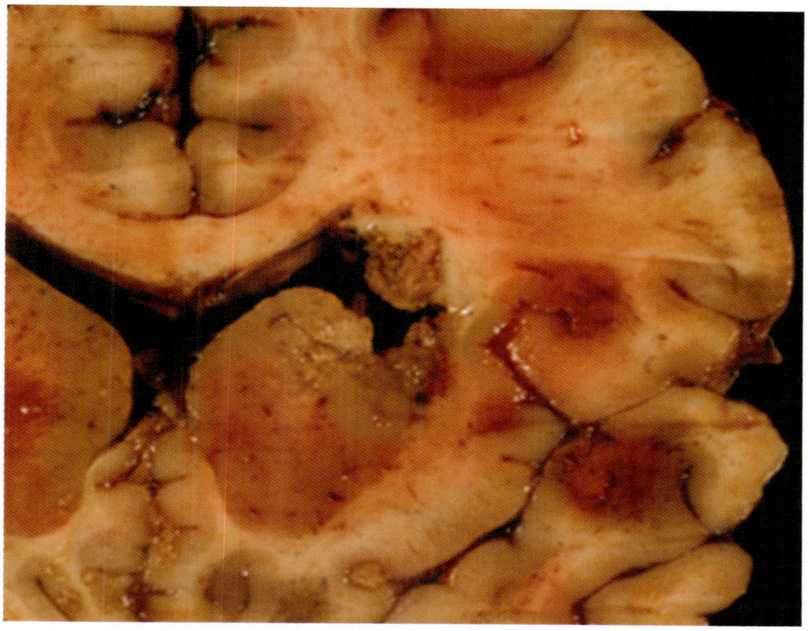

Figure 1-140. Multiple hemorrhagic, necrotic, ill-defined, and friable foci representing disseminated Aspergillosis in a transplant patient.

infections are typically seen in immunocompromised patients.[283] *Aspergillosis* causes hemorrhagic necrotic lesions. The lesions are ill-defined, soft, and friable similar to cerebritis **(Fig. 1-140)** in acute stage and may be walled-off like an abscess in chronic stage. *Zygomycosis*, also referred to as mucormycosis or phycomycosis, is caused by species of Mucor and Absidia, among others.[284] They tend to go to *basal ganglia* more often by hematologic spread. In the upper respiratory tract hemorrhagic necrotic mass-like presentation typically seen in diabetics and immunocompromised individuals, they tend to form *basal brain* lesions by invading the skull base. Pathology of these angioinvasive fungi is similar to aspergillosis. *Pseudallescheria boydii* is another angioinvasive fungus with hyphae and lesions similar to Aspergillus. *Granulomatous amebic encephalitis* caused by Acanthamoeba spp. and Balamuthia mandrillaris results in hemorrhagic necrotic lesions **(Fig. 1-141)**. *African trypanosomiasis* (sleeping sickness), caused by Trypanosoma brucei subspecies (rhodesiense: fulminant disease; gambiense: subacute–chronic meningoencephalitis), may be associated with a *hemorrhagic leukoencephalopathy*, which may or may not be related to melarsoprol treatment (which contains arsenicals), rather than the

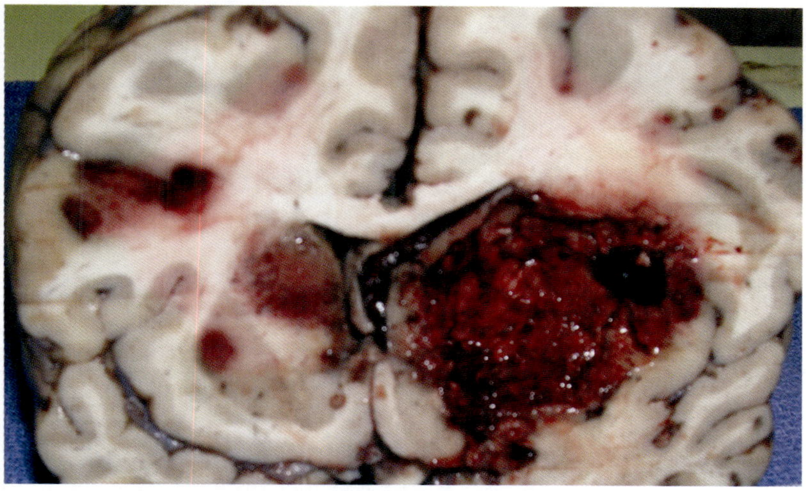

Figure 1-141. Numerous hemorrhagic, necrotic foci, in this patient due to Balamuthia mandrillaris infection. No other history of travel or immunosuppression, skin lesions, or involvement of other organs were present, although the small superficial lesions favor gray-white matter junction, supporting hematologic spread.

infection itself.[285] Petechial or larger hemorrhages can be seen in *trichinosis* (Trichinella spiralis)[286]

What may appear to be localized or widespread petechial hemorrhages may actually be extremely *congested vessels* in the white matter, or a *telangiectasia* in the case of focal grouping of such vessels. *Hemorrhagic infarcts* occur in the background of an infarct due to superimposed hemorrhage as a result of reperfusion of and hemorrhage from the necrotic vessels.[287] This may be a complication of thrombolytic therapy or a spontaneous event as a result of partial lysis or more distal propagation of the thrombus, allowing blood flow into necrotic brain tissue. It may be difficult to identify whether the hemorrhage or infarct came first. Hemorrhagic infarcts have a soft, solid tissue consistency rather than a pure blood clot and do not tend to fall apart as pure blood clot does. *Dural sinus thromboses*[288] result in diffuse *congestion* and eventually *hemorrhagic infarction* of the tissues they drain. Bilateral parasagittal regions are involved in superior sagittal sinus thrombosis. Involvement of lateral sinuses results in similar changes in the basal ganglia, and involvement of deep internal veins and the great vein of Galen results in such changes in the basal ganglia and brainstem.

In premature babies, *periventricular germinal matrix hemorrhages* are common indicators of *hypoxic/ischemic injury*.[289] They may dissect into the ventricular system. Likewise, white matter hemorrhages can be associated with periventricular leukomalacia (white matter necrosis). Hemorrhages are typically perinatal lesions and may be associated with other evidence of hypoxic/ischemic injury, hemorrhages in other structures, and even evidence of birth trauma, for example, dural tears indicating distortion of the head.

Parenchymal hemorrhage may be present in meningocerebral angiodysplasia and renal agenesis, which is characterized by very vascular leptomeninges, sometimes with subarachnoid hemorrhage, among other findings. Pancreas disease can cause a *pancreatic encephalopathy*[276] that is characterized by brain swelling, and some cases can show basal ganglion and periventricular petechiae. In *hyperthermic states* (including malignant hyperthermia), the brain is normal or mildly swollen, but some patients may have parenchymal and meningeal hemorrhages due to a bleeding diathesis.[290]

Ventricular System

The normal configuration of the ventricular system is altered in response to various factors.[291] *Normally*, the lateral ventricles have sharp and pointy corners extending into the centrum semiovale. The caudate nuclei bulge into the lateral ventricles to form a convex outline. The third ventricle has a slit-like configuration, with thalami on both sides, and a slight bulge in the midsection, before it narrows toward the aqueduct. The fourth ventricle has a peculiar complex configuration with a relatively flat base formed by pons and medulla oblongata, surrounded posteriorly by the cerebellum.

List of Features/Checklist for Ventricular System

AT A GLANCE

- *Ventricular shape*
  - Narrow/slit-like
  - Bat wing
  - Dilatation/hydrocephalus (uniform or irregular)
  - Compensatory dilatation (hydrocephalus ex vacuo)
  - Symmetry/asymmetry
  - Hydromyelia/hydrobulbia
  - Diverticulum
  - Septum pellucidum
  - Aplasia
  - Associated malformations/syndromes
- *Ventricular surfaces*
  - Smooth
  - Granular
  - Nodular
  - Necrotic/sloughing
  - Hemorrhagic
  - Adhesions
  - Aqueduct stenosis
- *Mass lesions*
  - Cysts
  - Neoplasms
  - Choroid plexus (see "Choroid Plexus")
  - Pineal region (see "Pineal Region")

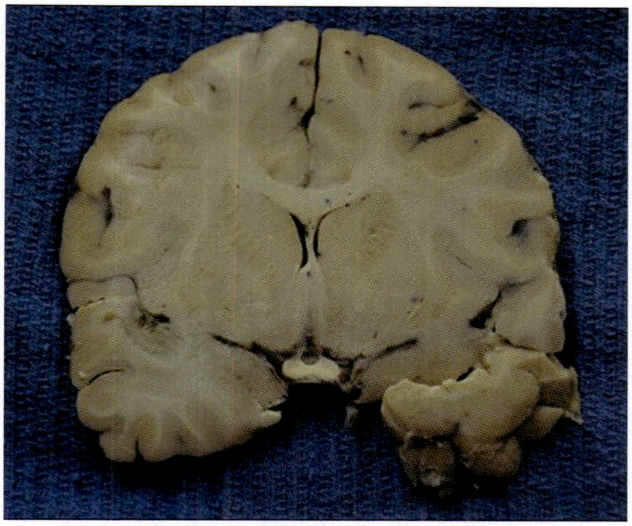

Figure 1-142. Diffuse brain swelling. The edema resulted in tightly packed gyri and slit-like lateral ventricles.

Especially the condition of the lateral ventricles can be very informative about the condition of the brain. In cases of brain swelling, lateral ventricles become squeezed and assume a *slit-like* semicircular configuration, rather than a cavity **(Fig. 1-142)**. *Bat-wing shape* of the lateral ventricles with their upper corners to be pointing upward is seen with agenesis of corpus callosum **(Fig. 1-98)**.[292]

Hydrocephalus ex vacuo or compensatory *dilatation* is a response to loss of brain tissue, due to degeneration in *generalized* form, or in the form of *focal and irregular distortions* in cases of parenchymal loss due to focal damage, such as cystic infarcts or healed hemorrhage cavities that communicate with the ventricular system. In cases of noncommunicating hydrocephalus, usually a lateral ventricle may rupture to form a fluid-filled lesion referred to as *ventricular diverticulum*.[293] It can be supra- or infratentorial and typically occurs at the medial wall of the trigone or the posterior wall of the third ventricle, although other locations are not necessarily spared. Sometimes, the rupture can advance to communicate with the subarachnoid space and creates a *spontaneous shunt*. These cavities are not lined by ependyma. In the *spinal cord*, dilatation of the central canal with intact ependymal lining is called hydromyelia. It can be focal or diffuse, may be an incidental finding, or may be associated with complex syndromes and other malformations, such as Arnold-Chiari malformation.[294] It should be distinguished from syringomyelia, which may be impossible on gross examination.

Many disorders with generalized tissue loss, especially white matter diseases, such as leukodystrophy, CADASIL, as well as neurodegenerative diseases such as AD and Huntington disease, can result in a *compensatory dilatation* of the ventricular system **(Fig. 1-143) (Table 1.20)**. In neurodegenerative diseases where there is relatively generalized involvement of the brain, such as AD,

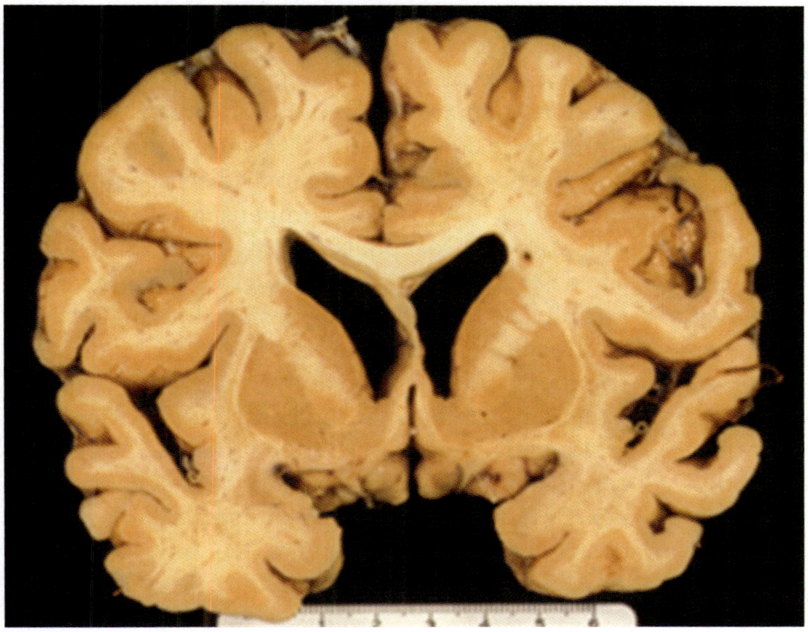

Figure 1-143. Dilatation of the lateral ventricles with blunting of their angles due to compensatory hydrocephalus secondary to brain atrophy seen as thinning of gyri and widening of sulci, especially prominent in the temporal lobe and Sylvian fissure.

TABLE 1.20 Common causes of hydrocephalus ex vacuo

Atrophy due to neurodegenerative disease
Leukodystrophies
Periventricular destructive lesions
Small vessel disease
CADASIL
Chemotherapy-induced leukoencephalopathy
DAI, chronic phase
Posttraumatic neurodegeneration (dementia pugilistica)
Chronic hypoglycemia
Gangliosidoses
Neuronal ceroid lipofuscinosis
Infections involving periventricular white matter
HIV encephalitis
Aging

the contours of the ventricular system tend to be preserved, except the ventricles are enlarged with blunting of the angles of the lateral ventricles. In Huntington disease, due to the atrophy of basal ganglia, especially of the caudate nucleus and putamen, the normally convex contours of the lateral walls of the lateral ventricles are flattened, and in advanced cases, they may actually become concave. Some degree of ventricular dilatation is seen with aging, usually represented as mild blunting of the angles of the lateral ventricles. White matter loss, such as leukodystrophies or periventricular leukomalacia, results in ventricular dilatation along with a decrease in the amount of white matter, which is identified by the reduced distance between the overlying cortex and the ventricular system. This is best appreciated in the centrum semiovale at the angles of the lateral ventricles. Hydrocephalus ex vacuo is also seen commonly with chemotherapy-induced leukoencephalopathy, as a compensatory response to decreased volume of the white matter. Similar changes are seen in the fourth ventricle, although to a lesser extent, when the posterior fossa structures are involved by a neurodegenerative process, such as pontocerebellar degeneration, resulting in dilatation of the fourth ventricle. Third ventricle dilatation can be due to thalamic atrophy or may be an indication along with the dilatation of lateral ventricles that an obstructive process is present at or below the level of aqueduct. Posttraumatic dilatations of the ventricles, especially lateral and third ventricles, can be the result of chronic changes of DAI in survivors. Other evidence of traumatic injury can be present as well as discolored and atrophic white matter, thin corpus callosum, atrophic brainstem, and cerebral peduncles and pyramids, depending on the extent of the damage. Posttraumatic neurodegeneration (dementia pugilistica, punch-drunk syndrome) due to long-term repetitive trauma is another common setting for dilated ventricles. Fenestrated interventricular septum and prominent cerebral atrophy due to neuron loss are common.[295] *Asymmetry* or dilatation of the ventricles has been investigated in connection with schizophrenia by radiologic and morphometric techniques; however, while significant results have been identified, their application to gross examination of the brain does not appear to be reproducible in practice. Same is true for generalized ventricular dilatation involving lateral and third ventricles, in the context of both affective disorders and schizophrenia.[296,297] In obstructive hydrocephalus, increased pressure within the ventricular system that is caused by the accumulation of CSF results in ventricular dilatation. This pressure on the brain tissue can cause subsequent degeneration and *softening of the white matter* due to fluid escaping into the tissues and may give the false impression of periventricular white matter disease. In normal-pressure hydrocephalus,[298] sometimes referred to as intermittently raised–pressure hydrocephalus, ventricular dilation is present without evidence of cortical atrophy. There is rarefaction of periventricular white matter and gliosis. Vascular problems should be ruled out in these cases. Some of these cases can be associated with subdural hematomas, especially in the elderly with shunts, as a complication.[299] A variety of metabolic, genetic, degenerative, and toxic diseases can result in various degrees of compensatory ventricular dilatation/hydrocephaly mainly as a result of tissue destruction. Chronic hypoglycemia cases show atrophy, neuron loss and gliosis, white matter loss, and resultant ventricular dilation.[300] Irregular ventricular surface of the caudate can be seen due to irregular shrinkage of the basal ganglia. GM1 and GM2 gangliosidoses, Batten's disease (neuronal ceroid lipofuscinosis), mucopolysaccharidoses, acute lead encephalopathy, infantile neuroaxonal dystrophy, and neuroaxonal leukodystrophy are some other examples.

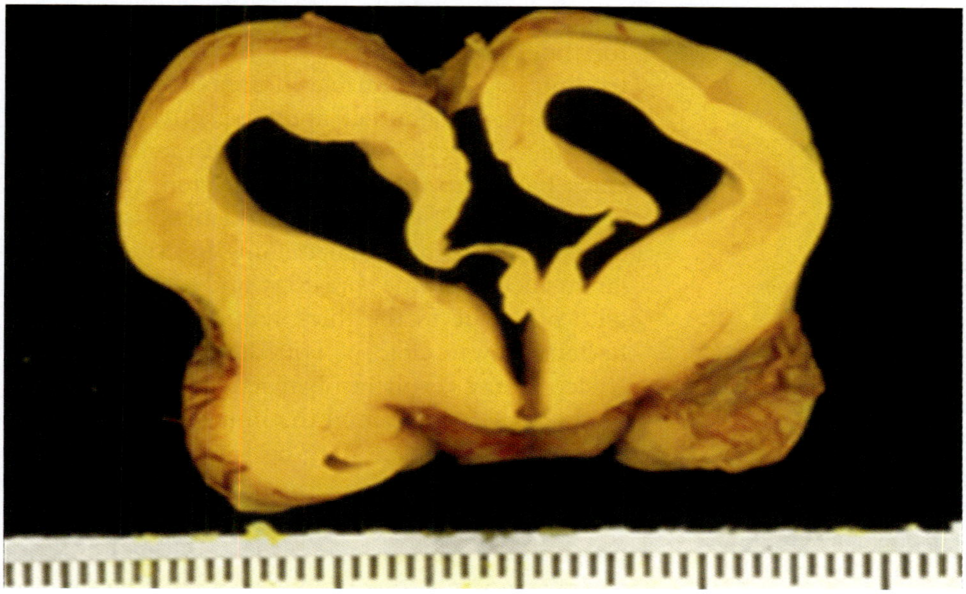

Figure 1-144. Prominent hydrocephalus involving lateral and third ventricles as a result of aqueductal stenosis in this fetal brain. Same case as in Figure 1-147.

Hydrocephalus **(Fig. 1-144)** can be a component of many *malformations and syndromes* involving the CNS **(Table 1.21)**. Walker-Warburg syndrome (cerebro-ocular dysplasia)[301] can have hydrocephalus, along with thin corpus callosum, lissencephaly II, multilayered or unlayered cortex, and glial and mesenchymal proliferation in the subarachnoid space resulting in thick leptomeninges obscuring sulcal–gyral pattern, and have variable combinations of ocular and cerebral dysplasias and muscular dystrophies. Optic nerves are thin. X-linked hydrocephalus may or may not be associated with aqueductal stenosis. Polygyria (not polymicrogyria), absence of pyramids, fusion of thalami, and corpus callosum agenesis are associated. Polygyria is typically associated with hydrocephalus that develops early in life. Cranial dysplasias and disorders may result in hydrocephalus by exerting pressure on venous return and CSF reabsorption.[302] Congenital cerebral lactic acidosis due to pyruvate dehydrogenase deficiency can have prominent hydrocephalus along with other abnormalities such as microcephaly, olivary heterotopias, and hypoplastic pyramidal tracts.[303] *Aplasia* of the fourth ventricle is characterized by the absence of the usual cavity to represent the fourth ventricle. Instead, a tissue composed of primitive cells is present in its place. It may be associated with occipital encephalocele and/or multiple other cerebral abnormalities.[214] Nonfusion of the leaves of septum pellucidum results in cavities called *cavum septi pellucidi* anteriorly **(Fig. 1-145)** and *cavum vergae* posteriorly. Although incidental findings typically with no significant implications, they may sometimes be associated with abnormalities.[304,305] *Septum pellucidum agenesis* can be an incidental

TABLE 1.21 Common causes of hydrocephaly

Hyersecretion of CSF
Choroid plexus neoplasm
Obstruction of CSF circulation
Mass lesions in the region of foramen Monro
Mass lesions in the third ventricle
Aqueductal obstruction (stenosis, hemorrhage, gliosis, inflammation/infection)
Mass lesions in the fourth ventricle
Occlusion of foramina of Magendie and Luschka (inflammation, cyst, neoplasm, gliosis)
Interference with CSF reabsorption
Meningitis
Leptomeningeal fibrosis, granulomatous inflammation
Meningeal carcinomatosis
Arachnoiditis
Idiopathic hypertrophic pachymeningitis
Syndromes/malformations
Arnold-Chiari malformation
Walker-Warburg syndrome
X-linked hydrocephaly
Cranial dysplasias
Cerebral lactic acidosis due to pyruvate kinase deficiency

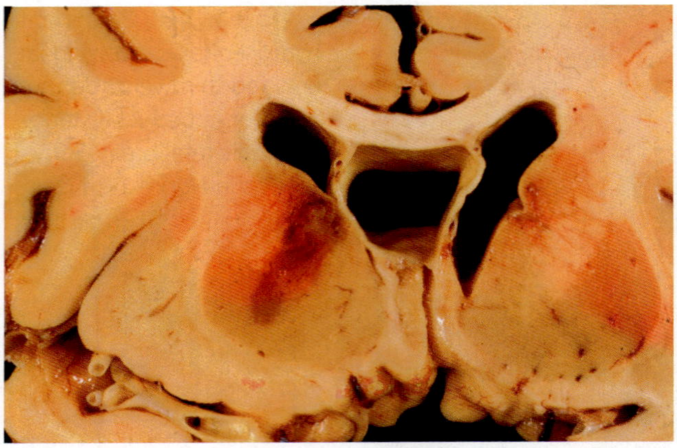

Figure 1-145. Nonfusion of the septum pellucidum resulting in cavum septi pellucidi, seen as an incidental finding in this autopsy. There are also hemorrhagic lesions in both basal ganglia due to angioinvasive fungal infection. The smaller one on the right is immediately under the ventricular surface, resulting in its collapse and irregular ventricular surface.

finding and may be associated with septo-optic dysplasia[306] or other syndromes.[307] If the *absence of septum pellucidum* is due to destruction as a result of inflammation, extensive hydrocephalus, porencephaly, or trauma, then irregular fenestrations or residual fragments of it can be seen.

Ventricular surfaces are normally smooth and glistening with the underlying vessels visible. They may become *granular and irregular* focally or diffusely in granular ependymitis **(Fig. 1-146)**, which is not necessarily an inflammatory/infectious process.[308] Ependymal granulation is a better term for these fine nodules of reactive glial tissue protruding into the ventricle in areas where ependymal lining is denuded and a reactive process is initiated. Infections of the leptomeninges may track back into the ventricular system to result in ventriculitis[309,310] and/or choroid plexitis. In such cases of acute bacterial meningitis, the ventricular surfaces become *congested* and may be covered with *pus*. Due to the thick nature of the pus and its tendency to clog the aqueduct and fourth ventricle, it may result in obstructive hydrocephalus. Ventricular surfaces and the immediately underlying neuroglial tissue may be friable, soft, *hemorrhagic, and necrotic* in cytomegalovirus (CMV) and varicella zoster virus (VZV) infections.[311] Other congenital infections such as rubella, syphilis, and toxoplasmosis also cause ventricular dilatation as a result of periventricular tissue destruction. They may appear as a *sloughing* layer over the ventricular walls. Brain abscess extending into ventricular system is another cause of bacterial ventriculitis.[312] Healed previous infections of the ventricles may leave behind *bands of glial tissue* or *adhesions*. When a *drain, shunt, or reservoir* is present, its location and tract should be noted. Whether its tip is at the intended target, that is, within the ventricle and whether it is patent or occluded by clot, choroid plexus, granulation tissue, pus, or neoplasm should be investigated. Ventriculitis is one of the most important complications of external ventricular drains. These are mainly bacterial infections with Gram-positive cocci and Gram-negative bacilli, with the risk of infection gradually increasing after the 4th day and peaking at around the 10th day of drain placement.[313] Sarcoidosis can result in hydrocephalus by involving the arachnoid granulations, as it can result in leptomeningeal granulomatous inflammation and fibrosis interfering with CSF reabsorption, or obstructing the flow of CSF within the ventricular system.[314]

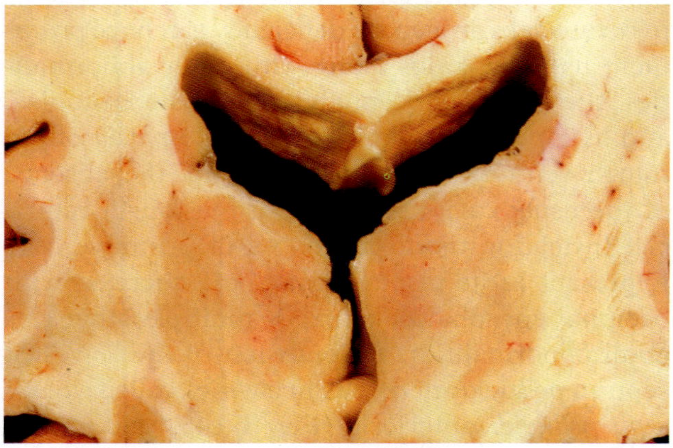

Figure 1-146. Prominent granular irregular surfaces of the lateral ventricles, both the roof and over the thalami, likely as a result of previous ventriculitis.

In *intraventricular hemorrhage*, especially in the germinal matrix hemorrhages in premature babies, hemorrhage into the ventricular system can result in clotting in and obstruction of the aqueduct, with subsequent obstructive hydrocephalus. The survivors may require permanent ventriculoperitoneal shunt to alleviate the pressure.[315] *Aqueduct* stenosis, atresia, gliosis, or septum may be suspected grossly as a pinpoint, if any, aqueduct **(Fig. 1-147)** and can

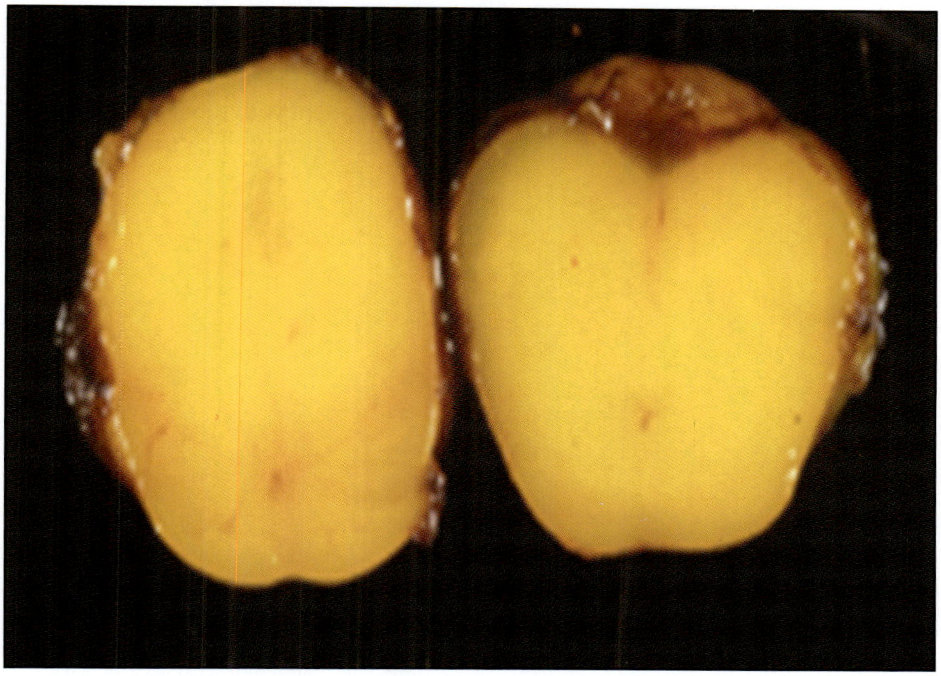

Figure 1-147. Aqueductal stenosis in a fetal brain, resulting in the hydrocephalus seen in Fig. 1-144. The aqueduct is barely visible as a pit.

be further characterized based on microscopic features. It may be sporadic, genetic, or associated with a variety of factors, such as previous infection or hemorrhage, Arnold-Chiari malformation, craniosynostosis, mumps meningoencephalitis, or hydranencephaly, among others.[308,316,317] In adults, intraparenchymal hemorrhage may dissect the neuroglial parenchyma to reach the ventricular system. Even aneurysmal hemorrhages from the basal arteries may dissect through the brain parenchyma to reach the ventricular system. Such cases are usually obvious by the epicenter of hemorrhage on the base of the brain, directing the attention to the basal vasculature; however, a thorough evaluation of all potential sources is required in any hemorrhage to accurately identify its origin.

A variety of *intraventricular neoplasms and nonneoplastic mass lesions* can be identified.[318] In tuberous sclerosis, *multiple firm nodules* of variable sizes protrude into the lumen from the ventricular surfaces. In the same context, SEGAs are larger with solid cut surfaces and can fill up and occlude an entire ventricle. They are most commonly seen in the region of foramen of Monro and lateral ventricles in children and young adults. SEGA, subependymal nodules, radial glioneuronal heterotopias, and cortical dysplasias (tubers) are seen in tuberous sclerosis complex. SEGA is usually solitary but may occasionally be multiple and involve more than one ventricle. Multiple subependymal nodules produce a ventricular surface appearance described as *candle guttering*[319,320] **(Fig. 1-148)**. Ependymoma can also protrude into the lumen as a well-circumscribed mass. Subependymoma[321,322] is a nodular neoplasms that bulges into the ventricle lumen and is typically identified incidentally during work-up for some other condition or at autopsy. Rarely, it can present with obstruction of CSF circulation and may be received as a surgical specimen or as a surprise at IOC. It can also be seen in the spinal cord, where it tends to be eccentric, rather than central. Ependymomas and choroid plexus neoplasms in the fourth ventricle may extend through foramina of Magendie and Luschka, creating a *"dumbbell" tumor*. These foramina can also be obstructed by reactive and nonneoplastic lesions such as gliosis and arachnoid cyst, resulting in noncommunicating hydrocephalus. Choroid plexus tumors are seen in association with choroid plexus. Central neurocytoma is also intraventricular with attachments to ventricular walls and/or septum pellucidum.[323] Colloid cyst of the third ventricle is a well-defined cyst with mucinous content and smooth surfaces **(Fig. 1-149)**. Rare intraventricular liponeurocytomas have been reported.[324] In the region of third

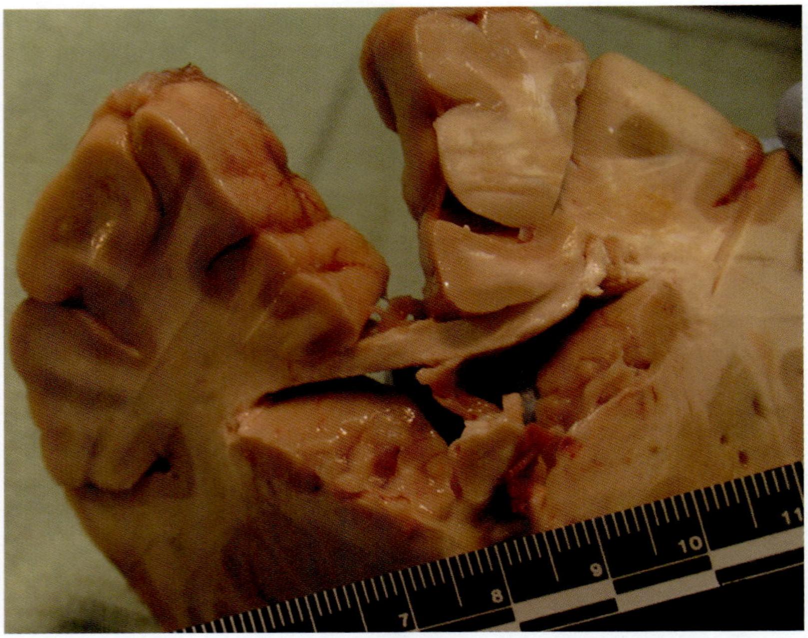

Figure 1-148. Irregular nodular surfaces of the lateral ventricles, mainly over the basal ganglia, due to subependymal nodules in a patient with tuberous sclerosis.

ventricle, mass lesions specifically arising from the anterior portion of the ventricle may represent chordoid glioma (thought to arise from organum vasculosum),[325] while one in the posterior aspect of the third ventricle may represent papillary tumor of the pineal region (PTPR; thought to arise from specialized ependyma of the subcommissural organ).[326] In the pineal region, pineal parenchymal tumors and germ cell tumors, the two most common neoplasms in this location, also tend to grow into the ventricle.[327] Pineal parenchymal tumors, regardless of the grade, and other mass lesions in the pineal region, especially germ cell neoplasms, also frequently result in hydrocephalus. Essentially, any of the intraventricular mass lesions can interfere with CSF circulation and result in hydrocephalus. In addition, hydrocephalus may simply occur due to overproduction of CSF without any interference with its flow in cases of large choroid plexus neoplasms or hyperplasias.[328] Therefore, ventricular system should be examined carefully, especially in cases of hydrocephalus, in an attempt to identify such lesions. Some of these neoplasms, such as pineoblastomas, germ cell tumors, and ependymomas, may also "coat" the ventricular surfaces, leptomeningeal surfaces, or cause drop metastases in the form of multiple nodules. *Parasitic cysts* can be identified within the ventricles. Cysticercosis may be numerous, mainly in the meninges, cortex, and ventricles.[329] When the organism is dead, it forms a firm white nodule, which eventually calcifies **(Fig. 1-150)**. Clear cysts may float in the ventricles or subarachnoid space. Coenurosis (Coenurus cerebralis) forms cysts that measure several centimeters within the ventricles, especially the fourth ventricle, and subarachnoid space.[214]

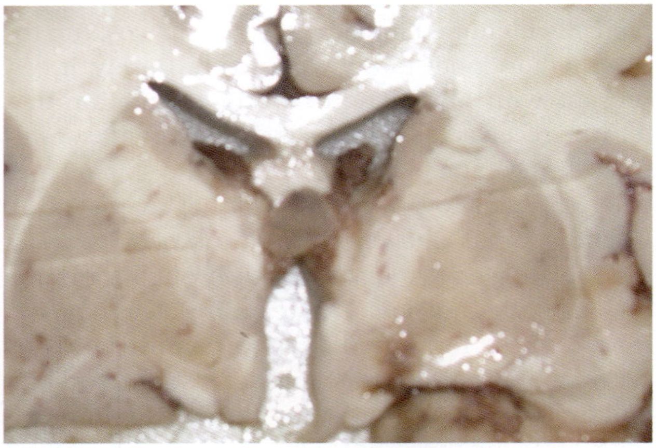

Figure 1-149. Incidental colloid cyst at the level of foramen of Monro, apparently with no obstruction, as the patient did not have history of syncope due to sudden obstruction. Lateral ventricles are not particularly dilated to indicate any long-term obstruction. Cut surface of the cyst appears tan and solid due to condensation of the mucinous contents during fixation.

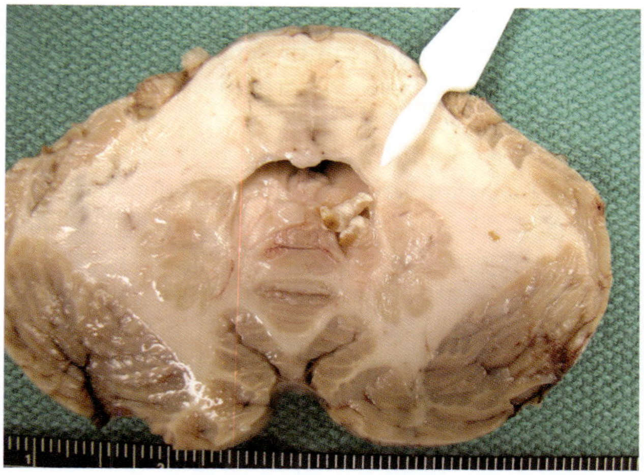

Figure 1-150. Multinodular calcified tan-white dead cysticerci on the surface of the fourth ventricle.

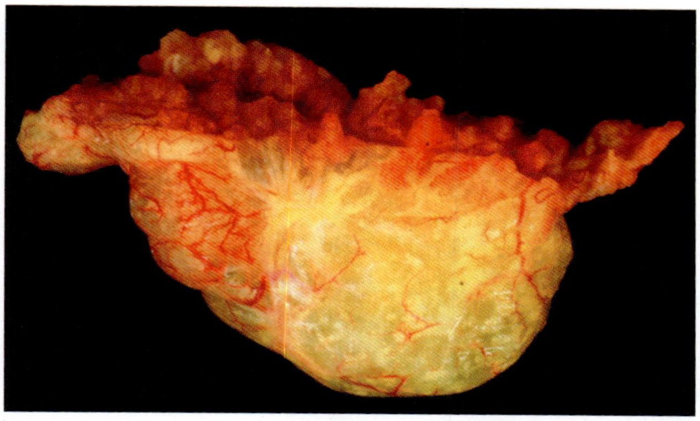

Figure 1-151. Incidental choroid plexus cyst is a common finding in adults but may be associated with syndromes in pediatric population.

Choroid Plexus

Choroid plexus can also be affected by the *infections* involving the ventricles (see also "Ventricular System" above). It is very common to see *cysts* as an incidental finding in autopsy cases **(Fig. 1-151)**. These vary from a few millimeters to usually about 1.0 cm, can be single or multiple, and are transparent with colorless to light yellow clear fluid content. Most common location is in the lateral ventricles. While they are of no known significance in adults, they may be associated with syndromes such as trisomy 18 or 21 in fetuses[330,331] **(Fig. 1-152)**. In older children and especially in boys, as well as in adults, some can grow larger to become symptomatic by obstructing foramen of Monro.[332,333] In premature and term infants, choroid plexus is a common location for *hemorrhages* and is a common source of intraventricular hemorrhages[334,335] **(Fig. 1-153)**. They are also common in cases of difficult delivery. Many, on the other hand, may not have any identifiable cause.

As for *mass lesions*, choroid plexus is a common location for xanthogranuloma and xanthoma.[336] Xanthogranuloma is usually bilateral in the trigone or atrium of lateral ventricle and can result in hydrocephalus **(Fig. 1-154)**. They are firm, well-circumscribed nodules of variable sizes with variegated cut surfaces due to hemorrhage, lipids, fibrosis,

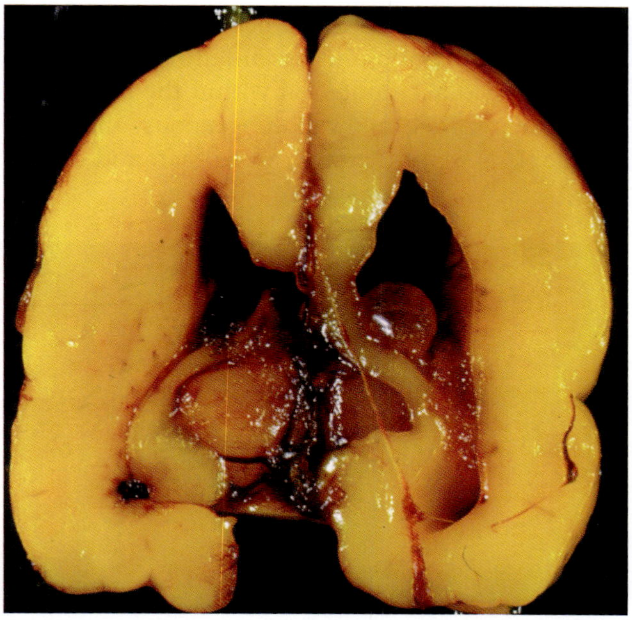

Figure 1-152. Choroid plexus cyst in the right ventricle in a fetus with multiple abnormalities and intrauterine demise.

List of Findings/Checklist for Choroid Plexus

AT A GLANCE

- Infection
- Cyst (incidental or syndromic)
- Hemorrhage
- Neoplasms (primary, associated with syndromes, metastatic)

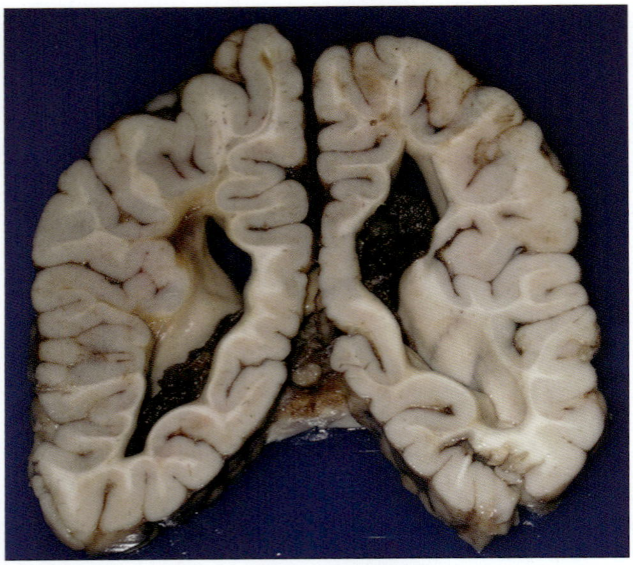

Figure 1-153. Prominent bilateral choroid plexus hemorrhage is seen in this infant's brain as well as subarachnoid hemorrhage is on the parasagittal region (top part of the picture), suggesting an acute/recent event. Extensive and widespread white matter loss is also present, along with rusty discoloration and cystic changes in the left periventricular areas, indicating a previous hemorrhagic, destructive process, such as periventricular leukomalacia. Altogether, these findings suggest a hypoxic/ischemic process.

inflammation, and cystic change. Xanthoma is typically asymptomatic and essentially entirely composed of lipid accumulation within the histiocytes and is therefore a yellow, homogeneous, and softer nodule. It is more common in women and can be associated with hypercholesterolemia.[337] Other nonneoplastic lesions can be seen, such as inflammatory pseudotumor.[338] Choroid plexus neoplasms commonly result in obstructive hydrocephalus, which is compounded by the excess CSF production by the voluminous neoplasm. Their papillary architecture, especially of papillomas, is reflected in their granular, cauliflower-like velvety surface. Large, bilateral papillomas may result in a hydrocephalus that cannot be alleviated by shunt. As papillomas develop more atypical features with solid areas and in choroid plexus carcinomas, due to the prominent loss of papillary architecture, their surfaces become smoother as the degree of malignancy increases. Carcinomas tend to be brain-invasive, and therefore, they may be difficult to separate from the neuroglial parenchyma. Choroid plexus neoplasms can sometimes be associated with various syndromes, for example, Aicardi syndrome,[339] Li-Fraumeni syndrome,[340] Down syndrome,[341] and von Hippel-Lindau syndrome.[342] Choroid plexus carcinoma is almost exclusively a neoplasm of childhood and is located in lateral ventricles. In adults, choroid plexus neoplasms are also equally common in the fourth ventricle.[343] They can grow out of the fourth ventricle through foramina of Luschka to present as cerebellopontine angle tumors, resulting in a dumbbell shape, raising the differential diagnostic possibility of ependymoma in this location and with this presentation. Other neoplasms can present as choroid plexus masses, for example, meningioma[344] or metastatic carcinomas[345] that can be the solitary presentation of

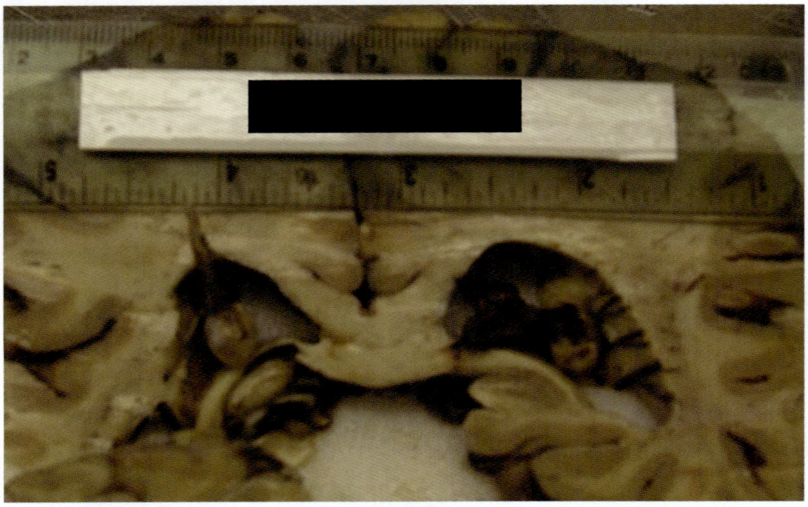

Figure 1-154. Bilateral xanthogranulomas in the choroid plexus, seen as round tan-yellow nodules, an incidental finding.

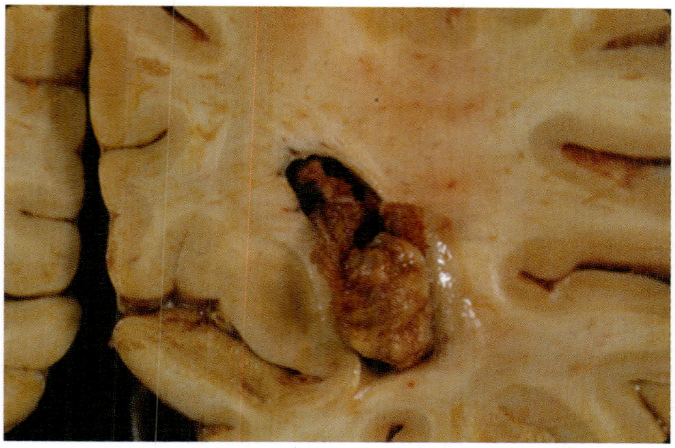

Figure 1-155. This lobular choroid plexus nodule was the only finding in the CNS and represented a metastatic ovarian papillary serous carcinoma. Such lesions can be seen as surgical specimens as metastatic carcinoma of unknown primary and can be challenging during IOC.

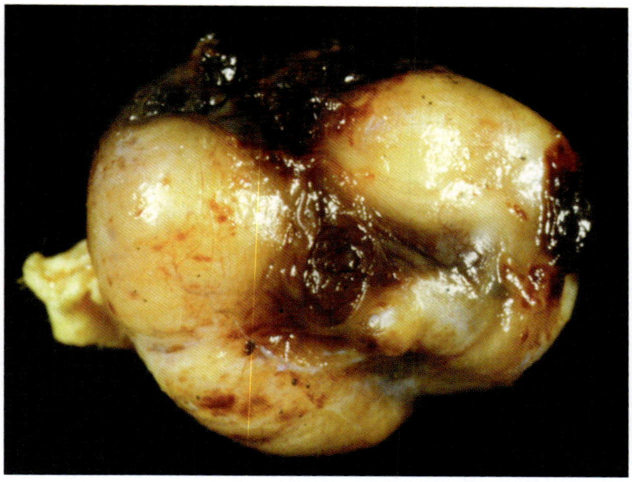

Figure 1-156. Mixed germ cell tumor in the pineal region. It is lobular with smooth surfaces and *tan-yellow* areas, suggesting the presence of adipose tissue.

an unknown primary **(Fig. 1-155)**. It can also be involved by the infiltration of a nearby neoplasm, mainly a high-grade glioma.

Pineal Region

Pineal gland is *normally* a tan-brown round, soft, well-circumscribed structure measuring approximately 1.0 cm and can easily be found by separating the brain and cerebellum from the posterior view. It is a common place for *calcifications* of various sizes that are normally present in the gland as an age-related change. When they are many and large, they are sometimes referred to as brain sand. Also common to see in the pineal parenchyma are one or more cysts of variable size, sometimes up to 1.0 cm to leave only a thin rim of pineal parenchyma surrounding it. They are filled with clear fluid and have smooth lining.

List of Findings/Checklist for Pineal Region

• AT A GLANCE

- Calcifications
- Cyst
- Neoplasms

In terms of *neoplasms*, pineal region and suprasellar region are the first two most common intracranial sites for GCT, followed by basal ganglia.[346] The cerebral hemispheres are more often involved in metastatic GCT and may be multifocal, just like in other metastatic neoplasms.[347] As such, calcifications and ossifications associated with these neoplasms can also be identified in these regions. Depending on the components of the neoplasm, a variety of appearances, cystic and solid areas, hair, and keratinous debris can be seen **(Figs. 1-156 and 1-157)**. The second most common

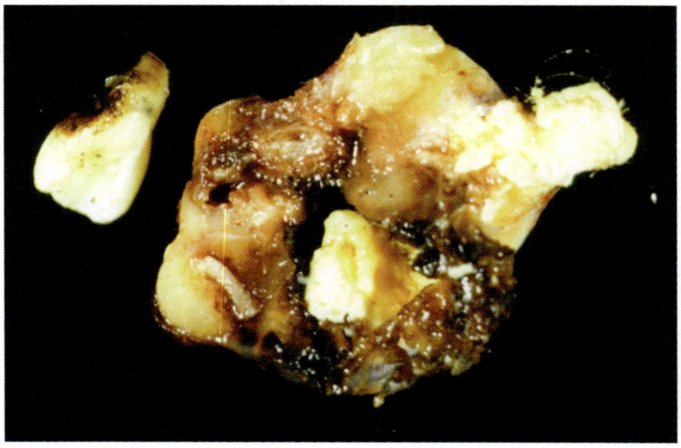

Figure 1-157. Cut surface of the neoplasm in Figure 1-156. Keratinous debris and hair are present in the teratoma, and solid areas contain other components.

neoplasms in this region are neoplasms that arise from the pineal parenchyma, that is, pineal parenchymal tumors including pineocytoma, pineal parenchymal tumor of intermediate differentiation, and pineoblastoma, the latter representing a PNET in this region.[327] They are fleshy, solid tan-white, and soft. Relatively rarely, glial neoplasms, such as glioblastoma and pilocytic astrocytoma, can also arise in this region.[348] A pigmented mass lesion may represent a melanotic neuroectodermal tumor of infancy (progonoma).[349] Papillary tumor of the pineal region[350] is specifically located close to the posterior commissure and, due to its papillary architecture, has a granular or lobulated surface. A number of rare neoplastic and nonneoplastic conditions, as well as metastatic neoplasms, can also be seen in the pineal region.

The neoplasms in the pineal region grow upward to protrude into the third ventricle due to the location of the pineal gland. Especially germ cell neoplasms and pineoblastomas then tend to seed the CSF and spread to the other areas of the CNS through subarachnoid space.[351–353]

Sellar/Suprasellar Region

The region of sella turcica is a very colorful area due to diverse tissues and a multitude of neoplastic and nonneoplastic lesions that occur there. Examination of this very small region grossly can be difficult and also requires particular attention during the removal of the brain at autopsy. Examination of skull base after removal of the brain should be routine and should include the sella before and after the pituitary gland is removed. In some cases, the bony structures forming the sella can be removed as a block cutting a roughly cubical block of bone around the sella. This allows for future evaluation of the pituitary gland and sella, and in some cases where a particular pathologic process is sought, cutting the block in whole in various planes after fixation can provide better views of the process. In addition, this way, the cavernous sinuses can also be evaluated on both sides of the sella, by cutting through the bone and exposing the cavernous sinus to sample for microscopic examination. Cavernous sinus can be involved by numerous, wide variety of reactive, inflammatory, infectious, neoplastic, and vascular disorders,[354] which can go undetected if not specifically sought.

List of Findings/Checklist for Sellar/Suprasellar Region

AT A GLANCE

- Cavernous sinuses
- Diaphragm
- Empty sella (primary or secondary)
- Pituitary stalk
- Posterior pituitary
- Cysts
- Necrosis/hemorrhage
- Pituitary adenoma
- Invasive adenoma
- Other neoplasms
- Sella and bones
- Suprasellar region
- Inflammatory/infectious processes

Empty sella syndrome[355] is the reduction of the volume of intrasellar contents, resulting in a partially or completely empty sella. In its primary form, arachnoid membrane, with accompanying CSF and its pressure, herniates through a defective diaphragm to result in pressure on and atrophy of the intrasellar structures. Secondary forms occur as a result of primary volume loss within the sella, such as postradiation necrosis, infarction of a pituitary adenoma, or as a result of removal or involution of a mass lesion.

Intrasellar lesions creating enough mass effect but are still confined to the sella can stretch the *diaphragm, with a dome shape* and are tense to palpation. Larger lesions, especially neoplasms, tend to infiltrate through the diaphragm to present as overt *mass lesions*. These include invasive adenomas of the anterior pituitary and neoplasms of the posterior pituitary, such as pituicytomas, meningiomas arising from the diaphragm or adjacent dura. Craniopharyngiomas and germ cell neoplasms are usually large and prominent enough to essentially always be readily visible in the suprasellar region. Suprasellar region is the second most common site in general for germ cell neoplasms but is the preferred site in females.[346] Craniopharyngioma is typically cystic with variegated cut surfaces due to hemorrhage, solid areas, and keratinous debris. Rathke's cleft *cysts* with their mucinous, opaque content are common and may be incidental findings. It is not unusual to find incidental pituitary adenomas and granular cell tumors.[356] They are usually identified upon microscopic examination.

Pituitary adenomas or hyperplasias and Rathke cleft cysts can have spontaneous *hemorrhage* in them, which can be identified grossly. Pituitary apoplexy is a neurosurgical emergency that presents with sudden and severe headaches,[357–359] eventually resulting in *necrosis*. In addition, hyperplastic or adenomatous pituitary gland can undergo ischemic infarction, creating a pale, soft appearance. A typical example is Sheehan syndrome, where hyperplastic pituitary undergoes ischemic necrosis due to peripartum or puerperal blood loss.[360] Pituitary adenomas can invade the surrounding structures, that is, *invasive adenoma*, regardless of their micro- or macroadenoma status, although this is commonly seen in association with macroadenomas, which expand the sella, then invade the diaphragm or capsule, to extend into bone, sphenoid sinus, nasopharynx, cavernous sinus, posterior pituitary, and cranial nerves and vascular structures. While this may occur with any type of adenoma, prolactinomas, silent subtype III adenomas, Nelson adenomas, Crooke cell adenomas, acidophil stem cell adenomas, TSH, and prolactin cell adenomas are particularly prone to become invasive adenomas.[361,362] Pituitary adenomas are classified, based on their size, as *microadenoma* if they are smaller than 1.0 cm and *macroadenoma* if larger.[363] Adenomas are tan, solid, and rarely with cystic areas, especially if there has been apoplexy. They are softer than the nonneoplastic gland. Prolactinomas, silent corticotroph cell adenomas, gonadotroph adenomas, TSH cell adenomas, null cell adenomas, and silent subtype III adenomas tend to be macroadenomas, while the corticotroph adenomas, with the exception of those associated with Nelson syndrome (Nelson adenomas), tend to be microadenomas.[363]

There may be irregular, firm, fibrous, nodular changes, and adhesion in and around the sella, as this region is favored by several *inflammatory and infectious processes*,[364] such as lymphocytic hypophysitis, granulomatous inflammations, and even hematolymphoid lesions such as Langerhans cell histiocytosis. In inflammatory conditions, the gland may initially become enlarged but later smaller and firm due to shrinkage associated with fibrosis.

Traumatic *transaction of the pituitary stalk*, as well as functional "transaction" due to compression from a mass lesion, results in dysfunction of the hypothalamic pituitary axis. Just like the cranial nerve avulsions, this should be evaluated on a case by case basis when there is history of trauma, but an attempt should be made to inspect it during removal of the brain. True traumatic transections are associated with evidence of fresh or remote hemorrhage and granulation tissue, depending on the time elapsed. There may be other evidence of traumatic injury in the neighboring structures.[365] In difficult cases, microscopic examination is helpful with distinguishing true traumatic injury from artifactual tissue tears, though even the subtle changes may not form in cases of instantaneous death.

Cystic Lesions

Very diverse lesions can present as a cyst or can have a cystic component. Some represent true cysts, some are degenerative in nature, and some assume a cystic appearance at some point in their evolution. Developmental, infectious, vascular, or neoplastic processes, among others, can result in cyst formation. Examination of the *scalp/skin* can reveal *subcutaneous nodules* of variable sizes that actually represent meningo- or meningoencephaloceles or meningomyeloceles.[366] Some such nodular soft skin masses can also be primary skin cysts, such as *epidermoid* or *trichilemmal* cysts. Both epidermoid and *dermoid* cysts can also present as subcutaneous cysts and may have connection to or origin from calvarial bones due to embryonic remnants entrapped within the bone.[367] Dermoid cysts are more often midline, subcutaneous, associated with a fontanelle or other sutures.[368] All of these cystic lesions can also be seen in the skin overlying the spine. *Spongy cystic space* within a bone or in the soft tissues may represent a *hemangioma* **(Fig. 1-158)**[369] or an *aneurysmal bone cyst*.[370] The latter can be a pure aneurysmal bone cyst or may represent a *secondary cyst formation* in another neoplasm, such as giant cell tumor of bone,[371] chondroblastoma,[372] osteoblastoma,[373] or fibrous dysplasia.[374] They are common in the spine and may cause spinal cord compression.[375] Cyst content is hemorrhagic. *Synovial* cysts arise commonly from

List of Findings/Checklist for Cystic Lesions

AT A GLANCE

- *Skin/subcutaneous*
  - Epidermoid
  - Dermoid
  - Trichilemmal/sebaceous
- *Bone*
  - Aneurysmal bone cyst (isolated or secondary)
  - Synovial
- *CNS*
  - Dural
  - Arachnoid
  - Glioependymal
  - Colloid
  - Rathke cleft cyst
  - Endodermal (enterogenous; neuroenteric)
  - Nerve root
  - Choroid plexus (see "Choroid Plexus")
  - Pineal (see "Pineal Region")
- *Neoplastic*
  - Germ cell neoplasm
  - Craniopharyngioma
  - Low grade with cyst and mural nodule
  - Schwannoma
  - Ependymoma
  - Glioblastoma
  - Meningioma
- *Parenchymal destruction*
  - Subependymal matrix cyst
  - Cystic encephalopathy
  - Syringomyelia
  - Others
- *Malformations*

the vertebral facet joints and are most commonly seen in the lumbar region.[376,377]

Dural cysts are rare lesions located within the dura mater layers **(Fig. 1-159)**. As such, they have fibrous tissue walls with an irregular, somewhat trabecular lining surface. They can be a few centimeters or can grow to large sizes. They can cause obstruction of a dural sinus.[378] *Arachnoid* cysts are seen as clear CSF-filled depressions of the brain surface and are covered by the thin, transparent arachnoid membrane.[379,380] They can represent true cysts that are of developmental origin and can be associated with other developmental abnormalities,[381,382] but some may also be associated with lesions of neoplastic, inflammatory, or traumatic origin,[383] suggesting a possible secondary compensatory CSF accumulation in response to tissue destruction **(Fig. 1-160)**. When an arachnoid cyst is opened or punctured, it collapses, and submitting orderly, well-oriented sections of its wall for microscopic examination is essentially impossible; however, the overlying clumped-up arachnoid membrane can be submitted as a whole, and its arachnoid nature can be confirmed that way. *Rathke cleft cyst*,[384] typically in the sella, *colloid cyst* of the third ventricle[385] **(Fig. 1-161)**, and *endodermal* (enterogeneous, enteric or neuroenteric) cysts **(Fig. 1-162)**, typically in the spinal

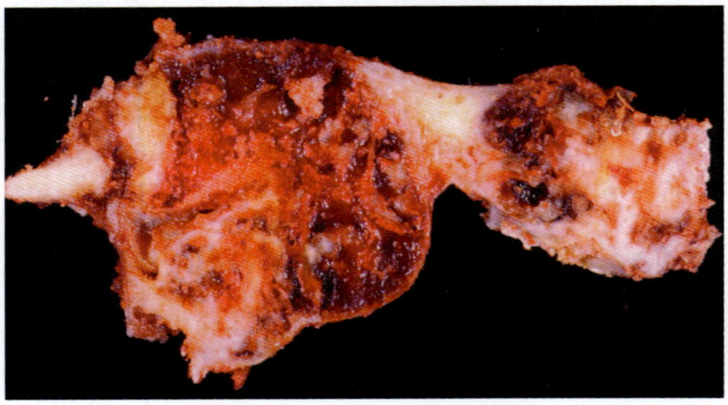

Figure 1-158. Cavernous hemangioma of calvarial bone appears like a spongy blood-filled cystic lesion.

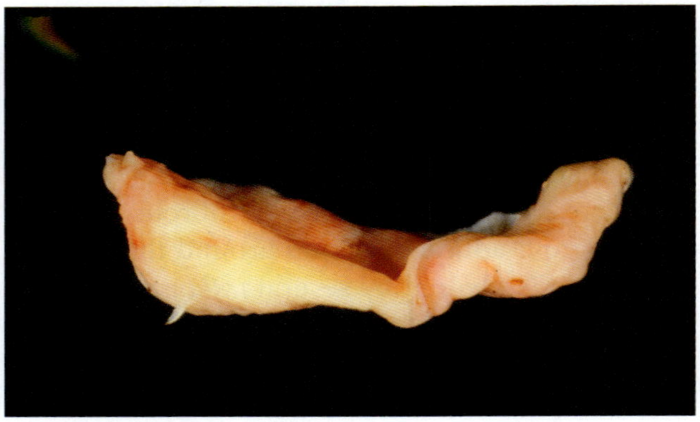

Figure 1-159. Collapsed dural cyst with thick fibrous walls.

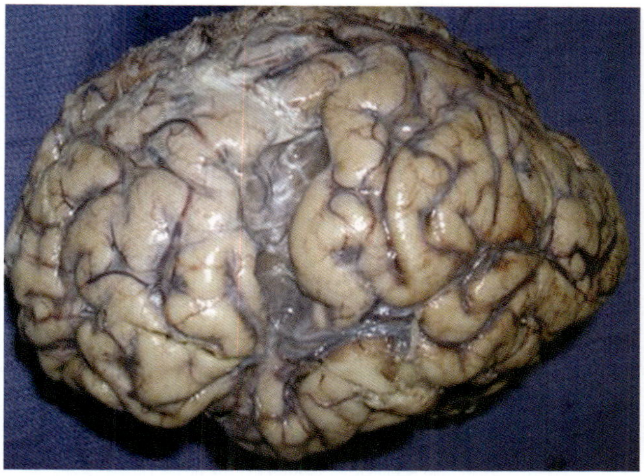

Figure 1-160. A CSF-filled cyst that is covered by arachnoid membrane has formed as a result of the collapse of the underlying parenchyma because of a large remote infarct.

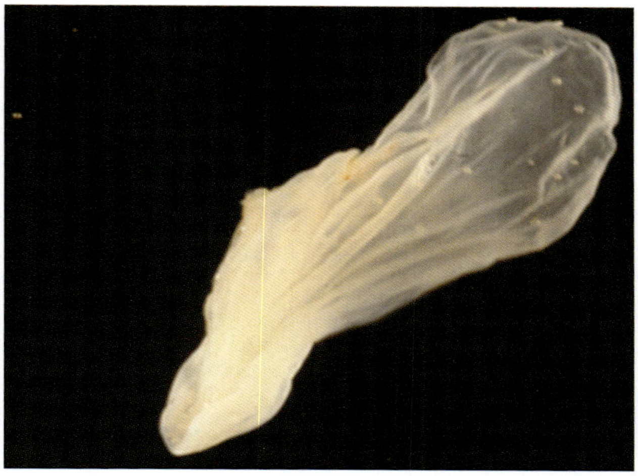

Figure 1-162. Spinal endodermal cyst surgically removed intact with clear contents and delicate wall.

canal[386] but rarely can be seen intracranially,[387] are other cystic lesions that are considered to be developmental in origin but are usually seen in the context of surgical neuropathology in practice as well as a rare incidental finding at autopsy. Endodermal cysts are typically located anterior to the spinal cord, in the subarachnoid space. Some, especially if located in the lumbosacral region, can be associated with other malformations such as spinal dysraphism, vertebral abnormalities, and internal organ malformations.[388,389] Occasionally, they can be intracranial at the cerebellopontine angle, within the ventricles, or even in cerebral hemispheres. *Craniopharyngioma* is typically a suprasellar neoplasm, which typically has a cystic component.[384] *Schwannoma* frequently undergoes degenerative changes to result in a cystic component. A cystic lesion, possibly of degenerative in nature, associated with spinal nerve roots is *Tarlov cyst* (nerve root cyst).[390] *Glioependymal* (ependymal) cysts are usually septated, variably sized cysts found in association with the ventricles, in cerebral hemispheres, brainstem, or spinal cord.[391,392] They can also be extra-axial[393] leading to the thought that they may arise from heterotopic neuroglial tissue. (See "Choroid Plexus" for choroid plexus cysts, "Pineal Region" for pineal cysts, and Chapter 2 for the microscopic features and differential diagnoses of the cystic structures discussed here.)

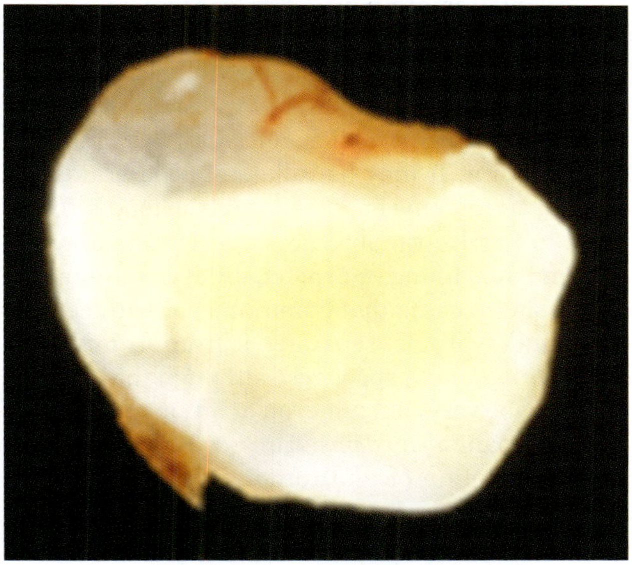

Figure 1-161. Colloid cyst that was surgically removed intact appears to have a solid cut surface due to condensation of its mucinous contents after fixation in formalin. Thin cyst wall is seen on the top part of the lesion.

In *hydranencephaly*, the entire brain becomes a large cyst with the brain parenchyma, if any, remaining as a thin rim surrounding the cavity **(Fig. 1-163)**. Destructive versus developmental nature of this abnormality is debatable; however, an extensive loss of parenchyma is the main feature.[394] *Malformations* can be accompanied by a cystic component, and their accurate classification may be complicated.[395] For instance, *Dandy-Walker malformation* has a cyst filled with CSF and

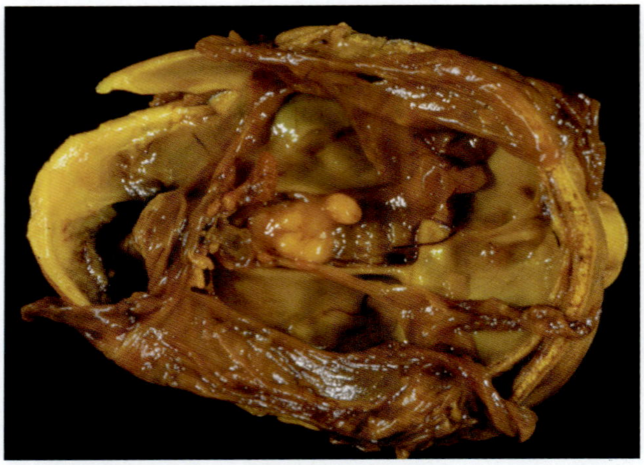

Figure 1-163. Hydranencephaly in a fetus with intrauterine demise, showing essentially entirely absent intracranial contents with only a thin membranous leptomeningeal and pial tissue remaining.

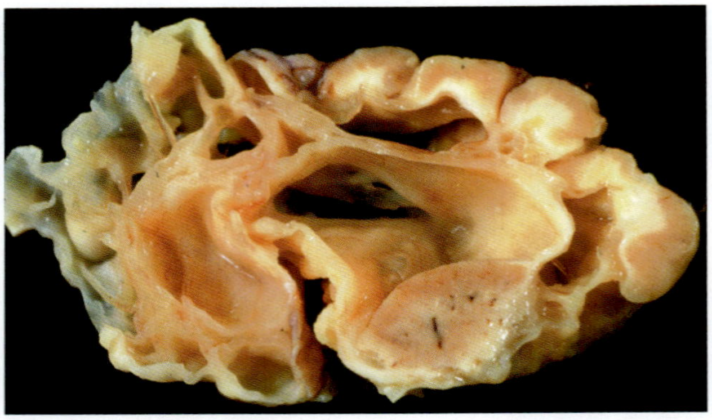

Figure 1-164. The entire brain has become a multicystic structure with very small amount of solid parenchyma left in this multicystic leukoencephalopathy due to extensive hypoxic/ischemic destruction.

covered by arachnoid membrane in place of the absent vermis. *Cavum septi pellucidi* and *cavum vergae* may appear like intraventricular cysts.

Cystic degeneration of the brain parenchyma can be the result of a degenerative process. Such cysts occur in larger lesions, while the actual lesions are usually in the form of irregular softening and friability of the parenchyma. For instance, *Leigh's disease*[396] and *mitochondrial disorders* can result in such cystic degenerations.[397] *Metabolic and neurodegenerative diseases of childhood*, such as megalencephalic leukoencephalopathy with subcortical cysts[398] and vanishing white matter disease,[399] can result in variable infarct-like cavities within the white matter. *Infarcts*, in their chronic/remote stages, tend to become cystic, as the necrotic debris is cleared out. They tend to have irregular, collapsed borders, which may show tan-yellow-brown discoloration if a hemorrhagic component was present. Likewise, in neonatal period, *periventricular leukomalacia*, depending on its extent and stage, can result in periventricular cysts within the white matter. They may vary from a few millimeters to many centimeters. The latter is termed cystic or multicystic leukomalacia or encephalopathy **(Fig. 1-164)**. They are similar to chronic infarcts where the resorption of the necrotic contents leaves behind a cyst.[400] Subependymal matrix cysts, also known as periventricular cysts, may form as a result of resolution of previous destructive lesions, such as hemorrhage. *Hypoxic/ischemic damage* in the developing brain can result in variable degree of tissue loss and cysts. Some examples are porencephaly, schizencephaly, and basket brain. *Syringomyelia* is a longitudinal cavity in spinal cord of variable length, typically involving several segments. It is usually seen in cervical and upper thoracic levels as a slit-like transverse cavity posterior to central canal and may be due to traumatic injury[401] or a variety of nontraumatic causes, such as vascular, neoplastic, and inflammatory disorders.[402] Many idiopathic cases may be associated with Chiari I malformation.[403] If it involves the medulla oblongata, then it is called *syringobulbia*. In the brainstem, the slit is behind the fourth ventricle and may be communicating with it. It may be isolated in the brainstem without syringomyelia. It can rarely extend into the brain to involve the internal capsule. The absence of ependymal lining, except focally at the communication site in cases that communicate with central canal and ventricle, separates it from *hydromyelia and hydrobulbia*, respectively, although this distinction may be very difficult even at autopsy.

Malignant *neoplasms* can become cystic due to the resorption of intratumoral hemorrhage and necrosis. *Germ cell neoplasms*, especially mature cystic teratomas, have keratinous hairy material in the cyst lumen. They are typically found in the pineal and suprasellar regions. Large metastatic *squamous cell carcinomas* can also appear cystic due to abundant necrosis and keratin content, which may even mimic pus to cause confusion with an abscess on gross examination. Of the primary neoplastic processes, several are well-known for their cystic nature. *Pilocytic astrocytoma, ganglioglioma, PXA, and hemangioblastoma* typically present with a cyst and mural nodule formation. The cystic component is usually difficult to appreciate in surgical resection specimens, both due to the fragmented nature of the specimen and due to the fact that the mural nodule is the main resected component. *Ependymomas* can frequently have cystic areas that can be identified grossly due to large ependymal canal formation by the neoplastic cells. Rarely, *GBM*[404] and *meningioma*[405] can be predominantly cystic.

One or more and usually multiple cystic lesions within the brain parenchyma may represent infectious processes. Better-known ones are cysticercosis,[406] which can be parenchymal, intraventricular, or subarachnoid; hydatid cysts[407]; amebic abscesses; and bacterial abscesses. Depending on the stage of development of the process, abscesses have granulation tissue wall and pus-filled lumen. Amebic abscesses have hemorrhagic, necrotic contents and an ill-defined border. Cysticercus and echinococcal cysts, unless complicated by rupture, hemorrhage, and inflammation, have clear white fluid, and the organisms can be seen in them. While Echinococcus granulosus has a solitary cyst, Echinococcus alveolaris (multilocularis) consists of multiple small cysts, creating a sponge-like interior. Coenurosis (Coenurus cerebralis) produces cysts that measure several centimeters, especially in the ventricles and subarachnoid space. The thin cyst wall is white, with no fibrous capsule.[214] Angioinvasive fungal microorganisms result in hemorrhagic necrotic, one or more lesions of variable sizes (see "Parenchymal Hemorrhage" above). In chronic stages, some of these may be walled-off to form cystic lesions with fibrotic walls. An artifact of delayed fixation and the result of growth of gas-forming bacteria is called "Swiss-cheese" artifact, as there are multiple cysts in the brain parenchyma. The cysts tend to occur in the deeper areas, where the fixative reaches the latest **(Fig. 1-165)**.

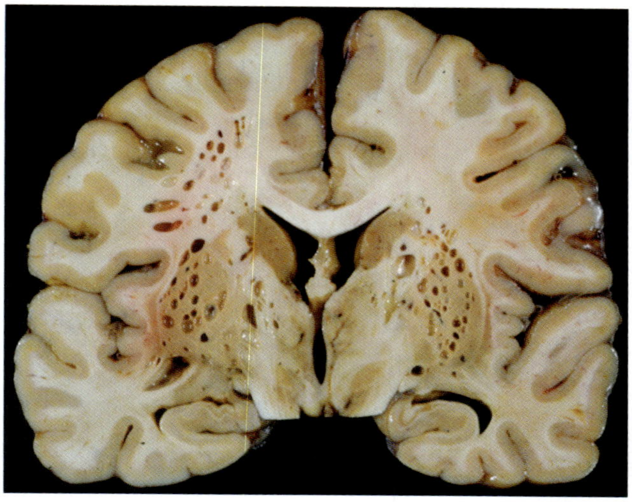

Figure 1-165. Swiss-cheese artifact with multiple cysts. They are located preferentially deeper in the parenchyma.

Surgical Specimens

The specimens received in surgical neuropathology practice are almost always in the form of irregular tissue fragments from resections or tissue cores from stereotactic biopsies. In addition, additional evaluations that are frequent in general surgical pathology practice, such as evaluation of resection margins or sampling particular areas for staging purposes, are not applicable to the neoplastic neuropathology specimens. Inking the specimens is not needed but may be useful for easier identification of small tissues in paraffin block. There are no specific, official

List of Findings/Checklist for Surgical Specimens

AT A GLANCE

- Bone curetting and resections (vertebral, skull base, calvarial)
- Intervertebral discectomy
- Hematoma evaluation
- Open biopsy
- Stereotactic biopsy
- Resection (parenchymal, dural, cavitron ultrasonic surgical aspirator, amygdalohippocampectomy, lobectomy, hemispherectomy, spinal cord)
- Cystic lesions and cyst contents
- Skeletal muscle biopsy (open biopsy, needle biopsy)
- Peripheral nerve biopsy (for medical or surgical disease)
- Cerebrospinal fluid (see Chapter 5)
- Autopsy

widely accepted guidelines or recommendations relating to the number of sections to be submitted for microscopic examination in certain specimens. In fact, in the great majority of specimens, due to the manageable amount of material, the entire specimen can be submitted for processing for microscopic evaluation in several cassettes, with not much more than sectioning the larger fragments is required for optimal processing and for possibly seeing the cut surfaces. Therefore, almost all descriptions and discussions of gross neuropathology are typically centered on autopsy material, with some points applicable to surgical specimens. Below are some comments on several common surgical specimen types received in most practices.

Bone curetting specimens mainly come from *vertebral bones*, such as corpectomy material. They are in the form of irregular, hemorrhagic bone fragments. There may be a soft tissue component that represents tendons, ligaments, and intervertebral or joint cartilage, or paraspinal soft tissues. They tend to stand out among the hemorrhagic bone fragments as gray-white and fibrous, elastic fragments. If skeletal muscle is present, it also appears red-hemorrhagic but is soft. These features are important to note if such a specimen is sent for intraoperative consultation and one is trying to select out the bone to freeze only the soft fragments and/or to prevent soft tissue fragments from being unnecessarily decalcified, which can potentially interfere with immunohistochemical and other special techniques. Optimum care of the specimen is important, especially in cases of metastatic neoplasms with unknown primary, which frequently require such subsequent work-up for diagnosis and prognosis. Preservation of cellular detail and architecture is also important for the diagnosis of primary bone and soft tissue lesions.

Similar specimens may also represent infections. Therefore, appropriate evaluation for selection of necrotic, granular, or friable areas for processing becomes important, especially to provide intraoperative guidance for cultures or other studies such as flow cytometry or electron microscopy. Depending on the clinical situation, suspected granulomatous diseases may preclude frozen sectioning and limit the examination to smear preparations, so that contamination of cryostats and laboratory environment is avoided as much as possible. Fracture repair is another common situation in which such bone and soft tissue fragments are received to rule out pathologic fracture. *Skull base* neoplasms may represent primary bone neoplasms, mainly chordoma and chondrosarcoma in clivus or those that infiltrate the bone from adjacent tissues. Bone fragments can be present among the fragments of skull base meningioma that invades the bone. Those should be decalcified and examined microscopically to identify invasion by meningioma. Similar situation with meningiomas is also true for the convexity meningiomas and calvarial bones.

Curetting material can originate from *calvarial bones* and can represent a variety of lesions similar to those elsewhere. More commonly, a roughly circular plate of bone is resected to remove the lesion. Such specimens should be serially sectioned with the saw perpendicular to the calvarium surface to obtain a cross section of the lesion. Most lesions cause a thickening of the bone in that region. Hematolymphoid processes, such as myeloma or Langerhans cell histiocytosis, and vascular lesions, such as hemangiomas, result in a relatively soft area due to bone destruction, with hemorrhagic cut surfaces. Metastatic carcinomas have solid gray-white cut surfaces. Depending on whether they are osteolytic or osteoblastic, their consistency can be variable.

Intervertebral disc material consists of fragments of fibrous cartilage with admixed fragments of fibrous tissue and sometimes bone. Their amount is variable but is usually only enough to fill one or two cassettes with early detection and microdiscectomy procedures, compared to bulkier amounts of the past. They can be submitted entirely, or in larger specimens; the fragments may be inspected, larger fragments sectioned to see the cut surfaces; and representative pieces are submitted for microscopic examination in cases of herniated nucleus pulposus. If there is a question of a specific pathologic process, such as discitis, an attempt should be made to submit the entire material for microscopic examination. Rarely, incidental microscopic findings, such as granulomas or gouty tophi, can be seen in an otherwise unremarkable intervertebral disc material removed for herniated nucleus pulposus, which may prompt examination of the remainder of the material, if it was not submitted in its entirety.

Hematoma evacuation specimens from various compartments in the cranial cavity consist of blood clot fragments. Larger fragments should be sectioned to examine the cut surfaces. There are usually irregular white linear zones representing fibrin. Depending on the age of the hematoma, gray-white and friable granulation tissue fragments, many times in the form of small membranous fragments mainly in subdural hematomas, can be seen. They represent the "pseudomembranes" in organizing hematomas, are more common and prominent in chronic cases, and can be submitted separately by the neurosurgeon, sometimes further separated into inner and outer membranes. Epidural hematomas, being arterial in origin, are too acute and rapidly progressing to develop any degree of organization before they have to be operated on.

Intraparenchymal hematomas should also be examined closely to identify any relatively solid or gray-white areas, as these may represent a metastatic, or rarely a primary neoplasm. Alternatively, such an effort will result in the identification of neuroglial tissue, which can be worked up for the potential cause of the hemorrhage, such as cerebral amyloid angiopathy.

Open biopsy is performed mainly for evaluation of leptomeningeal infiltrations; inflammatory, infectious, or neoplastic processes; vasculopathy; and rarely for neurodegenerative diseases, such as identification of Alzheimer pathology or transmissible spongiform encephalopathy. The specimens consist of multiple pyramidal fragments of superficial neuroglial tissue, the base of the pyramid at the surface and covered by leptomeninges, and the tip usually representing a smaller amount of subcortical white matter. They may vary from a few millimeters to about a centimeter in greatest surface dimension and larger fragments may need to be bisected, while smaller fragments may just be laid on their side, allowing appropriate orientation. While cutting the tissue, care should be taken to make sure the leptomeninges are not stripped off and both gray and white matter are properly demonstrated. The rare biopsies for possible spongiform encephalopathy are done under extreme precautions and should be handled appropriately according to prion disease protocols. In general, gross observations are very limited in these small tissue samples. Levels should be obtained and the skipped ribbons saved for possible future special stains, depending on the situation.

Stereotactic biopsy specimens are essentially needle core biopsy specimens obtained under computerized tomography guidance from focal lesions, which are usually deep-seated. The handling may be different depending on the approach of the neurosurgeon. In some situations, intraoperative consultation may be requested to confirm the diagnostic nature of the material, which is the recommended procedure. In others, the specimen is submitted directly for routine processing. The necrotic, hemorrhagic, pigmented, fragmented solid neoplastic quality and firm or soft consistency can provide some clues as to the abnormal and possibly neoplastic nature of the tissue. Levels should be obtained and the skipped ribbons saved for possible future special stains, depending on the situation.

Resection specimens are large specimens composed of irregular fragments of tissue, usually neoplastic, and may have variable color and consistency depending on the nature of the lesion. Since the specimens are not typically received in whole resections but rather in multiple fragments, and since the standard approach with margin evaluations, size of the neoplasm, lymph node and distant metastases are not applicable to the neoplasms of the CNS due to their very nature, the typical staging systems and procedures that are standard for the neoplasms of other organs and systems are not appropriate for the neoplasms of the CNS. Larger fragments may need to be sectioned to examine the cut surfaces and to trim the tissue for processing. The material is only rarely too large to be submitted entirely in several cassettes. Regardless, it is advisable to submit the entire material for microscopic evaluation in glioma specimens, due to the natural histopathologic heterogeneity of these neoplasms, so that accurate diagnosis and grading can be performed. Many such specimens are submitted by the surgeon divided into several parts, which makes the individual parts manageable even with abundant amount of material. In addition, in some cases, the surgeon may want to know the grades of the neoplasm separately for each part of the specimen, depending on the particular areas the neoplasm may be infiltrating and due to possible treatment and management implications. *Dura-based mass resection* specimens are also composed of fragmented tissue. Sometimes, they can be resected in toto and are received as intact mass lesions attached to a usually round or oval dura mater fragment. Especially in the larger meningioma specimens where the entirety of the neoplasm cannot be submitted for microscopic evaluation, one needs to make sure that the surfaces opposite to the dura are well-sampled, so that any attached brain tissue is included in the sections for the evaluation of brain invasion. Therefore, the specimen should be sectioned perpendicular to the dural surface. Hemorrhagic, necrotic appearing areas should be prioritized. Submitting additional sections from alternating slices provides good representation of the neoplasm. Again, as in the case of gliomas, most specimens can be submitted entirely for microscopic evaluation. During resection of especially meningiomas, a separate strip or piece of dura mater may be sent as *"dural margin"* for intraoperative consultation to evaluate for involvement by meningioma. These specimens are usually sent in cases where the meningioma is close to a dural sinus, so that sinus invasion can be evaluated. The specimen needs to be oriented on its side so that any attached meningioma can be seen microscopically, as it may be too small to be identified grossly. Critical areas of some of these specimens may be identified by the surgeon with a suture. Those may need to be further marked by ink so that they can be specifically evaluated. *Dura mater biopsy* specimens usually go along with open brain biopsy specimens, especially in cases of suspected infectious processes. Larger fragments should be sectioned. Fragments should be oriented on their side for optimal evaluation. *Cavitron ultrasonic surgical aspirator (CUSA)*[408] washings are received in large containers as several hundred milliliters of bloody fluid. They may sometimes be sent to cytopathology due to their mainly liquid nature. In spite of the huge amount of fluid, they yield relatively small amount of tissue fragments. The fluid should be filtered to collect the tissue fragments, which can then be submitted for routine processing. They tend to be soft and slimy if they remained in the fluid for more than several hours and also due to the artifacts produced by the procedure. *Hippocampectomy/amygdalohippocampectomy* procedures are done for seizures. While amygdala component is in the form of irregular fragments with no orienting features, hippocampectomy component deserves some attention. The resected portion of hippocampus is roughly a round, sausage-like structure, in which the hippocampus can be identified on cut surfaces after cross sectioning. If it is too short to be sectioned, it should be laid on its side to be able to visualize the hippocampus on microscopic sections. If specimen size allows, it can be serially sectioned. In cases where there is significant neuron loss and gliosis, the hippocampus appears shrunken and firm. If the specimen is fragmented and no hippocampus is obvious, then individual fragments should be inspected to identify the appearance of hippocampus so that they can be oriented appropriately. *Lobectomy/hemispherectomy* specimens are rare and are done for intractable seizures, usually in infants and young children. They should be fixed well, the surfaces should be inspected for abnormalities of sulcal–gyral pattern, and cut serially, perpendicular to the brain surface, similar to the examination of whole brain. The cut surfaces should be examined similar to that of the autopsy brain slices. *Spinal cord biopsy* specimens are necessarily very small fragments, and one has to be very selective if intraoperative consultation is requested. Otherwise, no specific gross features are expected in these irregular gray-white fragments.

It is very rare for *cystic lesions* to be resected and submitted to pathology intact. Usually, they are fragments of irregular membranous material. Their interior and exterior surfaces should be noted, any contents should be identified, and the cyst wall should be sectioned in strips to be submitted on edge for microscopic examination. If this is not possible due to the large amount of the material, or it has arrived already fixed in an irregular, clumped manner, submitting it as received should not cause a problem, as the cyst wall details and the nature of the cystic lesion will be seen in many areas microscopically, although one should be aware of the potentially worrisome and complex architecture resulting from tangential sectioning. Sometimes, especially when the *cyst contents* are liquid, they are aspirated before the actual resection of the cyst wall and submitted separately in a syringe. They can sometimes be routed to cytopathology as a "body fluid" specimen. They do not typically add much to the information that is gained from the microscopic examination of the cyst wall. However, they can provide an initial idea about the nature of the cyst, for example, "machinery oil" appearance in craniopharyngioma, clear fluid in arachnoid cyst, mucinous or keratinous/hairy in teratoma, mucinous or proteinaceous Rathke cleft cyst, and endodermal cyst. If they represent the only material that will be received from the lesion, then cytopathologic processing with centrifuging and preparation of cytospin slides and cell block sections should be carried out for optimal evaluation.

Skeletal muscle biopsy specimen can be sent in different ways, such as in metal (Price) or plastic (Rayport) clamp, stitched or pinned onto a tongue depressor, or wrapped in saline-soaked gauze. Floating in saline or formalin is not an acceptable way to submit skeletal muscle tissue. It is usually grossly quite unrevealing except in cases where the muscle is infiltrated by adipose tissue or has attached large amount of adipose tissue or skin submitted with it, as may be the case for inflammatory myopathies, especially dermatomyositis. The excisions/resections performed for neoplastic or other focal lesions of the skeletal muscle are the subject of soft tissue pathology and are not considered "muscle biopsy," which is performed for evaluation for medical diseases of the skeletal muscle, although rarely focal lesions that may present as mass lesions can be encountered in this setting as well, for example, focal myositis. Paying attention to the clinical situation assures optimal allocation and use of the tissue. Needle biopsy of the muscle is also becoming popular, mainly due to its surgical advantages. The specimens are typically in the form of tissue cores. *Peripheral nerve biopsy* specimens are also grossly quite unremarkable and consist of a segment of tan-white peripheral nerve with some attached epineurial connective tissue. The changes associated with peripheral nerve sheath tumors are the subject of soft tissue excision/resection material and are not considered "nerve biopsy," which is performed for evaluation for medical diseases of the peripheral nervous system. As with the skeletal muscle, paying attention to the clinical situation will prevent the rare situation of, for example, a traumatic neuroma excision to be processed for electron microscopy. For both muscle and nerve biopsy specimens, protocols for submitting the specimen, including long-distance transfer to consultation centers, and processing the specimens can be found in more detailed, specialized texts on the subject.

CSF is a cytopathology specimen and should be handled as such to prepare cytospin slides after centrifuging. CSF specimen originates most commonly from spinal tap, but also can be obtained by cisterna magna aspiration, ventricular shunt aspiration, or from the Ommaya reservoir. Especially in the latter, small tissue fragments representing granulation tissue, choroid plexus fragments, or pathologic tissue can be present. Therefore, depending on the gross appearance and source, cell block preparations should be considered in addition to cytospin slides. Typically, CSF is a clear, colorless fluid. It tends to be cloudy with inflammation, serosanguineous/red if there is blood (see Chapter 5).

Autopsy procedure is relatively more complicated and can be variable depending on the situation. Neurodegenerative diseases, prion diseases, forensic examination, pediatric cases, and infectious cases require an individualized approach to the specimen in most cases. In addition, which specific areas of the CNS to be sampled for microscopic evaluation is also guided by the particular question that is asked or a group of differential diagnostic possibilities that are being evaluated. For many of these situations, various recommendation protocols are available. In addition, in situations where the material needs to be transferred to another center for consultation or special testing, contacting that particular institution for their requirements is always a good idea and should ideally be done before the autopsy is started.

References

1. Drew LB, Drew WE. The contrecoup–coup phenomenon: a new understanding of the mechanism of closed head injury. *Neurocrit Care*. 2004;1:385–390.
2. Dawson SL, Hirsch CS, Lucas FV, et al. The contrecoup phenomenon. Reappraisal of a classic problem. *Hum Pathol*. 1980;11:155–166.
3. Puttgen KB, Lin DDM. Neurocutaneous vascular syndromes. *Childs Nerv Syst*. 2010;26:1407–1415.
4. Comi AM. Update on Sturge–Weber syndrome: diagnosis, treatment, quantitative measures, and controversies. *Lymph Res Biol*. 2007;5:257–264.
5. Lavin MF. Ataxia-telangiectasia: from a rare disorder to a paradigm for cell signaling and cancer. *Nat Rev Mol Cell Biol*. 2008;9:759–769.
6. Dayani PN, Sadun AA. A case report of Wyburn-Mason syndrome and review of the literature. *Neuroradiology*. 2007;49:445–456.
7. Dupuis-Girod S, Bailly S, Plauchu H. Hereditary hemorrhagic telangiectasia: from molecular biology to patient care. *J Thromb Haemost*. 2010;8:1447–1456.
8. Roach ES, DiMario FJ, Kandt RS, et al. Tuberous Sclerosis Consensus Conference: recommendations for diagnostic evaluation. National Tuberous Sclerosis Association. *J Child Neurol*. 1999;14:401–407.

9. Kandt RS. Tuberous sclerosis complex and neurofibromatosis type 1: the two most common neurocutaneous diseases. *Neurol Clin*. 2002;20:941–964.

10. Steiner J, Adamsbaum C, Desguerres I, et al. Hypomelanosis of Ito and brain abnormalities: MRI findings and literature review. *Pediatr Radiol*. 1996;26:763–768.

11. Ruggieri M, Pavone L. Hypomelanosis of Ito: clinical syndrome or just phenotype? *J Child Neurol*. 2000;15:635–644.

12. Frances C, Piette JC. The mystery of Sneddon syndrome: relationship with antiphospholipid syndrome and systemic lupus erythematosus. *J Autoimmun*. 2000;15:139–143.

13. Muzio LL. Nevoid basal cell carcinoma syndrome (Gorlin syndrome). *Orphanet J Rare Dis*. 2008;3:32–47.

14. Paraf F, Jothy S, Van Meir EG. Brain tumor-polyposis syndrome: two genetic diseases? *J Clin Oncol*. 1997;15:2744–2758.

15. Farooq A, Walker LJ, Bowling J, et al. Cowden syndrome. *Cancer Treat Rev*. 2010;36:577–583.

16. Palmeroa EI, Achatzb MIW, Ashton-Prollac P, et al. Tumor protein 53 mutations and inherited cancer: beyond Li-Fraumeni syndrome. *Curr Opin Oncol*. 2010;22:64–69.

17. Gutmann DH, Aylsworth A, Carey JC, et al. The diagnostic evaluation and multidisciplinary management of neurofibromatosis 1 and neurofibromatosis 2. *JAMA*. 1997;278:51–57.

18. Vezzosi D, Vignaux O, Dupin N, et al. Carney complex: clinical and genetic 2010 update. *Ann Endocrinol*. 2010;71:486–493.

19. Shah KN. The risk of melanoma and neurocutaneous melanosis associated with congenital melanocytic nevi. *Semin Cutan Med Surg*. 2010;29:159–164.

20. Kadonaga JN, Barkovich AJ, Edwards MS, et al. Neurocutaneous melanosis in association with the Dandy-Walker complex. *Pediatr Dermatol*. 1992;9:37–43.

21. Rahimi-Movaghar V, Karimi M. Meningeal melanocytoma of the brain and oculodermal melanocytosis (nevus of Ota): case report and literature review. *Surg Neurol*. 2003;59:200–210.

22. Malca SA, Roche PH, Thomassin JM, et al. An unusual cervical tumor: meningioma. Apropos of a case of petrous origin. Review of the literature of meningioma presenting as cervical mass. *Neurochirurgie*. 1994;40:96–108.

23. Penner CR, Thompson L. Nasal glial heterotopia: a clinicopathologic and immunophenotypic analysis of 10 cases with a review of the literature. *Ann Diagn Pathol*. 2003;7:354–359.

24. Khanna G, Sato Y, Smith RJ, et al. Causes of facial swelling in pediatric patients: correlation of clinical and radiologic findings. *Radiographics*. 2006;26:157–171.

25. Guggisberg D, Hadj-Rabia S, Viney C, et al. Skin markers of occult spinal dysraphism in children: a review of 54 cases. *Arch Dermatol*. 2004;140:1109–1115.

26. Sandler AD. Children with spina bifida: key clinical issues. *Pediatr Clin North Am*. 2010;57:879–892.

27. Copp AJ, Greene NDE. Genetics and development of neural tube defects. *J Pathol*. 2010;220:217–230.

28. Tubbs RS, Lyerly MJ, Loukas M, et al. The pediatric Chiari I malformation: a review. *Childs Nerv Syst*. 2007;23:1239–1250.

29. Dyste GN, Menezes AH, VanGilder JC. Symptomatic Chiari malformations. An analysis of presentation, management, and long-term outcome. *J Neurosurg*. 1989;71:159–168.

30. Gilbert JN, Jones KL, Rorke LB, et al. Central nervous system anomalies associated with meningomyelocele, hydrocephalus, and the Arnold-Chiari malformation: reappraisal of theories regarding the pathogenesis of posterior neural tube closure defects. *Neurosurgery*. 1986;18:559–564.

31. Alexiev BA, Lin X, Sun CC, et al. Meckel-Gruber syndrome: pathologic manifestations, minimal diagnostic criteria, and differential diagnosis. *Arch Pathol Lab Med*. 2006;130:1236–1238.

32. Samii M, Tatagiba M. Skull base trauma: diagnosis and management. *Neurol Res*. 2002;24:147–156.

33. Vignes JR, Jeelani NO, Dautheribes M, et al. Cranioplasty for repair of a large bone defect in a growing skull fracture in children. *J Craniomaxillofac Surg*. 2007;35:185–188.

34. Francel TJ, Birely BC, Ringelman PR, et al. The fate of plates and screws after facial fracture reconstruction. *Plast Reconstr Surg*. 1992;90:568–573.

35. Kim YO, Park BY. Reverse temporalis muscle flap: treatment of large anterior cranial base defect with direct intracranial-nasopharyngeal communication. *Plast Reconstr Surg*. 1995;96:576–584.

36. Uchil D, Arulkumaran S. Neonatal subgaleal hemorrhage and its relationship to delivery by vacuum extraction. *Obstet Gynecol Surv*. 2003;58:687–693.

37. Stergios K, Arulkumaran D, Arulkumaran S. Head injuries after instrumental vaginal deliveries. *Curr Opin Obstet Gynecol*. 2006;18:129–134.

38. Dolinak D, Matshes E. *Medicolegal Neuropathology: A Color Atlas*. Boca Raton, FL: CRC Press; 2002.

39. Kemp A, Dunstan F, Harrison S, et al. Patterns of skeletal fractures in child abuse: systematic review. *BMJ*. 2008;337:a1518.

40. Johnson K. Skeletal aspects of non-accidental injury. *Endocr Dev*. 2009;16:233–245.

41. Viel G, Gehl A, Sperhake JP. Intersecting fractures of the skull and gunshot wounds. Case report and literature review. *Forensic Sci Med Pathol*. 2009;5:22–27.

42. Voigt GE, Skold G. Ring fractures of the base of the skull. *J Trauma*. 1974;14:494–505.

43. Mohindra S, Kumar Mukherjee K, Chhabra R, et al. Orbital roof growing fractures: a report of four cases and literature review. *Br J Neurosurg*. 2006;20:420–423.

44. Kienstra MA, Van Loveren H. Anterior skull base fractures. *Facial Plast Surg*. 2005;21:180–186.

45. Abuabara A. Cerebrospinal fluid rhinorrhoea: diagnosis and management. *Med Oral Patol Oral Cir Bucal*. 2007;12:E397–E400.

46. Cohen MM Jr. The new bone biology: pathologic, molecular, and clinical correlates. *Am J Med Genet A*. 2006;140:2646–2706.

47. Stark A, Eichmann T, Mehdorn M. Skull metastases: clinical features, differential diagnosis, and review of the literature. *Surg Neurol*. 2003;60:219–226.

48. Rosahl S, Mirzayan M-J, Samii M. Osteolytic intraosseous meningiomas: illustrated review. *Acta Neurochir (Wien)*. 2004;146:1245–1249.

49. Shuangshoti S, Siriaungkul S, Suwanwela N. Primary meningioma intimately related to skull: case report and review of the literature. *Surg Neurol*. 1994;42:476–480.

50. Fujimaki T, Miyazaki S, Fukushima T, et al. Dermoid cyst of the frontal bone away from the anterior fontanel. *Childs Nerv Syst*. 1995;11:424–427.

51. Laigle-Donadey F, Taillibert S, Martin-Duverneuil N, et al. Skull-base metastases. *J Neurooncol*. 2005;75:63–69.

52. Nikolic S, Djonic D, Zivkovic V, et al. Rate of occurrence, gross appearance, and age relation of hyperostosis frontalis interna in females: a prospective autopsy study. *Am J Forensic Med Pathol*. 2010;31:205–207.

53. She R, Szakacs J. Hyperostosis frontalis interna: case report and review of literature. *Ann Clin Lab Sci*. 2004;34:206–208.

54. McRae DL. Bony abnormalities in the region of the foramen magnum: correlation of anatomic and neurologic findings. *Acta Radiol*. 1952;40:335–354.

55. Tracy M, Dormans J, Kusumi K. Klippel-Feil syndrome: clinical features and current understanding of etiology. *Clin Orthop Relat Res*. 2004;424:183–190.

56. Murphey MD, Andrews CL, Flemming DJ, et al. Primary tumors of the spine: radiologic-pathologic correlation. *Radiographics*. 1996;16:1131–1158.

57. Tehrani M, Friedman T, Pait TG, et al. The spectrum of spinal and paraspinal pathological processes encountered in neuropathology practice. *J Neuropathol Exp Neurol*. 2010;69:555–556.

58. Tyler KL. Acute pyogenic diskitis (spondylodiskitis) in adults. *Rev Neurol Dis*. 2008;5:8–13.

59. Jacobs WB, Fehlings M. Ankylosing spondylitis and spinal cord injury: origin, incidence, management, and avoidance. *Neurosurg Focus*. 2008;24:E12.

60. Krauss W, Bledsoe JM, Clarke MJ, et al. Rheumatoid arthritis of the craniovertebral junction. *Neurosurgery*. 2010;66:A83–A95.

61. Wang S, Wang C, Yan M, et al. Syringomyelia with irreducible atlantoaxial dislocation, basilar invagination and Chiari I malformation. *Eur Spine J*. 2010;19:361–366.

62. Yilmazlar S, Kocaeli H, Dogan S, et al. Traumatic epidural hematomas of nonarterial origin: analysis of 30 consecutive cases. *Acta Neurochir*. 2005;147:1241–1248.

63. Auer LM, Deinsberger W, Niederkorn K, et al. Endoscopic surgery versus medical treatment for spontaneous intracerebral hematoma: a randomized study. *J Neurosurg*. 1989;70:530–535.

64. Dolinak D, Matshes E. *Medicolegal Neuropathology: A Color Atlas*. Boca Raton, FL: CRC Press; 2002.

65. Pradilla G, Ardila GP, Hsu W, et al. Epidural abscesses of the CNS. *Lancet Neurol*. 2009;8:292–300.

66. Tompkins M, Panuncialman I, Lucas P, et al. Spinal epidural abscess. *J Emerg Med*. 2010;39:384–390.

67. An HS, Seldomridge JA. Spinal infections: diagnostic tests and imaging studies. *Clin Orthop Relat Res*. 2006;444:27–33.

68. Broner FA, Garland DE, Zigler JE. Spinal infections in the immunocompromised host. *Orthop Clin North Am*. 1996;27:37–46.

69. Tang HJ, Lin HJ, Liu YC, et al. Spinal epidural abscess—experience with 46 patients and evaluation of prognostic factors. *J Infect*. 2002;45:76–81.

70. Bose B. Thoracic extruded disc mimicking spinal cord tumor. *Spine J*. 2003;3:82–86.

71. Deshmukh VR. Rekate HL. Sonntag VK. High cervical disc herniation presenting with C-2 radiculopathy. Case report and review of the literature. *J Neurosurg*. 2004;100(3 suppl Spine):303–306.

72. Cohen MC, Scheimberg I. Evidence of occurrence of intradural and subdural hemorrhage in the perinatal and neonatal period in the context of hypoxic Ischemic encephalopathy: an observational study from two referral institutions in the United Kingdom. *Pediatr Dev Pathol*. 2009;12:169–176.

73. Castellano F, Guidetti B, Olivecrona H. Pterional meningiomas "en plaque." *J Neurosurg*. 1951;9:188–196.

74. Kupersmith MJ, Martin V, Heller G, et al. Idiopathic hypertrophic pachymeningitis. *Neurology*. 2004;62:686–694.

75. Hirunwiwatkul P, Trobe JD, Blaivas M. Lymphoplasmacyte-rich meningioma mimicking idiopathic hypertrophic pachymeningitis. *J Neuroophthalmol*. 2007;27:91–94.

76. Bertoni F, Unni KK, Dahlin DC, et al. Calcifying pseudoneoplasms of the neural axis. *J Neurosurg*. 1990;72:42–48.

77. Goutagny S, Kalamarides M. Meningiomas and neurofibromatosis. *J Neurooncol*. 2010;99:341–347.

78. Strojan P, Popovic M, Jereb B. Secondary intracranial meningiomas after high-dose cranial irradiation: report of five cases and review of the literature. *Int J Radiat Oncol Biol Phys*. 2000;48:65–73.

79. Saadatnia M, Fatehi F, Basiri K, et al. Cerebral venous sinus thrombosis risk factors. *Int J Stroke*. 2009;4:111–123.

80. McBane RD II, Tafur A, Wysokinski WE. Acquired and congenital risk factors associated with cerebral venous sinus thrombosis. *Thromb Res*. 2010;126:81–87.

81. Colli BO, Carlotti CG Jr, Assirati JA Jr, et al. Parasagittal meningiomas: follow-up review. *Surg Neurol*. 2006;66 (suppl 3):S20–S27.

82. Johnson MD, Powell SZ, Boyer PJ, et al. Dural lesions mimicking meningiomas. *Hum Pathol*. 2002;33:1211–1226.

83. Beall DP, Googe DJ, Emery RL, et al. Extramedullary intradural spinal tumors: a pictorial review. *Curr Probl Diagn Radiol*. 2007;36:185–198.

84. de Villiers JC, Cluver PF, Peter JC. Lipoma of the corpus callosum associated with frontal and facial anomalies. *Acta Neurochir Suppl*. 1991;53:1–6.

85. Lellouch-Tubiana A, Zerah M, Catala M, et al. Congenital intraspinal lipomas: histological analysis of 234 cases and review of the literature. *Pediatr Dev Pathol*. 1999;2:346–352.

86. Haines DE, Harkey HL, al-Mefty O. The "subdural" space: a new look at an outdated concept. *Neurosurgery*. 1993;32:111–120.

87. Wintzen AR. The clinical course of subdural haematoma. A retrospective study of aetiological, chronological and pathological features in 212 patients and a proposed classification. *Brain*. 1980;103:855–867.

88. Stone JL, Rifai MH, Sugar O, et al. Subdural hematomas. I. Acute subdural hematoma: progress in definition, clinical pathology, and therapy. *Surg Neurol*. 1983;19:216–231.

89. Rogers LR. Cerebrovascular complications in patients with cancer. *Semin Neurol*. 2004;24:453–460.

90. Oehmichen M, Auer RN, Konig HG. *Forensic Neuropathology and Associated Neurology*. Berlin, Germany: Springer-Verlag; 2009.

91. Squier W. Mack J. The neuropathology of infant subdural haemorrhage. *Forensic Sci Int*. 2009;187:6–13.

92. Osborn MK. Steinberg JP. Subdural empyema and other suppurative complications of paranasal sinusitis. *Lancet Infect Dis*. 2007;7:62–67.

93. Nassogne MC, Sharrard M, Hertz-Pannier L, et al. Massive subdural haematomas in Menkes disease mimicking shaken baby syndrome. *Childs Nerv Syst*. 2002;18:729–731.

94. Rogers LR. Cerebrovascular complications in cancer patients. *Neurol Clin*. 2003;21:167–192.

95. Pudenz RH, Foltz EL. Hydrocephalus: overdrainage by ventricular shunts. A review and recommendations. *Surg Neurol*. 1991;35:200–212.

96. Feigin VL, Rinkel GJ, Lawes CM, et al. Risk factors for subarachnoid hemorrhage: an updated systematic review of epidemiological studies. *Stroke*. 2005;36:2773–2780.

97. Patel KC, Finelli PF. Nonaneurysmal convexity subarachnoid hemorrhage. *Neurocrit Care*. 2006;4:229–233.

98. Yong-Zhong G, van Alphen HA. Pathogenesis and histopathology of saccular aneurysms: review of the literature. *Neurol Res*. 1990;12:249–255.

99. Dubey A, Sung WS, Chen YY, et al. Traumatic intracranial aneurysm: a brief review. *J Clin Neurosci*. 2008;15:609–612.

100. Opeskin K. Traumatic carotid artery dissection. *Am J Forensic Med Pathol*. 1997;18:251–257.

101. Kozniewska E, Michalik R, Rafalowska J, et al. Mechanisms of vascular dysfunction after subarachnoid hemorrhage. *J Physiol Pharmacol*. 2006;57(suppl 11):145–160.

102. Hughes DC, Raghavan A, Mordekar SR, et al. Role of imaging in the diagnosis of acute bacterial meningitis and its complications. *Postgrad Med J*. 2010;86:478–485.

103. Huskisson EC, Hart FD. Fulminating meningococcal septicaemia presenting with subarachnoid haemorrhage. *BMJ*. 1969;2:231–232.

104. Schmutzhard E, Boongird P, Vejjajiva A. Eosinophilic meningitis and radiculomyelitis in Thailand, caused by CNS invasion of Gnathostoma spinigerum and Angiostrongylus cantonensis. *J Neurol Neurosurg Psychiatry*. 1988;51:80–87.

105. Jones EM. Dawson A. Neuroleptic malignant syndrome: a case report with post-mortem brain and muscle pathology. *J Neurol Neurosurg Psychiatry*. 1989;52:1006–1009.

106. Kilpatrick MM, Lowry DW, Firlik AD, et al. Hyperthermia in the neurosurgical intensive care unit. *Neurosurgery*. 2000;47:850–855.

107. Valdivieso EM, Scholtz CL. Diffuse meningocerebral angiodysplasia and renal agenesis: a case report. *Pediatr Pathol*. 1986;6:119–126.

108. Teksam M, Casey SO, Michel E, et al. Subarachnoid hemorrhage associated with cyclosporine A neurotoxicity in a bone-marrow transplant recipient. *Neuroradiology*. 2001;43:242–245.

109. Lee GY, Gong GW, Vrodos N, et al. 'Ecstasy'-induced subarachnoid haemorrhage: an under-reported neurological complication. *J Clin Neurosci*. 2003;10:705–707.

110. Toossi S, Hess CP, Hills NK, et al. Neurovascular complications of cocaine use at a tertiary stroke center. *J Stroke Cerebrovasc Dis*. 2010;19:273–278.

111. Pagano L, Caira M, Falcucci P, et al. Fungal CNS infections in patients with hematologic malignancy. *Expert Rev Anti Infect Ther*. 2005;3:775–785.

112. Bariola JR, Perry P, Pappas PG, et al. Blastomycosis of the central nervous system: a multicenter review of diagnosis and treatment in the modern era. *Clin Infect Dis*. 2010;50:797–804.

113. Garg RK. Tuberculous meningitis. *Acta Neurol Scand*. 2010;122:75–90.

114. Terushkin V, Stern BJ, Judson MA, et al. Neurosarcoidosis: presentations and management. *Neurologist*. 2010;16:2–15.

115. Ghanem KG. Neurosyphilis: a historical perspective and review. *CNS Neurosci Ther*. 2010;16:e157–e168.

116. Valayannopoulos V, Nicely H, Harmatz P, et al. Mucopolysaccharidosis VI. *Orphanet J Rare Dis*. 2010;5:5.

117. Cuetter AC, Andrews RJ. Intraventricular neurocysticercosis: 18 consecutive patients and review of the literature. *Neurosurg Focus*. 2002;12:e5.

118. Ing MB, Schantz PM, Turner JA. Human coenurosis in North America: case reports and review. *Clin Infect Dis*. 1998;27:519–523.

119. D'Andrea G, Trillo G, Celli P, et al. Idiopathic intracranial hypertrophic pachymeningitis: two case reports and review of the literature. *Neurosurg Rev*. 2004;27:199–204.

120. Williams R, Swisher C, Jennings M, et al. Cerebro-ocular dysgenesis (Walker-Warburg syndrome): Neuropathologic and etiologic analysis. *Neurology*. 1984;34:1531–1541.

121. Wasserstrom WR, Glass JP, Posner JB. Diagnosis and treatment of leptomeningeal metastases from solid tumors: experience with 90 patients. *Cancer*. 1982;49:759–772.

122. Smith AB, Rushing EJ, Smirniotopoulos JG. Pigmented lesions of the central nervous system: radiologic-pathologic correlation. *Radiographics*. 2009;29:1503–1524.

123. Gutierrez J, Sacco RL, Wright CB. Dolichoectasia—an evolving arterial disease. *Nat Rev Neurosci*. 2011;7:41–50.

124. Potpara TS, Lip GY. Current therapeutic strategies and future perspectives for the prevention of arterial thromboembolism: focus on atrial fibrillation. *Curr Pharm Des*. 2010;16:3455–3471.

125. Bernard TJ, Manco-Johnson MJ, Goldenberg NA. The roles of anatomic factors, thrombophilia, and antithrombotic therapies in childhood-onset arterial ischemic stroke. *Thromb Res*. 2011;127:6–12.

126. Khimenko LP, Esham HR, Ahmed W. Spontaneous internal carotid artery dissection. *South Med J*. 2000;93:1011–1016.

127. Chang AJ, Mylonakis E, Karanasias P, et al. Spontaneous bilateral vertebral artery dissections: case report and literature review. *Mayo Clin Proc*. 1999;74:893–896.

128. Yasui T, Komiyama M, Nishikawa M, et al. Fusiform vertebral artery aneurysms as a cause of dissecting aneurysms. Report of two autopsy cases and a review of the literature. *J Neurosurg*. 1999;91:139–144.

129. Rhodes RH, Madelaire NC, Petrelli M, et al. Primary angiitis and angiopathy of the central nervous system and their relationship to systemic giant cell arteritis. *Arch Pathol Lab Med*. 1995;119:334–349.

130. Burke GM, Burke AM, Sherma AK, et al. Moyamoya disease: a summary. *Neurosurg Focus*. 2009;26:E11.

131. Kimura A, Tan CF, Wakida K, et al. Venous congestive myelopathy of the cervical spinal cord: an autopsy case showing a rapidly progressive clinical course. *Neuropathology*. 2007;27:284–289.

132. Rodriguez FJ, Crum BA, Krauss WE, et al. Venous congestive myelopathy: a mimic of neoplasia. *Mod Pathol*. 2005;18:710–718.

133. Puttgen KB, Lin DD. Neurocutaneous vascular syndromes. *Childs Nerv Syst*. 2010;26:1407–1415.

134. Ardeshiri A, Ardeshiri A, Beiras-Fernandez A, et al. Multiple cerebral cavernous malformations associated with extracranial mesenchymal anomalies. *Neurosurg Rev*. 2008;31:11–17.

135. Ho KC, Roessmann U, Straumfjord JV, et al. Analysis of brain weight. I. Adult brain weight in relation to sex, race, and age. *Arch Pathol Lab Med*. 1980;104:635–639.

136. Ho KC, Roessmann U, Straumfjord JV, et al. Analysis of brain weight. II. Adult brain weight in relation to body height, weight, and surface area. *Arch Pathol Lab Med*. 1980;104:640–645.

137. Witelson SF, Beresh H, Kigar DL. Intelligence and brain size in 100 postmortem brains: sex, lateralization and age factors. *Brain*. 2006;129:386–398.

138. Dekaban AS, Sadowsky D. Changes in brain weights during the span of human life: relation of brain weights to body heights and body weights. *Ann Neurol*. 1978;4:345–356.

139. Rabinowicz T, Macdonald-Comber J, Gartside P, et al. Structure of the Cerebral Cortex in Men and Women. *J Neuropathol Exp Neurol*. 2002;61:46–57

140. Singer DB, Sung CR, Wigglesworth JS. Fetal growth and maturation: With standards for body and organ development. In: Wigglesworth JS, Singer DB, ed. *Textbook of Fetal and Perinatal Pathology*. 2nd ed. Malden, MA: Blackwell Science; 1998:8–40.

141. Guihard-Costa A, Khung S, Delbecque K, et al. Biometry of face and brain in fetuses with trisomy 21. *Pediatr Res*. 2006;59:33–38.

142. Dawson TP, Neal JW, Llewellyn L, Thomas C. *Neuropathology Techniques*. London, UK: Arnold; 2003.

143. Ashwal S, Michelson D, Plawner L, et al. Practice parameter: Evaluation of the child with microcephaly (an evidence-based review): report of the Quality Standards Subcommittee of the American Academy of Neurology and the Practice Committee of the Child Neurology Society. *Neurology*. 2009;73:887–897.

144. Oostra RJ, van der Wolk S, Maas M, et al. Malformations of the axial skeleton in the museum Vrolik: II: craniosynostoses and suture-related conditions. *Am J Med Genet*. 2005;136A(4):327–342.

145. Sullivan PK, Melsen B, Mulliken JB. Calvarial sutural abnormalities: metopic synostosis and coronal deformation—an anatomic, three-dimensional radiographic, and pathologic study. *Plast Reconstr Surg*. 1990;86:1072–1077.

146. Ferrer I, Armstrong J. Microcephaly. In: Golden JA, Harding BN, eds. *Pathology and Genetics: Developmental Neuropathology*. Basel, Switzerland: ISN Neuropath Press; 2004:26–31.

147. Barkovich AJ, Ferriero DM, Barr RM, et al. Microlissencephaly: a heterogeneous malformation of cortical development. *Neuropediatrics*. 1998;29:113–119.

148. Cole G, Neal JW, Fraser WI, et al. Autopsy findings in patients with mental handicap. *J Intellect Disabil Res*. 1994;38:9–26.

149. Tucker ME, Garringer HJ, Weaver DD. Phenotypic spectrum of mosaic trisomy 18: two new patients, a literature review, and counseling issues. *Am J Med Genet*. 2007;143:505–517.

150. Mainardi C. Cri du Chat syndrome. *Orphanet J Rare Dis*. 2006;1:33.

151. Maas NM, Van Buggenhout G, Hannes F, et al. Genotype-phenotype correlation in 21 patients with Wolf-Hirschhorn syndrome using high resolution array comparative genome hybridisation (CGH). *J Med Genet*. 2008;45:71–80.

152. Cianchetti C, Sannio-Fancello G, Fratta AL, et al. Neuropsychological studies in families with fragile-X negative X-linked mental retardation. *Am J Med Genet*. 1992;43:505–509.

153. Olney AH. Macrocephaly syndromes. *Semin Pediatr Neurol*. 2007;14:128–135.

154. Gooskens RH, Willemse J, Bijlsma JB, et al. Megalencephaly: definition and classification. *Brain Dev*. 1988;10:1–7.

155. Uppal S, Mistry D, Coatesworth AP. Cowden disease: a review. *Int J Clin Pract*. 2007;61:645–652.
156. Di Rocco C, Battaglia D, Pietrini D, et al. Hemimegalencephaly: clinical implications and surgical treatment. *Childs Nerv Syst*. 2006;22:852–866.
157. Zahl SM, Wester K. Routine measurement of head circumference as a tool for detecting intracranial expansion in infants: what is the gain? A nationwide survey. *Pediatrics*. 2008;121:e416–e420.
158. Epps RE, Pittelkow MR, Su WP. TORCH syndrome. *Semin Dermatol*. 1995;14:179–186.
159. Winton MJ, Joyce S, Zhukareva V, et al. Characterization of tau pathologies in gray and white matter of Guam parkinsonism-dementia complex. *Acta Neuropathol*. 2006;111:401–412.
160. Miklossy J. Chronic inflammation and amyloidogenesis in Alzheimer's disease—role of Spirochetes. *J Alzheimers Dis*. 2008;13:381–391.
161. Praveen-kumar S, Sinha S, Taly AB, et al. Electroencephalographic and imaging profile in a subacute sclerosing panencephalitis (SSPE) cohort: a correlative study. *Clin Neurophysiol*. 2007;118:1947–1954.
162. Paisan-Ruiz C, Bhatia KP, Li A, et al. Characterization of PLA2G6 as a locus for dystonia-parkinsonism. *Ann Neurol*. 2009;65:19–23.
163. Savazzi GM, Cusmano F, Vinci S, et al. Progression of cerebral atrophy in patients on regular hemodialysis treatment: long-term follow-up with cerebral computed tomography. *Nephron*. 1995;69:29–33.
164. Bruggers CS, Friedman HS, Tien R, et al. Cerebral atrophy in an infant following treatment with ifosfamide. *Med Pediatr Oncol*. 1994;23:380–383.
165. Korogi Y, Takahashi M, Shinzato J, et al. MR findings in seven patients with organic mercury poisoning (Minamata disease). *Am J Neuroradiol*. 1994;15:1575–1578.
166. Harding B, Ellis D, Malcolm S. A case of Pelizaeus-Merzbacher disease showing increased dosage of the proteolipid protein gene. *Neuropathol Appl Neurobiol*. 1995;21:111–115.
167. Grindstaff P, Gruener G. The peripheral nervous system complications of HTLV-1 myelopathy (HAM/TSP) syndromes. *Semin Neurol*. 2005;25:315–327.
168. Koeppen AH. The pathogenesis of spinocerebellar ataxia. *Cerebellum*. 2005;4:62–73.
169. Brusse E, Maat-Kievit JA, van Swieten JC. Diagnosis and management of early- and late-onset cerebellar ataxia. *Clin Genet*. 2007;71:12–24.
170. Burk K, Farecki ML, Lamprecht G, et al. Neurological symptoms in patients with biopsy proven celiac disease. *Mov Disord*. 2009;24:2358–2362.
171. Lolin Y. Chronic neurological toxicity associated with exposure to volatile substances. *Hum Toxicol*. 1989;8:293–300.
172. Ziegler DK. Toxicity to the nervous system of diphenylhydantoin: a review. *Int J Neurol*. 1978;11:383–400.
173. Niethammer M, Ford B. Permanent lithium-induced cerebellar toxicity: three cases and review of literature. *Mov Disord*. 2007;22:570–573.
174. Cordoba J, Garcia-Martinez R, Simon-Talero M. Hyponatremic and hepatic encephalopathies: similarities, differences and coexistence. *Metab Brain Dis*. 2010;25:73–80.
175. Rosenbloom AL, Hanas R. Diabetic ketoacidosis (DKA): treatment guidelines. *Clin Pediatr*. 1996;35:261–266.
176. Hossain MA, Russell JC, Miknyoczki S, et al. Vascular endothelial growth factor mediates vasogenic edema in acute lead encephalopathy. *Ann Neurol*. 2004;55:660–667.
177. Clemedson C, Odland L, Walum E. Differential effect of carbon tetrachloride on the cell membranes of neurons and astrocytes. *Neurotoxicol Teratol*. 1990;12:597–602.
178. Hantson P, Vanbinst R, Mahieu P. Determination of ethylene glycol tissue content after fatal oral poisoning and pathologic findings. *Am J Forensic Med Pathol*. 2002;23:159–161.
179. Karayel F, Turan AA, Sav A, et al. Methanol intoxication: pathological changes of central nervous system (17 cases). *Am J Forensic Med Pathol*. 2010;31:34–36.
180. Terajima K, Igarashi H, Hirose M, et al. Serial assessments of delayed encephalopathy after carbon monoxide poisoning using magnetic resonance spectroscopy and diffusion tensor imaging on 3.0T system. *Eur Neurol*. 2008;59:55–61.
181. Sripathirathan K, Brown J III, Neafsey EJ, et al. Linking binge alcohol-induced neurodamage to brain edema and potential aquaporin-4 upregulation: evidence in rat organotypic brain slice cultures and in vivo. *J Neurotrauma*. 2009;26:261–273.
182. Buttner A, Mall G, Penning R, et al. The neuropathology of heroin abuse. *Forensic Sci Int*. 2000;113:435–442.
183. Varnell RM, Stimac GK, Fligner CL. CT diagnosis of toxic brain injury in cyanide poisoning: considerations for forensic medicine. *Am J Neuroradiol*. 1987;8:1063–1066.
184. Ferrari TC, Moreira PR, Cunha AS. Clinical characterization of neuroschistosomiasis due to Schistosoma mansoni and its treatment. *Acta Trop*. 2008;108:89–97.
185. Dobyns WB, Truwit CL, Ross ME, et al. Differences in the gyral pattern distinguish chromosome 17-linked and X-linked lissencephaly. *Neurology*. 1999;53:270–277.
186. Coto-Puckett WL, Gilbert-Barness E, Steelman CK, et al. A spectrum of phenotypical expression OF Neu-Laxova syndrome: Three case reports and a review of the literature. *Fetal Pediatr Pathol*. 2010;29:108–119.
187. Lindhard A, Graem N, Skovby F, et al. Postmortem findings and prenatal diagnosis of Zellweger syndrome. *APMIS*. 1993;101:226–228.
188. Williams D, Patel C, Fallet-Bianco C, et al. Fowler syndrome—a clinical, radiological, and pathological study of 14 cases. *Am J Med Genet*. 2010;152A:153–160.
189. Guadagni MG, Faggella A, Piana G, et al. Aicardi syndrome: a case report. *Eur J Paediatr Dent*. 2010;11:146–148.
190. Shevell MI. Clinical and diagnostic profile of agenesis of the corpus callosum. *J Child Neurol*. 2002;17:896–900.
191. Cohen MM Jr, Kreiborg S. Agenesis of the corpus callosum. Its associated anomalies and syndromes with special reference to the Apert syndrome. *Neurosurg Clin N Am*. 1991;2:565–568.
192. Hodgson BD, Davies L, Gonzalez CD. Acrocallosal syndrome: a case report and literature survey. *J Dent Child*. 2009;76:170–177.
193. Ahdab-Barmada M, Claassen D. A distinctive triad of malformations of the central nervous system in the Meckel-Gruber syndrome. *J Neuropathol Exp Neurol*. 1990;49:610–620.
194. Ten Donkelaar HJ, Lammens M. Development of the human cerebellum and its disorders. *Clin Perinatol*. 2009;36:513–530.
195. Bolduc ME, Limperopoulos C. Neurodevelopmental outcomes in children with cerebellar malformations: a systematic review. *Dev Med Child Neurol*. 2009;51:256–267.
196. Schulze KD, Braak H. Brain warts. *Z Mikrosk Anat Forsch*. 1978;92:609–623.
197. Pinar H, Tatevosyants N, Singer DB. Central nervous system malformations in a perinatal/neonatal autopsy series. *Pediatr Dev Pathol*. 1998;1:42–48.
198. Mariak Z, Mariak Z, Stankiewicz A. Cranial nerve II–VII injuries in fatal closed head trauma. *Eur J Ophthalmol*. 1997;7:68–72.
199. Reiter ER, DiNardo LJ, Costanzo RM. Effects of head injury on olfaction and taste. *Otolaryngol Clin North Am*. 2004;37:1167–1184.
200. Moller AR. The cranial nerve vascular compression syndrome: II. A review of pathophysiology. *Acta Neurochir*. 1991;113:24–30.
201. Rojana-udomsart A, Pulkes T, Viranuwatti K, et al. Idiopathic hypertrophic cranial pachymeningitis. *J Clin Neurosci*. 2008;15:465–469.
202. Magoun HI. Entrapment neuropathy of the central nervous system. 3. Cranial nerves V, IX, X, XI. *J Am Osteopath Assoc*. 1968;67:889–899.

203. Baba T. Minamida Y. Mikama T, et al. Entrapment neuropathy of the optic nerve due to hyperostosis associated with congenital anemia. *J Neurosurg*. 2005;103:917–919.

204. Binning MJ, Liu JK, Kestle JR, et al. Optic pathway gliomas: a review. *Neurosurg Focus*. 2007;23:E2.

205. Eddleman CS. Liu JK. Optic nerve sheath meningioma: current diagnosis and treatment. *Neurosurg Focus*. 2007;23:E4.

206. Jervis GA. Early familial cerebellar degeneration; report of 3 cases in one family. *J Nerv Ment Dis*. 1950;111:398–407.

207. Harding BN, Brett EM. Familial cerebellar cortical degeneration with early onset: 234. *J Neuropathol Exp Neurol*. 1995;54:469.

208. Dipti S, Childs AM, Livingston JH, et al. Brown-Vialetto-Van Laere syndrome; variability in age at onset and disease progression highlighting the phenotypic overlap with Fazio-Londe disease. *Brain Dev*. 2005;27:443–446.

209. Argyriou AA, Makris N. Neuromyelitis optica: a distinct demyelinating disease of the central nervous system. *Acta Neurol Scand*. 2008;118:209–217.

210. Pittock SJ, Lucchinetti CF. The pathology of MS: new insights and potential clinical applications. *Neurologist*. 2007;13:45–56.

211. Harley RD, Huang NN, Macri CH, et al. Optic neuritis and optic atrophy following chloramphenicol in cystic fibrosis patients. *Trans Am Acad Ophthalmol Otolaryngol*. 1970;74:1011–1031.

212. Pradhan M, Sharp D, Best S, et al. Drug-induced optic neuropathy-TB or not TB. *Surv Ophthalmol*. 2010;55:378–385.

213. Trouillas P, von Kummer R. Classification and pathogenesis of cerebral hemorrhages after thrombolysis in ischemic stroke. *Stroke*. 2006;37:556–561.

214. Ellison D, Love S, Chimelli L, et al. *Neuropathology. A Reference Text of CNS Pathology*. Philadelphia, PA: Elsevier; 2004.

215. Mott RT, Dickson DW, Trojanowski JQ, et al. Neuropathologic, biochemical, and molecular characterization of the frontotemporal dementias. *J Neuropathol Exp Neurol*. 2005;64:420–428.

216. McKhann GM, Albert MS, Grossman M, et al. Clinical and pathologic diagnosis of frontotemporal dementia: report of the work group on frontotemporal dementia and Pick's disease. *Arch Neurol*. 2001;58:1803–1809.

217. Kim SJ, Park YD, Hessler R, et al. Correlation between magnetic resonance imaging and histopathologic grades in Rasmussen syndrome. *Pediatr Neurol*. 2010;42:172–176.

218. Bao X, Wu Y, Wong LJ, et al. Alpers syndrome with prominent white matter changes. *Brain Dev*. 2008;30:295–300.

219. Sumi SM. Brain malformations in the trisomy 18 syndrome. *Brain*. 1970;93:821–830.

220. Bernauer TA. The radial bands sign. *Radiology*. 1999;212:761–762.

221. Choi BH, Lapham LW, Amin-Zaki L, et al. Abnormal neuronal migration, deranged cerebral cortical organization, and diffuse white matter astrocytosis of human fetal brain: a major effect of methylmercury poisoning in utero. *J Neuropathol Exp Neurol*. 1978;37:719–733.

222. Tuntiyatorn L, Laothamatas J. Acute Marchiafava-Bignami disease with callosal, cortical, and white matter involvement. *Emerg Radiol*. 2008;15:137–140.

223. Pearl GS. Traumatic neuropathology. *Clin Lab Med*. 1998;18:39–64.

224. Yamamoto Y, Craggs L, Baumann M, et al. Review: molecular genetics and pathology of hereditary small vessel diseases of the brain. *Neuropathol Appl Neurobiol*. 2011;37:94–113.

225. Poser CM. Notes on the pathogenesis of subacute sclerosing panencephalitis. *J Neurol Sci*. 1990;95:219–224.

226. Kohlschutter A, Bley A, Brockmann K, et al. Leukodystrophies and other genetic metabolic leukoencephalopathies in children and adults. *Brain Dev*. 2010;32:82–89.

227. Bugiani M, Boor I, Powers JM, et al. Leukoencephalopathy with vanishing white matter: a review. *J Neuropathol Exp Neurol*. 2010;69:987–996.

228. Filosto M, Tomelleri G, Tonin P, et al. Neuropathology of mitochondrial diseases. *Biosci Rep*. 2007;27:23–30.

229. Matsubayashi J, Tsuchiya K, Matsunaga T, et al. Methotrexate-related leukoencephalopathy without radiation therapy: distribution of brain lesions and pathological heterogeneity on two autopsy cases. *Neuropathology*. 2009;29:105–115.

230. Pande AR, Ando K, Ishikura R, et al. Disseminated necrotizing leukoencephalopathy following chemoradiation therapy for acute lymphoblastic leukemia. *Radiat Med*. 2006;24:515–519.

231. Bruck W, Heise E, Friede RL. Leukoencephalopathy after cisplatin therapy. *Clin Neuropathol*. 1989;8:263–265.

232. Anders KH, Becker PS, Holden JK, et al. Multifocal necrotizing leukoencephalopathy with pontine predilection in immunosuppressed patients: a clinicopathologic review of 16 cases. *Hum Pathol*. 1993;24:897–904.

233. Blaes AH, Santa-Cruz KS, Lee CK, et al. Necrotizing leukoencephalopathy following CHOP chemotherapy. *Leuk Res*. 2008;32:1611–1614.

234. Rosenblum MK, Delattre JY, Walker RW, et al. Fatal necrotizing encephalopathy complicating treatment of malignant gliomas with intra-arterial BCNU and irradiation: a pathological study. *J Neurooncol*. 1989;7:269–281.

235. Spriggs DR, Stopa E, Mayer RJ, et al. Fludarabine phosphate (NSC 312878) infusions for the treatment of acute leukemia: phase I and neuropathological study. *Cancer Res*. 1986;46:5953–5958.

236. Neiman J, Haapaniemi HM, Hillbom M. Neurological complications of drug abuse: pathophysiological mechanisms. *Eur J Neurol*. 2000;7:595–606.

237. Fasullo S, Cammarata A. On a case of cerebral embolism in atrial fibrillation in a patient with Friedreich's disease. *Acta Neurol*. 1973;28:560–565.

238. Charness ME. Brain lesions in alcoholics. *Alcohol Clin Exp Res*. 1993;17:2–11.

239. Gouw AA, Seewann A, van der Flier WM, et al. Heterogeneity of small vessel disease: a systematic review of MRI and histopathology correlations. *J Neurol Neurosurg Psychiatry*. 2011;82:126–135.

240. Jellinger KA. The pathology of ischemic-vascular dementia: an update. *J Neurol Sci*. 2002;203–204:153-157.

241. Ramaekers VTh, Lake BD, Harding B, et al. Diagnostic difficulties in infantile neuroaxonal dystrophy. A clinicopathological study of eight cases. *Neuropediatrics*. 1987;18:170–175.

242. Yang Y. Allen E. Ding J. Wang W. Giant axonal neuropathy. *Cell Mol Life Sci*. 2007;64:601–609.

243. Gerard A, Sarrot-Reynauld F, Liozon E, et al. Neurologic presentation of Whipple disease: report of 12 cases and review of the literature. *Medicine*. 2002;81:443–457.

244. Termine C, Uggetti C, Veggiotti P, et al. Long-term follow-up of an adolescent who had bilateral striatal necrosis secondary to *Mycoplasma pneumoniae* infection. *Brain Dev*. 2005;27:62–65.

245. Miyoshi K, Matsuoka T, Mizushima S. Familial holotopistic striatal necrosis. *Acta Neuropathol*. 1969;13:240–249.

246. Rinne JO, Daniel SE, Scaravilli F, et al. The neuropathological features of neuroacanthocytosis. *Mov Disord*. 1994;9:297–304.

247. Carrozzo R, Dionisi-Vici C, Steuerwald U, et al. SUCLA2 mutations are associated with mild methylmalonic aciduria, Leigh-like encephalomyopathy, dystonia and deafness. *Brain*. 2007;130:862–874.

248. Prockop LD, Chichkova RI. Carbon monoxide intoxication: an updated review. *J Neurol Sci*. 2007;262:122–130.

249. Gordon N. Pantothenate kinase-associated neurodegeneration (Hallervorden-Spatz syndrome). *Eur J Paediatr Neurol*. 2002;6:243–247.

250. Madry H, Prudlo J, Grgic A, et al. Nasu-Hakola disease (PLOSL): report of five cases and review of the literature. *Clin Orthop Relat Res*. 2007;454:262–269.

251. Aizawa H, Kwak S, Shimizu T, et al. A case of adult onset pure pallidal degeneration. I. Clinical manifestations and neuropathological observations. *J Neurol Sci*. 1991;102:76–82.

252. Sztriha L, Vos YJ, Verlind E, et al. X-linked hydrocephalus: a novel missense mutation in the L1CAM gene. *Pediatr Neurol*. 2002;27:293–296.
253. Steinlin M, Blaser S, Boltshauser E. Cerebellar involvement in metabolic disorders: a pattern-recognition approach. *Neuroradiology*. 1998;40:347–354.
254. Halliday GM, Fedorow H, Rickert CH, et al. Evidence for specific phases in the development of human neuromelanin. *J Neural Transm*. 2006;113:721–728.
255. Casals J, Elizan TS, Yahr MD. Postencephalitic parkinsonism—a review. *J Neural Transm*. 1998;105:645–676.
256. Winton MJ, Joyce S, Zhukareva V, et al. Characterization of tau pathologies in gray and white matter of Guam parkinsonism-dementia complex. *Acta Neuropathol*. 2006;111:401–412.
257. Wachter RM, Burke AM, MacGregor RR. Strongyloides stercoralis hyperinfection masquerading as cerebral vasculitis. *Arch Neurol*. 1984;41:1213–1216.
258. Takai K, Taniguchi M, Takahashi H, et al. Comparative analysis of spinal hemangioblastomas in sporadic disease and Von Hippel-Lindau syndrome. *Neurol Med Chir*. 2010;50:560–567.
259. Pollak L, Walach N, Gur R, et al. Meningiomas after radiotherapy for tinea capitis—still no history. *Tumori*. 1998;84:65–68.
260. Elijovich L, Patel PV, Hemphill JC III. Intracerebral hemorrhage. *Semin Neurol*. 2008;28:657–667.
261. Wityk RJ, Caplan LR. Hypertensive intracerebral hemorrhage. Epidemiology and clinical pathology. *Neurosurg Clin N Am*. 1992;3:521–532.
262. Yen CP, Lin CL, Kwan AL, et al. Simultaneous multiple hypertensive intracerebral haemorrhages. *Acta Neurochir*. 2005;147:393–399.
263. Tucker WS, Bilbao JM, Klodawsky H. Cerebral amyloid angiopathy and multiple intracerebral hematomas. *Neurosurgery*. 1980;7:611–614.
264. Chen YW, Lee MJ, Smith EE. Cerebral amyloid angiopathy in East and West. *Int J Stroke*. 2010;5:403–411.
265. Ishii T, Terao T, Komine K, et al. Intramedullary spinal cord metastases of malignant melanoma: an autopsy case report and review of the literature. *Clin Neuropathol*. 2010;29:334–340.
266. Wronski M, Arbit E, Russo P, et al. Surgical resection of brain metastases from renal cell carcinoma in 50 patients. *Urology*. 1996;47:187–193.
267. Vazquez E, Lucaya J, Castellote A, et al. Neuroimaging in pediatric leukemia and lymphoma: differential diagnosis. *Radiographics*. 2002;22:1411–1428.
268. Bitoh S, Hasegawa H, Ohtsuki H, et al. Cerebral neoplasms initially presenting with massive intracerebral hemorrhage. *Surg Neurol*. 1984;22:57–62.
269. Oldberg E. Hemorrhage into gliomas: a review of eight hundred and thirty-two consecutive verified cases of glioma. *Arch Neurol Psychiatry*. 1933;30:1061–1073.
270. Chanda A, Nanda A. Multiple cavernomas of brain presenting with simultaneous hemorrhage in two lesions: a case report. *Surg Neurol*. 2002;57:340–345.
271. Guardia SN, Bilbao JM, Murray D, et al. Fat embolism in acute pancreatitis. *Arch Pathol Lab Med*. 1989;113:503–506.
272. Kase CS, Pessin MS, Zivin JA, et al. Intracranial hemorrhage after coronary thrombolysis with tissue plasminogen activator. *Am J Med*. 1992;92:384–390.
273. Quinones-Hinojosa A, Gulati M, Singh V, et al. Spontaneous intracerebral hemorrhage due to coagulation disorders. *Neurosurg Focus*. 2003;15:E3.
274. Adams RJ. Stroke prevention and treatment in sickle cell disease. *Arch Neurol*. 2001;58:565–568.
275. Kang SS, McGavern DB. Microbial induction of vascular pathology in the CNS. *J Neuroimmune Pharmacol*. 2010;5:370–386.
276. Weathers AL, Lewis SL. Rare and unusual... or are they? Less commonly diagnosed encephalopathies associated with systemic disease. *Semin Neurol*. 2009;29:136–153.
277. Press MF. Lead encephalopathy in neonatal Long-Evans rats: morphologic studies. *J Neuropathol Exp Neurol*. 1977;36:169–193.
278. Caparros-Lefebvre D, Policard J, Sengler C, et al. Bipallidal haemorrhage after ethylene glycol intoxication. *Neuroradiology*. 2005;47:105–107.
279. Andersen KK, Olsen TS, Dehlendorff C, et al. Hemorrhagic and ischemic strokes compared: stroke severity, mortality, and risk factors. *Stroke*. 2009;40:2068–2072.
280. Geibprasert S, Gallucci M, Krings T, et al. Addictive illegal drugs: structural neuroimaging. *Am J Neuroradiol*. 2010;31:803–808.
281. Easton A. 48 year old male with sudden onset of right sided weakness. *Brain Pathol*. 2006;16:181–182, 187.
282. Haller L, Adams H, Merouze F, et al. Clinical and pathological aspects of human African trypanosomiasis (T. b. gambiense) with particular reference to reactive arsenical encephalopathy. *Am J Trop Med Hyg*. 1986;35:94–99.
283. Katz JM, Segal AZ. Incidence and etiology of cerebrovascular disease in patients with malignancy. *Curr Atheroscler Rep*. 2005;7:280–288.
284. Greenberg RN, Scott LJ, Vaughn HH, et al. Zygomycosis (mucormycosis): emerging clinical importance and new treatments. *Curr Opin Infect Dis*. 2004;17:517–525.
285. Rocha A, de Meneses AC, da Silva AM, et al. Pathology of patients with Chagas' disease and acquired immunodeficiency syndrome. *Am J Trop Med Hyg*. 1994;50:261–268.
286. Gay T, Pankey GA, Beckman EN, et al. Fatal CNS trichinosis. *JAMA*. 1982;247:1024–1025.
287. Bayramoglu M, Karatas M, Leblebici B, et al. Hemorrhagic transformation in stroke patients. *Am J Phys Med Rehabil*. 2003;82:48–52.
288. Beal MF, Wechsler LR, Davis KR. Cerebral vein thrombosis and multiple intracranial hemorrhages by computed tomography. *Arch Neurol*. 1982;29:437–438.
289. Hill A. Ventricular dilation following intraventricular hemorrhage in the premature infant. *Can J Neurol Sci*. 1983;10:81–85.
290. Cremer OL, Kalkman CJ. Cerebral pathophysiology and clinical neurology of hyperthermia in humans. *Prog Brain Res*. 2007;162:153–169.
291. Johnston I, Teo C. Disorders of CSF hydrodynamics. *Childs Nerv Syst*. 2000;16:776–799.
292. Larsen PD, Osborn AG. Computed tomographic evaluation of corpus callosum agenesis and associated malformations. *J Comput Tomogr*. 1982;6:225–230.
293. Huh JS, Hwang YS, Yoon SH, et al. Lateral ventricular diverticulum extending into supracerebellar cistern from unilateral obstruction of the foramen of monro in a neonate. *Pediatr Neurosurg*. 2007;43:115–120.
294. Wisoff JH. Hydromyelia: a critical review. *Childs Nerv Syst*. 1988;4:1–8.
295. McKee AC, Cantu RC, Nowinski CJ, et al. Chronic traumatic encephalopathy in athletes: progressive tauopathy after repetitive head injury. *J Neuropathol Exp Neurol*. 2009;68:709–735.
296. Swayze VW II, Andreasen NC, Alliger RJ, et al. Structural brain abnormalities in bipolar affective disorder. Ventricular enlargement and focal signal hyperintensities. *Arch Gen Psychiatry*. 1990;47:1054–1059.
297. Boronow J, Pickar D, Ninan PT, et al. Atrophy limited to the third ventricle in chronic schizophrenic patients. Report of a controlled series. *Arch Gen Psychiatry*. 1985;42:266–271.
298. Gallia GL. Rigamonti D. Williams MA. The diagnosis and treatment of idiopathic normal pressure hydrocephalus. *Nat Clin Pract Neurol*. 2006;2:375–381.
299. Governale LS, Fein N, Logsdon J, et al. Techniques and complications of external lumbar drainage for normal pressure hydrocephalus. *Neurosurgery*. 2008;63:379–384.
300. Ferguson SC, Blane A, Wardlaw J, et al. Influence of an early-onset age of type 1 diabetes on cerebral structure and cognitive function. *Diabetes Care*. 2005;28:1431–1437.
301. Vajsar J, Schachter H. Walker-Warburg syndrome. *Orphanet J Rare Dis*. 2006;1:29.
302. Steward CG. Neurological aspects of osteopetrosis. *Neuropathol Appl Neurobiol*. 2003;29:87–97.

303. Michotte A, De Meirleir L, Lissens W, et al. Neuropathological findings of a patient with pyruvate dehydrogenase E1 alpha deficiency presenting as a cerebral lactic acidosis. *Acta Neuropathol*. 1993;85:674–678.

304. Takahashi T, Yung AR, Yucel M, et al. Prevalence of large cavum septi pellucidi in ultra high-risk individuals and patients with psychotic disorders. *Schizophr Res*. 2008;105:236–244.

305. Winter TC, Kennedy AM, Byrne J, et al. The cavum septi pellucidi: why is it important? *J Ultrasound Med*. 2010;29:427–444.

306. Fard MA, Wu-Chen WY, Man BL, et al. Septo-optic dysplasia. *Pediatr Endocrinol Rev*. 2010;8:18–24.

307. Raybaud C. Di Rocco C. Brain malformation in syndromic craniosynostoses, a primary disorder of white matter: a review. *Childs Nerv Syst*. 2007;23:1379–1388.

308. Sarnat HB. Ependymal reactions to injury. A review. *J Neuropathol Exp Neurol*. 1995;54:1–15.

309. Salmon J. Ventriculitis complicating meningitis. *Am J Dis Child*. 1972;124:35–40.

310. Bakshi R, Kinkel P, Mechtler L, et al. Cerebral ventricular empyema associated with severe adult pyogenic meningitis: computed tomography findings. *Clin Neurol Neurosurg*. 1997;99:252–255.

311. Kleinschmidt-DeMasters BK. Gilden DH. The expanding spectrum of herpesvirus infections of the nervous system. *Brain Pathol*. 2001;11:440–451.

312. Maeda K, Sanada M, Kawai H, et al. Pyogenic ventriculitis with ruptured brain abscess. *Intern Med*. 2006;45:835–836.

313. Beer R, Lackner P, Pfausler B, et al. Nosocomial ventriculitis and meningitis in neurocritical care patients. *J Neurol*. 2008;255:1617–1624.

314. Westhout FD, Linskey ME. Obstructive hydrocephalus and progressive psychosis: rare presentations of neurosarcoidosis. *Surg Neurol*. 2008;69:288–292.

315. Scavarda D, Bednarek N, Litre F, et al. Acquired aqueductal stenosis in preterm infants: an indication for neuroendoscopic third ventriculostomy. *Childs Nerv Syst*. 2003;19:756–759.

316. Verhagen WI, Bartels RH, Fransen E, et al. Familial congenital hydrocephalus and aqueduct stenosis with probably autosomal dominant inheritance and variable expression. *J Neurol Sci*. 1998;158:101–105.

317. Senveli E, Altinors N, Kars Z, et al. Association of von Recklinghausen's neurofibromatosis and aqueduct stenosis. *Neurosurgery*. 1989;24:99–101.

318. Dumont AS, Farace E, Schiff D, et al. Intraventricular gliomas. *Neurosurg Clin N Am*. 2003;14:571–591.

319. Berhouma M. Management of subependymal giant cell tumors in tuberous sclerosis complex: the neurosurgeon's perspective. *World J Pediatr*. 2010;6:103–110.

320. Mizuguchi M, Takashima S. Neuropathology of tuberous sclerosis. *Brain Dev*. 2001;23:508–515.

321. Rushing EJ, Cooper PB, Quezado M, et al. Subependymoma revisited: clinicopathological evaluation of 83 cases. *J Neurooncol*. 2007;85:297–305.

322. Jabri HE, Dababo MA, Alkhani AM. Subependymoma of the spine. *Neurosciences*. 2010;15:126–128.

323. Schmidt MH, Gottfried ON, von Koch CS, et al. Central neurocytoma: a review. *J Neurooncol*. 2004;66:377–384.

324. Kuchelmeister K, Nestler U, Siekmann R, et al. Liponeurocytoma of the left lateral ventricle—case report and review of the literature. *Clin Neuropathol*. 2006;25:86–94.

325. Leeds NE, Lang FF, Ribalta T, et al. Origin of chordoid glioma of the third ventricle. *Arch Pathol Lab Med*. 2006;130:460–464.

326. Jouvet A, Fauchon F, Liberski P, et al. Papillary tumor of the pineal region. *Am J Surg Pathol*. 2003;27:505–512.

327. Dahiya S, Perry A. Pineal tumors. *Adv Anat Pathol*. 2010;17:419–427.

328. Fujimoto Y, Matsushita H, Plese JP, et al. Hydrocephalus due to diffuse villous hyperplasia of the choroid plexus. Case report and review of the literature. *Pediatr Neurosurg*. 2004;40:32–36.

329. Serpa JA, Graviss EA, Kass JS, et al. Neurocysticercosis in Houston, Texas: an update. *Medicine*. 2011;90:81–86.

330. Morcos CL, Platt LD, Carlson DE, et al. The isolated choroid plexus cyst. *Obstet Gynecol*. 1998;92:232–266.

331. McGahan JP. The fetal head: borderlines. *Semin Ultrasound CT MR*. 1998;19:318–328.

332. Nahed BV, Darbar A, Doiron R, et al. Acute hydrocephalus secondary to obstruction of the foramen of monro and cerebral aqueduct caused by a choroid plexus cyst in the lateral ventricle. *J Neurosurg*. 2007;107:236–239.

333. Radaideh MM, Leeds NE, Kumar AJ, et al. Unusual small choroid plexus cyst obstructing the foramen of monroe: case report. *Am J Neuroradiol*. 2002;23:841–843.

334. Mito T, Becker LE, Perlman M, et al. A neuropathologic analysis of neonatal deaths occurring in a single neonatal unit over a 20-year period. *Pediatr Pathol*. 1993;13:773–785.

335. Armstrong DL, Sauls CD, Goddard-Finegold J. Neuropathologic findings in short-term survivors of intraventricular hemorrhage. *Am J Dis Child*. 1987;141:617–621.

336. Muenchau A, Laas R. Xanthogranuloma and xanthoma of the choroid plexus: evidence for different etiology and pathogenesis. *Clin Neuropathol*. 1997;16:72–76.

337. Rabl W, Sigrist T. Xanthogranuloma of the choroid plexus of the lateral ventricle. *Fortschr Neurol Psychiatr*. 1992;60:305–307.

338. Miyahara K, Fujitsu K, Yagishita S, et al. Inflammatory pseudotumor of the choroid plexus. *J Neurosurg*. 2008;108:365–369.

339. Aicardi J. Aicardi syndrome. *Brain Dev*. 2005;27: 164–171.

340. Gonzalez KD, Noltner KA, Buzin CH, et al. Beyond Li Fraumeni Syndrome: clinical characteristics of families with p53 germline mutations. *J Clin Oncol*. 2009;27:1250–1256.

341. Hori A, Walter GF, Haas J, et al. Down syndrome complicated by brain tumors: case report and review of the literature. *Brain Dev*. 1992;14:396–400.

342. Blamires TL, Maher ER. Choroid plexus papilloma. A new presentation of von Hippel-Lindau (VHL) disease. *Eye*. 1992;6:90–92.

343. Wolff JE, Sajedi M, Brant R, et al. Choroid plexus tumours. *Br J Cancer*. 2002;87:1086–1091.

344. Bhatoe HS, Singh P, Dutta V. Intraventricular meningiomas: a clinicopathological study and review. *Neurosurg Focus*. 2006;20:E9.

345. Sung WS, Dubey A, Erasmus A, et al. Solitary choroid plexus metastasis from carcinoma of the oesophagus. *J Clin Neurosci*. 2008;15:594–597.

346. Lee D. Suh YL. Histologically confirmed intracranial germ cell tumors; an analysis of 62 patients in a single institute. *Virchows Arch*. 2010;457:347–357.

347. Nonomura N, Nagahara A, Oka D, et al. Brain metastases from testicular germ cell tumors: a retrospective analysis. *Int J Urol*. 2009;16:887–893.

348. Knierim DS, Yamada S. Pineal tumors and associated lesions: the effect of ethnicity on tumor type and treatment. *Pediatr Neurosurg*. 2003;38:307–323.

349. Rickert CH, Probst-Cousin S, Blasius S, et al. Melanotic progonoma of the brain: a case report and review. *Childs Nerv Syst*. 1998;14:389–393.

350. Fevre-Montange M. Hasselblatt M. Figarella-Branger D, et al. Prognosis and histopathologic features in papillary tumors of the pineal region: a retrospective multicenter study of 31 cases. *J Neuropathol Exp Neurol*. 2006;65:1004–1011.

351. Kim YH, Kim JW, Park CK, et al. Papillary tumor of pineal region presenting with leptomeningeal seeding. *Neuropathology*. 2010;30:654–660.

352. Chao CK, Lee ST, Lin FJ, et al. A multivariate analysis of prognostic factors in management of pineal tumor. *Int J Radiat Oncol Biol Phys*. 1993;27:1185–1191.

353. Shibamoto Y, Oda Y, Yamashita J, et al. The role of cerebrospinal fluid cytology in radiotherapy planning for intracranial germinoma. *Int J Radiat Oncol Biol Phys*. 1994;29:1089–1094.

354. Tang Y, Booth T, Steward M, et al. The imaging of conditions affecting the cavernous sinus. *Clin Radiol.* 2010;65:937–945.

355. Naing S, Frohman LA. The empty sella. *Pediatr Endocrinol Rev*. 2007;4:335–342.

356. Tomita T, Gates E. Pituitary adenomas and granular cell tumors. Incidence, cell type, and location of tumor in 100 pituitary glands at autopsy. *Am J Clin Pathol*. 1999;111:817–825.

357. Turgut M, Ozsunar Y, Basak S, et al. Pituitary apoplexy: an overview of 186 cases published during the last century. *Acta Neurochir*. 2010;152:749–761.

358. Chaiban JT, Abdelmannan D, Cohen M, et al. Rathke cleft cyst apoplexy: a newly characterized distinct clinical entity. *J Neurosurg*. 2011;114:318–324.

359. Nawar RN, AbdelMannan D, Selman WR, et al. Pituitary tumor apoplexy: a review. *J Intensive Care Med*. 2008;23:75–90.

360. Tessnow AH, Wilson JD. The changing face of Sheehan's syndrome. *Am J Med Sci*. 2010;340:402–406.

361. Kontogeorgos G. Classification and pathology of pituitary tumors. *Endocrine*. 2005;28:27–35.

362. Scheithauer BW, Gaffey TA, Lloyd RV, et al. Pathobiology of pituitary adenomas and carcinomas. *Neurosurgery*. 2006;59:341–353.

363. Kovacs K, Horvath E. *Tumors of the Pituitary Gland*. 2nd Series, Fascicle 21. Washington, DC: Armed Forces Institute of Pathology; 1986.

364. Berger SA, Edberg SC, David G. Infectious disease in the sella turcica. *Rev Infect Dis*. 1986;8:747–755.

365. Mark AS, Phister SH, Jackson DE Jr, et al. Traumatic lesions of the suprasellar region: MR imaging. *Radiology*. 1992;182:49–52.

366. Bale PM, Hughes L, de Silva M. Sequestrated meningoceles of scalp: extracranial meningeal heterotopia. *Hum Pathol*. 1990;21:1156–1163.

367. Wax MK, Briant TD. Epidermoid cysts of the cranial bones. *Head Neck*. 1992;14:293–296.

368. 382. Ruge JR, Tomita T, Naidich TP, et al. Scalp and calvarial masses of infants and children. *Neurosurgery*. 1988;22:1037–1042.

369. Naama O, Gazzaz M, Akhaddar A, et al. Cavernous hemangioma of the skull: 3 case reports. *Surg Neurol*. 2008;70:654–659.

370. O'Brien DP, Rashad EM, Toland JA, et al. Aneurysmal cyst of the frontal bone: case report and review of the literature. *Br J Neurosurg* 1994;8:105–108.

371. Ito H Kizu O, Yamada K, et al. Secondary aneurysmal bone cyst derived from a giant-cell tumour of the skull base. *Neuroradiology*. 2003;45:616–617.

372. Bertoni F, Unni KK, Beabout JW, et al. Chondroblastoma of the skull and facial bones. *Am J Clin Pathol*. 1987;88:1–9.

373. Han X, Dong Y, Sun K, et al. A huge occipital osteoblastoma accompanied with aneurysmal bone cyst in the posterior cranial fossa. *Clinl Neurol Neurosurg*. 2008;110:282–285.

374. Haddad GF, Hambali F, Mufarrij A, et al. Concomitant fibrous dysplasia and aneurysmal bone cyst of the skull base. Case report and review of the literature. *Pediatr Neurosurg*. 1998;28:147–153.

375. Daszkiewicz P, Roszkowski M, Grajkowska W. Aneurysmal bone cyst of skull and vertebrae in children. Analysis of own material and review of the literature. *Folia Neuropathol*. 2004;42:25–30.

376. Epstein NE. Lumbar synovial cysts: a review of diagnosis, surgical management, and outcome assessment. *J Spinal Disord Tech*. 2004;17:321–325.

377. Howington JU, Connolly ES, Voorhies RM. Intraspinal synovial cysts: 10-year experience at the Ochsner Clinic. *J Neurosurg*. 1999;91:193–199.

378. Ojemann JG, Moran CJ, Gokden M, et al. Sagittal sinus occlusion by intraluminal dural cysts. Report of two cases. *J Neurosurg*. 1999;91:867–870.

379. Arai H, Sato K. Posterior fossa cysts: clinical, neuroradiological and surgical features. *Childs Nerv Syst*. 1991;7:156–564.

380. Galassi E, Tognetti F, Gaist G, et al. CT scan and CT cisternography in arachnoid cysts of the middle cranial fossa: classification and pathophysiological aspects. *Surg Neurol*. 1982;17:363–369.

381. Galarza M, Lopez-Guerrero AL, Martinez-Lage JF. Posterior fossa arachnoid cysts and cerebellar tonsillar descent: short review. *Neurosurg Rev*. 2010;33:305–314.

382. Marin SA, Skinner CR, Da Silva VF. Posterior fossa arachnoid cyst associated with Chiari I and syringomyelia. *Can J Neurol Sci*. 2010;37:273–275.

383. Russo N, Domenicucci M, Beccaglia MR, et al. Spontaneous reduction of intracranial arachnoid cysts: a complete review. *Br J Neurosurg*. 2008;22:626–629.

384. Zada G, Lin N, Ojerholm E, et al. Craniopharyngioma and other cystic epithelial lesions of the sellar region: a review of clinical, imaging, and histopathological relationships. *Neurosurg Focus*. 2010;28:E4.

385. Lach B, Scheithauer BW, Gregor A, et al. Colloid cyst of the third ventricle: a comparative immunohistochemical study of neuraxis cysts and choroid plexus epithelium. *J Neurosurg*. 1993;78:101–111.

386. Agnoli AL, Laun A, Schonmayr R: Enterogenous intraspinal cysts. *J Neurosurg*. 1984;61:834–840.

387. Cheng JS, Cusick JF, Ho KC, et al. Lateral supratentorial endodermal cyst: case report and review of literature. *Neurosurgery*. 2002;51:493–499.

388. Paleologos TS, Thom M, Thomas DG. Spinal neurenteric cysts without associated malformations. Are they the same as those presenting in spinal dysraphism? *Br J Neurosurg*. 2000;14:185–194.

389. Rodrigues D, Behari S, Ismail A, et al. Giant presacral neuro-enteric cyst with anomalous sacrum in an adult patient. *Br J Neurosurg*. 2005;19:181–184.

390. Voyadzis JM, Bhargava P, Henderson FC. Tarlov cysts: a study of 10 cases with review of the literature. *J Neurosurg*. 2001;95:25–32.

391. Czervionke LF, Daniels DL, Meyer GA, et al. Neuroepithelial cysts of the lateral ventricles: MR appearance. *Am J Neuroradiol*. 1987;8:609–613.

392. Iwahashi H, Kawai S, Watabe Y, et al. Spinal intramedullary ependymal cyst: a case report. *Surg Neurol*. 1999;52:357–361.

393. Ranjan R. Tewari R. Kumar S. Cervical intradural extramedullary ependymal cyst associated with congenital dermal sinus: a case report. *Childs Nerv Syst*. 2009;25:1121–1124.

394. Marin-Padilla M. Developmental neuropathology and impact of perinatal brain damage. II: white matter lesions of the neocortex. *J Neuropathol Exp Neurol*. 1997;56:219–235.

395. Utsunomiya H, Yamashita S, Takano K, et al. Midline cystic malformations of the brain: imaging diagnosis and classification based on embryologic analysis. *Radiat Med*. 2006;24:471–481.

396. Topcu M, Saatci I, Apak RA, et al. Leigh syndrome in a 3-year-old boy with unusual brain MR imaging and pathologic findings. *Am J Neuroradiol*. 2000;21:224–227.

397. Lerman-Sagie T, Leshinsky-Silver E, Watemberg N, et al. White matter involvement in mitochondrial diseases. *Mol Genet Metab*. 2005;84:127–136.

398. van der Knaap MS, Lai V, Kohler W, et al. Megalencephalic leukoencephalopathy with cysts without MLC1 defect. *Ann Neurol*. 2010;67:834–837.

399. Pronk JC, van Kollenburg B, Scheper GC, et al. Vanishing white matter disease: a review with focus on its genetics. *Ment Retard Dev Disabil Res Rev*. 2006;12:123–128.

400. Back SA, Riddle A, McClure MM. Maturation-dependent vulnerability of perinatal white matter in premature birth. *Stroke*. 2007;38:724–730.

401. Bonfield CM, Levi AD, Arnold PM, et al. Surgical management of post-traumatic syringomyelia. *Spine*. 2010;35:S245–S258.

402. Srivatanakul K, Songsaeng D, Ozanne A, et al. Spinal arteriovenous malformation associated with syringomyelia. *J Neurosurg Spine*. 2009;10:436–442.

403. Koyanagi I, Houkin K. Pathogenesis of syringomyelia associated with Chiari type 1 malformation: review of evidences and proposal of a new hypothesis. *Neurosurg Rev*. 2010;33:271–284.

404. Maldaun MV, Suki D, Lang FF, et al. Cystic glioblastoma multiforme: survival outcomes in 22 cases. *J Neurosurg*. 2004;100:61–67.

405. De Jesus O, Rifkinson N, Negron B. Cystic meningiomas: a review. *Neurosurgery*. 1995;36:489–492.

406. Takayanagui OM, Odashima NS. Clinical aspects of neurocysticercosis. *Parasitol Int*. 2006;55:S111–S115.

407. Nourbakhsh A, Vannemreddy P, Minagar A, et al. Hydatid disease of the central nervous system: a review of literature with an emphasis on Latin American countries. *Neurol Res*. 2010;32:245–251.

408. Flamm ES, Ransohoff J, Wuchinich D, et al. Preliminary experience with ultrasonic aspiration in neurosurgery. *Neurosurgery*. 1978;2:240–245.

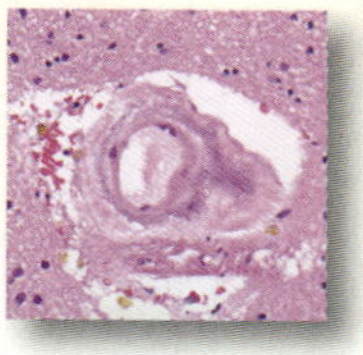
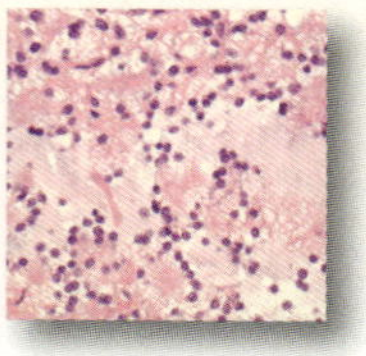
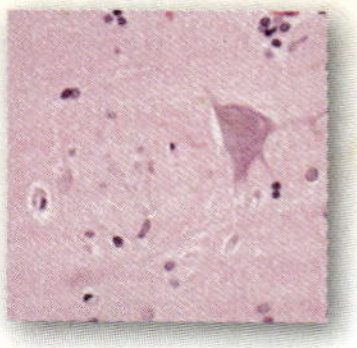

CHAPTER 2

Microscopic Features

Introduction

Although many ancillary techniques are utilized in the process of reaching a diagnosis and providing additional predictive and prognostic information that influence patient management, the basic microscopic evaluation using a light microscope and hematoxylin-eosin (H&E)-stained sections of formalin-fixed, paraffin-embedded tissue remains as one of the initial steps and the mainstay of this process. In addition, this evaluation also serves as a guide and paves the way for ancillary studies, when needed. On the other hand, what sounds like a simple step has constantly been becoming more and more complicated mainly due to two factors. One of these is the decrease in the amount of tissue with which the pathologist has to work, and the other is the increase in the number of considerations parallel to the increase in the number of new clinicopathologic entities that are being recognized. The frequent changes in nomenclature as the histogenesis, pathogenesis, and clinicopathologic implications of these entities are recognized only add to the difficulties associated with providing an accurate and clinically meaningful diagnostic interpretation. A brief look at the changes in the World Health Organization (WHO) classifications of the nervous system neoplasms provides an idea about how complicated this area has become.[1,2] Considering the additional areas such as nonneoplastic surgical neuropathology, neurodegenerative diseases, and neuromuscular pathology, the possibilities that the neuropathologist needs to keep up with and has to go over during daily work are numerous. This chapter, therefore, is intended to go over the individual microscopic findings and discuss their meaning in different settings. A brief differential diagnostic approach is also provided where necessary. Further steps to take, mainly limited to special stains, to distinguish particular entities from others are also mentioned. The details of special stains, additional microscopic features that are more relevant in intraoperative consultation (IOC), and neuromuscular pathology are discussed elsewhere in their respective chapters.

Apparently Unremarkable Tissue

In most cases, it is not a problem to tell normal tissue from abnormal; however, sometimes, the tissue may appear quite unremarkable even when there are significant pathologic changes. There are a few situations where this kind of appearance can be deceiving and may result in mistakes. The interpretation of such samples can be very difficult, because it is generally easier to prove the presence of pathology than to prove its absence in the tissue. Therefore, such samples should be investigated in detail and not rapidly given up on as "normal." Even if the sample truly has no pathologic features, the preferred wording should be *"no diagnostic histopathologic abnormality"* or other wording along similar lines, as essentially all samples that end up on a pathologist's microscope will have at least some changes, though they may not be diagnostic for any definitive pathologic condition, such as surgical changes, edema, tissue distortion, a mild gliosis, or microglial proliferation.

A particularly deceiving pattern is gliomatosis cerebri. By definition, it is a diffusely infiltrating glial neoplasm, most commonly astrocytic, without a distinct mass lesion, involving at least three

List of Findings/Checklist for Apparently Unremarkable Tissue

• AT A GLANCE

- No diagnostic histopathologic abnormality
- Mildly increased cellularity
  - Diffusely infiltrating neoplasm (gliomatosis, lymphomatosis)
  - Optic glioma
  - Satellitosis
  - Infiltrating periphery of a glioma
  - Reactive glial proliferation
  - Microglial proliferation
- Axonal spheroids
- Capillary damage
- Alzheimer type II astrocytes
- Opalski cells
- Perivascular macrophages
  - Fungal yeast forms
  - HIV encephalitis
- Vascular changes
- Neuropil irregularities
- Neurofibrillary tangles and other cytoplasmic inclusions (see "Cytoplasmic Inclusions")
- Nuclear inclusions (see "Nuclear Inclusions")
- Neuronal abnormalities
  - Dysmorphic ganglion cells
  - Abnormal orientation of cortical neurons
  - Hypothalamic neuronal changes
- Displaced neurons or gray matter
  - Neurons in cortical layer I
  - Gray matter islands in white matter
  - Tangential cuts of cortical gray matter
  - Neurons in white matter
- Hippocampus and dentate gyrus changes
  - Dysplasia, dispersion, duplication
- Olivary and/or dentate nucleus changes
  - Hypertrophy, dysplasia, heterotopia
- Status verrucosus
- Abnormalities of cortical layering
- Cerebellar heterotopias and dysplasia
- Atrophy, absence, atresia, or asymmetry
  - Pyramidal tracts
  - Aqueduct
  - Arcuate nuclei
- Pituitary gland
  - Adenohypophyseal hyperplasia versus normal
  - Reticulin and immunohistochemical stains
- Nerve fascicles
- Pacinian corpuscles
- Collapsed bone trabeculae

cerebral lobes.[3] Distinct mass lesions can develop in this particular background through localized proliferation of neoplastic cells. However, in the actual gliomatosis, the *scattered neoplastic cells* infiltrate the white matter without resulting in a significant increase in cellularity. Only upon close examination can they be identified as variably irregular nuclei with no apparent cytoplasm **(Fig. 2-1)**. When searched for, they can stand out in the background of the usual white matter cellularity as somewhat elongated nuclei with irregular nuclear borders and no prominent nucleoli. A few of them can form small aggregates. If there is gray matter infiltration, they can *satellite around neurons and capillaries*. It should be remembered that satellitosis can be a normal finding, especially in the temporal lobe. Therefore, one should also pay attention to the cytologic features of the satelliting cells. A pattern similar to gliomatosis cerebri can be seen in diffusely infiltrating lymphoma, that

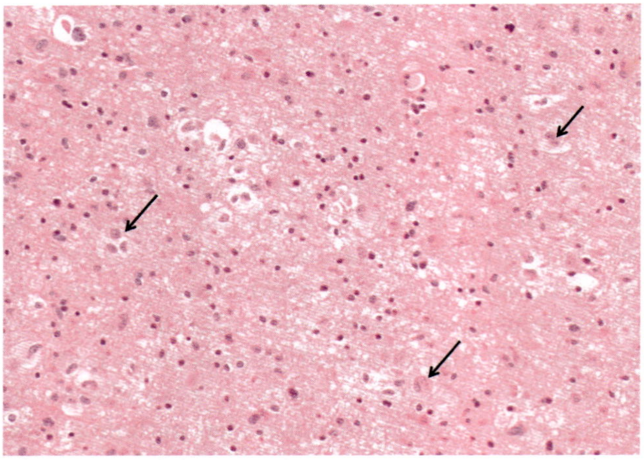

Figure 2-1. Gliomatosis cerebri: The tissue is at best mildly cellular but is otherwise unremarkable. Close examination, however, reveals scattered larger, irregular nuclei (*arrows*), sometimes forming vague grouping (H&E; original magnification: 200×).

is, lymphomatosis cerebri.[4] The cytologic features of these cells are quite different from infiltrating glioma cells with more open chromatin and prominent nucleoli (see "Nuclear Features"); however, this distinction may be difficult in a given case, and therefore, this possibility should be kept in mind for the differential diagnosis of gliomatosis cerebri. Optic glioma, while sometimes a loosely used term to refer to any glial neoplasm involving optic nerve, is typically a pilocytic astrocytoma (PA) involving the optic chiasm and nerves. Grossly and radiologically, the optic nerves are expanded and uniformly enlarged, but microscopic examination may not reveal prominent changes. The usual compartmentalized fascicular pattern of optic nerve on cross section is preserved, but it appears more cellular. The neoplastic cells also become elongated when they infiltrate this compact structure and appear round on cross section. They have very bland nuclear features. If *Rosenthal fibers* are present, they serve as alerting and supportive features for the diagnosis of PA in this setting. A prominent circumferential meningothelial proliferation that is commonly present in these cases is also useful to draw attention to the presence of an abnormality. A very subtle hypercellularity is present in reactive processes, mainly in mild astrocytosis and microglial proliferation. Especially the latter is very common as the microglial cells react to pretty much any type of insult, from hypoxic to inflammatory/infectious to neoplastic (see "Inflammation and Bone Marrow–Derived Cells"). In isolation, and although abnormal, microglial proliferation is highly nonspecific. Same comments are true for reactive gliosis. The importance of both of these reactive processes is to distinguish them from a low-grade glioma, or vice versa. The infiltrating periphery of a glial neoplasm also enters this differential diagnosis (see "Lesion Borders").

Diffuse axonal injury (DAI) can also be very subtle, especially in the early stages of the process, before the *axonal spheroids* have developed. The latter can be difficult to identify in subtle cases **(Fig. 2-2)** and if the *capillary damage* did not occur to result in the petechial hemorrhages to draw attention to the possibility of DAI. Nonetheless, knowledge of history of trauma or another event that may have resulted in rapid and angular acceleration of the head should alert one to search for the findings of DAI. Amyloid precursor protein immunohistochemistry can be positive as early as 2 to 4 hours postinjury and constitutes the earliest light microscopic change in DAI.[5] Axonal spheroids are also seen as part of chemotherapy/radiation-induced leukoencephalopathy; however, additional prominent pathologic changes such as white matter microinfarcts, myelin and axon loss, and microcalcifications are also present. Microvacuolation of the white matter neuropil can be present, which may appear like edema or poor fixation in mild cases. Hepatic encephalopathy causes subtle cellular changes in a diffuse manner. Hyperamonemia causes changes in astrocytes resulting in large nuclei with open chromatin pattern and prominent nucleoli, and no prominent cytoplasm, that is, *Alzheimer type II astrocytes* **(Fig. 2-3)**. In addition, *Opalski cells*, the origin of which is not clear, although they are thought to be astrocytic, appear especially in the basal ganglia. They are small cells with a small, round, and somewhat pyknotic nuclei and abundant eosinophilic granular cytoplasm, superficially resembling reactive astrocytes. Any type of pathologic process that is otherwise straightforward may become a problem if it is not represented appropriately in the sample or if it is very focal. Obviously, such a problem can be compounded by the small size of

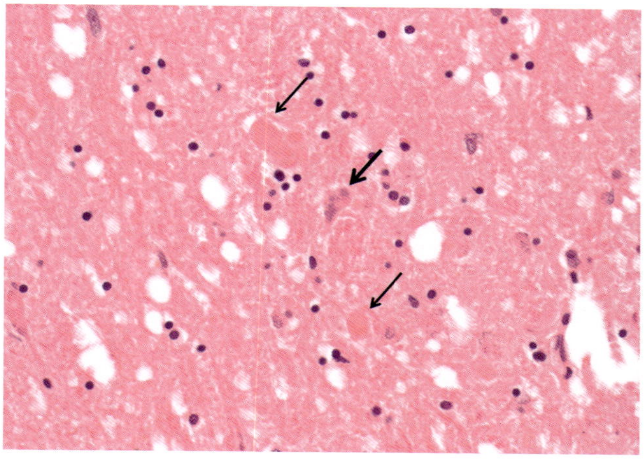

Figure 2-2. Axonal spheroids: Eosinophilic round structures of variable sizes and shapes (*thin arrows*), though typically round, are present in the neuropil in this case of DAI. There is also vacuolation of the neuropil, representing edema. This particular section is from the brainstem, and a neuron (*thick arrow*) still appears viable at this early stage (H&E; original magnification: 400×).

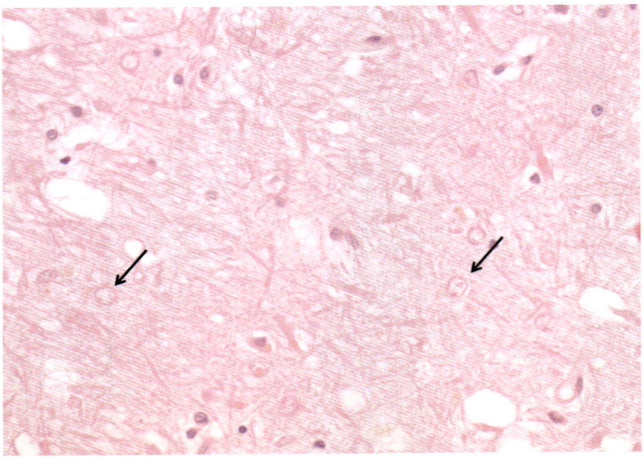

Figure 2-3. Alzheimer type II glia: Enlarged nuclei with open chromatin, small eosinophilic nucleoli, and no prominent perinuclear cytoplasm (*arrows*) are present in the basal ganglia in this case of hepatic encephalopathy. These cells can have lobulated irregular nuclei with similar chromatin pattern (H&E; original magnification: 400×).

the sample. For instance, white matter in human immunodeficiency virus (HIV) encephalitis can appear quite unremarkable except for some *myelin pallor*, and the *rare perivascular multinucleated macrophages* may be quite obscure. A few *fungal yeast forms* can be seen in perivascular spaces, as in *Cryptococcus* in Virchow-Robin spaces or as in *Histoplasma* within the macrophage cytoplasms, also favoring perivascular areas. In high-risk or suspected cases, they may be highlighted only by special stains. Blood vessels can have subtle changes that may be in their earlier phases and are not yet associated with significant tissue changes. A *bright eosinophilic appearance of superficial cortical and leptomeningeal vessels* may be an indication of amyloid accumulation, especially in those cases where plaques and tangles are also identified, since Alzheimer's disease (AD) pathology is associated with beta-amyloid accumulation. Other subtle vascular changes can be present in the white matter vessels without any other significant changes, except for some myelin pallor as a result of chronic ischemic changes. They may have *collagenous hyalinized thickening* as in hypertensive encephalopathy. They may also have basophilic granular material that is periodic acid-Schiff (PAS) positive, as seen in cerebral autosomal dominant arteriopathy with subcortical infarcts and leukoencephalopathy (CADASIL). Neurodegenerative diseases have very limited microscopic findings on routine sections. They can be as simple as *neuron loss and gliosis* and can be apparent only in well-developed or advanced cases. The other characteristic features of individual diseases, such as *various inclusions and accumulations*, can be identified only by special stains. Therefore, the routine sections can appear quite unremarkable upon initial evaluation. It is also important to be aware of the gross findings and the area that is being examined and that the section is representative of the area that is typically involved in a particular neurodegenerative disease, such as examining substantia nigra if the question is Parkinson's disease. In the most common dementing neurodegenerative disease, AD, it is not uncommon to identify microscopic features that at least suggest the possibility by a Bielschowsky silver stain in an otherwise unremarkable autopsy brain or in a brain that is being examined for another unrelated question. This kind of "screening" is typically initiated by the identification of some *irregularities in the neuropil* suggesting the presence of neuritic plaques **(Fig. 2-4)**, a few eosinophilic dense accumulations suggesting amyloid cores of neuritic plaques, or a few neurofibrillary tangles (NFTs) in an older patient. Therefore, evaluating the neuropil in the

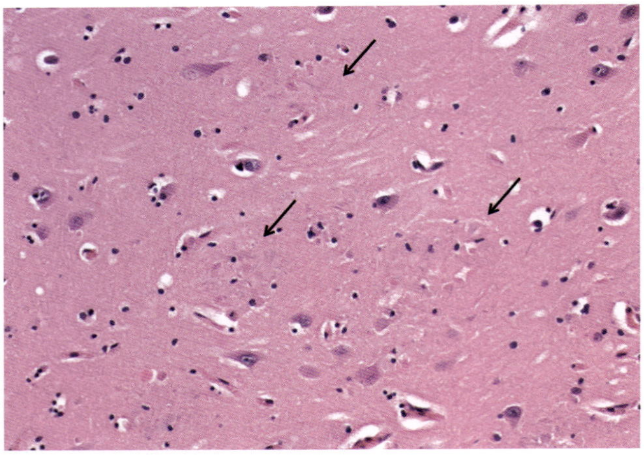

Figure 2-4. Neuritic plaques: The usual homogeneous finely granular texture of the neuropil seen in other areas of this picture is punctuated by vague irregularities with a roughly round outline and eosinophilic thickenings (*arrows*). Many of the plaques, including neuritic plaques, are difficult to identify on routine sections without special stains (H&E; original magnification: 200×).

cerebral gray matter, especially hippocampal/entorhinal cortex of such cases, may be very useful. Similar scenarios apply to other neurodegenerative diseases, although such further evaluations are typically the result of clinical question and correlation in such cases. In some cases, a rare Lewy body can be incidentally seen in the substantia nigra of an otherwise unremarkable brain. While the significance of such a finding is not clear, this condition is termed incidental Lewy body disease and is thought to represent a very early, subclinical stage of a developing Parkinson's disease.[6]

Gangliocytomas are ganglion cell neoplasms composed of *dysmorphic ganglion cells* with features similar to those seen in ganglioglioma but without a glioma component. In subtle cases, the neuronal density is simply more than that expected in a given region of the central nervous system (CNS), but diligent search should provide hints of ganglion cell abnormalities, in addition to the long-standing clinical history with seizures, cyst and mural nodule formation, predominantly temporal lobe location, and calvarial bone scalloping. Rarely, a binucleated neuron can be seen in otherwise unremarkable cerebral cortex. Apparently unremarkable cerebral cortex adjacent to the neoplasm can sometimes be slightly more cellular than expected in the subtle examples of gangliocytomas. Another histologically unremarkable-appearing lesion is hypothalamic hamartoma that occurs in the hypothalamic region, typically in the walls of the third ventricle, or less commonly in the parahypothalamic location inferior to the hypothalamus.[7] It is a nodular lesion composed of cytologically unremarkable neurons and glial cells, resembling normal gray matter. The *absence of the large neurons normally present in the hypothalamic region* may be a clue. Sometimes, differentiating these hamartomas from ganglioglioma may be challenging. However, the absence of dysmorphic forms and thick vascular network and the orderly distribution of neurons in the hamartoma are helpful. Correlation with radiologic features and knowledge of the exact location are also useful in this differential. Occasional hypothalamic hamartomas can be a component of Pallister-Hall syndrome that has skeletal and developmental stigmata.[8] *Gray matter heterotopias* in white matter can look like normal gray matter, and this should be considered in small islands of gray matter surrounded by white matter. They are commonly multiple and periventricular. The heterotopic gray matter can have some irregularities to the distribution of neurons and/or to their cytology, making it look different than the other areas of cortical gray matter. Various cerebral and cerebellar heterotopias, including *leptomeningeal glioneuronal heterotopias*, and cortical dysplasias[9] in the brain and cerebellum can be seen as part of neuronal migration disorders and various malformations as well as a result of some intoxications, such as mercury intoxication and fetal alcohol syndrome. They may also resemble *tangential cuts of gray matter* representing the base of the gyri. This situation usually arises in autopsy sections and can be clarified by noticing the topography and comparing the histologic and cytologic details. In a similar manner, apparently unremarkable cerebral cortex can show, upon closer evaluation, subtle features of cortical malformation. In the cortex, the neurons are aligned normally perpendicular to the pial surface, with axon hillock pointing toward the white matter. This orientation of neurons is altered in malformations of cortical development (MCD), with *neurons pointing to different directions*, creating variable degrees of haphazard appearances. Other features that indicate the presence of a cortical malformation are ballooning and dysplasia of the neurons. In addition, there may be *neurons within the molecular layer*, which is normally devoid of large neurons. Usually, careful microscopic examination will reveal such abnormalities, but additional special stains such as neurofilament and Bielschowsky can facilitate their identification by highlighting the neuronal and axonal population. Of the MCD, according to Palmini classification, the mildest form is type I and is characterized by the presence of neurons displaced to the molecular layer.[10] *Focal scattered individual neurons in the superficial white matter* is a common finding especially in the anterior temporal lobe and sometimes may be a part of a more significant abnormality in association with seizure disorders[11] **(Fig. 2-5)**. *Widespread presence of neurons within the white matter* is seen in diffuse neuronal heterotopia or radial glioneuronal heterotopia in tuberous sclerosis. Microdysgenesis is a poorly defined term that is variably used to describe heterotopias in molecular layer and white matter, layer II undulations, cortical disorganization, or perineuronal satelliting of glial cells in

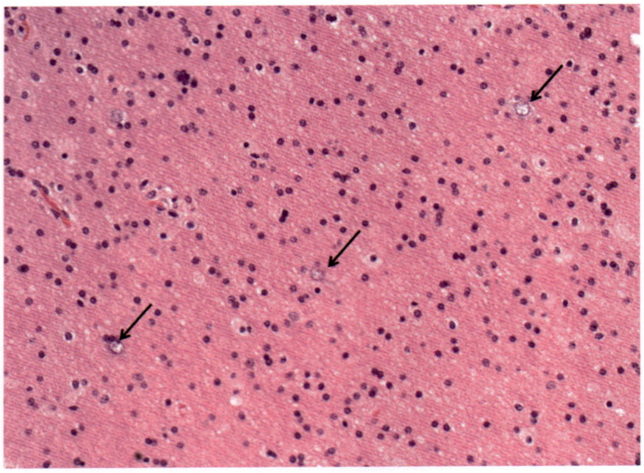

Figure 2-5. Neurons in white matter: A common finding in temporal lobe and seizure specimens; scattered larger nuclei with open chromatin pattern are seen in the white matter (*arrows*). They usually have only small amount of amphophilic cytoplasm (H&E; original magnification: 200×).

the temporal lobe.[12] As such, it does not indicate a specific diagnostic entity. Hemimegalencephaly, the asymmetrically enlarged cerebral hemisphere, microscopically can only show excess of neurons without any malformations in isolation or can be associated with other abnormalities such as pachygyria and polymicrogyria. A cortical malformation with features of focal cortical dysplasia (FCD) but in a diffuse manner is seen in unilateral cortical dysplasia with hemimegalencephaly. It is also seen in isolation or in association with various syndromes.

Inferior olivary hypertrophy **(Table 2.1)** may be noticed especially when compared to the other olivary nucleus, but may be bilateral, and subtle when the hypertrophic olivary nucleus is examined in isolation. It represents a form of transsynaptic degeneration due to the degeneration or destruction of the tracts associated with the olivary nucleus.[13] The gray matter ribbon is thickened with *enlarged and vacuolated neurons*. Dysplasias of various structures can be seen in various syndromes and disorders, such as *olivary nucleus dysplasia* in Miller-Dieker syndrome, *hippocampal disorganization* in thanatophoric dysplasia,[14] *dentate gyrus dysplasia* and *hypoplasia of hippocampus* in trisomy 18, or *duplication or dispersion of dentate gyrus* in temporal lobe epilepsy cases. A variety of other dysplastic appearances in olivary nuclei may be in seen in various combinations. Some examples include *dorsal thickening* in trisomy 18, *C-shape* without folding in Joubert,[15] *simplified folds, fragmentation*, dorsal thickening and C-shape in Zellweger syndrome,[16] and *excessive folding* in thanatophoric dysplasia. Horseshoe shape of the olivary nuclei in fetal stage is a normal finding. *Dentate nucleus hyperconvolution* can be seen in thanatophoric

TABLE 2.1 Changes in inferior olivary nuclei and their common associations

Microscopic Feature	Association	Other Findings
Hypertrophy	Transsynaptic degeneration	Thickened gray matter band, enlarged neurons with cytoplasmic vacuolation
Dysplasia	Miller-Dieker syndrome	Agyria, heterotopias
Dorsal thickening	Trisomy 18	Holoprosencephaly, dentate nucleus dysplasia, hippocampal abnormalities
C-shape	Joubert syndrome	Cerebellar vermis agenesis, dentate nucleus dysplasia, heterotopias
Fragmentation, C-shape, dorsal thickening, simplified folds	Zellweger (cerebrohepatorenal) syndrome	Various neuronal migration defects, dentate nucleus dysplasia, myelin loss, lipid deposition, adrenal cortical, hepatic and renal abnormalities
Horseshoe shape	Normal during fetal development	—
Loss of darkly myelinated sheath surrounding the olivary nucleus	Hypoplasias and dysplasias in general	—
Olivary heterotopia	Dandy-Walker malformation	Cerebellar vermis agenesis, midline cerebellar cyst
	Agyria/pachygyria	Variable
	Hemimegalencephaly	Variable

dysplasia; it is *simplified and segmented* in cerebellar hypoplasias and trisomy 13 and 18, or is in the form of a *thick plate without folding* in some other dysplasias.[17] *Dentate gyrus duplication or dispersion* can be seen in dysembryoplastic neuroepithelial tumor (DNET) of temporal lobe, "microdysgenesis," and Sturge-Weber syndrome and can be bilateral. In pontocerebellar hypoplasia[18] (or, more accurately, pontoneocerebellar hypoplasia, as primarily the neocerebellum is involved and paleocerebellum is relatively preserved), the *dentate nuclei are fragmented*, olivary nuclei are dysplastic, and *arcuate nuclei can be absent*, along with thin cerebellar folia with variable granule cell and Purkinje cell population. Dentate and olivary nuclear dysplasias are usually seen together. The normally thick, dark-staining, and dense *myelinated fiber sheath around dentate and olivary nuclei* is diminished in cases of hypoplasias and dysplasias of these structures. In *status verrucosus*,[19] layer II protrudes into the molecular layer in the form of microscopic verrucous projections, creating an undulated pattern while the brain surface remains flat. It is commonly seen between 10 and 28 gestational weeks. Whether it represents a normal stage in development or a true malformation is debatable. Microscopic examination of tissue from various grossly obvious malformations may show subtle changes. Cerebral cortex in holoprosencephaly may show status verrucosus. Nodular cortical dysplasia on the other hand, also known as "brain wart" due to wart-like protrusions of a few millimeters of cortex on brain surface, usually has layer II and III in it and a central blood vessel. A *four-layer cortex* can be present in holoprosencephaly.

Cerebellar heterotopias are usually incidental and common. They may be especially associated with trisomy 13[20] and other cerebellar hypoplasias and brainstem abnormalities. They consist of islands of disorganized mixture of granule cells and Purkinje cells. Focal *dysplastic cerebellar cortex*[21] is seen commonly especially in flocculonodular lobes as an incidental finding. In other areas, it can be prominent with cortical broadening, while the foliar layers seem to be orderly but thickened with apparent *fusing of folia*. *Folia are broadened* as the cerebral cortex is in cerebral cortical dysplasias. It can be isolated or associated with other abnormalities such as cerebro-ocular dysplasia. *Heterotopic olivary nuclei*[17] can be found close to the inferior cerebellar peduncle laterally or near the hypoglossal nucleus rootlets medially. The native olivary nuclei are usually dysplastic. Olivary nucleus heterotopias can be seen in agyria/pachygyria, Dandy-Walker malformation,[22] and megalencephaly, among others.

The *absence of certain structures* can be missed if not searched for specifically. *Pyramidal tracts are absent* in anencephaly, holoprosencephaly, porencephaly, hydranencephaly, and X-linked congenital aqueductal stenosis.[23] They may rarely be in the form of multiple fascicles in various cerebral malformations. Olivary heterotopias and hypoplastic pyramidal tracts can be associated with congenital cerebral lactic acidosis due to pyruvate dehydrogenase deficiency.[24] *Asymmetry* in these situations is common and may be together with spinal cord asymmetry. *Atrophy of many tracts in the brainstem and spinal cord* is associated with their degeneration or destruction at a more cranial location (see "Tract Degeneration"). *Aqueductal abnormalities*, namely, stenosis, gliosis, and atresia, can be subtle. Although these terms may be used interchangeably in practice, *aqueductal stenosis* is just small lumen with no gliosis in contrast to secondary damage. It can be sporadic or X-linked.[25] *Aqueductal atresia* shows many small channels, with no significant gliosis. It can be associated with Arnold-Chiari malformation, hydranencephaly, and meningoencephalitis (especially mumps)[26] or can be sporadic. In *aqueductal gliosis*, the aqueduct is obliterated by gliosis, typically due to previous injury—typically infectious/inflammatory.[27]

Pituitary hyperplasias may be difficult to recognize, especially in small samples. The main feature of hyperplasia is the *expansion of the normal acini* with increased numbers of cells. This can be better appreciated by a reticulin stain that shows the expansion of the reticulin pattern, which is somewhat irregular, but is not completely wiped out as would be expected in adenoma **(Fig. 2-6)**. Likewise, the cell groups representing the nesting pattern of nonneoplastic gland can be identified, though not as easily as in normal gland, and careful search reveals the presence of scattered admixed cell types other than those that became hyperplastic. Hyperplasias may be *nodular or diffuse*.[28] While nodular ones are easier to detect, as they stand out in the background of normal anterior pituitary parenchyma that provides comparison, the diffuse hyperplasias may be difficult to recognize. The absence of any radiologic

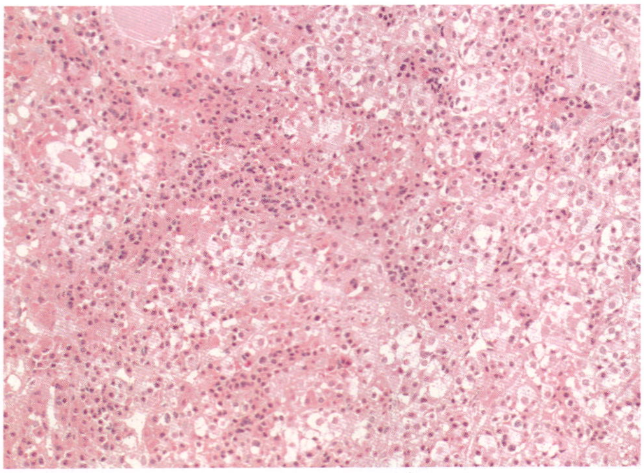

Figure 2-6. Pituitary hyperplasia: Whether the usual nesting pattern of the resting anterior pituitary parenchyma is preserved or distorted can be impossible to determine on routine sections, and a reticulin stain is necessary for this evaluation. The presence of a mixture of cell types helps exclude adenoma (H&E; original magnification: 200×).

or intraoperative distinct nodule and the alterations in the reticulin network, together with clinical, biochemical, and immunohistochemical features, at least allow one to suggest the diagnosis. Since acidophilic cells are most frequent in the lateral aspects of the gland, small tissue samples from these areas may appear to consist of predominantly acidophilic cells. Likewise, since basophilic cells tend to be larger, they appear to be the dominant cell type in an acinus, resulting in a false impression of hyperplasia or adenoma. Therefore, attention to the detail to identify the presence of other admixed cell types and the reticulin pattern is necessary to sort through normal, hyperplasia, or adenoma question, especially in small specimens. The possibilities of end-organ failure, as in cases of thyroidectomy or gonadectomy; hypofunction such as hypothyroidism or hypogonadism (e.g., in Klinefelter and Turner syndromes); ectopic releasing hormone production by neuroendocrine neoplasms in other parts of the body; unknown hypothalamic overstimulation; as well as physiologic states such as pregnancy should be considered as potential causes of hyperplasia. Adenoma formation in the background of hyperplasia is a rare occurrence and the link between them is not clear.[28] However, hyperplastic tissue may rarely be present adjacent to an adenoma, such as adrenocorticotropic hormone (ACTH) cell hyperplasia in association with ACTH cell adenoma or thyroid stimulating hormone (TSH) cell hyperplasia in association with prolactinoma. These rare situations may potentially complicate the decision making in some cases, especially in IOC. Again, communication with the surgeon and correlation with radiologic and intraoperative findings should help clarify such issues.

As for peripheral nerve lesions, traumatic-amputation neuroma is composed of *small groups of disorganized nerve fascicles* mimicking schwannoma or neurofibroma in some cases, but each group is surrounded by perineurium. Pacinian neuroma consists of one or more hypertrophic *pacinian corpuscles* that appear unremarkable other than being larger than normal. They are excised as a nodular lesion.

Some surgical bone curetting or core biopsy specimens appear as many irregular trabeculae with no significant amount of intervening bone marrow or stroma. They appear as though they represent a *collapsed bone fragment*. One possibility for this histologic appearance is the presence of a cavernous hemangioma within the bone, entirely occupying the intertrabecular space, which is destroyed during the procedure, leaving collapsed trabeculae behind. In such specimens, correlation with the radiologic findings and intraoperative observations is very useful to explain this situation and to distinguish it from surgical artifact.

Hypercellularity

This discussion is concerned with the mild increase in cellularity that is enough to realize that one is dealing with an abnormal tissue. The obviously hypercellular tissue seen in most straightforward lesions, such as the hypercellularity in a glioblastoma multiforme (GBM) or in an inflammatory process, is excluded. Assessment of cellularity is highly subjective, and even when the type of mild hypercellularity as discussed here is identified, that does not necessarily mean that a definitive diagnosis can be made. There are several situations where this assessment is critical.

Gliosis is a nonspecific reaction to pretty much any type of injury in the CNS. It is used interchangeably with *astrocytosis*, as astrocytes are the primary reacting cells in most situations and are easier to detect due to the fact that their cytoplasm and processes become prominent. In very mild

List of Findings/Checklist for Hypercellularity

AT A GLANCE

- Gliosis
- Astrocytosis (fibrillary, piloid)
- Low-grade glioma
- Infiltrating periphery of glioma
- Prominent cytoplasm
- Prominent processes
- Irregular grouping of cells
- Nuclear atypia
- Pleomorphism
- Mitotic activity
- Satellitosis
- Microcysts
- Microglial proliferation
- Inflammatory cells
- Immunohistochemistry (CD68, CD163, p53, Ki-67, WT-1, IDH1)
- Intraoperative consultations artifacts
- Hypoxic–ischemic changes

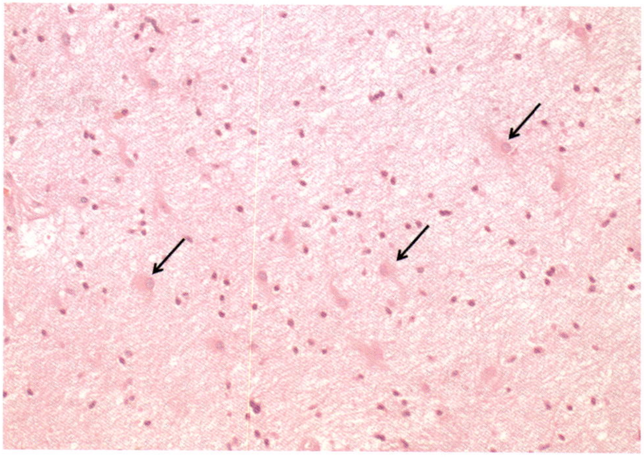

Figure 2-7. Fibrillary astrocytosis: Reactive astrocytes are easily identified because of their prominent cytoplasm (*arrows*). Many also have prominent cytoplasmic processes that can be easily identified by focusing up and down, and nuclei lack the hyperchromasia and irregularities associated with their neoplastic counterparts, that is, gemistocytes. They are somewhat regularly distributed in contrast to neoplastic processes. A reason, such as inflammation, for this reactive process is not always readily available, as is the case here (H&E; original magnification: 200×).

and subtle forms, it may even be difficult to identify the tissue as abnormal; however, close evaluation reveals scattered astrocytes with *prominent processes*. Glial fibrillary acidic protein (GFAP) immunohistochemistry can be useful in highlighting the astrocytes and evaluating their distribution, cytoplasms, and processes. Another related subject is the *type of astrocytic reaction*. By default, the term astrocytosis refers to the *fibrillary* type, which is described above **(Fig. 2-7)**. The presence of a dense, fascicular arrangement of elongated astrocytes, usually with Rosenthal fibers, is the *piloid* type **(Fig. 2-8)** and is associated with a more limited repertoire of etiologies. There are typically two main issues that arise in practice regarding gliosis: (a) is there gliosis and what caused it and (b) is it really gliosis or a *low-grade astrocytoma?* The answer to the first question either is usually readily apparent, in which case a diagnosis that is more definitive than just gliosis can be made and the issue becomes a topic other than "hypercellularity," or cannot be determined at all in most cases. The differential diagnosis of gliosis versus low-grade glial neoplasm is a difficult one with no straightforward answer. However, there are several features one can systematically sort through to at least favor one or the other especially in small tissue samples[29] **(Table 2.2)**, although admittedly, these features are also subjective. In addition, every effort should be shown to obtain any available information regarding the clinical, radiologic, and intraoperative findings. The cellularity in gliosis is theoretically

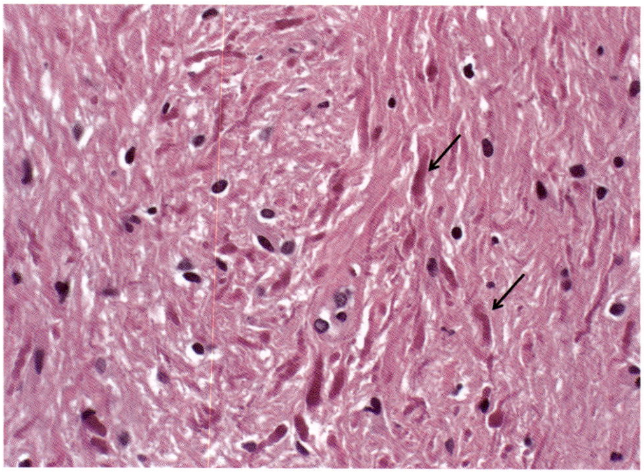

Figure 2-8. Piloid gliosis: Dense and thick, elongated fibrillarity forming a vague fascicular arrangement is seen. Rosenthal fibers (*arrows*) are usually present (H&E; original magnification: 400×).

TABLE 2.2 Differential diagnosis of reactive gliosis and low-grade glial neoplasm

Feature	Gliosis	Glioma
Cellularity	−/+	+
Nuclear atypia	−	+
Pleomorphism	−	+
Mitosis in glial cells	−	−/+
Satellitosis/cortical involvement	−	+
Uniform distribution of cells	+	−
Cytoplasmic prominence	+	−
Cytoplasmic processes	+	−
Macrophages/inflammation	+/−	−/+
Microglial proliferation	+	+
Microcysts	−	+
Mass lesion	−/+	+
Ki-67	−/+	+/−
WT-1	−	+/−
IDH1	−	−/+
P53	−	−/+[a]

+, present; −, absent; +/−, usually present; −/+, usually absent; WT-1, Wilms' tumor-1; IDH1, isocitrate dehydrogenase 1.
[a]Applies to astrocytic lesions.

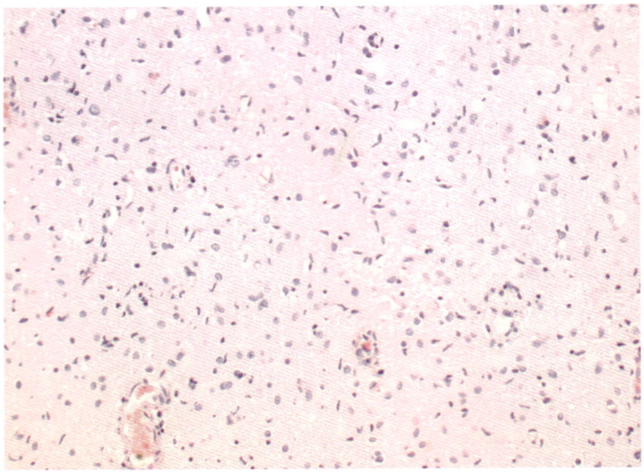

Figure 2-9. Microglial proliferation: An increased cellularity due to many spindled nuclei representing microglia is seen. Microglial proliferation may mimic low-grade astrocytoma or an infiltrating border of an astrocytic neoplasm. Considerable numbers of microglia may be present in glial neoplasms, also (H&E; original magnification: 200×).

not increased, as the astrocytes react and become prominent but do not necessarily *increase in number*, whereas a neoplastic process is expected to be more cellular. If there is a population other than the astrocytes, such as *inflammatory cells*, it will contribute to the cellularity. Likewise, *microglial proliferation* is almost always present, and the activated microglia, with their prominent and elongated nuclei, not only contribute to hypercellularity but also makes the lesion look like an infiltrating astrocytoma **(Fig. 2-9)**. Therefore, keeping microglial proliferation in mind, highlighting that population by immunohistochemical stains (e.g., CD68, CD163), and "subtracting" the microglial population from the rest of the cellularity should provide a more accurate assessment of cellularity. Likewise, the presence of an inflammatory population usually favors a reactive process; however, it should be remembered that it is not unusual for low-grade glial neoplasms to have perivascular small, round lymphocytes and even foamy macrophages; the latter can be especially prominent in oligodendrogliomas. Another subjective feature is *nuclear atypia*, based on the assumption that the neoplastic cells have more atypical nuclei than the nonneoplastic cells; however, it is well-known that sometimes the reactive changes can create more pronounced atypia than the neoplastic processes. Nonetheless, a coarse chromatin pattern, irregular nuclear membranes, and spindled or angulated nuclei, with or without nucleoli and no apparent cytoplasm or processes, favor a neoplastic process **(Fig. 2-10)**. *Pleomorphism* may not be obvious but, when present, favors a neoplastic process. The reactive astrocytes do not infiltrate the surrounding

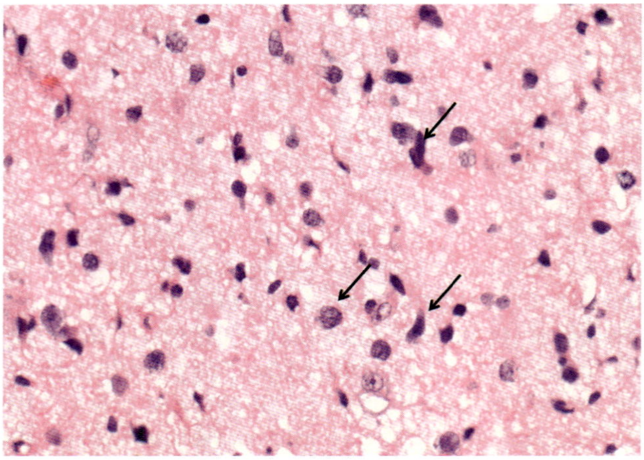

Figure 2-10. Astrocytoma: Nuclei are hyperchromatic and irregular (*arrows*) (H&E; original magnification: 400×).

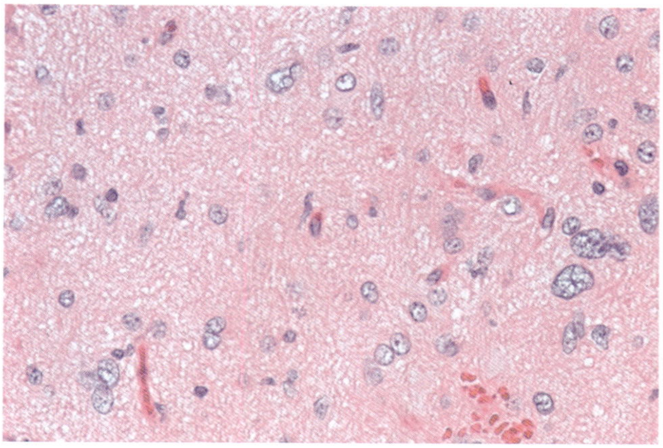

Figure 2-11. Astrocytoma: Nuclei show irregular distribution, resulting in small groups alternating with anuclear zones (H&E; original magnification: 400×).

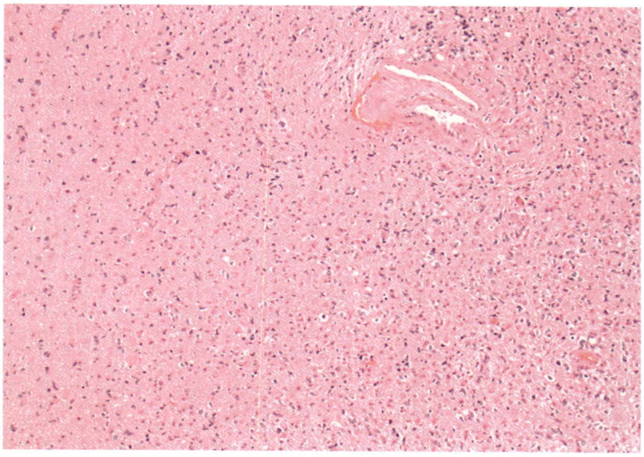

Figure 2-12. Infiltrative border of glial neoplasm: The cellularity of the neoplasm (**right side**) gradually fades into the surrounding tissues (**left side**), where it can create a low-grade appearance or where it can even be difficult to appreciate its neoplastic nature (H&E; original magnification: 100×).

tissues and stay where they are, creating an *orderly distribution of cells*, whereas neoplastic glial cells are infiltrative, resulting in *irregular distribution* with small groups or nuclei alternating with anuclear zones of neuropil **(Fig. 2-11)**. In addition, when the neoplastic cells infiltrate the gray matter areas, they tend to *satellite around neurons*, as well as capillaries. Since perineuronal satelliting is a common finding in nonneoplastic temporal lobe, the satelliting nuclei should be atypical neoplastic cells for this feature to be useful. A similar nonneoplastic *pericapillary satelliting* can be prominent by oligodendroglial cells in the white matter and should not be taken as evidence for malignancy. The identification of mitotic activity in the cell population of concern may be used in support of a neoplastic process; however, one has to make sure that the mitotic activity is not in the endothelial cells or in the inflammatory component. It is very unlikely to find convincing mitotic activity in such tissues with mild hypercellularity, unless one is dealing with the infiltrating periphery of a high-grade glioma, in which mitotic activity and nuclear atypia are already prominent. As for background neuropil, the presence of *microcytic changes* is a feature that favors a neoplastic process. The presence of a *mass lesion* by radiologic evaluation also favors a neoplastic process, although exceptions for both conditions occur. Obviously, this differential diagnosis is especially a challenge during IOC. In that context, the cellularity may be underestimated due to expansion of the tissue as a result of freezing artifact. On the other hand, the vacuolated appearance caused by the freezing artifact should not be interpreted as microcysts, unless basophilic mucinous or proteinaceous fluid is also seen. If there has been a previous diagnosis of glial neoplasm rendered and one is familiar with the histologic type and grade of the neoplasm, such interpretations become easier. For instance, if a high-grade glioma was diagnosed in a previous interpretation, one can now favor an infiltrating periphery of that glioma in this mildly hypercellular tissue.

In the context of neoplastic hypercellularity, the *infiltrating periphery of a glial neoplasm* also enters the differential diagnosis **(Fig. 2-12)**. Natural for infiltrating glial neoplasms, the cellularity gradually fades away as one moves away from the epicenter of the neoplasm, and there comes a point where only a few scattered extra cells are present to result in a mildly hypercellular tissue. As discussed above, knowledge of any previous diagnoses should facilitate this interpretation. Especially at IOC, but also in other settings, the identification of a clearly neoplastic process infiltrating the gray matter with satellitosis and in a mildly hypercellular fashion should prompt the comment that this tissue likely represents an infiltrating periphery of an underlying glioma, rather

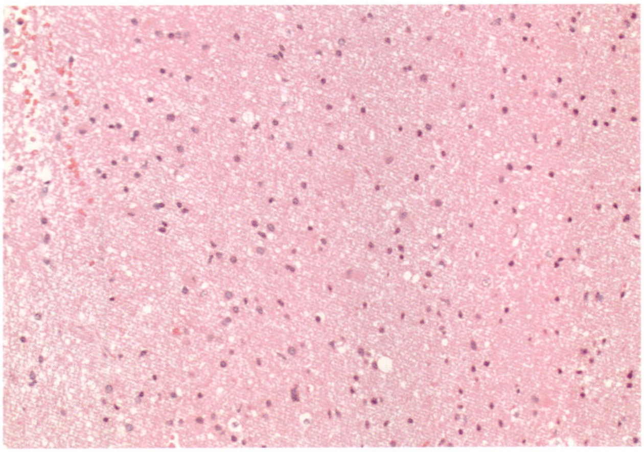

Figure 2-13. Atypical glial proliferation: The cellularity is worrisome but not diagnostic for a glioma. The distribution of cells is somewhat irregular. This interpretation, however, is highly subjective and comfort zones and accuracy vary widely among pathologists. Special stains can be helpful (see text) (H&E; original magnification: 200×).

than leaving the diagnosis at glioma. This can have significant implications for the neurosurgeon both during resections and stereotactic biopsies to retarget the approach so that diagnostic tissue is obtained. In general, if the reactive versus neoplastic nature of the process cannot be ascertained, descriptive terms such as "atypical glial proliferation" or "mildly hypercellular tissue" followed by a comment are appropriate **(Fig. 2-13)**. Another similar situation is when the main neoplastic process has been identified and diagnosed but the surgeon is sampling surrounding tissues to have an idea about the extent of the process. Sometimes loosely termed "margins," these tissue samples simply represent the infiltrating periphery of the neoplasm and should not pose a major problem in terms of identifying the neoplastic nature of even a few extra infiltrating cells in this context. Whether a bulky cellular neoplasm is present or an occasional infiltrating atypical cell is seen should be what is expected from these samples. A mutual understanding of the terms used and the familiarity with the limitations of each party are necessary for accurate communication. In difficult cases, reviewing the slides together with the surgeon may also provide a more objective view of the situation and facilitate the communication. The great majority of surgeons welcome such opportunities.

In both of the above circumstances, additional immunohistochemical studies may be useful. Nuclear p53 protein expression is identified in a significant subpopulation of neoplastic processes, although mainly in those with astrocytic nature, and essentially in none of the nonneoplastic lesions.[30] While similar results have been reproduced for neoplastic processes, some nonneoplastic lesions, such as progressive multifocal leukoencephalopathy (PML), have been found to be positive for p53.[31] WT-1 expression is found in the great majority of the neoplastic processes in contrast to none of the normal/reactive processes.[32] A little less than 50% of low-grade diffuse astrocytomas are positive for IDH1, while none of the reactive processes are immunoreactive for this antibody.[33] Ki-67 proliferation index is expected to be very low in reactive processes; however, it can be even higher than neoplastic processes in some reactive conditions,[34] while it can also be as low in neoplasms as in reactive conditions.[35,36]

A relatively easily explained hypercellularity situation arises in association with vascular malformations, especially arteriovenous malformation (AVM). Due to the *chronic hypoxic–ischemic changes* caused by the shunting of blood through the AVM, the admixed and surrounding neuroglial parenchyma collapses to appear hypercellular **(Fig. 2-14)**. The hypercellularity is also contributed by the

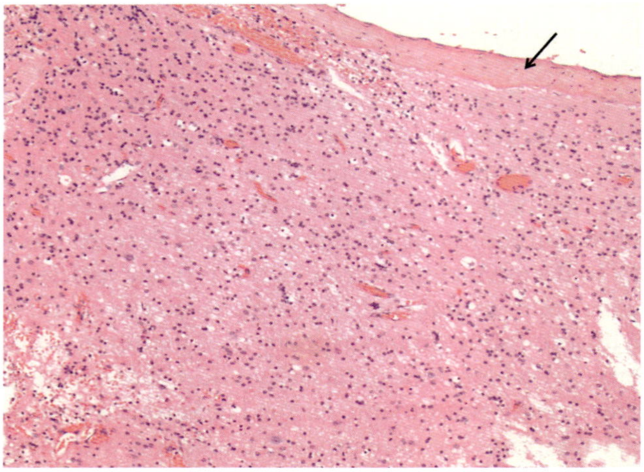

Figure 2-14. Increased cellularity: An increased cellularity of mainly oligodendroglial cells is seen and is due to the collapse of the white matter as a result of ongoing ischemia associated with AVM. A thick vessel wall is present (*arrow*) (H&E; original magnification: 100×).

associated macrophages and inflammatory cells. In some cases, this hypercellularity can be extremely pronounced and may be alarming for a neoplastic process, especially an oligodendroglioma.[37,38] Such a relative hypercellularity through a similar hypoxic–ischemic mechanism can also be seen in intractable seizure specimens in hippocampus.

Lesion Borders

Evaluation of the borders of a lesion, neoplastic or nonneoplastic, can provide valuable information. It can help differentiate high-grade glial neoplasms from metastatic neoplasms, provide prognostic and grading information as in the case of meningioma–brain border, or support the diagnosis as in the sharp borders of multiple sclerosis (MS) plaques in a small biopsy. The borders of the lesion can harbor more prominent diagnostic clues compared to the burnt-out center of the lesion, as in the identification of nuclear inclusions of PML.

One of the features that help with the differential diagnosis of *glial versus metastatic malignancy*, especially in high-grade neoplasms, is their borders. Glial neoplasms are infiltrative neoplasms and gradually fade into the surrounding, nonneoplastic neuroglial parenchyma **(Fig. 2-15)**, while metastatic neoplasms have *pushing borders* that create a *sharp demarcation* **(Fig. 2-16)**. Even if some metastatic carcinomas can have somewhat irregular borders that are due to several small groups of cells spreading into the neuroglial tissue, each such group has its own sharp border, whereas in glial neoplasms, literally individual cells diffusely *infiltrate the surrounding tissues*. In fact, the sharp border of metastatic carcinoma has been further confirmed by multiple needle biopsies of the resection cavity after initial resection, and the absence of any residual neoplastic cells has been shown.[39] One caveat in the interpretation of stereotactic needle biopsy specimens is the false sampling of the reactive glial tissue surrounding the well-circumscribed metastatic carcinoma nodules. This technical pitfall occurs especially with small

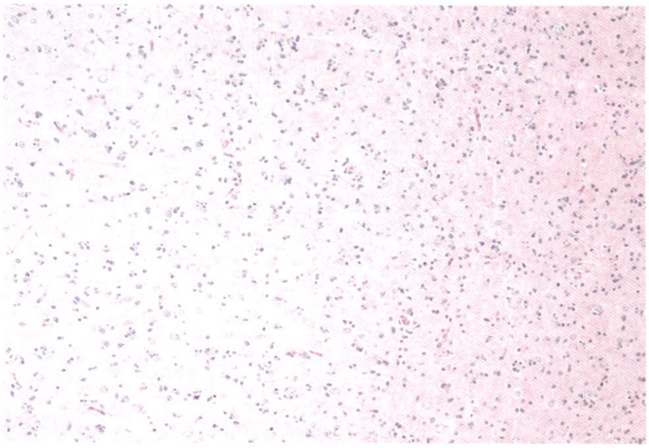

Figure 2-15. Infiltrative border of glial neoplasm: In this case, an oligodendroglioma in the white matter (**right side**) is fading into the overlying cortical gray matter (**left side**) (H&E; original magnification: 100×).

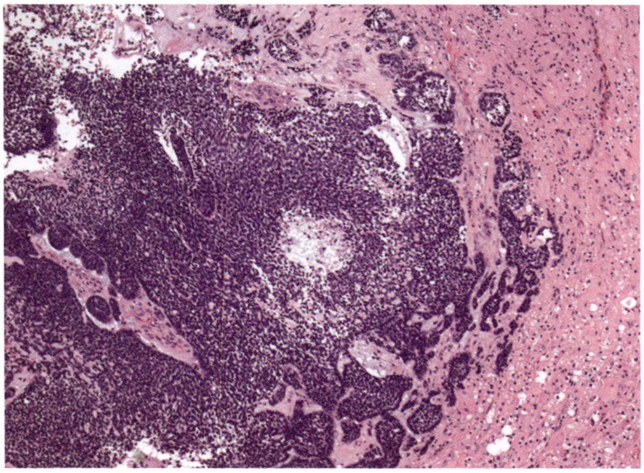

Figure 2-16. Sharp border of metastatic carcinoma: Even though there may be small islands of carcinoma cells infiltrating into the surrounding parenchyma (**right side**), its border is well-defined (H&E; original magnification: 40×).

List of Findings/Checklist for Lesion Borders

• AT A GLANCE

- Sharply defined borders
  - Pushing/expansile
- Infiltrative borders
  - Poorly defined (diffuse, gradually fading cellularity)
  - Irregular (finger-like projections)
- Neoplasms
- Nonneoplastic lesions

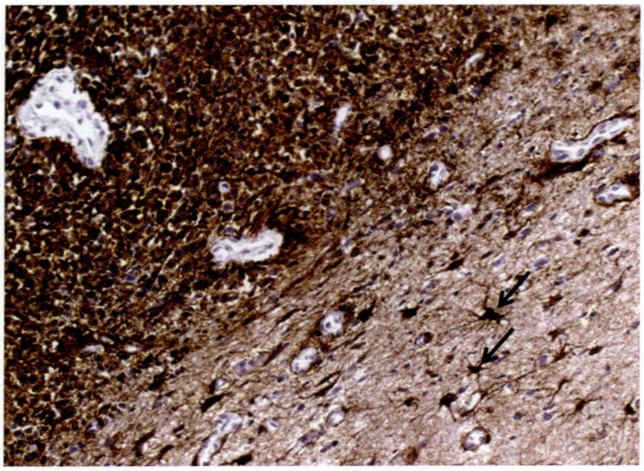

Figure 2-17. Glioblastoma with a well-defined border: Rarely, a glial neoplasm (**top**) can have a sharp border with the surrounding parenchyma (**bottom**), where scattered reactive astrocytes are present (*arrows*). This is usually due to the presence of dense and well-defined tracts in the parenchyma, which may be difficult to infiltrate (GFAP immunohistochemistry; original magnification: 100×).

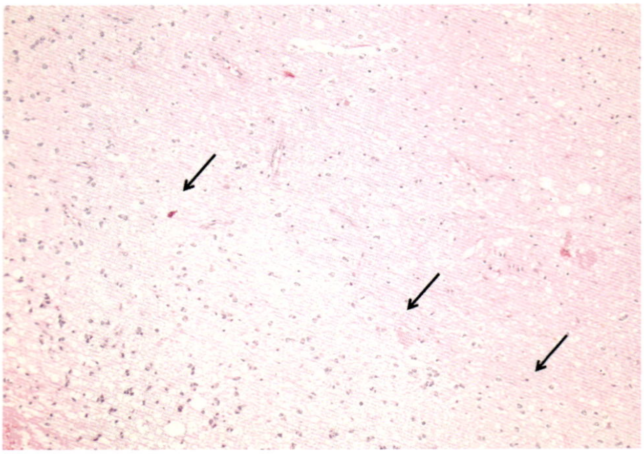

Figure 2-18. Well-circumscribed glioma: This PA (**lower left**), as an example of well-circumscribed gliomas, have a well-defined border (*arrows*) with the surrounding parenchyma (**upper right**) (H&E; original magnification: 100×).

lesions, where the needle radiologically may appear perfectly in the lesion but the reactive glial tissue is sampled as a result of small carcinoma sliding away from the needle. Therefore, in what appears to be radiologically and clinically metastatic carcinoma, this pitfall should be kept in mind if a stereotactic needle biopsy sample shows abnormal glial tissue. In contrast, there are exceptional situations where a glioblastoma can have well circumscription observed radiologically, intraoperatively, and microscopically, at least partially **(Fig. 2-17)**. The typically relative well circumscription of giant cell GBM may be responsible for the slightly better prognosis of this variant reported in some studies.[40] The GBM in the context of Turcot syndrome (brain tumor predisposition syndrome [BTPS]) has been reported to have a better prognosis and can have giant cell features.[41] Whether the prognosis is associated with the giant cell and/or better circumscribed nature of these neoplasms is not clear. The cytologic features of glial neoplasms and metastatic carcinomas are discussed in "Cytoplasmic Features" and "Nuclear Features." The above discussion takes into account the infiltrative gliomas. The so-called *well-circumscribed gliomas*, such as PA and ganglioglioma, have relatively well-defined borders as well **(Fig. 2-18)**. If examined in detail, their borders can also be shown to have a somewhat infiltrative nature. For instance, a *neurofilament immunohistochemistry* may highlight axons entrapped within a PA in the peripheral areas of the neoplasm.[29,42] However, this is different and more limited than the diffusely infiltrative nature of infiltrating gliomas, and for all practical intents and purposes, PA and similar neoplasms can be considered well-circumscribed. Hemangioblastoma, craniopharyngioma, pleomorphic xanthoastrocytoma (PXA), and desmoplastic infantile ganglioglioma (DIG) are examples of other neoplasms with relatively sharp borders. *Dysembryoplastic neuroepithelial tumor (DNT)* is a superficial, cortical–subcortical, multinodular lesion of debatable neoplastic or hamartomatous nature. Due to its round oligodendroglial-like cell population, in small specimens and in IOCs, it can be difficult to distinguish it from oligodendroglioma. Infiltrating borders of oligodendroglioma contrast with the well-circumscribed borders of the nodules of DNT **(Fig. 2-19)**. In spite of the cortical involvement, DNT does not show satellitosis, a feature that supports oligodendroglioma. *DIG/desmoplastic infantile astrocytoma (DIA)* has a dural connection with a pushing and sharp border with the brain parenchyma. A few finger-like extensions in to the brain parenchyma may be seen due to the neoplasm following the Virchow-Robin

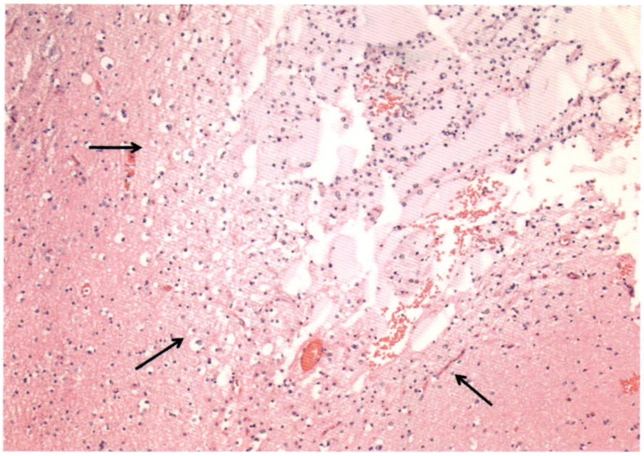

Figure 2-19. Dysembryoplastic neuroepithelial tumor (DNT): This DNT nodule (**center-upper right**) has a well-defined border (*arrows*) with the surrounding parenchyma (**bottom and left**), which can be an important clue in distinguishing it from oligodendroglioma (H&E; original magnification: 100×).

spaces, and are responsible for the adherent nature of the neoplasms to the parenchyma, but this is not an indication of a high-grade lesion. *Ependymomas*, including all variants, as well as anaplastic ependymomas, tend to be quite well-circumscribed from the surrounding tissue **(Fig. 2-20)**. Even in anaplastic ependymomas, only a mild degree of *finger-like projections* into the nonneoplastic neuroglial tissue are present. This feature may be useful in the differential diagnosis of especially clear cell ependymoma from oligodendroglioma, which has infiltrating borders. Extraventricular neurocytoma is also occasionally included in this differential and also has well-circumscribed borders. A low-grade neoplasm that may resemble ependymoma due to the perivascular arrangement of cells is angiocentric glioma. While its histogenesis is not clear, its immunohistochemical and ultrastructural features suggest ependymal differentiation.[43] In contrast to ependymomas, however, angiocentric glioma is an infiltrative neoplasm with admixed nonneoplastic neuroglial elements entrapped within the neoplasm. Astroblastoma, which may come into the differential diagnosis of ependymoma due to the presence of pseudorosettes (see "Perivascular Arrangements and Rosettes"), is also well-circumscribed. *Meningioma* borders are well-defined due to the neoplasm pushing the neuroglial tissue by abutting the brain surface. However, in meningiomas with brain invasion, the brain–meningioma border becomes irregular with finger-like projections of meningioma extending into the brain parenchyma **(Fig. 2-21)**. In extensively brain-invasive meningiomas, this feature may be difficult to identify but may be seen as islands of neuroglial tissue entrapped within the neoplasm. Meningioma

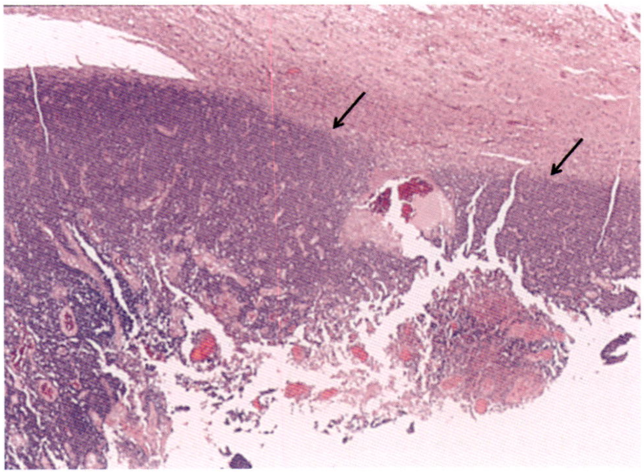

Figure 2-20. Ependymoma border: Although a glial neoplasm, ependymoma, and even anaplastic ependymoma as in this case, typically has a sharp border (*arrows*) with the surrounding parenchyma (**upper left**) (H&E; original magnification: 40×).

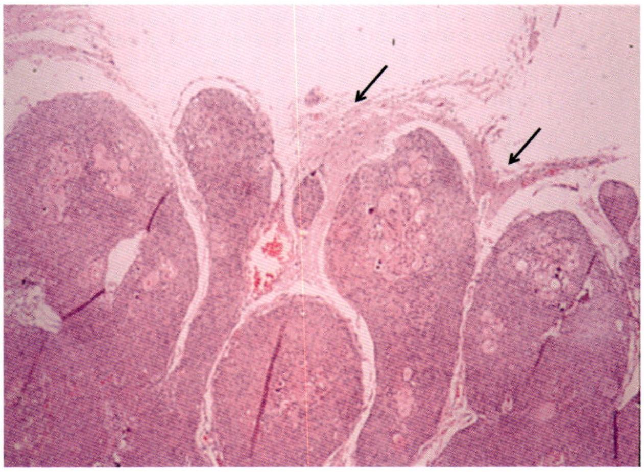

Figure 2-21. Brain invasion by meningioma: This meningioma (**bottom**) has an irregular border with the adjacent brain tissue (*arrows*) due to the finger-like projections into the neuroglial parenchyma, a high-grade feature (H&E; original magnification: 40×).

that tracks down along the Virchow-Robin spaces and appears to invade the brain should not be considered brain invasion. Therefore, the association of such invasive appearing groups with blood vessels is important to evaluate. In addition, the presence of reactive gliosis in the adjacent neuroglial parenchyma supports true invasion. Immunohistochemical stains for *GFAP or synaptophysin* are useful in the evaluation of brain invasion by meningioma by highlighting the neuroglial tissue. Accurate identification of brain invasion by meningioma is important, since it implies a greater likelihood of recurrence. WHO classification technically considers this feature as an independent feature, without direct effect on grading; however, in practice, it is often used as a feature of atypical (WHO grade II) meningioma.[44] Meningioangiomatosis is a lesion characterized by the proliferation of meningothelial cells around the vessels, along with fibroblastic and vascular proliferation, creating a superficial, intracortical, well-circumscribed, variably cellular, and collagenized lesion. If taken out of context in a small tissue sample, these intraparenchymal perivascular meningothelial proliferations may closely mimic an invasive meningioma. This is mainly a problem in the cellular rather than highly collagenized lesions. In contrast to meningioma, meningioangiomatosis does not form a dura-based mass with pushing border with the brain but rather an intraparenchymal lesion with intervening brain parenchyma. Some cases that are associated with meningioma have been described.[45,46] In *melanocytic neoplasms*, invasion of neuroglial parenchyma is a feature associated with malignancy and is helpful in distinguishing *melanocytoma* from *melanoma*, although it can be present in intermediate grade neoplasms, too.[47] The distinction of primary and metastatic melanoma is of great importance for prognostic and therapeutic considerations and is equally difficult. In general, metastatic melanomas tend to be multifocal and intraparenchymal, while primary melanomas are centered in the leptomeninges, even though they show considerable parenchymal invasion, and are in the form of a single mass lesion. Secondary foci from a primary melanoma can result in multifocality. The mitotic counts and proliferation indices of metastatic melanoma tend to be higher than those seen in primary melanoma, but there is considerable overlap. Therefore, a thorough clinical and radiologic work-up to identify or rule out a primary source elsewhere in the body becomes very important.

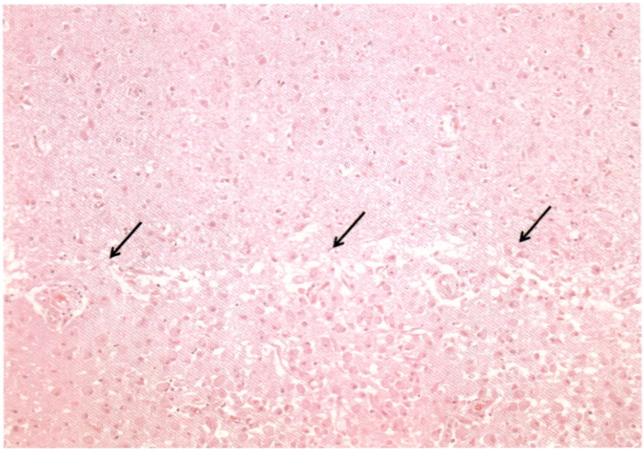

Figure 2-22. Infarct with sharp border: A subacute infarct with many macrophages (**bottom**) has a sharp border (*arrows*) with the adjacent viable parenchyma (**top**) (H&E; original magnification: 100×).

Demyelinating lesions typically have sharp demarcation of demyelination, although inflammation can spill into the surrounding parenchyma. This demarcation is more pronounced in the acute stages. In reality, the demyelination may extend into the surrounding parenchyma in the form of finger-like projections following vessels, that is, Dawson's fingers. They do not pose a diagnostic problem in terms of the evaluation of margins; however, in some cases, they may mimic acute disseminated encephalomyelitis (ADEM). In the chronic stage, the borders can become blurred as myelin regenerates into the lesion from the periphery, also known as the shadow plaque. Dysmyelinating processes (leukodystrophies) are diffuse processes with an ill-defined border, even by myelin stains. *Infarcts* become well-delineated from the surrounding tissue starting in their acute stage and into subacute stage and remote stages. This delineation is also highlighted by the contrast between the viable tissue and the pale, ghost-like appearance of the infarct **(Fig. 2-22)**.

Pituitary adenoma can show invasive characteristics, and adenoma cells can infiltrate the surrounding structures, such as pituitary capsule, bone, sphenoid sinus, and cavernous sinus, resulting in *"invasive adenoma"* **(Fig. 2-23)**, indicating a higher likelihood of recurrence; however, biologic

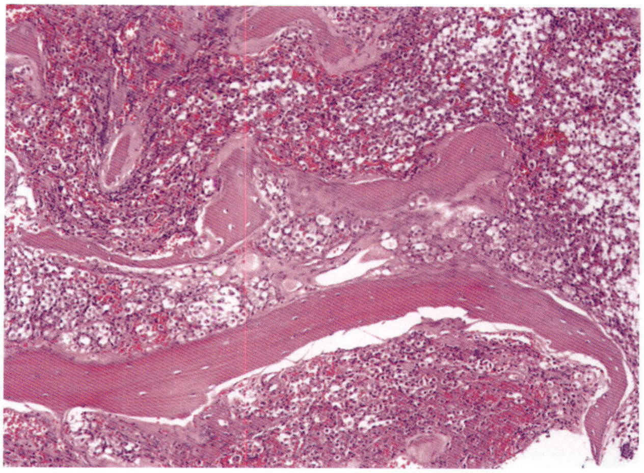

Figure 2-23. Invasive pituitary adenoma: This pituitary adenoma infiltrates the bone, entrapping trabeculae (H&E; original magnification: 100×).

behavior of pituitary adenoma appears to be dictated mainly by the hormonal subtype.[48] In cases of biopsy samples from extrasellar locations that show pituitary adenoma, especially in sphenoid sinus or nasopharynx, the possibility of ectopic adenoma should be considered before making a diagnosis of invasive adenoma. Correlation with radiologic findings, as well as with intraoperative observations, should clarify this issue. In the nonneoplastic gland, variable numbers of basophilic anterior pituitary cells can normally be present scattered in the neighboring areas of the neurohypophysis **(Fig. 2-24)**. This is called *basophil infiltration of posterior pituitary* and should not be mistaken for an invasive adenoma. Granular cell tumors and pituicytomas in the sellar region are well-circumscribed neoplasms.

In the *peripheral nervous system*, neurofibroma may be localized and nodular or may be diffusely infiltrative, especially along the adipose tissue septae, entrapping the skin adnexa.[49] This infiltrating variant can be deceptively bland. Plexiform and intraneural neurofibromas can, at some point, "spill" into the surrounding tissues and appear like a diffuse process. Schwannomas are well-circumscribed neoplasms. Nerve sheath myxoma consists of loosely scattered spindle cells in a myxoid background but is not encapsulated in contrast to other neoplasms with similar appearances, such as myxoid schwannoma and plexiform neurofibroma.

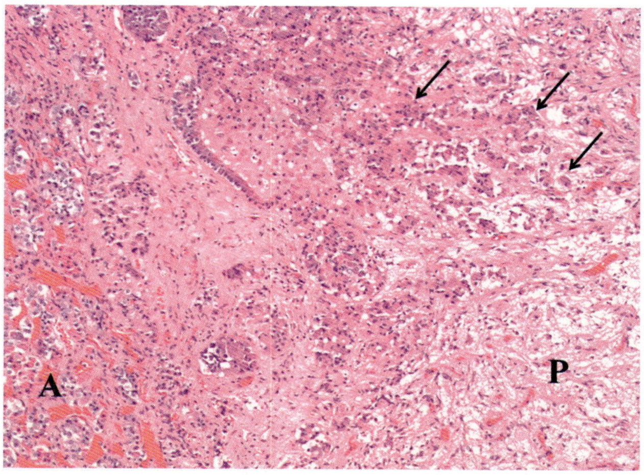

Figure 2-24. Basophil infiltration of posterior pituitary: The border between the anterior pituitary parenchyma (*A*) and the posterior pituitary parenchyma (*P*) has been breached, and many basophilic cells individually or in small groups (*arrows*) infiltrate into the posterior pituitary parenchyma, a normal finding that may cause confusion in small tissue samples and should not be interpreted as an invasive adenoma (H&E; original magnification: 100×).

Granular cell tumors are typically well-circumscribed, and malignant granular cell tumors, in addition to other features, may or may not have infiltrative borders. Malignant peripheral nerve sheath tumor (MPNST) is typically seen as a fusiform mass in association with the involved nerve, the latter showing thickening proximal and distal to the mass, corresponding to the infiltrative border of the MPNST with the adjacent nerve, even though the tumor soft tissue border can be quite well-defined. This transitional zone within the nerve, or the admixed nature of MPNST with the preexisting neurofibroma, as seen commonly in the setting of neurofibromatosis type 1 (NF1), causes a great deal of difficulty in the evaluation of resection margins in surgical pathology, especially during IOC.

Cytoplasmic Features

Cytoplasm is where the functions of the cell are performed; therefore, cytoplasmic features provide information about the differentiation and function of the cell. In the resting state, astrocyte cytoplasm is not easily identified at the light microscopic

List of Findings/Checklist for Cytoplasmic Features

• AT A GLANCE

- Thick eosinophilic cytoplasm
- Cytoplasmic processes
- Reactive astrocyte
- Gemistocyte
- Mini/microgemistocyte
- Opalski cells
- Myelination glia
- Rhabdoid cell
- Rhabdomyoblast
- Clear cell
- Foamy/xanthomatous/microvesicular cytoplasm
- Cytoplasmic vacuoles
- Signet ring cell
- Granulovacuolar degeneration
- Granular cytoplasm
- Oncocyte
- Eosinophilic granular bodies
- Hyaline globules
- Morular cell
- PAS-positive globules
- Acidophilic/basophilic/chromophobe cells
- Crooke's hyaline change
- Rosenthal fibers
- Distinct cytoplasmic borders
- Epithelioid cells
- Syncytial arrangement
- Cilia/microvilli
- Cytoplasmic swelling/ballooning
- Chromatolysis

level, since it is mainly in the form of processes admixed with the processes of other cell types in the neuropil. *Thick eosinophilic cytoplasm* refers to the cytoplasms of astrocytes that become prominent when *reactive or neoplastic*. There may be a small amount of discernible cytoplasm or it can be abundant. The astrocytic cytoplasm has a thick and glassy quality. Cytoplasmic processes become thick and more prominent. They are easily identified in the background of neuropil. In the case of astrocytomas, the increase in the amount of cytoplasm is referred to as *gemistocyte*. Although it is a descriptive term referring to an astrocyte with abundant cytoplasm, it is typically reserved for neoplastic cells. Their cytoplasms have a rounder contour with stubby and fewer processes **(Fig. 2-25)**. The processes are not as prominent as those of the

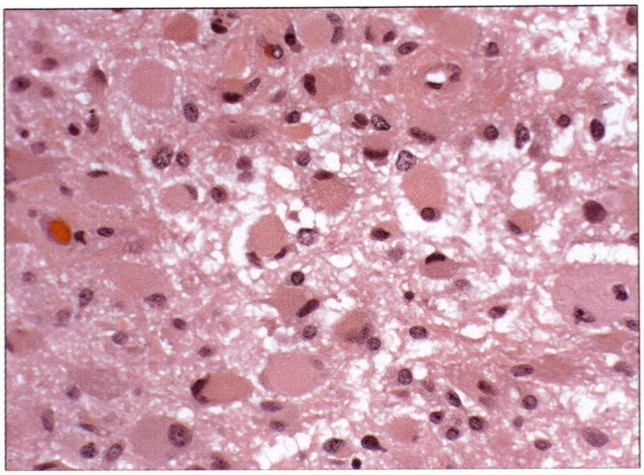

Figure 2-25. Gemistocytic astrocytoma: Many gemistocytes with prominent, somewhat rounded cytoplasm and irregular, hyperchromatic nuclei similar to other astrocytoma nuclei are present. Astrocytic processes of gemistocytes are less prominent compared to reactive astrocytes (H&E; original magnification: 400×).

reactive astrocytes. Depending on the cellularity of the neoplasm, they can be widely separated in the background of the neoplasm, or they may become crowded enough to form sheets, with only small distances between the cells. The presence of gemistocytic features arbitrarily in approximately 20% or more of the neoplastic cells is required to make a diagnosis of gemistocytic astrocytoma.[50] This type of reference cutoff is arbitrary and rarely needed for borderline cases, and the great majority of the cases are straightforward. The accurate terminology is important, as gemistocytic astrocytomas, although still WHO grade II, may have a tendency to show malignant progression more rapidly than the usual fibrillary astrocytomas.[51,52] *Minigemistocytes (microgemistocytes)* are smaller cells with small amount of eosinophilic cytoplasm, typically seen in oligodendrogliomas. Their cytoplasm is abundant enough to be identified but small enough to appear as barely hanging on to the nucleus, with the nucleus appearing to almost protrude from the cell **(Fig. 2-26)**. Their cytoplasms are not as bright eosinophilic and glassy as the gemistocytes or reactive astrocytes, with no definitive processes. They stand out in the background of typical oligodendroglioma cells and are usually sprinkled with some distance from each other. They should not be interpreted as a mixed oligoastrocytoma. *Opalski*

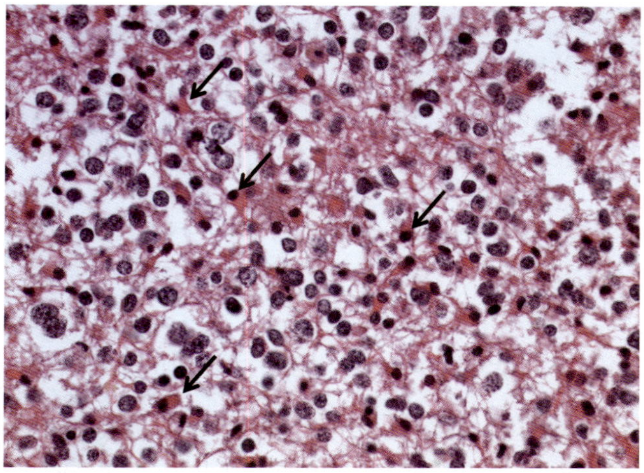

Figure 2-26. Minigemistocytes: Smaller versions of gemistocytes (*arrows*) are present in this oligodendroglioma. The nuclei of some minigemistocytes may appear to be protruding from the cytoplasm (H&E; original magnification: 400×).

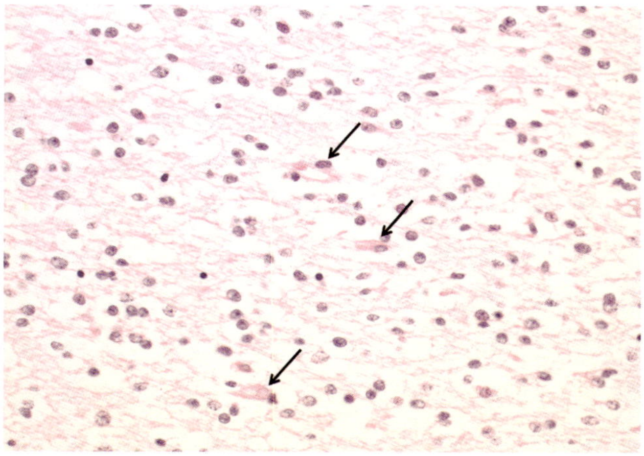

Figure 2-28. Myelination glia: Cells with irregular, small amount of wispy cytoplasm (*arrows*) are seen in pediatric brains in association with myelination process and should not be mistaken for reactive astrocytes to indicate a pathologic process (H&E; original magnification: 400×).

cells **(Fig. 2-27)** are seen in the setting of hepatic encephalopathy and somewhat more prominently in Wilson's disease (hepatolenticular degeneration), together with Alzheimer type II glia, and may be especially prominent in basal ganglia.[53] They tend to have hyperchromatic, round, small nuclei with a bright eosinophilic, polygonal, finely granular cytoplasm, without processes. While their origin is not entirely clear, they likely represent glial cells with a peculiar change in these

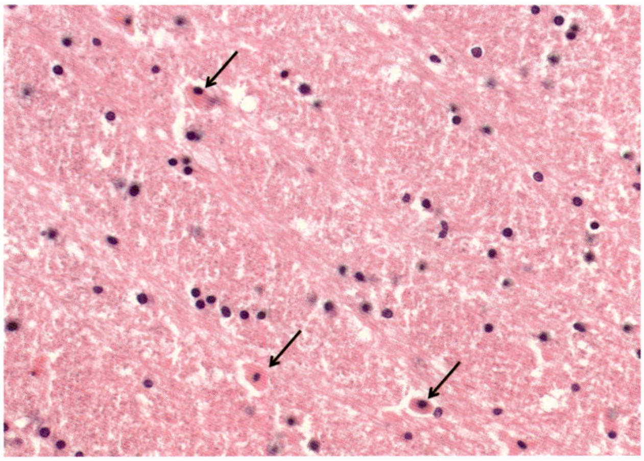

Figure 2-27. Opalski cells: Cells with small, pyknotic-appearing nuclei and abundant opaque eosinophilic cytoplasm (*arrows*) are seen (H&E; original magnification: 400×).

contexts.[54] In neonatal and pediatric brains, there is a relative increase in the number of glial cells in the white matter, in the period preceeding the start of myelination during normal development. These cells resemble smaller versions of reactive astrocytes and are GFAP positive. They are called *myelination glia*[55] **(Fig. 2-28)**. While it is debatable whether these cells are actual astrocytes or modified oligodendroglial cells in origin, their practical importance stems from the gliotic appearance they create in the normal developing white matter. The normal hypomyelinated state of the white matter adds to the confusion. Myelination glia tend to have somewhat more hyperchromatic and smaller nuclei and smaller and elongated cytoplasms compared to the reactive astrocytes.

The term *rhabdoid* refers to a dense, bright eosinophilic, somewhat whorled or fibrillary intracytoplasmic accumulation, typically formed by intermediate filaments, in a cell with eccentric nucleus, prominent nucleolus, and clear chromatin pattern. Typically, the entire cytoplasm is occupied by this accumulation, which appears to be about the same size as the nucleus and is located next to the nucleus. In some cases, the cytoplasm may have a pale, glassy appearance, which looks quite different than this typical description. The prototype of such a rhabdoid neoplasm is atypical teratoid/rhabdoid tumor (ATRT) **(Fig. 2-29)**. Rhabdoid change

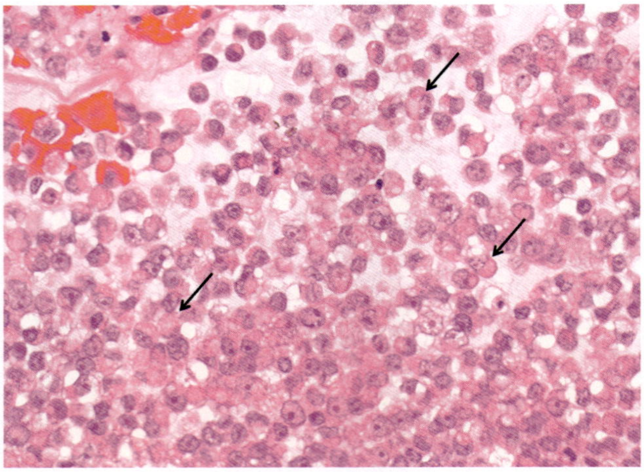

Figure 2-29. Rhabdoid cells: Variable amount of round, dense, and pale eosinophilic cytoplasm is present, along with an eccentric nucleus that typically has an open chromatin pattern and prominent nucleus in the rhabdoid cells of this atypical teratoid rhabdoid tumor (H&E; original magnification: 400×).

is not specific for ATRT and can also be seen in many other neoplasms. They are composite rhabdoid neoplasms such as rhabdoid meningiomas **(Fig. 2-30)**, rhabdoid melanomas, rhabdoid renal cell carcinomas, and rhabdoid tumors of the kidney

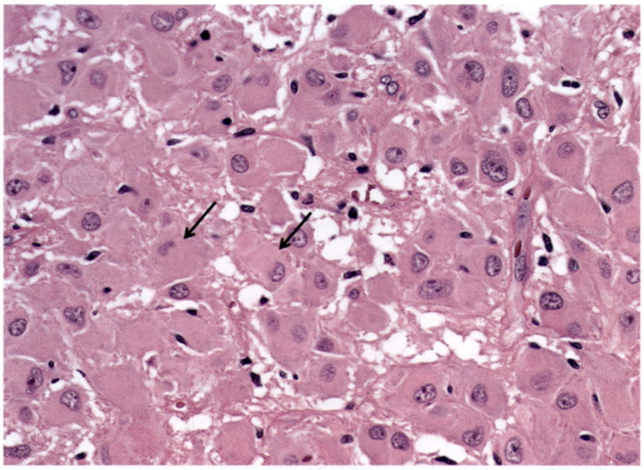

Figure 2-30. Rhabdoid meningioma: The rhabdoid cells of this meningioma have more abundant and pale cytoplasms, still creating a round cytoplasmic inclusion pushing the nucleus aside (*arrows*). With the separation of the cells from each other, a gemistocytic astrocytoma-like appearance is created, which can lead to confusion, especially during intraoperative consultations (H&E; original magnification: 400×).

and soft tissues seen in childhood. However, the characteristic loss of INI-1 expression seen in ATRT and malignant rhabdoid tumors of childhood is not present in these composite neoplasms.[56] Rhabdoid change in general implies a more aggressive biologic behavior. It can also be seen in choroid plexus carcinomas and should not be confused with ATRT. Retention of nuclear INI-1 expression helps identify the neoplasm as choroid plexus carcinoma.[57] In rhabdoid tumor predisposition syndrome, there is a familial tendency to develop rhabdoid tumors of the kidney and ATRT.[58] Rhabdoid features can be present as part of GBM.[59] Plump, rounded cells with abundant bright eosinophilic fibrillary or granular cytoplasm, with or without cross striations, may represent *rhabdomyoblastic differentiation* and are usually seen as a variable feature in another neoplasm in the CNS, most notably medulloblastoma, that is, medulloblastoma with myogenic differentiation. They can be seen in various sarcomas and sarcomatous areas in other neoplasms, such as gliosarcoma. Rare medulloepitheliomas can also show myoblastic elements, so can malignant meningiomas and triton tumors.

The term *clear cell* refers to cells with optically clear cytoplasm **(Table 2.3)**. It can be seen in a wide variety of cell types and in many lesions as a primary feature or as a minor change.[60] In most cases, this is caused by the presence of abundant glycogen and/or lipids in the cytoplasm and their subsequent removal by water, alcohol, and xylene during tissue processing, or as in the case of oligodendroglioma, the clearing is due to delayed fixation and resulting partial autolysis with hydropic degeneration of the cytoplasm. Clear cells, also referred to as "fried egg" appearance or perinuclear halos, although neither diagnostic nor specific for this entity, constitute a feature for which oligodendroglioma is best known. In cellular oligodendrogliomas in which the cells are back-to-back, the clear cytoplasms create a honeycomb appearance. As in many other entities, the diagnosis is one of a constellation of features, perhaps the most important one being the almost perfectly round nuclei. Nonneoplastic oligodendroglial cells in the white matter can also show similar clear cell features, with smaller and darker but still round nuclei and with no nucleoli. This change is again more prominent in cases of delayed fixation. Nonneoplastic oligodendroglial cells have a tendency to be arranged in single files along the

TABLE 2.3 Clear cell lesions

Oligodendroglioma
Nonneoplastic oligodendroglial cells
Neoplasms with oligodendroglioma component
- Glioblastoma multiforme with oligodendroglioma component
- Oligoastrocytoma/oligoependymoma
- Ganglioglioma with oligodendroglioma

Central neurocytoma
Clear cell ependymoma
Clear cell meningioma
Choroid plexus carcinoma
Metastatic carcinoma
Germinoma
Clear cell–like changes
- Hemangioblastoma
- PXA
- Metaplastic meningioma
- Chordoma
- Chondrosarcoma
- Macrophage-rich lesions (demyelinating lesion, subacute infarct, AVM)
- Granular cell astrocytoma
- CUSA artifact

Lesions with focal clear cell areas
- DNT
- PA
- PTPR
- Glioblastoma multiforme
- Medulloblastoma/PNET
- Pineal parenchymal tumors
- Paraganglioma
- Choroid plexus papilloma

capillaries or nerve fibers and appear orderly. The diffuse infiltration by oligodendroglioma, without the sheet-like growth pattern with chicken-wire vasculature, can be difficult to distinguish from nonneoplastic white matter **(Fig. 2-31)**. Neoplastic oligodendroglial cells have relatively larger nuclei with a somewhat open, finely granular chromatin pattern and small nucleoli, in contrast to dark, small, lymphocyte-like nuclei of their nonneoplastic counterparts with no or inconspicuous nucleoli. As with many other subtleties in neuropathology, becoming familiar with the normal appearances of different areas of the nervous system comes handy when one is faced with a difficult decision on a small sample. Oligodendroglial-like appearance is a common finding to a variable extent, and fortunately partially, in several other neoplasms. In neurocytic neoplasms, clear cytoplasm can be widespread, resulting in confusion with oligodendroglioma. In fact, until it was described and recognized as a separate entity, central neurocytoma used to be diagnosed as intraventricular oligodendroglioma based on its cytoplasmic features and round nuclei **(Fig. 2-32)**. Delicate, lacy background created by the neuritic processes of the neoplastic cells and irregular perivascular anuclear zones reminiscent of but quite different from ependymal pseudorosettes, along with diffuse synaptophysin positivity of the cells and the background, also aid in the diagnosis of central neurocytoma. Oligodendroglioma-like cells can be seen focally in

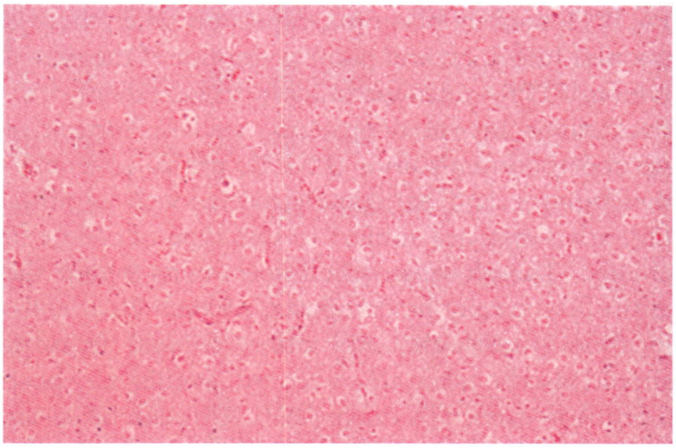

Figure 2-31. Oligodendroglioma: When oligodendroglioma is not very cellular and is diffusely infiltrating the white matter, it can be difficult to distinguish from a cellular appearing nonneoplastic white matter (H&E; original magnification: 100×).

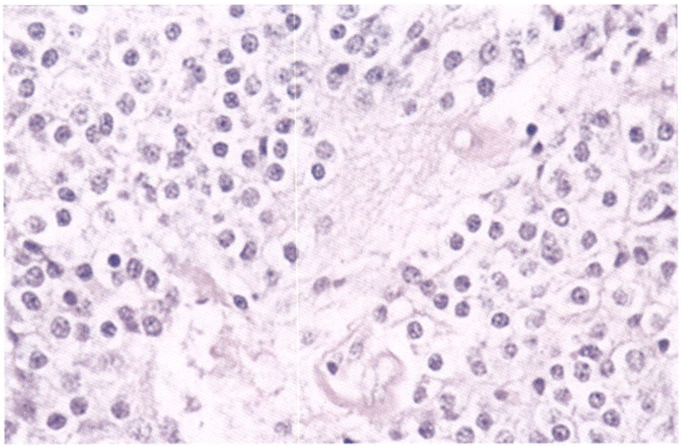

Figure 2-32. Central neurocytoma with oligodendroglial-like cells with clear cytoplasm and round nuclei (H&E; original magnification: 400×).

PA, DNT, medulloblastoma, especially when there is nodular histology, and papillary tumor of the pineal region (PTPR). As in medulloblastoma, other primitive and/or neural neoplasms, such as primitive neuroectodermal tumor (PNET), pineal parenchymal tumors, and paraganglioma, as well as pituitary adenoma, are subject to this type of clear cell change. Therefore, in small specimens where the entire tissue may be composed of such clear cells, location, radiologic, and other clinical features should also be taken into account, as this may pose a problem especially during IOC. This can be easier to work through in larger specimens with characteristic features of that particular entity and with the help of immunohistochemistry. In PTPR, the concern becomes more for central neurocytoma, due to the intraventricular location of both neoplasms. Nonetheless, all these neoplasms that can have oligodendroglial-like component have other prominent characteristic features that are readily identified. Even GBM can have areas with clear cells, which may be tempting for a diagnosis of glioblastoma with oligodendroglioma component, implying a better prognosis than the pure GBM; however, they are glioblastoma cells and, as such, their nuclei have astrocytic features, with irregular nuclear membranes and inconspicuous nucleoli **(Fig. 2-33)**. In addition to the similarity between oligodendroglioma and DNT, an additional differential diagnostic problem may arise in the context of so-called complex DNT, where there may be prominent areas with features of usual gliomas. A debatable nonspecific variant of DNT can be composed entirely of areas with features of low-grade glioma. In these two contexts,[61] differentiation from oligodendroglioma can become a challenge if the clinical history, radiologic features, and location are not taken into account. Specimens obtained by cavitational ultrasonic surgical aspiration (CUSA) are notorious for the artifactual clear cell appearance in the component cells, regardless of their origin. Therefore, any process may potentially appear like and be mistaken for oligodendroglioma in such specimens. Again, being aware of this artifact, paying attention to the nuclear features and, if at all possible, making such decisions in relatively intact areas of the tissue help avoid this pitfall. Clear cell ependymoma variant is predominantly seen in children in the supratentorial location and has sheets of cells with abundant clear cytoplasm and round nuclei. As such, it looks very similar to oligodendroglioma **(Fig. 2-34)**. Pseudorosettes may be subtle or absent, and true rosettes are absent. If the periphery of the neoplasm is present in the sample, the well circumscription of clear cell ependymoma in contrast to the infiltrative borders of oligodendroglioma is useful in this differential diagnosis. In

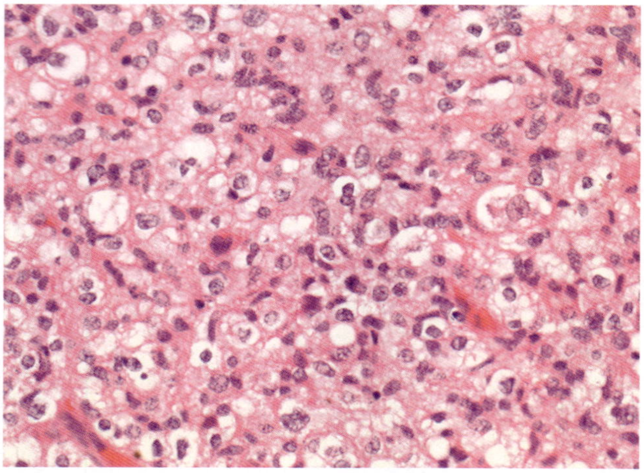

Figure 2-33. Glioblastoma with cells with clear cytoplasm: Although many cells may have nucleoli, their nuclei are irregular and of different sizes, shapes, and orientations, creating a hectic appearance, which should not be confused with an oligodendroglioma or a glioblastoma with oligodendroglioma component (H&E; original magnification: 400×).

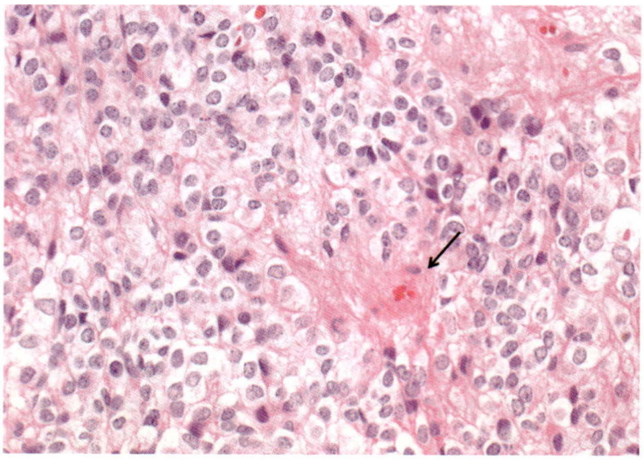

Figure 2-34. Clear cell ependymoma: Typical features of ependymoma are difficult to find. Even though perivascular anuclear zone may be present (*arrow*), well-developed pseudorosettes are not seen, potentially resulting in a diagnosis of oligodendroglioma (H&E; original magnification: 400×).

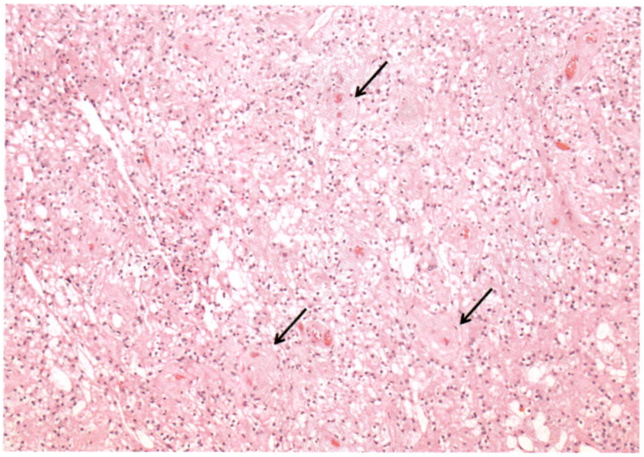

Figure 2-35. Clear cell meningioma: Sheets of clear cells are punctuated by hyalinized vessels (*arrows*), sometimes to a degree to obscure the cellularity. As in clear cell ependymoma, typical features of meningioma are usually difficult to find, necessitating the incorporation of location, clinical and radiologic information, as well as special studies (H&E; original magnification: 100×).

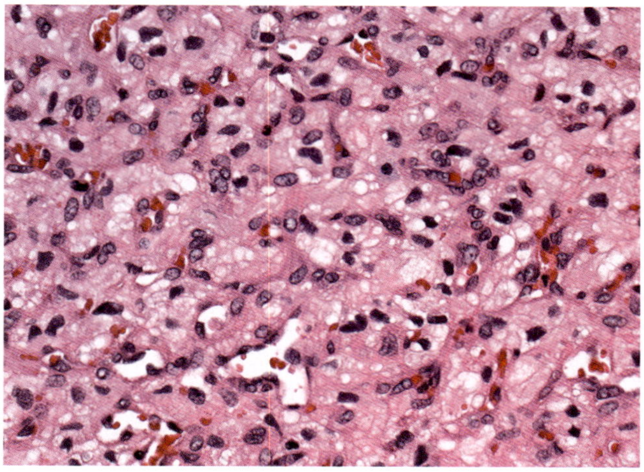

Figure 2-36. Hemangioblastoma: Clear cytoplasms have a microvesicular, bubbly quality. Many capillaries are present and some may only be noticed due to the erythrocytes in their lumens (H&E; original magnification: 400×).

larger specimens, typical ependymoma morphology may be present in other areas. Clear cytoplasm in ependymomas can also be the result of intracytoplasmic lumen formation, designated as signet ring cell ependymoma when extensive, and lipid accumulation, resulting in an appearance similar to mature adipose tissue and designated as lipidized ependymoma. Clear cell meningioma is also characterized by cells with abundant clear cytoplasm. The absence or paucity of typical meningioma features such as whorls and syncytial growth pattern makes the diagnosis difficult. Collagenized bands in the stroma and thick collagenized vessels may be very prominent and obscure the cellularity **(Fig. 2-35)**. However, consideration of this diagnosis as a possibility, preferred posterior fossa and upper cervical spinal cord location, immunohistochemical features of meningioma, and demonstration of intracytoplasmic glycogen by PAS stain with and without diastase treatment make this a relatively easy diagnosis. These cells in clear cell meningioma are different than the mature adipose tissue metaplasia and the xanthomatous change in metaplastic meningioma. The neoplastic cells of hemangioblastoma, referred to as stromal cells, have large, microvesicular, and foamy clear cytoplasms containing lipid **(Fig. 2-36)**. There are numerous delicate capillaries among the neoplastic cell groups, and a pericellular reticulin network is characteristic. Another primary neoplasm with a similar reticulin network and a xanthomatous quality to the cytoplasms, creating a somewhat clear cell appearance, is PXA. Cyst and mural nodule formation is typical for both of these neoplasms. Even though not to the degree seen in PXA, considerable nuclear pleomorphism can be seen in hemangioblastoma. The uniformly clear cytoplasms, delicate capillary network, and absence of a fibrillary background favor hemangioblastoma. In addition, cerebellum is a favored location for hemangioblastoma, while cerebral hemispheres are favored by PXA, usually with a connection to the leptomeningeal surface. Especially in the setting of von Hippel-Lindau syndrome, it is important to rule out metastatic clear cell renal cell carcinoma. Crisp borders of abundant clear cytoplasm, back-to-back arrangement of cells with no background fibrillarity, usually uniformly prominent nucleoli, and a tendency to crowd around the delicate capillaries are features to alert one to this possibility. In most cases, and especially if there is von Hippel-Lindau syndrome, where hemangioblastomas may be multiple to mimic metastasis, immunohistochemical workup is necessary for accurate diagnosis. Germinoma, in its typical locations in the pineal or suprasellar region, with solid sheet-like growth of its large epithelioid cells, divided by fibrovascular septa, is relatively easy to recognize. However, some germinomas can infiltrate the neuroglial tissue in the form of small groups or individual cells, where they may be difficult to distinguish from glioma or lymphoma. Embryonal carcinoma occasionally can have clear cytoplasm, although this tends to be a focal change. The main differential diagnostic consideration with these neoplasms is a metastatic carcinoma, where immunohistochemistry may be necessary. As for primary epithelial neoplasms of the CNS, clear cytoplasmic vacuoles can be frequent in choroid plexus papillomas, while clear cytoplasms can be seen more commonly in choroid plexus carcinoma. Chordoma is characterized by epithelioid cells with abundant clear or microvesicular cytoplasm, the latter referred to as physaliphorous cells. They can be arranged in single files, trabeculae, or groups in a myxoid background **(Fig. 2-37)**. The typical midline skull base intraosseous location, most commonly in the clivus, narrows the differential diagnosis to essentially between chordoma and chondrosarcoma, an important decision as chordomas are a lot more malignant and eventually fatal neoplasms compared to chondrosarcomas.[62] The differential diagnosis becomes complicated in cases of so-called chondroid chordoma, where, instead of the myxoid background, hyaline cartilage matrix is present and the cells reside in lacunae, mimicking chondrosarcoma. This change is typically partial, and classical chordoma can be identified elsewhere in the specimen. In small specimens or in difficult cases, immunohistochemistry is useful. Chondrosarcomas can have variably histologic appearance, but the hyaline cartilage matrix with atypical cells in small groups and collagenous stromal bands creating a lobular arrangement are typical features of chondrosarcoma. When chordoma grows in a confluent sheet-like pattern, metastatic carcinoma may be a consideration. Again, coexpression of cytokeratin, vimentin, epithelial membrane antigen (EMA) and S-100 protein, as well as nuclear positivity for brachyury, is diagnostic for chordoma. In the rare case of so-called poorly differentiated chordoma, where the typical chordoma features, including myxoid background, are not present, there is prominent cytologic atypia and sheet-like growth, and distinguishing it from metastatic carcinoma may be difficult.[63] The typical immunohistochemical features, as well as the presence or absence of expression of other markers that may be associated with specific organs of origin of a possible metastatic carcinoma, are useful in this differential diagnosis. Notochord remnants and related lesions such as benign notochordal cell tumor also contain vacuolated cells and are discussed in more detail in "Mucinous–Myxoid Material." In addition, poorly differentiated chordomas can have rhabdoid cytology,[63] which can mimic ATRT. To complicate the issue further, poorly differentiated chordomas

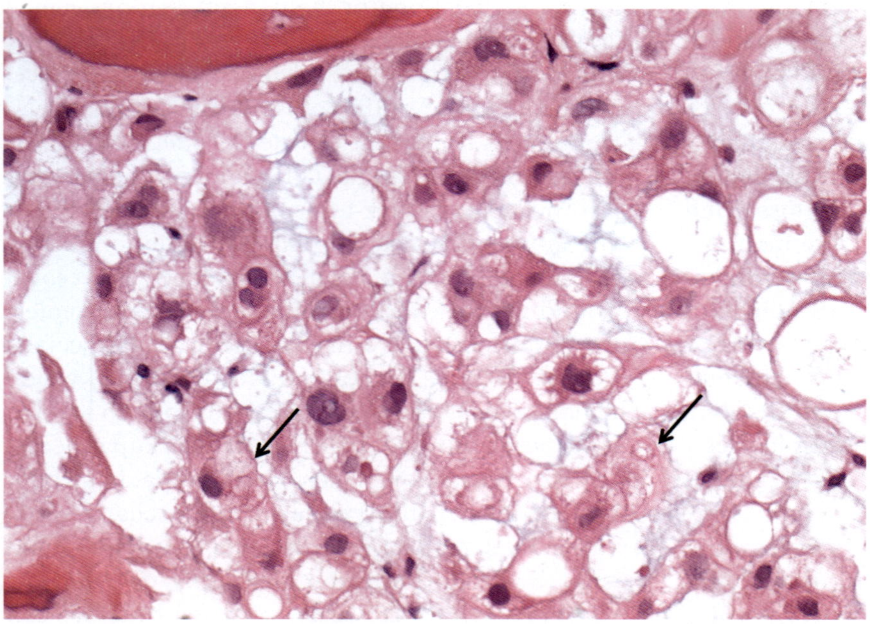

Figure 2-37. Chordoma: Cells with clear cytoplasm are floating in a mucinous background. They have multivesicular clear cytoplasm with multiple vacuoles of variable sizes, resulting in the term physaliphorous cells (*arrows*) (H&E; original magnification: 400×).

have been found to have loss of nuclear INI-1 expression.[64] A brief overview of microscopic features of commonly seen clear cell neoplasms is provided in **Table 2.4.** In regard to xanthomatous, microvesicular, foamy, or physaliphorous cytoplasmic appearances, macrophages should always be kept in mind. Macrophage-rich lesions such as demyelinating process and infarct, especially at its subacute stage, are notorious for causing diagnostic problems by mimicking clear cell lesions, especially during IOC. Reactive changes around AVM, due to the relative abundance of oligodendroglial cells due to chronic ischemic tissue collapse, as well as many macrophages, may mimic an oligodendroglioma if the entire lesion is not available for evaluation.[37,38]

Typically, *distinct cytoplasmic vacuoles* indicate glandular differentiation and may contain a wisp of mucin or an inspissated *mucin* globule that looks like a dot in the lumen. The presence of mucin can be confirmed by a mucin stain, such as mucicarmine. The fact that there is intra- or extracytoplasmic mucin indicates a glandular differentiation but not necessarily a glandular malignancy, that is, adenocarcinoma. For a diagnosis of adenocarcinoma, the cytologic and architectural features of malignancy must be present. Cytoplasmic vacuoles with mucin can also be seen in the lining cells of Rathke cleft cyst, colloid cyst, and endodermal cyst. They are bland columnar cells and it is clear that they form a lining on what is usually a membranous cyst wall (see "Cystic Lesions"). Similarly, in pituitary specimens, such cells may simply represent Rathke cleft remnants located in the intermediate lobe of the pituitary gland. Again, in the context of transsphenoidal resections or nasopharyngeal approaches, upper respiratory tract–type epithelium can be present in the specimen as a contaminant or may be intentionally submitted as a specimen part to evaluate for invasion by the suspected neoplastic or other pathologic process. Endodermal components of germ cell neoplasms should also be considered. Depending on the specific tissue represented, such cells may be abundant or may be scattered among others, as in the case of goblet cells. As for glial neoplasms, ependymoma cells may contain intracytoplasmic lumens. Some ependymomas may have overwhelming numbers of such intracytoplasmic lumens, resulting in an ependymal neoplasm with *signet ring cell* morphology **(Fig. 2-38)**, with

TABLE 2.4 Identifying microscopic features of main clear cell neoplasms

Oligodendroglioma	Uniformly round nuclei Fine chromatin pattern Inconspicuous nucleoli "Chicken-wire" vasculature Sheets or scattered cells Hypercellular foci Minigemistocytes Tendency to infiltrate cortex Satellitosis Subpial condensation of cells Microcalcifications Myxoid/microcystic background Infiltrative border S-100+ GFAP+ in minigemistocytes
Clear cell ependymoma	Round-to-oval nuclei Sharp cytoplasmic borders Rudimentary pseudorosettes Typical ependymoma areas GFAP+ in perivascular cells EMA+ Sharp demarcation
Clear cell meningioma	Intranuclear cytoplasmic invaginations Rudimentary whorls Hyalinization Glycogen EMA+ Progesterone receptor+
Germinoma	Nuclear atypia Prominent nucleoli Open chromatin Glycogen Lobular arrangement Fibrous bands Lymphocytic infiltrate Calcification Other germ cell components PLAP+, OCT4+, SALL4+
Metastatic clear cell carcinoma	Nuclear atypia Pleomorphism Open chromatin pattern Prominent nucleoli Mitotic activity Necrosis with pseudopapillae Sharp cytoplasmic border Epithelial mucin or glycogen Cytokeratin+, other markers for its origin

(Continued)

TABLE 2.4 Identifying microscopic features of main clear cell neoplasms *(Continued)*

Hemangioblastoma	Rich, delicate capillary network Microvesicular cytoplasms Pericellular reticulin Sharp demarcation Inhibin+, D2-40+, Brachyury+
Chordoma	Myxoid background Clear and physaliphorous cells Single files, groups, sheets of cells Bland nuclei Cytokeratin+, Vimentin+, S-100+, EMA+, Brachyury+

no prognostic implications, but potentially creating confusion with a metastatic adenocarcinoma. If typical ependymoma morphology is not apparent, absence of mucin and immunohistochemical workup will clarify this confusion. The presence of an intracytoplasmic lumen supports the diagnosis of ependymoma in an otherwise glial neoplasm. In cases where it is not visible by routine examination, immunohistochemistry for EMA or electron microscopy highlights its presence. Liponeurocytomas have a cell population with cytoplasmic vacuolation due to lipid accumulation.

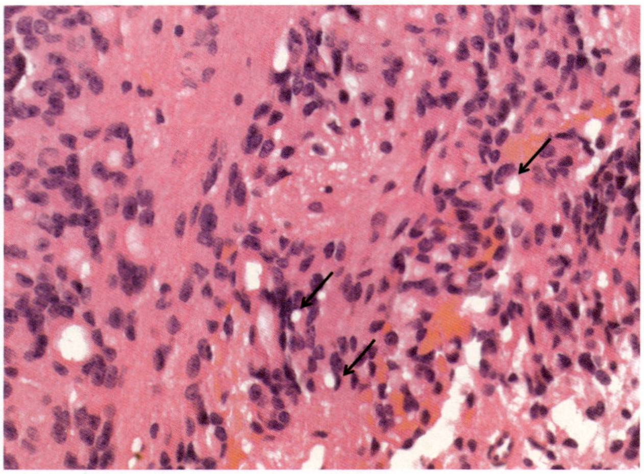

Figure 2-38. Ependymoma with vacuolar cells: Intracytoplasmic lumen formation may result in a vacuolar cytoplasm (*arrows*), which should not be confused with an adenocarcinoma together with the true rosettes mimicking gland formation (H&E; original magnification: 400×).

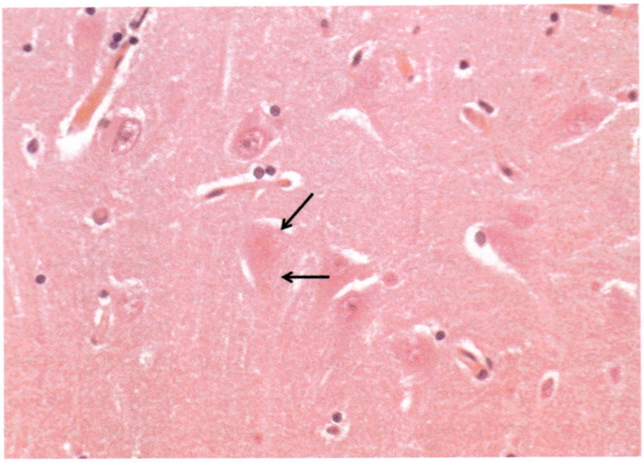

Figure 2-39. Granulovacuolar degeneration: Very small, usually multiple vacuoles with a dot-like granule are present in the cytoplasm of a neuron (*arrows*) (H&E; original magnification: 400×).

Granulovacuolar degeneration is a peculiar but nonspecific degenerative change seen in the cytoplasm of neurons. It consists of usually multiple minute vacuoles with a small dot-like granular structure in them, resulting in this descriptive name **(Fig. 2-39)**. It is positive for ubiquitin and is most prominent in the hippocampus. It should not be mistaken for viral inclusions. Granulovacuolar degeneration is especially frequent in AD and Pick disease. Neuronal cytoplasmic vacuolation can be seen as a nonspecific finding in other degenerative conditions. Inferior olivary hypertrophy is seen as a form of transsynaptic degeneration in olivary nuclei, where its neurons become hypertrophic with cytoplasmic vacuolation. Unverricht-Lundborg disease, a.k.a. Baltic myoclonus in reference to the region it is seen, is characterized by severe loss of Purkinje cells and swelling and cytoplasmic vacuolation in the remaining, along with Bergmann gliosis.[17] Vacuoles of variable size and shape can be seen in the neuron cytoplasm in spongiform encephalopathy, but they do not pose a problem as there is also prominent background *neuropil microvacuolation*. A delicate and subtle neuronal cytoplasmic microvacuolation is an early feature of hypoxic–ischemic change, before the characteristic eosinophilic neuronal necrosis (red neurons) forms. Lipidized or lipomatous meningioma is a metaplastic variant of meningioma with a mature *adipose tissue appearance*. It is usually a partial change and typical meningioma morphology is seen in other areas. One source of confusion may be in differentiating it from a meningioma that is widely infiltrating through the bone into subcutaneous fibroadipose tissue, a condition that should be easily clarified with the clinical and radiologic knowledge and the distinct delineation of meningioma and other components from each other. It should be remembered, however, that fibroadipose tissue is frequently present in association with dura mater. Nonetheless, this type of soft tissue and bone invasion or the lipidized nature of meningioma cells does not have prognostic significance and does not pose significant diagnostic or prognostic problems. Lipomas and liposarcomas are rare and are similar to their counterparts in other tissues. Lipoblasts are characterized by multivacuolated cytoplasm with indentation of the nuclei or a single vacuole creating a signet ring cell appearance. Epithelioid hemangioendothelioma has intracytoplasmic vacuoles of variable size and number, recapitulating primitive vascular lumen formation in an otherwise abundant eosinophilic epithelioid cytoplasm of the cells in a mucinous background. A small *paranuclear vacuole* is usually seen in the cytoplasm of choroid plexus cells with aging **(Fig. 2-40)**. A similar vacuole, representing a lysosome, is present in the ACTH-secreting, basophilic cells of the anterior pituitary gland. Scattered, variable-size cytoplasmic vacuoles are a feature of acidophil stem cell adenoma of the pituitary gland[65] **(Fig. 2-41)**. The cytoplasm can be variable from oncocytic to chromophobe. The vacuoles correspond to giant mitochondria. They are by definition aggressive adenomas regardless of any other criteria.

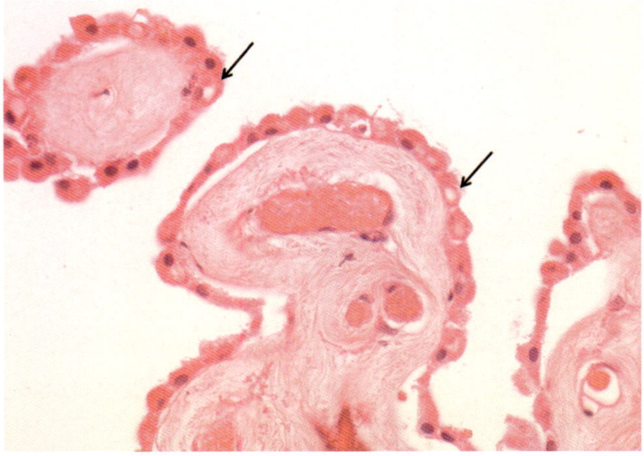

Figure 2-40. Cytoplasmic vacuole formation in choroid plexus epithelial cells is seen with increasing age (*arrows*) (H&E; original magnification: 400×).

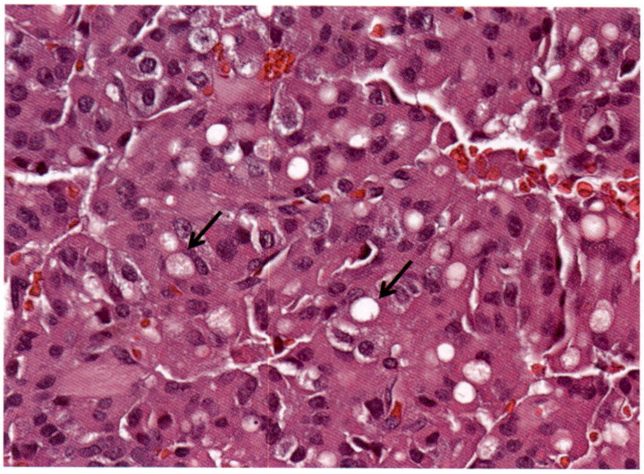

Figure 2-41. Acidophil stem cell adenoma: Cytoplasmic vacuoles of variable sizes are seen in the cytoplasm of the neoplastic cells (*arrows*) and correspond to enlarged vesicular mitochondria (H&E; original magnification: 400×).

Granular cytoplasm can be caused by various eosinophilic accumulations in the form of granules, which can be of various sizes and tinctorial qualities. Granular cell does not necessarily indicate a granular cell tumor. Just as popular in meaning is the cytoplasmic change seen in variable degrees in astrocytic neoplasms, that is, granular cell astrocytoma/glioblastoma **(Fig. 2-42)**. They are both due to lysosome accumulation in the cytoplasm, resulting in a fine dusty granularity, and tend to have an amphophilic quality. Granular cell change in astrocytic neoplasms implies a more aggressive biologic behavior.[66] These cells can easily be mistaken for macrophages due to their cytoplasmic features, as well as their bland nuclei. GFAP positivity and CD68 negativity confirm their glial origin in this context. However, the evaluation of immunohistochemistry may become a challenge due to the cross-reactivity and background-staining issues, resulting in an apparent positivity for both, especially if necrosis is present, in both astrocytic and histiocytic situations. CD163 is a more specific macrophage marker with less cross-reactivity and may be easier to interpret. Both cell types show PAS positivity that is diastase-resistant in the cytoplasm, due to lysosomes and debris.

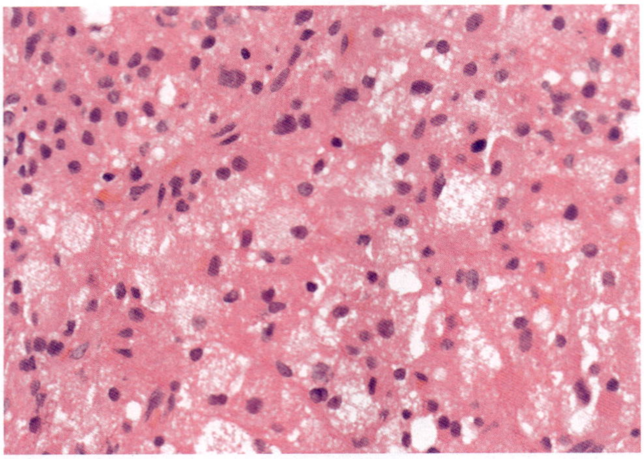

Figure 2-42. Granular cell astrocytoma: Granular to clear cytoplasms are seen in many cells in this astrocytoma and should not be confused with histiocytes (H&E; original magnification: 400×).

Granular cells of granular cell tumors are usually more uniformly and homogeneously packed with eosinophilic granules. These neoplasms are uniformly composed of these cells forming sheets. Granular cell tumors are typically found in the posterior pituitary and in the soft tissues, as they originate from peripheral nerves in the latter location. Granular cell tumor of the posterior pituitary originates from the pituicytes and, together with pituicytoma, they represent the two extremes of a morphologic spectrum. Granular cell tumors of the posterior pituitary are typically an incidental finding,[67] seen as a tumorlet identified during other studies or in autopsies. They are positive for S-100 protein in addition to PAS positivity that is diastase resistant. Granular cell tumor in the soft tissues can have PAS-positive and diastase-resistant *angulate bodies*.[68] Granular cell change can be present focally or widespread in schwannoma and neurofibroma. A malignant neoplasm that can rarely metastasize to CNS is alveolar soft part sarcoma. Its cells are arranged in a dyscohesive alveolar, organoid pattern and have abundant finely granular eosinophilic epithelioid cytoplasms. PAS-positive, diastase-resistant crystalloid inclusions in the cytoplasm support the diagnosis.

Another cell type where there is an eosinophilic granular quality to the cytoplasm is the *oncocyte*, in which the granularity is due to the accumulation of abundant mitochondria. The cytoplasm of the oncocyte is slightly more eosinophilic than the granular cell but still finely granular. In the nervous system, a variety of neoplasms can have oncocytic change.[69] Oncocytomas are seen in the pituitary region, that is, spindle cell oncocytoma of the adenohypophysis.[70] Rare choroid plexus tumors and ependymomas[71] can have oncocytic features, and rare cases of oncocytic meningiomas have been described[72] **(Fig. 2-43)**, although the experience is limited for a conclusion on the meaning of these changes in regard to prognosis.

Eosinophilic granular bodies (EGBs) are multiple, usually pleomorphic bright eosinophilic globules in the cytoplasm of astrocytic cells **(Fig. 2-44)**. They are considered as a feature that indicates the low-grade or long-standing nature of a lesion that is usually neoplastic, such as PA and ganglioglioma. They are especially helpful in a pleomorphic, high grade–appearing neoplasm to alert one to the possibility that one is dealing with a low-grade neoplasm, such as PXA. EGBs are PAS positive and diastase resistant and can be highlighted by this stain, although this is only rarely, if at all, necessary. Pilomyxoid astrocytoma (PMA) can rarely have EGBs and does not have Rosenthal fibers. Along with EGBs, Rosenthal fibers are more commonly seen in PA. Their presence in PMA should alert one to the possibility of a PA presence along with

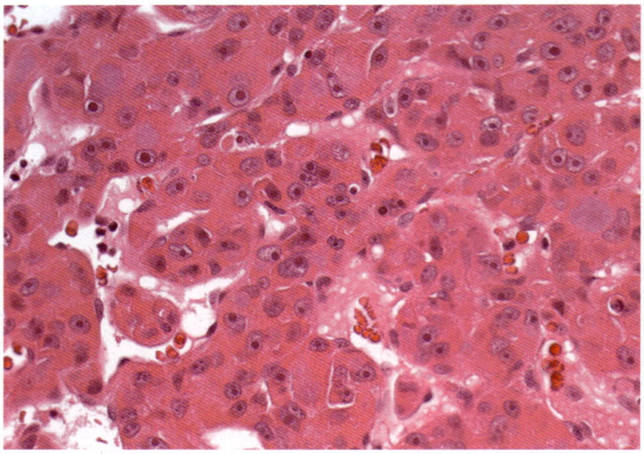

Figure 2-43. Oncocytic meningioma: Abundant eosinophilic granular cytoplasm is present along with prominent nucleoli, resulting in a melanoma-like appearance, making it difficult to recognize as meningioma. Typical meningioma morphology was present elsewhere in the neoplasm (H&E; original magnification: 400×).

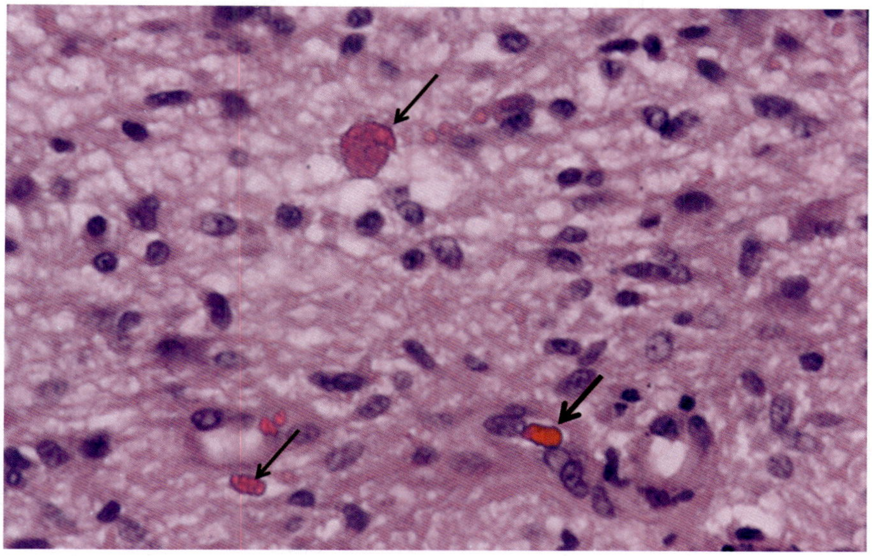

Figure 2-44. EGBs: Typically associated with low-grade neoplasms, EGBs may be of uniform or variable size and have a light eosinophilic, glassy refractile quality (*thin arrows*). Erythrocytes can be distinguished by their bright eosinophilia and squeezed stacked up appearance even if they may not be obviously intravascular (*thick arrow*) (H&E; original magnification: 400×).

PMA (see "Biphasic Pattern, Composite Lesions and Metaplastic Tissues"). Similar cytoplasmic or extracytoplasmic globular structures, though not as refractile and more hyaline, termed *hyaline globules*, are seen in yolk sac tumors and are positive for alpha-fetoprotein. Oligodendrogliomas sometimes have scattered neoplastic cells with more uniform eosinophilic granules in their cytoplasm. This is a rare finding in only scattered cells in an otherwise obvious oligodendroglioma and, as such, does not have significant diagnostic or differential diagnostic implications. African trypanosomiasis (sleeping sickness) results in a meningoencephalitis with perivascular and meningeal lymphocytes, plasma cells, and macrophages. Plasma cells with intracytoplasmic globules of immunoglobulin are seen. They are different than Russell bodies and are called *morular cells*.[73] They are not diagnostic but are considered characteristic in this context. Russell bodies are plasma cells with intracytoplasmic accumulation of immunoglobulin, creating one or multiple glassy refractile, bright eosinophilic globules, sometimes completely obliterating the cell. They are common in chronic inflammatory conditions that involve plasma cells. In the acute phase of American trypanosomiasis (Chagas' disease) *Trypanosoma cruzi*, amastigote parasites are present in the glial cells, creating a granular cytoplasm, which is not to be confused with *Toxoplasma* cysts. They can also be seen in the reactivation of chronic disease in glial cells and macrophages. Perivascular proteinaceous material accumulation, among other findings, and *PAS-positive globules* in this material and in astrocytes may be seen in acute lead encephalopathy.

Although the correlation between cytologic features and hormone secretion is not always accurate, generally, the granularity and tinctorial quality of the cytoplasm can provide some clues to the nature of pituitary adenomas. *Acidophilic cells* of the pituitary gland are considered to be growth hormone–secreting (somatotroph) cells. They are the most common cell type in the anterior pituitary and are most abundant in the lateral aspects of the gland. Therefore, small biopsy samples from these areas should not be mistaken for adenoma or hyperplasia, especially in intraoperative consultations. Attention to the nesting pattern of the nonneoplastic pituitary gland should help avoid this mistake; however, this may not be so easy in distorted tissues. Reticulin stain is very useful in highlighting the architecture and making this distinction. *Basophilic cells* of the anterior pituitary tend to have a larger cytoplasm and make the acini they reside in appear somewhat larger and expanded. These larger acini should not be interpreted as hyperplasia, especially in small biopsy samples. Likewise, since the great majority of ACTH cell adenomas are microadenomas of only a few millimeters, they may be difficult to identify both intraoperatively and histologically, necessitating extreme care, processing, leveling of tissue blocks, and special stains, especially ACTH and reticulin stains, to identify this microadenoma. Null cell adenomas tend to be *chromophobic*, with a subpopulation having oncocytic features. Oncocytic cytoplasm can be seen, in addition to null cell adenomas, in acidophil stem cell, silent ACTH cell, and gonadotroph cell adenomas. In general, prolactin cell adenomas (some may be amphophilic), sparsely granulated growth hormone cell adenomas, and acidophil stem cell adenomas (some may be acidophilic/oncocytic) tend to be chromophobic; densely granulated growth hormone cell adenomas tend to be acidophilic; and ACTH cell adenomas tend to be basophilic or amphophilic.[74] A peculiar cytoplasmic change in ACTH cell pituitary adenoma is *Crooke's hyaline change*. It is a peculiar perinuclear circular dense cytokeratin accumulation resulting in a pale, hyalinized appearance to the cytoplasm. Some ACTH cell adenomas are composed essentially entirely of such cells, called Crooke cell adenoma, an aggressive variant.[75] They are functional and behave aggressively. Scattered cells with Crooke's hyaline change can be seen in nonneoplastic pituitary parenchyma. Crooke's hyaline change, in nonneoplastic or adenomatous tissue, indicates glucocorticoid excess, which can be associated with adenomatous tissue, medical treatment, or adrenal gland pathology. This change is not seen in those nonneoplastic basophilic cells normally infiltrating the posterior pituitary.

Rosenthal fibers are accumulations in the cytoplasmic processes of astrocytes **(Fig. 2-45)**. They have an elongated ropy, glassy thick, and amorphous appearance with a dark red-to-burgundy color. They are composed of a mixture of components including alpha–beta crystalline, GFAP, and ubiquitin and are positive for these by immunohistochemistry. The identification of Rosenthal fibers should not prompt a diagnosis of PA. For the diagnosis of PA, a biphasic morphology with alternating piloid and loosely textured areas with round and bland nuclei and an admixture of thick vessels should be identified, although in small biopsies and intraoperative consultations, all features can be difficult to have altogether and it can turn out to be a difficult differential diagnosis without clinical and radiologic help. This issue can be further complicated by the fact that suprasellar/hypothalamic region is a common location for craniopharyngiomas and PAs, and cerebellum is a common location for both hemangioblastomas and PAs, since both craniopharyngiomas and hemangioblastomas tend to induce a piloid gliosis around them that can be rich in Rosenthal fibers. Rosenthal fibers are abundant and widespread in Alexander's disease, a genetic disease,[76] where they are most prominent around the vessels and on pial surfaces. In the younger children with this disease, astrocyte cytoplasm may contain eosinophilic granular structures, making the cytoplasm prominent, creating a granular appearance.[77] Increased Rosenthal fibers can be present in cortical dysplasias and in fucosidosis, especially around vessels, mimicking Alexander's disease. Rosenthal fibers are frequently present in the pineal region, as well as in the lining of pineal cysts, as part of the piloid gliosis forming the innermost layer of such cysts. Small tissue samples from pineal region, therefore, should not be confused with PA, even though PAs can occasionally involve the pineal region. The recognition of the fact that Rosenthal fibers can be present as part of the cyst lining in the pineal gland is useful in the evaluation of PPT in small tissue samples as well. The layer outside the gliotic cyst lining consists of a solid, disorganized layer of pineal parenchymal cells without the usual lobulated or organoid pattern of the normal pineal gland. This solid appearance should not be confused with the pineal parenchymal tumor of intermediate

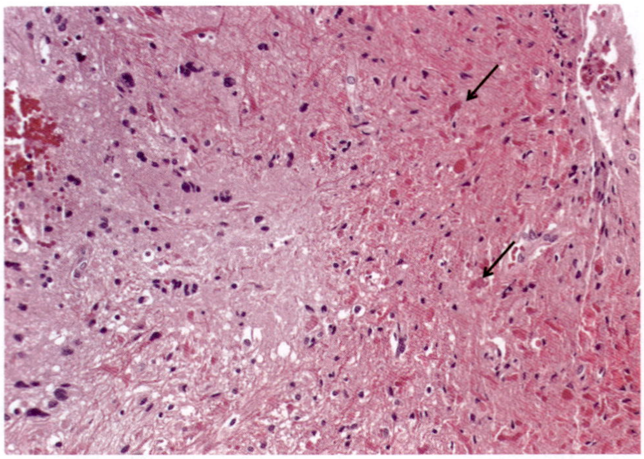

Figure 2-45. Rosenthal fibers: Many irregular, elongated, amphophilic ropy structures (*arrows*) are present in association with a PA (**left side**) but should not prompt such a diagnosis by themselves (H&E; original magnification: 200×).

differentiation (PPTID). The recognition of the gliosis with Rosenthal fibers next to such cellular layer should alert one to the possibility of nonneoplastic pineal parenchyma next to the cyst lining.

Evaluation of *cytoplasmic borders* can be useful in some cases. A *syncytial arrangement* where the cytoplasmic boundaries of individual cells are not distinct is typical in meningiomas. This is due to the interdigitating cell borders at the ultrastructural level, precluding their distinction at the light microscopic level. Meningioma cell borders can become distinctly visible when the tissue is stretched and the cells are separated from each other or when cellular changes, such as rhabdoid change, take place. Embryonal carcinoma cells can have somewhat syncytial arrangement that can be helpful in distinguishing that neoplasm from germinoma. Sharply demarcated cytoplasmic borders, on the other hand, create an *epithelioid appearance* in general. While this is typical for carcinomas, or epithelial lesions in general, some primary nervous system neoplasms can assume an epithelioid appearance. MPNST, epithelioid schwannoma, and anaplastic oligodendroglioma **(Fig. 2-46)**, as well as rare GBM referred to as epithelioid GBM,[59] are prominent examples. As such, clusters of atypical epithelioid cells in some schwannomas may be precursors of malignancy. If purely epithelioid, such neoplasms can create confusion with melanoma or carcinoma.

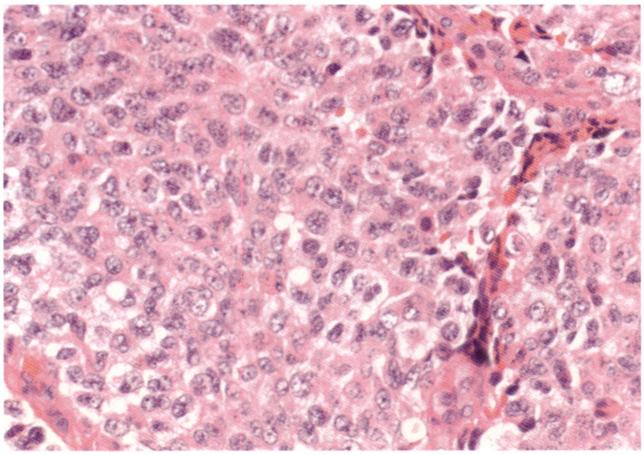

Figure 2-46. Anaplastic oligodendroglioma: Enlarged nuclei, prominent nucleoli, and abundant cytoplasms creating an epithelioid appearance (H&E; original magnification: 400×).

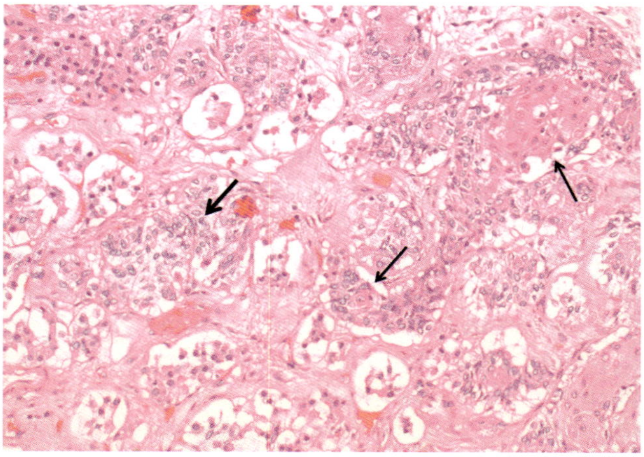

Figure 2-47. Erdheim rests: These squamoid islands are typically seen in the pituitary infundibulum and resemble the lacy pattern of a minute adamantinomatous craniopharyngioma (*thin arrows*). They are in close association with, and may even be seen in transition from, anterior pituitary cell groups (*thick arrow*) (H&E; original magnification: 200×).

Squamous islands are common in pars tuberalis of pituitary gland, where they are called Erdheim rests **(Fig. 2-47)** They are thought to arise through squamous metaplasia from glandular cells of the anterior pituitary gland. They should not be mistaken for squamous cell carcinoma, craniopharyngioma, or other squamous lesions, especially during IOC. Squamous cell carcinoma, especially nonkeratinizing/poorly differentiated one, can still be recognized in most cases by the thick quality of the cytoplasm with well-defined borders and desmosomes between the cells. Squamous epithelium is common in various types of cysts. Likewise, ciliated epithelial cells are seen in several cystic lesions (see "Cystic Lesions"). In addition, ependymal cells have both *cilia and microvilli*, although the latter are difficult to appreciate at the light microscopic level. Cilia are more prominent in pediatric brains and gradually diminish in adulthood, although are still easily identified. In fact, the identification of the basal bodies where the shafts of the cilia attach within the cytoplasm, that is, the *blepharoplasts*, by histochemical stains such as phosphotungustic acid-hematoxylin (PTAH), was used to support the diagnosis of ependymoma before the immunohistochemistry era.[78]

Cytoplasmic swelling or *ballooning* is a feature that can be seen in intracytoplasmic accumulations, resulting in a ballooned appearance, as seen in storage diseases,[79] such as GM1 and GM2 gangliosidosis, where the cytoplasms have a clear or foamy quality. In some disorders, the accumulation may be difficult to demonstrate, as it may be water-soluble as in mannosidosis, even with special stains such as PAS and Sudan. While the accumulations are generalized, they may be more prominent in certain areas; for example, vacuolated and enlarged neurons are widespread in fucosidosis but are more prominent in olivary nuclei and thalami. In Gaucher's disease, intracytoplasmic accumulation may not be seen in the neurons, but the macrophages with cytoplasmic needle-shaped crystals, that is, Gaucher cells, are characteristic. They tend to accumulate around blood vessels. Argyrophilic material can be seen in the cytoplasm of choroid plexus epithelial cells, glial cells, and especially neurons of the brainstem nuclei in aluminum intoxication. *Chromatolysis* also results in a swollen appearance of the cytoplasm with peripheral displacement of nucleus and Nissl substance. It is characteristic in the cell bodies of nerve cells, the axons of which have been transected, that is, as part of Wallerian degeneration or axonal reaction. Chromatolysis is typically localized to a group of neurons constituting a ganglion or nucleus associated with the damaged nerve fascicle. In arsenic intoxication, anterior horn cell chromatolysis and degeneration are seen due to peripheral neuropathy, whereas thallium intoxication is associated with chromatolysis of motor neurons and posterior column degeneration. Toxic oil syndrome[80] is a toxic cooking oil–related illness with chromatolysis, vacuolation, and neurofilament accumulations in large neurons of spinal cord, the latter also argyrophilic. Chromatolysis can be seen in association with the side effects of medications. Clioquinol[81] may result in chromatolysis of lumbosacral anterior horn neurons, dorsal root ganglia, and inferior olivary nuclei together with tract degenerations, while mainly the brainstem neurons are affected in vidarabine use.[82] Bright eosinophilic, somewhat smudgy, coagulated appearance of the neuron cytoplasm with disappearance of Nissl substance is called red neuron, shrunken neuron, or eosinophilic neuronal necrosis and indicates acute neuronal injury. Typically, the nucleus is also shrunken and the chromatin has lost its crispness. Red neurons develop gradually and variably 4 to 12 hours postinjury depending on the circumstances, are typically associated with hypoxic–ischemic injury, but can also be seen in other types of neuronal injury, and constitute the light microscopic evidence for irreversible neuron death.[83,84]

Cytoplasmic Inclusions

By definition, any abnormal accumulation in the cell constitutes an inclusion. This includes viral inclusions, accumulations that occur as a result of a genetic metabolic disease, such as neuronal storage diseases, and abnormal protein accumulations as seen in neurodegenerative diseases, among others. For the purposes of this discussion, mainly those accumulations that form a distinct inclusion that is characteristic, if not pathognomonic, for a particular disease or group of disorders are discussed here, while others are mentioned elsewhere. For instance, neuronal storage diseases are discussed under "cytoplasmic features" because such swollen cells are recognized in practice as swollen cells rather than inclusions. Cytoplasmic inclusions are commonly seen in the context of neurodegenerative diseases and have diagnostic implications in many cases[85,86] **(Table 2.5)**. They usually represent an abnormal accumulation of protein, which reflects an abnormality in the physiologic processes within the cell and results in the demise of the cell. Many of them require special stains for identification and appropriate characterization. Due to a significant overlap in the involvement patterns and histologic features in neurodegenerative diseases, clinical information needs to be incorporated in the evaluation of neuropathologic findings. To complicate the matter further, various diseases can be described by different names and may have significant overlapping features with others, while the characterization of the accumulations and the diseases with which they are associated is constantly evolving. In addition to the accumulations and inclusions associated with particular diseases, a broader classification takes into account the underlying molecular pathologic mechanism. That way, major neurodegenerative diseases can be classified into tauopathies, synucleinopathies, and trans-active response DNA-binding protein-43 (TDP-43) proteinopathies, and tauopathies can further be subclassified based on the type of tau protein that accumulates, such

List of Findings/Checklist for Cytoplasmic Inclusions

AT A GLANCE

Neuronal Cytoplasmic Inclusions
- Classical Lewy body
- Cortical Lewy body
- Pale body
- Bunina body
- Neurofibrillary tangles
- Hirano body
- Pick body
- Lyssa body
- Negri body
- Cytomegalovirus
- Collins body
- Papp-Lantos inclusion
- Biondi body/ring
- Age-related inclusions

Glial Cytoplasmic Inclusions
- Coils
- Grains
- Tufts
- Thorns

Others
- Fibrous body
- Endothelial inclusions

Lafora body, polyglucosan body, axonal spheroids, eosinophilic granular bodies, Russell bodies, storage diseases (see "Background and Neuropil Features")

TABLE 2.5 Summary of characteristic cytoplasmic accumulations or inclusions: Their immunohistochemical features and distribution in major neurodegenerative diseases

	Tau	Alpha-Synuclein	TDP-43	FUS	Location
AD	3R and 4R, NFT	—	—	—	CC, L
NFT dementia	3R and 4R, NFT	—	—	—	L
Pick's disease (FTLD with Pick bodies)	3R, Pick bodies	—	—	—	CC, L
CBD	Neuronal: 4R, pale body–like inclusions Glial: 4R (ubiquitin-negative), tufts, grains, coils	—	—	—	CC, BG
PSP	Neuronal: 4R, NFT Glial: 4R, tufts, thorns	—	—	—	BG, BS
AGD	Neuronal: 4R, NFT Glial: 4R, coils	—	—	—	L
PD	—	Neuronal: classical Lewy body Glial: filamentous	—	—	BS
DLB	—	Neuronal: cortical Lewy body Glial: filamentous	—	—	CC, L, BS
MSA	—	Neuronal and glial	—	—	BG, BS, C

(Continued)

TABLE 2.5 Summary of characteristic cytoplasmic accumulations or inclusions: Their immunohistochemical features and distribution in major neurodegenerative diseases *(Continued)*

FTLD-U, FTLD-MND/ALS, MND	—	—	Neuronal and glial: variable, some NF positive	Also positive	CC, BG, MN
FTLD-FUS, BIBD, NIFID	—	—	—	Neuronal and glial: variable, neurofilament positive in NIFID	CC

TDP-43, TAR [trans-active response] DNA-binding protein-43; FUS, fused in sarcoma protein; AD, Alzheimer's disease; R, repeat; NFTs, neurofibrillary tangles; CC, cerebral cortex; L, limbic; FTLD, frontotemporal lobar degeneration; CBD, corticobasal degeneration; BG, basal ganglia; PSP, progressive supranuclear palsy; BS, brainstem; AGD, argyrophilic grain disease; PD, Parkinson's disease; DLB, dementia with Lewy bodies; MSA, multiple system atrophy; C, cerebellum; FTLD-U, frontotemporal lobar degeneration with ubiquitin-immunoreactive inclusions; MND, motor neuron disease; ALS, amyotrophic lateral sclerosis; MN, motor neurons; NF, neurofilament; BIBD, basophilic inclusion body disease; NIFID, neuronal (neurofilament) intermediate filament inclusion disease.

as 3-repeat tau, 4-repeat tau, or both.[87] The great majority of them, as a rule, are ubiquitin positive.

Classical Lewy body is the diagnostic feature of Parkinson's disease.[88] It is a round, eosinophilic inclusion with a dense center and a pale, hazy halo **(Fig. 2-48)**. It may be single or multiple and is present typically in the substantia nigra and locus ceruleus but can also be seen in other nuclei such as dorsal motor nucleus of vagus, Edinger-Westphal nucleus, as well as thalamus and hypothalamus and intermediolateral column of the spinal cord. It is easily visible especially in the pigmented neurons since it pushes the neuromelanin aside to become more prominent. Rarely, they can be found in the neuropil by themselves, suggesting the death of the neuron, leaving them behind, or they may be in the axons. Rarely, during an otherwise unremarkable autopsy examination, an incidental Lewy body or two can be identified. This finding likely represents a subclinical and early phase of Parkinson's disease. Lewy bodies have been identified in peripheral and autonomic nervous systems also.[89,90] They are alpha-synuclein and ubiquitin positive by immunohistochemistry. Their immunohistochemical features are especially useful in the identification of *cortical Lewy bodies*, which, in spite of their name, have a different appearance with a pale, ill-defined condensation with no dense center or peripheral halo in the cytoplasm of deeper layer neurons of the cerebral cortex **(Fig. 2-49)**. They are commonly found in entorhinal cortex, periamygdaloid cortex, cingulate gyrus, insular cortex, and other cortical areas. The number and distribution pattern of Lewy body pathology affects the classification. Sampling standard areas and evaluation by alpha-synuclein are required for appropriate workup.[91,92] Cells with cortical Lewy bodies may look like reactive astrocytes, but they are neurons. Dementia with Lewy bodies frequently coexists with AD.

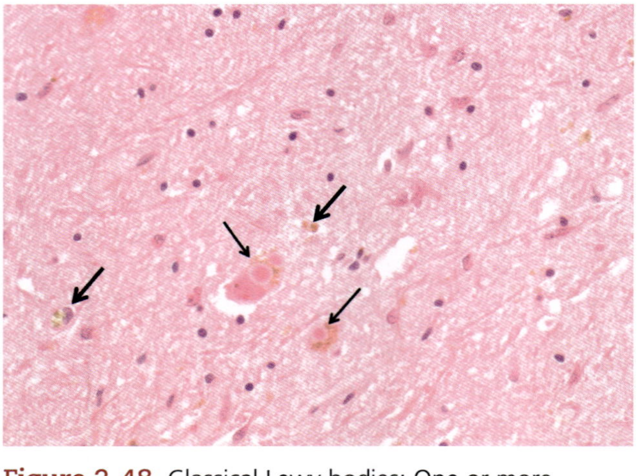

Figure 2-48. Classical Lewy bodies: One or more round eosinophilic neuronal cytoplasmic inclusions with a pale halo push the neuromelanin pigment aside in the substantia nigra (*thin arrows*). There is also neuron loss evidenced by free pigment in the neuropil (*thick arrows*), as well as a mildly increased cellularity due to gliosis (H&E; original magnification: 400×).

Pale bodies[93] are relatively well-defined, round, lightly eosinophilic areas apparently pushing the pigment in the cytoplasm of pigmented neurons aside **(Fig. 2-50)**. If the nucleus is not in the plane

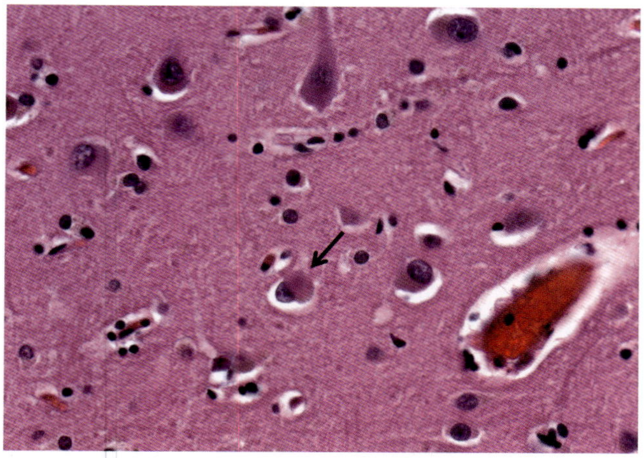

Figure 2-49. Cortical Lewy body: Homogeneous eosinophilic accumulation is present typically in the small neurons of the deeper layers of the cerebral cortex (*arrow*) and is different than the classical Lewy body (H&E; original magnification: 400×).

of section, they may appear as eosinophilic homogeneous structures in the neuropil. They are also positive for alpha-synuclein and ubiquitin. They are thought to represent an earlier developmental stage of Lewy body pathology. Therefore, if pale bodies are present, classical Lewy bodies should be searched for. If necessary, multiple sections should be examined before excluding the diagnosis. Lewy bodies can be found in sympathetic neurons of the spinal cord in autonomic failure, in dorsal motor nucleus of vagus in Lewy body dysphagia, and in substantia nigra and cerebral cortex in juvenile Parkinson's disease. Inclusions resembling Lewy bodies can be seen in substantia nigra neurons in ataxia-telangiectasia. In some cases of ataxia-telangiectasia, NFT can be present in the basal ganglia, hippocampus, and cerebral cortex. A variety of inclusions are seen in neuron cytoplasm in amyotrophic lateral sclerosis (ALS). *Bunina bodies*[94] are small eosinophilic inclusions, usually multiple and lined up in the cytoplasm. Other accumulations in ALS can be variable, ranging from large hyalinized structures filling the majority of the cytoplasm, displacing the organelles to the periphery, to rare round eosinophilic structures with a dense center and a pale periphery, resembling Lewy body of Parkinson's disease. By ubiquitin immunohistochemistry, these inclusions are highlighted as thread-like, skein-like, round with irregular margins, and irregular dot-like structures scattered within the cytoplasm. They are not always present nor are they found altogether, requiring immunohistochemistry and laborious search. Dot-like ubiquitin-positive inclusions can be found in the small neurons of the dentate gyrus in cases with extra-motor involvement.

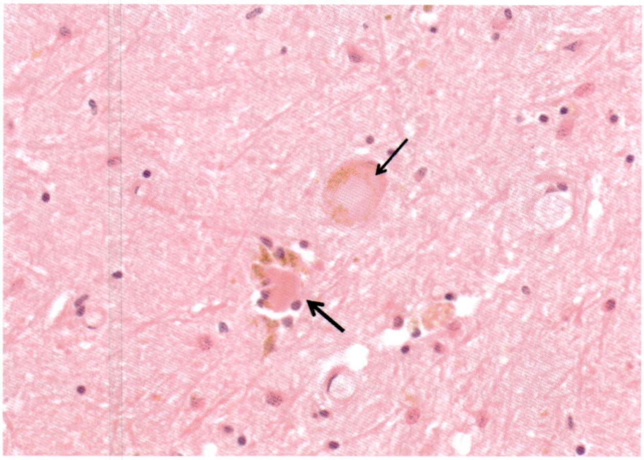

Figure 2-50. Pale body: Also present in the substantia nigra neurons, pale bodies are pale eosinophilic structures (*thin arrow*) that are not as well-defined as the classical Lewy bodies. Free classical Lewy bodies are also seen (*thick arrow*) in place of a degenerated neuron and are surrounded by the residual pigment both free and in the macrophages (H&E; original magnification: 400×).

Neurofibrillary tangles (NFT) are bundles of fibrillary amphophilic material that have a flame-shaped configuration in pyramidal neurons **(Fig. 2-51)**. In small neurons, they can form a globose mass with round outlines. They can be highlighted by silver impregnation techniques (Bielschowsky silver stain) and phosphorylated tau immunohistochemistry. In their later stages and when the neuron is degenerated, they may remain for some time in the neuropil as burnt-out tangles and lose their typical staining characteristics. They may then appear as pale brown fibrils by Bielschowsky silver stain. On H&E-stained sections, the intracortical fibers in the occipital cortex may appear as ghost NFT; however, their orderly distribution and prominence readily reveal their true nature. White matter bundles are well-organized and orderly distributed, while burnt-out tangles are scattered randomly and are present in small numbers in a given region. Their identification, frequency, and distribution are important for classification of the neurodegenerative disease and, where applicable,

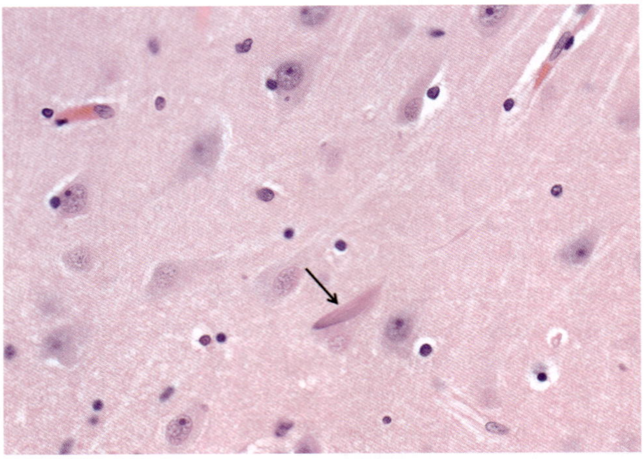

Figure 2-51. NFT: A thick, fibrillary, and amphophilic structure is seen and is described as "flame-shaped" (*arrow*). Although this particular tangle is oriented parallel to the long axis of the neuron, they can be round to fit in the shape of the cytoplasm of smaller neurons, forming "globose tangles" (H&E; original magnification: 400×).

for its staging and clinical application,[95,96] for example, as in Braak & Braak staging of AD.[97] Depending on the distribution of NFT and some other features, AD can have various variants. Many NFT are present in hippocampus and amygdala, in the presence of large numbers of neocortical plaques in limbic AD. Predominantly one hemisphere is involved in asymmetric AD. Predominantly occipital lobes are involved in posterior AD. Frontotemporal clinical features dominate in the presence of an otherwise typical AD pathology in frontal AD.[17] AD can coexist with other neurodegenerative diseases, such as dementia with Lewy bodies, and corticobasal degeneration (CBD), where swollen neurons can be present. Vascular dementia, or vascular pathology, can accompany AD and other neurodegenerative diseases. Rare cases may have no neuritic plaques or beta-amyloid pathology and are composed exclusively of NFT mainly in the hippocampus, entorhinal cortex, and amygdala, that is, tangle-only dementia. In aging, there may be mainly diffuse plaques and only a few neuritic plaques, and they are ubiquitin positive but are tau-negative. NFT are seen in small numbers only in the hippocampus and entorhinal cortex. NFT are present in progressive supranuclear palsy (PSP; Steele-Richardson-Olszewski syndrome) predominantly in the substantia nigra, periaqueductal gray matter, red nuclei, colliculi, loci cerulei, nuclei of cranial nerves X and XII, globus pallidus, hippocampus and subthalamic nuclei, dentate nuclei, and pontine nuclei. Neuropathologic criteria have been outlined for the evaluation of PSP.[98] Inferior olivary nuclei, putamen and caudate nuclei, and cerebral cortex can be involved. NFT can also be present in all these locations in an otherwise typical AD. NFT are predominantly in cortex and associated with neuritic plaques in AD. In a variant of Gerstmann-Straussler-Scheinker (GSS) disease, a type of prion disease that is associated with ataxia, cognitive decline, and parkinsonism, NFT are present in a distribution that is similar to that of AD. It is termed NFT GSS and also has amyloid plaques in the cerebral cortex, which may be confused with the amyloid cores of the neuritic plaques. The amyloid plaques of GSS are also present in the cerebellar cortex. NFT can occur in the hippocampal and neocortical neurons in some patients with long-standing subacute sclerosing panencephalitis (SSPE). NFT can also be seen in association with long-standing malformations or low-grade neoplasms, such as angiocentric glioma, meningioangiomatosis, and MCD, or in neurons adjacent to long-standing damage, such as radiation necrosis. Aside from Parkinson's disease, other conditions that involve and result in damage to substantia nigra, among others, can result in the clinical picture of parkinsonism. In postencephalitic parkinsonism, NFT are present in the substantia nigra and locus ceruleus, as well as in the hippocampus and cerebral cortex and mainly in a distribution with significant overlap with PSP, requiring incorporation of clinical findings in the differential diagnosis. They are also present in substantia nigra and locus ceruleus in the so-called tangle-only parkinsonism, without history of encephalitis. Guam parkinsonism–dementia complex is a neurodegenerative disease that is essentially always seen in the Pacific islands of Guam and Rota and is associated with NFT[99] in the hippocampus, amygdala, cerebral cortex, basal ganglia, thalamus, substantia nigra, tegmental nuclei, and anterior horn neurons of the spinal cord. Alpha-synuclein–positive accumulations can be present in amygdala. NFT, along with other features of AD, occur at an earlier age for the usual AD but toward the end of the lifespan of patients with Down syndrome. Chronic traumatic encephalopathy (posttraumatic neurodegeneration, dementia pugilistica or punch-drunk syndrome) due to long-term repetitive small trauma is characterized by neurodegenerative changes, including NFT and other changes in cerebral cortex along with neuron loss in substantia nigra, cerebral cortex, and cerebellum.[100] The disease referred to as diffuse NFT with calcification[101] may show Lewy bodies in the amygdala, hippocampus, and substantia nigra, along with alpha-synuclein–positive astrocytes in the hippocampus and temporal cortex. NFT are widespread, with neuron loss and gliosis, in the presence of calcifications in basal ganglia. In group II Niemann-Pick disease (i.e., without sphingomyelinase deficiency), ballooned neurons with finely granular eosinophilic material are present in the basal ganglia, brainstem, and spinal cord. In addition, NFT and neuroaxonal dystrophy are seen. NFT are tau positive and extend to dendrites and proximal axons, resulting in their thickening next to cell body. Some patients with neurodegeneration with brain iron accumulation type 1 (a.k.a., pantothenate kinase–associated neurodegeneration; formerly known as Hallervorden-Spatz disease), in addition to their typical pathologic features, may have NFT and Lewy body pathology. Sparse NFT can be present in argyrophilic grain disease,[102] which is characterized by dendrite-associated argyrophilic and tau-positive granules in the neuropil. NFT and Lewy bodies may be seen in infantile neuroaxonal dystrophies along with their typical features, as well as cerebral cortical degeneration.

Hirano bodies[103] are roughly rectangular bright eosinophilic neuronal intracytoplasmic actin-positive structures most commonly seen in the hippocampus **(Fig. 2-52)**. They are not pathognomonic for a particular disease process, but they are seen in older age and are more common in AD, Pick disease, and Guam parkinsonism–dementia complex. Similar inclusions may be present in thalamic neurons with increasing age but are especially common in myotonic dystrophy. Like other intracytoplasmic accumulations, they may remain by themselves in the neuropil when the neuron dies. *Pick bodies* are round, well-circumscribed eosinophilic or slightly basophilic structures that are about the size of the nucleus **(Fig. 2-53)**. They may resemble cortical Lewy bodies, are also seen in small neurons, but are better demarcated and are slightly more basophilic. They are predominantly present in the superficial layers of the cerebral cortex in contrast to the cortical Lewy bodies. They are tau positive and are positive by silver impregnation techniques. They are also commonly seen in dentate gyrus and pyramidal neurons of the hippocampus. Other areas of the brain can also have smaller numbers of Pick bodies. Frontotemporal lobar degenerations (FTLDs) other than Pick's disease also have different types of inclusions. FTLD linked to chromosome 17 can have NFT and inclusions that resemble Pick bodies.[104] FTLD with ubiquitin-only immunoreactive changes is characterized by ubiquitin-positive

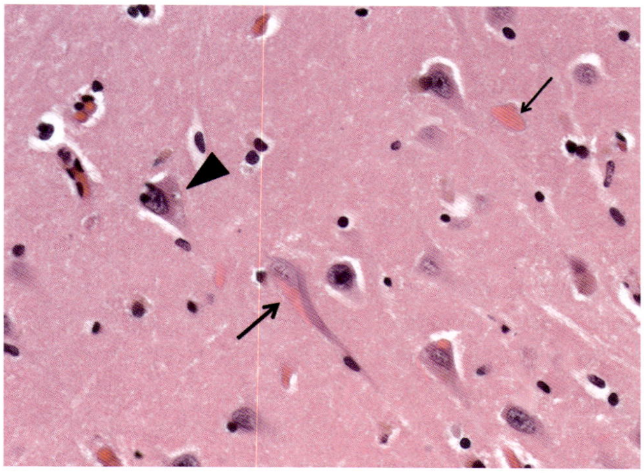

Figure 2-52. Hirano body: Rectangular eosinophilic glassy structures are present in the neuron cytoplasm (*thick arrow*) and free in the neuropil (*thin arrow*) after the neuron degenerates. A NFT is also seen in the neuron (*thick arrow*). Another neuron has granulovacuolar degeneration (*arrowhead*) (H&E; original magnification: 400×).

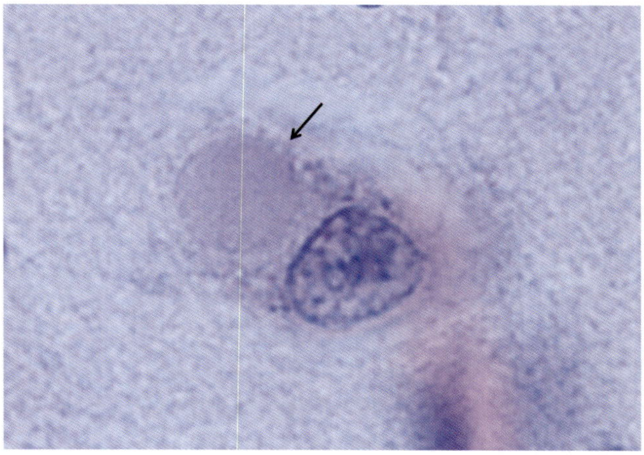

Figure 2-53. Pick body: Round, well-circumscribed, pale eosinophilic accumulation about the size of the nucleus (*arrow*) is present in this small neuron (H&E; original magnification: 600×).

neuronal inclusions. Neuronal cytoplasmic inclusions are small and round and are present in the dentate gyrus, amygdala, and cortex. Rarely, intranuclear inclusions may be present. FTLD with motor neuron disease shows motor neuron disease (MND)/ALS-type ubiquitin-positive neuronal cytoplasmic inclusions in the frontal and temporal cortex. FTLD with neurofilament inclusions has faint eosinophilic or slightly basophilic small intracytoplasmic inclusions in superficial cortical neurons. They can be larger in larger neurons such as Betz cells. They are neurofilament positive, weakly ubiquitin positive, and tau negative. Some may be positive for alpha–beta crystalline. The morphologic features of these inclusions on routine stains are similar to the inclusions in the disease called basophilic inclusion body disease, which arguably has some similarities and overlapping features with it.[105]

Motor neuron disease–inclusion dementia is characterized by *ubiquitin-positive cytoplasmic inclusions in the neurons* of the dentate gyrus, amygdala, and the involved areas of the cerebral cortex.[106] *Negri body* is an eosinophilic, round or slightly oval, well-circumscribed structure that is diagnostic for rabies infection **(Fig. 2-54)**. Somewhat less well-defined version is called *lyssa body*. There can be one or more Negri bodies in a neuron. Although widespread, they are best seen in Purkinje cells, brainstem, and pyramidal cells of the hippocampus.

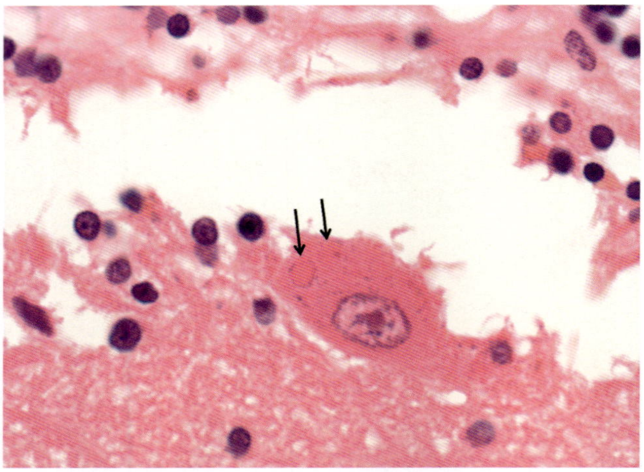

Figure 2-54. Negri body: Two well-circumscribed, erythrocyte-like round inclusions (*arrows*) are present in the cytoplasm of this Purkinje cell. Round, small nuclei of the internal granule cells are also seen, but inflammation is typically absent (H&E; original magnification: 400×).

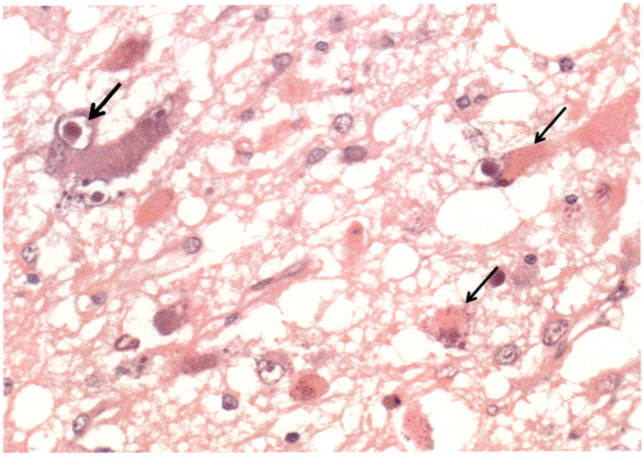

Figure 2-55. CMV inclusions: Infected cells show enlargement. Intranuclear inclusion (*thick arrow*) creates an owl-eye appearance, while intracytoplasmic inclusions (*thin arrows*) are in the form of eosinophilic or basophilic globules of variable sizes (H&E; original magnification: 400×).

Cytomegalovirus (CMV), in addition to its characteristic owl-eye intranuclear inclusions, can have intracytoplasmic inclusions in the form of bright eosinophilic, granular inclusions that are heterogeneous in size **(Fig. 2-55)**. MPTP (1-methyl-4-phenyl-1,2,3,6-tetrahydropyridine), a contaminant of illicit drug synthesis, results in parkinsonism due to striatal and nigral neuronal degeneration without Lewy bodies.[107]. Eosinophilic intracytoplasmic inclusions are seen in chronic administration. CBD inclusions are present in substantia nigra neuron cytoplasm. They are weakly basophilic, round structures, pushing neuromelanin aside, like pale bodies, but they are argyrophilic and tau positive. The glial inclusions seen in CBD can be in the form of grains, thorns, or coils next to the nucleus and differ from the inclusions of multiple system atrophy (MSA) in that they are negative for alpha-synuclein.[108] Dementia with neuroserpin accumulation (a.k.a. familial encephalopathy with neuroserpin inclusion bodies)[109] is characterized by neuronal inclusion bodies called *Collins bodies* that are found in neuronal cytoplasm or apparently free in the neuropil in deeper layers of the cortex, deep gray matter, substantia nigra, and some in the spinal cord and dorsal root ganglia. They are dark eosinophilic, round, well-defined, PAS positive, diastase resistant, and neuroserpin positive.

Glial filamentous inclusions in **PSP** are Bielschowsky- and tau-positive accumulations in the cell body. They may extend into cell processes to form neuropil threads. Glial cytoplasmic inclusions in MSA, a.k.a. *Papp-Lantos inclusions*,[110] are present in the oligodendroglia in gray and white matter, can be identified by Bielschowsky or Gallyas stains, and are tau, alpha-synuclein, and ubiquitin positive. They are small, elongated, flame-shaped, or curved structures next to the nucleus. MSA[111] also has *neuronal cytoplasmic and intranuclear inclusions*, as well as neuropil threads. Neuronal cytoplasmic inclusions are also present in MSA in neurons in affected regions, but especially in large numbers in putamen and basis pontis, are Gallyas, alpha-synuclein, and ubiquitin positive. MSA can additionally have motor neuron disease–type inclusions. Another inclusion that is not visible on routine sections but is highlighted by immunohistochemical stains is the *tau-positive inclusions in the glial cells* in the cerebral cortex in CBD. They can also be identified by silver impregnation techniques, especially Gallyas stain, but are negative for ubiquitin. They are in variable shapes described as *coils, grains, or tufts*. The cytoplasm of these cells is not abundant, and therefore, these inclusions are seen immediately adjacent to the nucleus and sometimes surrounding it completely. In PSP, various accumulations in the glial cells can be highlighted by tau immunohistochemistry and Gallyas stain and called *tufted astrocytes* and *thorn astrocytes*. Tufted astrocytes appear to be more commonly seen in PSP, while thorn astrocytes can be seen in other diseases. *Coiled bodies* are tau- and Gallyas-positive accumulations in oligodendroglial cell cytoplasm. PSP may occur together with vascular disease, Lewy bodies, CBD, and Creutzfeldt-Jakob disease (CJD), and it is not unusual to have overlapping and coexisting features of different neurodegenerative diseases in such conditions.[112] Neurofilament accumulation in neuron cytoplasm is a feature of cytosine arabinoside[113] and vincristine toxicity,[114] mainly in the brainstem and spinal cord neurons. Spinal motor neuron ballooning with neurofilament accumulation is also seen in ALS. Glial cytoplasmic filamentous inclusions have also been described in Parkinson's disease and dementia with Lewy bodies.[115]

Several apparently age-related intracytoplasmic inclusions can be seen in various cells. In caudate nucleus neuron cytoplasms, *spindled linear inclusions* are present with increasing age[116] but are more common in myotonic dystrophy. *Ill-defined eosinophilic intracytoplasmic inclusions* may be present in inferior olive neurons with increasing age. They may be difficult to identify in lipofuscin pigment but are ubiquitin positive. *Hyaline/colloid cytoplasmic inclusions* occur especially in hypoglossal nuclei.[117] They are well-circumscribed and homogeneous and appear similar to but not to be confused with others such as pale bodies of Parkinson's disease. *Biondi bodies*[118] are seen in ependymal and choroid plexus cells. They are fibrillary or ring-like (Biondi rings)

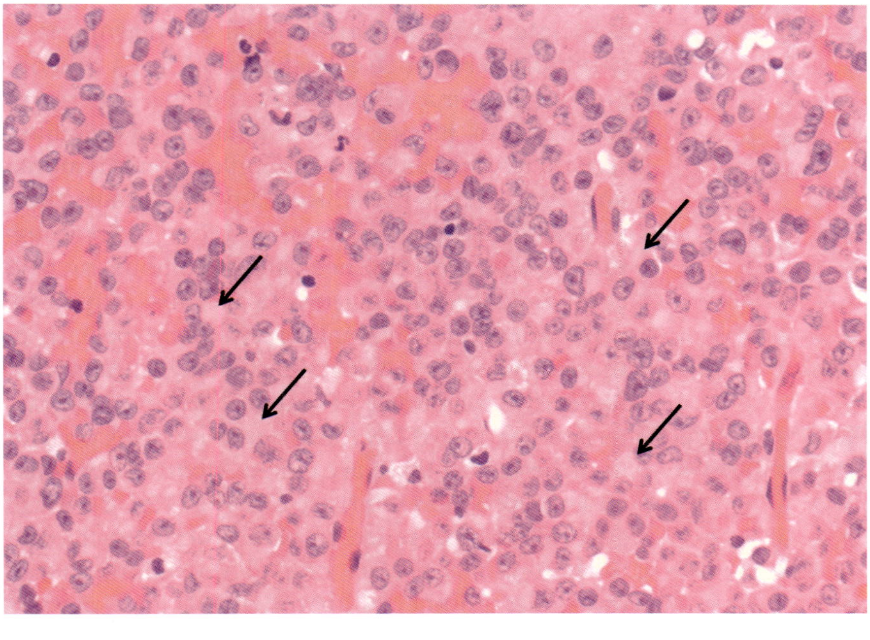

Figure 2-56. Fibrous bodies: Round, pale eosinophilic accumulations (*arrows*) are present in the cytoplasm of many cells and are about the size of the nucleus or smaller (H&E; original magnification: 400×).

and are positive for thioflavin-S, Congo red, and beta-amyloid.

Small intracytoplasmic, round homogeneous and hyaline structures are seen in the sparsely granulated growth hormone cell pituitary adenoma. They are about the size of the nucleus, occupy the majority of the cytoplasm, displace the nucleus, and sometimes indent it. They are called *fibrous bodies* and are positive for cytokeratin **(Fig. 2-56)**.[119] *PAS-positive intracytoplasmic inclusions in endothelial cells* are present in Fowler's syndrome (proliferative vasculopathy and hydranencephaly–hydrocephaly), which is characterized by a proliferative vasculopathy, among other features.[120] Other inclusions such as *Lafora body*, *Rosenthal fiber*, *spheroids*, seen in neuroaxonal dystrophy and accumulations as part of *storage diseases*, and *eosinophilic globules in Batten's disease* are discussed elsewhere. Some other intracytoplasmic structures such as *EGB* have been discussed previously. Ferritinopathy[121] and neurofilament inclusion body disease[122] also have cytoplasmic accumulations.

Mucinous–Myxoid Material

The wispy blue mucinous material can be seen in various settings, including primary and metastatic neoplasms, as well as nonneoplastic lesions, and is helpful in many cases to narrow down the differential diagnostic possibilities and direct one's attention to particular entities.

Variable amount of *epithelial mucin*, intracytoplasmic or extracytoplasmic, is associated with metastatic carcinomas, present in the lumens of glandular structures, or forming large pools. The identification of intracytoplasmic mucin is supportive of metastatic carcinoma in a poorly differentiated malignant neoplasm, which usually has a broad differential diagnosis. A metastatic poorly differentiated nonsmall-cell carcinoma of lung origin should further be qualified as squamous carcinoma or adenocarcinoma, as new treatment protocols are becoming available based on these components.[123] In that context, the presence of mucin should specifically be searched for, if necessary by mucin stains, in addition to the recommended additional immunohistochemical panels. The recognition of this material as mucin and its implication of confirming a glandular component in a carcinoma are straightforward. However, the presence of *mucinous–myxoid material* in nonepithelial lesions can be confusing in some settings. Adenocarcinoma, depending on its differentiation, shows variable degree of *gland formation*. Typically, these are the structures where mucin is identified. However, similar adenoid structures can be present in other types of neoplasms. Angiosarcomas can have vascular lumens lined by atypical endothelial cells, sometimes trapped within a collagenous stroma, mimicking metastatic adenocarcinoma. Some other neoplasms may have gland-like areas due to apoptosis or micronecrosis and subsequent clearing of necrotic debris, leaving a "lumen" behind. Some poorly differentiated neoplasms may have dyscohesive areas, also mimicking adenoid structure. Some choroid plexus papillomas can have mucinous degeneration and should not be confused with a metastatic papillary neoplasm.

Mucinous background has typically been associated with low-grade glial neoplasms. It is common to see such a background in PA and oligodendroglioma **(Fig. 2-57)**, among others. In some others, its presence is considered a characteristic feature, as in myxopapillary ependymoma and PMA. Such neoplasms, however, have their typical histologic features to allow their recognition, and the presence of a mucinous–myxoid component does not pose a serious diagnostic problem, except for small specimens, especially in the setting of IOC. A mucinous background resulting in the formation of mucin lakes is a characteristic feature of DNT. Scattered neurons present in these mucin lakes are called "floating neurons" and are also characteristic of DNT **(Fig. 2-58)**. In general, the presence of this mucinous–myxoid background can alert one to the possibility of low-grade glioma in an otherwise glial process

List of Findings/Checklist for Mucinous–Myxoid Material

• AT A GLANCE

- Intracytoplasmic mucin
- Extracytoplasmic mucin
- Mucin in glandular structures
- Background mucin

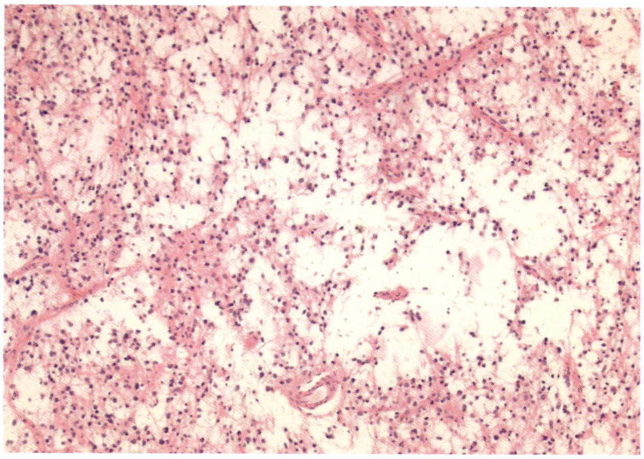

Figure 2-57. Oligodendroglioma with microcysts and mucinous background (H&E; original magnification: 200×).

and help narrow down the differential diagnosis. For instance, in the presence of round nuclei with bland cytologic features and long glial processes, its presence supports the possibility of a PA, especially in the right clinical and radiologic context. Paraganglioma can have a loosely textured histology with groups of cells floating in a mucinous background, resembling a chordoid morphology, as well as causing confusion with myxopapillary ependymoma. Since both myxopapillary ependymoma **(Fig. 2-59)** and paraganglioma in the CNS preferentially and almost exclusively involve

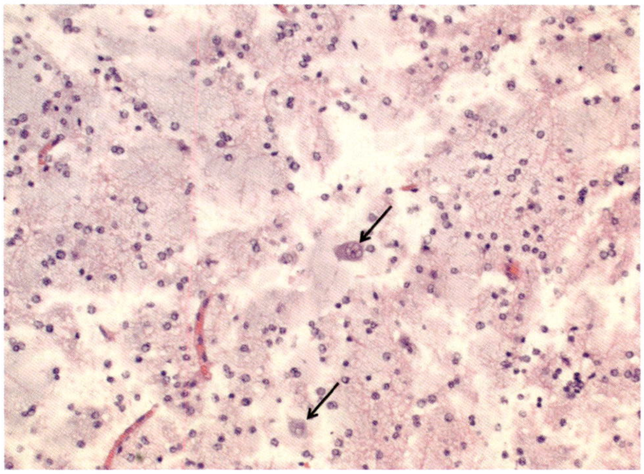

Figure 2-58. DNT: Two "floating neurons" (*arrows*) are present in a mucinous background along with oligodendroglial-like cells (H&E; original magnification: 200×).

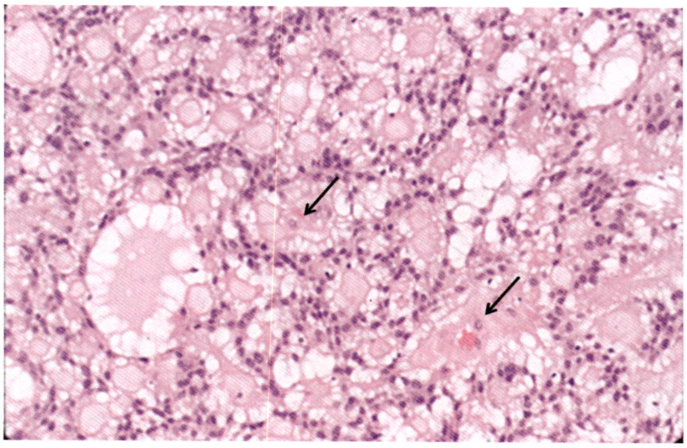

Figure 2-59. Myxopapillary ependymoma: A bubbly mucinous background is present, forming microcysts around hyalinized vessels (*arrows*) that can sometimes obscure the cellularity. Typical ependymoma features such as pseudorosettes and true rosettes are not present (H&E; original magnification: 200×).

the cauda equina region, immunohistochemical work-up may be necessary to confirm the diagnosis. Paragangliomas are typically positive for chromogranin and synaptophysin, with S-100 protein highlighting the sustentacular cells. Focal GFAP and cytokeratin positivity can create confusion with myxopapillary ependymoma and metastatic carcinoma, respectively.[124] In contrast, myxopapillary ependymomas are positive for S-100 protein and GFAP, while neural markers are negative.

Some glioblastomas can be extremely mucinous, although their glioblastoma nature is readily apparent due to the presence of a fibrillary background, hyperchromatic irregular or spindled nuclei indicating an astrocytic origin, and vascular proliferation and/or necrosis confirming the diagnosis of glioblastoma **(Fig. 2-60)**. The mucinous–myxoid background in such cases may raise suspicion for a sarcoma or, in the case of epithelioid or gemistocytic cells, a metastatic carcinoma. Focal mucinous degeneration is not uncommon in meningiomas and does not have any known clinical diagnostic significance. Myxoid pattern in meningioma is a metaplastic change **(Fig. 2-61)**; however, these meningiomas should not be confused with metastatic adenocarcinomas.[125] Mucinous change is also associated with microcytic meningiomas and chordoid meningiomas. In the former, this is in the form of small cystic spaces within a trabecular network of elongated cells **(Fig. 2-62)**.

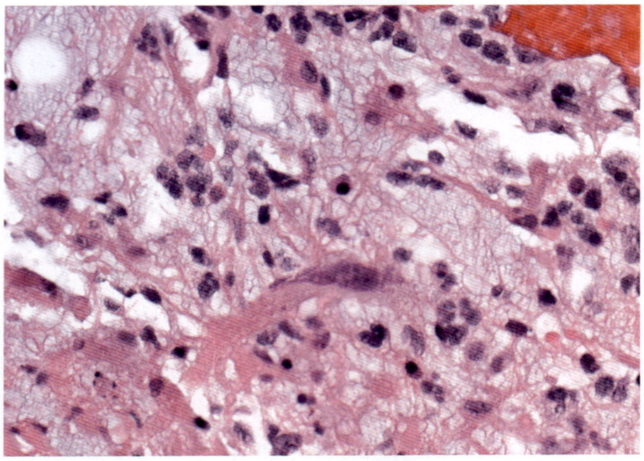

Figure 2-60. Glioblastoma with mucinous background: Typical features are usually present elsewhere and noticing the cytologic features with hyperchromatic elongated nuclei and cytoplasmic processes avoids confusion with metastatic carcinoma (H&E; original magnification: 400×).

Chordoid meningioma has a histology similar to chordoma and contains trabeculae or small groups of epithelioid cells in a background myxoid stroma. Distinction from other meningiomas containing mucinous material is important, as chordoid meningioma is a more aggressive form, WHO grade II.[44] Some chordoid meningiomas may be associated with prominent lymphoplasmacytic infiltrate and systemic Castleman's disease,[126] although this appears to be limited to pediatric population.[127] There may be considerable overlap among several

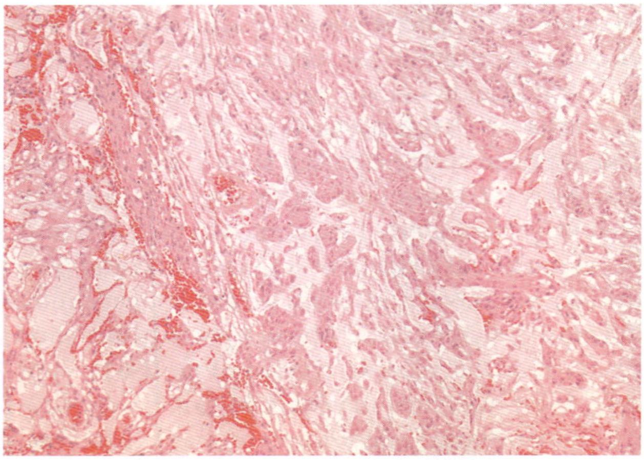

Figure 2-61. Myxoid meningioma: A mucinous material, a metaplastic change, separates large islands of meningioma cells (H&E; original magnification: 400×).

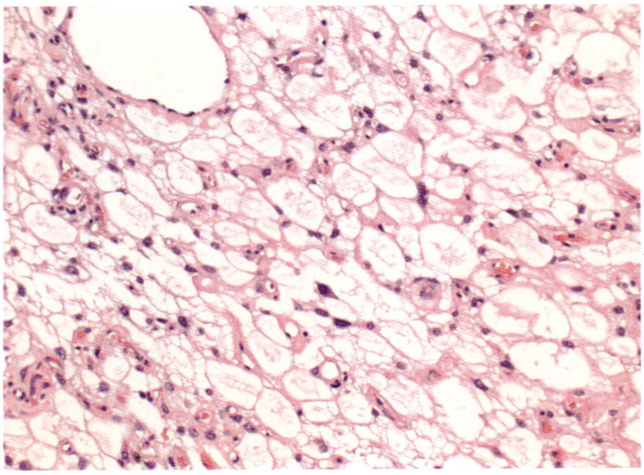

Figure 2-62. Microcystic meningioma: A lacy appearance is created by the thin, elongated cytoplasms of the meningioma cells, resulting in numerous microcysts filled with proteinaceous mucinous material (H&E; original magnification: 200×).

neoplastic categories mainly due to a chordoid pattern in a mucinous background. While the location and radiologic features are very helpful, they also differ in their immunohistochemical features[128] **(Table 2.6)**. ATRT may have myxoid foci or background in which the cells may form groups or trabeculae, imitating a metastatic carcinoma with mucin production. However, in the age group that the ATRT is seen, metastatic carcinoma is essentially not a differential diagnostic consideration. The presence of typical rhabdoid areas and, if necessary, immunohistochemistry should clarify this similarity.

Chordomas are characterized by groups or trabeculae of epithelioid cells floating in a mucinous background **(Fig. 2-63)**. In that sense, their main differential diagnosis in general and based solely on microscopical features is metastatic carcinoma. However, the histology of chordoma is highly characteristic and should at least be considered in the differential diagnosis, which can then further be supported by immunohistochemistry. Coexpression of diffuse and strong pancytokeratin and vimentin, and brachyury positivity, along with at least focal and weak S-100 protein and EMA positivity, is diagnostic of chordoma in this setting.[129] In addition, chordoma cells usually have a low nucleus-to-cytoplasm ratio. Nuclei are generally bland in most conventional chordoma cases,

TABLE 2.6 Typical location and immunohistochemical features of choroid/mucinous neoplasms

Neoplasm	Location	Immunohistochemistry
Chordoma	Skull base bones, midline /clivus	Vimentin+, Cytokeratin+, S-100+, EMA+, Brachyury+
Chordoid meningioma	Dura based, can be seen in skull base and may invade bone	Vimentin+, EMA+, PR+
Chordoid glioma	Third ventricle	GFAP+, S-100+, Cytokeratin+, EMA+
Chondrosarcoma	Skull base bones, clivus	Vimentin+, S-100+

(+), positive; EMA, epithelial membrane antigen; PR, progesterone receptor; GFAP, glial fibrillary acidic protein.

with a fine and uniform chromatin and a small nucleolus or chromocenter, in contrast to the large nucleus, open chromatic pattern, and prominent nucleolus of most carcinomas, even though there may be considerable overlap. The midline location of chordoma, vertebral/prevertebral in the spine and in the clivus in skull base, is characteristic, although a metastatic carcinoma to these locations is also a possibility. Especially in the clivus, the main differential diagnosis of chordoma is with chondrosarcoma, which also has a chondroid/myxoid matrix and can result in great difficulty in diagnosis, especially in high-grade lesions. Accurate diagnosis in this context is very important due to therapeutic and prognostic implications. The chondroid chordoma, a variant of chordoma with chondroid matrix production, may complicate this issue further. Brachyury positivity is very helpful in supporting the diagnosis of chordoma. Various sarcomas, most notably myxoid liposarcoma and myxoid malignant fibrous histiocytoma, can invade into or metastasize to the cranial/intracranial tissues. In such cases, there is typically a previous history and diagnosis that facilitate the work-up and accurate diagnosis. However, pleomorphic, myxoid, and round cell variants should not be confused with various types of glial neoplasms. The primarily dural/superficial/extra-axial location of the lipomatous neoplasms is also helpful in their recognition. Epithelioid hemangioendothelioma can rarely be seen in the skull bones or even within the neuroglial parenchyma. It has a myxoid background with small groups or cords of cells with cytoplasmic vacuolation, resembling chordoma.

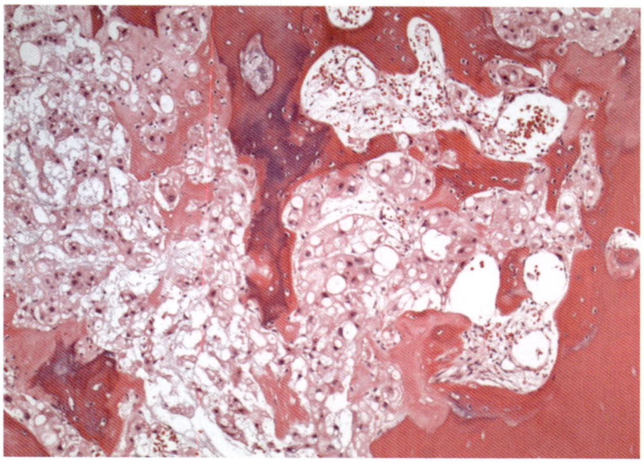

Figure 2-63. Chordoma: Trabeculae or small solid groups of clear cells lie in a mucinous background in the bone, potentially creating a pitfall for a misdiagnosis of metastatic carcinoma (H&E; original magnification: 200×).

Various cysts in the CNS have mucinous contents. These are nonneoplastic, developmental cysts and have a simple columnar or pseudostratified epithelial lining with a variable number of admixed mucinous cells. Colloid cyst of the third ventricle, endodermal cysts, and Rathke cleft cysts are prominent examples (see "Cystic Lesions").

Mucinous degeneration can be seen as part of degenerative changes in intervertebral disc material or may represent minute areas of notochordal cell remnants.[130] They are incidental findings and are histologically similar to chordoma; however, they can be easily distinguished from chordoma in this context. Likewise, two other lesions described in relation to notochord are benign notochordal cell tumor[131] and incipient chordoma, where an apparently early phase of infiltrating chordoma development is seen arising from a benign notochordal cell tumor.[132] A summary of these entities, including fetal notochord[130] **(Fig. 2-64)**, is given

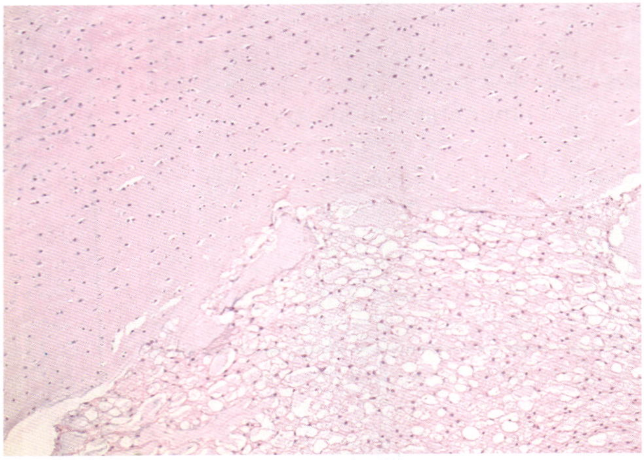

Figure 2-64. Notochord remnants: A round-to-oval group of clear cells in a mucinous background (**bottom**) are present in the center of an intervertebral disc (**top**) on this section prepared from the vertebral column in this fetus who died of unrelated causes (H&E; original magnification: 40×).

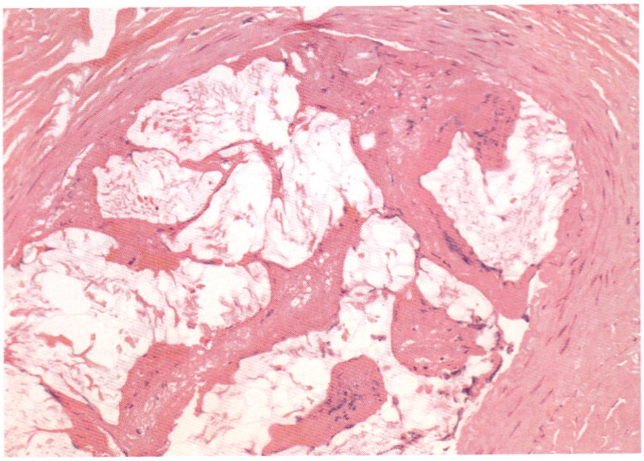

Figure 2-65. Embolized vessel: Amorphous mucinous material is present in the lumen of this artery and is surrounded by fibrin and foreign body giant cell reaction (H&E; original magnification: 200×).

in **(Table 2.7)**. Intervertebral disc material can be seen as embolic material in spinal vessels after spinal trauma, resulting in spinal cord infarcts.[133] In a similar setting, intervertebral disc fragments can break off to travel to other levels of the spine within the spinal canal, sometimes to come to attention later due to spinal cord compression, mimicking a neoplasm.[134] The cartilaginous nature of such fragments may not be readily obvious, except for some vague fibrillarity, unless chondrocytes are present. Myxoid material can embolize to the brain from cardiac myxomas and result in infarcts.[135] Intravascular myxoid-appearing material, usually associated with a histiocytic reaction including foreign body giant cells, is seen in lesions such as meningioma and vascular malformations preoperatively embolized by polyvinyl alcoholic agent **(Fig. 2-65)**.

Peripheral nerve sheath tumor (PNST) of various types can show prominent myxoid change,

TABLE 2.7 Summary of typical features of notochord and related lesions

Feature	Fetal Notochord	Notochordal Remnants	Benign Notochordal Cell Tumor	Incipient Chordoma	Chordoma
Location	Intervertebral disc	Intervertebral disc	Intervertebral disc	Bone, soft tissue, intervertebral disc	Bone, soft tissue, intervertebral disc
Growth pattern	Circumscribed, small groups, trabecular	Circumscribed, trabecular, solid	Circumscribed, single cells, solid	Infiltrative, single cells, trabecular, solid	Infiltrative, single cells, trabecular, solid
Stroma	Myxoid	Myxoid	Eosinophilic, colloid-like	Myxoid	Myxoid
Cytoplasm	No vacuoles	Vacuolar	Vacuolar, eosinophilic globules	Vacuolar	Vacuolar
CK18	+	+/−	+	+	+/−

CK, cytokeratin; (+), positive; (+/−), positive or negative.

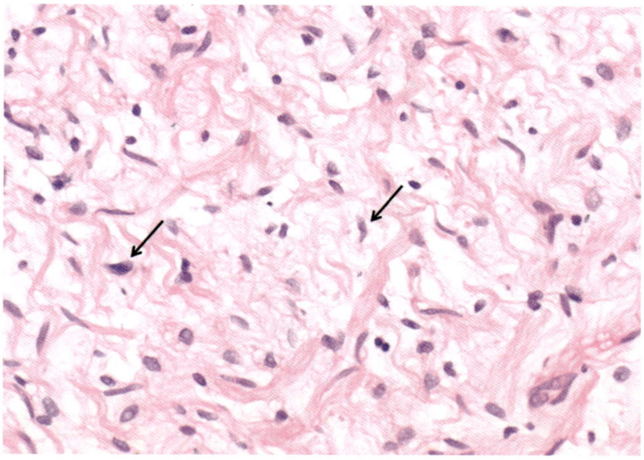

Figure 2-66. Neurofibroma: A loosely textured neoplasm is seen with spindled nuclei in a mucinous background. Many nuclei are wavy with one tip that is pointy compared to the other (*arrows*) (H&E; original magnification: 400×).

sometimes to a degree that obscures their true nature. Mucosal or cutaneous neurofibromas **(Fig. 2-66)**, the so-called nerve sheath myxoma and neurothekeoma, may be particularly rich in mucin, in which the wavy collagen and single cells or small bundles of spindle neoplastic cells can be identified. Their main differential diagnosis is with other myxoid lesions of subcutaneous and deep soft tissues.

Neuropil Features, Background, and Accumulations

The description of "background" is loose and, in practice, it usually refers to everything else other than the cellular component of a particular lesion. That

List of Findings/Checklist for Neuropil Features, Background, and Accumulations

AT A GLANCE

Vacuolations

- Coarse
- Fine
- Spongiform change (prion disease)
- Artifacts
  - Poor fixation
  - Freezing artifact
  - Sponge and tissue bag
- Edema
  - Hypoxic–ischemic change
- Predominantly cortical
  - Neuron loss and gliosis/neurodegenerative disease
  - Lyme disease
  - Rasmussen encephalitis
- Others
  - Toxic/metabolic encephalopathies
  - Lhermitte-Duclos disease
  - Chemotherapy/radiation therapy–related leukoencephalopathy
  - Unidentified bright objects
- Vacuolar myelopathy

Background Irregularities and Accumulations

- Neuritic plaques
- Astrocytic plaques
- Lewy neurites
- Neuropil threads
- Argyrophilic grains
- Grumose degeneration
- Corpora amylacea
- Lafora bodies
- Polyglucosan bodies
- Mulberries
- Refractile astrocytic inclusions
- Axonal spheroids/swellings, Herring bodies, dystrophic axons and neurites, torpedoes
- Background Fibrillarity
- Reactive astrocytosis (fibrillary, piloid, Chaslin's gliosis)
- Neoplasms

Extracellular Accumulations

- Collagen
- Amyloid
- Osteoid
- Keratin

TABLE 2.8 Major conditions associated with vacuolations

Artifacts
Triangular (sponge, gauze)
Linear (tissue bag)
Ice crystal artifact on frozen sections (slow freezing)
Poor fixation
Spongiform Encephalopathies
CJD
Protease-sensitive proteinopathy
Panencephalitic CJD
Variant CJD
Gerstmann-Straussler-Scheinker disease
Toxic, Metabolic and Mitochondrial Disorders
Alpers disease
Canavan's disease
MELAS
Kearns-Sayre syndrome
Mercury intoxication
Morel's laminar necrosis
Hepatic encephalopathy
Miscellaneous
Edema
Lyme disease
Rasmussen's encephalitis
UBO
Vacuolar myelopathy
HAM
Subacute combined degeneration

CJD, Creutzfeldt-Jacob disease; MELAS, mitochondrial myopathy lactic acidosis and stroke-like episodes; UBO, unidentified bright objects; HAM, HTLV-1-associated myelopathy

said, neuropil also contains cells in the form of the processes of neuronal and glial cells. Therefore, background and neuropil are used somewhat interchangeably in this discussion. Many findings can be present in the background in diverse lesions. Accumulations such as mucin and calcification are discussed in other sections, leaving some other findings that could not be included in more specific sections.

Various forms of *vacuolations* can occur in the neuropil **(Table 2.8)**. Although they superficially may all look the same, their distribution and appearance help favor certain conditions over others. In general, the vacuolation of neuropil is also referred to as *spongiform change*; however, since this term is closely associated with spongiform encephalopathies, that is, prion diseases, its use should best be restricted to that context (see below). A vacuolation involving both gray and white matter is seen as a result of *poor fixation* and is usually in the form

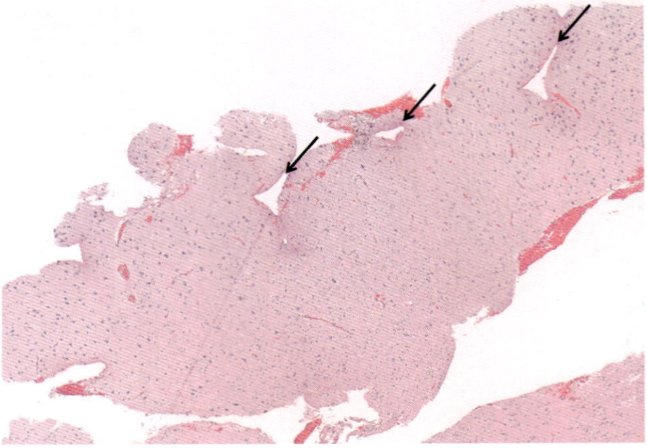

Figure 2-67. Sponge artifact: Roughly triangular holes are formed in the tissue by the fibers of the sponge or gauze in which the tissue was placed (*arrows*) (H&E; original magnification: 100×).

of large and coarse vacuoles that are spaced away from each other. It can be focal or diffuse depending on the nature of poor fixation and processing and is limited to autopsy material in practice. Another well-known artifact that results in extensive vacuolation and distortion of the tissue is *freeze artifact* due to ice crystal formation in the tissue as a result of slow freezing. This can be avoided by rapid freezing, but some specimens that have a microcystic or myxoid background are more prone to this artifact. It is more typical for frozen section in IOC, as well as muscle biopsy sections. Various *artifactual vacuolations*[136] distorting the tissues are easily recognized as artifacts. If brain tissue from surgical specimens is placed between sponges while being submitted for processing, roughly *triangular holes* with concave edges form due to the projections of the sponge **(Fig. 2-67)**. Biopsy bags result in *linear vacuoles* forming small squares of tissue in a grid pattern **(Fig. 2-68)**. *Edema* also results in vacuolation of the neuropil, both due to the presence of edema fluid in the parenchyma and by interfering with optimal fixation and processing. In addition to vacuolation, a rarified appearance of especially the white matter due to separation of axons and fascicles from each other can be present. Edema may be diffuse as seen in diffuse brain swelling or may be localized around mass lesions or associated with inflammatory processes. Likewise, vacuolation can be present diffusely in acute hypoxic–ischemic encephalopathy or in areas of focal hypoxic–ischemic change **(Fig. 2-69)**.

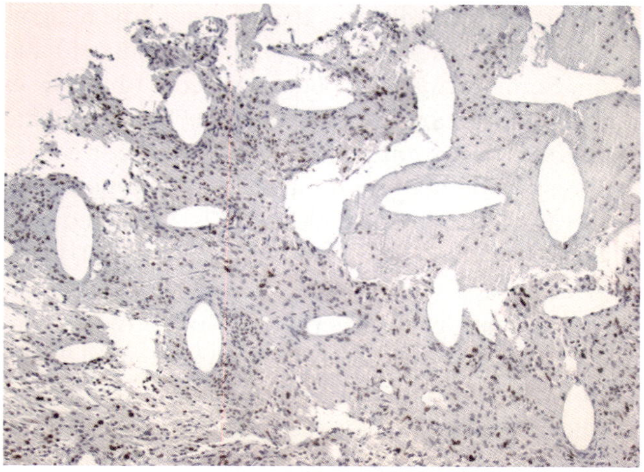

Figure 2-68. Tissue bag artifact: Oval holes in a rectangular configuration are made in the tissue by the fibers of the biopsy bag (H&E; original magnification: 100×).

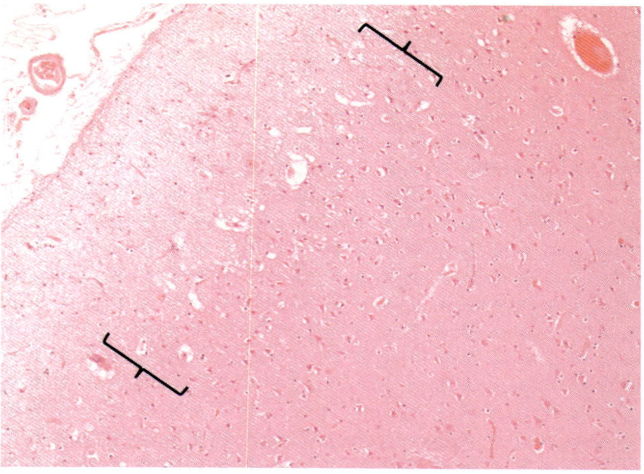

Figure 2-70. Superficial cortical vacuolation: A peculiar microvacuolation involving the superficial layers of the cerebral cortex (*brackets*) associated with neuron loss in some neurodegenerative diseases (H&E; original magnification: 100×).

Conditions associated with neuron loss and *gliosis*, as seen in neurodegenerative disease, create a vacuolar background, especially in the later stages of these diseases. This type of vacuolation is somewhat coarser than seen in other conditions. More prominently in dementia with Lewy bodies, a selective vacuolation of the cerebral cortex can be present **(Fig. 2-70)**. It typically involves the superficial layers of the cortex but can also involve its entire thickness in some cases, making it difficult to distinguish from the vacuolation of prion disease. However, in such circumstances, the history of rapidly progressing dementia resulting in death in 1 to 2 years favors CJD, while long history and gradual decline are features of neurodegenerative diseases. In addition, identification of additional microscopic features, such as cortical Lewy bodies, will aid in this differential. In more difficult cases, immunohistochemistry and ancillary tests for prion protein and the neurodegenerative disease in question are useful. Other neurodegenerative diseases that may be relatively prominently associated with dementia and vacuolation of the cortex are FTLD, CBD, dementia with motor neuron inclusions, Pick disease, and ALS. Progressive subcortical gliosis results in gliosis of frontal and temporal white matter, neuron loss, and superficial microvacuolation in frontal and temporal lobes, creating a picture similar to FTLD.[104,137]

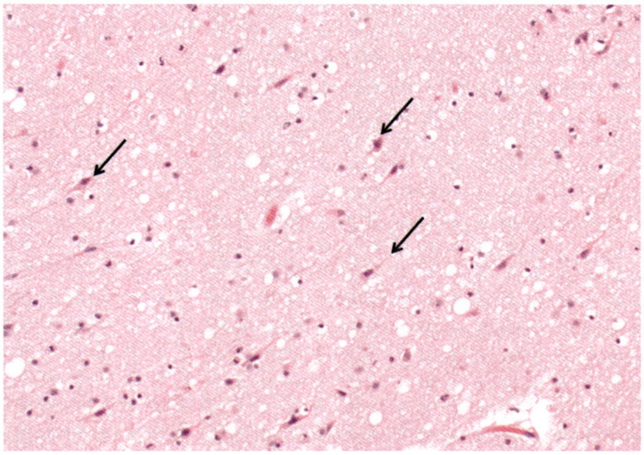

Figure 2-69. Neuropil vacuolation in ischemia: One of the earliest ischemic changes is the vacuolation of the neuropil. Eosinophilic neuronal necrosis ("red neurons") is also seen (*arrows*) (H&E; original magnification: 200×).

The microvacuolation or spongiform change in prion disease **(Fig. 2-71)**, the prototype of which is CJD, is the main type of vacuolation with significant diagnostic implications. It is a delicate and uniform vacuolation composed of vacuoles of more or less similar size and quality. They are actually intracytoplasmic vacuoles within the cell bodies and processes and contain granular and membranous material. It involves the gray matter, especially cerebral cortex, but can also involve deep gray matter structures. Cortical involvement may be full

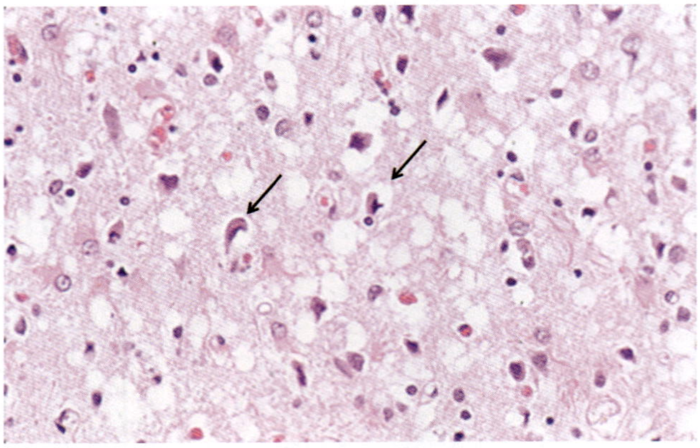

Figure 2-71. Spongiform change: A microvacuolation is present in the cortical gray matter. The vacuoles are intracytoplasmic and distort some of the neurons (*arrows*) (H&E; original magnification: 400×).

thickness or may be limited to deeper layers of the cortex. Although cerebral and cerebellar cortices are consistently involved, this involvement may be diffuse or variable and patchy. While the typical clinical picture is one of rapidly progressing dementia, there is a recently described group of patients that present with behavioral and psychiatric symptoms and distinct immunohistochemical and histopathologic features. It is termed protease-sensitive proteinopathy[138] and many of such cases may be classified as non–Alzheimer-type dementia. The vacuoles are a mixture of small and large ones and the cerebellum is usually spared. In addition, small plaque-like eosinophilic structures surrounded by a halo are also present in the cerebellum. They are negative for amyloid. Panencephalopathic CJD shows extensive involvement of entire brain, including white matter. In addition to spongiform change in the cortex, basal ganglia, and thalamus, there is extensive neuron loss and gliosis. White matter is extremely pale with diffuse loss of myelin, resulting in a spongy and cavitated appearance.[139,140]

The eosinophilic microstructures described above and seen in protease-sensitive proteinopathy are different than the cerebellar plaques of another prion disease, GSS disease.[141] GSS plaques are typically seen in the cerebellar cortex and contain amyloid. They are densely eosinophilic and granular accumulations in the neuropil, are of variable sizes, and are generally round but can be irregular. Depending on the subtype of this disease, spongiform change may be absent, present, or may not be prominent. These plaques are present in the neocortex, as well as in white matter, in the telencephalic form. Some forms may be associated with NFTs in a distribution similar to that of AD. To complicate matters further, some forms of GSS produce a slowly progressive dementia and are associated with vascular amyloid accumulation, NFTs, and neuropil threads in the neocortex. Variant CJD (vCJD)[142] is also associated with plaques, in addition to spongiform change. They are present in both cerebral and cerebellar cortices and contain amyloid. They are of variable sizes and have a denser center and a paler periphery. They are termed florid plaques when they are surrounded by vacuoles forming a rim around them. Spongiform change, neuron loss, and astrocytosis are most prominent in the basal ganglia and thalamus, however. Microvacuolation of cortex can be seen in some cases of Lyme disease, along with the inflammatory changes.

Metabolic encephalopathies, such as Alpers-Huttenlocher syndrome (Alpers disease) and aminoaciduria, can also show neuropil vacuolation in gray and white matter. Alpers-Huttenlocher syndrome (progressive neuronal degeneration of childhood)[143] shows a thin, friable, dusky cortex especially prominent in calcarine cortex. There is superficial microvacuolation, along with neuron loss and gliosis. Prion disease may be a consideration due to microvacuolation and the presence of granulomembranous debris in the vacuoles by electron microscopy; however, lipid accumulation as seen by oil red O, typical distribution of vacuolation, and associated liver disease help easily differentiate these two entities.

Diffuse and prominent vacuolation of white matter is a feature of Canavan's disease (spongiform leukodystrophy). The vacuolation is more prominent at the gray–white matter junction. There is diffuse myelin loss and the U-fibers are not spared. Cerebral cortex is devoid of vacuolation and neuron loss, but there may be Alzheimer type II astrocytes in the cortex. A peculiar vacuolation of the superficial white matter, at the junction of gray and white matter, is seen in disorders associated with hepatic encephalopathy, where Alzheimer type II glia are also present. In MELAS (Mitochondrial Encephalomyopathy Lactic Acidosis and Stroke-like Episodes),[144] foci of necrosis and cavitation of different stages are seen in cortex, predominantly in the crests of gyri and predominantly in occipital lobe. Basal ganglia, thalamus, and cerebellum may be involved less often. Rarely, a spongy vacuolation of cerebral and cerebellar white matter is present, along with vascular changes. Kearns-Sayre syndrome[145] also shows spongy vacuolation in white matter due to myelin vacuolation, mainly in the brainstem but less commonly in the cerebellum and cerebrum. It also has vascular changes such as thickening, fibrosis, and calcification of the vessel walls. Mercury intoxication[146] results in variable calcarine and cerebellar atrophy in survivors. Small neurons are affected more, such as internal granule cells and sensory, visual, and auditory cortices. This may be severe and associated with spongiform change. Acute lesions may have macrophage infiltration. Dorsal root ganglion cell degeneration and dorsal column degeneration may be seen. Purkinje cell sprouting occurs in long term. Mercury may be shown by special histochemical techniques in neurons, astrocytes, and microglia. Morel's laminar sclerosis[147] mainly involves cortical layer II and sometimes deeper layers with microvacuolation and gliosis, especially in frontal and temporal lobes. It is seen in alcoholics or those with Marchiafava-Bignami disease. Alzheimer type II glia are also present. It should not be confused with CJD or neurodegenerative disease due to the presence of cortical microvacuolation. Extensive neuron loss and gliosis, regardless of the cause, result in a prominent and widespread vacuolation that is called *status spongiosus*. It is essentially an end-stage condition.

Vacuolation of cerebellar white matter is common in cases of Lhermitte-Duclos disease (dysplastic cerebellar gangliocytoma) **(Fig. 2-72)**. A focal and variable degree of vacuolar change in both gray and white matter is typically limited to the involved areas in Rasmussen encephalitis.[148] The cortical ribbon is thin with neuron loss and gliosis, but there are also perivascular lymphocytic infiltrates and microglial nodules, resembling viral encephalitis. Vacuolation of neuropil in the white matter is seen as part of the chemotherapy/radiation-induced leukoencephalopathy. The exact histologic correlate of radiologic finding of "unidentified bright objects" (UBO) is not clear; however, neuropil vacuolation or edema in white matter has been described. They can be seen in the white matter, basal ganglia, cerebellum, and brainstem.[149]

In the spinal cord, vacuolar myelopathy[150] seen in association with HIV infection involves the white matter of the spinal cord, predominantly the posterior columns **(Fig. 2-73)**. Histologically, it is identical to the changes seen in subacute combined degeneration seen in spinal cord associated with B_{12} deficiency. HTLV-1-associated myelopathy (HAM) also results in vacuolar change in the spinal cord white matter, though it is not as prominent

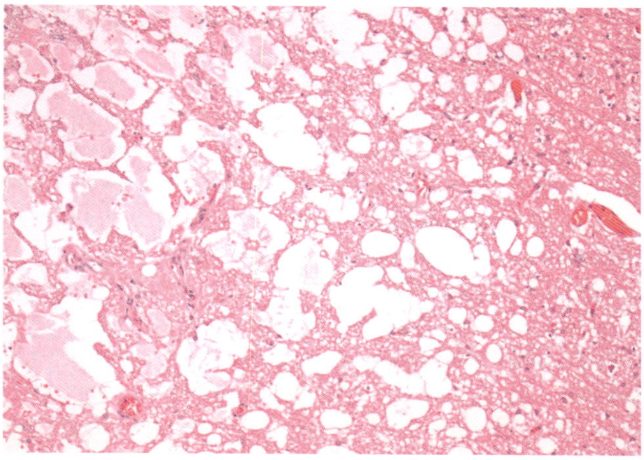

Figure 2-72. Cerebellar white matter vacuolation in Lhermitte-Duclos disease: Vacuoles of variable sizes and shapes, some creating microcystic spaces, can be seen in the white matter underlying the dysplastic gangliocytoma of the cerebellum (not shown) (H&E; original magnification: 100×).

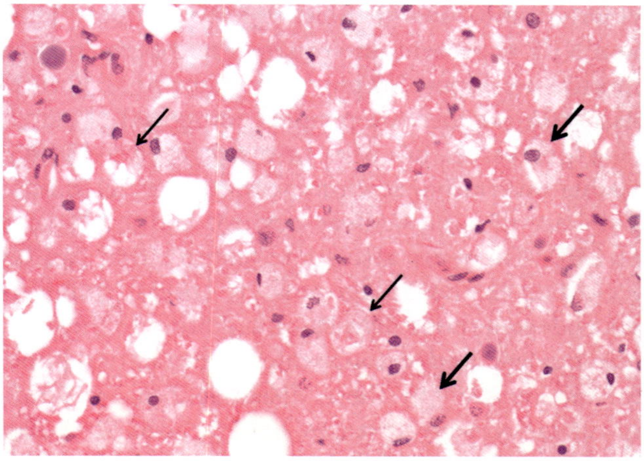

Figure 2-73. Vacuolar myelopathy: Numerous vacuoles are formed as a result of myelin swelling around the axons (*thin arrows*), which are seen as darker eosinophilic dots in the center of swollen myelin, and subsequent degeneration, leaving vacuoles behind. Macrophages are also present (*thick arrows*) (H&E; original magnification: 400×).

and is associated with prominent inflammation and thickening of vessel walls.

Plaques are microscopic localized structures composed of a mixture of beta-amyloid, astrocytes, microglia, and dystrophic neurites. On routine sections, they are difficult to identify; however, the usual homogeneous, finely granular or fibrillary appearance of the neuropil becomes coarse and irregular in some areas, and this should prompt a more focused search for neuritic plaques and other associated findings depending on the disease process, such as the common NFTs in AD. *Neuritic (mature) plaques* may be seen upon careful search because of their amyloid core and irregularities they cause in the usual homogeneous, finely granular texture of neuropil. They have diffuse, primitive, neuritic, and burnt-out stages, all of which can be highlighted by Bielschowsky silver stain and beta-amyloid and phosphorylated tau stains. Their identification, typing, frequency, and distribution are important especially in the diagnosis of AD, as utilized in Consortium to Establish a Registry for Alzheimer's Disease (CERAD) criteria.[151] Burnt-out plaques are devoid of the dystrophic neurites and appear on routine sections as an eosinophilic amorphous amyloid accumulation. Mainly diffuse plaques are seen in aging and only a few neuritic plaques. Some plaques may have chromogranin-A and ubiquitin positivity but may be negative for tau. This is usually seen in sparse plaques in elderly individuals without cognitive impairment, and NFT, if present, are in small numbers and are limited to hippocampus and entorhinal cortex. *Astrocytic plaques* are plaques composed of astrocyte processes, but they are not even remotely visible on routine sections without special stains. They are tau and Gallyas positive and are typical of CBD. There are also some features that can be identified in the background by special stains in neurodegenerative diseases, in addition to the various nuclear and cytoplasmic accumulations and inclusions seen in these diseases. *Lewy neurites* in all Lewy body diseases have beaded irregular swellings. They are alpha-synuclein positive and are typically present in substantia nigra, CA2 and CA3 regions of the hippocampus, dorsal motor nucleus of vagus, nucleus basalis of Meynert, and amygdala. *Neuropil threads* are tau-positive neurites in the background of tauopathies such as PSP and AD in the involved areas. In argyrophilic grain

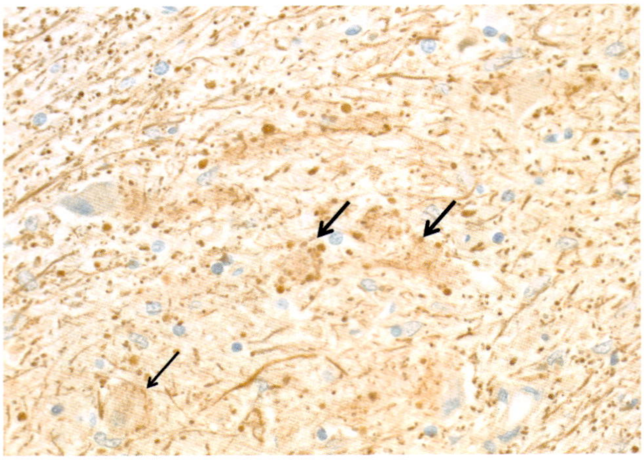

Figure 2-74. Grumose degeneration: This peculiar type of degeneration is seen as eosinophilic granular aggregates and can be further highlighted by special stains mainly around apparently degenerated neurons (*thick arrows*), in contrast to another that is still intact (*thin arrow*) (neurofilament immunohistochemistry; original magnification: 400×).

dementia,[102] hippocampus, entorhinal cortex, and some subcortical nuclei have *coils or grains of argyrophilic material* that are also tau positive. In the context of neurodegeneration, a peculiar type of degeneration in the dentate nucleus is seen as an accumulation of variably sized eosinophilic granules surrounding the dentate nucleus neurons and is termed *grumose degeneration*[152] **(Fig. 2-74)**. It is typically associated with PSP, although it has been described in several other conditions, such as CBD,[153] ornithine transcarbamylase deficiency,[154] dentatorubropallidoluysian atrophy (DRPLA),[155] Ramsey-Hunt syndrome,[156] Huntington's disease,[157] and juvenile AD with myoclonus.[158]

Several distinct and peculiar structures can be identified in the background normally or in certain diseases. *Corpora amylacea* are round, light blue to purple structures within the astrocyte processes **(Fig. 2-75)**. Depending on the thickness of the section and staining quality, some may have a concentric circular interior, somewhat resembling a psammoma body, while others may have a denser core or are more homogeneous or may have peripheral radially arranged fibrillary appearance. Careful observation or GFAP immunohistochemistry shows a thin rim of eosinophilic astrocyte cytoplasm encircling them. They are commonly found in increasing numbers with increased age and are considered an age-related change; however, they

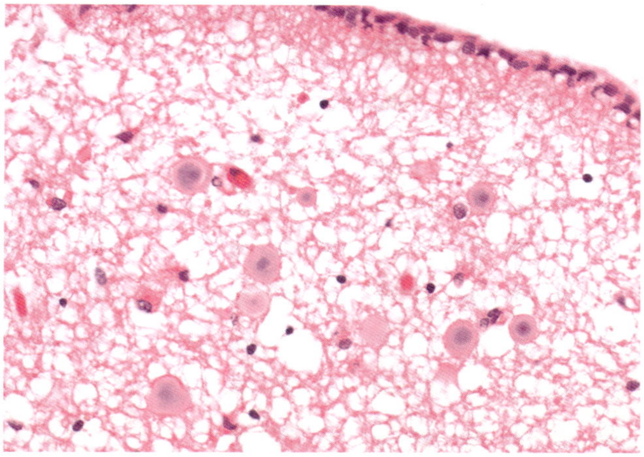

Figure 2-75. Corpora amylacea: Round, basophilic structures with denser centers and lighter periphery are seen. Some may have circular laminated interior but are not as crisp and dark as psammoma bodies. They are surrounded by a thin rim of eosinophilic cytoplasm, since they are intracytoplasmic. Ependymal surface is seen in the top right corner (H&E; original magnification: 400×).

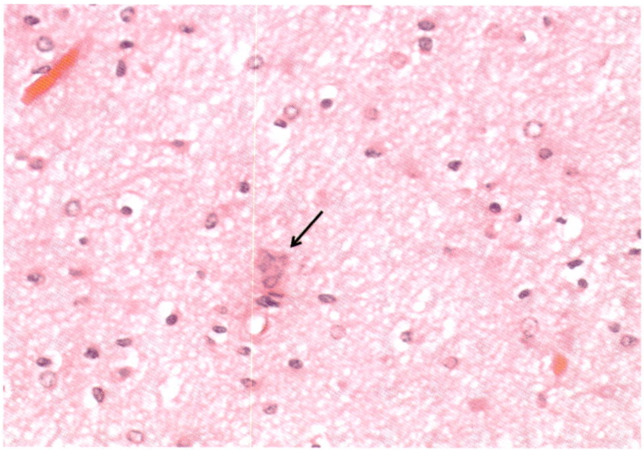

Figure 2-76. Mulberries: Leakage of plasma proteins into the tissue creates dense, multilobular, darkly eosinophilic accumulations typically around capillaries (*arrow*). They gradually become basophilic as they calcify. They are nonspecific indicators of vascular tissue damage and are typically associated with periventricular leukomalacia or perinatal telencephalic leukoencephalopathy (H&E; original magnification: 400×).

can be more frequent than normal aging in AD. They are typically associated with the pial surfaces, such as the brain surface and perivascular areas. They are PAS positive and diastase resistant and do not stain with Congo red.

There are other similar round structures with similar light and electron microscopic and staining features, such as Lafora bodies and Bielschowsky bodies. The general term polyglucosan body is sometimes preferred to cover all similar structures. *Lafora bodies* are intraneuronal structures within the cytoplasm. Lafora body disease is characterized by Lafora bodies abundantly present in the cytoplasm of neurons and astrocytes in the cerebral cortex, diffusely in the CNS, but fewer in the brainstem and spinal cord. Similar to corpora amylacea in composition and staining features, they are PAS positive with dense center and pale periphery. They are associated with neuron loss and gliosis. They can be found in the liver, muscle, and heart and also in apocrine gland myoepithelial cells and eccrine gland cells, allowing skin biopsy to be used as a diagnostic tool. *Polyglucosan bodies*,[159] while similar to Lafora bodies, are used for the inclusions seen in adult polyglucosan body disease and progressive familial myoclonic epilepsy where they are present in axon hillock and axons in the peripheral nerve. *Mulberries* are dark eosinophilic, amphophilic, or basophilic, small, round or irregular accumulations in the neuropil **(Fig. 2-76)**. They seem to represent a stage between the leaked plasma from the vessels and their eventually calcified/mineralized stage that results in microcalcifications, and therefore, they are typically perivascular. As such, they are also associated with a hypoxic–ischemic or other insult that resulted in damage to the endothelial cells. They are more commonly seen in cases of periventricular leukomalacia but are not diagnostic or specific for any particular entity. They may also have somewhat laminated or layered interior, depending on their stage of development. Peculiar accumulations within the astrocyte cytoplasm, apparently representing a form of astrocytopathy, have been described in a group of pediatric epilepsy patients.[160] These inclusions are amorphous, pale eosinophilic, and refractile structures seen as accumulations in the background neuropil **(Fig. 2-77)**.

Various types of distortions, irregularities, and swellings can be seen in axons, with various implications **(Table 2.9)**. *Axonal spheroids* are eosinophilic, roughly spherical structures within the axons and are seen as such standing out in the fibrillary background of the neuropil. When they are scarce, they may be difficult to identify, unless specifically sought for. They indicate disruption of axonal

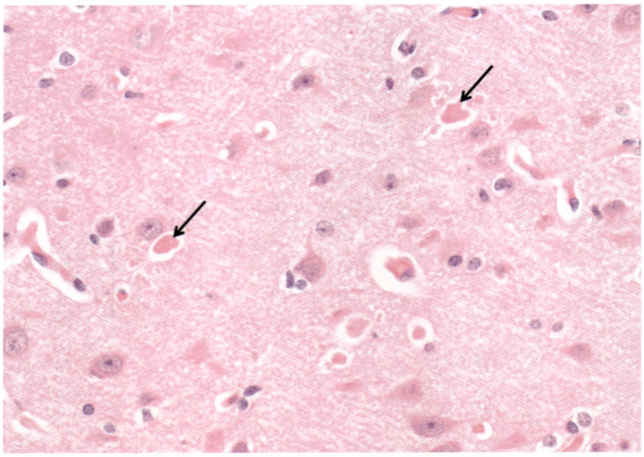

Figure 2-77. Astrocytic accumulations (astrocytopathy): Amorphous eosinophilic accumulations in the astrocyte cytoplasm are seen as accumulations in the neuropil (H&E; original magnification: 400×).

TABLE 2.9 Axonal swellings

Herring bodies
DAI
TAI
Neurodegeneration with brain iron accumulation type 1 (pantothenate kinase-associated neurodegeneration; Hallervorden-Spatz disease)
Vitamin E deficiency
Acrylamide intoxication
ALS
Nasu-Hakola disease
Giant axonal neuropathy
Niemann-Pick disease
Peroxisomal disorders
Infantile osteoporosis
Torpedoes
Cerebellar degeneration
Menkes disease
Pelizaeus-Merzbacher disease
Metabolic disorders
Mitochondrial disorders
Tay-Sachs disease
Mercury intoxication
Dystrophic neurites
Neurodegenerative diseases
AD (plaques and neuropil threads)
Lewy body pathology (neuropil threads)
Huntington disease
Multifocal necrotizing leukoencephalopathy

DAI, diffuse axonal injury; TAI, traumatic axonal injury.

transport and, as such, serve as the identifiers of a problem with axon integrity. For instance, they are frequent at the edges of an infarct, due to the transaction of axons at that point and subsequent accumulation of axonal transport material. In that context, they are useful in distinguishing such ill-defined infarcts from demyelination. In the latter, even though the myelin is lost, axonal transport is intact and axonal spheroids do not form. In DAI, axonal spheroids are more diffusely spread in the white matter, especially in areas of long, organized tracts such as corpus callosum, centrum semiovale, and brainstem. They result from the mechanical damage exerted in the axons due to shearing forces created by angular acceleration of the head. Beta-amyloid precursor protein immunohistochemistry can be used to identify early lesions. It is positive within 2 to 4 hours of injury, before the axonal spheroids develop. Axonal distortions and varicosities are seen in about 12 to 24 hours and typical axonal spheroids are seen at 24 hours and last about 2 months. After 2 months, they become difficult to find. In remote cases, scattered microglial nodules, thin corpus callosum, and myelin pallor remain. In traumatic injury with lacerations, and especially in pontomedullary tears, axonal spheroids support the lesion's true nature, as opposed to various artifacts. One should be careful with removing the brain as artifactual tears may occur in especially pontomedullary junction. Distinguishing them from true tears may become impossible in some cases as axonal swellings cannot be seen as this injury is rapidly fatal and petechial hemorrhages may not develop in some cases of such instant death.

Since axonal spheroids can result from a variety of insults, one of which is trauma, it is suggested that DAI is kept as a general descriptive term for this process and traumatic axonal injury (TAI) is used specifically to refer to the traumatic axonal spheroids. When the question is if the DAI is due to trauma or to a nontraumatic event, the most likely differential diagnosis is with hypoxic–ischemic injury. Especially in the early stages, this differentiation can be difficult. Petechial hemorrhages, widespread distribution, presence of axonal spheroids in the brainstem and upper cervical cord, and absence of neuronal ischemia favor traumatic origin. Beta-amyloid precursor protein immunohistochemistry, while highlighting the injured axons, can further help with this differential. The pattern of staining has been evaluated to identify overlapping but somewhat useful patterns,[161,162] though it was not found useful in infant brains.[163] The patterns were described as diffuse multifocal, linear (outlining the lesion), and a mixture of the two. While there was overlap among patterns and etiologies, the mixed pattern favored severe traumatic damage.[162] The axonal swellings in nutritional or metabolic disorders, and in neuroaxonal dystrophies, are referred to as dystrophic axons. Neurodegeneration with brain iron accumulation type 1 (a.k.a. pantothenate kinase-associated neurodegeneration, formerly referred to as Hallervorden-Spatz disease),[164] in addition to its other features, has axonal spheroids in globus pallidus and substantia nigra. Spheroids are especially prominent in gray matter connections between putamen and caudate. In infantile neuroaxonal dystrophy, axonal spheroids are present diffusely in the CNS, including gray and white matter, along with gliosis, though they may be more prominent in the cerebellum, brainstem, and spinal cord. They are also seen in peripheral nervous system (PNS) along with degeneration of corticospinal and corticobulbar tracts. Skin and conjunctiva are also involved. Therefore, skin, muscle, and nerve biopsies may be used for diagnosis, but if they cannot be found, diagnosis is eventually made by brain biopsy or autopsy. There is cerebellar atrophy. Spheroids are extremely small, requiring special stains. Also present are myelin pallor and degeneration in cerebral and cerebellar white matter. NFT, cerebral cortical degeneration, and Lewy bodies may be seen especially in the late infantile, juvenile, and adult forms. Some cases may overlap with neurodegeneration with brain iron accumulation type 1. Vitamin E deficiency is also associated with the formation of numerous axonal spheroids in several areas of the CNS, including posterior columns, corticospinal and spinocerebellar tracts. Axonal spheroids are of variable sizes and shapes. They can only have peripheral positivity by neurofilament. There is degeneration of especially gracile but also in cuneate nuclei, as well as in brainstem nuclei and basal ganglia.[165] These findings can be seen in cystic fibrosis, abetalipoproteinemia, and pancreas and biliary dysfunction. Cerebellar ataxia with isolated vitamin E deficiency also results in the formation of axonal spheroids and degeneration of posterior columns, along with Purkinje cell loss, similar to vitamin E deficiency due to malabsorption. Intoxication with acrylamide,[166] a compound with industrial use and use as a food additive, can cause axonal swellings in the distal posterior spinal, spinocerebellar, and corticospinal tracts. In ALS, axonal spheroids can be seen in anterior horns of the spinal cord. Variable numbers of axonal swellings can be seen as a physiologic change in aging in gracile and cuneate nuclei, substantia nigra, inner segment of globus pallidus, and peripheral sympathetic ganglia. Other conditions that are associated with widespread axonal spheroids are Nasu-Hakola disease (polycystic lipomembranous osteodysplasia with sclerosing leukoencephalopathy),[167] giant axonal neuropathy, Niemann-Pick disease type C,[168] peroxisomal disorders such as Zellweger syndrome,[169] and some cases of infantile osteopetrosis.[170]

Another form of axonal swelling, called *torpedo* due to its shape, is a fusiform expansion of the degenerating Purkinje cell axons. They may be rare depending on the case, but they are relatively easy to identify among the basophilic background of internal granule layer cells **(Fig. 2-78)**. Like axonal spheroids, they are also argyrophilic and neurofilament positive. They are seen in degenerative diseases involving the cerebellum, such as cerebellar cortical degeneration and Menkes (kinky hair) disease. The latter

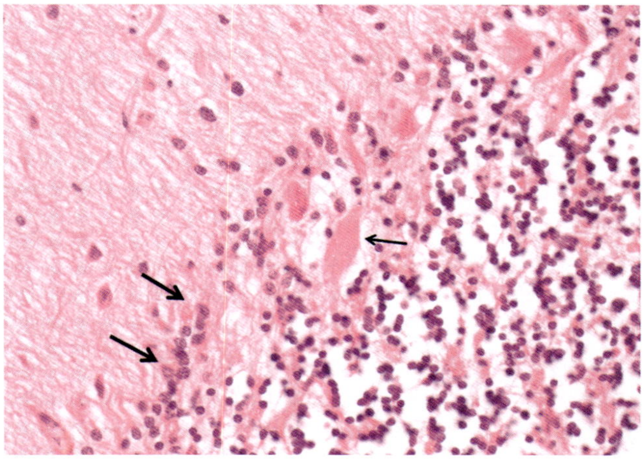

Figure 2-78. Torpedo: A fusiform axonal swelling (*thin arrow*) is easily identified in the cellular background of internal granule layer cells in the cerebellum, associated with Purkinje cell degeneration, as evidenced by the Bergmann gliosis forming a distinct cellular layer in place of the degenerated Purkinje cells (*thick arrows*) (H&E; original magnification: 400×).

is associated with low copper and ceruloplasmin levels, frequent subdural hematomas, cerebellar atrophy, neuron and myelin loss in temporal cortex and hippocampus, and granule cell loss in the cerebellum. Purkinje cells are displaced into the molecular layer. They have increased dendritic sprouting and arborization, as well as torpedoes. Cerebellar degeneration with similar cerebellar changes, including torpedoes, is also seen as part of Pelizaeus-Merzbacher disease. Similar changes, that is, torpedoes, along with Purkinje cell changes characterized by increased arborization, can be seen in familial hemiplegic migraine with cerebellar atrophy, as well as the other metabolic diseases, Tay-Sachs-type disease, organic mercury intoxication, and mitochondrial encephalopathies.[171] *Dystrophic neurites* are irregular swellings and distortions of axons, rather than the more obvious axonal spheroids. They may be difficult to appreciate on routine sections but may be seen as thickened eosinophilic, tortuous lines in the background. They are common in aging, AD (neuropil threads), Lewy body pathology (Lewy neurites), Huntington disease, and frontal lobe dementias. They can be highlighted by special stains such as tau, alpha-synuclein, ubiquitin, neurofilament, and Bielschowsky, depending on the nature of the pathologic process. Multifocal necrotizing leukoencephalopathy is characterized by multiple, typically microscopic, infarcts with calcifications in the white matter. It is associated with AIDS, leukemia, radiation therapy, and methotrexate and other drugs. Swollen and fragmented axons, which then calcify, are seen in areas of necrosis. Dystrophic axonal swellings are also seen with increasing age, as well as a result of diabetes mellitus, in dorsal root ganglia.[172]

Background fibrillarity provides clues to the nature of a pathologic process, as well as whether a pathologic process is actually present. Fibrillary appearance of the background is an indication that one is dealing with a primary brain parenchymal process. The fibrillary appearance is similar to that of normal neuropil in that it is composed of cellular processes as in normal neuropil. In normal neuropil, it is due to an admixture of glial and neuronal processes, that is, axons and dendrites. In the white matter where myelinated axons are organized in fascicles, it has a relatively regular appearance where fibrils lie parallel for the most part. Due to their myelin sheaths, white matter is bright eosinophilic, in contrast to gray matter neuropil, where the axons are arranged in various directions and are diluted by dendrites, resulting in a pale and relatively finely fibrillary neuropil. Regardless, "normal" neuropil has a homogeneous, finely granular appearance. *Reactive fibrillary (anisomorphic) astrocytosis* contains many very prominent coarse and glassy eosinophilic fibrillarity, and they can be identified as originating from the astrocytes with prominent cytoplasm with similar tinctorial quality. *Piloid (isomorphic) astrocytosis* also has fibrillarity of similar quality, except that the processes are thinner and better organized roughly in fascicles. They may also be associated with irregularly thickened segments and obvious *Rosenthal fibers*. While fibrillary astrocytosis can be associated with pretty much any kind of process, from inflammatory to metastatic to hemorrhagic to infarcts, piloid astrocytosis is more limited to around long-standing processes, such as nonneoplastic cysts, or low-grade neoplasms, such as craniopharyngioma and hemangioblastoma. Developmental cysts, syrinx formation, and even ependymomas can be associated with piloid gliosis and Rosenthal fibers. It can also be seen normally on pial surfaces, especially in the brainstem, or on the pial surfaces overlying MCD, known as *Chaslin's gliosis* **(Fig. 2-79)**. This type of piloid fibrillarity, especially when associated with Rosenthal fibers, should not be

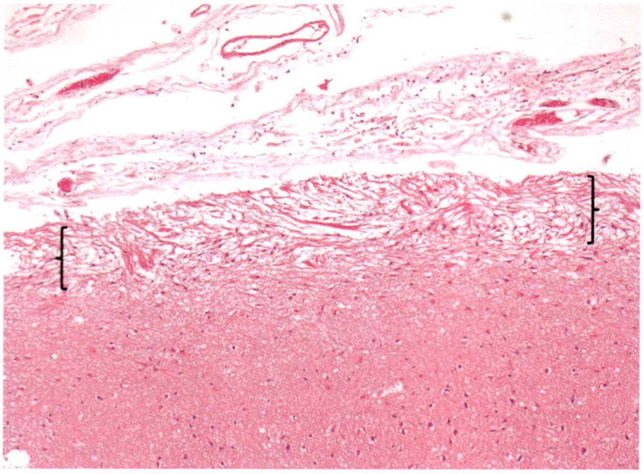

Figure 2-79. Chaslin's gliosis: A dense layer of piloid gliosis is seen in the subpial region (*brackets*) (H&E; original magnification: 100×).

misdiagnosed as PA. For the diagnosis of PA, a biphasic morphology with alternating piloid and loosely textured areas with round and bland nuclei and an admixture of thick vessels should be identified, although in small biopsies and IOC, all features can be difficult to have and it can turn out to be a difficult differential diagnosis. This issue can be further complicated by the fact that suprasellar/hypothalamic region is a common location for craniopharyngiomas and PAs, and cerebellum is a common location for both hemangioblastomas and PAs. Since hypothalamic region is a common location for PAs, the normal histology of neurohypophysis is in the differential diagnosis. Neurohypophysis has complex, fibrillary, and spindled histology. The vascular channels made prominent by a condensation of pituicytes around them, that is, Gomitoli, and the axonal transport material seen as eosinophilic swellings, that is, Herring bodies, may simulate EGBs, all contributing to the PA-like appearance of the neurohypophysis **(Fig. 2-80)**. In neurohypophysis, axonal transport material in the axons of the neurons in the hypothalamic nuclei can be seen as Herring bodies, in this case, carrying oxytocin and ADH. Needless to say, this can easily be confused with a PA in small tissues, especially those sent for IOC. This can be avoided by first keeping this possibility in mind and being familiar with the normal histology in hypothalamic/sellar region specimens. In addition, if present, a biphasic appearance with denser piloid background alternating with loosely textured, microcystic areas; Rosenthal fibers; and EGBs in this context favor PA. The exact location that the tissue was taken may be investigated by communicating with the surgeon.

The fibrillarity of the *neoplastic processes* also reflects the nature of the cells. In low-grade diffusely infiltrating gliomas, astrocytic or oligodendroglial, the background may be similar to nonneoplastic white matter since the neoplasm is not cellular enough to override the white matter. As the cellularity increases, the nature of the background changes depending on the cell type. In astrocytomas, it is bright eosinophilic but has a glassy quality due to the relatively coarse astrocytic processes **(Fig. 2-81)**. Ependymomas do not display a significant background fibrillarity in cellular areas but have processes similar to those of astrocytomas around the vessels, forming pseudorosettes. They are arranged in a peculiar manner to extend from cell bodies to the vessel wall, forming a circular anuclear perivascular zone. The cells of oligodendroglioma, as their name implies, have fewer processes, which are also thinner. Therefore, the background of oligodendroglial neoplasms has a paucifibrillary

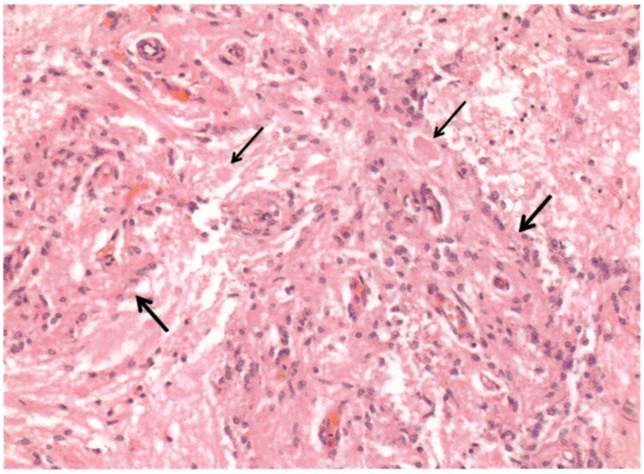

Figure 2-80. Herring bodies: Eosinophilic granular structures (*thin arrows*) reminiscent of axonal swellings are seen normally in the posterior pituitary parenchyma and represent axonal transport material. They may be mistaken for EGBs in this region that is already normally cellular due to Gomitoli, that is, coiled vessels surrounded by cellular zones (*thick arrows*) and spindle cell morphology, mimicking PA (H&E; original magnification: 200×).

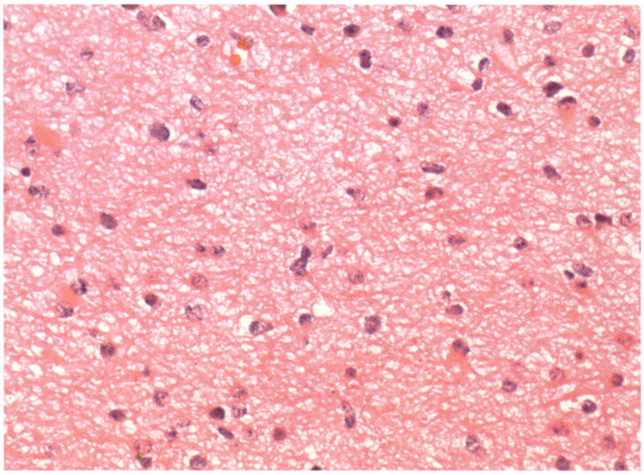

Figure 2-81. Astrocytoma: Thick and bright eosinophilic processes are seen in the background of an astrocytoma. Also note the irregular contours and distribution of hyperchromatic nuclei (H&E; original magnification: 400×).

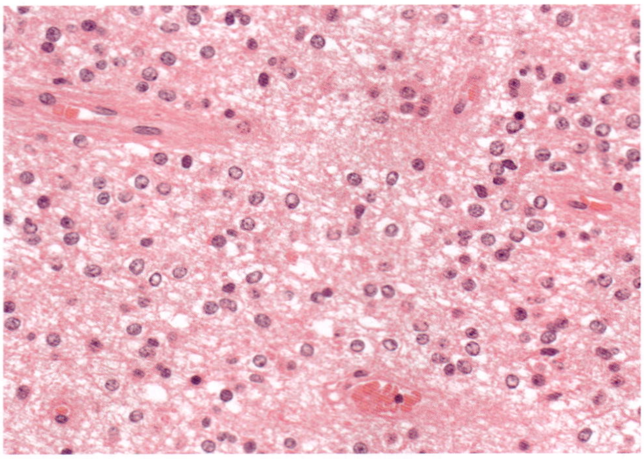

Figure 2-82. Oligodendroglioma: The background contains many processes, but not as thick, as bright eosinophilic, and as dense as in astrocytoma. Also note the round and more uniform nuclei (H&E; original magnification: 400×).

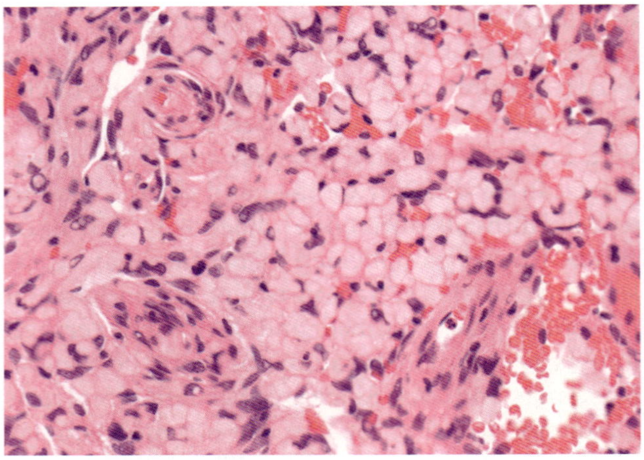

Figure 2-83. Collagen: Cross sections of collagen bundles are seen as round, pale eosinophilic structures, among which the nuclei are squeezed, mimicking rhabdoid cells in this otherwise unremarkable meningioma. A trichrome stain reveals their collagenous nature (H&E; original magnification: 400×).

and pale appearance **(Fig. 2-82)**. The most delicate end of the spectrum where the fibrillarity is very delicate and relatively homogeneous is neurocytomas. They have neuritic processes that are shorter and somewhat wavy. The absence of glial fibrillarity in the background is useful in distinguishing astroblastoma from ependymoma by favoring astroblastoma. These two neoplasms can appear similar due to the presence of pseudorosettes, well circumscription, and variable EMA positivity in both, though the latter is not as prominent in astroblastoma as in ependymoma. The glial fibrillarity of the background is not prominent in chordoid glioma, although the neoplastic cells have the processes, and this feature further adds to the confusion if this entity is not considered based on its location.

Several *extracellular accumulations* can be seen in the CNS. Sometimes these accumulations are coincidental bystanders and sometimes they may have diagnostic implications. No fibroblasts are present in the CNS parenchyma, except for meninges and vascular adventitial connective tissue. The repair process in the CNS is through reactive astrocytosis, hence the term glial scar. Therefore, *collagen* is not produced in the CNS parenchyma unless these structures are involved in the process. The changes involving vessel walls are discussed in "Vascular Changes." Extensive collagenization and hyalinization of the stroma and/or vessels can be seen in some neoplasms and can obscure the neoplasm. This phenomenon can be seen more commonly in meningioma, PA, ependymoma, myxopapillary ependymoma, astroblastoma, and ganglioglioma. It is especially prominent in clear cell meningioma and in the vessels of angiomatous meningioma. Some meningiomas can be essentially entirely hyalinized/collagenized to result in the term sclerosing meningioma, leaving only scattered entrapped neoplastic cells available for diagnosis. The so-called meningeal fibroma is likely an extensively collagenized meningioma. Small bundles of collagen may mimic rhabdoid change in meningioma **(Fig. 2-83)**. As the name implies, DIG/DIA has abundant collagen in the spindle cell/mesenchymal areas. Collagen is commonly found in spindle cell lesions. Thick, keloid-like collagen is typical for solitary fibrous tumor (SFT), alternating with more cellular areas, resulting in a so-called patternless pattern. Collagen can also be seen in a delicate, lacy pattern among the cells. Leptomeningeal fibrosis is a nonspecific finding that may be associated with aging or may indicate previous injury. In the case of age-related change, it is commonly and more prominently seen bilaterally in the parasagittal areas. In cases of healed meningitides, it may be more diffuse or patchy in the most severely affected areas. If arachnoid granulations are entrapped, hydrocephalus may result. Leptomeningeal fibrosis may also accompany

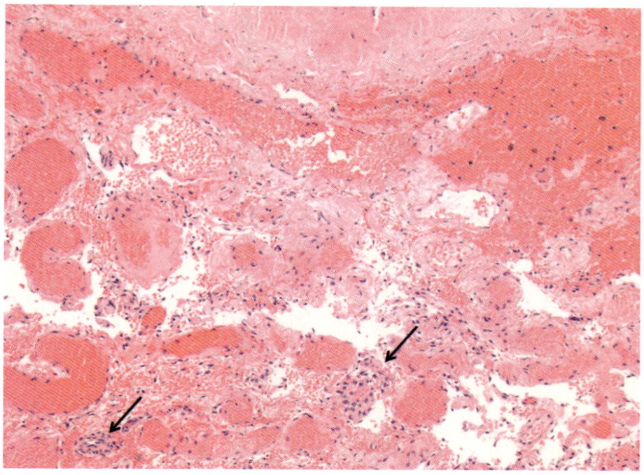

Figure 2-84. Vascularity in idiopathic hypertrophic pachymeningitis: Many congested capillaries form a vascular layer under the dura mater (**top**). Proliferating meningothelial cell groups are also present (*arrows*) (H&E; original magnification: 100×).

cortical malformations. Idiopathic hypertrophic pachymeningitis is characterized by a diffuse collagenous thickening and chronic inflammation of dura mater. Increased vascularity is frequently seen **(Fig. 2-84)**. Although a subpopulation of cases can be associated with fungal or acid-fast microorganism infections, collagen vascular diseases, and diffuse involvement of dura mater with malignancies, many are idiopathic and it is a diagnosis of exclusion. Clinical, radiologic, and pathologic features may overlap and can be associated with spontaneous intracranial hypotension syndrome (a.k.a. low cerebrospinal fluid [CSF] pressure syndrome).[173]

Round, pale eosinophilic structures with a peripheral spiculation are sometimes present in the mucinous background of myxopapillary ependymomas and are termed collagen balloons or collagen balls. They are variably positive for PAS after diastase digestion, trichrome, and reticulin. Interstitial fibrosis occurs in prolactinomas after long-term treatment with dopamine agonists. The adenoma cells also have a shrunken, small cell appearance. These changes should not be confused with an invasive adenoma or metastatic small cell carcinoma or other small blue cell neoplasm.

Some glioblastomas may have extensive vascular proliferation and an inflammatory component, resembling an abscess wall in small, fragmented specimens. Likewise, abscess specimens can be extremely cellular with cytologic atypia of the component cells, resembling a GBM. In such difficult cases, the collagenous component of the granulation tissue of the abscess can be highlighted by trichrome or reticulin stains to help with the differential diagnosis. In addition, the reticulin fibers in the outer layers of collagenous capsule of the abscess tend to be aligned parallel to the abscess cavity surface. This contrasts with the pattern of collagen restricted to perivascular areas in GBM. An example of a rare but peculiar situation where the collagen in the granulation tissue is useful is sparganosis, caused by Spirometra mansonoides or erinacei. The lesions consist of a degenerating central worm, surrounding fibrous capsule, lymphocytic inflammation, edema, and gliosis. Cavities lined by granulation tissue indicate larva migration.

An unusual and prominent collagenous fibrosis within the brain parenchyma in response to deep brain stimulation electrode has been reported, whereas the typical reaction to these electrodes is in the form of gliosis.[174] In tethered cord specimens, an ependyma-lined canal may be seen with little, if any, surrounding parenchyma, but with prominent surrounding fibroadipose tissue. In soft tissues and peripheral nervous system, a widely collagenized spindle cell neoplasm, with or without a myxoid matrix and with spindled and wavy nuclei, should prompt one to consider the diagnosis of neurofibroma, no matter how paucicellular it may appear.

Amyloid is a homogeneous, pale eosinophilic amorphous protein that accumulates as a result of a wide variety of processes, from infectious to endocrine to neoplastic, to name a few. Specifically beta-amyloid is well-known in the CNS in association with Alzheimer pathology. It can be a component of other pathologic conditions, some of which have been previously mentioned above, for example, spongiform encephalopathies and DAI. Amyloid may be difficult to tell apart from collagen, especially hyalinized homogeneous collagen, when collagen's fibrillary nature is not readily visible. In addition, amyloid accumulation may be focal and mild, although this is more of a problem in the muscle and nerve biopsy specimens, where abundant accumulation is only occasionally seen. Therefore, in such cases, the interpretation of special stains can be challenging.

Amyloid accumulation rarely occurs in pituitary adenoma but is a peculiar feature, especially in prolactin-producing adenomas. Round,

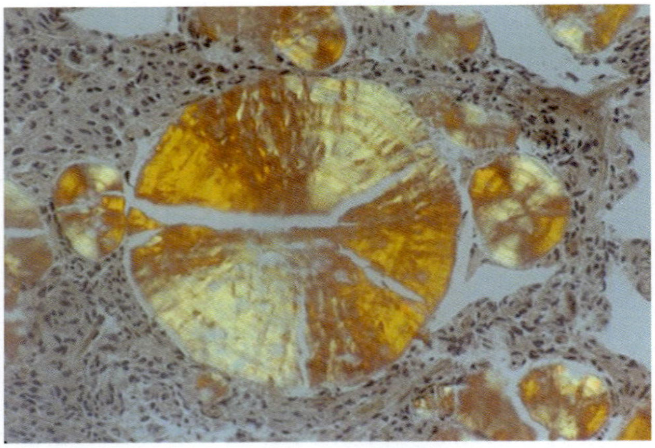

Figure 2-85. Prolactinoma: Peculiar amyloid accumulation resembling psammoma bodies are present. They show the "apple-green" birefringence by polarized light examination of Congo red-stained sections (Congo red; polarized light; original magnification: 400×).

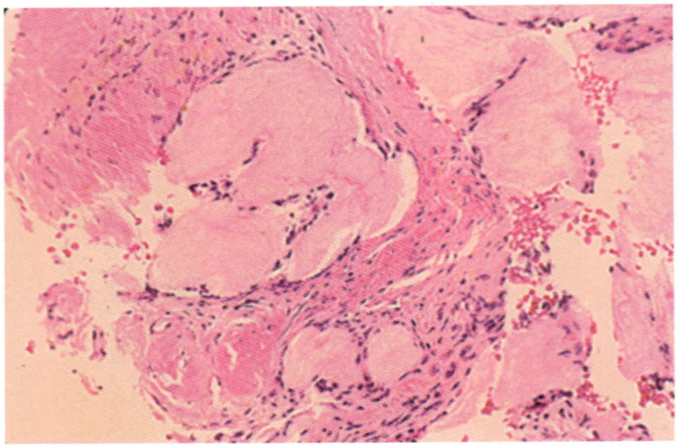

Figure 2-86. Gouty tophi: Amorphous acellular pale eosinophilic accumulations are surrounded by multinucleated foreign body giant cells (H&E; original magnification: 200×).

psammomatous accumulations have features of amyloid by Congo red stain **(Fig. 2-85)**. Amyloid accumulation is rare in ACTH adenoma and may be perivascular in growth hormone (GH) adenoma. Amyloid accumulation has been described in the stroma of meningiomas, especially the psammomatous variant.[175] It can also be seen in the context of plasma cell myelomas and solitary plasmacytomas. Amyloid accumulation can result in a mass lesion, that is, amyloidoma, even without definitive association with an inflammatory or neoplastic plasma cell.[176] Somewhat homogeneous eosinophilic microscopic accumulations with a nodular arrangement, usually surrounded by a foreign body giant cell reaction, can be an incidental finding in discectomy specimens and represent gouty tophi **(Fig. 2-86)**.

While metaplastic bone formation can be seen in several neoplasms, an irregular accumulation of *osteoid* in association with a malignant neoplasm should prompt consideration of osteosarcoma. This should be differentiated from a malignant neoplasm infiltrating and entrapping bone trabeculae. An orderly increase in the number of trabeculae rimmed by osteoblasts is seen in osteoid osteoma and osteoblastoma. This area is consistent with the nidus of the osteoma that is surrounded by a sclerotic bone. In osteoblastoma, which is considered as a diagnosis when the lesion is >1.0 cm, this distinction is not as well-defined. Nonetheless, the facial bones, especially paranasal sinuses, are common places for these lesions and should not be confused with osteosarcoma because of the busy histology of the nidus. The osteoid is disordered and is not rimmed by osteoblasts in osteosarcoma. As with bone lesions in general elsewhere in the body, correlation with radiologic features should be made to avoid mistakes. The irregular shapes of trabeculae, described as alphabet soup, in a fibrous, dense intertrabecular background and without osteoblastic rimming are characteristic of fibrous dysplasia.

Although *keratin* is an intracellular protein, it is briefly included here to discuss the keratin accumulation and keratinous debris seen in several lesions. Keratin is the most obvious indicator of squamous differentiation in cells. In adamantinomatous craniopharyngiomas, the keratin has a waxy, hyalinized appearance (as opposed to flaky keratin seen in epidermis or in other keratinizing stratified squamous epithelia) called wet keratin. It usually is seen in the form of small collections, rather than individual cells, and is one of the hallmarks of adamantinomatous craniopharyngioma. Wet keratin is not seen in papillary craniopharyngioma.

Calcifications

Calcifications are usually found *normally* in several areas of the CNS **(Table 2.10)**. Parasagittal regions are common locations for psammomatous

List of Findings/Checklist for Calcifications

AT A GLANCE

- Normal
- Neoplastic
- Vascular
- Parenchymal
- Infectious
- Toxic-metabolic
- Artifact

calcifications associated with arachnoid granulations. They can also be seen in other areas of the brain, associated with arachnoid cap-cell clusters. The stroma of the papillae of the choroid plexus commonly contains variable numbers of psammomatous calcifications. Smaller and fewer psammomatous calcifications can be found within anterior pituitary parenchyma, usually within the epithelial cell nests. In the pineal gland, calcifications are more variable and, with increasing age, they form larger chunky dystrophic aggregates that frequently crack or dislodge from the section during microsectioning to leave a hole in their place. They are sometimes referred to as corpora arenacea, or brain sand. Dura mater can undergo dystrophic calcification and even ossification, which is usually in the form of a thin flat layer attached to it. Commonly in falx cerebri, they can form somewhat irregular aggregates of variable size. Many of them represent extensively psammomatous incidental meningiomas. Pituitary capsule is another area where psammomatous calcifications can be seen. Especially in the lumbosacral leptomeninges, flat, delicate, flaky, variably fibrous, calcified, or ossified structures can be identified. They are usually multiple and are attached to leptomeninges. These are called fibrohyaline plaques and are of no known significance. With increasing age, especially in the basal ganglia, vascular wall calcifications can be seen. These can be extensive enough to involve the entire vessel wall. In this context, they are of no known significance; however, they can be a part of arteriosclerotic changes and/or hypertensive changes. In the hippocampus, very fine granular calcifications can be seen impregnating the capillary walls as a normal change with aging. Small psammomatous calcifications should not be confused with corpora amylacea, or vice versa. Focusing up and down will yield the concentric laminations of microcalcifications and the cloudy interior of the corpora amylacea, as well as the thin astrocyte cytoplasm surrounding the latter.

Calcifications can also be seen in association with *neoplasms*. While it is not unusual to find calcifications in many neoplasms, some are particularly recognized to have prominent calcifications **(Table 2.11)**. Usually, these are low-grade neoplasms, as they had to have existed long enough time to allow calcifications to develop. PA, low-grade oligodendroglioma and ganglioglioma commonly harbor variable amounts of microcalcifications. They are typically scattered throughout the neoplasm or

TABLE 2.10 Locations where calcifications can normally be seen

Dura mater
Arachnoid granulations
Anterior pituitary
Pineal gland
Basal ganglionic vessel walls
Hippocampus
Choroid plexus
Spinal leptomeninges (fibrohyaline plaques)

TABLE 2.11 Neoplasms with calcifications

Glial/neuronal
PA
Oligodendroglioma
Gangliocytoma/ganglioglioma
Subependymal giant cell astrocytoma
Astroblastoma
PXA
Ependymoma/subependymoma
Central neurocytoma
Pineal parenchymal tumors
Supratentorial PNET
Medulloblastoma
Pituitary adenoma
Craniopharyngioma
Meningioma
Calcifying pseudoneoplasm of the neuraxis
Psammomatous melanotic schwannoma
Metastatic neoplasms

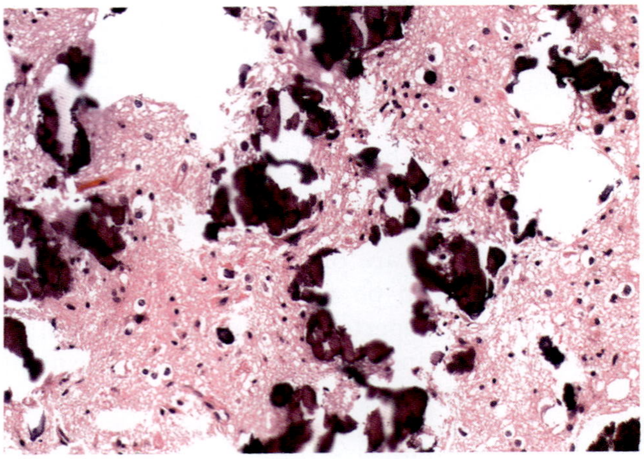

Figure 2-87. Oligodendroglioma with abundant calcifications that is partially obscuring the cellularity. Calcifications are more commonly seen in the form of microcalcifications (H&E; original magnification: 400×).

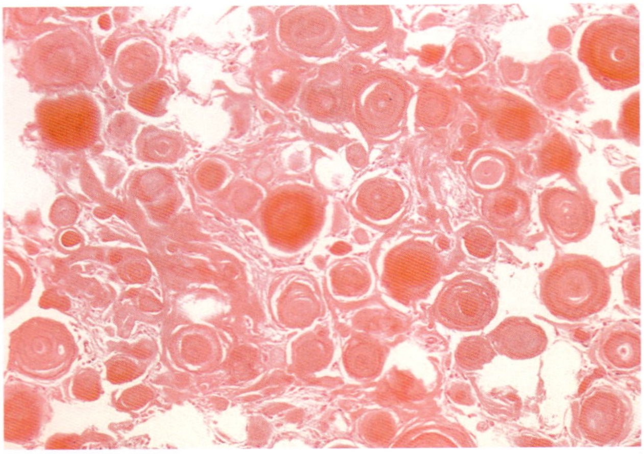

Figure 2-88. Psammomatous meningioma: Numerous psammoma bodies with their typical concentric laminations are present in this meningioma identified as an incidental finding at autopsy and had to be decalcified for sections to be prepared (H&E; original magnification: 100×).

may aggregate in some areas but occasionally can be extensive **(Fig. 2-87)**. Subependymal giant cell astrocytoma (SEGA), central neurocytoma, and astroblastoma are frequently and heavily calcified, whereas PXA can be calcified in some cases. Ependymomas and subependymomas can have foci of calcifications. Pineal parenchymal tumors are frequently calcified; however, nonneoplastic pineal gland can also have abundant calcification and their presence cannot be used for identification of a neoplasm or for distinguishing among the pineal parenchymal tumor grades, although they are more frequent in pineocytomas. Calcifications are frequent in supratentorial primitive neuroectodermal tumor (S-PNET) but rare in medulloblastomas; however, calcification of the falx cerebri in the presence of a medulloblastoma may be an indication of nevoid basal cell carcinoma syndrome (Gorlin syndrome).[177] Scattered psammomatous calcifications are not uncommon in meningiomas; when they constitute a prominent feature, they are then termed psammomatous meningioma **(Fig. 2-88)**. They can be seen as incidental calcified nodules attached to dura mater in autopsies and may need decalcification so that they can be sectioned. Some meningiomas can have dystrophic calcifications and may even develop metaplastic ossifications, sometimes creating confusion with invasion of bone by meningioma, especially on histologic grounds alone. Another peculiar lesion that may grossly resemble a meningioma with calcification is calcifying/ossifying pseudoneoplasm of the neuraxis. The latter is a peculiar lesion with granular calcified debris, fibrillary amphophilic material, and a histiocytic reaction to them. It may ossify. A prominent reactive meningothelial proliferation may accompany it, resulting in confusion with meningioma. In pituitary adenomas, calcification may be abundant, especially in prolactinomas, sometimes termed pituitary stones. Prolactinomas can also have psammomatous amyloid accumulations. Psammomatous melanotic schwannoma is a schwannoma variant with melanin pigment and psammomatous calcifications, creating differential diagnostic pitfalls with meningioma and melanocytic neoplasms. It can be a component of Carney's complex, along with cardiac myxomas, endocrine abnormalities, and pigmented skin lesions.[178] Otherwise, its histochemical and immunohistochemical features are those of schwannoma. Craniopharyngioma typically has abundant calcification and helps identify a suprasellar cystic lesion with abundant calcification as craniopharyngioma. Other low-grade neoplasms, such as DNT, as well as malformations, such as FCD and meningioangiomatosis, also show variable degrees of calcifications. Metastatic neoplasms, especially those with papillary features, can have prominent calcifications, mainly in the form of psammoma bodies. Prominent examples are papillary thyroid carcinoma, though it rarely metastasizes to the brain, and serous papillary

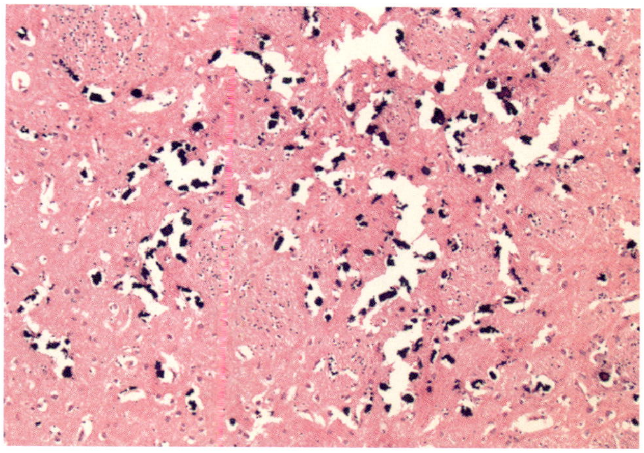

Figure 2-89. Basal ganglionic calcifications: Numerous calcifications are associated mainly with vessels and can be associated with many disorders (H&E; original magnification: 100×).

carcinoma of the ovary. Calcification and ossification are naturally present in a variety of bone neoplasms and malignancies with sarcomatous components, such as malignant mixed mullerian tumor with heterologous elements or carcinosarcomas with chondroid and/or osseous components.

Vascular calcifications may indicate an underlying condition. Fahr disease is a familial condition with widespread and symmetrical calcifications of the basal ganglia, dentate nuclei, and brain parenchyma[179] **(Fig. 2-89)**. *Basal ganglionic calcification* **(Table 2.12)** due to other causes is sometimes referred to as Fahr syndrome.[180] The disorder diffuse NFTs with calcification also show diffuse involvement similar to Fahr disease.[101] In addition, there is widespread involvement with NFTs. Numerous alpha-synuclein–positive neuronal and astrocytic inclusions; Lewy bodies in substantia nigra, dorsal motor nucleus of vagus, hippocampus, and amygdala; and Lewy neurites in hippocampus and subiculum are seen. In both conditions, there is variable degree of neuron loss and gliosis, likely at least partially contributed to by vascular insufficiency resulting from obliteration of the vessel lumens. Basal ganglia calcifications can also be seen in mitochondrial encephalopathies, Kallman syndrome,[181] tuberous sclerosis,[182] myotonic muscular dystrophy,[183] and systemic lupus erythematosus involving the CNS.[184] Vascular changes consisting of calcification, fibrous thickening, and narrowing of lumen occur in MELAS and are mainly seen in globus pallidus but may also involve the white matter, thalamus, dentate.[185] Similar changes are also present in Kearns-Sayre syndrome.[186] Mineralization of vessels in the basal ganglia and white matter is seen in myoclonal epilepsy with ragged red fibers (MERRF).[187] AVMs and cavernous angiomas can have variable amounts of dystrophic calcifications due to organization of repeated hemorrhages. As part of complex atherosclerotic changes, intimal and mural calcifications are seen in the basal arteries with severe atherosclerosis. In fact, they can grossly be felt like metal pipes. In such cases, if a cross section needs to be submitted in order to examine a possible thrombus in the lumen, or for arterial dissection, they should not be cut forcefully but should be gently decalcified by light decalcification first to preserve the integrity of tissue during gross sectioning. Nasu-Hakola disease (polycystic lipomembranous osteodysplasia with sclerosing leukoencephalopathy), in addition to axonal spheroids and myelinated fiber loss in the white matter and systemic findings, causes neuron loss, gliosis, and mineralization of the basal ganglia.[188] Thalamus may be involved. Meningocerebral angiodysplasia and renal agenesis[189] is characterized in the CNS by very vascular leptomeninges, sometimes with hemorrhage and calcification. Angiodysplasia consists of ectatic capillaries and veins. They are present in leptomeninges brain, cerebellum, and brainstem. Calcifications, hemorrhage, thrombosis, infarcts, and hemosiderin-laden macrophages can be seen in these locations.

Calcification of the *cerebral cortex* in a linear manner is typical in Sturge-Weber syndrome in the atrophic cortex. The overlying venous angiomatosis

TABLE 2.12 Basal ganglionic calcifications

Fahr disease/Fahr syndrome
Diffuse NFTs with calcification
MELAS
MERRF
Kearns-Sayre syndrome
Nasu-Hakola disease
Human immunodeficiency virus infection
Tuberous sclerosis
Myotonic muscular dystrophy
Systemic lupus erythematosus
Kallman syndrome

MELAS, mitochondrial encephalomyopathy, lactic acidosis and stroke-like episodes; MERRF, myoclonal epilepsy with ragged red fibers.

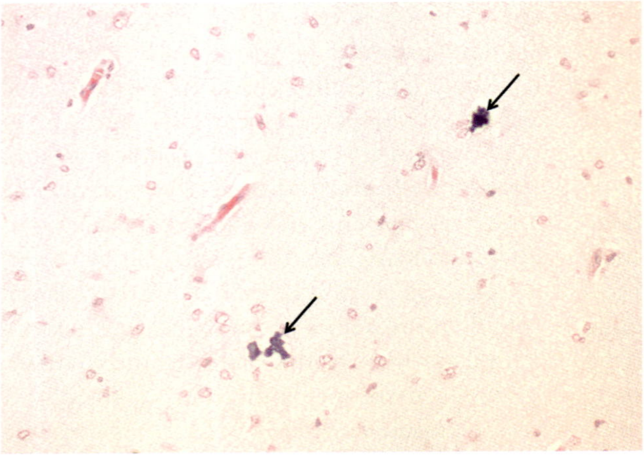

Figure 2-90. White matter microcalcifications (*arrows*): Especially around capillaries, they typically represent the calcified versions of mulberries. White matter is thin and pale, supporting previous damage (H&E; original magnification: 400×).

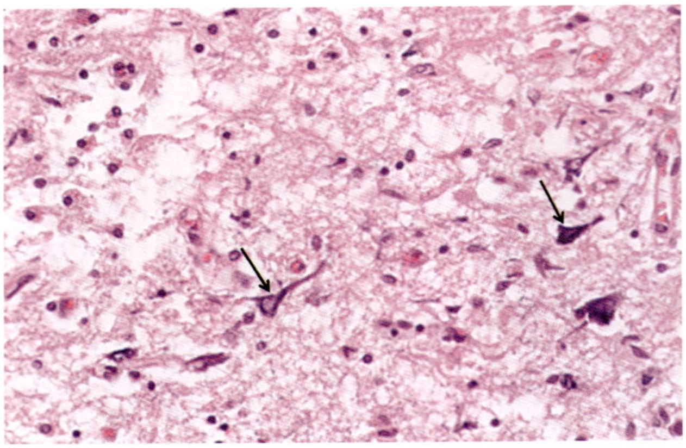

Figure 2-91. Mineralized neurons: The dead neurons did not disintegrate and are impregnated by a dusty mineralization mainly composed of calcium and iron, highlighting their outlines and processes (*arrows*) and indicating previous hypoxic–ischemic injury (H&E; original magnification: 400×).

in the leptomeninges also shows extensive calcifications in the vessel walls, resulting in a tram-track appearance on radiologic evaluation. Many cortical tubers, subependymal nodules, and SEGA in tuberous sclerosis complex also show variable amounts of calcifications. In perinatal telencephalic leukoencephalopathy (periventricular leukomalacia) associated with prenatal and perinatal injury, there is vascular leakage initially resulting in the formation of perivascular amorphous amphophilic proteinaceous material called mulberries, which later become mineralized, including calcification, to form perivascular laminated structures. They can be found in the periventricular regions and in the white matter **(Fig. 2-90)**. Mineralization of neurons is a peculiar delicate finely granular impregnation of dead neuron cytoskeletons, a component of which is calcium **(Fig. 2-91)**. It can be seen in association with perinatal hypoxic–ischemic injury, as well as in infarcts. Mobius syndrome is characterized by aplasia or hypoplasia of cranial nerve nuclei, which may be isolated or associated with other brainstem malformations.[190] Necrosis and calcifications of brainstem nuclei, suggesting infection or anoxia, peripheral nerve involvement, and myopathy are also present. orthochromatic leukodystrophy (OLD) with calcification (Aicardi-Goutieres leukoencephalopathy) has calcifications in WM and basal ganglia,[191] while in Cockayne disease, calcifications are around vessels in the cortex and basal ganglia.[192] Fowler syndrome (proliferative vasculopathy and hydranencephaly–hydrocephaly) is characterized by a diffuse vascular proliferation in the CNS, accompanied by numerous calcifications, which can be large, chunky or small, and widespread.[193] In celiac disease, cortical and subcortical calcifications occur in parietal and occipital lobes.[194] Calcium accumulation in tissues occurs in hypercalcemic states as a result of disorders of calcium metabolism, especially in hyperparathyroid states, as well as part of the disturbances associated with end-stage renal disease. Such calcifications are referred to as metastatic calcifications.

Infectious processes and especially TORCH (toxoplasma, rubella, cytomegalovirus, herpes virus) group are typically associated with microcalcifications, especially in the periventricular destructive areas **(Table 2.13)**.[195] Prominent

TABLE 2.13 Infections typically associated with calcifications
CMV
Varicella
Rubella
Toxoplasma
Human immunodeficiency virus
Tuberculosis
Cysticercosis

examples are fetal varicella infection with cystic destruction, hydrocephalus, and microcephaly; CMV ventriculitis, encephalitis, and congenital infection with periventricular calcifications, viral inclusions, destruction, and microcephaly; and congenital rubella infection, microcephaly, calcifications, hydrocephalus, and cystic destructive lesions in the parenchyma, especially in the basal ganglia and thalamus. In congenital toxoplasmosis, there are multiple, especially periventricular and subpial areas of necrosis, hydrocephalus, and even hydranencephaly. Calcifications tend to be throughout the brain, in contrast to preferably periventricular areas as in CMV. Microcephaly and mineralization of lesions also occur. A similar presentation but with negative serology for TORCH infections has been termed pseudo-TORCH syndrome.[196] In children, HIV infection causes, in addition to the usual findings, additional prominent perivascular lymphocytes and dystrophic calcifications in vessels and parenchyma but especially in basal ganglia.[197] Older lesions of tuberculosis may show large dystrophic calcifications. Cysticercosis is typically multiple and may be numerous, located mainly in meninges, cortex, and ventricles. Once the organism is dead, the lesions degenerate and become firm white nodules, which eventually calcify. They are usually surrounded by an intense inflammatory reaction, including eosinophil polymorphonuclear (PMN) leukocytes and granulomas. Dusty granular calcifications associated with degenerative processes, such as fibrosis, or organizing hemorrhage can have an appearance mimicking fungal yeast forms **(Fig. 2-92)**. Such overlapping calcifications may even mimic budding. Calcifications, however, are highly pleomorphic and larger ones can show concentric laminations upon closer examination. In difficult situations, special stains will resolve this issue.

Toxic effects of *medications* can be associated with calcifications. Intrathecal gentamycin may result in white matter necrosis and calcification in midbrain and pons. Methotrexate toxicity can cause multifocal necrotizing leukoencephalopathy. The lesions in the shrunken and gliotic white matter later calcify.[198] There may also be vessel wall calcifications, most prominent in the basal ganglia. BCNU (bis-chloroethyl nitrosourea) can also cause methotrexate-like multifocal necrotizing leukoencephalopathy, vascular injury, and calcification.[199] Multifocal necrotizing leukoencephalopathy can also be associated with AIDS, leukemia, and radiation.[200] Swollen and fragmented axons, which then calcify, are seen in areas of necrosis. The lesions may have a predilection for brainstem.[201] Necrotizing leukoencephalopathy in HIV is characterized by necrotic white matter lesions with numerous macrophages and variable lymphocytes primarily in perivascular location. The lesions later become gliotic and calcify.

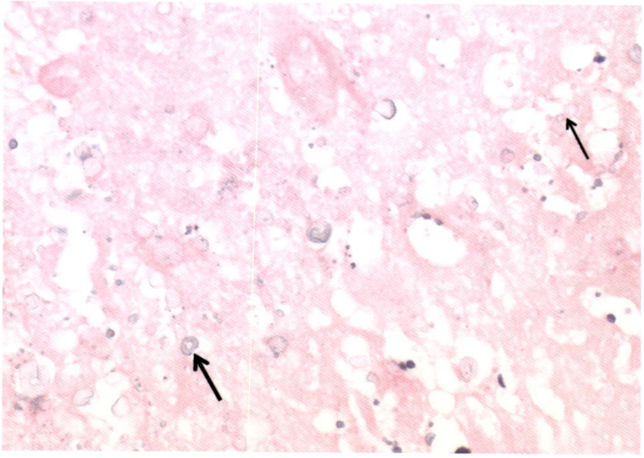

Figure 2-92. Dystrophic microcalcifications: These pale basophilic round microcalcifications of various sizes are usually associated with necrosis, hyalinization of previous areas of tissue damage, or burnt-out infectious granulomas. They may mimic fungal yeast forms due to double contour (*thick arrow*) or budding appearance due to overlapping structures (*thin arrow*) (H&E; original magnification: 400×).

Irregular dystrophic calcifications can be scattered commonly within the necrotic, degenerative, and long-standing reactive processes. Irregular fragments of densely basophilic bone fragments as an *artifact* may be seen buried into the tissue, mimicking calcification **(Fig. 2-93)**. They represent bone dust resulting from the drilling of bone during craniotomy or from the bone saw during autopsy. Those originating from surgical procedures and contaminating biopsy specimens may be more difficult to recognize in some cases, resulting in difficulty in interpretation. Bone dust may also mimic necrotic bone, especially if it was implanted in the tissue during a previous procedure and seen in subsequent surgical specimens together with some degeneration and inflammatory reaction.

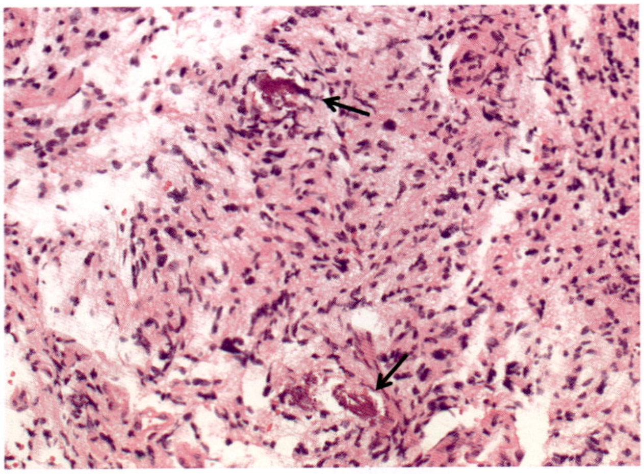

Figure 2-93. Bone dust: Contamination of bone chips from drilling or sawing of cranial bones can mimic calcifications. They have an amorphous, irregular, and smudgy quality (H&E; original magnification: 200×).

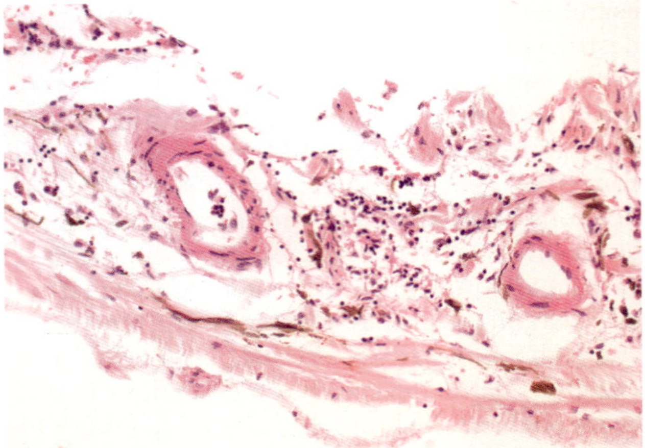

Figure 2-94. Leptomeningeal melanocytes: These elongated dendritic cells with dusty brown-green melanin pigment are normally present in the leptomeninges and should not be confused with a melanocytic lesion or hemosiderin pigment (H&E; original magnification: 200×).

Pigments

A variety of pigments can accumulate or normally be found in the nervous system. Even though they all may have colors that represent shades of brown-yellow, they need to be differentiated from each other, as each has separate implications. As with all the brown pigments in general, one has to be careful with the interpretation of *immunohistochemical stains* so that these pigments are not misinterpreted as positive staining of immunohistochemistry using brown chromogen such as DAB (3,3′ diaminobenzidine). As long as this pitfall is remembered, it does not become a problem in practice; however, if it does in a rare situation where interpretation becomes complicated, immunohistochemistry can be performed using a chromogen yielding another color, such as AEC (aminoethyl carbazole), or an alkaline phosphatase-based system with chromogens other than brown can be used.

List of Findings/Checklist for Pigments

AT A GLANCE

- Melanin
- Neuromelanin
- Lipofuscin
- Hemosiderin
- Bile
- Copper
- Sulfatide
- Hematin
- Gunpowder
- Amorphous material
- Formalin pigment

Melanin pigment is normally present in the CNS in the leptomeningeal melanocytes that appear as dendritic cells scattered in variable numbers **(Fig. 2-94)**. They are more prominent in naturally darker skinned individuals on the anterior surfaces of the brainstem and may give the leptomeninges a darker appearance. They are thought to be the origin of primary CNS melanocytic neoplasms, that is, melanocytomas and primary melanomas, and the intermediate grade melanocytic neoplasms.[47] These melanocytes and the melanin pigment should not be confused with hemosiderin pigment indicating a previous subarachnoid hemorrhage and can easily be distinguished by the dendritic processes of the former, as well as the uniform finely granular darker brown nature of the melanin pigment. Melanocytosis and melanomatosis represent the benign and malignant ends of diffuse melanocytic proliferation, respectively, of the leptomeninges and are typically heavily pigmented.[202] Malignant transformation of benign melanocytic lesions can rarely occur.[203] Other neoplasms can have melanin pigment[204] and may rarely cause confusion when the pigment is widespread. Melanotic schwannoma,[204] psammomatous melanotic schwannoma,[178] subependymoma and ependymoma with melanin formation,[205] medulloblastoma with melanotic differentiation,[206] melanotic neuroectodermal tumor of infancy (a.k.a. progonoma or retinal anlage tumor),[207] pineal anlage tumor,[208] medulloepithelioma,[209] PA,[210] ganglioglioma,[211] and choroid plexus papilloma[212] can have melanin pigment but this usually does not cause significant diagnostic problems, as the true nature of the neoplasm is readily obvious. Recognizing the particular variant may be of importance in some situations, however, as in the case of psammomatous melanotic schwannoma and Carney's complex association.[178] *Neuromelanin* accumulates as a metabolic by-product in dopaminergic neurons and has histochemical and electron microscopic properties resembling both melanin and lipofuscin. It is prominent in substantia nigra and locus ceruleus and can be seen grossly in adult brains when it reaches a significant level in the neurons. In contrast, these structures do not appear pigmented in children, even though the pigment is present but in smaller amounts, as it takes time to accumulate,[213] and appear pale or completely nonpigmented in individuals with neurodegenerative diseases involving these structures and resulting in neuron loss and pigment loss varying depending on the degree of involvement.[214,215] Sometimes, especially with a relatively faster and prominent degeneration of neurons, they can grossly appear normally pigmented in spite of significant neuron loss because the remaining pigment tends to linger in the neuropil and within the macrophages until it is cleared. Neuromelanin is also present in smaller amounts in dorsal motor nucleus of vagus, dorsal root ganglia, and sympathetic ganglia.

Another pigment that is normally present in the CNS is *lipofuscin* **(Fig. 2-95)**. It is a lighter brown-to-yellow pigment compared to melanin and has a dusty appearance with indistinct or very fine granules, creating a brown-yellow hue in the cytoplasm. It is positive by PAS and Ziehl-Neelsen stains and is autofluorescent by ultraviolet light. These features should be kept in mind to avoid confusion while interpreting such preparations. It too accumulates within the neuron cytoplasm over time with aging[216] and is diffusely present in the CNS in the pyramidal neurons of the cerebral cortex, and more prominently in the thalamus, lateral geniculate nucleus, amygdala, dentate nucleus of the cerebellum, inferior olivary nuclei, and anterior horn cells of the spinal cord, as well as dorsal root ganglia. It can be present in glial cells, though not as prominent as in the neurons. It is increased in neurodegenerative diseases such as AD, a feature that appears to be too subjective and difficult to use in practice. It accumulates abundantly and diffusely in neuron cytoplasms in storage diseases associated with accumulation of lipofuscin, that is, neuronal ceroid lipofuscinosis (Batten disease),[217] which, as is the case with the genetic metabolic diseases (inborn errors of metabolism) in general, has infantile, late infantile, juvenile, and adult clinicopathologic forms, as well as a number of variants based on the gene involved and the enzyme defect. Abundant granular intracytoplasmic PAS-positive accumulation material is seen diffusely in the neuron cytoplasm, both in the CNS and in the autonomic nervous system. The pigment may be associated with eosinophilic globules representing enlarged mitochondria in the cytoplasm.[218] OLD with pigmented glia and macrophages[219] has Sudan- and PAS-positive macrophages and glia, giving the white matter grossly a green hue. The pigment is mostly lipofuscin but is also positive with Pearl's iron and Fontana-Masson stains. Vitamin E deficiency, along with widespread axonal spheroids, also has neuronal cytoplasmic lipofuscin

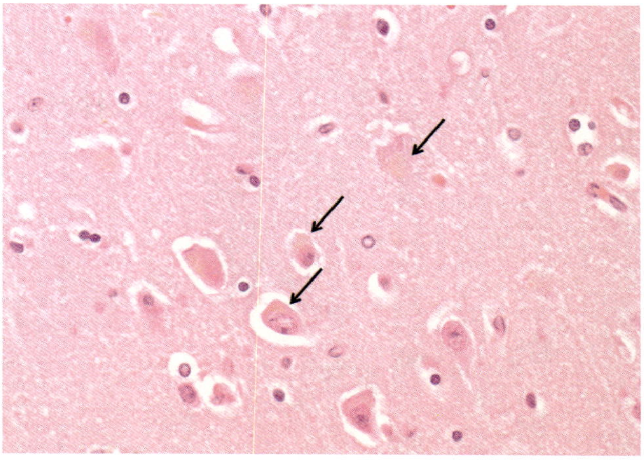

Figure 2-95. Lipofuscin pigment is present in neuron cytoplasm as a finely granular yellow-brown pigment. It can be very prominent or may create a mild discoloration (*arrows*) (H&E; original magnification: 400×).

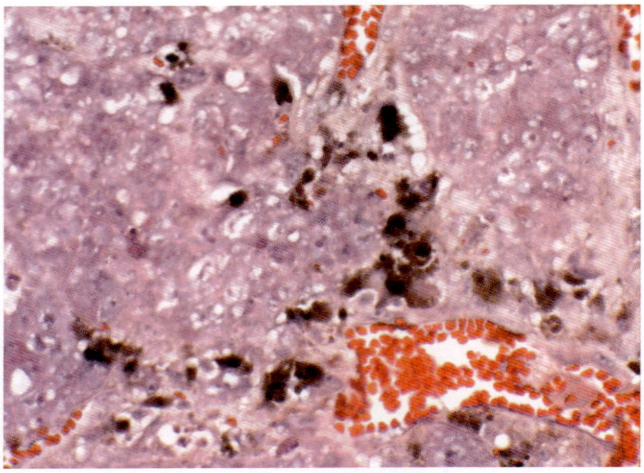

Figure 2-96. Hemosiderin pigment: As a result of hemorrhage in this metastatic carcinoma, hemosiderin pigment can be present and, together with the prominent nucleoli of carcinoma cells, may lead to confusion with melanoma. Hemosiderin pigment typically has large and pleomoprhic globules with a golden-brown color, rather than the more uniform, finely granular green-brown quality of melanin pigment (H&E; original magnification: 400×).

pigment accumulation.[220] Likewise, neuroaxonal dystrophy cases may have brown dusty lipofuscin pigment and iron in the neurons.[221] Striatonigral degeneration shows, among other findings, atrophy and gray-tan discoloration of putamen due to lipofuscin-like pigment accumulation in glial cells.

Hemosiderin pigment **(Fig. 2-96)** forms in about 48 hours after hemorrhage and serves as evidence of previous hemorrhage in cases where the fresh blood is no longer obvious. It has a golden-brown, somewhat refractile quality and is in the form of larger and variably sized globules, in contrast to the uniform, fine and green-brown granules of melanin pigment. It is seen in the subarachnoid space, usually within macrophages, as evidence of a previous subarachnoid hemorrhage. In the parenchyma, its presence indicates a previous hemorrhage, and in association with a remote infarct, it suggests a hemorrhagic component. It is not unusual to see a small amount of hemosiderin pigment in the Virchow-Robin spaces of some vessels in the white matter and more commonly in basal ganglia in adult autopsy brains, even if they are otherwise unremarkable and are sometimes referred to as brain microbleeds. Whether this is a finding that is common enough to accept as normal can be debated,[222] as they likely indicate a subclinical small leak from the vessels. In cases of healed vasculitis, hemosiderin serves as a supportive feature of previous vessel wall damage, along with other features, such as fibrosis and recanalized thrombus. Other situations in which hemosiderin pigment is commonly seen as evidence of previous hemorrhage are AVMs, radiation change, and previous surgery sites. It can be seen in mammillary bodies as part of the vascular injury associated with Wernicke's encephalopathy. Neurodegeneration with brain iron accumulation type 1 (a.k.a. pantothenate kinase–associated neurodegeneration, or formerly Hallervorden-Spatz disease)[221] is characterized by iron-containing pigment and lipofuscin and neuromelanin in pars reticularis of substantia nigra and in globus pallidus. Similar pigment can also be present in renal tubular epithelium. It should be noted that a minimal amount of pigment can be identified in glial cells in the basal ganglia of many otherwise unremarkable autopsy brains as an age-related change or sometimes as free pigment from degenerated neurons in other diseases. Gamma-Gandy bodies are fibrotic nodules with abundant hemosiderin pigment and have been historically described in the spleen. They represent organized small hemorrhagic areas and, although relatively rare in the CNS, are associated with a wide variety of neoplastic and nonneoplastic lesions.[223] In general, iron accumulation frequently accompanies other accumulations, including various mineralization and calcifications, such as mineralized neurons in hypoxic–ischemic lesions and microcalcifications in periventricular leukomalacia. In such situations, iron is not readily visible but can be identified by an iron stain, and its identification is not diagnostically significant.

Bile pigments are composed of conjugated and unconjugated bilirubin, biliverdin, and hematoidin; however, their specific distinctions from each other and their limited involvement in neuropathology are of no known practical significance. Bile pigments can be seen in tissues in cases of hyperbilirubinuria as a pale yellow pigment and can be difficult to appreciate unless specifically searched for. It can be seen as a bright yellow-green discoloration in the cytoplasm of neurons and glia.[224] Usually, its presence neither comes as a surprise nor has any significant diagnostic contributions, as the clinical jaundice and its cause is readily apparent. In a patient with jaundice, the CNS parenchyma is spared of the yellow-green discoloration due to the blood–brain barrier, while dura mater, pineal gland, pituitary gland, and choroid plexus are involved. However, in cases of kernicterus (bilirubin encephalopathy), where there is damage to the blood–brain barrier, parenchyma is also affected.[225] There is preferential discoloration of globus pallidus, subthalamic nucleus, hippocampus (especially CA2), subiculum, lateral geniculate nucleus, substantia nigra and other brainstem nuclei, and dentate nucleus of the cerebellum. Although unconjugated bilirubin is toxic, it does not reach such high levels in this day and age as a result of better perinatal care, but toxicity can be seen in association with hypoxic–ischemic conditions resulting in vascular endothelial injury, that is, disruption of blood–brain barrier. Bile pigments, especially hematoidin, can be present along with hemosiderin pigment in association with remote hemorrhages **(Fig. 2-97)**. If needed, mainly as might be the case in kernicterus cases where pigment and discoloration are not obvious, several special stains are available. *Copper* pigment can accumulate in Wilson's disease (hepatolenticular degeneration) in cells that are apparently reactive astrocytes and are similar to Alzheimer type II astrocytes in basal ganglia and substantia nigra. Copper pigment is finely granular and has an orange-brown color.[226] Copper and iron accumulation in brain, especially in basal ganglia, red nucleus, and dentate nucleus with neuron loss and gliosis, is seen in hereditary ceruloplasmin deficiency.[17] While not a pigment, *sulfatide* accumulations in oligodendroglia, Schwann cells, neurons, and macrophages in metachromatic leukodystrophy yield a brown color when stained with toluidine blue or cresyl violet, that is, metachromasia. They are seen as PAS-positive, diastase-resistant granular material in a background of myelin loss with an luxol-fast blue LFB/PAS stain.

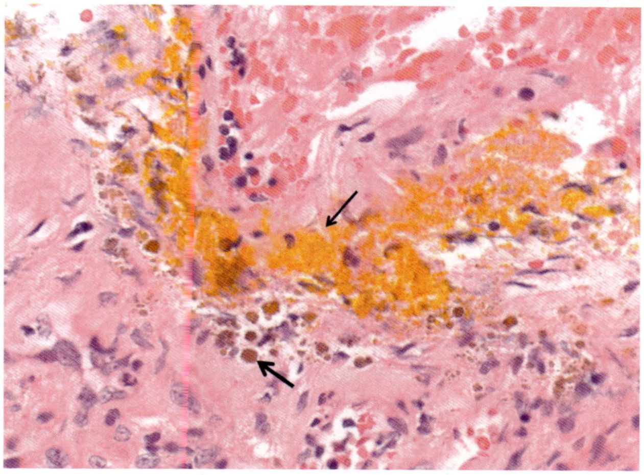

Figure 2-97. Hematoidin forms in the early stages of erythrocyte breakdown and creates a yellow-brown haze associated with the hemorrhage (*thin arrow*), while some hemosiderin has already formed (*thick arrow*) (H&E; original magnification: 400×).

Some *infectious agents* can produce a pigment that allows their easier identification. Phaeohyphomycosis is infection by a pigmented (dematiaceous) fungus. Chromoblastomyces is a pigmented fungus[227] with a brown discoloration of its lesions, which need to be distinguished from hemorrhage. It prefers frontal lobe parenchyma and may extend to meninges and ventricles. The lesions are essentially necrotic abscesses. The microorganism has conidia with hyphae, both of which are pigmented. There may be PMNs, lymphocytes, macrophages, giant cells, fibrosis, and gliosis.[228] Malaria can be seen as a pigmented dot in the erythrocytes or as a pigmented rim around them. It resembles formalin pigment and is likewise birefringent.[229] Microglia contain iron pigment and the microglial nodules they form are referred to as Durck granuloma. Schistosoma infections can be associated with a pigment similar to formalin and malaria pigments but has a chunky quality.[229]

Soot and gunpowder, simply known as gunpowder residue, is a pigment with nonrefractile black granules and larger tan polygonal crystals, respectively. It can be seen grossly as granular dark discoloration around gunshot wounds but can be identified and confirmed easier in subtle cases. Its identification and distribution provide information regarding the contact—close (a few inches), intermediate (from a few inches up to a few feet), and distant range of the wound. Also depending on multiple factors, such as the weapon used and clothing, gunpowder can be identified deeper in the tissues as the weapon is closer or may not be present at all in distant range wounds.[230] *Amorphous pigmented material* is typically seen as surgical material used for embolizations of hemorrhagic lesions, such as vascular malformations and meningiomas, or to minimize hemorrhage during surgery. One type of embolization material (Onyx) used for preoperative

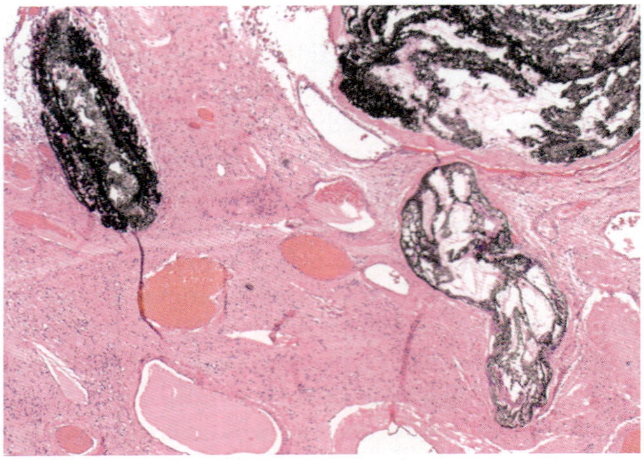

Figure 2-98. Onyx embolization material is seen in the vessels as black granular material in this AVM (H&E; original magnification: 100×).

embolization of vascular malformations and neoplasms can be seen as a black granular pigment, with alternating confluent black areas where the granules coalesce, and vacuoles, associated with giant cells **(Fig. 2-98)**. *Formalin pigment* is a brown-black precipitate that preferably accumulates in bloody areas as well as in large congested vessels. It occurs with acidic formalin fixation.[229] It has a crystalline structure that is birefringent. Although neurologic manifestations are seen in some types of *porphyrias*, with the exception of a rare case report,[231] typically no specific morphologic findings, including pigment accumulation, have been identified in the CNS, except for chromatolytic neurons.[17] The inherent instinct in the surgical pathology laboratory to ink specimens may result in various colors around the tissue sections when applied to brain biopsy tissue. It is actually a good idea to selectively ink the surfaces of small biopsy samples, so that the tissue is not inadvertently trimmed away while the paraffin block is being faced and levels are being obtained in the histology laboratory.

White Matter Changes and Myelin Loss

Myelin loss simply refers to the absence of myelin and does not specify *demyelination*, which is the loss of already formed intact myelin, or *dysmyelination*, which is the myelin loss due to the

List of Findings/Checklist for White Matter Changes and Myelin Loss

AT A GLANCE

- Myelin loss
  - Demyelination
  - Dysmyelination
  - Myelin pallor
  - White matter vacuolation
- Multiple Sclerosis
  - Active lesion
  - Chronic lesion
  - Classical (Charcot) type
  - "Variants"
  - Tumefactive demyelination
- Progressive multifocal leukoencephalopathy
- Subacute sclerosing panencephalitis
- Varicella-zoster virus infection
- Lymphoma sentinel lesion
- Osmotic demyelination syndrome
  - Central pontine myelinolysis
  - Extrapontine myelinolysis
- Marchiafava-Bignami disease
- Treated lymphoma
- Langerhans cell histiocytosis
- Leigh's disease
- Thiamine deficiency
- Acute disseminated encephalomyelitis
- Acute hemorrhagic leukoencephalopathy
- HIV encephalitis
- Fat embolism
- Arbovirus infections
- Mumps
- Leukodystrophies
- Storage diseases
- Lysosomal and peroxisomal disorders
- Carbon monoxide poisoning
- Subacute arteriosclerotic leukoencephalopathy
- Sequelae of previous lesions
- Panencephalopathic Creutzfeldt-Jakob disease
- Therapy-induced leukoencephalopathy
- Neuroaxonal dystrophies
- Nasu-Hakola disease
- Menkes disease
- Periventricular leukomalacia/perinatal telencephalic leukoencephalopathy
- Hypomyelinated state of normal developmental
- Vacuolar myelopathy
- Subacute combined degeneration
- HTLV-1-associated myelopathy
- Tabes dorsalis
- Hypermyelination
  - Etat fibromyelinique
  - Status marmoratus

defective formation or breakdown of the myelin that is defective from the beginning, as in leukodystrophies. Myelin can be lost secondary to other processes such as in an infarct; however, this type of situation is not considered a myelin problem and is not discussed here. Therefore, in an area with myelin loss, it is important to identify the process as one of primary myelin problem or a secondary myelin loss. Also important is to note that, with some subtle differences in some processes, it is not possible to identify the disease entity simply by microscopic examination. The identification of myelin loss should then be interpreted in the context of location, pattern, distribution, and clinical features.

The prototype demyelinating disease is *multiple sclerosis (MS)*[232] **(Table 2-14)**, where demyelination occurs as a result of autoimmune attack. The lesion is sharply demarcated from the surrounding tissue. The lesion, called a plaque, is seen on routine sections as a pale eosinophilic area and the adjacent tissues are bright eosinophilic just like how the normal white matter is seen. By a myelin stain such as LFB, the loss of myelin and the sharp demarcation of the lesion become more obvious. In the acute stage, the lesion is cellular with a prominent lymphohistiocytic infiltrate **(Fig. 2-99)**. Histiocytes have blue-staining myelin debris that they have ingested and are called *gitter cells* **(Fig. 2-100)**. In later stages of demyelinating conditions, this myelin debris assumes a PAS-positive quality. Small T lymphocytes are scattered throughout the lesion and also form perivascular infiltrates along with some histiocytes. In spite of this busy and destructive appearance of the lesion, a stain for axons,

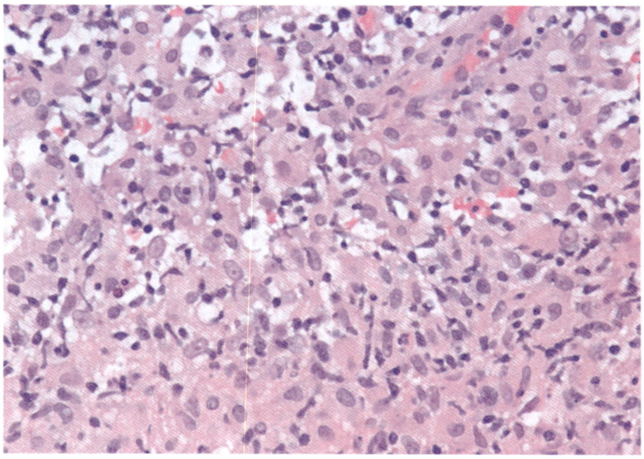

Figure 2-99. Demyelinating lesion: Numerous histiocytes and admixed lymphocytes create an inflammatory picture and may mimic a neoplastic process due to high cellularity and irregular nuclei of histiocytes (H&E; original magnification: 400×).

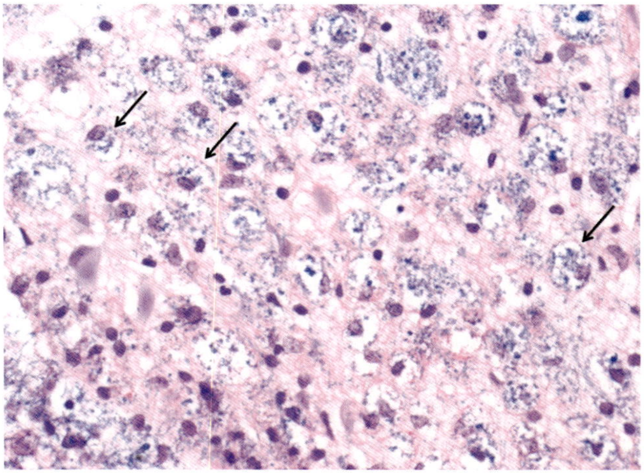

Figure 2-100. Gitter cells: Cytoplasmic myelin debris in the histiocytes is seen as blue granules (*arrows*) in the acute stage of demyelination and becomes mainly PAS positive as it is degraded in later stages. No myelin is left in the background due to demyelination (LFB/PAS/CV; original magnification: 400×).

TABLE 2.14 Diseases with unifocal or multifocal myelin loss

Immunologic
Multiple sclerosis
Tumefactive demyelination
Neoplasm-Associated
Sentinel lesion preceeding lymphoma
Treated lymphoma
Recurrent Langerhans cell histiocytosis–associated demyelination
Therapy-induced leukoencephalopathy
Infectious
PML
SSPE
VZV infection
HAART-associated demyelination
Metabolic
Osmotic demyelination syndrome
Central pontine myelinolysis
Extrapontine myelinolysis
Marchiafava-Bignami disease
Thiamine deficiency
Wernicke's encephalopathy
Korsakoff syndrome

HAART, highly active antiretroviral therapy.

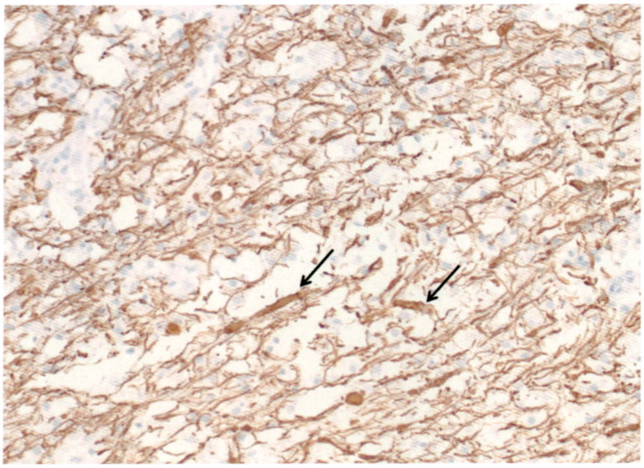

Figure 2-101. Relative preservation of axons: There may be some degree of axon loss and some of the remaining ones may show dystrophic changes in the form of irregularities and swellings (*arrows*), but the axons are preserved relative to the degree of myelin loss (neurofilament immunohistochemistry; original magnification: 200×).

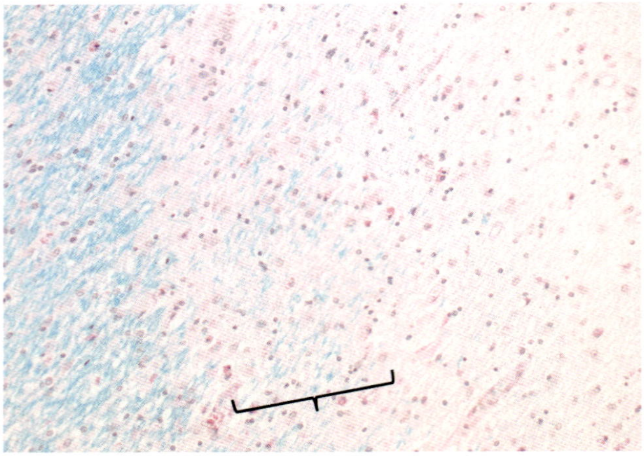

Figure 2-102. Shadow plaque: In long-standing chronic plaques, remyelination starts from the periphery of the lesion, using the preexisting axons as a template. This newly formed myelin is relatively pale and thin and can be seen as a separate zone (*bracket*) between the lesion (**right side**) and the surrounding unaffected parenchyma (**left side**) (LFB/PAS/CV; original magnification: 200×).

such as Bielschowsky silver stain or neurofilament immunohistochemistry, shows a remarkable preservation of axons, though they may be reduced in number and some may be distorted **(Fig. 2-101)**. As the plaque becomes chronic, reactive astrocytes start to appear, while the inflammation subsides. Meanwhile, a regenerative attempt to remyelinate the lesion starts with the ingrowth of regenerating myelin from the periphery of the lesion, following the remaining axons. This myelin is relatively pale and thin **(Fig. 2-102)**. This remyelination corresponds to the shadow plaque. Eventually, the inflammation essentially entirely disappears and a pale gliotic area remains. Even at this stage, many intact axons can be demonstrated in the plaque, even though there has been significant axon loss due to the degeneration of axons that were devoid of their myelin sheaths. Therefore, a key phrase in the description of demyelinating lesions in general is "myelin loss with relative preservation of axons." This is in contrast to complete loss of axons in addition to myelin loss seen in infarcts. For this reason, performing concurrent stains for the evaluation of myelin and axons is useful in the evaluation of pale, focal lesions with histiocytic infiltrates, especially in small biopsy specimens. Such demyelinating lesions can mimic neoplasms clinically and radiologically and can be biopsied with an IOC request. Another pitfall is the *tumefactive demyelination* (tumefactive MS; demyelinating pseudotumor),[233] presenting as a single mass lesion in the brain, mimicking a neoplastic process. The edema it induces and the ring enhancement complicate the situation further. The enhancement is in the form of an incomplete, C-shaped ring, with the open side pointing toward the cortex. A stereotactic biopsy with IOC request reveals a cellular lesion. If the inflammatory nature of the lesion and the presence of macrophages are not appreciated, an erroneous diagnosis of glial neoplasm may be rendered. Sharp demarcation of this type of lesion is helpful, in contrast to the ill-defined and infiltrative nature of a glial neoplasm **(Fig. 2-103)**. Many of these cases presenting as a mass lesion progress to become typical MS over time. Demyelinating lesions are predominantly in the white matter, but gray matter is not immune and it is not unusual to have demyelinating lesions involving the cortex and deep gray matter areas. Optic nerves and spinal cord are also commonly involved. In the spinal cord, extensive involvement by active demyelinating plaques may induce secondary ischemic changes due to edema and swelling, compromising circulation. In such cases, depending on the severity and stage of the process, evidence of acute neuronal injury in the form of eosinophilic neuronal necrosis or overt infarcts can be seen. This condition may further interfere with the accurate diagnosis, especially in necessarily small tissue samples from the spinal

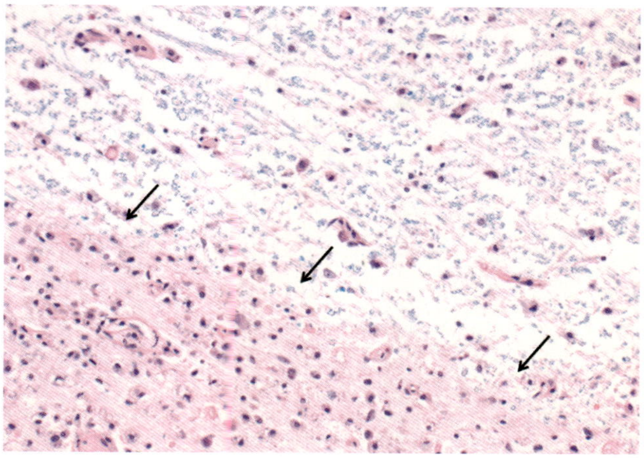

Figure 2-103. Sharp border of demyelinating lesion (*arrows*) is seen between the myelinated unaffected parenchyma (**top**) and the lesion devoid of myelin (**bottom**) (H&E; original magnification: 200×).

cord, as the differential diagnosis is between demyelination and infarct to start with.

The typical MS is termed *classical MS* or *Charcot type MS* there are a number of so-called MS variants that are based on clinical, pathologic, radiologic, and molecular features.[232] Some, such as primary progressive MS, are not well-defined clinical entities; however, others, mostly considered acute MS variants, are better established. Whether they are truly variants of MS are also debatable. *Concentric sclerosis (of Balo)* is characterized by large plaques with a peculiar circular or concentric myelinated and demyelinated layer pattern. They may show central necrosis, but their cellular composition is similar to classical MS plaque. In *Schilder disease (myelinoclastic diffuse sclerosis)*, histologic appearance is similar to the typical active MS plaque, but the lesions are large and confluent, sometimes with involvement of an entire hemisphere, rather than multiple plaques. In that regard, it may resemble a leukodystrophy; however, the U-fibers are involved, at least focally (see below). *Marburg disease (acute MS)*, not to be confused with the acute stage of classical MS, is histologically similar to the acute plaques of MS; however, the clinical course is rapidly progressive and may result in death within months. *Concentric lacunar leukoencephalopathy*[234] has a concentric laminated arrangement of its lesions, similar to concentric sclerosis of Balo, except that there is prominent axon loss and the layers are formed by bands of necrosis and demyelination **(Table 2.15)**.

TABLE 2.15 Diseases associated with myelin loss and a necrotic component

Concentric lacunar leukoencephalopathy
Acute necrotizing myelopathy
Neuromyelitis optica (Devic's disease)
Leigh's disease
Therapy-induced leukoencephalopathy
Periventricular leukomalacia

Acute necrotizing myelopathy is characterized by an isolated necrotic lesion of the spinal cord and a relapsing clinical course.[235] *Devic disease (neuromyelitis optica)* is the type that is most controversial as an "MS variant"[236] and is considered as a separate entity. The lesions are of necrotic nature and involve exclusively the optic nerves and spinal cord, where they are typically central, involving both gray and white matter. Only occasional cases have typical MS lesions in other areas of the CNS parenchyma. The inflammatory infiltrate in the lesions of neuromyelitis optica also contains neutrophil and eosinophil PMN leukocytes.

Progressive multifocal leukoencephalopathy (PML) has multiple predominantly periventricular white matter demyelinating lesions.[237] In addition to the variable lymphohistiocytic infiltrate and sharply demarcated demyelination, there are reactive astrocytes that show prominent atypia due to viral cytopathic effect **(Fig. 2-104)**, which constitute a pitfall causing confusion with an astrocytic

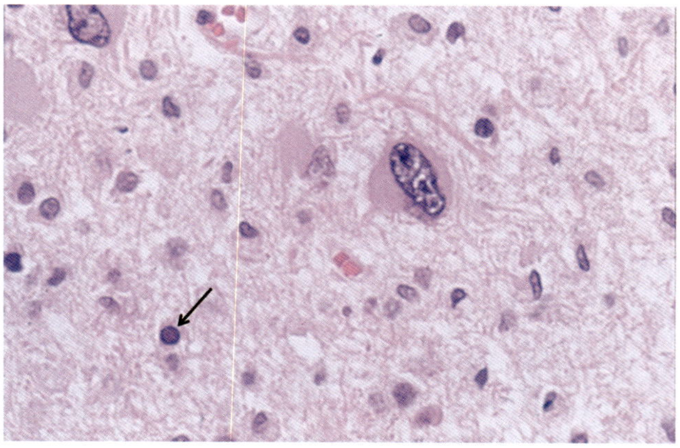

Figure 2-104. PML: An atypical astrocyte as a result of viral cytopathic effect is seen in a pale and rarified background of demyelination. A purple round nucleus (*arrow*) represents an oligodendroglial nucleus with viral inclusion (H&E; original magnification: 400×).

neoplasm, especially in small biopsies that are interpreted out of clinical context of immunosuppression. In addition, there are enlarged, plum-colored ground-glass oligodendroglial nuclei due to the presence of intranuclear viral inclusions filling up the nucleus. These should be specifically looked for but may be difficult or impossible to find as they are usually present at the periphery of the demyelinating lesions and those areas may not always be sampled. In stereotactic biopsies, not only for PML but also in general for any type of lesion, examining the borders of the lesion can provide important clues to the diagnosis. Therefore, if at all possible, tissue representing the border of the lesion should be requested at the time of IOC during these procedures. *SSPE* is another viral infection that can cause extensive demyelination, as well as neuronal degeneration. Dark eosinophilic-to-amphophilic inclusions in the enlarged nuclei of oligodendroglia and neurons result in a ground-glass appearance with margination of the chromatin.[238,239] *Varicella-zoster virus (VZV) infection*[240] may produce patchy, subtle, multifocal white matter lesions with myelin pallor and ischemic features, as oligodendroglia are infected and there is damage to small, medium, or large vessels. The latter may result in hemorrhagic necrotic lesions, similar to Herpes virus infection. *Lymphoma* that has been previously treated with corticosteroids may appear as acute demyelination on biopsy. Lymphoma responds to corticosteroid treatment dramatically and the malignant cells become essentially impossible to find. Only a reactive population of small, round, reactive T cells, macrophages, and reactive astrocytes and myelin loss mimic the active MS plaque or, more likely in single mass lesions, tumefactive MS. These cases recur as lymphomas and eventually declare their true nature. In addition, some cases of primary CNS lymphoma are apparently preceded by a demyelinating lesion and have no indication of lymphoma. They have been termed *"sentinel lesion"* and their nature is identified in retrospect when eventually lymphoma presents itself at a future time[241] **(Fig. 2-105)**. *Osmotic demyelination syndrome* (central pontine and extrapontine myelinolysis)[242] typically occurs due to rapid correction of hyponatremia, resulting in demyelination in the center of basis pontis **(Fig. 2-106)**. It is also seen in association with conditions that may interfere with electrolyte balance, such as alcoholism, diabetes mellitus, and malnutrition. The lesion has a characteristic butterfly shape, but this is highly variable depending on the extent of the lesion. In general, there is demyelination with relative preservation of axons and many macrophages and only minimal, if any, lymphocytic infiltrate. The cell bodies of the neurons of pontine nuclei are also intact. Older lesions may resemble infarcts due to subsequent

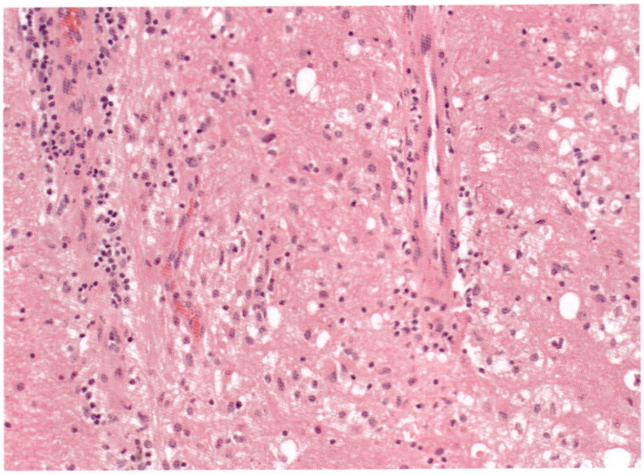

Figure 2-105. Sentinel lesion: A lesion (**bottom left**) with rarified and pale background due to myelin loss, perivascular lymphocytes, and reactive astrocytes and a sharp border with the surrounding parenchyma that has a darker eosinophilic background (**top right**) is seen. Subsequent biopsy revealed a lymphoma (H&E; original magnification: 200×).

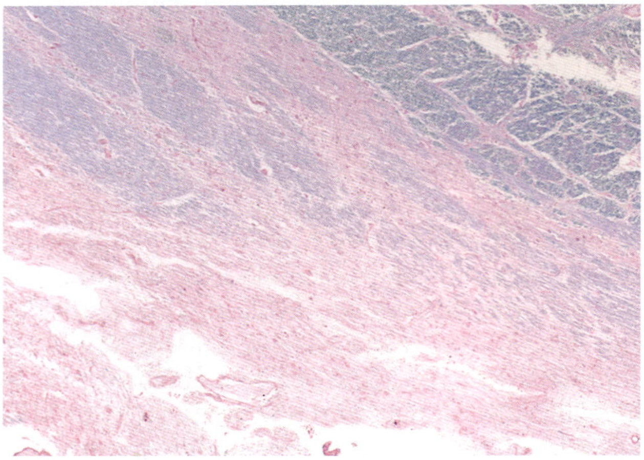

Figure 2-106. Central pontine myelinolysis: Prominent myelin loss is seen in pontine tracts (**bottom left**) where intact neurons can still be identified (LFB/PAS/CV; original magnification: 40×).

degeneration of axons and neuron cell bodies. Extrapontine lesions can coexist with or can occur without pontine involvement. They have a predilection for sites where there is intimate association of gray and white matter areas. Common extrapontine sites are internal, external, and extreme capsules; basal ganglia; thalamus; lateral geniculate body; gray–white matter junction; cerebral subcortical white matter; and cerebellum. When multiple, the lesions are at the same stage of development, in contrast to MS lesions, which tend to be at different stages at a given time. MS lesions involving the brainstem tend to be eccentric and asymmetric and have a connection with the surface. In addition, the inflammatory component is not present or very subtle in osmotic demyelination compared to MS. *Marchiafava-Bignami disease* is characterized by demyelinating lesions of the corpus callosum, associated with chronic alcoholism with or without malnutrition.[243] The lesions tend to be central in the corpus callosum surrounded by intact tissue. They are predominantly in the genu and body of the corpus callosum. They may be composed of demyelination and necrosis and may result in cavitation in older lesions. In addition to typical demyelination, there are many macrophages especially in the early stages with essentially no lymphocytic infiltrate. A peculiar hyalinization and proliferation of small vessels can also be present. Sometimes, there is also involvement of anterior and posterior commissures, optic chiasm, and middle cerebellar peduncles. It may also be accompanied by striatal necrosis and with Morel's laminar sclerosis in some cases.[244,245] A rare situation that may be mistaken for a demyelinating disorder can be seen in *Langerhans cell histiocytosis*.[246,247] The demyelination is the predominant feature, while the Langerhans cell population is scarce. The lesions may have a predilection for cerebellum, may precede the presentation, may be primary demyelination, or may be secondary to axonal degeneration. Since this situation tends to arise as a late recurrence, the previous history may not be available or may appear unrelated, resulting in a potential pitfall. *Leigh's disease (subacute necrotizing encephalomyelopathy)* has multiple symmetrical and typically vasculocentric lesions. They may be at different stages of development at a given time. Early stages are rich in macrophages with eosinophilic neuronal necrosis in an edematous background, resembling an infarct. Midstage

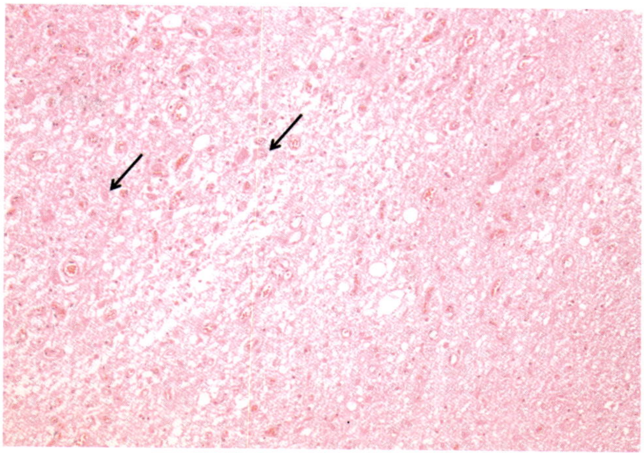

Figure 2-107. Leigh's disease: This basal ganglionic lesion shows a pale and rarified neuropil due to loss of myelin (**left side**). Neurons (*arrows*) are intact within the lesion, which has a sharp border with the surrounding parenchyma (**right side**) (H&E; original magnification: 100×).

is the most typical with associated gliosis, macrophages, prominent capillaries with congestion, and collapsed neuropil with a few residual neurons **(Fig. 2-107)**. Striatum, subthalamic nucleus, substantia nigra, inferior olives, and brainstem tegmentum are typically involved. Cerebellar degeneration is commonly present. Periventricular white matter, optic nerves, spinal cord, and cerebellar white matter may have vacuolation and myelin loss. *Thiamine deficiency*[243] results in Wernicke's encephalopathy and Korsakoff psychosis characterized by lesions that resemble the lesions of Leigh's disease located in the mammillary bodies, hypothalamus, medial thalamic nuclei, periaqueductal region, and floor of the fourth ventricle. Medial thalamic nuclei are also additionally involved in Korsakoff psychosis. The lesions are commonly associated with, but not necessarily limited to, chronic alcoholism. Gastrointestinal disorders and total parenteral nutrition are other common conditions that can result in thiamin deficiency. Microscopically, tissue necrosis sparing neurons, petechiae, prominent capillaries with endothelial hyperplasia, and perivascular macrophages are seen in the acute stage. Reactive astrocytes, mild neuron loss, vacuolation, and myelinated fiber loss are seen later **(Fig. 2-108)**. Both Leigh's disease and thiamine deficiency lesions can closely resemble a demyelinating process if taken in isolation out of their clinical context and typical distribution.

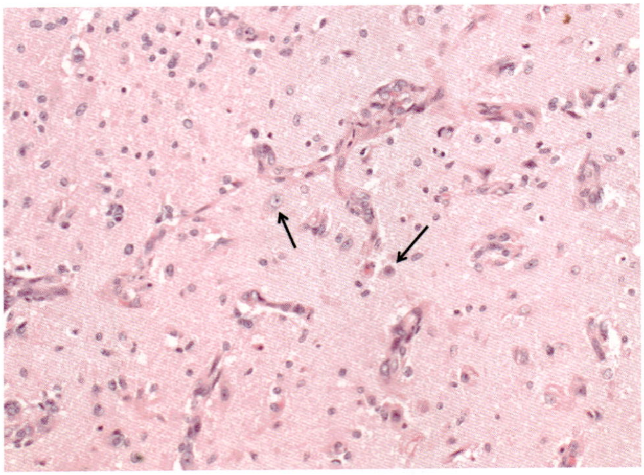

Figure 2-108. Wernicke's encephalopathy: Mammillary body parenchyma is pale and has a shrunken appearance. Neurons are present (*arrows*) and vessels are prominent (H&E; original magnification: 200×).

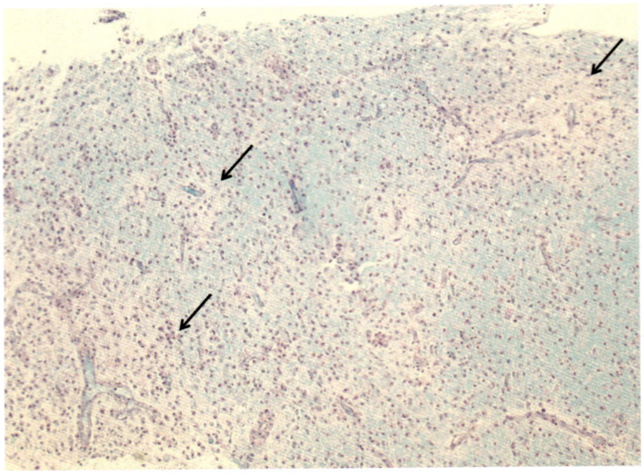

Figure 2-109. Acute demyelinating encephalomyelitis: Myelin loss is centered around the vessels as pale areas (*arrows*) (LFB/PAS/CV; original magnification: 100×).

Acute disseminated encephalomyelitis (ADEM), also known as perivenous encephalomyelitis and postinfectious encephalomyelitis, occurs after several weeks of an infection or vaccination, suggesting a cross immunity, although many cases may not have this history. Demyelination has a multifocal perivenous pattern **(Table 2.16)** and is associated with a perivascular lymphohistiocytic infiltrate with scattered plasma cells **(Fig. 2-109)**. One caveat, especially in small tissue samples obtained to evaluate the plaques in MS, is that, if the tissue samples represent the periphery of the MS plaque, as in a tangential sampling by stereotactic biopsy, the perivascular extensions of the MS plaque, that is, Dawson's fingers, may mimic ADEM **(Fig. 2-110)**. Therefore, it is important to interpret the microscopic findings in the context of clinical and radiologic features. A related condition, *acute hemorrhagic leukoencephalopathy (AHL)* or acute hemorrhagic and necrotizing leukoencephalopathy, is also preceded by an infection in many cases. It is also multifocal but its lesions consist of small vessels with fibrinoid necrosis, surrounding necrosis and hemorrhage. The circular perivascular pattern of hemorrhage is termed ring- and ball-shaped

TABLE 2.16 Diseases associated with perivascular myelin loss

Acute demyelinating encephalomyelitis
Acute hemorrhagic leukoencephalitis (AHL)
Periphery of multiple sclerosis plaques (Dawson's fingers)
HIV encephalitis
Fat embolism
Arbovirus infections
Mumps
Leigh's disease

HIV, human immunodeficiency virus.

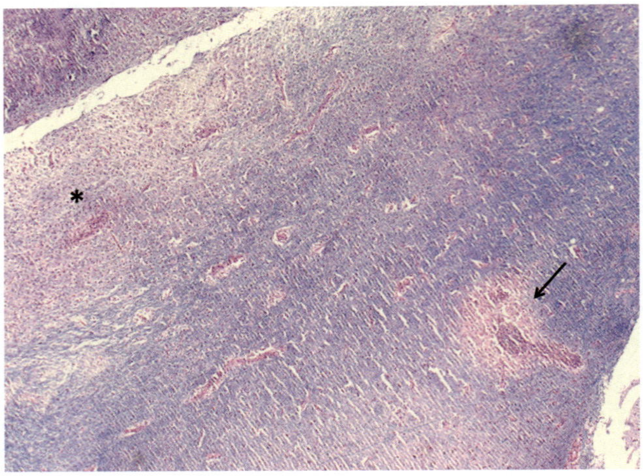

Figure 2-110. Dawson's fingers: In multiple sclerosis lesions, demyelination may extend from the well-defined main lesion (*asterisk*) toward the periphery along the vessels (*arrow*), creating a pitfall for acute demyelinating encephalomyelitis in tangential biopsy samples (LFB/PAS/CV; original magnification: 40×).

hemorrhage. Some vessels may be intact with a perivascular inflammatory infiltrate composed of neutrophil PMN leukocytes and lymphocytes, along with demyelination. Due to the perivascular tissue destruction there is associated axon damage, identified as axon loss by axon stains, such as Bielschowsky, Bodian, or neurofilament, as well as axonal spheroids at the edge of the lesions; however, there is relative preservation of axons compared to the severity of myelin loss. In some cases of *HIV encephalitis*, the myelin loss can be diffuse or predominantly perivascular, mimicking ADEM or AHL; however, although there may be some lymphocytic infiltrate, vascular and axonal damage are not features of HIV encephalitis. In addition, there is a prominent, mainly perivascular multinucleated giant cell infiltrate that shows positivity for HIV antigens. Microglial nodules are also present. Variable degrees of white matter atrophy can be seen in patients who survive *fat embolism*. However, the typical lesions in the acute stage include perivascular myelin loss and axonal degeneration, together with axonal spheroids, which may progress to overt microinfarcts. Lack of inflammation and vascular damage help differentiate it from ADEM/AHL. Clear, round fat globule spaces pushing the erythrocytes aside within the blood vessels are left by the fat globules dissolved during processing **(Fig. 2-111)**. Oil red O stain can be performed on frozen tissue if this condition was suspected grossly and frozen

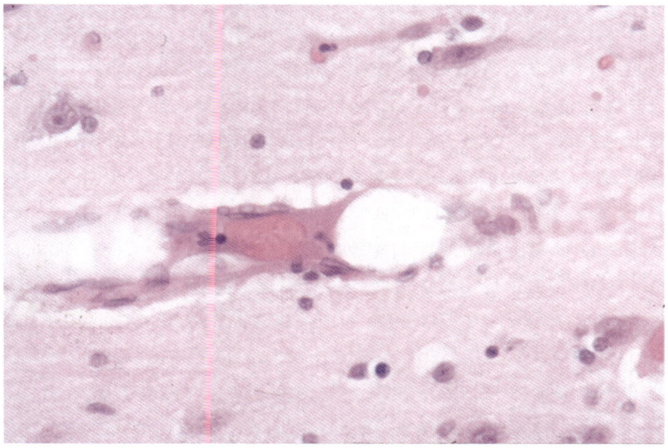

Figure 2-111. Fat embolism: A round vacuole is present in the lumen of this capillary, pushing the erythrocytes and fibrin aside and expanding the vessel (H&E; original magnification: 400×).

TABLE 2.17 Conditions characterized by diffuse absence of myelin

Leukodystrophies
Storage diseases
Lysosomal and peroxisomal disorders
Neuroaxonal dystrophies
Nasu-Hakola disease
Menkes disease
HIV encephalitis
Panencephalopathic Creutzfeldt-Jakob disease
Neurodegenerative diseases
Subacute arteriosclerotic leukoencephalopathy (Binswanger's disease)
Perinatal telencephalic leukoencephalopathy
Carbon monoxide poisoning
Therapy-induced leukoencephalopathy
Normal developmental stage

HIV, human immunodeficiency virus.

tissue was saved. *Arboviruses* tend to more prominently involve the brainstem, thalamus, and basal ganglia, and some also additionally involve the spinal cord, such as West Nile virus and Japanese encephalitis. In addition to typical encephalitis picture, they may also cause perivascular hemorrhages and perivascular destruction of myelinated fibers, reminiscent of ADEM. *Mumps* can result in transverse myelitis, as well as a picture reminiscent of ADEM.[17]

Leukodystrophies are inborn errors of metabolism, are usually seen in pediatric population, although many have adult forms, and involve the white matter diffusely **(Table 2.17)**. There may be subtle variations in this diffuse involvement pattern in some diseases. For instance, adrenoleukodystrophy predominantly involves the occipital lobes. Another common feature of leukodystrophies is the sparing of the U-fibers that lie in the superficial, subcortical white matter. Some leukodystrophies have distinguishing microscopic features. For instance, in globoid cell leukodystrophy (Krabbe's disease), many histiocytes with intracytoplasmic PAS-positive material are seen throughout the white matter but with a preferential accumulation around the vessels **(Fig. 2-112)**. In metachromatic leukodystrophy, the metachromatic sulfatide accumulation seen by toluidine blue stain is in the macrophages, and in the Schwann cells in the peripheral nerve.

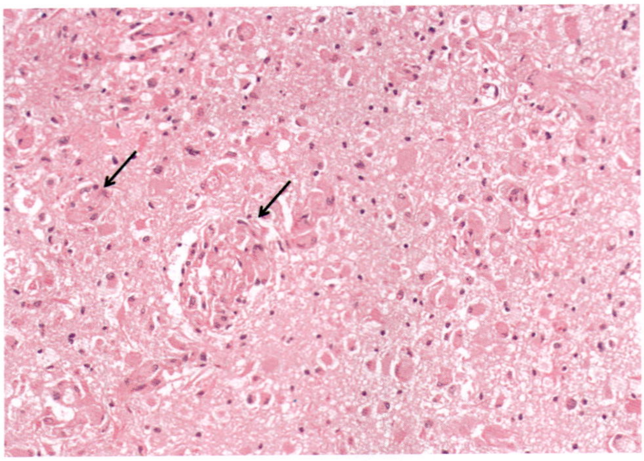

Figure 2-112. Krabbe's disease (globoid cell leukodystrophy): Many macrophages are present in the white matter, with a tendency to aggregate around the vessels (*arrows*). The neuropil is pale and rarified due to myelin loss (H&E; original magnification: 200×).

In adrenoleukodystrophy, needle-shaped spaces can be identified in the cytoplasm of histiocytes and there are perivascular lymphocytic infiltrates **(Fig. 2-113)**. Prominent descending tract involvement is seen in adrenomyeloneuropathy. The common denominator of all is a diffuse myelin loss with sparing of the U-fibers. Even though the primary process is a leukodystrophy, eventually axonal degeneration accompanies the severe myelin loss. The definitive diagnosis of this group of diseases is biochemical testing of fresh tissue and genetic testing, underscoring the advance planning for tissue allocation in correlation with all the findings. Alexander's disease is characterized by numerous Rosenthal fibers in perivascular and subpial areas and in a background of myelin loss. Canavan's disease is characterized by extensive vacuolation in the white matter with myelin loss. The subcortical U-fibers are not spared. Alzheimer type II glia are also present. In Pelizaeus-Merzbacher disease, there is discontinuous myelin loss with relative sparing of perivascular myelin, resulting in a *tigroid pattern*. Peripheral nerves are spared and this can also be seen dramatically and grossly in spinal cord examination, with white nerves contrasting with dusky and shrunken cord. Cerebellar degeneration is common. Cockayne disease has discontinuous myelin loss, as well as calcifications around vessels in cortex and basal ganglia. A number of leukodystrophies are termed OLDs based on the positivity on frozen sections of the lipid debris within the macrophages for Sudan stains. They are further characterized based on additional features, mainly in a descriptive manner.[17] OLD, not otherwise specified, even with biochemical, clinical, and morphologic/electron microscopic means, simply has Sudan-positive macrophages. OLD with calcification (Aicardi-Goutieres leukoencephalopathy) in addition has calcifications in the white matter and basal ganglia. OLD with meningeal angiomatosis is associated with increased vascularity in the leptomeninges. OLD with cavitation and oligodendroglial proliferation shows massive cavities and increased numbers of oligodendroglia. This oligodendroglial crowding should not be interpreted as inflammation. OLD with pigmented glia and macrophages has accumulations in glia, as well as in macrophages, which are also positive by Perls (Prussian) blue stain and Fontana-Masson stain. The pigment is mostly composed of lipofuscin, and grossly, the white matter has a greenish hue due to this accumulation. Myelin loss, white matter pallor, and gliosis are commonly seen in *storage diseases and lysosomal and peroxisomal disorders*, along with their more characteristic features. GM1 and GM2 gangliosidoses, Niemann-Pick disease, Batten's disease (neuronal ceroid lipofuscinosis), Gaucher's disease, mannosidosis, fucosidosis, Zellweger syndrome (cerebrohepatorenal syndrome), and pseudo-Zellweger

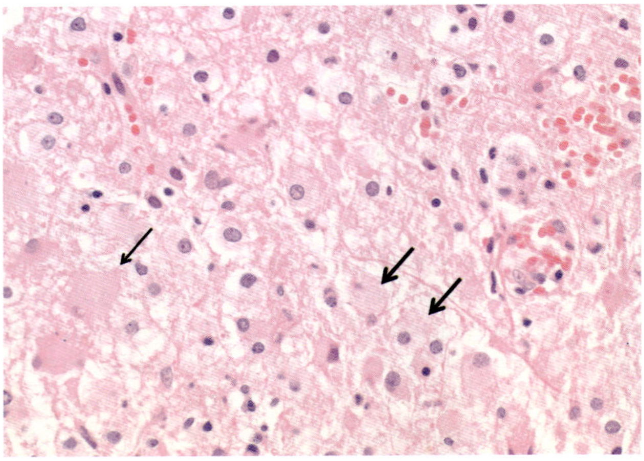

Figure 2-113. Adrenoleukodystrophy: White matter is pale and rarified, with a busy appearance due to reactive astrocytes (*thin arrow*) and pale macrophages (*thick arrows*) (H&E; original magnification: 400×).

syndrome (which has similar pathologic features while peroxisomes are present in the liver) are some prominent examples that are associated with diffuse myelin loss. Myelin components that accumulate within the neuron cytoplasm can be shown by LFB stain in Batten's disease and GM2 gangliosidosis.

A mild and subtle myelin loss can be present in large areas of white matter with gradual transition from normal to abnormal areas. This can be seen on routine sections and by a myelin stain as pale areas and is termed *myelin pallor*. Such a picture is seen in *HIV encephalitis*.[237] There is diffuse myelin pallor and macrophages may be rare. In addition, a demyelinating process with severe inflammation can be seen in AIDS patients receiving highly active antiretroviral therapy (HAART), mimicking acute MS lesion.[248] Immunohistochemical stains for HIV can help accurately identify such lesions; however, a high degree of suspicion incorporating the clinical context is needed in such cases. Multifocal or diffuse myelin pallor can also be a feature of *carbon monoxide poisoning*, in addition to its other and more typical features, as may be seen depending on the length of survival, such as necrosis and/or hemorrhage due to anoxic/ischemic damage in the areas involved, and subsequent macrophage infiltration with eventual cavitation. There is preservation of U-fibers in diffuse demyelinating-type lesions where there is extensive and confluent involvement of the white matter, also known as Grinker's disease or Grinker's myelinopathy.[83] Diffuse myelin pallor with white matter volume loss and small vessel disease, usually associated with dementia, is seen in *subcortical arteriosclerotic leukoencephalopathy (Binswanger disease or Binswanger encephalopathy)*. Similar findings can be seen in association with *neurodegenerative diseases*, such as AD, and likely represent coexisting vascular disease. Small vessel disease is seen as hyaline arteriosclerosis and arteriolosclerosis and consists of collagenized thickening of vessel walls. Hypertension and diabetes mellitus are usually present. White matter has ischemia with a collapsed and pitted appearance and associated ventricular dilation. Virchow-Robin spaces are dilated, resulting in etat crible. There is myelin pallor, gliosis, and axon loss. Widespread sampling, especially of deep white matter, is needed, as subcortical white matter is usually preserved. Myelin pallor later in life can be seen as a *sequela of previous white matter lesions* such as perinatal telencephalic leukoencephalopathy/periventricular leukomalacia or DAI in its chronic stage, especially after a few months postinjury. In *panencephalopathic CJD*, there is extensive and diffuse involvement of entire brain, including white matter, resulting in extensive myelin loss, pallor, and cavitation.[249] Spongiform change, neuron loss, and gliosis are present in cortical and deep gray matter areas, as well as in the cerebellar cortex. Such an appearance in the white matter may mimic a leukodystrophy, especially since panencephalopathic CJD also contains lipid-laden macrophages in the white matter; however, additional findings such as spongiform change and the recent history of rapidly progressive dementia are useful in favoring CJD. *Chemotherapy-induced leukoencephalopathy* is typically attributed to methotrexate as it is the best known chemotherapeutic agent associated with this process, especially with intrathecal administration, in which case, the lesions tend to be periventricular; however, other chemotherapeutic agents can also cause this leukoencephalopathy, for example, 5-fluorouracil (5-FU), which can also result in significant inflammatory reaction, alone or in combination with radiation treatment.[250–252] A more descriptive term for this condition is *diffuse necrotizing leukoencephalopathy*, although the leukoencephalopathy is not always diffuse or necrotic. A similar picture can be seen after radiation treatment alone. The leukoencephalopathy is characterized by variable degrees and extent of myelin and axon loss, vacuolation of neuropil, focal infarcts, axonal fragmentation and spheroids, and microcalcifications **(Fig. 2-114)**. White matter is gliotic and shrunken in later stages. There may be fibrinoid necrosis of vessel walls, which may result in hemorrhagic infarcts.[253] Vessel wall calcifications can be seen and are most prominent in basal ganglia. This process tends to resemble an infarct rather than a demyelinating lesion in its full-blown microscopic picture; however, early and subtle lesions may mimic demyelination. Spinal cord can also be involved. Myelin pallor and degeneration in cerebral and cerebellar white matter can be a feature of *infantile neuroaxonal dystrophy*[17]; U-fibers are spared. *Neuroaxonal leukodystrophy*[254] also results in similar changes with prominent myelin loss and gliosis in the white matter and distal degeneration of corticospinal and posterior columns. U-fibers

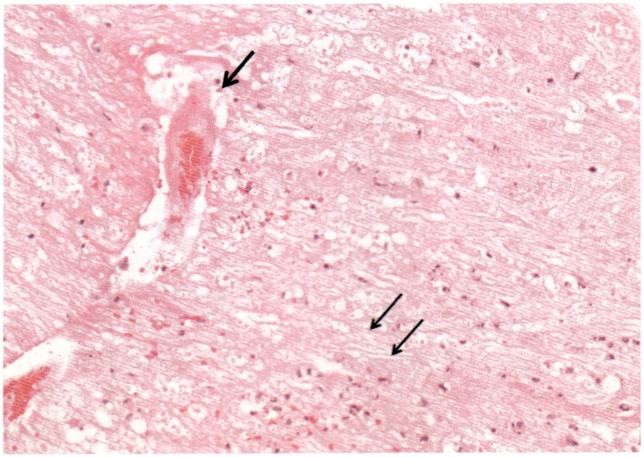

Figure 2-114. Necrotizing leukoencephalopathy: White matter is necrotic; however, linear outlines of axons can still be identified (*thin arrows*) and can be further highlighted by special studies, such as neurofilament immunohistochemistry. Vessel wall shows fibrinoid necrosis (*thick arrow*). No significant inflammation is present (H&E; original magnification: 200×).

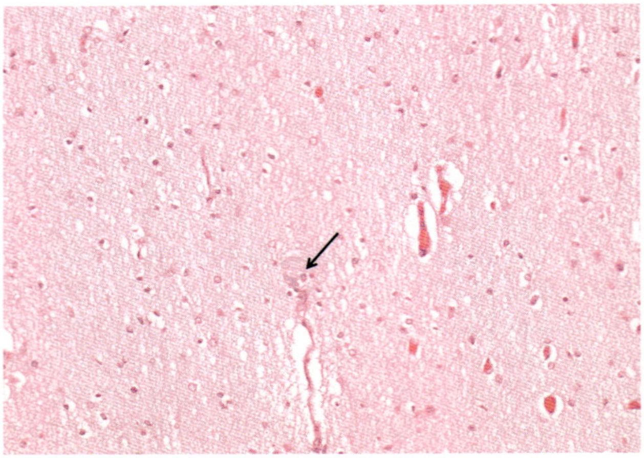

Figure 2-115. Perinatal telencephalic leukoencephalopathy: White matter is pale and rarified with a lacy and microvacuolated appearance in this remote case. An ill-defined mulberry is present next to a capillary (*arrow*) (H&E; original magnification: 200×).

are spared. Myelin pallor in white matter can be seen in neurodegenerative diseases, especially in advanced stages due to degeneration of neurons and their axons. For instance, in CBD, there can be myelinated fiber loss in cerebral white matter under the affected cortex and sometimes in corticospinal tracts. White matter can be rarified and gliotic in FTLD and in progressive subcortical gliosis. *Nasu-Hakola disease* (polycystic lipomembranous osteodysplasia with sclerosing leukoencephalopathy) is also associated with myelinated fiber loss from cerebral white matter, with sparing of U-fibers.[255] In cases of *hypoplasia or dysplasia of dentate and olivary nuclei*, the thick, dark, and dense myelinated fiber sheath around these nuclei is diminished. Myelin pallor can be seen in cases of reversible posterior leukoencephalopathy syndrome[256] as a result of tissue edema, although the detailed neuropathologic findings are not available in this mainly clinicoradiologic entity. In addition, it is not always reversible or necessarily posterior or limited to white matter. Nonetheless, an association with hypertension, chemotherapeutic agents including methotrexate, and high-dose corticosteroids has been noted. Neuron and myelin loss can be prominent in the temporal cortex and hippocampus in *Menkes (kinky hair) disease*,[257] in addition to its cerebellar atrophy with degenerations and changes in internal granule cells and Purkinje cells.

Periventricular leukomalacia results in destructive lesions[258] along with decreased myelination in the periventricular white matter and in internal capsule. In subtle cases, in addition to showing the decreased myelination, LFB/PAS stain outlines the lesion better as a pale center and increased staining at the edges, due to PAS-positive debris in the macrophages around the lesion, or as a patch if there are sheets of many macrophages. Perinatal telencephalic leukoencephalopathy,[259] a term sometimes used interchangeably with periventricular leukomalacia, but preferably referring more to those lesions without cavitation and tissue destruction, but rather with diffuse gliosis, white matter rarification and decreased myelin, and scattered mulberries, also shows myelin pallor **(Fig. 2-115)**. Myelin can normally be identified microscopically by myelin stains in the deep and intermediate white matter in about 1 month of age and in the subcortical white matter in about 2 months of age.[55] Therefore, the *normal hypomyelinated state* of the white matter can create confusion in the interpretation of these pediatric cases **(Fig. 2-116)**. Sequential myelination starts in different areas of the brain and is associated with myelination glia, which closely resemble reactive astrocytes in a background of pale myelin. Searching for other features of periventricular white matter injury, such as mulberries, microcalcifications, macrophages, cavitation, and mineralization, helps distinguish the pathologic cases. There may also be additional findings attributable

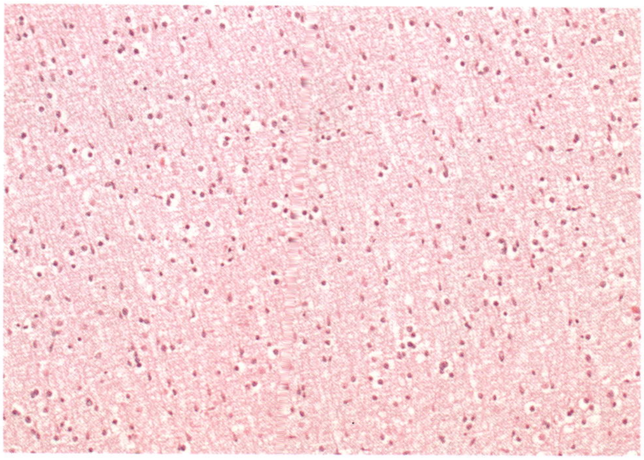

Figure 2-116. Fetal brain with hypomyelination: White matter is normally pale, and an orderly alignment of glial cell processes and axons can be seen. No other findings, such as calcifications, histiocytes, or reactive astrocytes, to indicate a previous injury are seen. Myelin stain will also show pallor of white matter. Knowledge of the exact location of the tissue being examined and of age of the patient is important to avoid mistaking normal hypomyelinated state from a pathologic process (H&E; original magnification: 200×).

to hypoxic–ischemic injury in these cases, such as hemorrhages in germinal matrix and other areas.

White matter vacuolation and myelin loss mainly as a result of myelin edema and subsequent degeneration are associated with a variety of conditions. These range from intoxications to toxic effects of medications to infectious etiologies. Triethyltin,[260] hexachlorophene/hexachlorophane, lithium,[261] 5-FU (see above), mitochondrial encephalopathies, Canavan's disease, B_{12} deficiency, vacuolar myelopathy, and HAM are some prominent examples for myelin edema and vacuolation. Organic pentavalent arsenicals are present in insecticides and in some medications such as melarsoprol used to treat trypanosomiasis.[262] In addition to myelin loss, they may cause AHL with fibrinoid necrosis of white matter vessels and perivascular hemorrhages. Anterior horn cell chromatolysis and degeneration can be seen due peripheral neuropathy. Fluid accumulation in myelin sheaths occurs with triethyltin exposure,[83] while trimethyltin causes neuron loss from the hippocampus, basal ganglia, entorhinal cortex, and amygdala, with apoptotic destruction of neurons in CA3 and other limbic structures rather than such myelin vacuolation.[263] Hexachlorophene/hexachlorophane causes white matter vacuolation[264] due to myelin edema most prominently in the brainstem. Optic nerve, optic chiasm, and optic tract necrosis may occur.[17] Cyclosporine A[265] can result in white matter edema, especially in parietal and occipital lobes; vacuolation of subcortical white matter; foamy macrophage infiltration; as well as rare subarachnoid and parenchymal hemorrhages. Cytosine arabinoside[17] can cause cerebellar cortical degeneration, brainstem tegmental neuron degeneration, spinal motor neuron degeneration, perikaryal neurofilament accumulation, and white matter vacuolation that is prominent in the spinal cord. Cerebellar cortical and dentate nucleus degeneration and vacuolation of cerebellar white matter can be seen with lithium toxicity. In cases of so-called normal pressure hydrocephalus, or perhaps more appropriately termed intermittently [high-, raised-] pressure hydrocephalus, as there may be fluctuations in CSF pressure, there is ventricular dilation without evidence of cortical atrophy. In that regard, it is different from hydrocephalus ex vacuo. White matter appears to have been secondarily affected due to the increased pressure, though temporary. There may be periventricular white matter edema, rarification, myelin pallor, and gliosis, though no consistent pathologic changes have been identified, while some cases showed arachnoid fibrosis, suggesting interference with CSF circulation.[266] The white matter changes may result from the interference of increased pressure with perfusion of the parenchyma, as well as mechanical effect.[267]

White matter involvement in the spinal cord and the pattern of involvement are characteristic in some diseases. *Vacuolar myelopathy* associated with HIV infection and *subacute combined degeneration* of vitamin B_{12} deficiency involve posterior and lateral columns and are essentially histologically identical. Lower cervical and thoracic segments are more severely involved in these conditions. Shrunken posterior and lateral columns may be grossly seen. Initially, the myelin vacuolation is seen in dorsal columns. Lateral columns (corticospinal and spinocerebellar tracts) are involved in later stages. Axonal degeneration, macrophages, and gliosis eventually take place. In some cases, perivascular macrophages with demyelination and axon loss are seen in cerebral white matter and optic nerves. Vitamin B_{12} deficiency can be associated with gastrointestinal problems that interfere with its absorption, such as pernicious anemia, intestinal malabsorption, intestinal blind loops or diverticular disease with bacterial overgrowth, fish tapeworm infection, nitrous oxide abuse, folate deficiency, and methylation defects. *HTLV-1-associated myelopathy (HAM)*,[268] also known as tropical spastic paraparesis, is characterized by spinal cord atrophy and leptomeningeal and parenchymal vascular fibrosis. Especially the lower thoracic region is involved. Degeneration of anterior and, more prominently, lateral funiculi is involved, as well as posterior columns. As in vacuolar myelopathy and subacute combined degeneration, myelin degeneration is initially seen in these funiculi, while axonal degeneration and gliosis subsequently take place. *Adrenomyeloneuropathy* (see above "adrenoleukodystrophy") involves the gracile and lateral corticospinal tracts.[269] In *tabes dorsalis*, as part of the parenchymatous neurosyphilis in the tertiary stage of syphilis, there is degeneration of the posterior spinal nerve roots, dorsal root ganglia, and subsequent degeneration of the dorsal columns, which are shrunken and depleted of nerve fibers; however, this is due to the degeneration of axons and is not a myelin problem. There is also associated lymphocytic inflammation.

Exceptionally, excess and disorganized production of myelin can also be seen and is present typically in gray matter areas. *Hypermyelination* in cerebral cortex (etat fibromyelinique) is associated with glial scars after healing of hypoxic–ischemic damage during development. A similar lesion called status marmoratus (marbling), showing a mixture of gray matter with admixed linear hypermyelination areas, is seen in the thalamus and basal ganglia after the lesions damaging these areas.

Neuron Loss and Gliosis

Neuron loss and gliosis **(Fig. 2-117)** are nonspecific microscopic findings that correspond grossly to atrophy, especially as they apply to neurodegenerative diseases. In advanced stages of this atrophy, there may be prominent shrinkage, tan-light brown discoloration, and even cavitation of the affected areas. Any process that results in injury, for example, infarct, can be associated with neuron loss and gliosis as an end-stage manifestation of that injury; however, the term typically implies an unknown or not well-defined cause. In well-developed cases, the atrophic areas can usually be identified or suspected on gross examination. The involved anatomical structures are atrophic and are histologically described to have neuron loss and gliosis. This involvement pattern, together with clinical features, guides the subsequent pathologic evaluation. Many of these diseases have additional findings, such as calcifications, vascular changes, and systemic findings, and they can then be incorporated into the evaluation. In addition to the degeneration of particular areas as a result of involvement by specific disorders, neuron degeneration and gliosis can also be secondary to transsynaptic degeneration in certain nuclei, without the direct involvement by the disease process, but as a result of involvement of their afferent connections. **Tables 2.18 to 2.21** highlight the main features of some of the disorders

List of Findings/Checklist for Neuron Loss and Gliosis

AT A GLANCE

- Cerebral cortex
- Basal ganglia
- Thalamus
- Cerebellum
- Brainstem
- Spinal cord

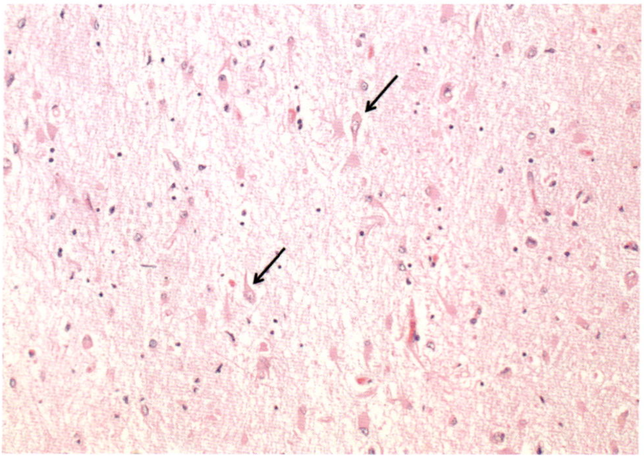

Figure 2-117. Neuron loss and gliosis: This basal ganglion section shows only a few remaining neurons (*arrows*) and many reactive astrocytes in pale and thin neuropil. Taken out of context, it may resemble a chronic demyelinating lesion (H&E; original magnification: 200×).

TABLE 2.18 Disorders commonly affecting the cerebral cortex

Disorder	Predominant Pattern	Other Features
AD	Hippocampus, diffuse cortical	Beta-amyloid, neuritic plaques, NFT
FTLD	Frontotemporal	Inclusions and staining based on subtype
PSCG	Frontotemporal	Subcortical nuclei involved
Posttraumatic neurodegeneration	Cerebrum, cerebellum, substantia nigra	History of repetitive trauma, beta-amyloid, neuritic plaques, NFT
Alpers-Huttenlocher syndrome	Calcarine cortex	Lipid accumulation, microvacuolation
Aluminum	Diffuse cerebral, brainstem	Microglial proliferation, argyrophilic material
Mercury	Sensory, visual, and auditory cortices	Internal granule cells, DRG
Trimethyltin	Hippocampus, limbic areas	Apoptotic debris
Morel's laminar sclerosis	Frontotemporal, layer II	Can be with Marchiafava-Bignami disease, Alzheimer type II glia
Lyme disease	Generalized	Inflammation
Syphilis	Generalized	Inflammation, rarely spirochetes
Hypoxic–ischemic injury and hypoglycemia	Hippocampus, generalized	Acute neuronal injury
Pontosubicular necrosis	Subiculum and pons	Hypoxic–ischemic damage, also in other areas

AD, Alzheimer's disease; NFT, neurofibrillary tangles; FTLD, frontotemporal lobar degeneration; PSCG, progressive subcortical gliosis; DRG, dorsal root ganglia.

TABLE 2.19 Disorders commonly affecting the basal ganglia

Disorder	Predominant Pattern	Other Features
CBD	Basal ganglia, substantia nigra, locus ceruleus, cerebral cortex	Enlarged neurons, asymmetric involvement
Leigh's disease	Striatum, subthalamic nucleus, brainstem tegmentum, inferior olivary nuclei	Symmetrical, necrosis, myelin loss
Thiamine deficiency	Medial thalamic nuclei, mammillary bodies, hypothalamus, periaqueductal gray	Petechiae and myelin loss
Fahr disease	Basal ganglia, red nuclei, dentate nuclei	Calcifications
Manganese toxicity	GP, thalamus	Substantia nigra preserved
Neuroacanthocytosis	Basal ganglia, thalamus, substantia nigra, anterior horns	Cortical atrophy, acanthocytes
McLeod syndrome	Striatum	Myopathy, Kell protein absence
Neuroaxonal dystrophy	GP	Axonal swellings
DRPLA	GP, dentate and red nuclei, subthalamic nuclei	—
MSA	Striatum and substantia nigra, thalamus	Inclusions
Isolated pallidal degenerations	GP	No or minimal other pathology
NDBIA	GP, substantia nigra	Pigment
Nasu-Hakola disease	Basal ganglia, thalamus	Adipocyte and bone pathology
Isolated thalamic degenerations	Thalamus	No or minimal other pathology
Huntington disease	Striatum, thalamus, cerebral cortex	—
CJD	Basal ganglia, thalamus, cerebral cortex	Microvacuolation

CBD, corticobasal degeneration; GP, globus pallidus; DRPLA, dentatorubropallidoluysian atrophy; MSA, multiple system atrophy NDBIA, neurodegeneration with brain iron accumulation type 1; CJD, Creutzfeldt-Jakob disease.

TABLE 2.20 Disorders commonly affecting the cerebellum, brainstem, and cranial nerve nuclei

Disorder	Predominant Pattern	Other Features
Parkinson's disease	Substantia nigra, locus ceruleus	Lewy bodies, cerebellar cortex in DLB
Postencephalitic parkinsonism	Substantia nigra, locus ceruleus	Mild generalized atrophy
PSP	Substantia nigra, locus ceruleus, periaqueductal gray, dentate nucleus, globus pallidus, subthalamic nucleus, hippocampus	Globose NFTs
Pontocerebellar hypoplasia	Pons, cerebellar hemispheres	Vermis relatively spared, dentate nuclei fragmented, arcuate nuclei absent, olivary nuclei hypoplastic
Granule cell aplasia	Cerebellum	Variable Purkinje cell loss
Pelizaeus-Merzbacher disease	Cerebellum	Asteroid structures by silver stains
Menkes disease	Cerebellum	Myelin loss in temporal lobe and hippocampus
Ataxia-telangiectasia	Cerebellum	Posterior column degeneration, ataxia, telangiectasia
CDG-1	Cerebellum, pons	Inferior olivary nuclei, middle cerebellar peduncles, pontine nuclei
Cerebellocortical degeneration (of Jervis)	Cerebellum	Visual system
ADCA II	Cerebellum, internal olivary nuclei, pontine nuclei	Ataxia, visual problems
Paraneoplastic cerebellar degeneration	Cerebellum	Inflammation
Unverricht-Lundborg disease	Cerebellum, medial thalamic nuclei	Cytoplasmic vacuolation in remaining cells
Celiac disease	Cerebellum, inferior olivary nuclei, dentate nuclei	Myelin loss, parietal and occipital calcifications
Mannosidosis	Cerebellum, brainstem, spinal cord	Cytoplasmic vacuolation
Fucosidosis	Cerebellum, inferior olivary nuclei, thalamus	Cytoplasmic vacuolation
MERRF	Dentate nuclei, inferior olivary nuclei, substantia nigra, red nuclei, basal ganglia	Gracile and cuneate nuclei, Clarke's column
Cyanide	Cerebellum in long-term survivors	—
Ethanol	Cerebellar vermis	—
MPTP	Substantia nigra, striatum	No Lewy bodies
Medications	Variable cerebellum, brainstem, dentate nuclei, inferior olivary nuclei	—
Mobius syndrome	Brainstem nuclei	Calcifications
Hereditary bulbar palsies	Cranial nerve motor nuclei	Anterior horn cells
TCE	Cranial nerve nuclei	
Fazio-Londe disease	Cranial nerve nuclei	Anterior horn cells
Brown-Vialetto-van Laere syndrome	Ventral cochlear nuclei, other cranial nerve nuclei	Cerebellum, Clarke's column
Kennedy's disease	Facial and hypoglossal nuclei, anterior horn cells	Oculomotor, trochlear and abducens nuclei spared
MSA	Olivopontocerebellar atrophy, substantia nigra	Inclusions
Guam parkinsonism–dementia complex	Substantia nigra, cerebral cortex	Anterior horn cells

DLB, dementia with Lewy bodies; PSP, progressive supranuclear palsy; NFT, neurofibrillary tangles; CDG-1, carbohydrate-deficient glycoprotein syndrome type 1; ADCA II, autosomal dominant cerebellar ataxia type II; MERRF, myoclonal epilepsy with ragged red fibers; MPTP, 1-methyl-4-phenyl-1,2,3,6-tetrahydropyridine; TCE, trichlorethylene; MSA, multiple system atrophy.

TABLE 2.21 Disorders commonly affecting the spinal cord and dorsal root ganglia

Disorder	Predominant Pattern	Other Features
SMA types 1-3	Anterior horn cells, DRG	Motor nerve root atrophy
ALS	Anterior horn cells, basal ganglia, motor cortex	Inclusions
Clioquinol	Spinal and optic tract degeneration, DRG, inferior olivary nuclei	
Stiff man syndrome	Anterior horn medial neurons	Brainstem in stiff man plus syndrome
Friedreich's ataxia	Gracile, cuneate, dentate, vestibular, cochlear, superior olivary nuclei, Clarke's column, DRG	Spinal cord tract degeneration, hypoxic–ischemic changes in brain if cardiomyopathy present
Paraneoplastic ganglioneuronopathy	DRG	Lymphocytic infiltrates, dorsal column degeneration

SMA, spinal muscular atrophy; DRG, dorsal root ganglia; ALS, amyotrophic lateral sclerosis.

according to areas they commonly involve with neuron loss and gliosis. There is some overlap among these tables, as many of the disorders mentioned have relatively minor components involving other structures. Therefore, these tables are not exclusive and only serve as a brief guide.

In *neurodegenerative diseases*, the pattern of involvement by neuron loss and gliosis is especially helpful, and subsequent evaluation especially with immunohistochemical stains, to identify more definitive findings, such as various accumulations and inclusions, is needed to further classify the process **(Table 2.18)**. AD in its initial stages predominantly involves the hippocampus and entorhinal cortex and eventually becomes generalized to cause cerebral cortical atrophy, with some degree of occipital sparing. FTLD typically has selective involvement of frontal and temporal cortices with neuron loss and gliosis and subsequent atrophy. Basal ganglia and substantia nigra may also be affected. Progressive subcortical gliosis results in gliosis of frontal and temporal white matter, neuron loss, and superficial microvacuolation in frontal and temporal lobes, creating a picture similar to FTLD. Cortical atrophy is prominent in DLB (see below). There is also variable but significant involvement of subcortical nuclei. Spongiform encephalopathies result in a rapidly progressive neuron loss and gliosis. Alpers-Huttenlocher syndrome (progressive neuronal degeneration of childhood) especially involves calcarine cortex.[143] There is superficial microvacuolation along with prominent neuron loss and gliosis. Lipid accumulation can be demonstrated by oil red O stain. Lipid accumulation, typical location, and the presence of liver pathology help distinguish it from prion diseases, where the spongiform change tends to be more widespread, and hypoxic–ischemic encephalopathy, which is associated with vascular zones, sparing the crests of the gyri. Posttraumatic neurodegeneration (dementia pugilistica; punch-drunk syndrome) occurs due to long-term repetitive small trauma. NFT and plaques with beta-amyloid positivity are present in cerebral cortex.[100] Fenestrated interventricular septum and neuron loss in the substantia nigra, cortex, and cerebellum are also present. Aluminum exposure is usually seen in the context of dialysis and as part of antiacid medications. Aluminum or dialysis encephalopathy can be manifested as mild cortical gliosis and mild microglial proliferation; argyrophilic material can be identified in the choroid plexus epithelium, glial cells, and neurons, especially in the brainstem nuclei. Although neuronal changes can be seen, significant neuron loss is not may not be present.[270–272] Mercury intoxication affects the small neurons more, such as internal granule cells and sensory, visual, and auditory cortex neurons, resulting in variable calcarine and cerebellar atrophy in survivors. Purkinje cell sprouting occurs in the long term. Dorsal root ganglion cell degeneration and dorsal column degeneration may be seen.[146,273] Morel's laminar sclerosis involves cortical layer II.[147] Sometimes, deeper layers show microvacuolation and gliosis in frontal and temporal lobes. It can be seen as an isolated finding in alcoholics or in association with Marchiafava-Bignami disease. Alzheimer type II glia are present. It should not be confused with spongiform encephalopathies due to microvacuolation and neuron loss. Some *infectious diseases*, such as general paresis in the tertiary stage of syphilis, result in cortical neuron loss and gliosis, along with fibrotic meninges, atrophic and firm brain, scattered meningeal and parenchymal perivascular lymphoplasmacytic cells, and microglial proliferation. Spirochetes can be seen by silver stain in some cases in the cortex. Similar changes can also be seen in Lyme disease. In *hippocampal sclerosis*, hippocampus shows neuron loss and gliosis mainly in the most vulnerable CA1 region (Sommer's sector) **(Fig. 2-118)**. CA3 and CA4 regions are less vulnerable, while CA2 region is the least vulnerable and is usually spared except in the most devastating conditions. There is some degree of neuron loss in the dentate gyrus as well. Neuron loss and gliosis in the hippocampus may be associated with long-standing seizures or is the result of a previous hypoxic–ischemic episode.

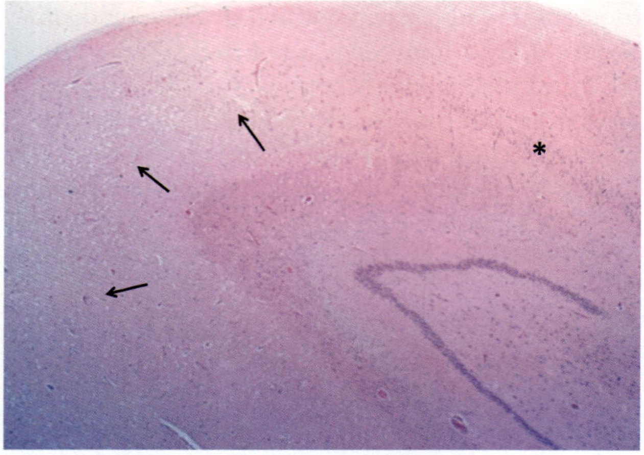

Figure 2-118. Sommer's sector neuron loss: This panoramic view of hippocampus shows that the pyramidal neurons (*asterisk*) are lost in CA1 region (Sommer's sector) (*arrows*), leaving a vacuolar neuropil behind (H&E; original magnification: 40×).

Depending on the severity and extent of the insult, basal ganglia and cortical gray matter are also involved. Hypoglycemia also causes similar findings. Pontosubicular necrosis is usually seen in association with other hypoxic–ischemic damage in other areas. Neuron loss and gliosis occur, but rather than an actual infarct, the damage tends to be in the form of apoptotic debris.[274] Trimethyltin causes not such myelin vacuolation as triethyltin but neuron loss from the hippocampus, basal ganglia, entorhinal cortex, and amygdala. Apoptotic destruction of neurons is seen especially in CA3 and other limbic structures.[146]

A predominant involvement of *basal ganglia and thalamus* is seen in some other diseases **(Table 2.19)**. Leigh's disease (subacute necrotizing encephalomyelopathy).[275] shows symmetrical involvement of striatum, subthalamic nucleus, substantia nigra, inferior olives, and brainstem tegmentum. Cerebellar degeneration is commonly present. Periventricular white matter, optic nerves, spinal cord, and cerebellar white matter may have vacuolation and myelin loss. Older lesions may be cavitary. Different stages of lesions can be seen simultaneously. Thiamine deficiency affects mammillary bodies, hypothalamus, medial thalamic nuclei, periaqueductal region, and floor of the fourth ventricle. In addition, there may be petechial hemorrhages and hemosiderin pigment. Gliosis can be prominent, but neuron loss is relatively mild. In Fahr disease,[179] neuron loss and gliosis in the involved areas, such as the basal ganglia, dentate nucleus, and red nucleus, may be due to hypoxic–ischemic injury. In manganese toxicity, while presenting clinically with parkinsonism, substantia nigra is preserved.[276] Globus pallidus, subthalamic nucleus, and, to a lesser extent, caudate nuclei and putamen show neuron loss and gliosis. Neuroacanthocytosis is a group of neurodegenerative disorders associated with acanthocytes.[277,278] Characteristic features are atrophy, neuron loss and gliosis in affected CNS regions, and acanthocytes in the blood. The latter may be difficult to find and may require advanced techniques such as scanning electron microscopy in suspected cases. Typically, basal ganglia are affected, associated with ventricular dilation and variable cortical atrophy. Thalamus, substantia nigra, and anterior horns may also be involved. Some cases of acanthocytosis may be associated with abetalipoproteinemia and vitamin E deficiency. McLeod syndrome[279] is the association of striatal degeneration, myopathy, and the absence of Kell blood group precursor protein. Basal ganglia are also involved in CBD. Posterior frontal, parietal, and perirolandic cortices are also involved but not necessarily symmetrically, along with substantia nigra and locus ceruleus. Globus pallidus may be involved in a variety of diseases such as neuroaxonal dystrophy, DRPLA, MSA, and ALS. Isolated pallidal degeneration is diagnosed in the absence of other pathology.[280] In juvenile and acute pallidal degeneration, and in pallidoluysian degeneration, in addition to neuron loss and gliosis in globus pallidus, there is involvement of subthalamic nucleus. Pallidonigroluysian degeneration involves globus pallidus, subthalamic nucleus, substantia nigra, and ventrolateral thalamic nuclei. Pallidonigrospinal degeneration involves globus pallidus, substantia nigra, and anterior horns, with variable involvement of subthalamic nucleus and pontine tegmentum. There are also variable degrees of corticospinal tract degeneration. Neurodegeneration with brain iron accumulation (a.k.a., pantothenate kinase–associated neurodegeneration; formerly known as Hallervorden-Spatz disease) has involvement primarily of globus pallidus and substantia nigra. Nasu-Hakola disease (polycystic lipomembranous osteodysplasia with sclerosing leukoencephalopathy) involves primarily the basal ganglia, but the thalamus may also be involved.[281] The thalamus may be involved in various neurodegenerative diseases, and thalamic degeneration with neuron loss and gliosis can be seen as part of a wide variety of diseases such as MSA, spinocerebellar ataxias (SCA), Wernicke's encephalopathy,[282] Huntington disease, CJD,[283] Menkes disease,[284] membranous lipodystrophy, neuroaxonal dystrophy, and fatal familial insomnia.[285] It can rarely be seen as pure thalamic degeneration, that is, in the absence of any other pathology, although inferior olivary nuclei may be involved.

Atrophy of the posterior fossa contents indicates selective primary involvement of the cerebellum and brainstem **(Table 2.20)**. Pontocerebellar hypoplasia (a.k.a. pontoneocerebellar hypoplasia, as primarily the neocerebellum is involved and paleocerebellum is relatively preserved) is characterized by atrophic posterior fossa contents with a disproportionately small cerebellum.[286] Mainly the hemispheres are small, while the vermis is normal. The cerebellum has a flattened appearance. The brainstem is small and especially the bulge of basis pontis is diminished. Microscopically, the folia are thin with variable losses of granule cell and Purkinje cell population. Dentate nuclei are fragmented. Olivary nuclei are dysplastic and arcuate nuclei are absent. Granule cell layer is absent in granule cell aplasia. Folia are thin. Purkinje cells are randomly distributed in molecular layer along with ectopic residual granule cells in molecular layer. Numerous torpedoes are also seen. Gliosis is present in gray and white matter. Dentate and olivary nuclei may be relatively mildly involved. In general, cerebellar degeneration of various types has in common variable losses of Purkinje and/or internal granule layer cells Bergmann gliosis, thinning of the folia, and diminished white matter **(Fig. 2-119)**. Cerebellar degeneration is a component of a large group of disorders included under the term SCA.[287] Cerebellar degeneration is common in Pelizaeus-Merzbacher disease with variable Purkinje cell loss, torpedoes, displaced Purkinje cells into molecular layer, decreased granule cell layer, and asteroid structures by silver stain. Menkes (kinky hair) disease[288] is another disease associated with cerebellar atrophy with granule cell loss and displacement of Purkinje cells into the molecular layer. Torpedoes, increased Purkinje

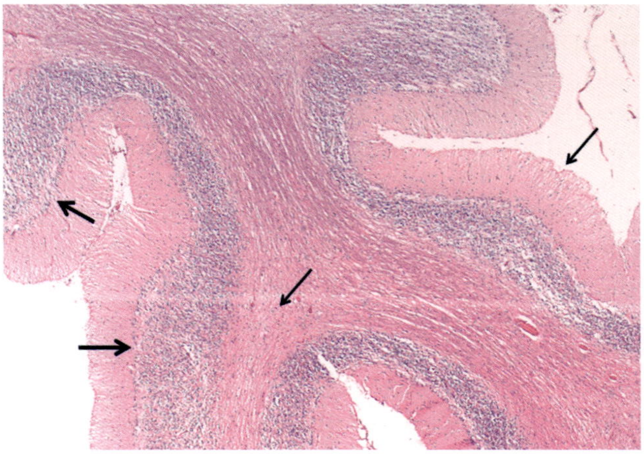

Figure 2-119. Cerebellar degeneration: This cerebellar folium is thin due to neuron loss, resulting in the pale and vacuolated appearance of the molecular layer and white matter (*thin arrows*). There is extensive Purkinje cell loss and prominent Bergmann gliosis forming a distinct layer (*thick arrows*) (H&E; original magnification: 40×).

cell dendritic sprouting/arborization with abnormal swelling, are present. Neuron and myelin loss can be present in temporal cortex and hippocampus. Ataxia-telangiectasia[289] shows cerebellar atrophy with prominent loss of Purkinje cells and internal granule layer cells. Telangiectasia in skin and sclera can appear by the end of the first decade, but ataxia is noted from the beginning of walking in ataxia-telangiectasia. Purkinje cell and internal granule cell loss in the cerebellum and neuron loss in the inferior olivary nuclei are present. Posterior column degeneration, especially of gracile, is present. There is ganglion cell loss in dorsal root ganglia, with the remaining ones being small, as well as scattered atypical forms. Anterior horn cell loss is seen in some cases. In some other cases, NFT in the basal ganglia, hippocampus, and cerebral cortex, with some degree of neuron loss, is also identified. Carbohydrate-deficient glycoprotein syndrome type I (CDG-1) is characterized by cerebellar and pontine atrophy.[290] All layers show reduced number of cells, but dentate nuclei and superior cerebellar peduncles appear unremarkable, while inferior olivary nuclei and middle cerebellar peduncles, pontine transverse fibers, and pontine nuclei are depleted. In cerebellocortical degeneration (of Jervis), cerebellar cortex, olives, and visual system, including optic nerves, superior colliculi, lateral geniculate bodies, and visual cortex, show neuronal degeneration, sparing pons. Autosomal dominant cerebellar ataxia type II (ADCA II)[291] is characterized by ataxia and visual failure. Atrophy of the cerebellum with more prominent loss of Purkinje cells compared to internal granule cells, olivary nuclei, and pontine nuclei are seen. Paraneoplastic cerebellar degeneration[292] is usually grossly undetected. Severe loss of Purkinje cells, variable granule cell loss, Bergmann gliosis, and microglial proliferation are present. Lymphocytic infiltrates in the cortex, perivascular and meningeal, may be present. Inflammation may not correlate with areas of neuron loss. There may be some overlap with paraneoplastic encephalomyelitis. Unverricht-Lundborg disease (a.k.a. Baltic myoclonus, referring to the region it is seen)[293] is associated with severe loss of Purkinje cells, swelling and cytoplasmic vacuolation in the remaining ones, and Bergmann gliosis. Neuron loss and gliosis are also seen in medial thalamic nuclei. Celiac disease[294] can result in cerebellar atrophy with Purkinje cell loss, Bergmann gliosis, and granule cell loss with rarefaction of and myelin loss in the white matter. Neuron loss and gliosis in dentate and olivary nuclei are also present. Sometimes, it is associated with perivascular lymphocytes in the cerebellum. In addition, cortical, subcortical, parietal, and occipital calcifications may occur. Cerebellar degeneration can be seen in mannosidosis.[295] Cerebral cortex, brainstem, and spinal cord neurons, as well as astrocytes, endothelial cells, and pericytes, are vacuolated and neurons eventually degenerate. Gliosis accompanies areas of neuron loss. Fucosidosis, similar to mannosidosis, causes widespread vacuolated and enlarged neurons, including Purkinje cell loss, but especially in olives and thalamus. MERRF[296] is associated with neuron loss and gliosis in dentate nuclei, inferior olives, substantia nigra, red nuclei, and basal ganglia. Gracile and cuneate nuclei and Clarke's column may be involved. Cyanide poisoning[83] causes swelling, subarachnoid hemorrhages, and petechial hemorrhages within a few hours. Pallidal and white matter necroses are also seen. Longer survivors suffer from Purkinje cell loss and cerebral cortical gliosis. A number of medications can show side effects and toxicity on the cerebellum and brainstem. Vidarabine causes chromatolysis and degeneration of neurons, especially in the brainstem. Cytosine arabinoside can cause cerebellar cortical degeneration, brainstem tegmental neuron degeneration, and spinal motor neuron degeneration, while Purkinje cell, dentate nucleus, and inferior olivary nucleus degeneration can be seen with 5-FU.[17] Cerebellar cortical and dentate nucleus degeneration can be seen with lithium as well.[297] Phenytoin[298] can cause cerebellar vermis and hemisphere atrophy with loss of Purkinje cells with Bergmann gliosis, as well as internal granule cell degeneration. Acute ethanol intoxication results in congestion, edema, and petechial hemorrhages, while chronic alcoholism can cause a variety of findings, including thiamine deficiency states (see above). Degeneration of superior vermis, where crests tend to be affected more than the depths in contrast to hypoxic–ischemic damage, is another well-recognized finding. In addition, dorsal layer of inferior olivary nucleus can have neuron loss and gliosis. MPTP (*N*-methyl-4-phenyl-1,2,3,6-tetrahydropyridine),[83] a contaminant of illicit drug synthesis, results in parkinsonism due to striatal and nigral neuronal degeneration without Lewy bodies. However, eosinophilic intracytoplasmic inclusions can occur in chronic administration. Cerebellar ataxia with isolated vitamin E deficiency[299] is associated with Purkinje cell loss, together with axonal spheroids in and degeneration of posterior columns.

Aplasia or hypoplasia of cranial nerve nuclei can be isolated or associated with other malformations. Necrosis and calcifications of brainstem nuclei, suggesting an infectious or anoxic etiology, peripheral nerve involvement, and myopathy indicate Mobius syndrome.[300] Hereditary bulbar palsies (hereditary motor neuropathy),[301] types I and II, have degeneration of cranial motor nerve nuclei in the brainstem and anterior horn neurons in the spinal cord. In type I, there is also sensory vestibulocochlear nerve and ventral cochlear nucleus involvement. Trichlorethylene (TCE)[302] causes neuron loss in the cranial nerve nuclei in the brainstem. Fazio-Londe disease is characterized by loss of neurons from facial, motor vagal, hypoglossal, motor trigeminal, and oculomotor nuclei, as well as from anterior horns of the spinal cord. Brown-Vialetto-van Laere syndrome is characterized by neuron loss primarily in ventral cochlear nuclei, as well as in other motor nuclei. Purkinje cell and anterior horn cell loss, loss of cells from Clarke's column, and degeneration of posterior columns and spinocerebellar tracts are also seen.[303] Spinobulbar muscular atrophy (Kennedy's disease; X-linked bulbospinal neuronopathy)[304] involves facial and hypoglossal nerves and spinal motor neuron, sparing the oculomotor, trochlear, and abducens cranial nerves. Parkinson's disease predominantly affects substantia nigra and locus ceruleus, resulting in grossly pale appearance due to the degeneration of the pigmented neurons, as well as substantia innominata, thalamus, hypothalamus, dorsal motor nucleus of vagus, Edinger-Westphal nucleus, and intermediolateral column of the spinal cord. In dementia with Lewy bodies, primarily deeper layers of frontal and parietal cortices, entorhinal cortex, periamygdaloid cortex, cingulate gyrus temporal cortex, and insular cortex are affected Postencephalitic parkinsonism refers to the condition seen in survivors of encephalitis lethargica (von Economo's disease). Substantia nigra and locus ceruleus degenerations are present. Mild generalized atrophy may be seen with neuron loss in the hippocampus, entorhinal cortex, insular cortex, and other cortical areas. PSP (Steele-Richardson-Olszewski syndrome) involves predominantly brainstem structures, including substantia nigra and locus ceruleus, periaqueductal gray, red nuclei, colliculi, pontine tegmentum, the 10th and 12th cranial nerve nuclei, dentate nucleus, globus pallidus, subthalamic nucleus, hippocampus, and globus pallidus. MSA[305] encompasses olivopontocerebellar atrophy (involving predominantly cerebellum, middle cerebellar peduncles, basis pontis, and olivary nuclei), Shy-Drager syndrome (involving predominantly substantia nigra and locus ceruleus), and striatonigral degeneration (involving predominantly basal ganglia and substantia nigra) in addition to their typical inclusions with their staining properties, as in other neurodegenerative diseases. Shy-Drager syndrome is the association of autonomic failure and parkinsonism. In addition to being part of MSA, it can be associated with Lewy body pathology. Either way, there is neuron loss in the intermediolateral column of the spinal cord, but multiple sections should be evaluated because of the highly variable numbers of neurons in this region normally. Cases associated with MSA have ubiquitin- and tau-positive glial inclusions in this region, too. Otherwise, other features of MSA or Lewy body pathology are found in other areas. There is generalized brain atrophy in Guam parkinsonism–dementia complex, with involvement of substantia nigra and locus ceruleus. Neuron loss and gliosis also involve the hippocampus, amygdala, and anterior horn cells.

In the *spinal cord* **(Table 2.21)**, spinal muscular atrophy including acute infantile (SMA type 1; Werdnig-Hoffmann disease), intermediate (SMA type 2; chronic infantile), and chronic (SMA type 3; chronic proximal; Kugelberg-Welander syndrome) forms, shows anterior horn neuron loss and gliosis with resultant anterior spinal nerve root and nerve atrophy. It may involve brainstem cranial nerve nuclei and dorsal root ganglia. Some variants may be associated with cerebellar atrophy or hypoplasia. Dorsal roots and ganglia are affected in tabes dorsalis in the tertiary stage of syphilis. There is lymphoplasmacytic inflammation in the meninges and dorsal root ganglia. General features of dorsal root ganglion degeneration, such as ganglion cell loss and nodules of Nageotte, characterized by

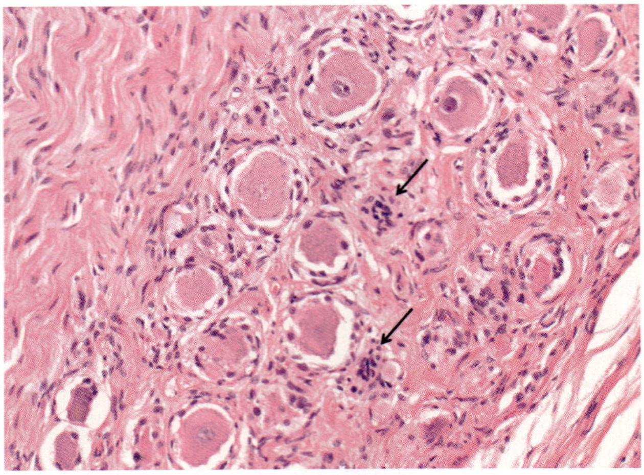

Figure 2-120. Dorsal root ganglion cell loss: The former sites of degenerated ganglion cells are marked by nodules of Nageotte (*arrows*) (H&E; original magnification: 200×).

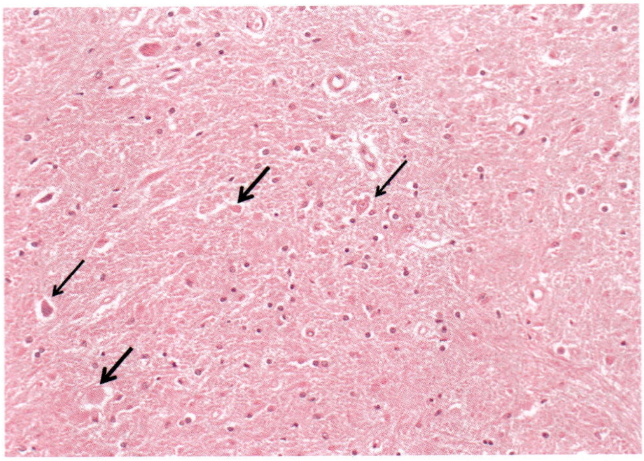

Figure 2-121. ALS: This spinal cord section shows prominent neuron loss in the anterior horn with only a few neurons (*thin arrows*) remaining in a gliotic background. Scattered axonal swellings (*thick arrows*) are also present (H&E; original magnification: 200×).

proliferation of satellite cells in place of lost ganglion cells, as well as loss of nerve fibers in the dorsal root ganglia **(Fig. 2-120)**, are seen. Posterior column degeneration in the spinal cord is most prominent in the lumbar segments. Clioquinol[306] affects the distal parts of spinal corticospinal tracts (i.e., in lumbar), posterior columns (i.e., in cervical), and optic tracts (i.e., near lateral geniculate body), resulting in degeneration. Also there may be chromatolysis of lumbosacral anterior horn cells, dorsal root ganglion cell degeneration with nodules of Nageotte, neuron loss and gliosis in inferior olives, edema, and white matter gliosis. Motor neuron loss and gliosis in anterior horns of the spinal cord, brainstem nuclei, and motor cortex are typical of ALS **(Fig. 2-121)**. As a result, the anterior nerve roots are thin and spinal cord and precentral gyrus are atrophic. There is spinal motor neuron ballooning with neurofilament accumulation. Anterior and lateral corticospinal tract degeneration, as well as degeneration of internal capsule and pyramids, can be present. There may also be frontal and temporal atrophy in cases associated with dementia. Axonal spheroids are seen in anterior horns.

Stiff man syndrome[307] is associated with neuron loss and gliosis, especially in the anterior horn medial motor nuclei, along with perivascular lymphocytic inflammation. Stiff man plus syndrome[307] also shows neuron loss, gliosis, and perivascular lymphocytic inflammation in the spinal cord but, in addition, has involvement of the brainstem. Friedreich's ataxia is associated with degeneration in gracile and cuneate nuclei in the medulla; vestibular, cochlear and superior olivary nuclei; and cerebellar dentate nuclei. Cerebellar cortex is unremarkable, but white matter is astrocytic. Posterior column degeneration, distal degeneration of pyramidal and spinocerebellar tracts, and a typical severe neuron loss in Clarke's column are also seen. Superior cerebellar peduncles are atrophic. There is ganglion cell loss in dorsal root ganglia, with nodules of Nageotte. Hypoxic–ischemic changes and associated neuron loss and gliosis can be seen anywhere, especially in cerebral and cerebellar cortex due to cardiomyopathy.[17] Paraneoplastic ganglioneuronopathy[308] is characterized by degeneration of dorsal root ganglion cells with lymphocytic infiltrate and nodules of Nageotte. There is dorsal column degeneration in the spinal cord.

Tract Degeneration and Spinal Cord Patterns

White matter involvement in the spinal cord and the pattern of involvement are characteristic in many diseases. Identification of this tract involvement pattern helps narrow the differential diagnostic possibilities. It may also become important

List of Findings/Checklist for Tract Degeneration and Spinal Cord Patterns

AT A GLANCE

Predominantly Posterior Column Involvement
- Infectious
  - Vacuolar myelopathy
  - HTLV-1-associated myelopathy
  - Tabes dorsalis
- Nutritional
  - Subacute combined degeneration
  - Niacin deficiency
  - Vitamin E deficiency
- Toxic
  - Mercury
  - Thallium
  - Cisplatin
  - Fludarabine
- Neurodegenerative
  - Brown-Vialetto-van Laere syndrome
  - Corticobasal degeneration
  - Friedreich's ataxia
- Others
  - Paraneoplastic ganglioneuronopathy
  - Ataxia-telangiectasia

Predominantly Corticospinal Tract Involvement
- Adrenomyeloneuropathy
- Neurolathyrism
- Pallidal degenerations
- Neuroaxonal dystrophies
- Amyotrophic lateral sclerosis

Predominantly Spinocerebellar Tract Involvement
- Idiopathic late-onset cerebellar ataxia
- Dentatorubropallidoluysian atrophy
- SCA3
- SCA7

Predominantly Distal Tract Involvement
- Acrylamide
- Carbon disulfide
- Hexacarbons
- Organophosphates
- Clioquinol
- Hepatic porphyrias

Others
- Multiple system atrophy
- Basal ganglionic and internal capsule lesions
- Hexachlorophene

to know which levels of the spinal cord are more prone to involvement by particular disorders. Therefore, sampling and examination of the entire length of the spinal cord should be performed whenever possible. The identification of exact site of involvement requires knowledge of anatomy of the spinal tracts. Evaluation of microscopic cross sections is greatly facilitated by the use of an LFB/PAS stain to highlight gray and white matter, myelin vacuolation, and early degenerations. An axon stain such as Bielschowsky or neurofilament immunohistochemistry further helps with axonal degeneration. Myelin and axon stains are also useful in the simultaneous evaluation of the spinal nerve roots represented on the section. GFAP immunohistochemistry is useful in highlighting the reactive astrocytosis in the involved areas. Immunohistochemistry for CD68 or CD163 for macrophages also indicates the microglial proliferation and macrophage infiltration in the injured areas. Therefore, it is possible to identify the exact tracts involved in a pathologic process in the great majority of cases, although early and subtle changes may be difficult to identify and distinguish from technical artifact, especially with myelin vacuolation.

Vacuolar myelopathy associated with HIV infection **(Fig. 2-122)** and *subacute combined degeneration* of vitamin B_{12} (cobalamin) deficiency involve posterior and lateral columns and are essentially histologically identical but can easily be distinguished based on the clinical and other laboratory information.[309] The involvement is most prominent in the lower cervical and thoracic segments. Vitamin B_{12} deficiency can be seen in association with gastrointestinal/stomach problems (e.g., pernicious

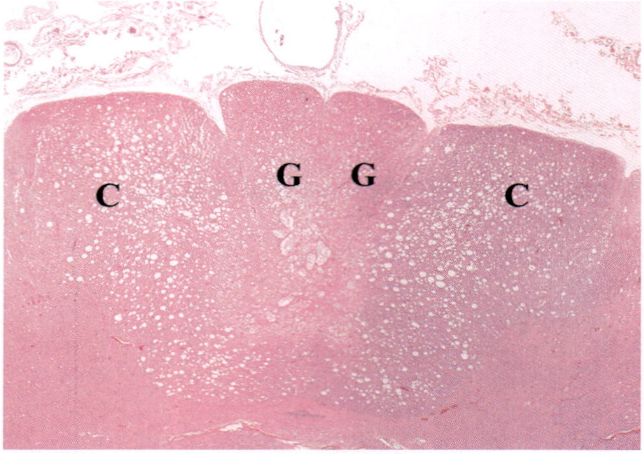

Figure 2-122. Vacuolar myelopathy: Gracile (*G*) and cuneate (*C*) fasciculi are involved and show prominent vacuolation (H&E; original magnification: 20×).

anemia), intestinal malabsorption, intestinal blind loops or diverticular disease with bacterial overgrowth, fish tapeworm infection, nitrous oxide abuse, folate deficiency, and methylation disorders. *HTLV-1-associated myelopathy* (HAM) (a.k.a. *tropical spastic paraparesis*)[268] involves especially the lower thoracic region. There is degeneration of the anterior and lateral columns, the latter being more prominent **(Fig. 2-123)**. Involvement of posterior columns may also be seen. *Nicotinic acid (niacin, vitamin B_3) deficiency (Pellagra)* results in dorsal column degeneration, especially in the gracile, and lesser degree of corticospinal tract degeneration. These changes are seen mainly in the late stages. In addition, there are chromatolysis in Betz cells, pontine nuclei, dentate nucleus, and anterior horn.[310] Chronic alcoholism; Hartnup disease; antituberculosis medications, especially isoniazid; and intestinal malabsorption are some of the conditions that are associated with nicotinic acid deficiency. In *vitamin E deficiency*, posterior columns and corticospinal and spinocerebellar tracts show axonal swelling with axonal spheroids of variable sizes and shapes and eventual degeneration. In the spinal cord, the changes are especially prominent in gracile but are also present in cuneate fasciculi. Similar changes are also present in brainstem nuclei and basal ganglia.[165] Vitamin E deficiency is especially pronounced in cystic fibrosis, abetalipoproteinemia, and pancreatic and biliary dysfunction. Similar changes are seen in *cerebellar ataxia with isolated vitamin E deficiency*.[311] *Adrenomyeloneuropathy*[269] involves predominantly the gracile and lateral corticospinal tracts, with the latter being more prominently affected. Posterior column degeneration in the spinal cord in *tabes dorsalis* is most prominent in the lumbosacral segments. There is fiber loss in the dorsal spinal nerves and dorsal root ganglia. Spinal cord posterior column degeneration is also associated with *ataxia-telangiectasia*.[289] Cerebellar atrophy with prominent loss of Purkinje cells and internal granule layer cells and telangiectasias of conjunctiva and skin are also present. *Mercury intoxication*, along with other changes in the brain, cerebellum, and brainstem discussed elsewhere, may result in dorsal root ganglion cell degeneration and dorsal column degeneration.[312] *Paraneoplastic ganglioneuronopathy* results in dorsal column degeneration in the spinal cord.[308] *Thallium* can cause chromatolysis of motor neurons and posterior column degeneration.[313] *Cisplatin* rarely causes posterior column degeneration.[314] *Fludarabine* can be associated with necrotizing leukoencephalopathy predominantly in the occipital lobes, which may also involve the pyramids and posterior columns of the spinal cord.[315] *Lathyrus toxin (neurolathyrism)*[316] causes corticospinal tract degeneration, most prominent in lumbosacral and less prominent in thoracic region. Mainly distal degeneration of long tracts in the spinal cord, that is, mainly lumbar in corticospinal

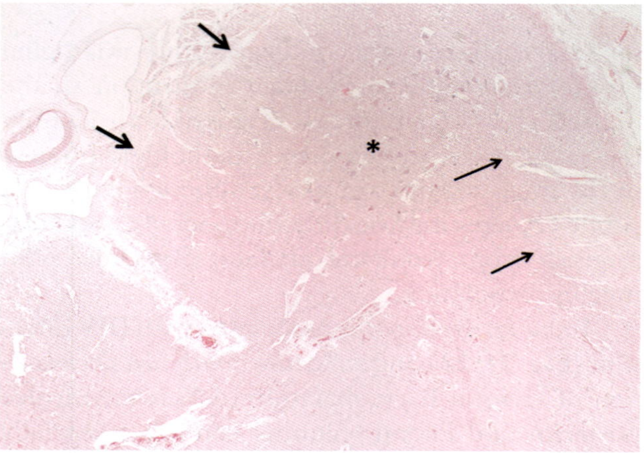

Figure 2-123. HTLV-1-asociated myelopathy (HAM): Anterior (*thick arrows*) and lateral (*thin arrows*) columns of the spinal cord are thin and pale with some vacuolation as a result of degeneration. Anterior horn (*asterisk*) is well populated by neurons (H&E; original magnification: 20×).

tracts and cervical in dorsal columns, is associated with several toxic substances. Typically, there is axonal swelling and subsequent degeneration in the involved segments. *Acrylamide*[317] exposure can cause posterior column and spinocerebellar and corticospinal tract degeneration. The involvement is usually distal in relation to the anatomical orientation of these tracts and is associated with axonal swellings and eventual degeneration. *Carbon disulfide* exposure also shows swelling of distal spinocerebellar tracts.[318] *Hexacarbons*[319] involve distal parts of posterior columns and spinocerebellar tracts as well as corticospinal tracts. *Organophosphates*[320] result in posterior column and spinocerebellar and corticospinal tract distal swelling and degeneration. Among the porphyrias, CNS involvement is seen mainly in *hepatic porphyrias*. There is degeneration of distal posterior columns in some cases.[17] Chromatolysis of spinal and brainstem motor neurons is also seen. There may be hemorrhages due to hypertensive attacks. *Clioquinol*[306] affects the distal parts of spinal corticospinal tracts and posterior columns, as well as optic tracts (i.e., near lateral geniculate body), resulting in degeneration.

In *ALS*, there is anterior and lateral corticospinal tract degeneration, along with degeneration of motor neurons. Anterior root axon loss and endoneurial fibrosis are seen. There can be some degree of degeneration of the internal capsule and pyramids, as a transsynaptic degeneration secondary to the cortical motor neuron loss. Macrophages can be associated with degenerating tracts. Posterior column and spinocerebellar tract degeneration can be a component of *Brown-Vialetto-van Laere syndrome,*[303] associated with neuron loss and other changes in other areas. *Multiple system atrophy*[321,322] shows atrophy and subsequent myelin pallor due to degeneration of various tracts associated with the degenerating neurons depending on the components involved. Corresponding tracts such as external capsule, cerebellar white matter, middle cerebellar peduncle, striatopallidal fibers, and transverse pontine fibers are affected. However, in neurodegenerative diseases in general, the identification of the sites of neuron degeneration and any associated inclusions or accumulations, usually with the help of special stains, is the key, and evaluation of tracts is usually an associated finding. Myelinated fiber loss can be present in cerebral white matter under the affected cortex, and sometimes in corticospinal tracts, in *corticobasal degeneration*, and in *PSP*.[323,324] *Friedreich's ataxia*[325] is associated with posterior column degeneration that is more prominent in gracile than in cuneate fasciculus. There is also distal degeneration of pyramidal and spinocerebellar tracts. Superior cerebellar peduncle is atrophic. *SCA3 (Machado-Joseph disease)*[326] has neuron loss in dentate nucleus, with sparing of cerebellum and olivary nuclei. Superior cerebellar peduncle and spinocerebellar tract degeneration are seen. There is also neuron loss in Clarke's column, substantia nigra, and anterior horn of the spinal cord. Ataxin-3 and ubiquitin-positive neuronal intranuclear inclusions are seen. *SCA7*[327] is associated with cerebellar cortical atrophy and spinocerebellar and olivocerebellar tract degeneration. Motor neurons of the brainstem and spinal cord are involved. Substantia nigra and subthalamic nucleus neuron losses are seen. Neuronal intranuclear inclusions with expanded polyglutamine repeats are found in inferior olives. Superior cerebellar peduncles are atrophic in *dentatorubropallidoluysian atrophy (DRPLA)*.[328] Spinocerebellar tract and posterior column degeneration may be seen. *Idiopathic late-onset cerebellar ataxia*[329] is characterized by cerebellar atrophy that is most prominent in the superior part of the cerebellum, especially the vermis. Inferior olivary nuclei and especially their dorsal parts are atrophic. Spinocerebellar tract degeneration is variable. *Juvenile and acute pallidal degenerations*, in addition to the presence of neuron loss and gliosis in the globus pallidus, have myelinated fiber loss in pallidoluysian tract, as well as gliosis of the subthalamic nucleus. There is variable corticospinal tract degeneration in *pallidonigrospinal degeneration*, along with neuron loss and gliosis in globus pallidus, substantia nigra, and anterior horns of the spinal cord. Variable involvement of subthalamic nucleus and pontine tegmentum is also seen.[17] *Infantile neuroaxonal dystrophy* is associated with prominent degeneration of corticospinal and spinobulbar tracts,[254] while *neuroaxonal leukodystrophy* shows distal degeneration of corticospinal tracts and posterior columns.[330]

Tract degeneration in the brainstem usually indicates destruction of cerebral structures associated with those particular tracts **(Fig. 2-124)**. Cerebral peduncles as seen on the midbrain section

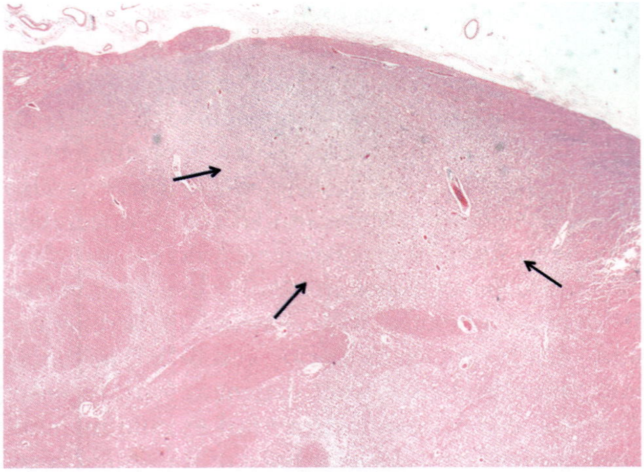

Figure 2-124. Tract degeneration: A well-defined area (*arrows*) in the crus cerebri on this midbrain section is pale relative to the surrounding parenchyma as a result of degeneration of this particular tract due to a cerebral infarct (H&E; original magnification: 20×).

can become atrophic secondary to cerebral *lesions involving basal ganglia and internal capsule*. There is atrophy of the tracts on affected side and hypertrophy on the contralateral side in large cerebral lesions involving basal ganglia and internal capsule. Contralateral cerebellar hemispheric atrophy may occur as a result of extensive cerebral destructive lesions. *Hexachlorophene (hexachlorophane)*[264] mainly affects white matter, resulting in vacuolation due to myelin edema that is most prominent in the brainstem. Optic nerve, chiasm, and optic tract necrosis may occur.

Vascular Changes

Vessels can draw attention due to various peculiar arrangements, such as in the pseudorosettes of ependymomas (see "Perivascular Arrangements and Rosettes"). Here, the changes that directly concern the vascular components, such as vascular proliferation or accumulations, and perivascular changes that occur mainly outside the neuroglial parenchyma that are associated with the vascular component, such as perivascular inflammation, are discussed. Vascular patterns can provide clues to the nature of a lesion, such as the so-called "hemangiopericytomatous" vascular pattern.

Some processes tend to affect preferentially the intima and cause *intimal thickening*. Variable stages and degrees of *atherosclerotic changes* are commonly seen in the arteries of the basal circulation and their branches in the leptomeninges and in the parenchyma. These range from minimal intimal thickening to complex changes with calcification, hemorrhage, endothelial erosion, and thrombus formation with severe narrowing of the lumen. Obliteration of the lumen should be evaluated on cross section both grossly and microscopically and should be stated that way. Angiographic evaluation does not always show the vessels on cross section, and therefore, the degree of lumen obliteration may not always correlate. This type of large vessel disease can be associated with global hypoxic–ischemic changes, hippocampal sclerosis, and watershed zone infarcts, likely secondary to hypotensive episodes as a result of extensive atherosclerosis. Large infarcts due to atheroemboli are also common. *Meningovascular syphilis*[331,332] is *characterized by an arteritis* involving all sizes of arterial vessels by a lymphoplasmacytic infiltration of adventitia and media and collagenous thickening of intima (Huebner's endarteritis). It may occlude the lumen to result in infarcts. Inflammation is also present around veins and cranial nerves. Perivascular inflammation and gliosis are seen in periventricular white matter. *Lyme disease* can also produce a vasculopathy similar to syphilis and may result in infarcts.[333] *Tuberculous endarteritis*[334] characterized by intimal thickening and lymphocytic infiltrates can also result in brain infarcts. Intimal and medial thickening without atherosclerosis in medium and small arteries can be seen in *fibromuscular dysplasia*,[335] where elastic laminae are irregular or disrupted. *Moyamoya disease* mainly involves basal vessels and results in intimal thickening in arteries.[336] This thickening is due to fibromuscular hyperplasia of the intima. It can be associated with mild atherosclerotic changes and elastic membrane disruption, as well as with thrombus formation in the lumen. Media becomes thinner and internal elastic lamina fragmented. *Coccidioidomycosis* may cause an endarteritis resulting in infarcts and leukomalacia. *HIV-associated arteriopathy*[197] produces a fibromuscular hyperplasia of the intima along with fragmentation of the internal elastic lamina, resulting in aneurysmal dilatations of the vessels. It

List of Findings/Checklist for Vascular Changes

AT A GLANCE

Intimal Thickening
- Atherosclerosis
- Syphilis
- Tuberculosis
- Lyme disease
- Coccidioidomycosis
- HIV-associated arteriopathy
- Whipple disease
- Fibromuscular dysplasia
- Neurofibromatosis
- Moyamoya disease

Infectious Vascular Injury
- Candidiasis
- Pseudallescheriasis
- Zygomycosis
- Angiostrongylosis

Aneurysms
- Saccular
- Mycotic
- Fusiform
- Dissecting
- Traumatic
- Miliary
- Cerebral autosomal recessive arteriopathy with subcortical infarcts and leukoencephalopathy

Thromboses
- Postmortem clot
- Thromboemboli
  - Infective endocarditis
  - Noninfective endocarditis
- Atherosclerosis
- Cytomegalovirus
- Antiphospholipid antibody syndrome
- Protein-C deficiency
- Factor V Leiden mutation
- Antithrombin III disorders
- Carbohydrate-deficient glycoprotein synthase-I deficiency
- Platelet glycoprotein polymorphisms
- Thrombotic thrombocytopenic purpura
- Hemolytic uremic syndrome
- Disseminated intravascular coagulation
- Venous thromboses
  - Hypernatremia
  - Carbon tetrachloride poisoning
  - L-Asparaginase
  - Rickettsia
- High-grade glial neoplasm

Emboli
- Thromboemboli
- Atheroemboli
- Cardiac valve calcifications
- Fat emboli
- Neoplastic cells
- Septic emboli
- Intervertebral disc
- Iatrogenic material

Giant Cells
- Primary angiitis of the CNS
- Giant cell arteritis
- Takayasu arteritis
- Reaction to vascular amyloid
- Sarcoidosis
- HIV encephalitis

Perivascular Inflammation and/or Vascular Necrosis
- Kawasaki disease
- Varicella Zoster Virus infection
- Adrenoleukodystrophy
- Microbleeds
- Vasculitis
  - Primary angiitis of the CNS
  - Polyarteritis nodosa
  - Churg-Strauss syndrome
  - Wegener's granulomatosis
- Lymphomatoid granulomatosis
- Lymphoma
- HIV infection
- Trichinosis
- Schistosomiasis
- Meningitis
- Malaria
- Toxins, Medications, Drugs
  - Arsenic
  - Methotrexate
  - BCNU
  - Amphetamines
  - Cocaine
- Infiltrating glial and primitive neoplasms
- Malignant hypertension
- Radiation treatment

(Continued)

List of Findings/Checklist for Vascular Changes *(Continued)*

• AT A GLANCE

Thickening and Accumulations
- Arteriosclerosis
- Hypertension
- Marchiafava-Bignami disease
- Healed acute disseminated encephalomyelitis
- Mitochondrial encephalopathy lactic acidosis and stroke-like episodes
- Kearns-Sayre syndrome
- Neoplasms
- Vascular malformations
    - Cavernous angioma
    - Arteriovenous malformation
    - Venous malformation
    - Venous congestive myelopathy
- Cerebral amyloid angiopathy
- Cerebral autosomal dominant arteriopathy with subcortical infarcts and leukoencephalopathy
- Systemic lupus erythematosus
- Fabry disease
- Pompe disease
- Acute lead encephalopathy
- Ethylene glycol
- Heroin
- Azzopardi effect
- Calcifications (see "Calcifications")

Proliferation, Endothelial Prominence, and Hypertrophy
- Glial neoplasms
- Other primary neoplasms
- Hypoxic–ischemic injury
- Subacute diencephalic angioencephalopathy
- Abscess
- Papillary endothelial hyperplasia
- Sturge-Weber syndrome
- Meningocerebral angiodysplasia and renal agenesis
- Idiopathic hypertrophic pachymeningitis
- Fowler syndrome
- Mitochondrial DNA depletion syndrome

Vascular Pattern
- Staghorn pattern
    - Hemangiopericytoma/solitary fibrous tumor
    - Meningioma
- Chicken-wire pattern
    - Oligodendroglioma

Blood Cells
- Nucleated erythrocytes
- Megakaryocytes
- Sickling
- Malaria
- Sepsis
- Leukemic blasts
- Intravascular lymphoma

can have variable degrees of foamy histiocyte infiltration, with a picture similar to atherosclerotic plaque. The histiocytes can be positive for HIV immunohistochemically, and the HIV-positive status of the patient should help in the consideration of HIV-associated arteriopathy. HIV-associated vasculopathy mainly involves meningeal arteries and can result in infarcts and/or hemorrhages in HIV. Aneurysmal changes are also seen.[337] *Whipple disease*[338] is characterized by parenchymal macrophage clusters with PAS-positive material, representing intracytoplasmic microorganisms, which are also GMS positive. The microorganisms, *Tropheryma whipplei,* are also gram-positive, although this may be difficult to demonstrate in the tissue due to bacterial degeneration. It may lead to thickening of arterioles and subsequent microinfarcts. The aggregates may be associated with scant lymphocytic infiltrate. *Vascular dysplasia* in the form of a fibromuscular intimal thickening can be seen in neurofibromatosis[339] **(Fig. 2-125)**. In *vessels entrapped within a chronic inflammatory process*, a reactive intimal proliferation may occur. It may be extensive enough to result in significant lumen obliteration and strokes. In general, with fungal microorganisms, hyphae tend to invade and occlude vessels and produce large infarcts, while yeasts form meningitis and cerebritis. Eventually, granulomas can form in all fungal infections, depending on immune status. *Candida* spp. can occlude small parenchymal vessels with microinfarcts around the vessels and subsequent

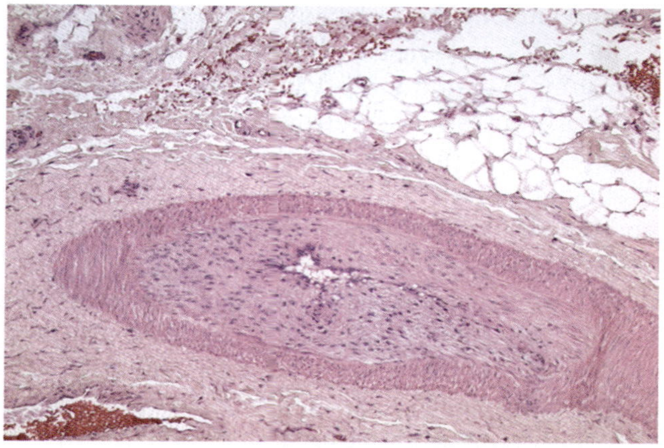

Figure 2-125. Vascular dysplasia in neurofibromatosis type 1: This artery in the soft tissue adjacent to a neurofibroma shows prominent thickening of the intima, obliterating the lumen (H&E; original magnification: 100×).

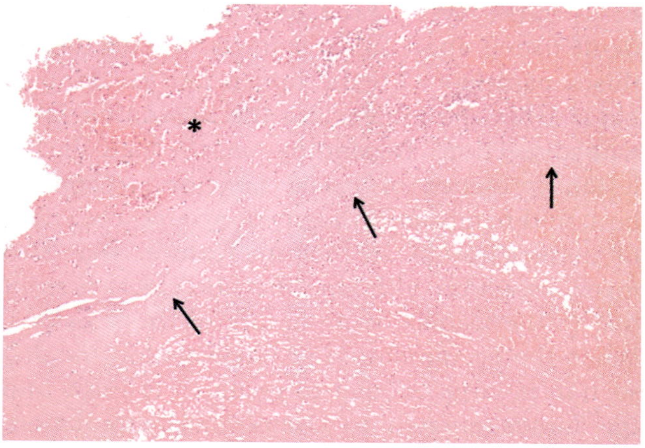

Figure 2-126. Aneurysm rupture: While it may be difficult to pinpoint the exact rupture site in a given aneurysm, the rupture can be indirectly identified by the presence of hemorrhage and PMN leukocytic reaction (*asterisk*) in the acute stage outside the extremely thin and degenerated aneurysm wall (*arrows*), which can be highlighted by special stains (H&E; original magnification: 100×).

microabscesses. *Aspergillus* spp. is the prototype of angioinvasive fungal pathology.[340] *Fusarium infection* is rare in the CNS and can result in meningitis, abscesses, mononuclear infiltrate, and microglial nodules in parenchyma. It is also angioinvasive and may not be distinguished from *Aspergillus* without culture. *Pseudallescheria boydii* hyphae are similar to *Aspergillus*. Meningeal, parenchymal, and vascular invasion and more prominent granuloma formation are seen. *Zygomycosis*,[341] formerly referred to as phycomycosis, is commonly used interchangeably with mucormycosis and typically refers to the infection caused by any of the fungi in the order of Mucorales, which include Mucor, Rhizopus, and Absidia, among others. Hematogenous spread tends to go to the basal ganglia more often, with a pathologic picture similar to aspergillosis, occluding and invading the vessels, resulting in extensive infarcts. Angiostrongylosis (*Angiostrongylus cantonensis*) causes an eosinophilic meningoencephalitis and can have vascular necrosis, thrombosis, hemorrhages, and infarcts.[17]

The most common aneurysm is *saccular (berry) aneurysm*, which can be multiple in 25% to 35% of cases. Gross examination and submission of appropriate sections should provide a good look at the microscopic features, with the normal vessel wall phasing into the aneurysmal dilation with gradual loss of medial smooth muscle layers and gradual thinning of the aneurysm wall as it progresses into the aneurysm, eventually resulting in a thin layer of fibrous tissue or a layer of fibrin and inflammation, if a rupture site is present **(Fig. 2-126)**. Again, as in the case of dissection, because aneurysm rupture is an acute and catastrophic event in the great majority of the cases, such secondary changes may not have developed and one has to rely on gross observations and appropriate handling of the specimen, especially in small aneurysms. In regard to saccular aneurysms, they develop from the weak points in the bifurcations of arteries where smooth muscle has an interruption. This feature is sometimes possible to observe as an incidental finding in unrelated cases where random sections happen to show arterial branching points. As in bacterial meningitis, blood in the subarachnoid space results in spasm of arteries, leading to parenchymal infarcts as a complication in surviving cases. If there have been previous attempts for *endovascular coiling*, there may be variable degrees of clot formation, inflammation, hemosiderin pigment, granulation tissue formation, recanalization, and hyalinization of the clot in the lumen.

Arterial dissection[342] may be difficult to assess unless one is prepared from the beginning of the autopsy to answer this question. The vessels of interest should have been carefully removed and delicately handled because subtle separation between the layers of the arterial wall may be difficult to tell apart from artifacts. Connection of this separation with the lumen and tracking of blood from the lumen into the separation favor true dissection. Depending on the age of the lesion, presence of tissue reaction, inflammation, and hemosiderin pigment around the edges of the separation are helpful features that also favor dissection, although they are rarely present due to the usually acute nature of these lesions. When the accumulation of blood within the dissection is large enough to result in a bulge into the lumen enough to compromise circulation, then it is called *dissecting aneurysm*. The *dissecting aneurysms* show intramural hemorrhage and variable degrees of internal elastic lamina fragmentation. The actual intimal defect is difficult to identify, but the intramural hemorrhage is typical and encircles the lumen as a layer **(Fig. 2-127)**. The dissection typically occurs between intima and media or in the inner one-third of the media. There are usually accompanying prominent atherosclerotic changes, although atherosclerosis is not necessary for dissection. It may be difficult in some cases to distinguish whether the hemorrhage is part of complex atherosclerotic changes or a true dissection. Since these lesions are examined in autopsy, hemorrhage due to surgical intervention is usually not in question. Fresh hemorrhage in the right location, examination of serial cross sections of the artery, and a history of trauma, including head and neck manipulation as in a chiropractor setting or hyperextension, support dissection. When the dissection causes expansion of arterial wall, obliterates the lumen, and bulges outward due to large amount of blood, dissecting aneurysm, rather than arterial dissection, is more appropriate. In chronic cases who survive the initial event or in those cases treated with stent, the usual clot formation and organization stages can be seen, including intramural neovascularization, indicating a past event. *Fusiform aneurysm* is an elongated expansion of the artery diameter and can be seen as a result of diffuse damage to the vessel wall, resulting in the loss of its structural integrity. While atherosclerosis and associated conditions such as hypertension and disorders of collagen and elastic tissues such as Marfan's syndrome and Ehlers-Danlos syndrome can result in fusiform aneurysms, dissecting aneurysms also result in this type of fusiform expansion of the vessel.[343] Therefore, fusiform aneurysm and dissecting aneurysm are sometimes used interchangeably. When destruction of the vessel wall is due to infection, bacterial or fungal, especially angioinvasive ones such as *Aspergillus* spp. resulting in small focal aneurysms, they are termed *infective or mycotic aneurysms*. They may result in hemorrhages and hemorrhagic infarcts. Inflammation and microorganisms can be seen in the vessel wall. Surviving cases show hyalinization of the vessel wall. A history of infection in the region, such as cavernous sinus infections, or procedures, such as lumbar puncture, can explain this process. The aneurysms are typically multiple. Angioinvasive fungi are typically hyphal forms rather than yeast-forming fungi. *Traumatic aneurysms* may develop as a result of traumatic injury of the superficial vessels.[344] They represent destruction of the vessel wall resulting in tears and expansions, and as such, many are actually pseudoaneurysms formed by the injured vessel wall covered by surrounding organizing hemorrhage. They should be easily distinguished from saccular aneurysms by their typical location and the history of trauma; however, some cases may prove difficult in that regard. They tend not to have a well-defined neck and occur with no association with branching point of the vessels.[345]

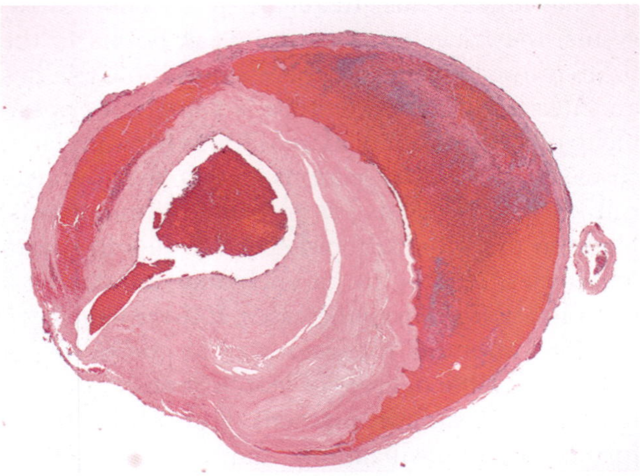

Figure 2-127. Arterial dissection: Fresh hemorrhage is present in the media outside the undulated internal elastic lamina, while the intima has atherosclerotic changes on this cross section of basilar artery (H&E; original magnification: 40×).

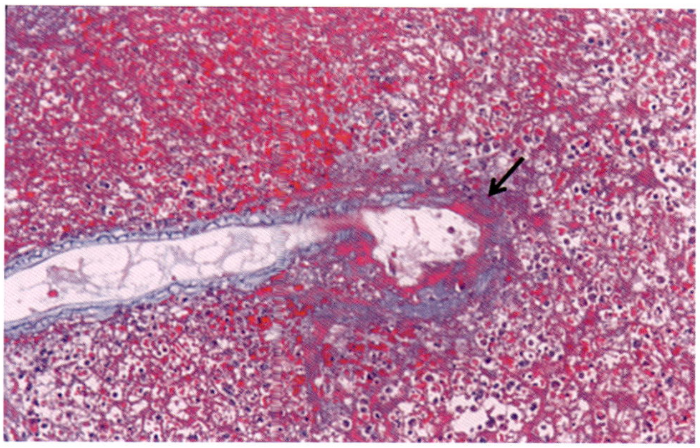

Figure 2-128. Charcot-Bouchard microaneurysm: An arteriole is highlighted in the background of this intracerebral hemorrhage evacuation material and shows a small bulge with bright red fibrin at one tip, representing the microaneurysm *(arrow)* (Masson's trichrome; original magnification: 200×).

Charcot-Bouchard microaneurysms, also known as *miliary aneurysms*, are microscopic outpouchings of intraparenchymal small arteries and arterioles.[346] They usually also show evidence of acute or previous hemorrhage. Healed ones may have hyalinized walls and perivascular hemosiderin pigment with an irregular vascular contour. They can be identified if sought in many intraparenchymal hematoma evacuation specimens. Vessels, with or without these aneurysms, may not be obvious in the background of hemorrhage but can be identified by Verhoeff-van Gieson and Masson's trichrome stains. **(Fig. 2-128)** Although they are commonly seen in hemorrhages, a causal relationship is debatable. *HIV arteriopathy* (also see above) can result in aneurysmal dilation, rather than true aneurysms, of the vessels due to internal elastic lamina damage. Damage to the elastic membranes resulting in aneurysmal dilatations in the white matter arterioles is also described in *cerebral autosomal recessive arteriopathy with subcortical infarcts and leukoencephalopathy (CARASIL)*,[347] not to be confused with its autosomal dominant counterpart (see below, CADASIL), as the presumed pathologic process is different in spite of the similarity in their names. The vessels in CARASIL do not have the PAS-positive granular material by light microscopy or granular osmiophilic material (GOM) by electron microscopy, nor is the skin biopsy useful.

Thrombus forms when there is endothelial damage and the coagulation cascade is activated. In other cases, thrombi represent emboli, that is, *thromboemboli, or a systemic clotting problem* that results in formation of generalized thrombi. *Postmortem clot* formation in vessels is common and sometimes can be difficult to differentiate from especially early thrombus formation. The layering of fibrin with leukocyte aggregation, attachment of the clot to the vessel wall, growth of endothelium over and into the clot, or any other evidence for organization favors true thrombus formation. On the other hand, postmortem clots are loose and easily removed from the vessel and tend to fragment. *Atherosclerosis*, especially when complicated, as well as any other condition that results in disruption of endothelial integrity, can result in thrombus formation. Therefore, whenever a thrombus is identified, the vessel should be evaluated for any evidence of a *vasculopathy*, which is self-evident in most cases. *Atheroemboli* are seen as cholesterol clefts and come from proximal foci of complicated plaques, usually in the internal carotid arteries **(Fig. 2-129)**. *Endocarditis* is a common source of thromboemboli. These can be nonbacterial thrombotic endocarditis or infectious endocarditis; in the latter case, it may be possible to identify bacterial or fungal microorganisms in them. Usually, these septic emboli are associated with PMN leukocytes. In cases of severe sepsis, bacteria with or without PMNs

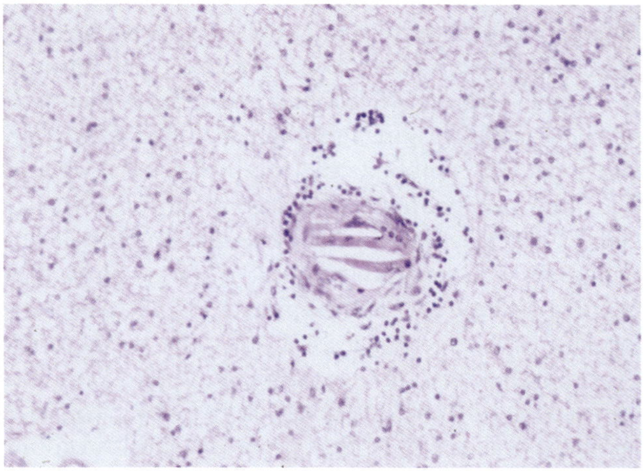

Figure 2-129. Atheroembolus: Complete occlusion by an atheroembolus of the lumen of this arteriole next to an infarct is seen and is characterized by cholesterol clefts and foreign body giant cell reaction among them (H&E; original magnification: 200×).

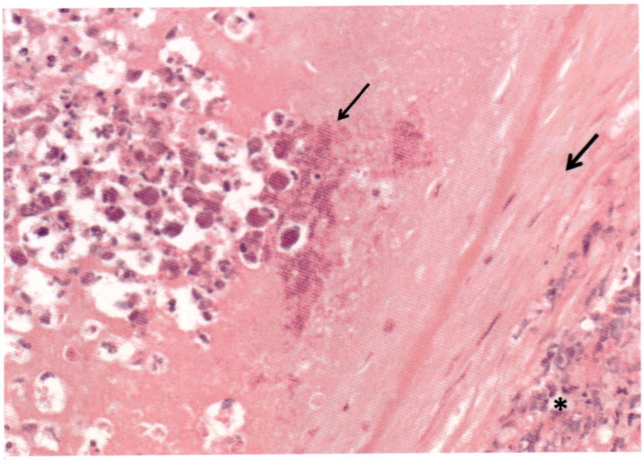

Figure 2-130. Septic embolus: The lumen is occluded by a fibrin thrombus with many PMN leukocytes and bacterial colonies (*thin arrow*). Inflammation (*asterisk*) is also present outside the vessel wall (*thick arrow*) (H&E; original magnification: 400×).

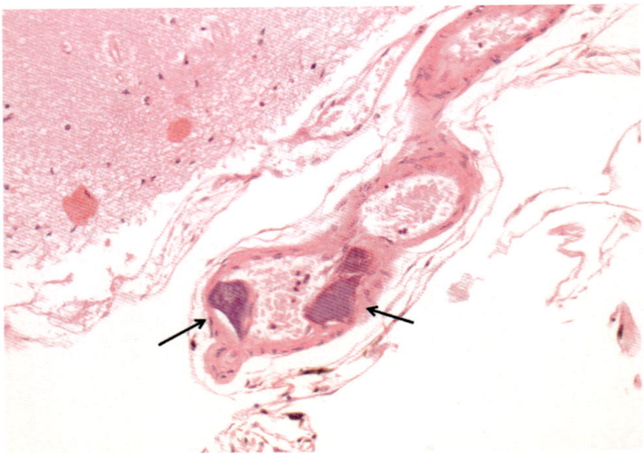

Figure 2-131. Embolization of mitral annulus calcification: Leptomeningeal arterioles contain irregular basophilic fragments of dystrophic calcifications *(arrows)* in a patient with extensive calcification in the mitral valve and with many infarcts in other organs, as well as in the brain (H&E; original magnification: 200×).

can be seen in the vessels **(Fig. 2-130)**. This is more generalized than septic emboli and similar findings are present in other organs of the body. Postmortem bacterial growth may be difficult to differentiate from premortem sepsis. Both lack the thromboembolus component associated with septic emboli, such as those originating from bacterial endocarditis. The presence of prominent PMN infiltration is helpful in favoring sepsis, but this infiltrate is not always present. In those cases, one should assess the focal versus widespread nature and the clinical and other laboratory findings to make that judgment. *Libman-Sacks endocarditis* in systemic lupus erythematosus is another source of nonbacterial thromboemboli of endocardial origin. Fragments of *dystrophic calcifications* can embolize the cerebral arterial system from the calcifications of mitral or aortic stenoses **(Fig. 2-131)**. Other cardiac sources for emboli are myxomas and mural thrombi. *CMV myelitis and meningoradiculitis*[348] can be associated with a vasculopathy with microthrombi around the nerve roots. Thrombi that form in the setting of antiphospholipid antibody syndrome, protein-C deficiency, protein-S deficiency, factor V Leiden mutation, antithrombin III abnormalities, carbohydrate-deficient glycoprotein synthase type I deficiency, and platelet glycoprotein polymorphisms, thrombotic thrombocytopenic purpura, among many other *inherited disorders that affect coagulation system*, are associated with generalized fibrin thrombi resulting in brain infarcts in children and young adults and should be considered in such clinical settings **(Fig. 2-132)**. *Disseminated intravascular coagulation* is also a common cause of bland fibrin thrombi. *Hemolytic uremic syndrome*[349] is associated with platelet thrombi, which are hyalinized-appearing eosinophilic thrombi in small arteries and arterioles, which result in multiple microinfarcts in cerebral and cerebellar gray matter. The endothelium is swollen.

The thrombi in these conditions may not be readily apparent and should be sought for based

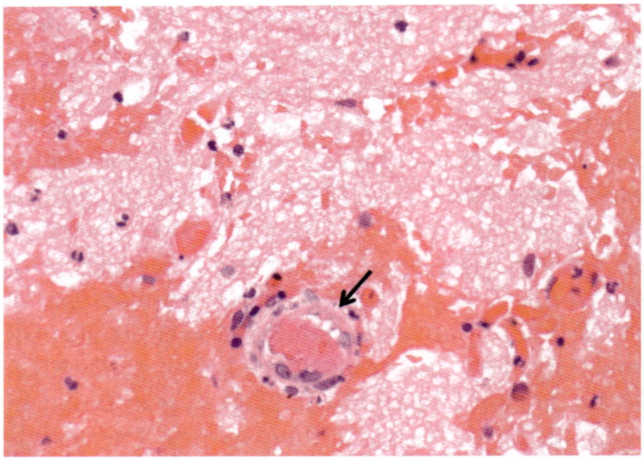

Figure 2-132. Fibrin microthrombi: Multiple fibrin microthrombi, one of which is shown here (*arrow*), were identified in this 37-year-old woman who presented with brain infarcts (H&E; original magnification: 400×).

on suspicion and clinical clues. *Hypernatremia* can be complicated by venous thrombosis due to fluid loss. Hemorrhages may occur, likely due to tissue shrinkage in the acute phase. *Carbon tetrachloride poisoning* is characterized by brain edema, hemorrhages, venous thromboses, and hemorrhagic infarcts.[17] *L-asparaginase* can cause coagulation problems, superior sagittal sinus thrombosis, and hemorrhages.[350] *Rickettsiae* are seen as small gram-negative coccobacilli. They cause neuropathology in typhus and Rocky Mountain spotted fever. Brain is swollen with petechial hemorrhages. Perivascular mononuclear inflammation, thrombosis, and microinfarcts, without fibrinoid necrosis of vessel wall, are seen.[351] Microglial nodules are present in gray matter. *Strongyloidiasis* (*Strongyloides stercoralis*) can be associated with microinfarcts if the larvae occlude the vessels[352] and, when multiple, may clinically mimic vasculitis.[353] *Formic acid treatment of tissues*, used in tissues with the suspicion of prion disease, creates a homogenized and somewhat basophilic appearance of the erythrocytes, resulting in a fibrin thrombus-like appearance within the capillaries **(Fig. 2-133)**. However, the nature of the tissue and the treatment are usually known beforehand, avoiding the confusion.

Embolism by other material can cause significant pathology.[354] *Fat embolism* can be subtle but typically presents with petechial hemorrhages in

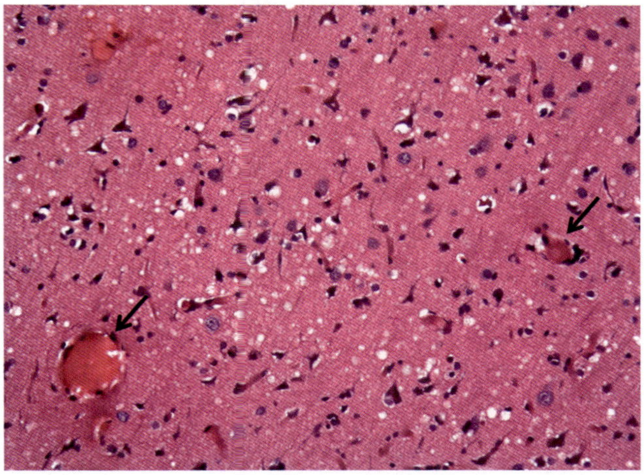

Figure 2-133. Formic acid artifact: Formic acid treatment of tissues suspicious for prion disease results in a smudgy and somewhat basophilic appearance of erythrocytes, mimicking microthrombi (*arrows*). Note the spongiform change in the neuropil in this case of Creutzfeldt-Jakob disease (H&E; original magnification: 200×).

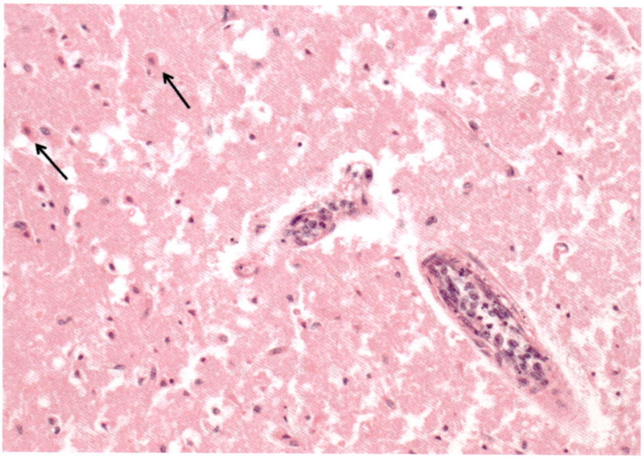

Figure 2-134. Neoplastic emboli: Many neoplastic microemboli were present in the vessels, resulting in multiple microinfarcts in this patient with a history of intra-abdominal primitive sarcoma. Neurons with eosinophilic neuronal necrosis are also seen (*arrows*), while the tissue immediately adjacent to the embolized vessels show more advanced hypoxic–ischemic damage with granular, fragmented, and pale appearance (H&E; original magnification: 200×).

the white matter. Microscopic examination reveals a round "space" within the vessel lumen among the erythrocytes. If suspected by clinical history and/or gross findings, fresh frozen tissue can be stained for oil red O to confirm the presence of fat globules within the vessel lumen. Neoplastic cells within the vessel lumen represent *neoplastic emboli* **(Fig. 2-134)**. These are in clusters and may be attached to the vessel wall, rather than circulating individual cells. Extremely increased cellularity in blast crisis of an acute leukemia is complicated by the embolization and occlusion of vessels by the sluggish cellular aggregates, resulting in infarcts. *Iatrogenic material*, intentionally as in the case of preoperative embolization of vascular malformations or unintentionally as in postcardiac surgery, can be seen.[355] These can be the complication of cardiovascular surgical procedures or angiographic procedures and are typically birefringent by polarized light examination. Cotton fibers are common. Other types of particulate material can also be seen. Especially in the spinal cord, traumatic fragmentation of intervertebral disc and vascular tissues may result in embolization of *intervertebral disc fragments* and acute infarct.[356] **(Fig. 2-135)**. They are associated with traumatic injury to the spine. As for the air emboli that can be associated with cardiac surgery or decompression sickness and that

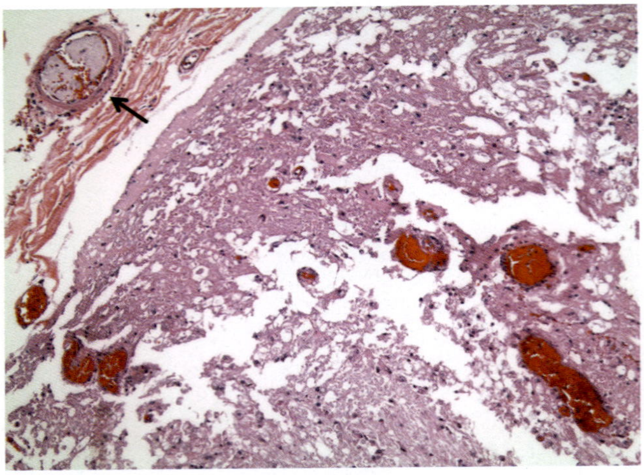

Figure 2-135. Intervertebral disc embolization: A fragment of cartilage is present in a leptomeningeal vessel (*arrow*) causing infarct of the spinal cord. This was identified at autopsy in an individual after multiple severe injuries sustained during an accident (H&E; original magnification: 100×).

can result in acute infarcts, especially in the spinal cord, one has to rely on clinical history and gross techniques as we currently have no stains for air! Fibrin thrombi are common in *high-grade glial neoplasms* **(Fig. 2-136)**. It has been suggested that their identification in anaplastic astrocytoma indicates a more aggressive biologic behavior, even though the diagnostic features of glioblastoma are not yet present.[357] Likewise, it is not uncommon to find larger

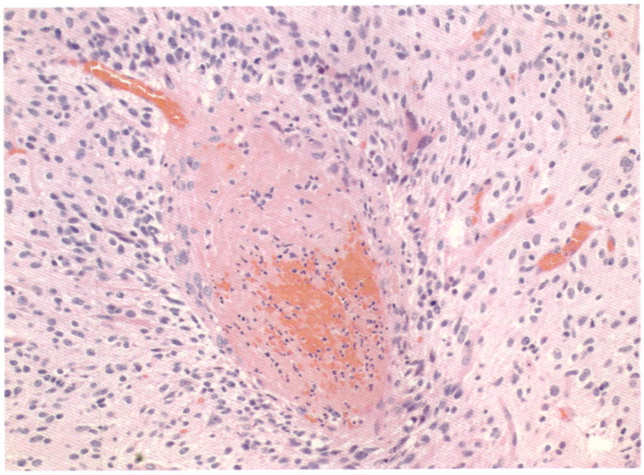

Figure 2-136. Thrombosed vessel in astrocytoma: Complete occlusion of a vessel is seen in this oligoastrocytoma, although no definitive necrosis was present (H&E; original magnification: 200×).

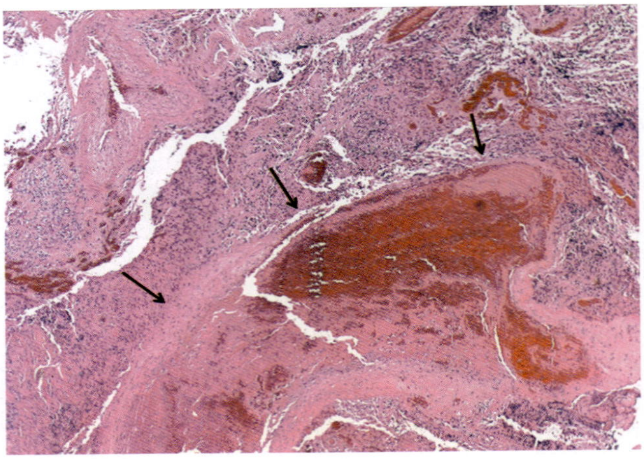

Figure 2-137. Thrombosis in glioblastoma: Identification of a thrombosed vein (*arrows*) on the surface of the brain or within the neoplasm is sometimes used as an indirect evidence for glioblastoma by some neurosurgeons (H&E; original magnification: 40×).

thrombosed vessels in glioblastomas, which can also be identified intraoperatively **(Fig. 2-137)**.

Vessels may be involved by *inflammatory processes*, with or without *giant cells*. Multinucleated giant cells associated with vessels, perivascular and/or intramural, are seen in giant cell arteritis/primary angiitis of the CNS (PACNS); the latter may or may not be associated with giant cells but is a vasculitis limited to the CNS.[358] *Giant cell arteritis* changes are similar to those of the temporal arteritis and are highly focal and variable in quality and amount depending on the phase of the lesion, with fibrosis, fragmentation of internal elastic lamina, and lymphocytic and histiocytic infiltration. Giant cells are associated with internal elastic lamina **(Fig. 2-138)**. It involves the large- and medium-sized arteries. These are usually the basal arteries and their main branches. An elastic tissue stain, for example, Verhoeff-van Gieson, may highlight any elastic lamina fragments within the giant cells. Foreign body type giant cells can be present within the vessel wall or around the vessels as a *foreign body giant cell reaction to amyloid* in vessels involved by amyloid accumulation. These should not be mistaken for giant cell arteritis. Intramural granulomatous inflammation involving aorta and the large arteries arising from it, including internal carotid arteries, and resulting in vessel wall damage and fibrosis is called *Takayasu arteritis*.[359] *Sarcoid granulomas* may be vasculocentric, causing confusion with granulomatous angiitis. Rarely vascular damage may

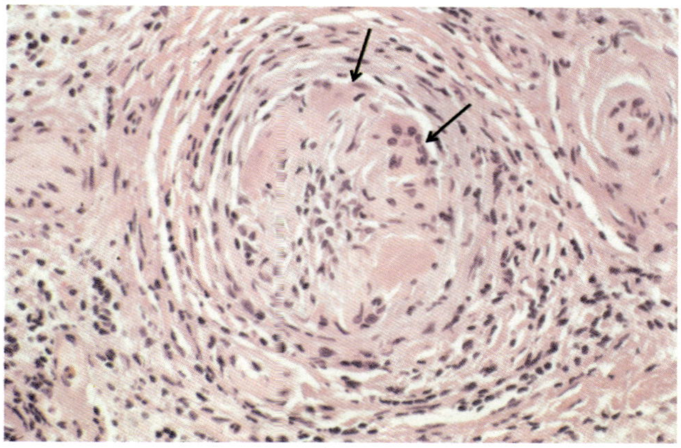

Figure 2-138. PACNS Several multinucleated giant cells (*arrows*) are present in the vessel wall, associated with internal elastic lamina, and also occlude the lumen of this arteriole (H&E; original magnification: 400×).

be present. They typically involve the base of the brain but can be anywhere, including parenchyma, choroid plexus, spinal nerves, and cranial nerves. They may cause hydrocephalus. Variable numbers of multinucleated or mononuclear histiocytes around the vessels, especially in the white matter, are seen in *HIV encephalitis*.[237] These histiocytes can be extremely bland and can be difficult to identify unless specifically searched for in some cases. The process is also associated with generalized white matter pallor due to myelin loss.

Mycoplasma pneumonia infection in the brain is characterized by leptomeningeal acute inflammation extending to the brain parenchyma following Virchow-Robin spaces, creating perivascular and parenchymal acute inflammatory cell collections. Cerebral vessels may be involved in *Kawasaki's disease* by arteritis and aneurysms.[360] *VZV vasculitis* can occur without parenchymal involvement as an isolated process; shows fibrinoid necrosis of the vessel wall, lymphocytes, macrophages, and giant cells; and may result in infarcts. *Perivascular lymphocytic infiltrate* is one of the characteristic features of adrenoleukodystrophy, along with the myelin loss, macrophage infiltration, and gliosis in the white matter. Even though there should not be any inflammatory cells normally in the brain parenchyma, it is not unusual to find *a few lymphocytes around scattered vessels*, usually in the basal ganglia. Their significance is not clear, but they appear to be present even in brains that are completely unremarkable on routine evaluation. One may argue that they are usually seen in autopsy cases and that the brain may have been affected by some generalized condition. At any rate, these are small, round lymphocytes and are not associated with any other cell types, except for a few, possibly hemosiderin-laden histiocytes. They do not infiltrate the vessel wall or are associated with any evidence of vessel wall damage. They are sometimes referred to as *brain microbleeds* and their clinical significance is debatable.[361] In true vasculitis,[362] and depending on the type and phase of the process, there is usually an admixture of plasma cells, larger lymphocytes, possibly giant cells, nuclear debris, PMN leukocytes, including eosinophils, vessel wall necrosis, vessel wall fibrosis, hemosiderin pigment as evidence of vessel wall damage, and thrombosis in the lumen at various stages of evolution or completely recanalized. The perivascular inflammatory infiltrate may raise the differential diagnostic possibility of a lymphoma in some cases. Immunohistochemical workup to identify the predominantly B-cell population as well as the large cell morphology are useful, as the great majority of CNS lymphomas are diffuse large B-cell-type lymphomas. Rarely, the B-cell predominance can be seen in a nonneoplastic/inflammatory population, as in the case of B-cell dominant PACNS[363]; however, the component cells are small lymphocytes with no monoclonality in such cases **(Fig. 2-139)**. *Polyarteritis nodosa (PAN)* affects small- and medium-sized arteries with

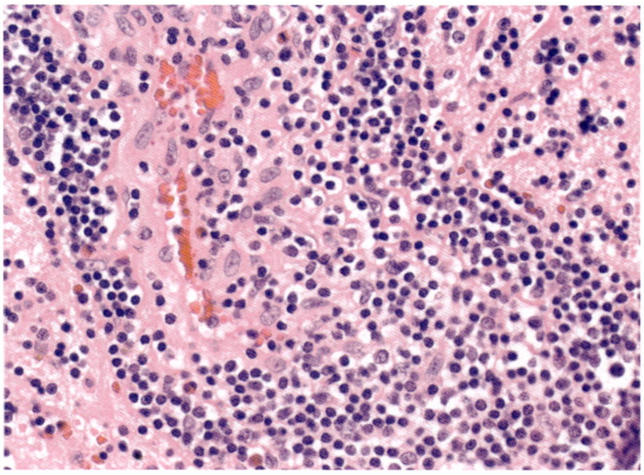

Figure 2-139. PACNS: This vasculitis is characterized by a prominent small lymphocytic infiltrate in and around the vessel wall, resulting in reactive swelling of the endothelial cells, even though thrombosis is not present. The lymphocytic population proved to be predominantly of B-cell type but was polyclonal (H&E; original magnification: 400×).

neutrophil PMN and fibrinoid necrosis of the wall in its acute stage. Patients should be investigated for hepatitis B and C, as well as HIV infections, as a PAN-like vasculitis can be seen in these settings. *Churg-Strauss syndrome (allergic angiitis and granulomatosis)* has fibrinoid necrosis with eosinophil PMNs and giant cells and/or granulomas in the small- and medium-sized arteries and veins, as well as in capillaries. *Wegener's granulomatosis* also has fibrinoid necrosis and chronic inflammation of arterioles and venules, as well as giant cells and/or ill-defined granulomas. *Lymphomatoid granulomatosis* involves arteries and arterioles by a transmural infiltrate of polymorphous lymphocytic population along with fibrinoid necrosis. The lymphocytes have atypical features. It may look like primary CNS lymphoma and, with the atypia and polymorphism of the infiltrate, it may also mimic an angiocentric T-cell lymphoma. Due to the variable presence of plasma cells, small lymphocytes, macrophages, and even PMN leukocytes including eosinophils in the mix, it may be mistaken for an inflammatory process. It is typically associated with immunosuppression and may present with infarcts due to the vascular damage. Vasculitides, with the exception of PACNS, are systemic diseases and these patients either already have a previously established diagnosis or a thorough clinical and laboratory investigation is needed to establish one. *HIV infection in children* can be associated with, in addition to the usual findings, additional prominent perivascular lymphocytes and dystrophic calcifications in parenchyma and vessels, but especially in basal ganglia. Perivascular and leptomeningeal inflammation may be associated with *trichinosis* (*Trichinella spiralis*). *Schistosomiasis* (*Schistosoma japonicum*, *Schistosoma haematobium*, *Schistosoma mansoni*) usually involves lumbosacral spinal cord segments and is rarely seen in thoracic and cervical cord. Brain parenchyma is also involved by numerous granulomas, which may rarely be single, forming mass lesions. Involved cord segment is swollen. Arteritis may be present. Eosinophil PMN leukocytes are typically present. The Schistosoma eggs can be seen in the inflammatory response **(Fig. 2-140)**. They are typically elongated fusiform structures. *S. mansoni* has a lateral and *S. haematobium* has a terminal spine, while the smaller *S. japonicum* egg's lateral spine may be obscure and difficult to identify. Perivascular

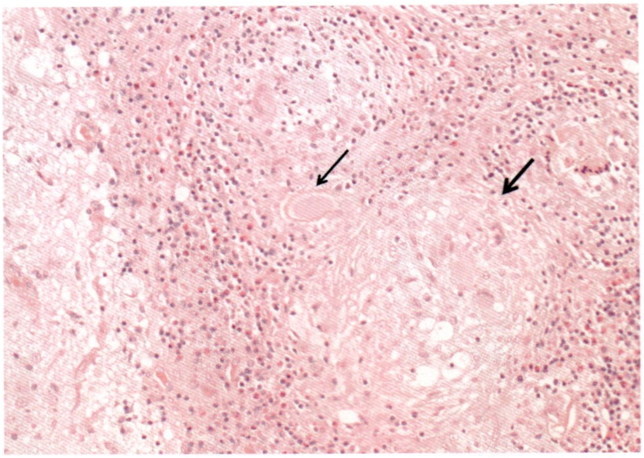

Figure 2-140. Schistosomiasis: Multiple granulomas (*thick arrow*) with multinucleated giant cells are present in the cerebral parenchyma and contain irregular tan-yellow membranous fragments (*thin arrow*) representing degenerating organisms. Many eosinophils are also present in the inflammatory infiltrate (**left side)** (H&E; original magnification: 200×).

inflammation in Virchow-Robin spaces may represent *meningitis* infiltrating along the vessels into the neuroglial parenchyma. This infiltrate may be composed of PMN leukocytes, mononuclear inflammatory cells, or a combination of both, depending on the type and phase of the meningitis. *Perivascular microglial proliferation*, the so-called *Durck granuloma,* can be seen as a result of *malaria* damage to the vessels, resulting in ring-and-ball hemorrhage with a necrotic vessel in the center and surrounding tissue damage. *Organic pentavalent arsenicals* are present in insecticides and in some medications such as melarsoprol for trypanosomiasis.[262] They may cause AHL with fibrinoid necrosis of white matter vessels and perivascular hemorrhages, without inflammation. There may be fibrinoid vessel wall necrosis as a complication of *methotrexate* treatment, with or without concurrent radiation treatment, resulting in multifocal necrotizing leukoencephalopathy. *BCNU* (bis-chloroethyl nitrosourea) treatment can be complicated by a leukoencephalopathy as seen with methotrexate,[364] vascular injury, and calcification. *Amphetamines, methamphetamine, and methylenedioxymethamphetamine (ecstasy)* can sometimes result in necrotizing vasculitis involving various types of vessels.[365] Arterial and venous infarcts and subarachnoid and parenchymal hemorrhages can be seen. *Cocaine* can cause perivascular mixed inflammatory infiltrate but usually without fibrinoid necrosis of vessel wall.[366] Arterial infarcts and subarachnoid and parenchymal hemorrhages are seen.[367] They may be due to a combination of vasospasm or emboli from the heart secondary to cardiomyopathy. If there is saccular aneurysm, it may rupture secondary to acute hypertensive episode. Likewise, fatal parenchymal hemorrhages can be seen. Perivascular lymphocytic infiltrates can be seen in a variety of low-grade or high-grade *glial neoplasms*. Especially in low-grade astrocytomas and in the infiltrative periphery of the neoplasm, this picture may mimic encephalitis with microglial proliferation, especially in small samples. Another perivascular small blue cell accumulation occurs frequently in *medulloblastoma/PNET* but rarely causes a diagnostic problem, as the nature of the process is usually quite obvious. Due to the tendency of medulloblastoma/PNET to involve leptomeninges, the infiltrating cells then spread back into the parenchyma following the Virchow-Robin spaces of the penetrating vessels and appear like perivascular infiltrates. In cases where the actual leptomeningeal infiltration is not represented in the tissue, these perivascular infiltrates suggest indirectly the presence of such involvement.

A *hyalinized collagenous thickening of the vessel walls*, especially in the deep white matter, is seen as a result of *arteriolosclerosis and hypertension*.[368] *Small vessel disease* is seen as hyaline arteriosclerosis and arteriolosclerosis and consists of collagenized thickening of vessel walls.[346] Hypertension and diabetes mellitus are usually present. Their walls have a layered fibrillary appearance. They can be hyalinized and referred to as lipohyalinosis[346] **(Fig. 2-141)**. In advanced stages, they are associated with leukomalacia and loss of white matter. Widespread sampling, especially of deep white matter, is needed, as subcortical white matter is usually preserved. Similar changes are also seen commonly in the basal ganglia vasculature. The increased thickening and tortuosity of these vessels result in expanded Virchow-Robin spaces **(Fig. 2-142)**, corresponding to etat lacunaire and etat crible in the basal ganglia and white matter, respectively. In *malignant hypertension*, in addition to similar changes in vessel walls, there is fibrinoid necrosis and even fibrin thrombi in the lumen. There may be perivascular lymphocytes, hemosiderin pigment, and macrophages. Dilation of Virchow-Robin spaces, especially in the white matter, is seen in conditions where there is loss of neuroglial parenchyma, as in neurodegenerative diseases, Binswanger's disease (subacute arteriosclerotic leukoencephalopathy), and in specimens excised for intractable seizures **(Fig. 2-143)**. Perivascular microinfarcts may be present. Remote microinfarcts, gliosis, and even microglial nodules may be

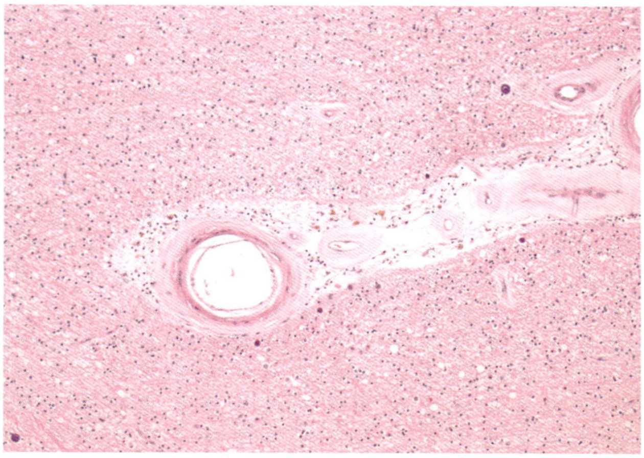

Figure 2-141. Small vessel changes: Changes associated with arteriolosclerosis and hypertension consist of a variable hyalinized collagenous thickening of deep white matter vessels and expansion of Virchow-Robin spaces. Scattered perivascular lymphocytes and siderophages can also be seen, the latter indicating microbleeds (H&E; original magnification: 100×).

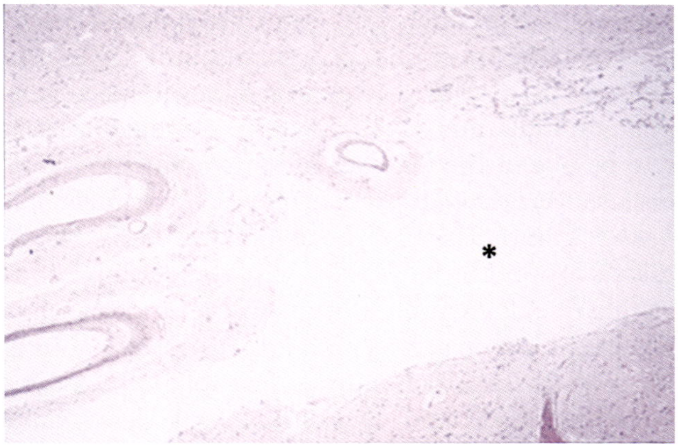

Figure 2-142. Dilated Virchow-Robin spaces: Extensive dilation of Virchow-Robin spaces (*asterisk*) due to thickening and tortuosity of arteries is commonly seen in the basal ganglia in association with hypertension (H&E; original magnification: 40×).

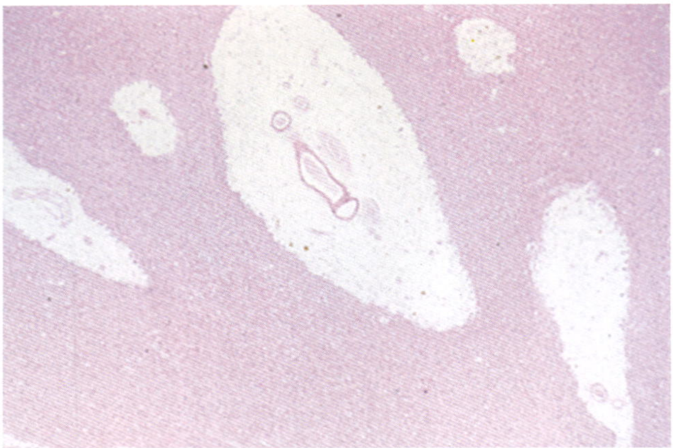

Figure 2-143. Dilated Virchow-Robin spaces can be due to parenchymal loss and/or vascular changes in the deep white matter as in this case of intractable seizures (H&E; original magnification: 40×).

seen in older cases. The presence of perivascular lymphocytes and microglial nodules should not be confused with encephalitis. A clinicopathologic picture with the above findings has also recently been termed as *reversible posterior leukoencephalopathy syndrome*,[256] but this picture is not necessarily associated with hypertension, is not always reversible, is not always posterior, and can be seen in other settings such as medication use, illegal drug use, and pregnancy. Therefore, its accuracy as a term to describe the hypertensive changes is debatable. Such changes are prominent and widespread in Binswanger's subcortical arteriosclerotic leukoencephalopathy, which can result in clinical dementia. Usually, there are prominent atherosclerotic changes in arteries, as well as lacunes in basal ganglia and thalamus. Hyalinized thickening of vessels can be one of the features of *Marchiafava-Bignami disease. Perivascular fibrosis may be the sequela of a healed ADEM*. This may be associated with a vague gliosis around these vessels. Vascular changes consisting of calcification, fibrous thickening, and narrowing of lumen are seen mainly in globus pallidus in *MELAS* (Mitochondrial Encephalomyopathy Lactic Acidosis and Stroke-like Episodes)[185] and *Kearns-Sayre syndrome*[186] but may also involve the white matter, thalamus, and dentate nucleus.

Some *neoplasms* can have prominent vascular hyalinization, obscuring the actual neoplasm in extreme cases. A consistent presence of hyalinized vessels is a feature of *astroblastomas*, aiding in their differential from neoplasms with similar histologic features, such as ependymomas. An extensive hyalinization and thickening of vessels can occur in some *pilocytic astrocytomas* and may be in such a diffuse manner that it obscures the neoplasm in the background. *Myxopapillary ependymoma* is another neoplasm that can have thick, hyalinized vessels. This feature can pose a problem when prominent and widespread enough to obscure the true nature of the neoplasm in an occasional case. However, this becomes an issue in small tissue samples, and the true nature of the lesion should be apparent in other areas or should be suspected based on the location and gross findings, that is, typically a sausage-like, gelatinous expansion of the conus medullaris. *Cavernous angioma* has essentially uniformly hyalinized collagenous vessel walls with no smooth muscle or internal elastic lamina. This change is partial and focal in *AVM*, alternating with smooth muscle layer.

Similar thickening in vessel walls is present in *cerebral amyloid angiopathy (CAA; congophilic angiopathy)*.[369] Rather than a hyalinized collagenous fibrillary appearance, they have a somewhat bright eosinophilic, homogeneous quality. Sometimes, a double-barrel appearance is also present due to a peculiar separation of the layers in the vessel wall **(Fig. 2-144)**. As with amyloid accumulation in general, they are pink-red by Congo red stain and show the peculiar birefringence described as

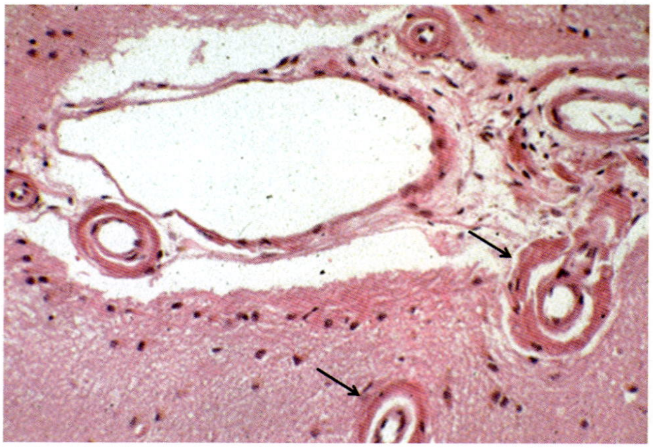

Figure 2-144. CAA: Vessel walls become bright eosinophilic as a result of amyloid accumulation, and some may assume a double-barrel appearance (*arrows*) (H&E; original magnification: 100×).

"apple-green" birefringence by polarized light examination of that stain, typical for amyloid. This amyloid is of beta-amyloid type and can be identified as such by immunohistochemistry. CAA is frequently associated with AD. It involves the leptomeningeal and cerebral cortical, that is, superficial, vessels in a widespread manner. Therefore, the hemorrhages associated with CAA typically tend to be multiple and superficial, in contrast to basal ganglionic hemorrhages of hypertensive etiology. The parenchymal hemorrhage evacuation material therefore should be examined meticulously in an attempt to identify the tissue fragments that may harbor such vessels so that they can be evaluated for the presence of amyloid, as well as for any other vasculopathy. Amyloid accumulation in cerebral vessels can also occasionally be present as part of systemic amyloidosis. A lymphoplasmacytic and histiocytic inflammatory reaction around the vessels involved by CAA may be seen, may be pronounced, and may include foreign body type giant cells, resulting in a picture sometimes termed A-Beta-related angiitis. If cerebral cortex is represented in the evacuation specimen, beta-amyloid immunohistochemistry may highlight the presence of plaques of various stages of development. Additional work-up may also be performed by Bielschowsky silver stains to identify neuritic plaques and NFT, or tau immunohistochemistry may be used to identify tau pathology. However, the diagnosis of AD requires detailed examination of different areas of the brain, as well as close clinical correlation, especially with a history of dementia. Therefore, one should refrain from making a definitive diagnosis of AD in such surgical specimens, although the findings, if any, should be reported and a suspicion may be raised as indicated.

A granular, somewhat amphophilic granular quality to the walls of the white matter vessels is seen in *cerebral autosomal dominant arteriopathy with subcortical infarcts and leukoencephalopathy (CADASIL)* **(Fig. 2-145)**. These granular accumulations correspond to the GOM by electron microscopy and are associated with the smooth muscle cells of the vessel. The diagnosis can now be facilitated by the electron microscopic examination of a skin biopsy for similar findings, as this process is systemic, rather than brain biopsy. Identification of Notch3 gene mutation is also diagnostic. Thickening of small arteries and arterioles in a hyalinized and sometimes somewhat cellular manner has been described in *systemic lupus erythematosus*. They can be associated with vasculitis or perivascular lymphocytic infiltrates. In *Fabry disease*,[370] endothelium and smooth muscle of vessels have birefringent accumulation. They are best seen on frozen sections, are PAS and Sudan positive, and may lead to small infarcts due to vascular accumulation. In *Pompe disease* (acid alpha-glucosidase deficiency; acid maltase deficiency),[371] glycogen accumulation is additionally seen in endothelial and smooth muscle cells of the vessels. *Acute lead encephalopathy* results in endothelial swelling, vascular necrosis, and perivascular proteinaceous material accumulation with PAS-positive globules in this material and in astrocytes. There is also tissue edema and swelling, petechial hemorrhages, and congestion.[17] *Ethylene glycol* is identified as birefringent calcium oxalate crystals[372] in vessel walls and perivascular areas in the parenchyma, meninges, and choroid plexus. There are also hypoxic changes in neurons, congestion, edema, and petechial hemorrhages. *Heroin* can be associated with laminar, bilateral globus pallidus, watershed infarcts, ischemic myelopathy, global hypoxic–ischemic damage, congestion, and edema. Rarely, refractile particles in spinal cord vessels are seen.[373] A basophilic smudgy accumulation in vessel walls can be seen in association

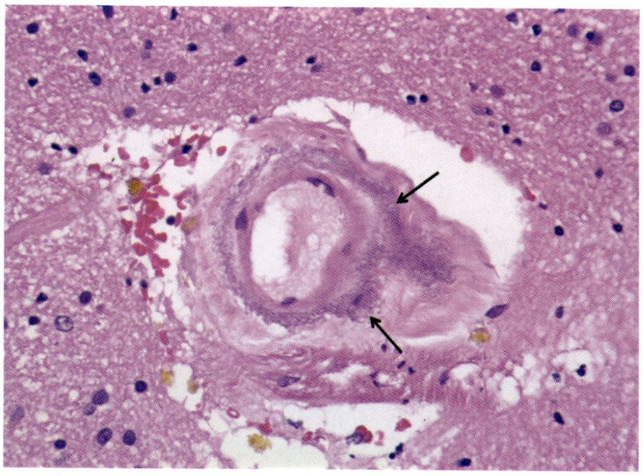

Figure 2-145. CADASIL: Basophilic granular accumulations are present in the vessel wall (*arrows*) and can also be seen as PAS-positive diastase-resistant material by PAS (H&E; original magnification: 400×).

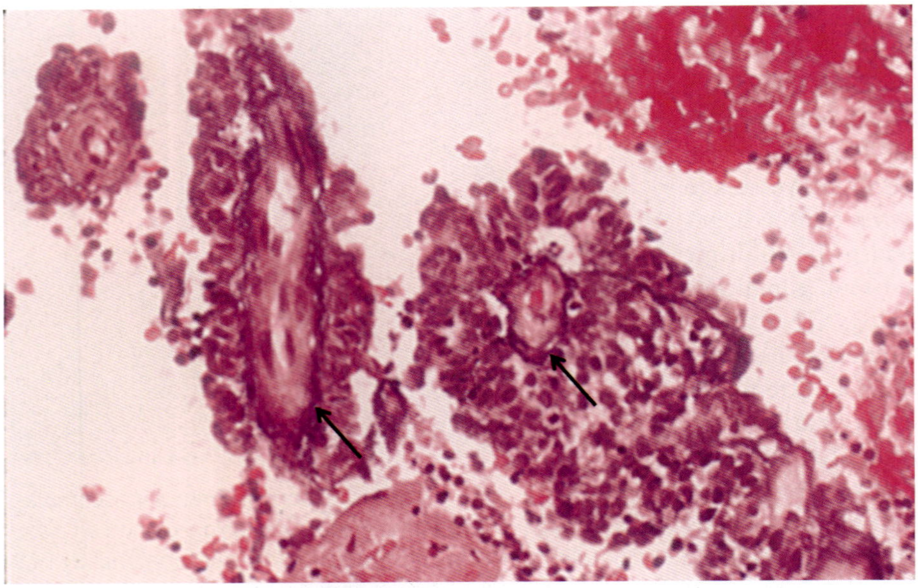

Figure 2-146. Azzopardi effect: Basophilic accumulations around the vessels (*arrows*) in small cell carcinoma due to accumulation of nuclear material from the necrotic neoplastic cells (H&E; original magnification: 400×).

with high-grade neuroendocrine carcinoma (small cell carcinoma) **(Fig. 2-146)**. It is also common in retinoblastoma and can be seen in other small blue cell tumors. It is due to filtering of DNA from degenerating cells of the neoplasm and is called Azzopardi effect. It may appear as crush artifact. The presence of the neoplasm is obvious and its recognition is not problematic. The condition that is commonly seen as a "normal" finding in otherwise unremarkable cases and termed siderocalcinosis, and ferrugination of vessel walls is common in basal ganglia and in hippocampus, specifically dentate fascia. Their components can further be elucidated by histochemical stains for calcium and iron, but this is not necessary.

In cases with focal or widespread *congestion*, the vessels become readily apparent and give a false impression that they are increased in number. A focal aggregate of apparently congested and somewhat dilated capillaries may represent a *telangiectasia*. There is considerable amount of unremarkable neuroglial parenchyma among the vessels. It is typically an incidental autopsy finding, commonly located in the brainstem and temporal lobe, and it is easy to pass over it thinking that it is a small area of congestion **(Fig. 2-147)**. A similar scenario, but with larger vessels with muscular walls usually in the deep white matter, applies to venous malformation. Since these two vascular malformations do not pose a significant risk of complications, such as risk of hemorrhage or seizures, they rarely come to attention during life or are seen in surgical specimens.

In regard to small groups of ectatic capillaries, especially in the white matter, a component of changes associated with *radiation treatment* should also be mentioned.[374] In that setting, such ectatic capillaries are easily recognized as part of the spectrum of radiation change in the background of necrosis, cytologic changes with bizarre cells, fibrosis, hemorrhage, hyalinization or fibrinoid necrosis of some other vessel walls, astrocytosis, which may be difficult to differentiate from

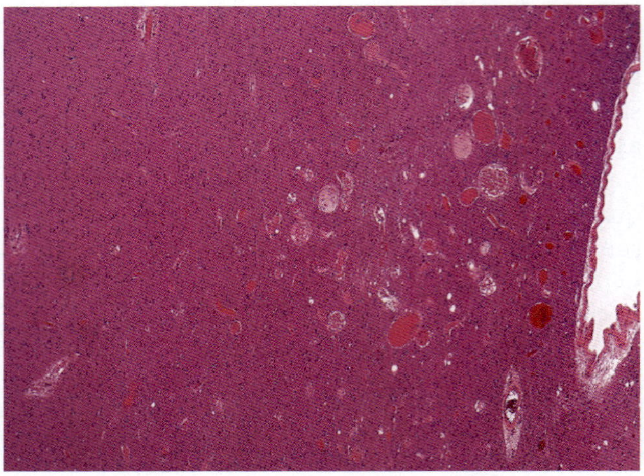

Figure 2-147. Telangiectasia: Many dilated and congested vessels are grouped in and are separated by unremarkable parenchyma (H&E; original magnification: 40×).

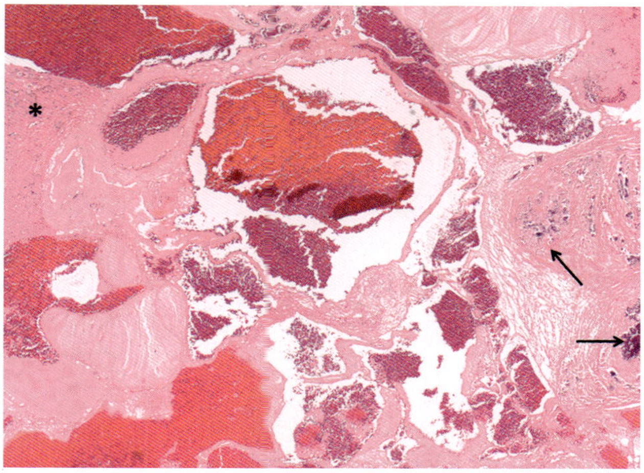

Figure 2-148. Cavernous angioma: Back-to-back vascular channels with hyalinized walls are seen well-demarcated from the surrounding parenchyma (*asterisk*). Dystrophic calcification (*arrows*) is common (H&E; original magnification: 40×).

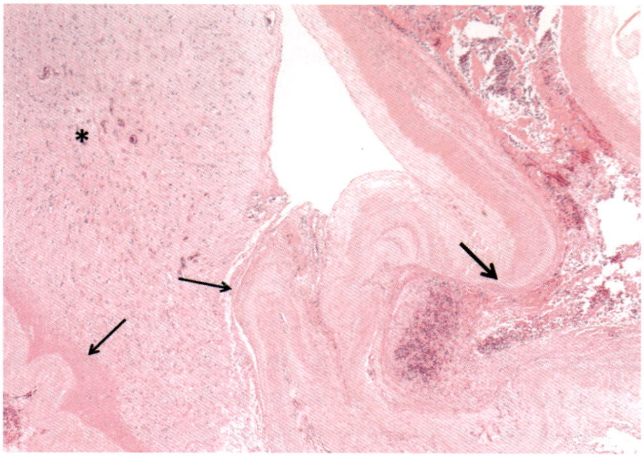

Figure 2-149. AVM: Vascular structures of various sizes, shapes, and wall thicknesses (*thin arrows*) are present with intervening parenchyma (*asterisk*). Transition from thick muscular to thin venous quality (*thick arrow*) can be seen in some (H&E; original magnification: 40×).

residual/recurrent glioma, and possibly an overt glial neoplasm. Radiation injury typically involves small- and medium-sized vessels. The atypia and prominence in endothelial cells associated with radiation treatment may result in confusion and possibly a diagnosis of recurrent neoplasm or unnecessary upgrading of a low-grade glioma. True vascular proliferation typically has multiple layers of cells and channels in its wall. Changes associated with gamma knife radiosurgery are similar but have been reported to occur earlier than the changes of traditional radiation treatment.[375] A well-circumscribed aggregate of tightly packed dilated vessels of variable sizes and shapes with hyalinized fibrotic walls represents a *cavernous angioma (cavernoma)* **(Fig. 2-148)**. Although they are typically devoid of intervening neuroglial parenchyma, small amount of parenchyma may be present in some cases and does not rule out the diagnosis. With a Verhoeff-van Gieson stain, the vessels show no internal elastic lamina. They also do not have muscle layer and show a hyalinized vessel wall for the most part, lined by endothelial cells. Dystrophic calcifications are common and evidence of previous hemorrhage can be seen. A similar lesion that is less well-circumscribed with admixed variable amount of neuroglial tissue, typically with ischemic changes and evidence of hemorrhage, is *arteriovenous malformation (AVM)*. The component vessels are irregularly shaped with variable wall thicknesses. They are hybrids with partially arterial and partially venous features **(Fig. 2-149)**. A Verhoeff-van Gieson stain helps identify this hybrid morphology by highlighting the internal elastic lamina. It also helps differentiate AVM from cavernoma in some cases with limited material and distorted vessels due to surgical and thermal artifact. It is also possible to have composite malformations with features of both and even with a component of telangiectasia. Especially AVMs can be embolized preoperatively, resulting in foreign material and giant cell reaction within the lumen (see above emboli-thrombi). The chronic ischemia and subsequent parenchymal loss may result in condensation of cells and a relative increase in cellularity, which sometimes can mimic a glioma, mostly oligodendroglioma. Saccular aneurysms may develop in the feeding vessels and may coexist with AVM. The *aneurysm of vein of Galen*[376] is a large arteriovenous fistula, which may also be considered an AVM and, when large enough, may result in congestive heart failure, especially in children. The chronic ischemic lesion formed in the spinal cord as a result of *Foix-Alajouanine syndrome* or other vascular malformation can be cellular and can have prominent vascular component, potentially causing misdiagnosis as a glioma in small biopsies and IOC. The picture termed venous congestive myelopathy represents relatively new terminology for Foix-Alajouanine syndrome, simply referring to the dural arteriovenous fistula typically over the lower spinal cord segments, and is composed of prominent gliosis, variable chronic inflammatory infiltrate, and vessels with thick, hyalinized walls.[377] While the diagnosis is a clinicopathologic one, it is important to appreciate the reactive nature of this lesion. Capillary changes with congestion and endothelial prominence are one of the histologic features of *Leigh's disease* and *Wernicke's encephalopathy. Drowning* does not have any specific pathologic findings but can result in extensive congestion, especially in the gray matter.[230]

Aside from the thickening of vessel walls as described above, especially capillaries, arterioles, and venules may become prominent due to *endothelial reactions*. Endothelial cells may become swollen as a nonspecific reaction to a broad spectrum of pathologic processes; however, this prominence is best recognized in the context of neoplasms and hypoxic–ischemic states. *Vascular proliferation* is a high-grade feature in *glial neoplasms*. It is easily recognized and its implication is straightforward in contrast to the earlier changes such as *endothelial hypertrophy* **(Fig. 2-150)**, which is thought to represent an earlier light microscopic change associated with these neoplasms. The endothelial cells become prominent and create a thickened eosinophilic appearance to the vessel wall. The endothelial cells may have enlarged nuclei and prominent nucleoli. These changes make the capillaries stand out. They may indicate an impending transformation to a high-grade glioma. The distinction between endothelial hypertrophy and hyperplasia has been arbitrarily set as more than two layers of cells for hyperplasia. The other end of the spectrum is the fully developed vascular proliferation forming glomeruloid structures and large strips or epithelioid islands standing out in the background of the neoplasm **(Fig. 2-151)**. They have multiple channels that may be small enough to be identified only by the presence of an erythrocyte in the lumen. Although it may start as an endothelial process, vascular proliferation is the preferred term over endothelial proliferation, since it has been shown that all components of the vessel contribute to this proliferation.[378] It should be noted that even though such umbrella terms are used interchangeably to refer to the proliferation of vessels, they may have different implications.[379] In the grading of oligodendroglioma, endothelial hypertrophy has been identified as one of the significant features in univariate analysis, though not in multivariate analysis.[380] Foci of vascular proliferation can be seen in medulloblastoma and PNET—a rare occurrence and is not a prominent feature as in glioblastoma and other high-grade gliomas. Although presence of scattered mitotic figures in them is not

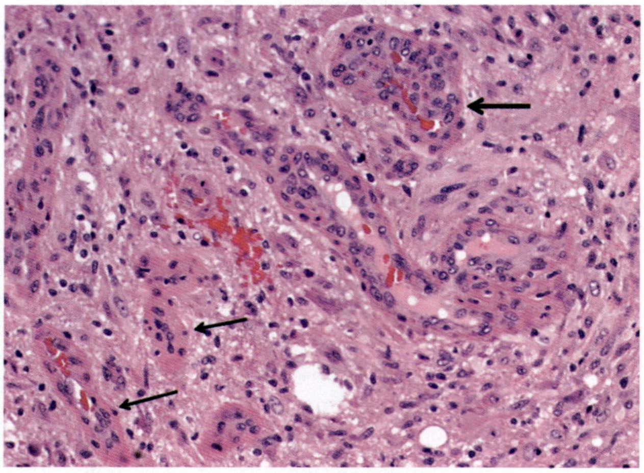

Figure 2-150. Endothelial hypertrophy: Thickened and prominent but not proliferating endothelial layer (*thin arrows*), typically less than two layers in thickness, can be identified due to eosinophilic cytoplasm of the endothelial cells. Gradual transition to a more obvious vascular proliferation (*thick arrow*) can be seen (H&E; original magnification: 200×).

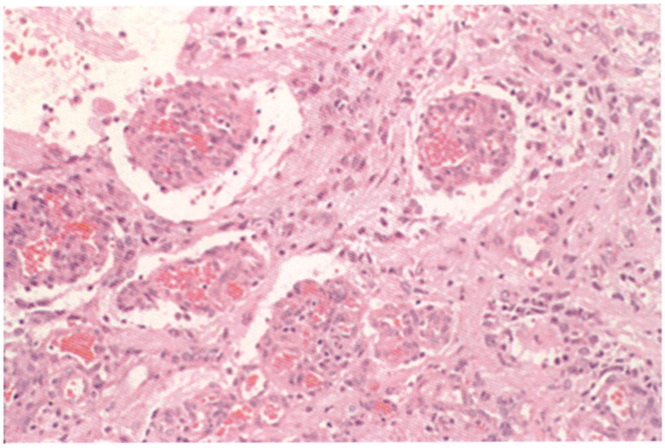

Figure 2-151. Glomeruloid vascular proliferation: Many round foci of vascular proliferation are present and resemble renal glomeruli due to their shape and multiple vascular channels (H&E; original magnification: 200×).

unusual, when these vascular proliferation areas are abundant, widespread, and cellular, they should be evaluated for sarcomatous changes, including spindling, increased mitotic count, and cytologic atypia. There is no definitive mitotic count, size, or any other feature to make the diagnosis of *gliosarcoma* over glioblastoma; however, this kind of information is not necessary in practice since it is clear that one is dealing with a gliosarcoma when the sarcomatous component is present. Endothelial proliferation, microvascular hyperplasia, and endothelial hyperplasia are synonyms for vascular proliferation. These terms should not be used to imply a simple increase in the number of vessels within a lesion, or even within a neoplasm, to avoid misunderstanding. *Sulfonamides* may result in endothelial swelling and necrosis as well as gray and white matter necrosis with or without hemorrhage. *Subacute diencephalic angioencephalopathy* is a rare condition characterized typically by symmetrical bilateral thalamic changes, including a peculiar vascular thickening, endothelial prominence, and microcalcifications.[381]

Endothelial reaction and even mild degrees of vascular proliferation can be seen in *hypoxic–ischemic conditions* as an attempt of the vasculature to provide more perfusion and oxygenation to the area. These changes are more widespread in generalized ischemic conditions but are limited to the sites of infarct. Vascular changes are visible as early as the first few days of an acute infarct but become prominent especially in the subacute stage, when they can contribute to the significant potential pitfall of mistaking a subacute infarct with a glial neoplasm, especially on small biopsy specimens during IOC. Attention to the presence of more than an occasional macrophage should allow one to at least consider the possibility of a nonneoplastic process. Development and evolution of *abscess* is associated with a prominent vascular proliferation as part of the granulation tissue capsule formation. In the first 1 to 2 days, acute focal suppurative cerebritis is seen; 2 to 7 days, confluent central necrosis develops and macrophages and lymphoplasmacytic infiltrate come in; 5 to 14 days, early encapsulation occurs, with early granulation tissue formation; and 14 days and later, late encapsulation with well-developed capsule is formed. If abscess heals without surgical treatment, a fibrous cyst with scattered macrophages in the lumen may be all there is left.

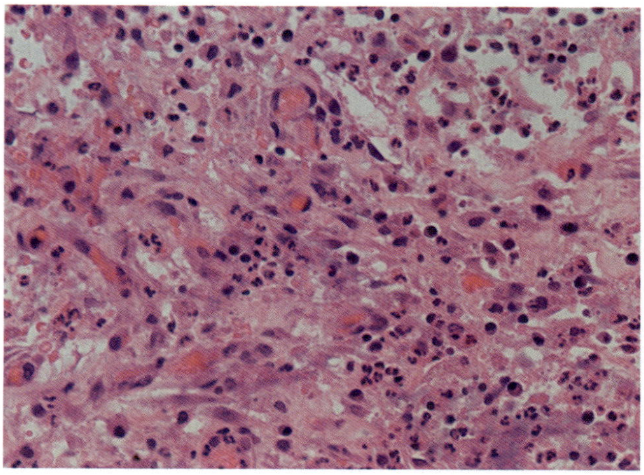

Figure 2-152. Granulation tissue: A common example of granulation tissue in the context of mass lesions in surgical neuropathology is abscess wall, which contains numerous proliferating endothelial cells and fibroblasts with active nuclei, mimicking a high-grade glioma due to atypia and vascularity (H&E; original magnification: 400×).

This prominent granulation tissue and the vessels associated with it and the vascular proliferation in *GBM* can be mistaken for each other, especially in small tissue samples and during IOC, and this pitfall should be kept in mind **(Fig. 2-152)**. The presence of collagen and rich reticulin network by special stains widespread in the background of an abscess, in contrast to collagen and reticulin being limited to the vascular structures in GBM, is a helpful finding in this distinction. Immunohistochemistry to show the atypical cells to be GFAP-positive cells supports the diagnosis of GBM, while reactive fibroblasts in the abscess wall are negative. The occasional possibility of the so-called inflammatory GBM may complicate the matter further. Attention to the presence of at least a suggestion of layering effect by fibrinoid necrosis and pus, surrounded by spindle cell granulation tissue areas composed of prominent vessels and fibroblasts, usually with acute and chronic inflammation, and a dense fibrotic outer layer should clarify the issue at the light microscopic level. Any admixed fibrotic leptomeningeal tissue should not be overinterpreted in favor of an abscess wall. These specimens are typically in the form of strips of membranous material as the surgeon removes the abscess wall, and this zonation can be appreciated along some of these fragments. It should be noted that both GBM and abscesses may have similar radiologic features in some cases, creating radiologic uncertainty.

Some glial neoplasms may have an abundance of vessels, prominent due to congestion and dilation, without or in addition to the actual vascular proliferation. The loosely applied term *angioglioma* is sometimes used for either of these situations, with no prognostic or diagnostic implications. In addition, some vascular malformations may have an increased oligodendroglial cellularity that is worrisome for a neoplastic process, apparently due to the collapse of ischemic tissue and an artificially increased cellularity.[37] Some *neurocytomas*, central or extraventricular, can have more than an occasional mitotic figure, are associated with vascular proliferation and necrosis, and have been designated as *atypical neurocytomas*, without a WHO grade. They also tend to have a Ki-67 proliferation index of more than 2%. An anaplastic version of neurocytoma has not been designated and is debatable. Vascular proliferation is used as one of the features to identify *anaplastic (malignant) astroblastoma*, although it can be seen in an occasional well-differentiated astroblastoma. A WHO grade I neoplasm that can rarely have foci of "vascular proliferation" is *DIG/DIA*, with no prognostic implications. Likewise, prominent and increased numbers of vessels can be present in *pilocytic astrocytoma*, sometimes creating a pitfall for GBM **(Fig. 2-153)**.

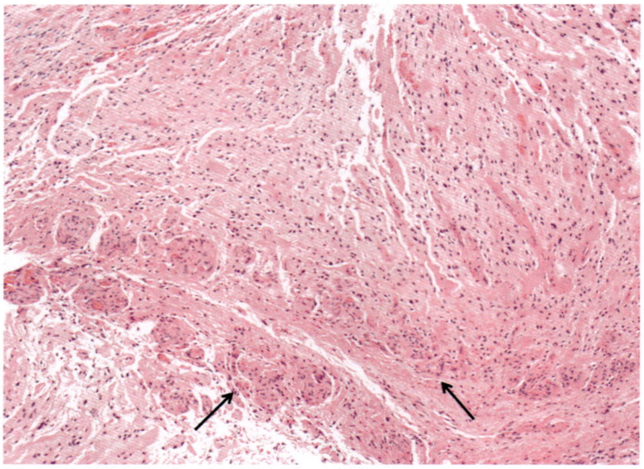

Figure 2-153. Prominent vessels in PA: Extremely prominent vessels (*arrows*) may cause confusion with a high-grade glial neoplasm if the discrepancy between these vessels and the bland features of the neoplasm is overlooked (H&E; original magnification: 100×).

In *angiomatous meningioma*, numerous hyalinized vessels may predominate and even obscure the neoplastic cells. Areas among the vessels may have a microvacuolated appearance, which may imitate a hemangioblastoma or clear cell meningioma. Vascular channels are obviously increased in number in *angiosarcoma*, although a sarcomatous appearance, rather than the vessels, is the main feature of these neoplasms. Vascular channels are delicate and can be difficult to appreciate, especially in cellular and solid variants. Angiosarcoma can develop rarely in schwannoma. A nonneoplastic condition that can have very exuberant anastomosing vascular channels and may sometimes be confused with angiosarcoma is *papillary endothelial hyperplasia*.[382] It is common in organizing hematomas and thrombi **(Fig. 2-154)**. The recognition of the setting and the bland appearance of endothelial cells should avoid any confusion.

An increase in the number of vessels can be associated with syndromes. For instance, diffusely increased number of *vessels in the leptomeninges* can be present as a component of syndromes such as *Sturge-Weber syndrome*. OLD with meningeal angiomatosis is associated with increased vascularity in the leptomeninges. The syndrome of *meningocerebral angiodysplasia and renal agenesis*[189] has very

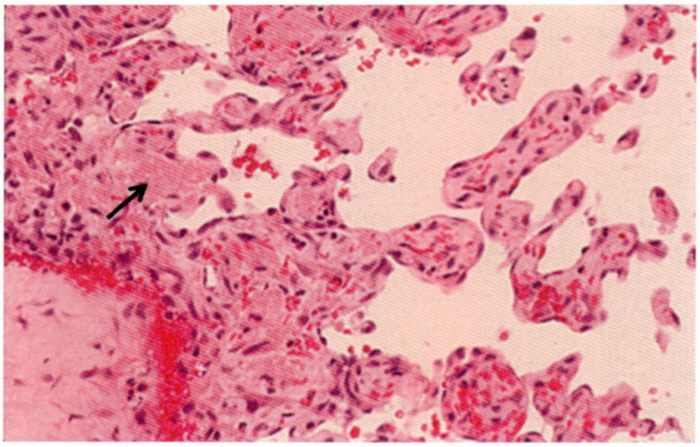

Figure 2-154. Papillary endothelial hyperplasia: Commonly seen in organizing hematomas or thrombi, papillary endothelial hyperplasia consists of growth of endothelial cells into the hemorrhage, encircling lysed erythrocytes and fibrin (*arrow*), creating papillary structures, which later hyalinize. Together with complex channels and the active endothelial cells, this process should not be confused with a more significant one, such as angiosarcoma (H&E; original magnification: 200×).

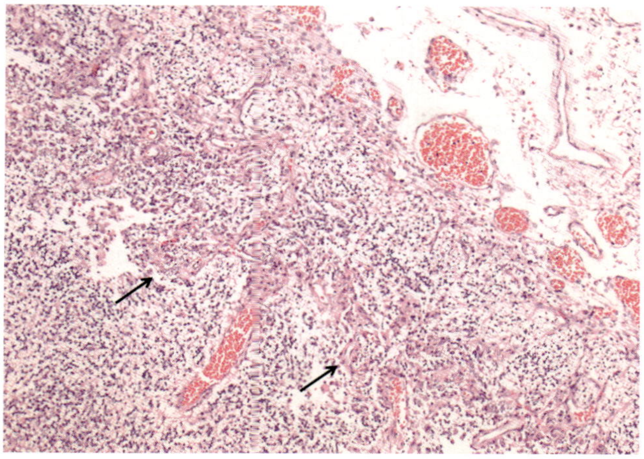

Figure 2-155. Fowler syndrome: Numerous proliferating capillaries (*arrows*) are seen in the cerebral cortex and pial surface. Calcifications are commonly present (not shown). Leptomeninges are seen in the top right corner (H&E; original magnification: 100×).

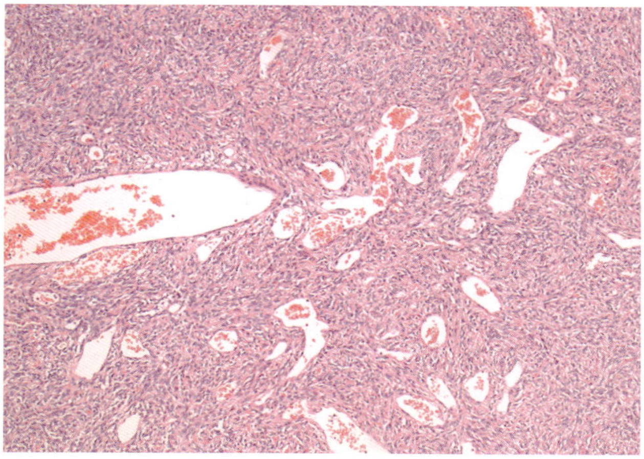

Figure 2-156. Staghorn vasculature: Many sharply defined, thin-walled, branching vessels are seen in this hemangiopericytoma (H&E; original magnification: 100×).

vascular leptomeninges, sometimes associated with subarachnoid hemorrhage. Angiodysplasia is in the form of ectatic capillaries and veins and can be seen in leptomeninges, as well as in the brain, cerebellum, and brainstem. A diffuse numerical increase in the leptomeningeal vessels can be seen in association with *idiopathic hypertrophic pachymeningitis*. *Fowler syndrome* (proliferative vasculopathy and hydranencephaly–hydrocephaly) is characterized by glomeruloid vascular proliferation diffusely in the CNS **(Fig. 2-155)**. There are also numerous calcifications and hydrocephaly/hydranencephaly. Endothelial cells have PAS-positive intracytoplasmic inclusions.[193] In the hepatocerebral form of *mitochondrial DNA depletion syndrome*, in addition to the changes attributable to hepatic failure (such as Alzheimer type II astrocytes), vacuolation and cavitation of putamen and vascular proliferation in affected areas can be seen.[17]

A *vascular pattern* composed of sharply demarcated, branching, thin-walled vessels is called *hemangiopericytomatous vascular pattern* **(Fig. 2-156)**, or staghorn vascular pattern, as it was initially described in association with hemangiopericytoma and was thought to be quite characteristic for it. While this is true, other neoplasms with similar vascular pattern have also been recognized, most notably *solitary fibrous tumor (SFT)*. In fact, due to their frequently overlapping histologic features and similar vascular patterns, it has been suggested that SFT and hemangiopericytoma may represent histologic variations of the same entity.[383] Both present as well-circumscribed dural-based mass lesions mimicking meningioma clinically and radiologically, and even histologically in some cases. In the earlier editions of the WHO classification, hemangiopericytoma was classified as a subtype of meningioma before it was recognized as a separate neoplasm. In addition, this pattern can occasionally be seen in an unexpected neoplasm and may result in misdiagnosis. This vascular pattern can rarely be seen in *malignant meningiomas*; however, attention to cytologic features and the general meningioma features should help resolve this issue. In cases where the histologic features are not clear, EMA positivity in meningioma, and pericellular reticulin pattern, as well as CD99 and BCL-2 positivity in hemangiopericytoma should be useful in this differential diagnosis. SFT is characterized, in addition to cellular areas that can have a similar vascular pattern, by less cellular areas with thick, keloid-like collagen, creating a picture described as "patternless pattern." The overlap and association between hemangiopericytoma and SFT are also seen in their immunohistochemical profile,[383] with both neoplasms variably positive for CD34, CD99, EMA, BCL-2, and SMA, although less so in hemangiopericytoma. A rich network of branching delicate capillaries described as *"chicken-wire" vasculature* is typically seen in *oligodendroglioma* **(Fig. 2-157)**.

While examining the vessels and evaluating what is in or around them, it is a good idea to pay

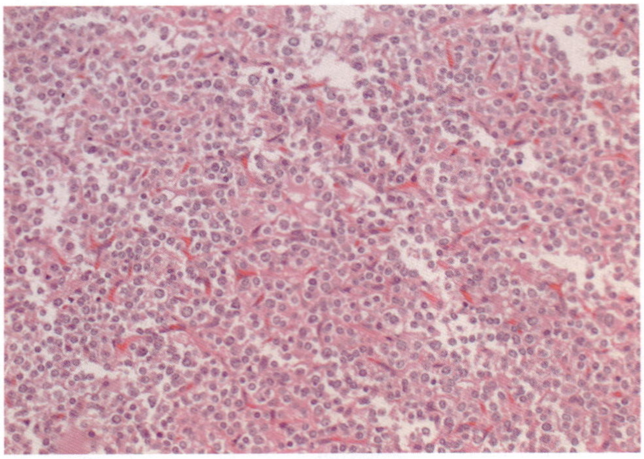

Figure 2-157. Chicken-wire vasculature: Many thin, branching capillaries form a network reminiscent of chicken-wire in the cellular background of this oligodendroglioma (H&E; original magnification: 200×).

some attention to *blood cells*. *Erythrocytes* can show subtle changes that provide valuable clues to the clinicopathologic process at hand. *Sickling* can be identified in cases of sickle cell disease or trait and may explain mental status changes and ischemic changes **(Fig. 2-158)**. Various distortions in erythrocytes should not be confused with sickling, and truly sharply angulated, spiked edges should be seen rather than random irregularities. Erythrocytes may harbor microorganisms, namely *malaria*, which results in the formation of black dots in them due to changes in hemoglobin. Inflammation is not present; however, in some cases, due to margination of infected erythrocytes, vascular damage, occlusion, and hemorrhage, especially in the form of ring-and-ball hemorrhages, can occur.[384] *Erythrocyte precursors* may be prominent in premature or newborns and are seen as nucleated forms. They may be normal for the gestational age or may represent a stress or accompany an anemic condition in older individuals. *Leukocytes* tend to aggregate and form cellular islands within the blood vessel among the erythrocytes, especially in congested vessels. If the lumen is engorged by PMN leukocytes as a consistent finding in many vessels, this may be an indication of *sepsis*, and even bacteria may be identified in such vessels. *Leukemic blast crisis* results in leukemic cell emboli occluding the lumen and may be associated with infarcts. Otherwise, depending on the peripheral cell count and status of the patient, *leukemic cells* can be present in the blood. *Intravascular lymphoma*[385] is a large B-cell lymphoma that can present with infarcts and skin lesions and may be very subtle **(Fig. 2-159)**. An occasional hyperchromatic large cell that seems to be trying to squeeze through capillaries may stand out in the neuropil in an otherwise unremarkable case or in a case unrelated to other pathologic processes. They represent *megakaryocytes* in circulation and are of no known significance **(Fig. 2-160)**.

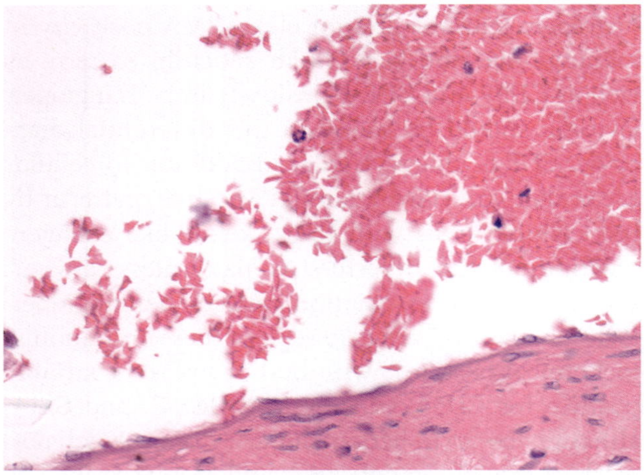

Figure 2-158. Erythrocyte sickling: Many erythrocytes have collapsed appearance with sickle-shaped and spiky contours. This patient presented with mental status changes due to multiple microinfarcts as a result of this sickling and vascular occlusion (H&E; original magnification: 400×).

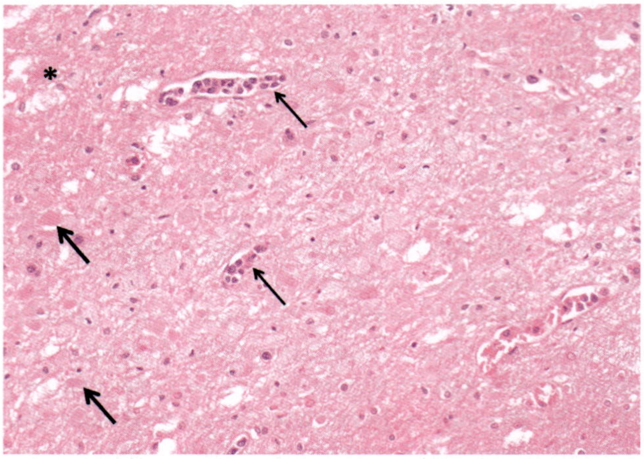

Figure 2-159. Intravascular lymphoma: Capillaries are studded with large lymphoid cells (*thin arrows*). The immediately adjacent parenchyma is pale due to a microinfarct at its acute stage. It is well-demarcated from the darker eosinophilic surrounding parenchyma (*asterisk*), and axonal spheroids (*thick arrows*) are present at its periphery (H&E; original magnification: 200×).

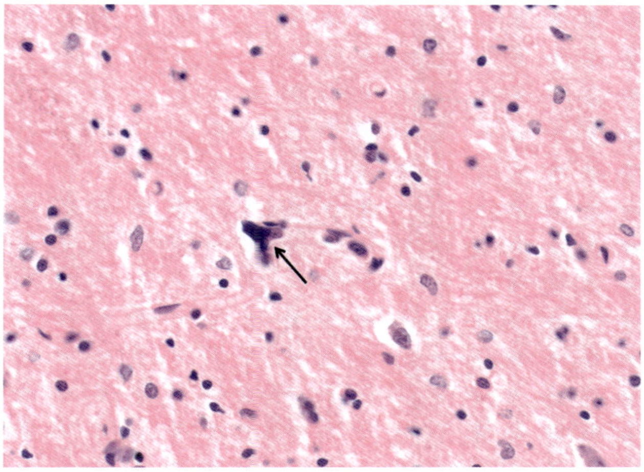

Figure 2-160. Megakaryocyte: A large cell with dark nucleus and chromatin is wedged in the branching capillary *(arrow)* (H&E; original magnification: 400×).

As with other bone marrow elements, including adipose tissue component of the marrow, they may be more common in patients who underwent resuscitation, resulting in bone marrow elements getting into the circulation from the injured costae.

Perivascular Arrangements and Rosettes

There are peculiar arrangements of cells around the vessels that can draw attention to the vessels, even though the vessels themselves may be unremarkable. In addition, rosettes can be present unrelated to vessels and provide important diagnostic clues.

List of Findings/Checklist for Perivascular Arrangements and Rosettes

AT A GLANCE

Pseudorosettes
- Ependymoma
- Astroblastoma
- Papillary glioneuronal tumor
- Rosette-forming glioneuronal tumor of the fourth ventricle
- Angiocentric glioma
- Pilomyxoid astrocytoma
- Pilocytic astrocytoma
- Subependymal giant cell astrocytoma (SEGA)
- Pituitary adenoma
- Paraganglioma

True Rosettes
- Ependymoma
- Primitive neuroectodermal tumor (PNET)
- Embryonal tumor with abundant neuropil and true rosettes (ETANTR)
- "Ependymoblastoma"
- Pineoblastoma
- Retinoblastoma
- Medulloblastoma
- Medulloepithelioma
- Atypical teratoid/rhabdoid tumor (ATRT)
- Immature neuroepithelial component in germ cell neoplasms

Wright Rosettes
- PNET
- Embryonal tumor with abundant neuropil and true rosettes
- "Ependymoblastoma"
- Pineoblastoma
- Retinoblastoma
- Medulloblastoma

Other Rosettes
- Fleurettes
  - Retinoblastoma
  - Pineoblastoma
- Pineocytomatous rosettes
  - Pineocytoma
  - Atypical pineocytoma
  - Pineal parenchymal tumor of intermediate differentiation
- Neurocytic rosettes
  - Rosette-forming glioneuronal tumor of the fourth ventricle

Other Perivascular Arrangements and Rosette mimickers
- Ependymal cells entrapped in the parenchyma
- Lymphoma (see also "Vascular Changes")
- Schiller-Duval bodies
- Schwannosis
- Meningioangiomatosis

They are also discussed here. Some other perivascular processes, such as inflammation and neoplastic infiltration in Virchow-Robin spaces, are discussed in the following section on inflammation. True rosettes (or simply rosettes) were originally described as those rosettes with a central lumen, as described by Flexner in retinoblastoma[386,387]; hence, they are also known as Flexner-Wintersteiner rosettes or retinoblastomatous rosettes. They were then grouped together with the true rosettes of ependymoma (a.k.a. ependymal canals) under "rosettes" by Bailey and Cushing, while the pseudorosettes (i.e., those with a central vessel), as well as the Homer Wright rosettes (or simply Wright rosettes to go with only the last name) that are composed of a solid, anuclear center without a lumen or vessel, formed by the neuritic processes of the surrounding cells, as seen in medulloblastoma, PNET, or neuroblastoma, were called "pseudorosettes." The latter apparently historically resulted in some confusion as some medulloblastomas were interpreted as ependymomas based on the presence of "pseudorosettes," which were in fact Wright rosettes. At any rate, there are three basic types of rosettes: *perivascular pseudorosettes, true rosettes* with a central lumen, and *Wright rosettes*, each with their own implications.

Pseudorosettes are rosettes formed by cells around a central vessel. They are best known in association with *ependymoma* and are formed by the extensions of glial processes of the cells from cell body to the vessel wall creating a radial arrangement **(Fig. 2-161)**. The nuclei are placed at a uniform distance from the vessel, creating a seam-like appearance on cross section. Similar pseudorosettes are also present in *astroblastoma*. Astroblastoma, although considered to be a controversial entity, can be difficult to differentiate from ependymoma. The pseudorosettes of astroblastoma have thicker and shorter processes and the vessel walls tend to show hyalinization. *Papillary glioneuronal tumor* has perivascular arrangements of glial cells around hyalinized vessels.[388] They are more closely associated with the vessel walls than they are in ependymoma; the fibrillary anuclear zone is narrower than in ependymoma or central neurocytoma. Together with the several layers of surrounding nuclei, they form pseudopapillary structures. Although they are not typically referred to as pseudorosettes, such perivascular condensation of cells

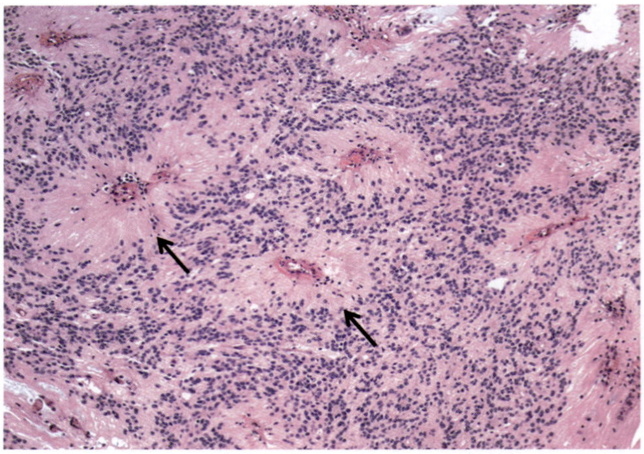

Figure 2-161. Ependymoma: The cellularity is punctuated by pseudorosettes consisting of circular anuclear fibrillary zones around vessels *(arrows)*, an easily recognized pattern at low power that is typical for ependymoma (H&E; original magnification: 100×).

is present in angiocentric glioma,[42,389] where the neoplastic cells appear to cling to the vessel walls but with no anuclear zone. The neoplastic cells have oval to somewhat spindled bland nuclei and point to different directions, creating a haphazard appearance. They tend to be aligned parallel, rather than perpendicular, to the vessel wall **(Fig. 2-162)**. *Pilomyxoid astrocytoma (PMA)* also has an angiocentric arrangement of its piloid cells radially around the vessels, in a myxoid background[390] **(Fig. 2-163)**. In contrast to angiocentric glioma, and as the name implies, PMA has a loose, myxoid background, while nonneoplastic neuroglial elements are present in between the vascular structures of angiocentric glioma. Focal and somewhat subtle perivascular arrangement of cells can be seen in an otherwise typical *pilocytic astrocytoma (PA)* and should not be confused with PMA. In the light of PMA having histologic features of PA partially or entirely in subsequent resections, it is not clear whether this arrangement represents a point in the spectrum of a maturation phenomenon.[391] PA may rarely and focally have cellular and vascular arrangements resembling pseudorosettes[392]; however, these should not cause any diagnostic problems with the rest of the tissue having typical features of PA. Although not a typical feature of *SEGA*, a perivascular rosette-like arrangement of epithelioid, elongated cells of SEGA can be present and provides an important clue in some

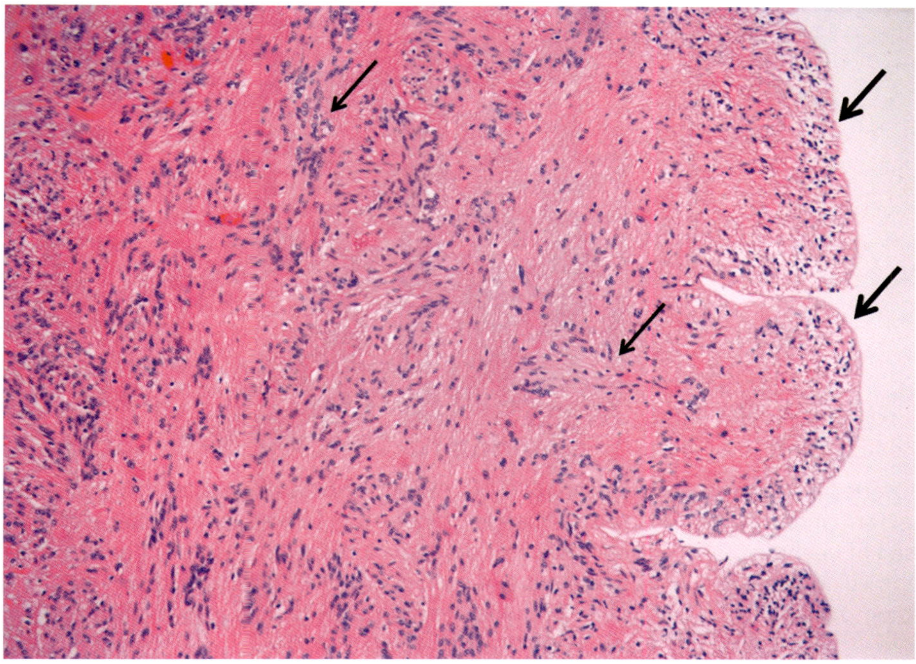

Figure 2-162. Angiocentric glioma: Bland, somewhat spindled cells tend to aggregate around vessels (*thin arrows*), as well as under the pial surface (*thick arrows*) (H&E; original magnification: 400×). (Courtesy of Sakir Humayun Gultekin, M.D., Department of Pathology, Oregon Health & Science University, Portland, OR.)

cytologically highly atypical cases. A perivascular arrangement of cells mimicking pseudorosettes that can at times cause considerable difficulty especially during IOC can be seen in some *pituitary adenoma* **(Fig. 2-164)** and *paraganglioma*. The similarity becomes more prominent if the cells are somewhat columnar or are artifactually stretched. Noting that the seams are formed by actual thin cytoplasm, rather than the thick glial cytoplasmic processes, and the distinct cytoplasmic borders helps rule out ependymoma. Especially gonadotroph cell adenomas have a tendency to form such pseudorosettes.

True rosettes can be present in *ependymoma*, although not as commonly as the pseudorosettes. They are also referred to as ependymal canal formation, as they imitate an attempt to form central canal

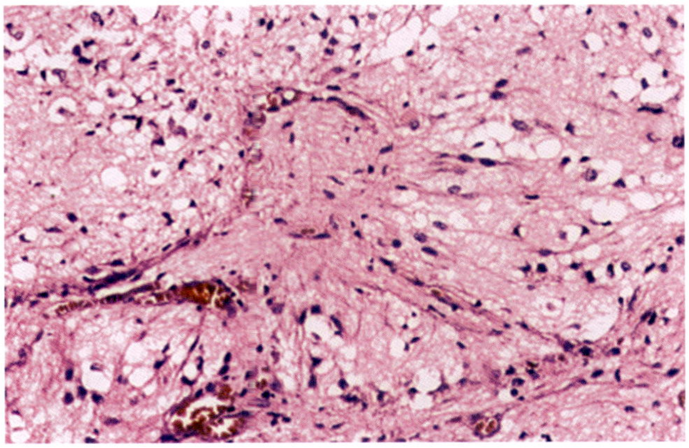

Figure 2-163. PMA: Elongated neoplastic cells are radially arranged around a vessel in a myxoid background (H&E; original magnification: 400×).

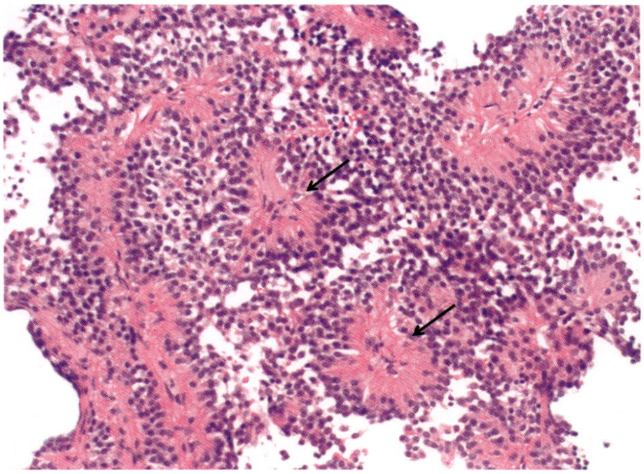

Figure 2-164. Pituitary adenoma: Adenoma cells formed pseudorosette-like structures (*arrows*), reminiscent of ependymoma. The perivascular anuclear zones are formed by the elongated cytoplasms of the adenoma cells. A pseudopapillary pattern formed as a result of dehiscence of cellularity (H&E; original magnification: 200×).

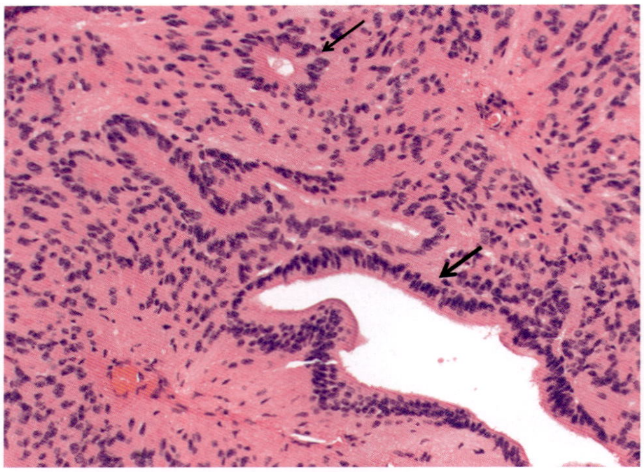

Figure 2-165. Ependymoma: True rosettes that are round (*thin arrow*) or ependymal canal formations that are irregular (*thick arrow*) are composed of ependymal cells lining a lumen, reminiscent of ventricular lining or central canal (H&E; original magnification: 200×).

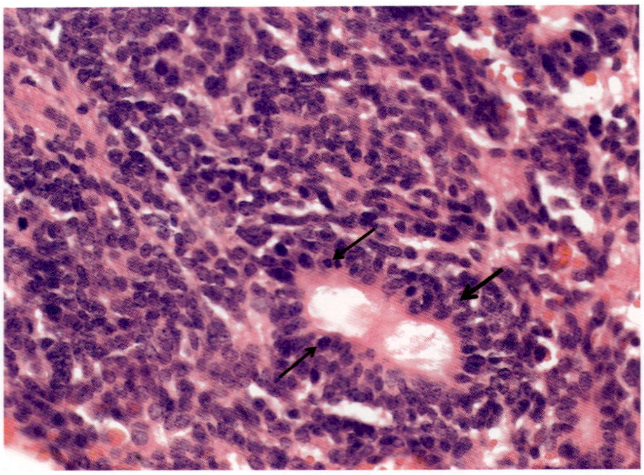

Figure 2-166. "Ependymoblastic rosettes": A round-to-oval rosette (*thick arrow*) formed by multiple layers of primitive cells around a lumen, reminiscent of primitive neural tube, is seen in this PNET. The component cells show prominent mitotic activity (*thin arrows*) (H&E; original magnification: 400×).

and ventricles. True rosettes are of variable sizes and shapes and can even be in abortive forms consisting of only a few cells, or in complex branching channels, or as irregular cystic spaces **(Fig. 2-165)**. Sometimes referred to as ependymal rosettes, they should not be confused with the so-called ependymoblastic, multilayered rosettes of CNS *PNET*. *Ependymoblastic* (ependymoblastomatous) rosettes are similar to the true rosettes in that they have a well-defined central lumen, but they are lined by multiple layers of primitive cells, imitating neural tube formation **(Fig. 2-166)**. There may be cilia and basal bodies, known as blepharoplasts, on the luminal surface. This structure represents an abortive attempt to form neural tube. It has historically been associated with a PNET that shows ependymal differentiation, that is, *ependymoblastoma*, which is considered to be a controversial entity due to the presence of such rosettes in various other neoplasms.[393] One such relatively recently recognized neoplasm is *embryonal tumor with abundant neuropil and true rosettes (ETANTR),*[394] which is a peculiar small blue cell tumor with PNET-like features and, as the name implies, abundant neuropil due to neural differentiation **(Fig. 2-167)**. Likewise, ependymoblastic rosettes or similar structures have also been identified in *medulloblastoma* and *ATRT*.[393] Similar rosettes in a neuropil-like background or a cellular background with features of germinal matrix can be a part of *germ cell tumors with immature neuroepithelial component*. Although other germ cell components are typically present and the nature of the process is readily apparent, especially in the pineal region, which is the most common location for intracranial germ cell neoplasms, the possibility of a pineoblastoma should also be considered in limited material if no other germ cell components are present. In these situations, correlation with radiologic and intraoperative findings is useful. In *pineoblastomas*, these

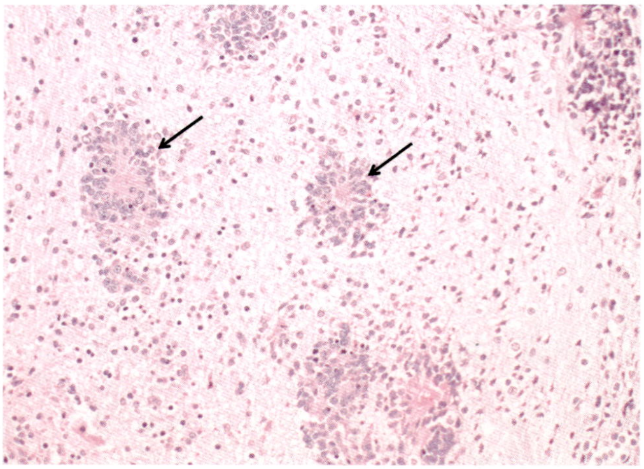

Figure 2-167. Embryonal tumor with abundant neuropil and true rosettes (ETANTR): As the name describes, a neuropil-like delicate background is punctuated by cellular true rosettes (*arrows*) in this peculiar neoplasm (H&E; original magnification: 200×).

rosettes may also display evidence of photoreceptor-like differentiation, similar to rods and cones of the retina, resulting in crowded columnar cell aggregates partially or entirely involving a rosette. They are sometimes referred to as fleurettes, as they may resemble a bouquet of flowers. They are also commonly present in retinoblastoma. To further reiterate the similarities between the retinoblastoma and pineoblastoma, a condition with bilateral retinoblastomas can be associated with a similar neoplasm in the pineal or parasellar region and is called trilateral retinoblastoma.[395] Trilateral retinoblastoma should be distinguished from bilateral retinoblastoma with intracranial metastasis, and the absence of rosettes and fleurettes in the intracranial neoplasm favors a metastasis.[396] Ependymoblastic rosettes or similar structures resembling neural tube are abundant in various forms in a variant of CNS PNET called *medulloepithelioma*. They can be in longitudinal orientation, in the form of trabeculae, or lining irregular lumens; nonetheless, they have the multilayered columnar PNET-type small blue cell population with prominent mitotic activity. They can show differentiation along multiple cell lines.

Another type of rosette is the *Wright rosette* **(Fig. 2-168)**. It is typically seen in *PNET* and *medulloblastoma*, as well as any primitive neoplasm that may have some degree of neural differentiation. As such, it may be present, just like true rosettes, in retinoblastoma and pineoblastoma. It is composed of an acinar arrangement of neoplastic cells. In the center, instead of a lumen, however, is a solid tangle of their neuritic processes filling the central area. A similar rosette is *pineocytomatous or pineocytic rosette* **(Fig. 2-169)**, consisting of round nuclei of *pineocytoma* surrounding a central fibrillary area that contains the processes of these cells. However, the rosettes are irregular with a geographic shape and not perfectly circular. The club-shaped terminal processes of the neurites may be highlighted by neurofilament or Bielschowsky and may even be noted on H&E as small eosinophilic dots. These rosettes are retained and are useful in the identification of the *atypical/pleomorphic pineocytoma*, where there is nuclear atypia (the small, round pineocytoma nuclei are slightly enlarged and have open chromatin, small nucleoli, and irregular nuclear membranes, and there may be scattered multinucleated giant cells).[397] Their identification avoids confusion with a high-grade neoplasm because of these cytologic features. These rosettes are few or less prominent in *pineal parenchymal tumors of intermediate differentiation*, which are mainly composed of sheets of cells. Pineal parenchymal tumors of intermediate differentiation can have sheets of uniform round cells that result in an oligodendroglioma- or neurocytoma-like appearance. Alternatively, they can be in a lobular arrangement, divided by fibrovascular septae. Only a few, if any, pineocytomatous rosettes can be seen, however.

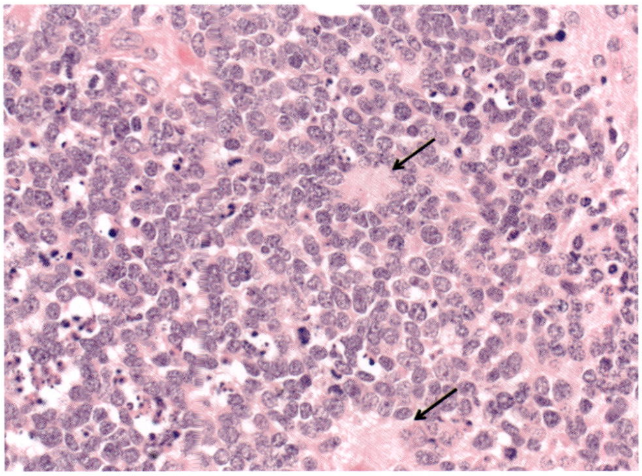

Figure 2-168. Wright rosettes (*arrows*): Rosettes with no true lumen and no central vessel but with an eosinophilic tangle composed of the neuritic processes of the component cells are seen in this PNET (H&E; original magnification: 400×).

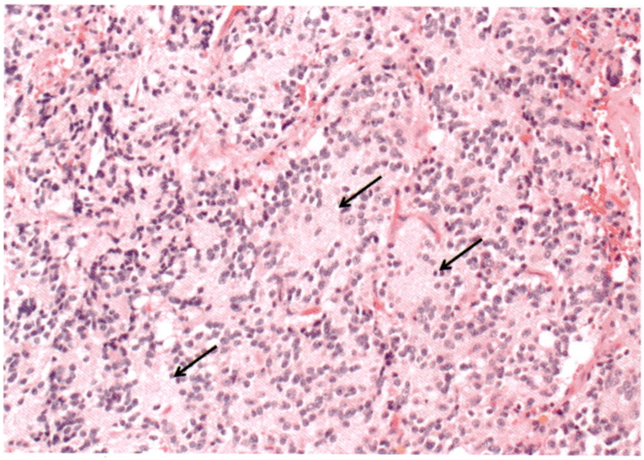

Figure 2-169. Pineocytomatous rosettes: Rosettes with irregular outlines are formed by this pineocytoma. The component cells are not as primitive and hyperchromatic as in the PNET. These rosettes can be thought of as similar to the Wright rosettes in that there is no central vessel or true lumen but a neuropil-like fibrillary center (*arrows*) (H&E; original magnification: 200×).

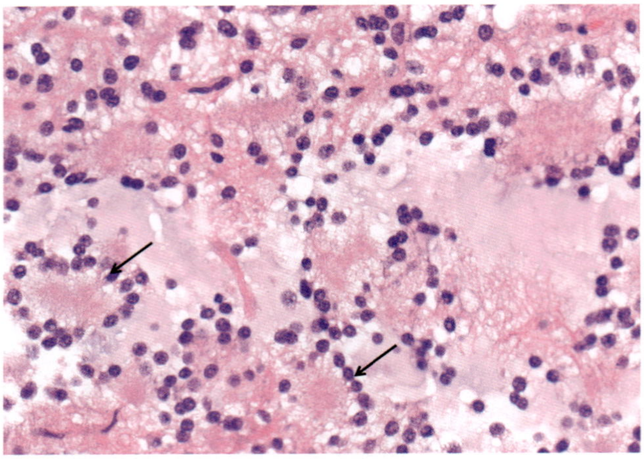

Figure 2-170. Rosette-forming glioneuronal tumor of the fourth ventricle: Neurocytomatous rosettes (*arrows*) are seen in a mucinous background as part of this peculiar neoplasm that has different components. The rosettes are formed by round neurocytic cells that are better differentiated than neuroblasts or cells of primitive neuroectodermal tumor and have a fine chromatin and chromocenters. Their eosinophilic fibrillary neuritic processes fill the center of the rosette (H&E; original magnification: 400×).

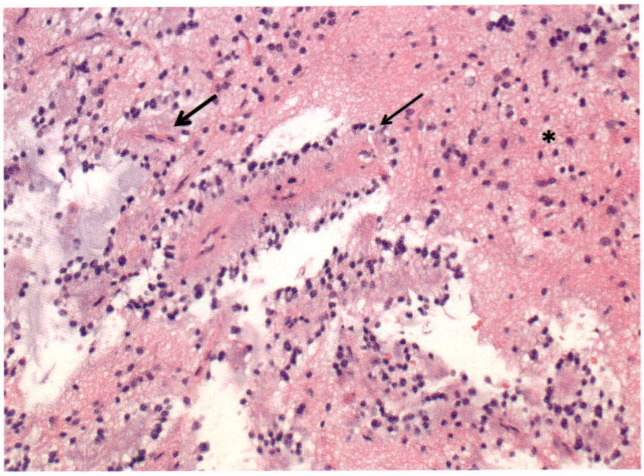

Figure 2-171. Rosette-forming glioneuronal tumor of the fourth ventricle: Another feature of this neoplasm is the presence of perivascular pseudorosettes, seen on cross- (*thick arrow*) and longitudinal (*thin arrow*) section, (*arrows*), which are formed by the delicate neuritic processes of the component cells, in contrast to the thick glial processes of the ependymoma. Solid areas of the neoplasm (asterisk) may have PA or oligodendrglioma-like appearance (H&E; original magnification: 200×).

This roundness and uniformity are also seen in the smaller cells of pineocytomas, but they are punctuated by pineocytomatous rosettes and are easy to recognize as a pineal parenchymal tumor.[398] Even in the atypical variant of pineocytoma, in which the nuclei are slightly enlarged, have open chromatin pattern, small nucleoli, and irregular nuclear membranes, the presence of rosettes makes its recognition easier. *Rosette-forming glioneuronal tumor of the fourth ventricle*[399] has peculiar delicate rosettes formed by small, round neurocytic cells with a small central vessel or fibrillary material composed of neurites originating from these cells. In that sense, they are reminiscent of Wright rosettes and are referred to as *neurocytic rosettes* **(Fig. 2-170)**.This neoplasm also has perivascular pseudorosettes, though not as prominent as in ependymoma. Typically, a single layer of neurocytic cells surrounds the vessel, and the thin rim of acellular fibrillary area is composed of their neuritic processes **(Fig. 2-171)** and is therefore synaptophysin positive. Carcinomas with neuroendocrine features can have rosette-like arrangements resembling Wright rosettes, although rosettes are not a common feature of these neoplasms, and especially high-grade neuroendocrine carcinomas with such rosettes, such as small cell carcinoma, may mimic primary neoplasms when they metastasize to the CNS sites.

Ependymal cell proliferation in the occipital and frontal white matter is normally present as trapped groups of ependymal cells, especially at the corners of occipital and frontal horns of the lateral ventricles **(Fig. 2-172)**. They can be in the form of individual cells, small or larger groups of cells, or occasionally,

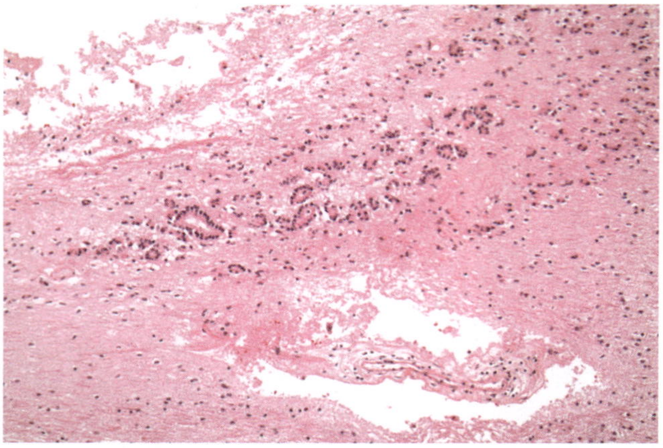

Figure 2-172. Ependymal proliferation: Commonly seen in the periventricular white matter, this ependymal proliferation entrapped within the parenchyma can sometimes be alarming for the unwary and should not be mistaken for a metastatic carcinoma or ependymoma due to the rosette- or gland-like structures (H&E; original magnification: 100×).

they can form acinar structures just like the true rosettes of an ependymoma. Although they are easy to recognize as such in large autopsy sections, they can become a source for confusion for ependymoma or even metastatic carcinoma in small and unoriented tissue samples, especially in IOC.

An *angiocentric pattern* is characteristic of lymphoma in the CNS, although diffusely infiltrating and compact growth patterns, or a mixture of these patterns are not uncommon. Since the great majority of primary CNS lymphomas are of diffuse large B-cell lymphoma (*DLBCL*), these infiltrates are relatively easy to distinguish from inflammatory infiltrates (see "Inflammation and Bone Marrow–Derived Cells"). In cases of lymphoma previously treated with corticosteroids, due to the dramatic response of lymphoma to therapy, only a reactive population of small T lymphocytes may remain, making the recognition of lymphoma essentially impossible. On the other hand, the knowledge of a lesion that responded to corticosteroid treatment is supportive of lymphoma, keeping in mind that there are other processes that show a similar response to corticosteroid treatment, such as demyelinating disease and sarcoidosis. *Schiller-Duval bodies* are formed by a perivascular layer of neoplastic cells separated from the vessel wall by an edematous stroma. They are seen in the endodermal sinus pattern of yolk sac tumors.

Mainly in spinal cord sections, microscopic aggregates of intraparenchymal perivascular spindle cells may be seen. They may also be present around the spinal nerve roots, may be incidental findings, or may be widespread and grossly visible. They represent Schwann cell proliferations, also known as *schwannosis or Schwann cell tumorlets*. This is different than schwannomatosis, which indicates multiple schwannomas in nonvestibular locations without other features of neurofibromatosis type 2 (NF2). Schwannosis may be seen in an otherwise unremarkable autopsy as an incidental finding **(Fig. 2-173)**. In others, it may be associated with NF2 and potentially with the development of multiple schwannomas.[400] They may also explain the rare occurrence of intraparenchymal schwannomas.[401] However, their reactive versus neoplastic nature has not been clarified. It has a high incidence in association with spinal cord injury.[402] *Meningioangiomatosis* is a peculiar lesion that shows proliferation of vessels and meningothelial cells, typically extending into the cerebral cortical parenchyma, forming a nodular mass lesion of variable size or a superficial plaque-like lesion. The meningothelial proliferation is typically around the vessels, resulting in a trabecular appearance dividing the parenchyma into nodules or compartments. The parenchyma is usually distorted with disorganized neurons, which, together with the thickened appearance of the vessels, may create confusion with a ganglion cell neoplasm **(Fig. 2-174)**. Meningioangiomatosis may be sporadic[403] or may be associated with NF2.[404] They can coexist with overlying meningiomas or can give rise to

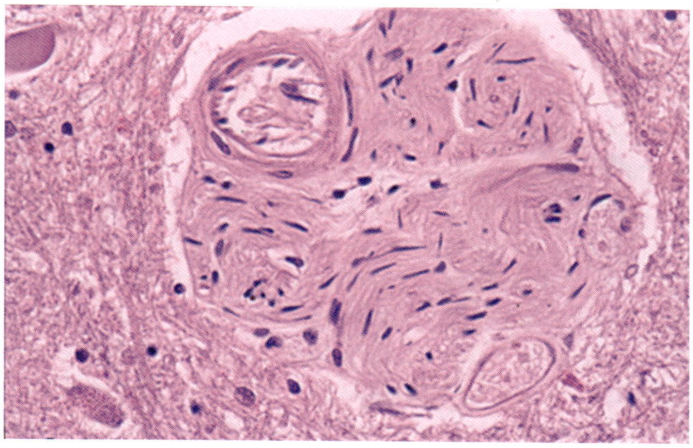

Figure 2-173. Schwannosis: A microscopic perivascular nodule of Schwann cells is seen in the spinal cord parenchyma as an incidental autopsy finding in an otherwise unremarkable CNS in this patient who died of cardiac problems (H&E; original magnification: 400×).

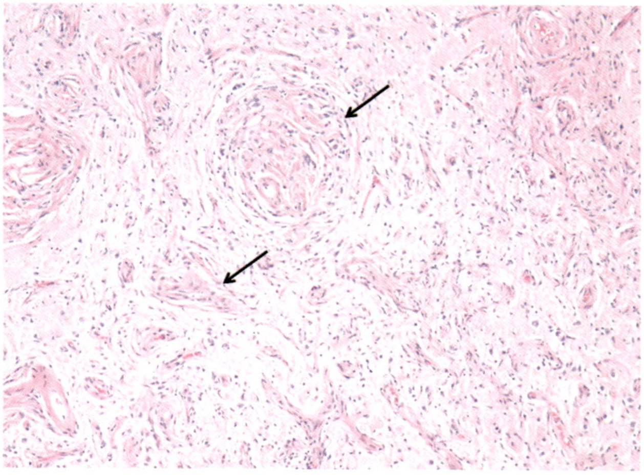

Figure 2-174. Meningioangiomatosis: Vessels are prominent (*arrows*) due to the variable amount of perivascular meningothelial and fibroblastic proliferation (H&E; original magnification: 100×).

meningiomas.[45,46] Their differential diagnosis also includes brain-invasive meningioma, which can be distinguished by close attention to the extensive and mass-forming nature of meningioangiomatosis and the absence of an overlying meningioma. In addition, the close association of meningothelial proliferation with vessels speaks against true brain invasion and should prompt consideration of meningioangiomatosis. Large numbers of *Rosenthal fibers* can be seen in *cortical dysplasias*, especially around vessels, mimicking Alexander's disease. *Mycobacterium avium-intracellulare* often has perivascular foamy macrophages filled with bacteria, with only mild parenchymal injury. Its nature may not be appreciated without special stains and subtle cases may be easily missed.

Inflammation and Bone Marrow–Derived Cells

This discussion is about the bone marrow–derived cells that participate in various disorders that affect the CNS, whether they are residents of the CNS, that is, microglia, or come through the circulation. The type and the location of the inflammatory infiltrate can be important in further defining the disorder. An inflammatory component may be present along with neoplasms. Distinguishing them from their neoplastic counterparts can also be challenging.

Microglia are the monocytic phagocyte system representatives in the CNS with diverse functions.[405,406] In spite of their name, they are of bone marrow origin. They are normally difficult to find and can be seen after some search with the help of their small, curved nuclei with condensed chromatin **(Fig. 2-175)**. When they react, they increase in number and also become more prominent with elongated nuclei. Their reaction is quite nonspecific and can even be seen in light microscopically unremarkable CNS tissue samples, surgical or autopsy **(Fig. 2-176)**. In certain situations, they can transform into actual macrophages with abundant foamy cytoplasm and eccentric nuclei. In addition, macrophages can also come from the circulation when needed and it is not possible morphologically to tell microglial versus circulatory origin of the macrophages apart. Immunohistochemically, macrophage markers, specifically both CD68 and

List of Findings/Checklist for Inflammation and Bone Marrow–Derived Cells

AT A GLANCE

Microglia
- Microglial proliferation
  - Nonspecific/ubiquitous
  - Neurodegenerative diseases
  - Neoplasms
- Microglial nodules
  - Viral infections
  - Paraneoplastic syndromes
  - Rasmussen's encephalitis
  - Spinal muscular atrophy
  - Chronic malignant hypertension
  - Rickettsial infections
  - Malaria (Durck granuloma)
  - Syphilis (general paresis)
  - Lyme disease
- Neuronophagia
- Viral infections
- Microglioma

Histiocytes
- Nonspecific/ubiquitous
- Infections
- Demyelination
- Dysmyelination
- Infarct
- Tract degeneration
- Siderophages
- Erythrophagocytosis
- Perivascular histiocytes
- Radiation changes
- Langerhans cell histiocytosis
- Rosai-Dorfman disease
- Erdheim-Chester disease
- Histiocytic sarcoma
- Epithelioid histiocytes/granulomas
  - Infectious
  - Necrotizing
  - Nonnecrotizing

(Continued)

List of Findings/Checklist for Inflammation and Bone Marrow–Derived Cells *(Continued)*

AT A GLANCE

- Rheumatoid nodule
- Neoplasms
- Foreign body reaction
- Angiitis
- Wegener's granulomatosis
- Granulomatous hypophysitis

- Multinucleated giant cells (see "Cellular Enlargement and Multinucleation")

Polymorphonuclear Leukocytes
- Bacterial meningitis
- Reactive meningitis
  - Hemorrhage
  - Chemical
  - Sensitivity to medications
- Aseptic meningitis
  - Viral infections
  - Syphilitic meningitis
  - Lyme meningitis
  - Behcet's disease
  - Medication reactions
  - Mollaret meningitis
- Cerebritis
- Abscess
- Eosinophil polymorphonuclear leukocytes
  - Parasitic infections
  - Churg-Strauss syndrome
  - Coccidioidomycosis
  - Neuromyelitis optica

Lymphocytes and Plasma Cells
- Mainly mixed
  - Chronic inflammation
  - Aseptic meningitis
  - Treated/subacute meningitis
  - Idiopathic hypertrophic pachymeningitis
  - Toxoplasma cerebritis
  - Lymphoplasmacyte-rich meningioma
- Lymphocyte-predominant
  - Viral infections
  - Demyelinating diseases
  - Dysmyelinating diseases
  - Lymphoma (including intravascular)
  - Treated lymphoma
  - Sentinel (demyelinating) lesion of lymphoma
  - Immune reconstitution inflammatory syndrome (IRIS)
  - Neoplasms
  - Granulomatous infections
  - Paraneoplastic ganglioneuronopathy
- Plasma cell predominant
  - Plasma cell myeloma
  - Syphilis
  - Rheumatoid arthritis
  - Plasma cell granuloma/inflammatory pseudotumor

Mast Cells
- Peripheral nerve sheath neoplasms
- Soft tissue neoplasms

Bone Marrow Elements
- Extramedullary hematopoiesis
- Nucleated erythrocyte precursors
- Bone marrow fragments
- Megakaryocytes
- Leukemic infiltrates
- Neuroacanthocytoses

CD163, stain both microglia and blood-borne macrophages. While their positivity does not help the differentiation of these two cell populations, CD163 appears to be more sensitive and specific in marking both of these populations, and its crisper membranous staining round-to-oval macrophage outlines contrasts with the dendritic and granular staining pattern of microglia, providing a means to differentiate them. In practice, however, identifying these populations without nonspecific background staining is more important than distinguishing the two populations. CD163 has been recommended as a better choice for this purpose.[407]

Microglia are further named based on their appearances and the development of their processes, such as ameboid or ramified microglia, or based on the appearance of their nuclei, such as rod cells or lamellar microglia. However, in diagnostic practice, these differences are too subtle and are difficult to reproduce. The important point for practical purposes is to appreciate the presence and *proliferation of microglia* in the environment.

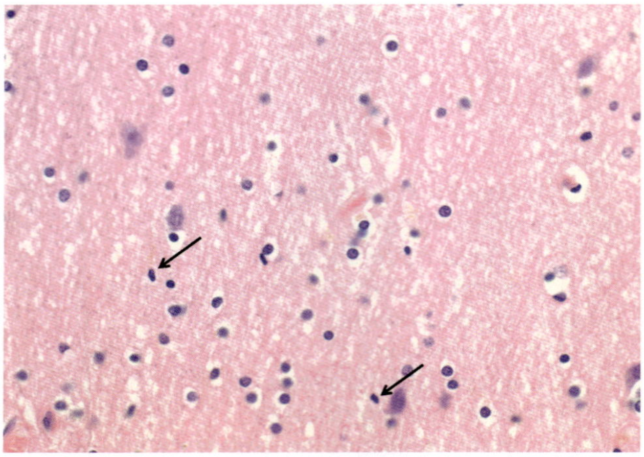

Figure 2-175. Microglia: Slightly elongated and comma-like nuclei are seen in the neuropil and are normally difficult to find (*arrows*) (H&E; original magnification: 400×).

Perhaps the best known histologic finding associated with microglia is the formation of *microglial nodules* **(Fig. 2-177)**. They too are nonspecific findings associated with diverse etiologic factors as a reactive proliferation; however, the main pathologic process they are best known for is viral infection of the neuroglial parenchyma, that is, *encephalitis or encephalomyelitis*.[408,409] Typically, other components of this process are perivascular

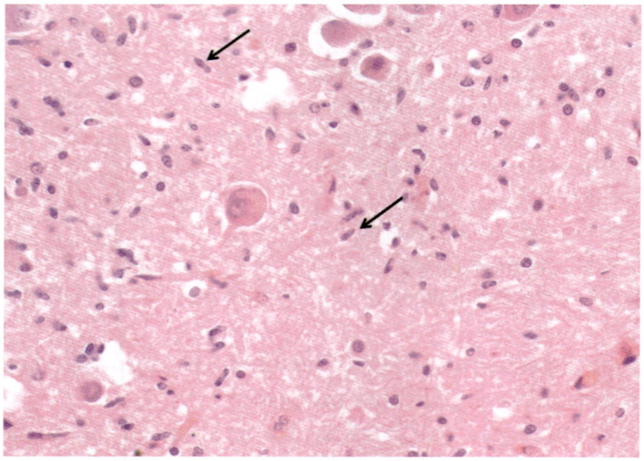

Figure 2-176. Microglial proliferation: Microglial cells can easily be identified due to their increased numbers and elongated nuclei (*arrows*). Many times, they represent a nonspecific reaction to many types of injury and a specific reason cannot be ascertained. Microglial proliferation should not be mistaken for an infiltrating glial neoplasm (H&E; original magnification: 400×).

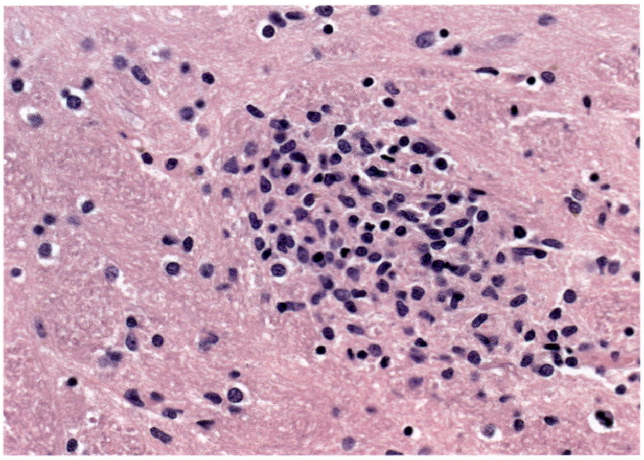

Figure 2-177. Microglial nodule: Many microglial cells form this nodular aggregate. While some are small and others are large, round contours are likely due to cross section of their nuclei (H&E; original magnification: 400×).

lymphocytic infiltrate **(Fig. 2-178)**, which can also be leptomeningeal in cases of meningoencephalitis, and *neuronophagia,* where microglia surround and attack a neuron **(Fig. 2-179)**. When the neuron is destroyed, microglia remain as a microglial nodule. Although this type of encephalitis histologic picture is nonspecific, some viral infections may have additional findings. For instance, arboviruses such as West Nile virus and Japanese encephalitis tend to more prominently involve the brainstem, thalamus, and basal ganglia; some also additionally involve the spinal cord.[410] In addition

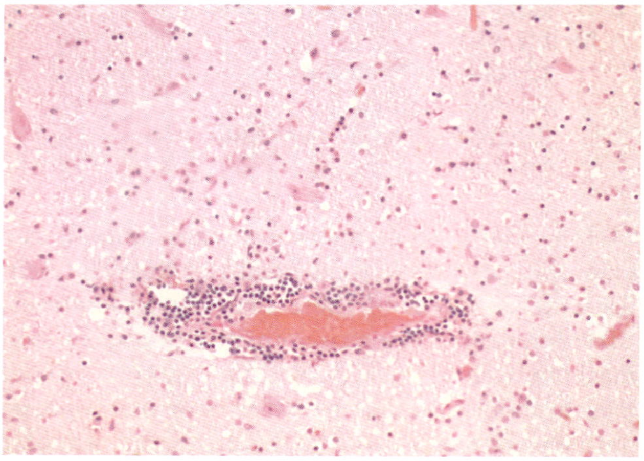

Figure 2-178. Perivascular lymphocytes in encephalitis, not to be confused with vasculitis (H&E; original magnification: 200×).

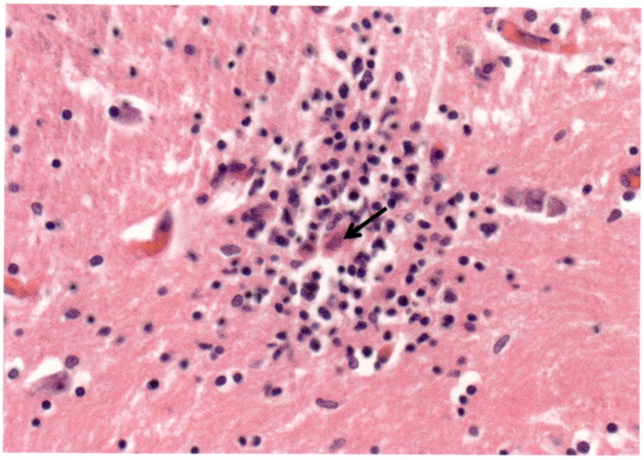

Figure 2-179. Neuronophagia: A degenerating, apparently unhappy eosinophilic neuron (*arrow*) is surrounded by microglial cells, which will remain as a microglial nodule after the neuron is destroyed (H&E; original magnification: 400×).

to typical encephalitis picture, they may also cause perivascular hemorrhages and perivascular destruction of myelinated fibers, reminiscent of ADEM. Microglial proliferation and microglial nodule formation are seen in HIV encephalitis[408] and have a predilection for gray matter. They are seen in later stages of HIV infection, while HIV encephalitis is seen in earlier stages of HIV infection, predominantly involves white matter, and is characterized by diffuse myelin loss and perivascular macrophages, and the microglial changes are limited. Anterior horns of the spinal cord are involved in poliomyelitis, and medial temporal lobe in Herpes encephalitis. Herpes viruses tend to produce a myeloradiculitis in addition to destructive lesions in the brain.[411] Neonatal Herpes simplex virus (HSV) infection shows more diffuse involvement of the CNS. Rabies infection has a tendency to involve the cerebellum and hippocampus. There is an absence of or relatively limited inflammation in rabies, but Negri bodies are present, especially in Purkinje cell and hippocampal pyramidal neuron cytoplasms. Lyssa bodies are less well-defined inclusions seen in rabies. The microglial nodules remaining after neuronophagia are termed *Babes' nodules*. Virus can be identified in corneal and skin biopsies.[412] Neonatal enterovirus encephalitis (commonly coxsackie and echovirus strains) causes hemorrhagic and necrotic areas with mixed inflammatory infiltrates and tissue destruction that can be widespread but more prominent in the anterior horn and brainstem. In any case with a suspicion of viral infection, frozen tissue should be saved for further studies in an attempt to characterize the specific virus. Relatively limited immunohistochemical and molecular diagnostic studies can also be performed on formalin-fixed, paraffin-embedded tissue. These examples also attest to the importance of thorough sampling of autopsy cases due to such selective vulnerability to gain maximum information from the examination. The pattern of distribution in any process provides additional insight to its nature. The changes associated with gene therapies for neoplasms using viral vectors, such as Herpes virus and adenovirus, have not been well-defined. A variable amount of predominantly perivascular lymphoplasmacytic infiltrate can be seen in the case of adenovirus vector, with no definitive evidence of the virus.[413]

Paraneoplastic syndromes can be great mimickers of viral infections due to the involvement of lymphocytic inflammation and microglial proliferation, including microglial nodules. There are a variety of paraneoplastic syndromes that are seen in association with a variety of malignancies. Paraneoplastic encephalomyelitis[414] is commonly seen in the setting of small cell carcinoma of the lung, prostate carcinoma, neuroblastoma, and some sarcomas. Other forms may be in the form of limbic encephalitis, predominantly affecting medial temporal lobes, inferior frontal lobes, insular cortex, and cingulate gyrus, or brainstem encephalitis, affecting mainly medulla. In the cerebellum, inflammation is leptomeningeal and/or deep, involving dentate nuclei but sparing the cortex. Spinal cord involvement may be complete or predominantly cervical and lumbar. Paraneoplastic cerebellar degeneration[415] shows severe loss of Purkinje cells, variable granule cell loss, Bergmann gliosis, and microglial proliferation. Lymphocytic infiltrates are present in the cerebellar cortex and in perivascular and meningeal locations. Inflammation may not correlate with areas of neuron loss, which may indicate some degree of overlap with paraneoplastic encephalomyelitis. *Rasmussen encephalitis* has features similar to viral encephalitis, including perivascular lymphocytic infiltrates and microglial nodule formation[416] **(Fig. 2-180)**. There are neuronal degeneration and gliosis, also. The changes are typically

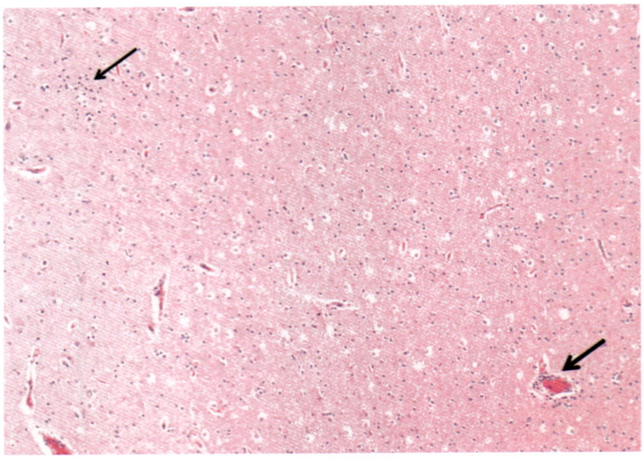

Figure 2-180. Rasmussen's encephalitis: A microglial nodule (*thin arrow*) and a vessel with perivascular lymphocytes (*thick arrow*) are present in a background where some of the cells with clear cytoplasm are oligodendroglia and others are histiocytes (H&E; original magnification: 100×).

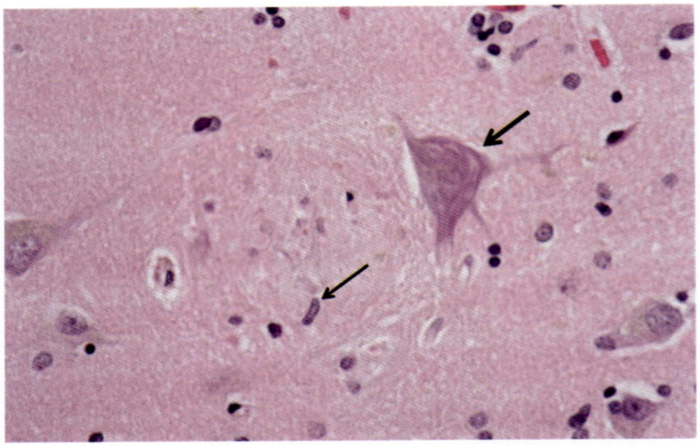

Figure 2-181. Neuritic plaque: The irregular area with round contours in the neuropil represents a neuritic plaque, which can be shown by special stains to be formed by contributions from beta-amyloid, dystrophic axons, reactive astrocytes, and microglial cells. A microglial cell (*thin arrow*) is seen in this particular plaque. A NFT is also present in a neuron (*thick arrow*) (H&E; original magnification: 400×).

seen in the involved areas of the brain. In addition, a vacuolar, spongiform change is present involving both gray and white matter in these areas.

An example for microglia's involvement in widely diverse processes is their involvement in neurodegenerative diseases. Chromatolysis and microglial nodules are seen in early lesions of *spinal muscular atrophy*, including acute infantile (SMA type 1; Werdnig-Hoffmann disease), intermediate (SMA type 2; chronic infantile), and chronic (SMA type 3; chronic proximal; Kugelberg-Welander syndrome) forms, and may also involve brainstem cranial nerve nuclei and dorsal root ganglia. Some variants may be associated with cerebellar atrophy or hypoplasia. In AD, *neuritic plaques* contain microglia as one of their component cells **(Fig. 2-181)**. Microglial proliferation is seen in association with ALS, as well as others.[405,417] Rarely, microglial nodules may be seen along with perivascular lymphocytes, perivascular gliosis, and hyalinization of vessel walls in the deep white matter, as part of *chronic hypertensive damage*.[418] Typically, microglial reaction is a constant component of any type of tissue injury. In pretty much any tissue injury and even in infectious processes, possibly with the exception of viral infections where it is the predominant finding, microglial proliferation is present in the background of the more prominent other findings that may be associated with that particular infection. Along with petechial hemorrhages, perivascular mononuclear inflammation, thrombosis, and possible microinfarcts, microglial nodules are seen in the gray matter in *Rickettsial infections*.[419] Microglia participate in the formation of *Dürck granuloma* in malaria[420] and may contain iron, as this granuloma apparently forms in relation to the resorption of petechial hemorrhages in malaria. It also contains reactive astrocytes and lymphocytes. *General paresis* (chronic meningoencephalitis) in the tertiary stage of syphilis infection is associated with scattered meningeal and parenchymal perivascular lymphoplasmacytic infiltrates, a microglial proliferation, and cortical neuron loss and gliosis. Spirochetes can be seen by silver stain in some cases in the cortex. Lymphoplasmacytic infiltrates, microglial nodules, neuron loss, and gliosis are present in *Lyme disease* in meninges and parenchyma.[421] There may be microvacuolation of cortex and an endarteritis similar to that of syphilis, which may result in infarcts. *Fusarium infection* is rare in the CNS. It can cause meningitis and abscesses and may be associated with mononuclear infiltrates and microglial nodules in the parenchyma. It is also angioinvasive like *Aspergillus* spp. but may not be distinguished from *Aspergillus* without cultures.[422]

In small biopsy samples, the spindled nuclei representing microglial proliferation may mimic diffuse infiltration of a glioma, especially the infiltrating periphery of a glioma or gliomatosis cerebri. A prominent microglial proliferation is usually present accompanying glial neoplasms, contributing to the cellularity.[423] This can particularly become problematic in the differential diagnosis of reactive gliosis versus low-grade glioma. In such cases, microglial cells may be stained by immunohistochemical markers, and that cellularity can be "subtracted" from the picture, giving a better idea about the actual glial component. To further complicate this issue, microglial and inflammatory cells may contribute to Ki-67 proliferative index and may yield falsely high counts. In this context, it should also be remembered that some low- and high-grade gliomas may be associated with perivascular lymphocytic infiltrates, further mimicking encephalitis with microglial proliferation. *Microglioma* is a peculiar and rare neoplastic proliferation of microglia[424]; however, its specific characteristics and even true existence have not been well-established.

Histiocytes/macrophages in the CNS can come from the general circulation or can be the result of microglial transformation. Like microglia, they too can be seen in a very broad spectrum of conditions; however, infections, demyelinating processes, and infarcts are the main conditions to consider initially. In addition, like microglia, macrophages can be a part of diverse pathologic processes such as necrotizing leukoencephalopathy and the lesions of Wernicke's syndrome.

Typically, they have a large cytoplasm, which can be described as multivacuolated or foamy and can have intracytoplasmic debris, and an eccentric nucleus, which can be round to oval, usually with an indentation creating what is described as kidney-, bean-, or slipper-shaped nucleus depending on the taste, interest, and imagination power of the pathologist. However, macrophages are highly variable in appearance. Their importance comes from the fact that identification of a prominent population of macrophages in a specimen should sway one away from a neoplastic process toward a reactive, inflammatory or demyelinating process. In general, macrophages are present in any type of *tissue destruction* and/or when *microorganisms* are involved. In *demyelinating processes*, histiocytes are abundant in the acute phase, along with a small lymphocytic infiltrate. Although not so prominent in the acute phase of these lesions, reactive astrocytes can also be present in variable numbers and, together with the overall high cellularity, these lesions can be mistaken for a glial neoplasm, especially in those cases presenting as demyelinating pseudotumors.[233] Therefore, the identification of histiocytes in such cases can be very important. They usually also have ingested myelin debris in their cytoplasm, easily highlighted by a LFB/PAS stain as blue in earlier stages and PAS positive in later stages, supporting the demyelinating nature of these lesions. This stain also shows the myelin loss, typically with a sharp border with the surrounding tissues if available in the specimen, with a relative preservation of axons as seen on an axon stain such as Bielschowsky silver stain or neurofilament immunohistochemistry (see "White Matter Changes and Myelin Loss"). While a nonspecific finding, it is not unusual to find Creutzfeldt astrocytes in association with demyelinating lesions. In *dysmyelinating diseases* (leukodystrophies), the clinical presentation and radiologic findings are quite different; however, histologic appearance is again that of a myelin loss with macrophages and may not be definitively distinguished from demyelinating lesions on histologic grounds alone. There are a few dysmyelinating diseases with special features to at least allow them to be considered as a differential diagnostic possibility, such as Krabbe's disease (globoid cell leukodystrophy, where macrophages with intracytoplasmic PAS-positive material tend to accumulate around the white matter vessels), metachromatic leukodystrophy (with metachromatic material within the macrophages as seen by a toluidine blue stain), or adenoleukodystrophy (with vague needle-shaped crystalloid spaces left from the dissolved lipids in the cytoplasm of histiocytes, along with a perivascular small lymphocytic infiltrate). OLDs have Sudan-positive macrophages. Macrophages may show clues to identify specific *infections*. They may contain intracytoplasmic tachyzoites in toxoplasmosis, along with a microglial proliferation in the background. Mycobacterium avium-intracellulare infection often has perivascular foamy macrophages filled with bacteria, with only mild parenchymal injury. The bacteria can be seen packing the macrophage cytoplasm, by Ziehl-Neelsen or Fite stain. The spindle-shaped histiocytes with foamy cytoplasm forming a mass lesion may not

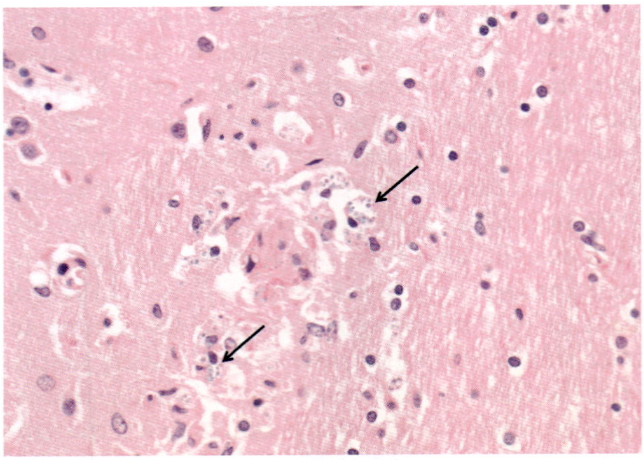

Figure 2-182. Histoplasma infection: On an otherwise unremarkable section, close examination revealed scattered histiocytes with intracytoplasmic yeast forms of 3 to 5 micrometers (*arrows*) (H&E; original magnification: 400×).

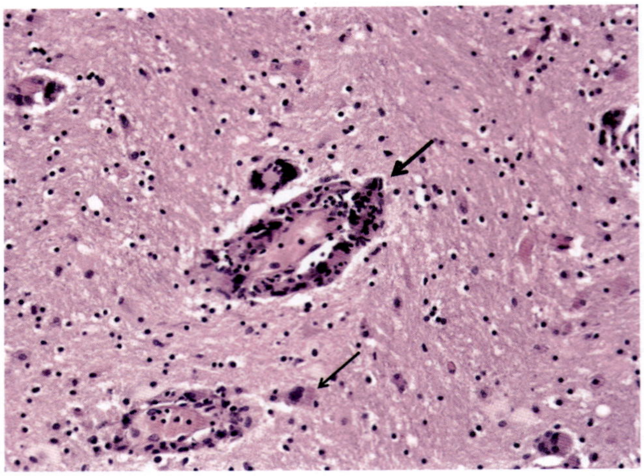

Figure 2-183. HIV encephalitis: Many multinucleated histiocytes tend to aggregate around white matter vessels (*thick arrow*), although they are also present away from the vessels (*thin arrow*) (H&E; original magnification: 200×).

be recognized as histiocytes in the mycobacterial pseudotumor of Mycobacterium avium-intracellulare or other mycobacteria,[425] especially in association with AIDS. A Ziehl-Neelsen or Fite stain shows their cytoplasm to be packed with acid-fast bacteria. A few histiocytes with intracytoplasmic *Histoplasma* yeast forms can be present around the vessels **(Fig. 2-182)**, form small groups within the parenchyma, or be found scattered in the leptomeninges. Another condition that can be represented by subtle or not so subtle perivascular histiocytes is HIV encephalitis.[426] These may be mononuclear or multinuclear histiocytes in variable numbers and can be very difficult to appreciate in some cases, unless specifically searched for around the white matter vessels **(Fig. 2-183)**. Immunohistochemical stain for HIV proteins may highlight them, as they carry the virus. HIV encephalitis is also associated with variable degrees of diffuse white matter pallor. Therefore, in addition to a history of HIV positivity, such a diffuse pallor in white matter should initiate such a search for their presence, as no other inflammatory infiltrate should be expected. As is the case with immunocompromised conditions, more than one infection can coexist. Therefore, in such cases, viral, fungal, and protozoal infections should also be searched for. Amebic trophozoites can be difficult to distinguish from histiocytes **(Fig. 2-184)**. Trophozoites are usually more monomorphous and uniform in appearance, with a round, eccentric nucleus and sharp cytoplasmic borders, whereas histiocytes are more variable in appearance in terms of their cytoplasmic borders, size, cytoplasmic quality, and nuclear features. Both amebae and histiocytes can have intracytoplasmic erythrocytes and other debris. In a typical case, the tendency of amebae to accumulate in the leptomeninges and in Virchow-Robin spaces is helpful. In more difficult cases, and in cases where the amebae are not as prominent but are suspected, immunohistochemistry can help with their accurate identification.

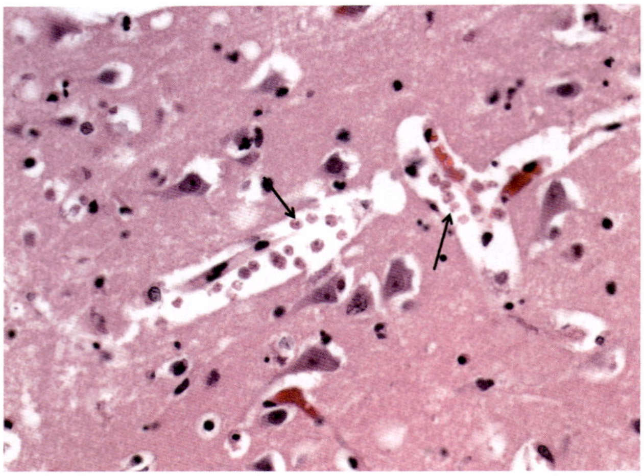

Figure 2-184. Amebic encephalitis: Many histiocyte-like amebae *(arrows)* are present around the vessels and can be mistaken for histiocytes (H&E; original magnification: 400×).

In *infarcts*, an abundance of histiocytes constitute the hallmark of subacute stage and predominate the picture after 1st week and up to the end of the first moth postinjury. This stage can be associated with a prominent edema around the lesion, which, especially in the subclinical infarcts, can result in a sudden and dramatic presentation as a mass lesion, mimicking a malignant neoplasm. Especially on frozen sections, when the fragile cytoplasms of histiocytes and their cytoplasmic borders are not readily visible, the sea of nuclei punctuated by somewhat prominent vessels that are also typical for this stage of infarcts may result in an erroneous diagnosis of a glial neoplasm. Alternatively, if the cytoplasms and cytoplasmic borders are visible, together with the clear nature of the cytoplasms of these foamy histiocytes, differentiation from oligodendroglioma can be difficult. Therefore, appreciation to the presence of a prominent macrophage population is crucial in avoiding such mistakes, especially in IOC. In such situations, well-prepared cytologic preparations are especially useful. Oligodendrogliomas can sometimes have a quite prominent perivascular foamy histiocyte population, although this should not cause any difficulties with the diagnosis due to the presence of obvious neoplasm **(Fig. 2-185)**. However, in small biopsy specimens that do not represent the actual neoplastic areas, these perivascular histiocytes should not be interpreted as the clear cells of an oligodendroglioma. Macrophages are frequently associated with degenerating tracts and can mark the areas of that degeneration at first glance (see "Tract Degeneration").

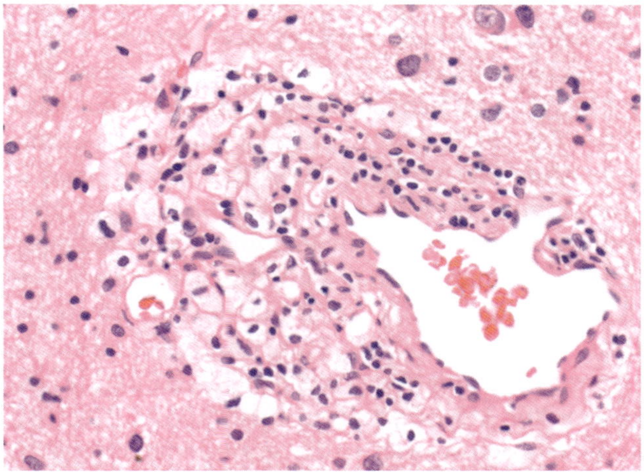

Figure 2-185. Perivascular foamy histiocytes: Oligodendroglioma was present nearby (H&E; original magnification: 400×).

By nature, macrophages phagocytose any debris in the environment, be it necrotic cellular debris from an infarct, myelin breakdown products, microorganisms, or foreign material, and in areas of hemorrhage, it is not unusual to see *hemosiderin pigment* (i.e., siderophages) and erythrocytes in their cytoplasm. In a particular disorder, hemophagocytic syndrome or *hemophagocytic lymphohistiocytic disorder*, histiocytes phagocytose erythrocytes.[427] Many histiocytes with their cytoplasm packed with erythrocytes are predominantly seen around vessels. This process may be triggered by viral infections or may have a genetic component. It is not unusual to find a few *perivascular histiocytes* in the white matter and especially in the basal ganglia in an otherwise unremarkable case. A few may be hemosiderin-laden. While their presence is abnormal, they are so common and do not have any associated obvious pathology that their significance is not clear. They likely represent a reaction to a small amount of previous leakage from those vessels (see "Vascular Changes"). Same is true for an occasional macrophage in the leptomeninges.

Foamy histiocytes can also be prominent as part of *radiation necrosis*.[374] They can be scattered throughout the tissue, be concentrated around vessels, or form diffuse sheets. They usually have a dusty pigment representing lipofuscin and hemosiderin in their cytoplasm. Together with the previous history of a high-grade glioma, radiation treatment, and other changes, such as cellular changes, fibrinoid necrosis of vessel walls, telangiectatic capillaries, fibrosis, and hemorrhage associated with radiation, this process does not pose a diagnostic problem in most cases (see also "Necrosis" and "Cellular Enlargement and Multinucleation"). A similar histiocytic infiltration can also be present in previous surgery sites. The granular cell change associated with some astrocytomas can be difficult to distinguish from histiocytes.[428] The intimate admixture of granular cells with the more obvious neoplastic cells, the absence of other reactive changes, and, if necessary, immunohistochemical stains make this differential relatively easy. Nuclear features of histiocytes and astrocytes are also helpful, as at least a subpopulation of neoplastic cells with this granular change still have atypical astrocytic nuclei. Scattered macrophages distributed in the white matter that may show some degree of myelin pallor and neuropil vacuolation may represent a mild case of chemotherapy-induced leukoencephalopathy. These macrophages and scattered axonal spheroids can be highlighted by CD68 or CD163 and neurofilament, respectively, and the process may be accurately identified with the right clinical history.

Some *specific histiocytic disorders* are clearly malignant, such as histiocytic sarcoma, while the neoplastic versus reactive nature of others, such as Rosai-Dorfman disease, is debated. In many of these disorders, it may be difficult to identify the component cells as histiocytes. *Langerhans cell histiocytosis* is characterized by Langerhans cells with typical coffee bean–shaped nuclei due to a nuclear groove. Multinucleated or mononuclear histiocytes, with abundant pale cytoplasm and intracytoplasmic small, round lymphocytes with a halo around them, giving them the appearance that they are in an intracytoplasmic vacuole (emperipolesis), are characteristic for *Rosai-Dorfman disease* (sinus histiocytosis with massive lymphadenopathy) **(Fig. 2-186)**. In *Erdheim-Chester disease*,[429] many histiocytes with foamy cytoplasm are present in sheets, which may be difficult to recognize as histiocytes in parenchymal lesions as they may be distorted and appear like spindle cells, mimicking glial

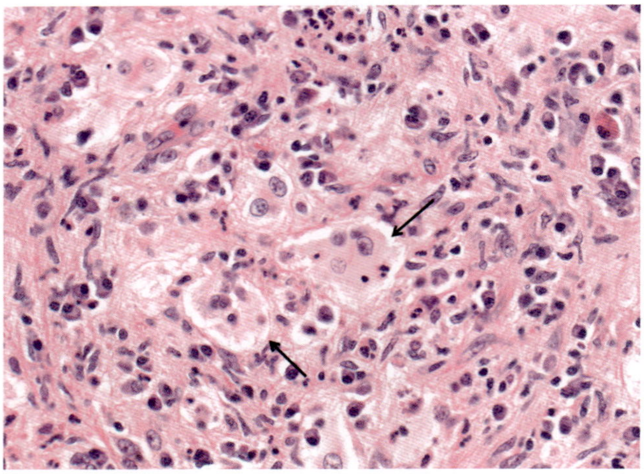

Figure 2-186. Rosai-Dorfman disease: Peculiar large histiocytic cells with abundant pale cytoplasm and one or more nuclei are present in a lymphoplasmacytic background. Intact small lymphocytes are seen in their cytoplasm (emperipolesis) (*arrows*) (H&E; original magnification: 400×).

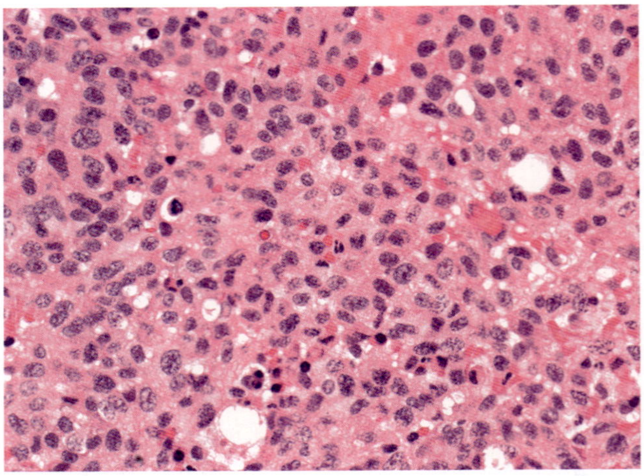

Figure 2-187. Histiocytic sarcoma: The malignant cells are difficult to recognize as of histiocytic origin, necessitating high degree of suspicion and the use of special stains for the diagnosis of this rare neoplasm (H&E; original magnification: 400×).

neoplasm. *Histiocytic sarcoma*[430] has clearly malignant cells with a high-grade morphology complete with areas of necrosis, prominent mitotic activity, and high proliferative index **(Fig. 2-187)** and is difficult to appreciate as being histiocytic without a high degree of suspicion. Therefore, it can easily be mistaken for a lymphoma, such as anaplastic large cell lymphoma or even a metastatic carcinoma or sarcoma. It is positive for CD68 and CD163, while markers for other categories of neoplasms are negative. As with many unusual lesions, a high degree of suspicion is needed to further work such cases up and identify this neoplasm accurately.

As is the case elsewhere in the body, *epithelioid histiocytes* can form *granulomas* and provide some clues for the type of granulomatous inflammation. *Multinucleated giant cells* that can be seen in granulomas or around necrotic foci are also macrophages. For multinucleated giant cells and additional information on granulomatous diseases, see also "Cellular Enlargement and Multinucleation." Granulomas with caseating necrosis, that is, *necrotizing granulomas*, are considered highly suspicious for Mycobacterium tuberculosis. Necrosis may be microscopic in the granuloma or maybe large and geographic due to the coalescence of multiple granulomas, surrounded by epithelioid histiocytes. Similar granulomas can also be associated with fungal infections. Meningovascular syphilis, in addition to its other findings, such as fibrous thickening of meninges, lymphocytes, and plasma cells, can have *gummas*, which are granulomas similar to tuberculous granulomas. Likewise, they can present as mass lesions.[431] The central reticulin is preserved in the necrotic area in a gumma, in contrast to a caseating tuberculous granuloma. Well-circumscribed granulomas with no necrosis, that is, *nonnecrotizing granulomas*, are typically seen in sarcoidosis, where they also have a thin peripheral small lymphocytic rim. Some of them can have a small, central fibrinoid necrosis, but necrosis is absent as a rule.[432] Granulomas may not be present or prominent in immunocompromised patients. Sarcoidosis is a clinicopathologic diagnosis of exclusions and can only be suggested as one of the possibilities by the pathologist after the special stains for microorganisms are negative. Sarcoid granulomas tend to be in close association with vessels and may induce an inflammatory reaction in the vessel wall, mimicking a granulomatous angiitis.[433] This may result in ischemic tissue damage in the parenchyma. Granulomatous inflammation in the leptomeninges tends to involve the basal surfaces and is typically associated with mycobacterial and fungal infections, as well as with sarcoidosis. The term *granulomatous amebic encephalitis* is not entirely accurate, as granuloma formation is not a typical feature of this process, which is rich in macrophages.

Epithelioid histiocytes and the granulomas they form may look like gemistocytic astrocytes or vice versa. The typical nuclear features of histiocytes in granulomas and their bland chromatin pattern are in stark contrast with the atypical and pleomorphic astrocyte nuclei. In addition, the cytoplasms of gemistocytes are thick and glassy due to GFAP accumulation, in contrast to the thin, vacuolated cytoplasms of histiocytes with debris. Reactive or neoplastic astrocytes are diffusely distributed in the tissue, in contrast to the aggregates forming the granulomas. Granulomas with central necrobiotic collagen and peripheral palisading of histiocytes, as well as multinucleated giant cells, are typical for the nodules of rheumatoid arthritis. Rheumatoid arthritis is also frequently associated with a plasma cell–rich inflammatory infiltrate. Some of these patients, especially those on steroid treatment, may have superimposed fungal infections, and GMS may highlight fungal microorganisms in these granulomas in some cases, although the distinction from a primary fungal infection becomes difficult. Rheumatoid arthritis granulomas, that is, *rheumatoid nodules,*[434] are seen more commonly in leptomeninges and dura mater and may present as mass lesions when large enough. Granulomas can be associated with some *neoplastic processes*, most notably germinomas (as in seminomas)[435] and Hodgkin lymphomas.[436] When abundant, they can obscure these neoplasms and may result in misdiagnoses. These granulomas can be well-circumscribed or ill-defined and may appear like an abundance of macrophages throughout the tissue. An ill-defined granulomatous reaction can be seen as part of a *foreign body giant cell reaction* process in reaction to the keratinous debris of craniopharyngiomas, epidermoid or dermoid cysts when they rupture, surgical material, or against foreign material implanted after penetrating trauma. These reactions also contain foreign body giant cells engulfing the material they are reacting to.

In *granulomatous angiitis and in temporal arteritis*, multinucleated giant cells are seen in association with and phagocytosing the fragments of internal elastic lamina, a feature that can be seen on routine H&E stain but better highlighted by an elastic tissue stain, such as Verhoeff-van Gieson stain. *Wegener's granulomatosis* is, in spite of its name, not only associated with ill-defined granulomas but rather has large areas of fibrinoid necrosis with scattered multinucleated giant cells. It involves the leptomeninges and dura mater and only rarely the parenchyma. It is associated with a mixed inflammatory infiltrate, in addition to granulomas. In the anterior pituitary gland, *granulomatous hypophysitis*[437,438] is characterized by noncaseating granulomas, and giant cells, as well as a minor population of lymphocytes. These are noninfectious granulomas with no microorganisms identified by special stains or cultures. Similar lesions may be seen in other endocrine organs. In contrast to sarcoidosis and infectious granulomas, extension outside the anterior pituitary is not present. A rare and poorly understood giant cell/granulomatous response may also be seen in *pituitary adenomas*, possibly through a mechanism similar to those seen in other neoplasms that can have granulomas, such as germinomas.

Polymorphonuclear (PMN) leukocytes are acute inflammatory cells that are the first responders to

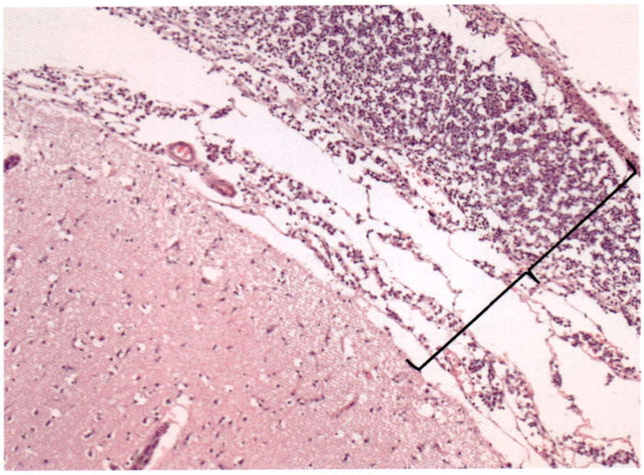

Figure 2-188. Acute (bacterial; suppurative) meningitis: The subarachnoid space is filled with PMN leukocytes (*bracket*) (H&E; original magnification: 100×).

injury. In *acute* (bacterial, purulent) *meningitis*, neutrophil PMNs are abundant in the subarachnoid space **(Fig. 2-188)**. They can track down the vessels along Virchow-Robin spaces to extend into the parenchyma and may result in cerebritis and abscesses as a complication. In addition, they can cause damage to the vessels in the subarachnoid space **(Fig. 2-189)**, resulting in thrombosis, or spasm, to cause infarcts. In severe cases, there may be an admixture of immature forms, which should not be mistaken for leukemic infiltrate. The presence of linear basophilic debris in the background represents pus and supports inflammation. They are also seen in the acute phase of cerebritis within the neuroglial parenchyma **(Fig. 2-190)**. In cases where infection involves the meninges by direct invasion from neighboring structures, such as mastoid cells or paranasal sinuses, the inflammation tends to be localized in that region at least in its earlier stages or may predominantly involve the basal meninges. These types of infections also tend to have an epidural component. Meningitis in general may involve the cranial nerve roots to cause cranial nerve palsies and permanent nerve damage. Mycoplasma pneumonia infection mimics acute meningitis in that there is leptomeningeal acute inflammation extending to brain parenchyma following Virchow-Robin spaces, creating perivascular and parenchymal acute inflammatory cell collections. A *reactive acute inflammatory infiltrate* can be seen in conditions that irritate the leptomeninges, such as subarachnoid hemorrhage, chemical meningitis as seen in association with keratinous debris from epidermoid cysts[439] and craniopharyngiomas spilling into the subarachnoid space, and reactions to various medications, either as a sensitivity reaction or direct effect of intrathecal medications.[440] Aseptic meningitis is a term used to describe meningitis in which no microorganisms are identified

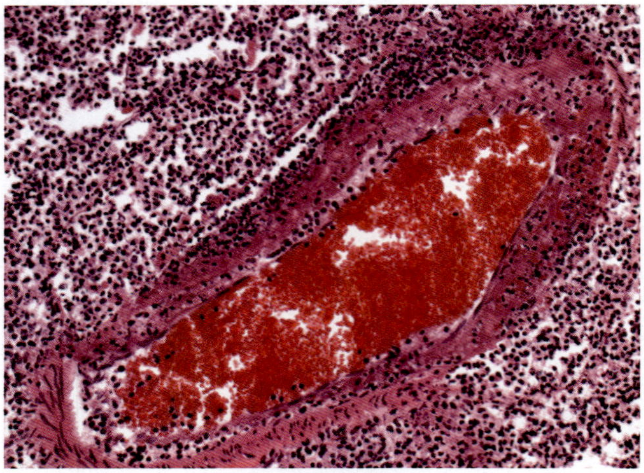

Figure 2-189. Acute meningitis: A subarachnoid artery is entrapped within and infiltrated by the inflammation, sustaining damage as evidenced by the fibrinoid necrosis in its wall. This can result in subarachnoid hemorrhage or thrombus may develop in its lumen, resulting in parenchymal infarct (H&E; original magnification: 200×).

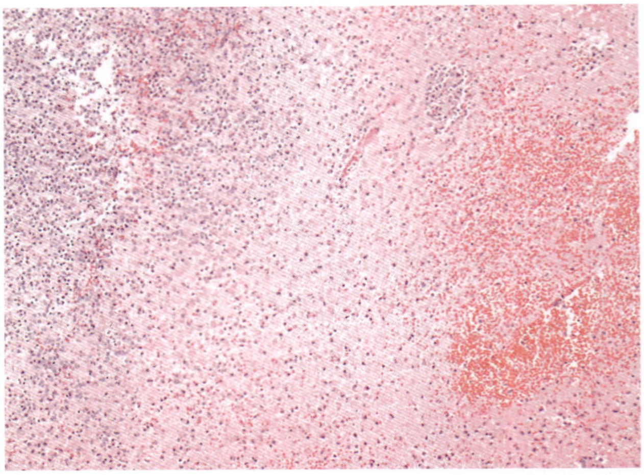

Figure 2-190. Cerebritis: Neuroglial parenchyma is diffusely infiltrated by PMN leukocytes and shows hemorrhage. This may progress to abscess formation (H&E; original magnification: 100×).

or microorganisms are difficult to identify. For this reason, viral meningitides are commonly referred to as being aseptic. Uncommon bacterial infections such as syphilis and Lyme disease, inflammatory disorders such as Behcet's, and drugs such as ibuprofen also result in aseptic meningitis. Mollaret meningitis,[441] also known as recurrent aseptic meningitis, may be related to HSV infection.[442] Usually, these conditions are diagnosed based on clinical and radiologic features and do not require tissue examination for diagnosis. *Abscess* development can mimic early infarct. In the first 1 to 2 days, there is acute focal suppurative cerebritis; 2 to 7 days, confluent central necrosis develops and macrophages and lymphoplasmacytic infiltrate appear; 5 to 14 days, early encapsulation, with early granulation tissue formation, takes place; and 14 days and later, late encapsulation with well-developed capsule develops. A prominence of *eosinophil PMN leukocytes* is seen typically in association with parasitic infections. Among fungi, *Coccidioides immitis* tends to cause prominent eosinophil PMN leukocyte infiltration. A robust eosinophil PMN leukocyte response is seen in tissues that contain microfibrillar collagen,[443] an amorphous, fibrillary, or filamentous substance used for embolization and hemostasis. In necrotizing angiitis, neutrophil PMN leukocytes are predominant and are admixed with other inflammatory cells. Eosinophil PMN leukocytes are prominent in Churg-Strauss syndrome (allergic angiitis and granulomatosis) along with lymphocytes and plasma cells. The inflammatory infiltrate in the lesions of neuromyelitis optica may also contain neutrophil and eosinophil PMN leukocytes.[444]

Lymphocytes and plasma cells, usually present in variable numbers, in the context of inflammation generally indicate chronicity, a slowly evolving process, or a viral infection. Lymphocytes are typically small and round, although in some inflammations, a polymorphous population can also be seen. In encephalitis and aseptic meningitis, a predominantly lymphocytic infiltrate is present. It is perivascular in encephalitis and leptomeningeal in meningitis. In encephalitis, additional findings to support a viral etiology are microglial nodules and neuronophagia (see above). Lymphocytes are also present in the CSF in aseptic meningitis. This inflammatory picture should not cause any confusion with a lymphoma, as the great majority of lymphomas of the CNS are diffuse large B-cell type and are relatively easy to suspect on histologic/cytologic grounds. In addition, inflammatory/reactive processes are T-cell predominant, although there are exceptions, such as the B-cell-predominant form of PACNS that can potentially raise concern for a small lymphocytic lymphoma or CNS involvement by a chronic lymphocytic leukemia (see also "Perivascular Arrangements and Rosettes"). In diffuse large B-cell lymphoma that has been treated with corticosteroids, only a reactive small lymphocytic population of T cells may remain around the vessels, making the recognition of lymphoma essentially impossible, mimicking an inflammatory process.[445] Lymphomas previously treated with corticosteroids may appear as acute demyelination on biopsy. Lymphoma responds to corticosteroid treatment dramatically and the malignant cells become essentially impossible to find **(Fig. 2-191)**. Only a reactive population of small, round reactive T cells, macrophages, and reactive astrocytes and myelin loss mimic the active MS plaque or, more likely in single mass lesions, tumefactive MS. These cases recur as lymphomas and eventually declare their true nature.

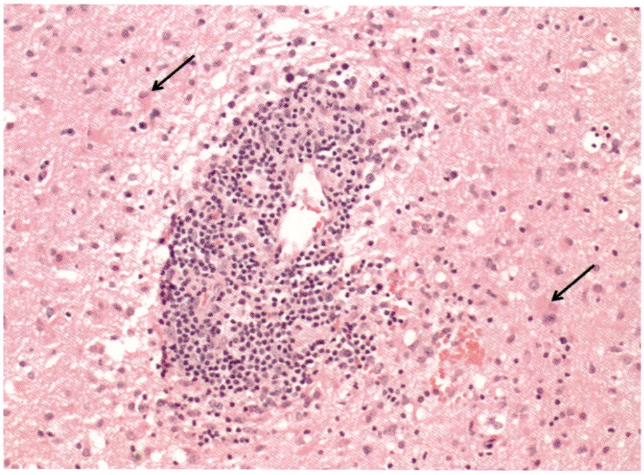

Figure 2-191. Treated lymphoma: Only perivascular small, round lymphocytes remain after steroid administration before the biopsy was performed. Scattered reactive astrocytes (*arrows*) are also present. A definitive pathologic diagnosis is not possible based on these nonspecific findings, but this picture should not be mistaken for another pathologic process, such as vasculitis or demyelination, emphasizing the importance of checking the clinical information (H&E; original magnification: 200×).

Sometimes, a truly demyelinating lesion may be the initial presentation of a CNS lymphoma only to eventually recur as a frank diffuse large B-cell lymphoma. Such demyelinating lesions have been referred to as "sentinel lesions."[241] A perivascular lymphocytic infiltrate can also be seen in adrenoleukodystrophy, in which they are predominantly CD8-positive T cells. Demyelinating diseases are also associated with a lymphocytic infiltrate both perivascular and within the parenchyma, in addition to histiocytes, mainly in the acute stage. Lymphoplasmacytic infiltrate is a prominent component of meningovascular syphilis and rheumatoid arthritis (see above). Lymphoplasmacytic inflammation is present in dorsal spinal nerve roots and dorsal root ganglia in tabes dorsalis.

Immune reconstitution inflammatory syndrome (IRIS) is the reconstitution of immune response after HAART, resulting in an exuberant inflammatory reaction to infections previously familiar to the immune system. As such, a prominent lymphocytic infiltrate is seen in the parenchyma and/or around the vessels and may mimic lymphoma, except that the lymphocytes are CD8-positive small T lymphocytes.[446] Microorganisms can be obscured by this intense inflammatory infiltrate. Although this inflammatory pattern is not specific for IRIS, in the right clinical context and with the knowledge of this syndrome, both the diagnosis of IRIS can be suggested and any microorganisms can be sought for.

A lymphoplasmacytic infiltrate with an admixture of histiocytes in a necrotic background is seen in toxoplasma cerebritis and is highly suspicious for it especially in the typical setting of immunosuppression and multiple periventricular lesions.[447] Tachizoites may be difficult to appreciate and confused with nuclear debris; however, immunohistochemistry can be useful in this situation to confirm the diagnosis. If it is not available or is difficult to interpret due to high background staining associated with necrosis, the diagnosis can be suggested based on this histologic appearance together with the typical radiologic and clinical features. If cyst forms are identified, the diagnosis can be made easily. The importance of these lesions, aside from making the accurate diagnosis, is not to mistake them for an infarct or a high-grade glial neoplasm due to the presence of necrosis and prominent vessels that are part of the reactive/inflammatory process, especially in small specimens, as stereotactic biopsy is a common approach.

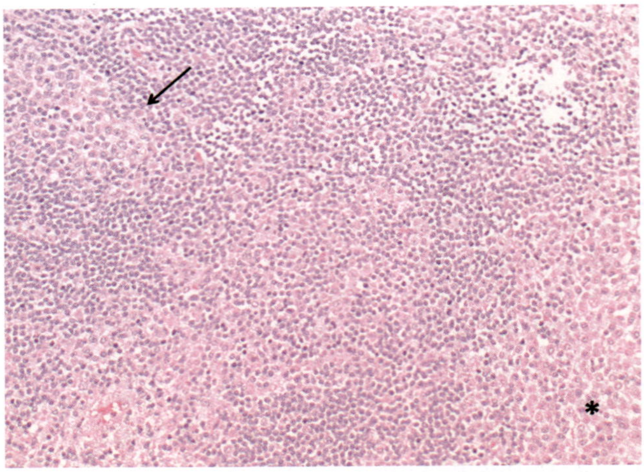

Figure 2-192. MALToma: This plasmacytoid subtype of mucosa-associated lymphoid tissue (MALT)-type lymphoma may mimic a reactive inflammatory process due to lymphoid follicle formation (*arrow*) and the presence of plasma cells (*asterisk*), creating a polymorphous population (H&E; original magnification: 200×).

Involvement by lymphoma or plasma cell myeloma **(Fig. 2-192)** can be in the form of diffuse involvement of leptomeninges or as focal mass lesions in epidural and subdural spaces, in leptomeninges, or in the neuroglial parenchyma. A wide variety of lymphomas and reactive/inflammatory conditions, such as Rosai-Dorfman disease, Castleman's disease, inflammatory myofibroblastic tumor, and inflammatory pseudotumor/ plasma cell granuloma, can involve the CNS and present as dural-based masses clinically and radiologically mimicking meningiomas.[448] Otherwise, they have features similar to those of their counterparts elsewhere. Intravascular lymphoma[385] is a large B-cell lymphoma that presents clinically with skin lesions and neurologic findings due to occlusion of capillaries and subsequent microinfarcts. It can be easy to miss as only a few cells within the vessels may be all that is present. Involvement of CNS by plasma cell myeloma is rare; however, scattered individual atypical plasma cells or small groups of such cells can be present in the leptomeninges or in the pituitary region in those cases.[449]

The so-called plasma cell granuloma or inflammatory pseudotumor is an inflammatory/reactive

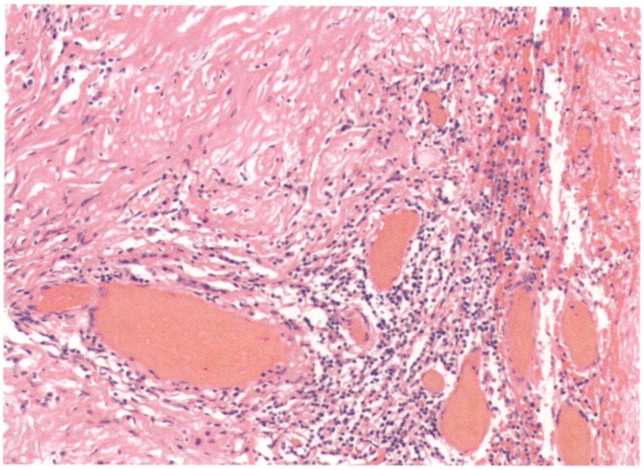

Figure 2-193. Inflammatory pseudotumor: Fibrosis, hyalinization, and a mixed lymphoplasmacytic inflammatory infiltrate are seen in this meningeal mass lesion clinically mimicking a meningioma (H&E; original magnification: 100×).

lesion with fibrosis and lymphoplasmacytic infiltrate **(Fig. 2-193)**. It is typically associated with the meninges and may have prominent meningothelial cell proliferation. Idiopathic hypertrophic pachymeningitis also shows fibrous thickening of dura mater and chronic inflammatory infiltrate composed of lymphocytes, plasma cells, macrophages, and even granulomas and giant cells **(Fig. 2-194)**. This process diffusely involves the meninges and is

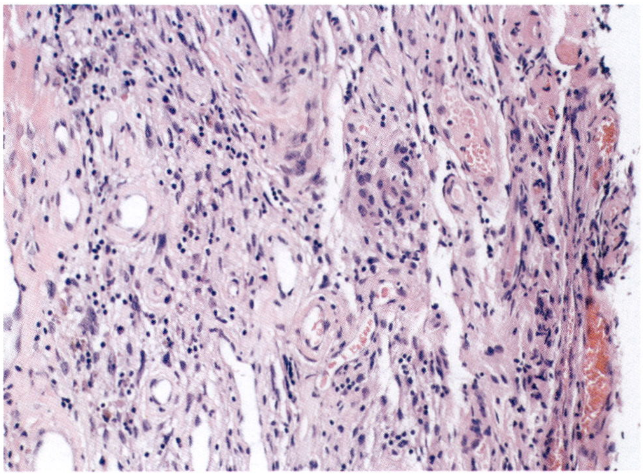

Figure 2-194. Idiopathic hypertrophic pachymeningitis: Diffusely fibrotic and thickened meninges show increased number of vessels and an inflammatory infiltrate (H&E; original magnification: 200×). (Courtesy of Mahtab Tehrani, M.D., Inova Pathology Institute, Fairfax, VA.)

a diagnosis of exclusion. Foci of chronic inflammation can be present in specimens resected as part of seizure surgery and are due to the seizure work-up with electrodes. They may be associated with leptomeningeal fibrosis and small, rounded or linear infarcts as a result of electrode placement. Such specimens may be otherwise essentially entirely unremarkable or may show subtle gliosis, while others may show prominent neoplastic or malformative abnormalities. Lymphoplasmacyte-rich meningioma[450] is characterized by an intense lymphoplasmacytic infiltration within and around the neoplasm, sometimes obscuring the meningothelial cell population. Its nature as a true meningothelial neoplasm versus a primarily inflammatory process with secondary and exuberant meningothelial hyperplasia is debatable, as some may show spontaneous regression. A predominantly lymphoplasmacytic infiltrate with an admixture of rare PMN leukocytes, including eosinophils, accompanying a spindle cell proliferation with bland cytologic features should bring to mind inflammatory myofibroblastic tumor. Inflammatory pseudotumor/plasma cell granuloma also has a mixed inflammatory infiltrate and should not be confused with inflammatory myofibroblastic tumor.[451] Inflammatory myofibroblastic tumor is ALK-1-positive and is neoplastic, while inflammatory pseudotumor is a reactive process that can be associated with systemic symptoms and is considered in the group of IgG4-positive lesions.

A lymphocytic infiltrate is associated with germinoma, mainly located in the fibrovascular septae separating the neoplastic cell groups into compartments. In fact, the presence of these septae, the lymphocytic infiltrate, and granulomas are useful in distinguishing germinoma from embryonal carcinoma by favoring the former. In difficult cases, immunohistochemistry may be needed. A mixed lymphoid background is a characteristic feature of Hodgkin lymphoma, in which the diagnostic Reed-Sternberg cells can be extremely rare, potentially resulting in a misdiagnosis of inflammatory process. In many neoplasms, it is not unusual to have variable degrees of inflammatory infiltrates as a reaction. In some, this reactive infiltrate may be more prominent and consistent, adding to the typical features to support the diagnosis for that particular neoplasm. For instance, in chordoid glioma, a prominent lymphoplasmacytic infiltrate, together with Russell

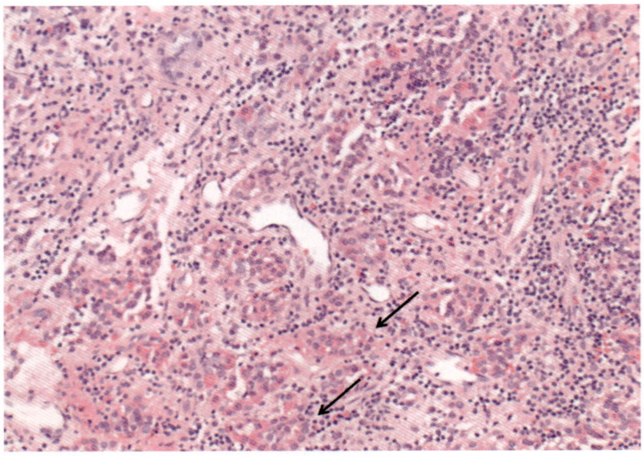

Figure 2-195. Lymphocytic hypophysitis: Anterior pituitary parenchyma is infiltrated by many lymphocytes, effacing the parenchyma, which remains in the background as scattered nests composed of a mixture of cell types (*arrows*). This process can closely mimic pituitary adenoma clinically (H&E; original magnification: 200×).

bodies, can be present within and at the borders of the neoplasm.[452] Lymphocytic hypophysitis is characterized by a prominent small, round lymphocytic infiltrate in the pituitary gland and should not be confused with pituitary adenoma **(Fig. 2-195)**.

In partially treated acute meningitis and in subacute–chronic cases, a mononuclear infiltrate dominates the leptomeningeal inflammation. Likewise, in the acute phase of some viral meningitides, PMN leukocyte dominance may be seen. In treated acute meningitis, this occurs typically within a few days of treatment, and therefore, the presence of a mononuclear component should not rule out suppurative meningitis. The granulomatous meningitis associated with tuberculosis tends to be patchy, with foci of granulomas alternating with areas of variable amount of lymphocytes. Therefore, the diagnostic yield of open brain biopsies may vary due to sampling variation and, as in cases of vasculitis, multiple sections should be examined to identify any granulomas. Search for acid-fast bacilli should be carried out in cases with clinical concern even if there are no granulomas, using special stains and molecular techniques, such as polymerase chain reaction (PCR). A similar picture is also seen in fungal infections, necessitating additional special stains for their search. Viral meningitis is also characterized by a lymphocytic infiltrate that can be quite subtle. This is especially true in rapidly fatal cases. Paraneoplastic ganglioneuronopathy[308] is associated with dorsal root degeneration with lymphocytic infiltrate and nodules of Nageotte. Dorsal column degeneration is seen in spinal cord.

Another pitfall in regard to lymphocytic infiltrate is the collapsed neuroglial tissue, resulting in an artificial crowding of oligodendroglia, mimicking lymphocytic infiltrate. Likewise, oligodendroglial proliferations may also appear as a lymphocytic infiltrate or an oligodendroglioma (see "Nuclear Features").

Mast cells can be identified more prominently in several lesions. The presence of mast cells in neurofibromas is well-recognized. They can also be seen in various soft tissue neoplasms with no known diagnostic or prognostic significance. As for primary intraparenchymal neuroepithelial neoplasms, mast cells can be quite frequent in SEGA and can be highlighted by CD117 (c-kit).

Bone marrow elements can be seen in a variety of conditions in the CNS, and their identification is important to avoid mistaking them for leukemic involvement or inflammation. In *extramedullary hematopoiesis* (EMH), all three lineages are represented with cells at various stages of maturation, although one lineage may predominate. EMH can be seen especially in the leptomeninges in addition to other locations in the body as part of a generalized hematologic condition.[453] EMH is common in the granulation tissue associated with chronic subdural hematomas[454] **(Fig. 2-196)**. A subpopulation of hemangioblastomas also shows EMH.[455] *Nucleated*

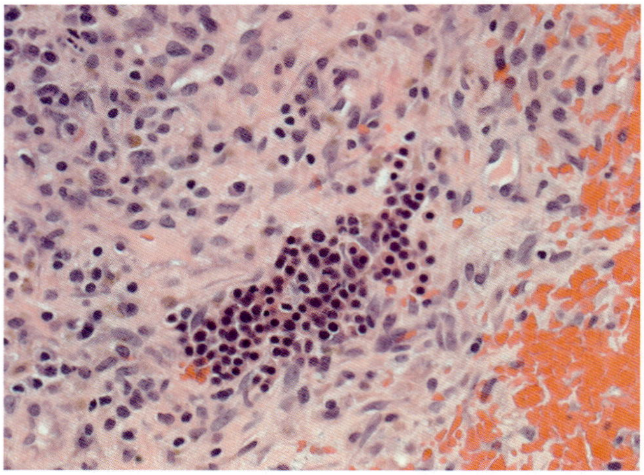

Figure 2-196. A focus of EMH in an organized (chronic) subdural hematoma, not to be confused with a leukemic infiltrate (H&E; original magnification: 400×).

erythrocyte precursors can be seen in the blood in premature infants, as well as in association with hematologic abnormalities involving erythrocyte production and destruction. *Bone marrow fragments* can be identified within the vessels after fractures due to trauma or aggressive resuscitation. Rare hyperchromatic large cells stuck in some capillaries represent *megakaryocytes* and are common findings in autopsy tissues with no known significance. *Leukemic involvement* of the brain can be in the form of diffuse leptomeningeal infiltration; epidural, subdural, or intraparenchymal mass lesions; and hemorrhages or infarcts due to occlusion of vessels by blastic cells, especially in cases with blast crises.[456] The cell population is variable depending on the type of leukemia and can range from primitive blasts in acute leukemias to fairly mature myeloid cells, resembling acute inflammation in chronic myeloid leukemia and chronic inflammation in chronic lymphocytic leukemia. Therefore, especially in hematoma evacuation material, checking the patient's history for any such condition that can metastasize to or involve the CNS and result in hemorrhage as well as thorough gross examination, sampling, and microscopic examination are warranted. *Neuroacanthocytoses*[277] are a group of neurodegenerations associated with acanthocytes. They are characterized by atrophy, neuron loss and gliosis in affected CNS regions, and acanthocytes in the blood. Acanthocytes may be difficult to find and may require advanced techniques such as scanning electron microscopy in suspected cases. Typically basal ganglia are affected, associated with ventricular dilation and variable cortical atrophy. Thalamus, substantia nigra, and anterior horns may be affected. *McLeod syndrome* consists of striatal degeneration and myopathy. Kell blood group precursor protein is missing. Some cases of acanthocytosis may be associated with *abetalipoproteinemia/vitamin E deficiency*.[457]

Hemorrhage

Grossly and microscopically, the identification of hemorrhage is straightforward; however, it is important to show an attempt to incorporate its pattern, distribution, potential causes, and clinical context to further characterize the hemorrhage. Many of the changes associated with vessel walls

List of Findings/Checklist for Hemorrhage

AT A GLANCE

- Large hemorrhages
  - Hypertension
  - Cerebral amyloid angiopathy
  - Angioinvasive fungi
  - Herpes virus encephalitis
  - Methanol
  - Carbon monoxide
  - Carbon tetrachloride
  - Amphetamines
  - Primary and metastatic neoplasms
- Multiple small hemorrhages
  - Contusions
  - Arsenicals
  - L-Asparaginase
  - Duret hemorrhage
- Petechial hemorrhages
  - Fat embolism
  - Diffuse axonal injury
  - Acute disseminated encephalomyelitis
  - Arbovirus infections
  - Vasculitides
  - HIV arteriopathy
  - Pancreatic encephalopathy
  - Acute lead poisoning
  - Cyanide
  - Sulfonamides
- Subarachnoid hemorrhage
  - Aneurysms
  - Vascular trauma
  - Meningocerebral angiodysplasia and renal agenesis
  - Vasculitides
  - HIV arteriopathy
  - Dissection of parenchymal hemorrhage
  - Trauma
  - Extension from ventricular hemorrhage
- Intraventricular hemorrhage
  - Germinal matrix hemorrhage
  - Choroid plexus hemorrhage
  - Extension from subarachnoid space
- Subdural, dural, intradural hemorrhage
  - Perinatal hypoxic–ischemic injury
  - Trauma
- Pituitary gland
  - Pituitary apoplexy

resulting in hemorrhage are discussed in "Vascular Changes." Here, they are briefly mentioned mainly in regard to their microscopical features to provide a correlation between these changes and the hemorrhage pattern, as it pertains to the thought process when hemorrhage is identified. See Chapter 1 for gross images of some of these patterns.

Hypertensive hemorrhage typically occurs in the basal ganglia (*ganglionic hemorrhage*) and is usually seen at autopsy in the form of fresh hemorrhage. Detailed examination with extensive sampling can reveal the presence of Charcot-Bouchard microaneurysms in the background. They are small outpouching of arteriolar walls, some with actual fibrinoid necrosis and rupture. On routine sections, all one can see may be the hemorrhage, but vessels, strands of fibrous tissue associated with them, and Charcot-Bouchard microaneurysms can be highlighted by elastic tissue stains such as Verhoeff-van Gieson and trichrome stains. The latter shows the vessel wall damage and fibrin as bright red. They are neither necessary for diagnosis nor are diagnostic for hypertensive hemorrhage and their relation to intracranial hemorrhage is also debatable however, and they have been described as a feature in other conditions, namely, CAA, and in normotensive individuals.[346,458,459] Other common location for hypertensive hemorrhage is pons, where it is seen typically as a single large expansile hemorrhage. Duret hemorrhages are multiple hemorrhages in the brainstem and are due to the tearing of penetrating parenchymal vessels when the brainstem is pushed away by the herniating medial temporal lobe. In cases where uncal herniation is difficult to evaluate, such as extensive infarct or ventilator brain, or hemorrhage disrupting tissue integrity, *Duret hemorrhage* can serve as an indirect finding for the presence of transtentorial herniation. Hemorrhages in the basal ganglia can be due to hypertensive attacks in hepatic porphyrias. Petechial hemorrhages and most typically bilateral putamen and claustrum hemorrhagic infarctions can be seen in *methanol intoxication*.[460] After 1 to 2 days, *carbon monoxide poisoning*[461] results in widespread white matter petechiae and larger hemorrhages in globus pallidus, usually bilaterally and symmetrically. After several days, the pallidal lesions gradually become cavitary, and white matter foci of necrosis may be present, sparing the U-fibers. *Cerebral amyloid angiopathy*[346,459] is the most common cause of nonhypertensive intraparenchymal hemorrhage and has a tendency to cause multiple simultaneous or metachronous superficial cerebral hemorrhages, also referred to as *lobar hemorrhage*. Multiple, usually *superficial parenchymal hemorrhages* of variable sizes and shapes, at least some of which connect with the leptomeningeal surface and associated with corresponding subarachnoid hemorrhage, grouped especially in the basal frontal and anterior temporal aspects of the brain, are seen in *contusion*. The inclusion of leptomeninges in the injury favors a traumatic origin, rather than a parenchymal vascular injury of other causes, indicating that the impact came from outside the brain. However, some parenchymal hemorrhages may dissect into the leptomeninges and some hemorrhages originate in the subarachnoid space, such as aneurysmal hemorrhages. The sparing of leptomeninges and subpial neuroglial tissue is useful in favoring a medical cause for a superficial hemorrhage rather than a traumatic brain injury–related parenchymal hemorrhage. In distinguishing primary intraparenchymal hemorrhage from traumatic hemorrhage, the presence of axonal swellings and absence of vascular pathology favor traumatic origin. Contusions can also be present along the lacerations due to penetrating injuries, such as bullet tracts, and are not necessarily related to external blunt trauma. *Contusional tears*[462,463] or hemorrhagic tears are seen in association with trauma in children and are commonly seen in orbitofrontal and temporal white matter. *Gliding contusions*[464] are typically bilateral, but are not necessarily symmetrical, and are located in parasagittal gray matter and subcortical white matter. They appear as multiple curvilinear petechiae, arranged in groups or streaks. They tend to curve downward toward the corpus callosum. They are thought to arise from gliding of the brain against its dural attachments and injuring the veins within the parenchyma on their way to the dural sinuses. *Aspergillus* infection, due to its angioinvasive nature, results in hemorrhagic, necrotic lesions that may be multiple and of variable sizes. Similar lesions are also seen in *Pseudallescheria boydii* infection, which is also angioinvasive with hyphae similar to those of *Aspergillus*. *Carbon tetrachloride poisoning* can result in brain edema, hemorrhages, hemorrhagic infarcts, and venous thromboses.[17] *Amphetamines*, methamphetamine, and methylenedioxymethamphetamine (ecstasy) are associated with arterial and

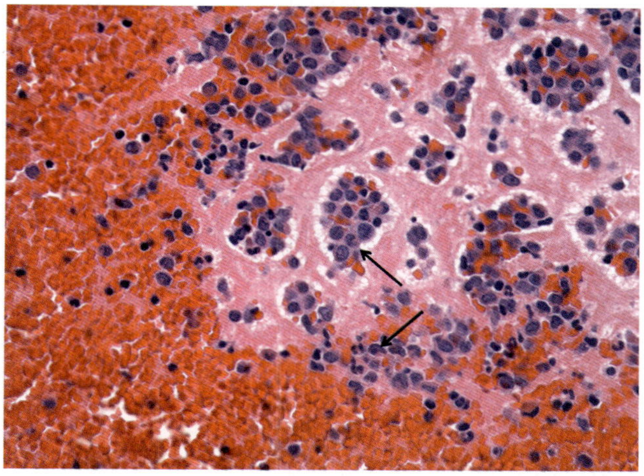

Figure 2-197. Acute myeloblastic leukemia presenting with subdural hemorrhage: Groups of atypical hematolymphoid cells with curved, myeloid nuclei (*arrows*) are present (H&E; original magnification: 400×).

venous infarcts, subarachnoid and parenchymal hemorrhages, and sometimes necrotizing vasculitis involving various types of vessels.[365]

In any hemorrhagic material, one should keep the possibility of a *neoplastic process* in mind.[465] Hematolymphoid malignancies, especially leukemic infiltrates, can present as intraparenchymal, subarachnoid, or subdural hemorrhage **(Fig. 2-197)**. Melanoma **(Fig. 2-198)**, renal cell carcinoma, and, although relatively rare, choriocarcinoma

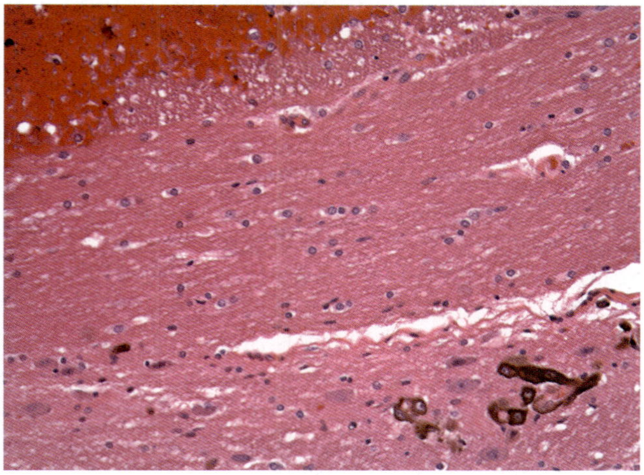

Figure 2-198. Metastatic melanoma: This acute intraparenchymal hemorrhage (**top**) resulted in the setting of metastatic melanoma. Scattered groups of pigmented melanoma cells are present in the surrounding parenchyma (**bottom**) (H&E; original magnification: 200×).

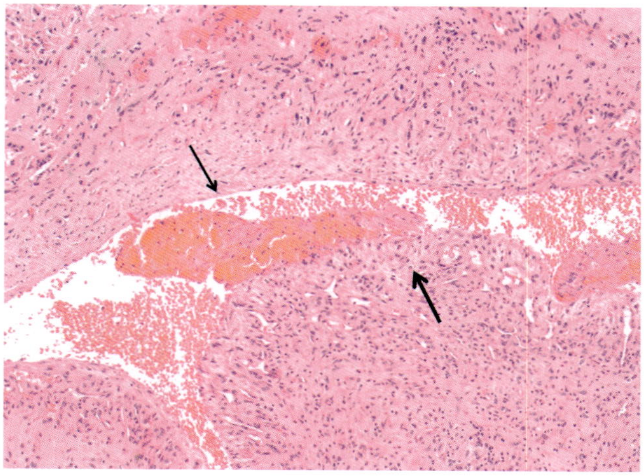

Figure 2-199. Glioblastoma with hemorrhage: Previous hemorrhage in this glioblastoma formed a hematoma with hyalinized, granulation tissue–like lining (*thin arrow*), which also contains neoplastic cells (*thick arrow*) (H&E; original magnification: 200×).

are especially notorious for presenting, sometimes for the first time, with brain hemorrhage. Among primary CNS neoplasms, glioblastoma, oligodendroglioma, and PA can present with hemorrhage **(Fig. 2-199)**. While a previous history, radiologic and intraoperative findings avoid unpleasant surprises in most cases, one has to be on the lookout for this possibility while evaluating a hemorrhagic specimen. *Hemorrhagic, necrotic, and inflammatory debris* may be seen in *Herpes virus infections*, typically in the medial temporal lobe. In those cases, the hemorrhage is not pure and is spread within the necroinflammatory tissue, in which intranuclear viral inclusions should be sought **(Fig. 2-200)**. African trypanosomiasis (sleeping sickness), caused by *Trypanosoma brucei* subspecies *T. brucei rhodesiense*, results in fulminant disease, while *T. brucei gambiense* results in subacute–chronic meningoencephalitis. *Arsenicals* are present in insecticides and in some medications such as melarsoprol used for the treatment of trypanosomiasis. They may cause AHL with fibrinoid necrosis of white matter vessels, and perivascular hemorrhages.[262] *L-asparaginase* interferes with the coagulation system, resulting in superior sagittal sinus thrombosis and hemorrhages.[350]

Multiple widespread *petechial white matter hemorrhages* are usually in the form of so-called ring-and-ball hemorrhage as a ring around the

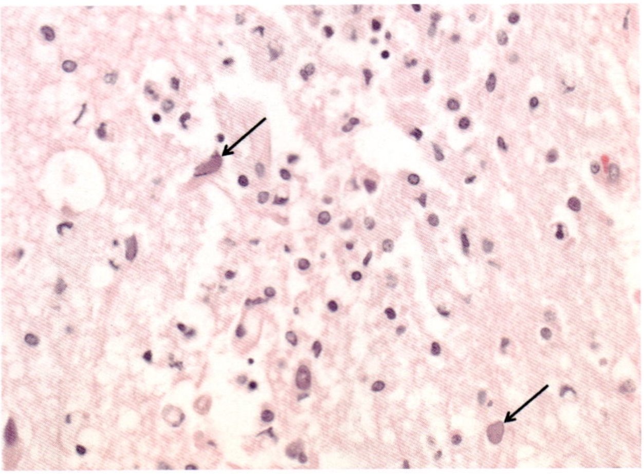

Figure 2-200. HSV encephalitis: Neurons with ground-glass nuclei containing intranuclear inclusions (*arrows*) are seen in a necroinflammatory background. They may be difficult to find without immunohistochemistry. Hemorrhagic areas were present elsewhere, resulting in a picture mimicking a hemorrhagic infarct or cerebritis (H&E; original magnification: 400×).

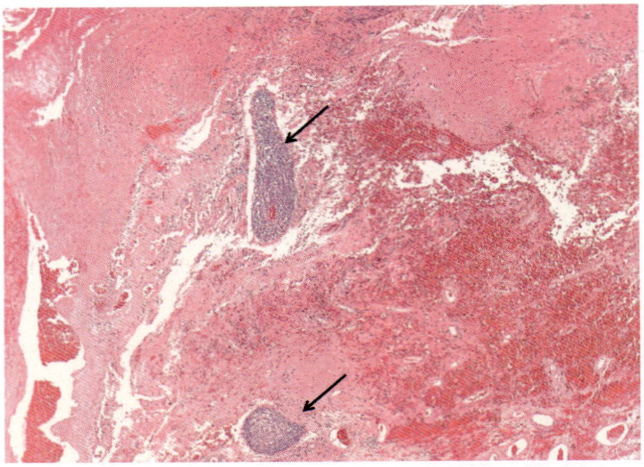

Figure 2-201. Hemorrhage due to vasculitis: Vessels with prominent perivascular lymphocytic infiltrates (*arrows*) are seen in association with the hemorrhage. Evaluation of the lymphocytic population showed it to be composed of polyclonal small, round lymphocytes predominantly of T cells (H&E; original magnification: 40×).

small vessels. This pattern is mainly seen in *fat embolism*, *diffuse axonal injury*, and *acute hemorrhagic encephalomyelitis*. In the latter, there is also fibrinoid necrosis of the vessel wall, a lymphohistiocytic inflammatory infiltrate with admixed plasma cells, and demyelination. DAI is also associated with axonal spheroids, but if the death is sudden, only petechial hemorrhages can be present, as axonal distortions and spheroids take about 12 to 24 hours to form. *Arboviruses* tend to more prominently involve the brainstem, thalamus, and basal ganglia, and some also additionally involve the spinal cord, such as West Nile virus and Japanese encephalitis. In addition to typical encephalitis picture, they may also cause perivascular hemorrhages and perivascular destruction of myelinated fibers, reminiscent of ADEM. Vessels affected by *vasculitis* that causes damage in the vessel wall can result in multifocal *perivascular hemorrhage* or, in some cases, frank large hemorrhages[358] **(Fig. 2-201)**. In older, healing, or treated lesions, in addition to recanalized thrombus in the lumen of a fibrotic vessel, evidence of previous hemorrhage in the form of hemosiderin pigment can be seen to support the diagnosis. Small amount of perivascular hemosiderin pigment and a few hemosiderin-laden macrophages are commonly present as an incidental finding in the basal ganglionic and white matter vessels in an otherwise unremarkable autopsy brain, and their significance is debatable. They may simply indicate small leaks in these vessels due to unknown reasons. Infarcts and hemorrhages in the setting of HIV infection may be the result of *HIV arteriopathy*, which may involve the parenchyma and leptomeninges.[197] *Hypernatremia* may result in venous thrombosis due to fluid loss and hemoconcentration and predisposes to parenchymal hemorrhages likely due to tissue shrinkage and tearing of vessels in the acute phase. *Pancreatic encephalopathy*[466] may be associated with swelling and basal ganglionic and periventricular petechiae, which are pericapillary hemorrhages. *Acute lead encephalopathy* is associated with swelling, petechial hemorrhages, congestion, and hydrocephalus. Vessels show endothelial swelling, vascular necrosis, and a perivascular proteinaceous material within which PAS-positive globules can be seen.[17] *Cyanide poisoning*[467] causes swelling, subarachnoid hemorrhages, and petechial hemorrhages within a few hours. *Sulfonamides* are associated with endothelial swelling and necrosis, which may result in hemorrhages.[17]

The presence of an *aneurysm* is usually easily recognized clinically, radiologically, and pathologically by its presentation and the resultant *subarachnoid hemorrhage* predominantly involving the basal surface of the brain. Traumatic aneurysms can be difficult to identify, and although rare, they should be considered as a possibility with subarachnoid hemorrhages. They are aneurysms that develop from a weakened vessel wall after the vessel is damaged by traumatic injury and tend to occur on the convexities. Hyperextension injuries can result in basilar and vertebral artery tears and subarachnoid hemorrhages,[468] as well as arterial dissections. *Meningocerebral angiodysplasia and renal agenesis*[189] is associated with very vascular leptomeninges of the brain, cerebellum, and brainstem, sometimes with subarachnoid hemorrhage, small brain with atrophic gyri, and gray and white matter necrosis. Hemorrhage and calcification may be present. Angiodysplasia consists of ectatic capillaries and veins present in leptomeninges. Calcifications, hemorrhage, thrombosis, infarcts, and hemosiderin-laden macrophages can be seen.

Intraventricular hemorrhage in adults usually results from the dissection of a parenchymal hemorrhage into the ventricular system. Such dissection can occur toward the brain surface to result in a subarachnoid component, as well. In infants, especially in premature infants, intraventricular hemorrhage typically originates from a *germinal matrix hemorrhage* **(Fig. 2-202)** or *choroid plexus hemorrhage* associated with *hypoxic episodes* and

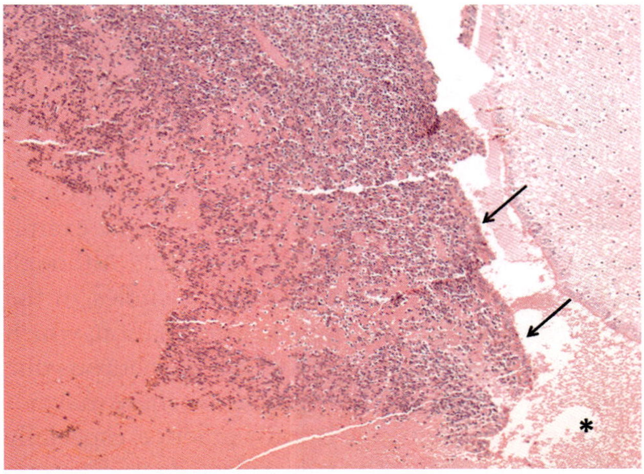

Figure 2-202. Germinal matrix hemorrhage: Hemorrhage underneath the ependymal lining (*arrows*) made its way into the ventricular system (*asterisk*) (H&E; original magnification: 100×).

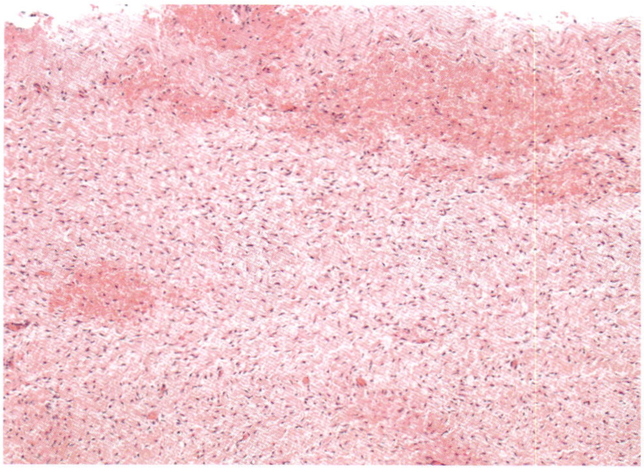

Figure 2-203. Intradural hemorrhage: Hemorrhagic foci are present within the dura mater in this premature neonate who suffered extensive hypoxic–ischemic injury to the brain (H&E; original magnification: 100×).

constitutes common autopsy findings. If the child survives, the intraventricular hemorrhage can extend into aqueduct to organize there and occlude the CSF flow, resulting in noncommunicating hydrocephalus, necessitating a shunt. Other forms of hemorrhage in this context are subarachnoid, subdural, and *intradural hemorrhage*,[469] that is, within the dural fibrous tissue layers **(Fig. 2-203)**. The latter represents the most subtle form of hemorrhage in the context of hypoxic–ischemic injury in premature infants and can be an isolated finding. Ventricular hemorrhages may spread into subarachnoid space or vice versa following the CSF circulation.

Subdural hemorrhage can become chronic by organization forming the so-called membranes or pseudomembranes of granulation tissue. This granulation tissue is cellular in its earlier stages with proliferating fibroblasts and neovascularization, complete with mitotic activity, which should not be mistaken for some kind of spindle cell neoplasm **(Fig. 2-204)**. There is usually variable numbers of predominantly chronic inflammatory cells and macrophages. Many eosinophil PMN leukocytes can be present. These changes should not be taken for an infectious process. EMH is not unusual and should not be mistaken for leukemic involvement.[454,470]

In pituitary adenoma, hemorrhage known as *pituitary apoplexy* results in a rapid enlargement of

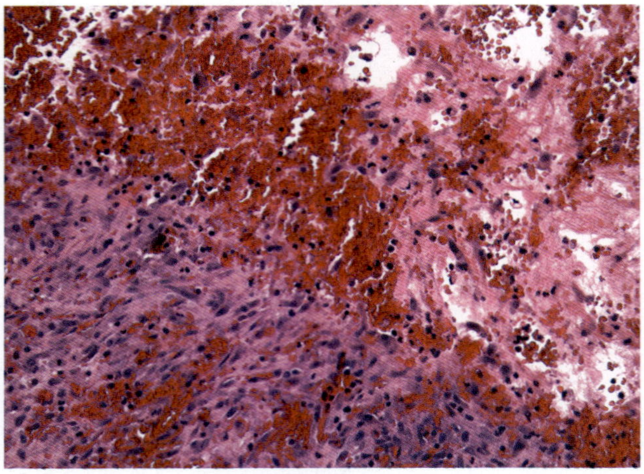

Figure 2-204. Granulation tissue: Ingrowth of neovascularization and fibroblastic proliferation (**bottom**) into the hematoma (**top**) is seen in this organizing subdural hematoma (H&E; original magnification: 200×).

the adenoma and a decrease in or disappearance of the function of adenoma. There is usually associated infarction of the adenoma. The specimen consists of largely hemorrhagic and necrotic fragments that are difficult to recognize as adenoma or even pituitary gland **(Fig. 2-205)**. However, the reticulin network is typically preserved and reticulin stain should highlight the nature of the pituitary lesion. Immunohistochemical work-up should not be done, as results are not accurate in such tissues.

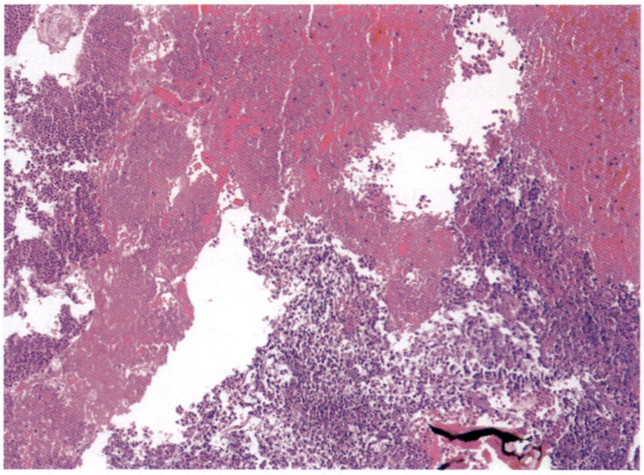

Figure 2-205. Pituitary apoplexy: Eosinophilic hemorrhagic fibrinous areas and basophilic necrotic cellular areas are seen (H&E; original magnification: 100×).

Necrosis

Necrosis simply indicates the loss of viability of the tissue and may take different definitions depending on the context it occurs, such as infarct, and/or based on its appearance, such as fibrinoid necrosis. It also can be classified based on the mechanism involved in its development, such as liquefactive necrosis, resulting in different appearances and implying different pathogeneses. It may be very useful to recognize the nature of the necrosis in cases where the tissue may be limited, so that additional workup can be initiated and appropriate recommendations are made, especially at the time of IOC.

Infarct is the term used in embolic stroke to refer to this type of anoxic/ischemic injury. Although in general pathologic terms this kind of injury results in coagulative necrosis and in the acute neuronal injury stage dying neurons resemble coagulative necrosis, necrosis in the CNS is typically in the form of liquefactive necrosis, where the proteins are digested rapidly, resulting in a viscous liquid material. Depending on the stage of development, it can take different appearances, although in practice and traditionally, infarct is more commonly used to refer to the fully developed tissue death as seen after the complete disintegration of the tissue. While the stages of an infarct are well-characterized, its chronologic assessment is not, especially in the later stages, because it is dependent on various factors, such as the severity of the insult, the extent of the injury, reperfusion, collateral circulation, and metabolic activity of the tissue. In general, however, infarcts follow a quite constant histologic evolution pattern (see below; **Table 2.22**).[471] The most sensitive cells to hypoxic/ischemic damage are neurons, and the earliest morphologic finding is mitochondrial swelling seen by electron microscopic examination as early as 1 hour postinjury.[472] Although they may be represented as small vacuoles in the cytoplasm by light microscopic examination, which may also show *vacuolation* around the neurons due to the swelling of astrocyte processes, these may not prove to be reproducible in daily practice, especially with autopsy tissue. The use of electron microscopy is not a practical approach, and mitochondrial swelling is a nonspecific finding that can also commonly develop as an artifact of the problems associated with tissue fixation and processing. In practice, *acute neuronal injury*, also referred to as eosinophilic neuronal necrosis, red neurons, or shrunken

List of Findings/Checklist for Necrosis

AT A GLANCE

Infarct
- Acute neuronal injury
- Acute
- Subacute
- Chronic
- Lacunar
- Laminar necrosis
- Watershed zone infarct
- Hemorrhagic infarct
- Venous infarct
- Microinfarcts
  - Vasculopathy
  - Embolic shower
  - Infections
  - Fabry's disease
- Spinal cord infarct

White Matter Necrosis
- Periventricular leukomalacia
- Infections
- Cerebral autosomal dominant arteriopathy with subcortical infarcts and leukoencephalopathy (CADASIL)
- Mitochondrial encephalomyopathy, lactic acidosis and stroke-like episodes (MELAS)
- Myoclonal epilepsy with ragged red fibers (MERRF)
- Orthochromatic leukodystrophy
- Multifocal necrotizing leukoencephalopathy
  - Radiation
  - Chemotherapy
  - Other medications
  - HIV

Bilateral Basal Ganglionic Necrosis
- Heroin (globus pallidus)
- Carbon monoxide (globus pallidus)
- Cyanide (globus pallidus)
- Holotopistic striatal necrosis (striatum)
- Leber's hereditary optic neuropathy (striatum)
- Methanol (putamen)

Fibrinoid Necrosis
- Vessel walls
  - Vasculitis
  - Radiation change
- Radiation
- Abscess

Infections
- Tuberculosis (caseation)
- Abscess (fibrinoid necrosis)
- Angioinvasive fungi
  - *Aspergillus spp.*
  - Zygomycetes
  - *Pseudoallescheria spp.*
- Parasitic infections
  - Toxoplasmosis
  - Amebiasis
  - Others

Neoplasms
- Infarct-like necrosis
  - Embolization
  - Glioblastoma
  - Pituitary adenoma
- Palisading necrosis
  - Glioblastoma
  - Other high-grade gliomas
  - Malignant peripheral nerve sheath tumor
- Pseudonecrosis
- Radiation necrosis

Apoptosis
- Premature internal granule cells
- Pontosubicular necrosis
- Trimethyltin
- Neoplasms with high cellular turnover rate

neurons based on their microscopic appearance on routine examination, is the earliest light microscopic sign of irreversible neuron death. It is seen in a gradual manner anywhere from as early as 4 hours postinjury and develops fully in about 10 to 12 hours postinjury. At this stage, the cytoplasm is eosinophilic and dull with loss of Nissl substance and crisp granularity. The crispness of chromatin is lost and the nucleus assumes a smudgy appearance and subsequently disintegrates **(Fig. 2-206)**. This neuronal change should not be confused with the purple, shrunken neurons, in spite of the similarities in their names, seen in surgical specimens **(Fig. 2-207)**. The latter is formed by a shrinkage reaction of the vital neurons to surgical manipulation.

In about 24 hours, the tissue completely disintegrates into pale eosinophilic, granular, necrotic material and neutrophil PMN leukocyte infiltration

TABLE 2.22 Microscopic features of infarct evolution

Time Postinjury	Microscopic Changes
Acute Stage (0–15 d)	
1 h	Neuronal and perineuronal microvacuolation
4–12 h	Red neurons
15–24 h	PMN leukocyte infiltration, karyorrhexis
2–3 d	Macrophage infiltration and vascular proliferation start
5 d	Reactive astrocytosis starts
Subacute Stage (2–6 wk)	
2–6 wk	Vascular prominence, gradual macrophage predominance, gradual increase in reactive astrocytosis
Chronic Stage (6 wk and on)	
6 wk and on	Gradual cystic change, decrease/disappearance of macrophages, reactive astrocytosis

d, day; h, hour; wk, week

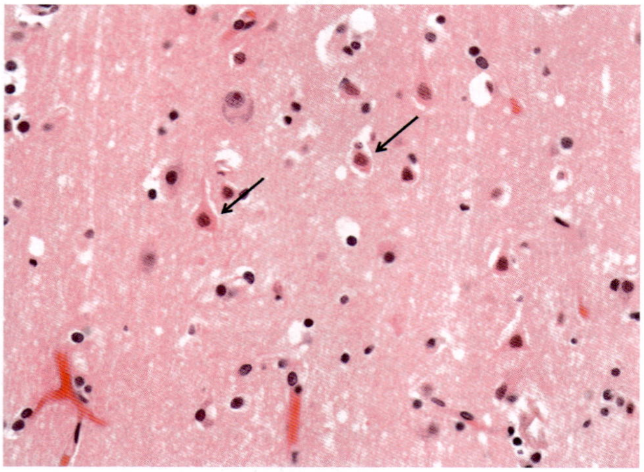

Figure 2-206. Eosinophilic neuronal necrosis (*red neurons*): Acute hypoxic–ischemic injury shows red neurons with their eosinophilic cytoplasm and smudgy nuclei (*arrows*). Viable-appearing neurons are also seen in this area, but they may not have had enough time elapsed since they were subjected to the hypoxic–ischemic episode and, therefore, may not yet show the typical light microscopic features of such irreversible injury (H&E; original magnification: 400×).

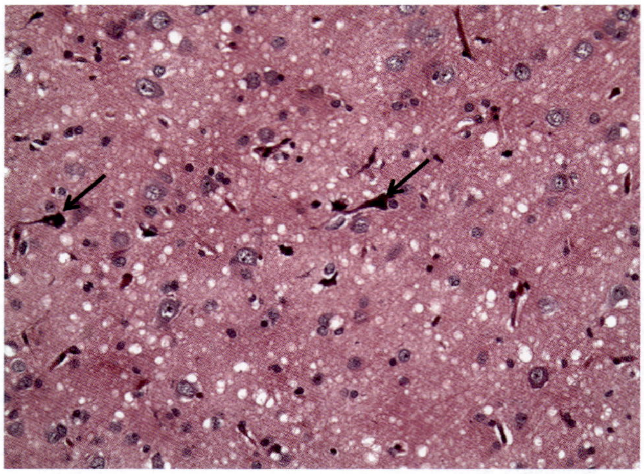

Figure 2-207. Basophilic (*purple*) neurons (*arrows*): Commonly seen in surgical specimens, neurons show this peculiar shrinkage artifact in reaction to surgical manipulation in situ. This biopsy specimen was obtained from a suspected Creutzfeldt-Jakob disease patient and shows the spongiform change (H&E; original magnification: 200×).

starts. At this stage, it may be confused with a cerebritis or necrotic material associated with an inflammatory/infectious process **(Fig. 2-208)**. In about 48 hours, macrophages appear, gradually become abundant, and may remain up to months depending on the size of the infarct. Meanwhile, neutrophil PMN leukocyte infiltration ceases at

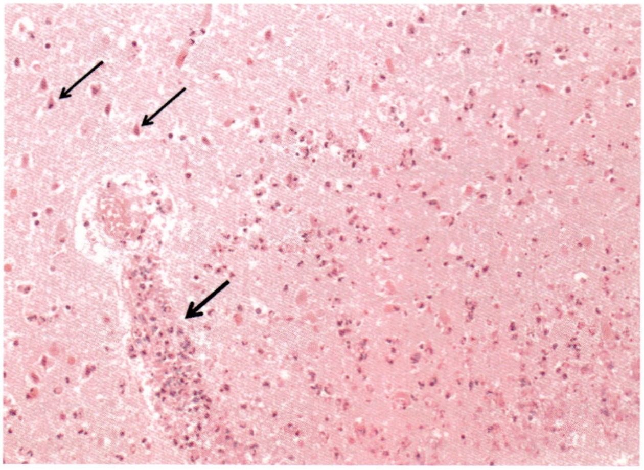

Figure 2-208. Acute infarct: Although a few red neurons (*thin arrows*) are present, other areas are disintegrating and show PMN leukocyte infiltration around the vessels (*thick arrow*), as well as within the necrotic parenchyma (H&E; original magnification: 200×).

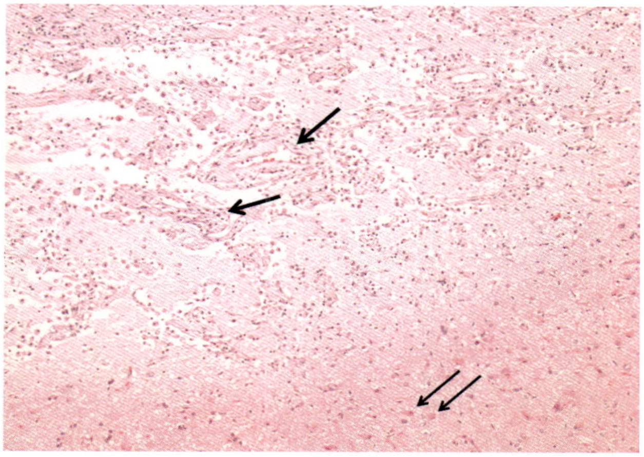

Figure 2-209. Subacute infarct: Vessels are prominent (*thick arrows*) and there are numerous histiocytes in this subacute infarct that is well-circumscribed from the surrounding parenchyma that contains scattered reactive astrocytes (*thin arrows*) (H&E; original magnification: 100×).

day 5 and astrocytes gradually start proliferating around the lesion. About this time, vessels also show endothelial hyperplasia and neovascularization **(Fig. 2-209)**. Eventually, the debris is cleared and macrophages disappear to leave a gliotic cystic lesion **(Fig. 2-210)**. All these changes are gradual, overlapping, and variable; however, in general, the *acute phase* is characterized by neuronal changes, tissue disintegration, and neutrophil PMN leukocyte infiltration; *subacute phase* by prominent macrophage infiltration and vascular changes; and *chronic or remote phase* by reactive astrocytes and cystic lesion. At the chronic stage, which may take weeks to months depending on the size of the lesion, it is not possible to judge the age of the lesion any further with any degree of accuracy. The subacute stage of an infarct may cause serious problems in surgical neuropathology practice and especially in IOC due to the abundant macrophage infiltration and vascular changes, imitating a glial neoplasm. The cytoplasm of these foamy macrophages are fragile and cytoplasmic borders disappear during the preparation of smears and frozen sections, creating a sea of nuclei punctuated by prominent and even proliferating vessels, which may result in a diagnosis of high-grade glial neoplasm. These deceiving changes are focal for the most part and the presence of macrophages can be appreciated at least in some areas of the preparations. Touch preparations can be especially useful in preserving the macrophage cytoplasms, and the yield is high in contrast to actual glial neoplasms where the neoplastic cells are difficult to obtain simply by touching the slide due to the rich network of processes.

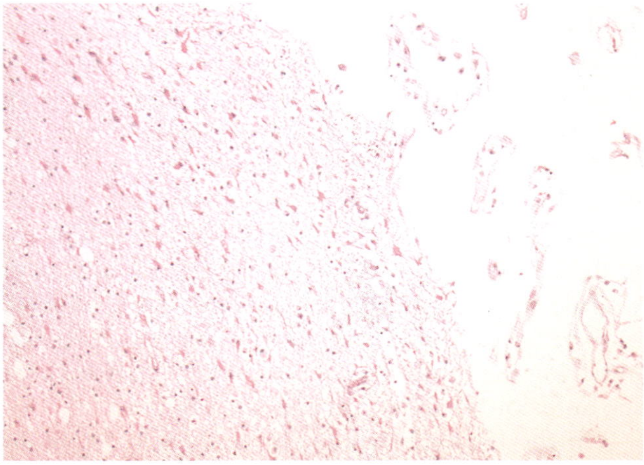

Figure 2-210. Chronic (remote) infarct: The necrotic tissue has been cleared, leaving a cystic cavity (**right side**) surrounded by gliotic parenchyma (**left side**) (H&E; original magnification: 100×).

Lacunar infarcts or lacunes are infarcts that are seen mainly in the basal ganglia, thalamus, cerebellum, and brainstem and that, by definition, measure less than 1.5 cm. They can be seen in the superficial cerebral hemispheres, are typically multiple and of variable sizes, and are associated with atherosclerotic disease.[473] They are common findings in autopsies. Their microscopic features are similar to those of other infarcts stage by stage. Sometimes, dilated Virchow-Robin spaces around vessels as a result of atherosclerotic and hypertensive changes may look like lacunae, but the vessel can be seen within the cavity grossly and microscopically. *Laminar infarct/laminar necrosis* or, if more than one layer of the cerebral cortex is involved, *pseudolaminar necrosis*, although these terms are used interchangeably in practice, refers to hypoxic–ischemic damage to cerebral cortex, preferentially involving layers III, V, and VI, layer III being the most sensitive to this type of injury[474] **(Fig. 2-211)**. The typical setting is one of generalized hypoxic–ischemic encephalopathy in association with systemic disease interfering with perfusion and oxygenation of the brain. The early changes consist of microvacuolation of the cortical neuropil, and may be confused with the

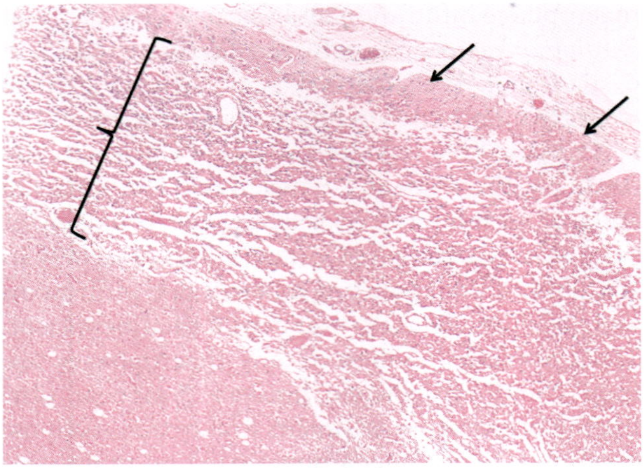

Figure 2-211. Pseudolaminar necrosis: The entire thickness of cerebral cortex is involved (*bracket*), at this point sparing the underlying white matter as well as leaving the subpial layer intact (*arrows*) (H&E; original magnification: 40×).

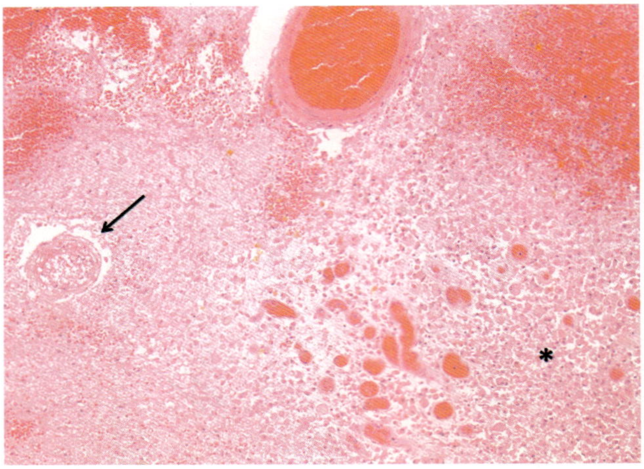

Figure 2-212. Hemorrhagic infarct: Fresh hemorrhage is present in the background of an infarct with many histiocytes (*asterisk*) and necrotic vessels (*arrow*), likely originating from such vessels (H&E; original magnification: 100×).

spongiform changes of CJD, in which the vacuolation may also be laminar or diffuse. In CJD, the neuron loss and gliosis are minimal until its later stages; eosinophilic neuronal necrosis is not present, unless there is superimposed hypoxic–ischemic injury; and the clinical scenarios are very different between the two conditions. Sometimes, an end-stage histologic picture may be seen as a result of diverse insults and result in extensive neuron loss, gliosis, and tissue destruction. The etiology in such cases may not be further elucidated. Laminar necrosis also goes through similar stages of evolution as described above and may result in a laminar cavitation in chronic cases. Laminar necrosis may be more prominent in the watershed zones. *Watershed zone infarcts* are typically associated with a relatively brief and transient drop in the perfusion pressure,[475] resulting in the hypoxic–ischemic injury to these areas between the major arterial territories supplied by the end-capillaries from these territories. Their microscopic features and evolution are also similar to those described above. *Hemorrhagic infarct* is typically an embolic or thromboembolic infarct in which reperfusion occurs, resulting in secondary hemorrhages from the infarcted and weakened vessels. It may be a complication of thrombolytic therapy[476] **(Fig. 2-212)**. Relatively recent hemorrhagic foci can be identified in a background of more advanced and predominant infarct. *Venous infarcts* are mainly large areas of congestion and hemorrhage within the softened tissue, rather than large hematomas in contrast to hemorrhages. The main diagnostic evaluation of hypoxic–ischemic lesions is gross examination, since their location and gross appearances, as well as clinical correlation, are important to further characterize them. They are commonly associated with venous sinus thrombosis.[477] *Spinal cord* can also suffer from similar pathologic processes. The watershed zone of the spinal cord is roughly in the midthoracic region, corresponding to T6-T8, where watershed zone infarcts develop in hyoperfusion states.[478] Other infarcts typically occur as a result of problems with the aorta, such as atherosclerotic narrowing, dissection, and embolization, while hemorrhagic infarctions are rare. Microscopic features and evolution of the lesions are similar to those described above. Usually in premature infants, spinal cord infarcts may be in the form of central necrosis especially involving the lumbosacral cord or diffusely involve the anterior horn neurons, in term infants.

In the brain, histologic appearance of remote infarct is seen also in infarcts that occur earlier in development. For instance, the histologic appearance of *porencephaly* is essentially a remote infarct with a cystic space lined by gliotic tissue. Since such early destruction interferes with the development

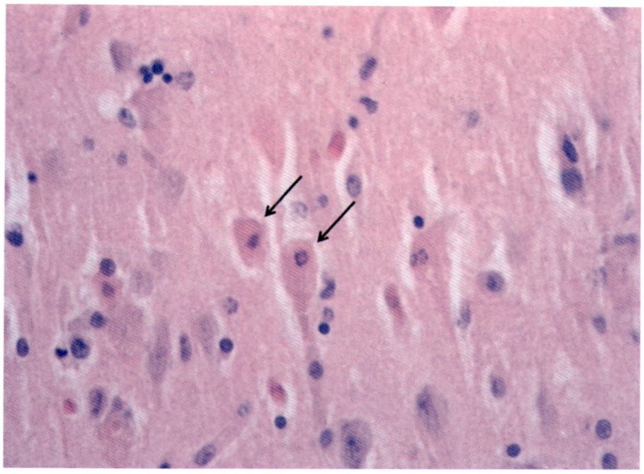

Figure 2-213. Eosinophilic neuronal necrosis (*red neurons; arrows*): This section is from the Sommer's sector (CA1) of the hippocampus, and similar changes can also be seen in hypoglycemia (H&E; original magnification: 400×).

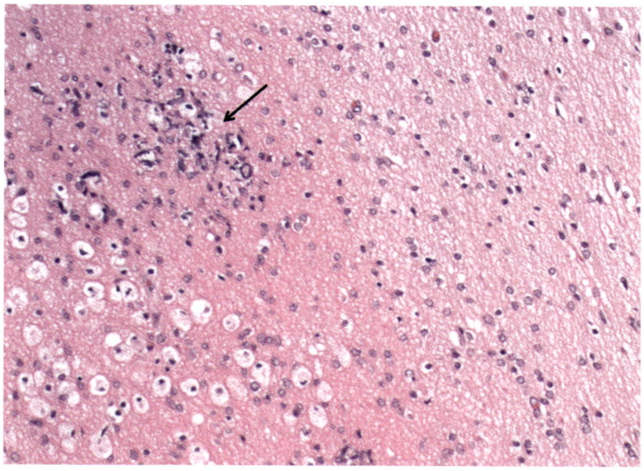

Figure 2-214. Periventricular leukomalacia: Histiocytes (**bottom left**) and mineralized neurons (*arrow*) are seen along with a pale white matter (**right side**) (H&E; original magnification: 200×).

of adjacent tissues, foci of polymicrogyria, MCD, or periventricular heterotopic gray matter foci are commonly found in association with such lesions. The most sensitive area of the brain to hypoxic/ischemic injury is CA1 region of the hippocampus (*Sommer's sector*). Purkinje cells are also sensitive. Therefore, in most mild cases of brain anoxia, the earliest changes can be seen in these areas **(Fig. 2-213)**. In pediatric brains, the damage presents as variable degrees of *periventricular white matter injury*, which can be as mild as a mild gliosis and rarification with scattered mulberries to overt periventricular leukomalacia with cystic changes, calcifications, and macrophages **(Fig. 2-214)**. Overt necrosis is not typically prominent in these lesions. A similar tissue loss with resultant variable degrees of cavitation may rarely be seen after any kind of destruction. Severe *encephalitides*, especially those associated with necrosis and hemorrhagic lesions, such as Herpes encephalitis, may result in a similar multicystic leukomalacia picture. Typically, such destruction is patchy and cannot be explained by a vascular territory, in contrast to vascular infarcts. In survivors of temporal lobe Herpes virus infections, there may be cavitated lesions in temporal lobes like remote infarcts, with gliosis. Residual small lymphocyte aggregates may still be seen in parenchyma and meninges. Virus can still be identified in these lesions at this stage by polymerase chain reaction. In addition, Herpes viruses may cause necrotizing myelopathy.VZV also involves vessels of various calibers to result in hemorrhagic and necrotic lesions. Congenital toxoplasmosis is also very destructive.

Evaluation of vessels is important in any infarct to identify any *vasculopathy* (see "Vascular Changes") that may have resulted in that infarct, although it is not always possible to identify the exact problem in every case. However, vasculitis, lymphomatoid granulomatosis, intravascular lymphoma, CAA, atheroembolic, or other types of occlusions, among others, may be seen. Meningocerebral angiodysplasia and renal agenesis is associated with highly vascular leptomeninges, among other features, and can have gray and white matter necrosis.

Multifocal white matter infarcts are seen in later stages of CADASIL and CARASIL.[347] They are usually perivascular, ill-defined lesions of variable stages in a background of myelin pallor as part of the leukoencephalopathy. Other recognized syndromes that can have such white matter ischemic lesions and infarcts are MELAS,[479] MERRF,[480] and familial hemiplegic migraine,[481] which is associated with a genetic defect in collagen gene. In moyamoya disease, the occlusion is gradual and is due to intimal proliferation and thickening. Subsequent thrombus formation also contributes to luminal obstruction. By definition, no atherosclerotic changes or inflammation are present. In the pure, congenital form, the process is referred to as moyamoya disease, but similar changes may occur secondarily as part of various syndromes, such as NF1 and Down syndrome, as well as due to various forms of vascular damage, such as radiation therapy, trauma, or vasculitis, in which case it is referred to as moyamoya syndrome.[482] OLD with cavitation and oligodendroglial proliferation results in massive cavities with Sudan-positive macrophages and increased oligodendroglia, mimicking an inflammatory process.[17] Necrotizing leukoencephalopathy in HIV[483] involves the white matter and pons and is characterized by numerous macrophages and variable numbers of lymphocytes, primarily perivascular location, and in later stages astrocytosis and calcifications. HIV-associated arteriopathy mainly involves meningeal arteries and can result in infarcts and/or hemorrhages in the parenchyma.[484,485] Hemorrhage or infarcts can be seen in porphyrias due to hypertensive attacks. Multifocal necrotizing leukoencephalopathy can also be seen in leukemia,[486] radiation, chemotherapy[252,487–489] especially with methotrexate, as well as other drugs, such as amphotericin-B, BCNU, fludarabine, cisplatin, and cytosine arabinoside (see "White Matter Changes and Myelin Loss"). The lesions of fludarabine tend to involve predominantly the occipital lobes, also involving pyramids and posterior columns of spinal cord. White matter lesions may be perivascular or more confluent and may involve overlying cortex. The lesions of multifocal necrotizing leukoencephalopathy in general tend to be better circumscribed and are associated with axonal damage, axonal swellings, and calcifications, in contrast to those seen in those associated with carbon monoxide, cyanide, methanol, global hypoxia, and mitochondrial disorders. Necrotic lesions in the white matter can also be associated with intrathecal gentamycin, along with calcifications in the midbrain and pons; nimorazole, which also has Leigh's-like lesions in the brainstem and dentate nuclei; and sulfonamides, which can also involve the gray matter. Various hemorrhagic and necrotic lesions can be seen in association with various medications and toxic states along with their other findings.[17,83] Some examples are carbon tetrachloride (venous thromboses and hemorrhagic infarcts), amphetamines, methamphetamine, methylenedioxymethamphetamine (ecstasy) (arterial and venous infarcts), and heroin (laminar, bilateral globus pallidus, and watershed infarcts, global hypoxic–ischemic damage, ischemic myelopathy).

Infarcts can occur in particular situations in particular locations. Knowledge of such patterns is useful in the interpretation of the overall pathologic picture. Gross examination is once again very important in the identification of these patterns, as microscopic clues are limited. Holotopistic striatal necrosis (familial striatal degeneration) is associated with softening, necrosis, and cavitation in caudate nuclei and putamina.[490] There may also be atrophy with neuron loss and gliosis in these structures in some cases. Cortical gray matter and cerebellar degeneration may or may not be present. Bilateral striatal necrosis is usually seen together with features of Leber's hereditary optic neuropathy. Putamen, caudate nucleus, and parts of internal capsule between them, as well as white matter, are bilaterally cavitated. There are lipid-laden macrophages and surrounding gliosis.[17,491] Methanol intoxication[83] most typically causes bilateral putamen and claustrum hemorrhagic infarctions. There may also be white matter necrosis and global hypoxic–ischemic changes. Carbon monoxide intoxication[83] typically results in bilateral globus pallidus hemorrhage and necrosis, which eventually become cavitary **(Fig. 2-215)**.

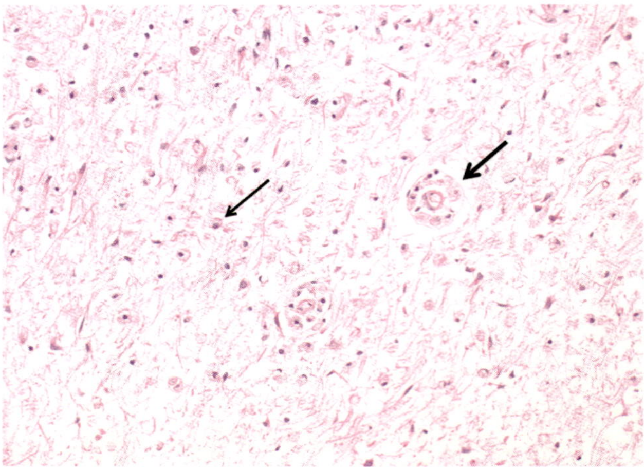

Figure 2-215. Carbon monoxide poisoning: This survivor had bilateral soft, partially cavitary lesions in the basal ganglia. They histologically are similar to subacute or chronic infarcts with histiocytes in the parenchyma (*thin arrow*) and around the vessels (*thick arrow*) in a gliotic background (H&E; original magnification: 200×).

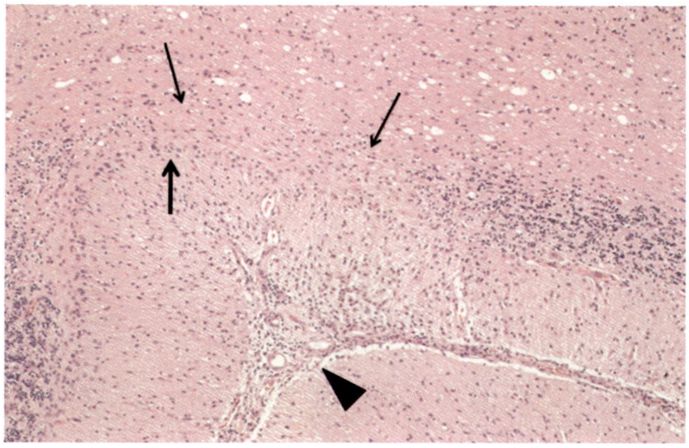

Figure 2-216. Cerebellar microinfarct: There is loss of Purkinje cells and internal granule layer cells (*thin arrows*). Purkinje cell layer has been replaced by Bergmann gliosis (*thick arrow*). Several thick vessels are present in the fibrotic and inflamed leptomeninges (*arrowhead*) in this area of healed vasculitis (H&E; original magnification: 100×).

There may also be necrotic foci in the white matter, sparing the U-fibers. Similar bilateral globus pallidus and white matter necrosis is also seen in cyanide poisoning. Posterior cerebral artery territory infarction in occipital lobes and brainstem can occur as a complication in uncus herniation. Optic nerve, chiasm, and tract necrosis may occur in association with hexachlorophene.[17]

Microinfarcts are usually a sign of a systemic or generalized CNS vasculature problem, such as vasculitis or embolic showers. They may be at different stages of evolution if this process has been continuing off and on with recurrences. Small vessel disease and embolic showers can result in multiple microinfarcts **(Fig. 2-216)**. Very small infarcts that may have linear or rounded contours depending on the orientation of the section can be seen in tissues resected during seizure surgery. They occur as a result of electrode placement during their preoperative work-up. They are usually also associated with variable degrees of fibrosis in the leptomeninges and chronic inflammation. Multiple microinfarcts in cerebral and cerebellar gray matter can occur in hemolytic uremic syndrome as a result of the platelet thrombi, which are hyalinized-appearing eosinophilic thrombi, in small arteries and arterioles. Tuberculous endarteritis, which is characterized by intimal thickening and lymphocytic infiltrate, may also result in brain infarcts. A similar endarteritis, resulting in infarcts, is also seen in syphilis,[492] coccidioidomycosis,[493] and Lyme disease.[333] Arteriolar thickening with microinfarcts can be seen in Whipple's disease.[338] While in general hyphae tend to occlude vessels and produce large infarcts and yeast forms tend to produce meningitis,[494] Candida can occlude small parenchymal vessels and may be associated with microinfarcts around vessels and subsequent microabscesses.[495] Perivascular necrosis, along with atrophy, gliosis, and macrophages, can be seen in uremic encephalopathy. There are PAS-positive and Sudan-positive material accumulation in the vessel walls in Fabry's disease, along with neuronal storage. Microinfarcts can occur due to vascular involvement.[496]

Necrosis is an important finding in the evaluation of *neoplasms* and, in general, indicates a high-grade malignancy. In surgical specimens and especially small ones with various *artifacts*, it is important not to mistake areas of hemorrhage and admixed fibrin for necrosis. A peculiar distortion of tissue fragments can be seen in specimens obtained by CUSA, termed *pseudonecrosis*, where tissue appears hypereosinophilic and distorted and the distorted nuclei appear as nuclear debris **(Fig. 2-217)**. Likewise, cauterized or crushed edges of the tissue may appear as necrosis. Crush artifact can occur during handling of tissue carelessly with a forceps. Poor staining, especially understaining

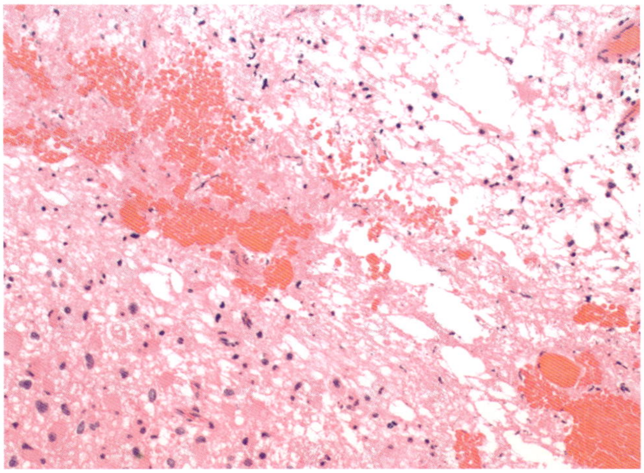

Figure 2-217. Pseudonecrosis: Artifactually crushed tissue (**top right**) has a smudgy appearance with admixed smeared nuclear material, mimicking necrosis in this glial neoplasm (**bottom left**) (H&E; original magnification: 200×).

by hematoxylin and overstaining by eosin, or lack of hematoxylin staining due to low dye level in the container leaving one edge of the tissue more eosinophilic may result in a necrotic appearance. Bony specimens that have been overly decalcified subsequently tend to stain eosinophilic and not take up hematoxylin. The tissue architecture is still preserved albeit as a ghost in the background, however, and should not be mistaken for coagulative necrosis. Using excessive force to smear tissue fragments that are naturally resistant to smearing, such as mesenchymal lesions or densely gliotic tissues, may result in crush artifact with fragmentation of nuclei in a proteinaceous background formed by cytoplasmic debris. In glial neoplasms, recognizing such artifacts and distinguishing them from true necrosis is especially important, as it directly influences grading by making them high-grade in most instances, and in the case of fibrillary astrocytomas, resulting in a diagnosis of glioblastoma. Necrosis that is associated with neoplasms is typically coagulative necrosis, at least in the earlier stages, where the necrotic tissue outlines, as well as individual cells, can be identified as eosinophilic ghosts. In later stages, as the proteins are digested, it assumes a "dirty" appearance with granular debris and without any further details. Necrosis is also commonly present in metastatic carcinomas, creating a pseudopapillary appearance resulting from several layers of neoplastic cells remaining viable around the vessels, a feature sometimes called peritheliomatous pattern, and in the right context, helps favor a metastatic origin in contrast to a glioblastoma with epithelioid cells (see "Papillary and Pseudopapillary Structures"). Sarcomas and high-grade lymphomas, especially those associated with immunodeficiency states, also commonly show large areas of necrosis. In glioblastoma,[497] necrosis can be confluent and infarct-like, affecting large areas **(Fig. 2-218)**, or can be in the form of typical *pseudopalisading (or palisading) necrosis* **(Fig. 2-219)** that is characteristic for, but not diagnostic of, glioblastoma.[498] In the former, only small islands of largely perivascular viable tissue can remain but still demonstrate a glial morphology with irregular nuclei, variable amount of cytoplasm, and a fibrillary background separating the cells/nuclei. In the case of pseudopalisading necrosis, necrosis is seen in a serpentine pattern rimmed by a zone of concentrated nuclei forming a pseudopalisading arrangement.

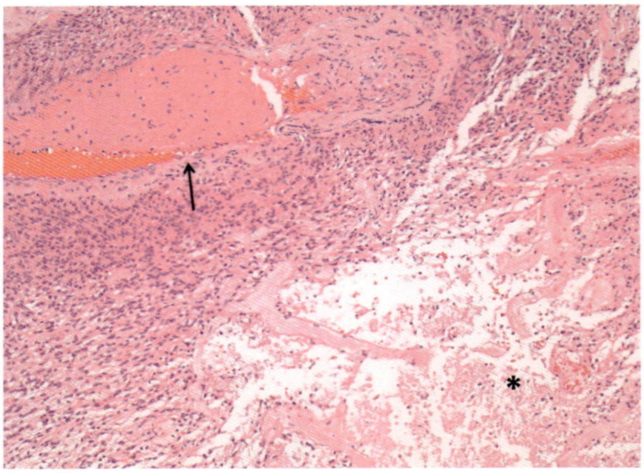

Figure 2-218. Infarct-like confluent necrosis (*asterisk*) in glioblastoma: A thrombosed vessel (*arrow*) is also present adjacent to necrosis (H&E; original magnification: 100×).

It can be seen in other high-grade glial neoplasms, namely, anaplastic oligodendroglioma, as well as in medulloblastoma, PNETs, and MPNSTs, bringing these neoplasms into the differential diagnosis of glioblastoma, especially when it is composed predominantly of small, bipolar cells. It is a rare occurrence in medulloblastoma, however. Especially in the case of PNET or medulloblastoma, additional considerations become glioblastoma with PNET component or a PNET with glial differentiation

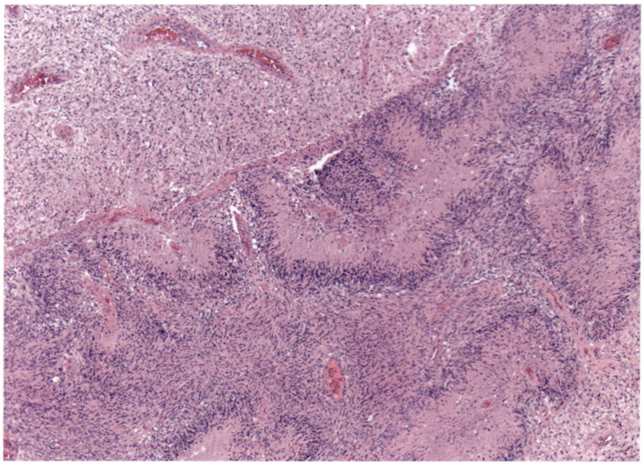

Figure 2-219. Pseudopalisading necrosis: A typical finding for glioblastoma, but can also be seen in other neoplasms, pseudopalisading necrosis is typically geographic with crowded nuclei at its periphery (H&E; original magnification: 40×).

(see "Small Blue Cells"). Some neurocytomas, central or extraventricular, can have more than an occasional mitotic figure, are associated with vascular proliferation and necrosis, and have been designated as atypical neurocytomas, without a WHO grade.[499,500] They also tend to have a Ki-67 proliferation index of more than 2%. An anaplastic version of neurocytoma has not been designated and is debatable. In choroid plexus neoplasms, focal necrosis is one of the features of atypical choroid plexus papilloma (WHO grade II), while choroid plexus carcinomas (WHO grade III) show more prominent necrosis. Immunohistochemistry can further help delineate the degree of various differentiations and their extent. Usually, this rarely becomes a practical problem, and in most cases, the neoplasm declares its predominant character. Necrosis, associated with at least two other features out of hemorrhage, cytologic atypia, and hypercellularity, is a feature of anaplastic (WHO grade III) hemangiopericytoma.[501] Necrosis may be extensive in some neoplasms and may make especially the small tissue fragments impossible to evaluate. Same is true for the neoplasms in the overdecalcified bone specimens. The interpretation of immunohistochemical stains should be done with extreme caution, if they are performed at all. In some situations, at least a general idea about the nature of the lesion may be obtained by immunohistochemistry in spite of their necrotic nature.[502] Necrosis in schwannoma can be seen as part of the hemorrhagic degenerative change that commonly results in the cystic appearance, and has no prognostic implications, except that it should not be mistaken for a malignancy. Necrosis is rarely seen in cellular schwannoma and is without palisading, while especially palisading necrosis is common in MPNST. Necrosis may be one of the several features to qualify a granular cell tumor as malignant, where three of marked cellularity, pleomorphism, high nucleus-to-cytoplasm ratio, nucleoli, brisk mitotic activity, spindle cells, and necrosis are needed.[503]

Some low-grade neoplasms can also have necrosis. Its significance may not be as straightforward in such cases. For instance, in meningiomas, necrosis is only one of the features that, if found in combination with others, upgrades a WHO grade I meningioma to atypical, that is, WHO grade II.[44] In the context of meningioma, one should be careful with previously embolized meningiomas, which can show large areas of confluent necrosis **(Fig. 2-220)**. In truly atypical meningiomas, it usually is not a problem to find additional features to support the high-grade nature of the neoplasm. History of embolization and identification of embolization material within the vessels are also helpful. In addition, although not always a reliable feature, the coagulative, infarct-like appearance of embolization necrosis contrasts with the "dirty" appearance of true tumor necrosis. Some PAs can have necrosis, which is not always a clinically significant feature, unless it is also associated with high proliferation index as identified by Ki-67 immunohistochemistry and/or increased mitotic activity. Same comments are applicable to radiation necrosis seen especially in recurrent meningiomas. Anaplastic transformation in PA, which usually occurs years after initial diagnosis and radiation treatment, also includes necrosis.[504] The necrosis associated with malignancy in PA typically is in the form of pseudopalisading necrosis, rather than infarct-like areas. PXAs with anaplastic features are those PXAs with necrosis, with or without pseudopalisading, and increased mitotic activity, designated as 5 or more mitotic figures in 10 high power fields (HPFs)[505] (see "Mitotic Activity"). Pseudopalisading necrosis is one of the features that help identify anaplastic (malignant) astroblastomas, although in occasional cases, it can be seen in well-differentiated astroblastomas. Necrosis in

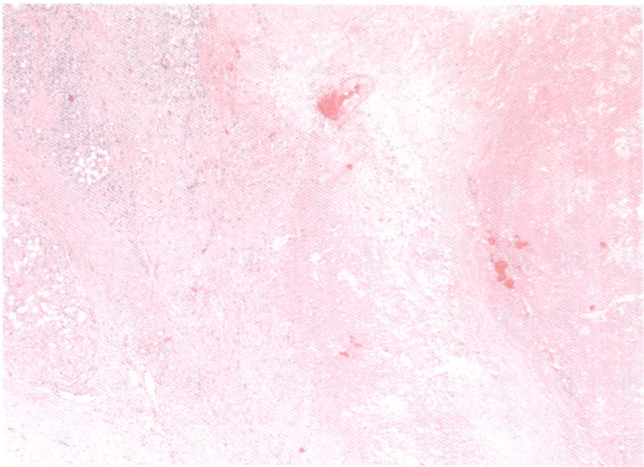

Figure 2-220. Embolized meningioma: Large, confluent infarct (**right side**) is present, leaving a rim of viable cellular meningioma (**left side**) (H&E; original magnification: 40×).

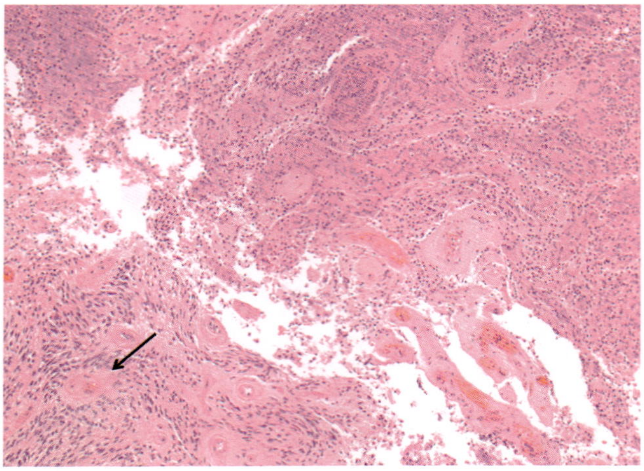

Figure 2-221. Ependymoma: Confluent necrosis (**top right**) is present in this otherwise unremarkable ependymoma (**bottom left**) with typical pseudorosettes (*arrow*) and does not necessarily imply anaplasia (H&E; original magnification: 100×).

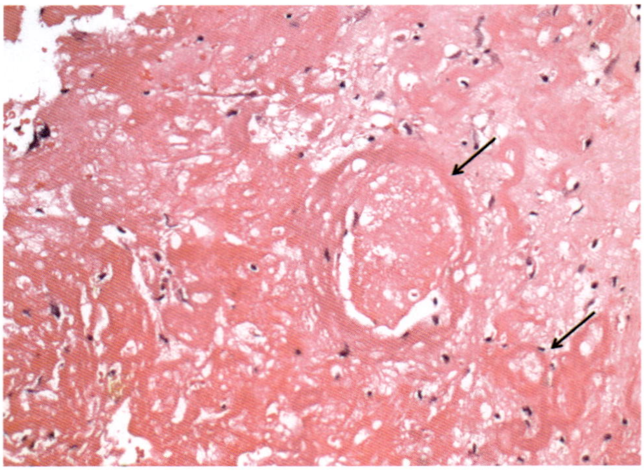

Figure 2-222. Radiation necrosis: A peculiar bright red appearance is associated with fibrinoid necrosis seen in association with radiation treatment, both in the tissue and in the vessel walls (*arrows*) (H&E; original magnification: 200×).

low-grade ependymoma[506,507] is a common finding and does not appear to have an impact on prognosis when it is in the form of geographic, infarct-like necrosis **(Fig. 2-221)**. On the other hand, pseudopalisading necrosis is significant for the designation of anaplastic ependymoma. In melanocytic neoplasms, necrosis is an important feature to separate melanocytoma and intermediate grade neoplasms from melanoma. Another WHO grade I neoplasm that can rarely have foci of necrosis is DIG/DIA, with no prognostic implications. SEGA is a WHO grade I neoplasm that is essentially entirely composed of large cells with neuron-like nuclei and astrocyte-like cytoplasm. It is well-circumscribed in spite of its cytologically atypical and worrisome appearance, contrasting with the infiltrative nature of high-grade glial neoplasms. Rare cases may have mitotic activity and foci of necrosis. In pituitary adenoma, hemorrhage known as pituitary apoplexy results in a rapid enlargement of the adenoma and a drop in the function of adenoma. There is usually associated infarction of the adenoma. The specimen consists of largely hemorrhagic and necrotic fragments that are difficult to recognize as adenoma or even pituitary gland. However, the reticulin network is typically preserved and reticulin stain should highlight the nature of the pituitary lesion. Immunohistochemical work-up should not be done, as results are not accurate in such tissues.

In the context of neoplasms, *radiation necrosis* should also be considered. It has a fibrinoid quality, which is especially prominent in the vessel walls **(Fig. 2-222)**. Large areas of necrosis can be difficult to distinguish from tumor necrosis, but the presence or absence of recurrent/residual neoplasm is more important rather than the necrosis. While this distinction is not always possible or accurate, in general, radiation necrosis tends to have a large geographic distribution without the pseudopalisading. It may contain dystrophic calcifications. In addition, other changes associated with radiation treatment, such as fibrosis, hemosiderin pigment, telangiectatic changes in vessels, fibrinoid necrosis of vessel walls, bizarre nuclei with smudgy chromatin, and reactive astrocytosis, are helpful in this distinction. There will always be scattered atypical cells that represent residual neoplasm, even if a significant amount of neoplasm is not present **(Fig. 2-223)**. However, an idea of how much of radiation change and viable neoplasm is present should be provided as much as possible. The appearance of the current neoplasm can be compared to the histology of the original neoplasm to have an idea about residual versus recurrent nature. This distinction can be somewhat facilitated in glioblastomas if a cellular neoplasm with pseudopalisading necrosis is present, which favors a recurrence.[42]

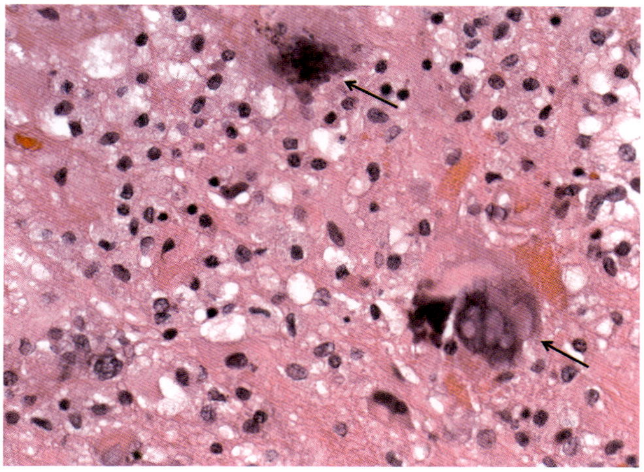

Figure 2-223. Radiation atypia: Bizarre changes are seen in residual neoplastic cells and are characterized by various combinations of multinucleation, nuclear and cytoplasmic enlargement, and smudgy chromatin (*arrows*). Many histiocytes are also present in the background (H&E; original magnification: 400×).

Some infectious processes are characterized by necrosis, among other features. *Fibrinoid necrosis* with a prominent acute inflammatory cell component may represent abscess content **(Fig. 2-224)**. Bacteria may or may not be identified in this material even with special stains, such as a Gram-Twort stain. Abscess development can mimic early infarct. In the first 1 to 2 days, there is acute focal suppurative cerebritis; 2 to 7 days, confluent central necrosis develops and macrophages and lymphoplasmacytic infiltrate appear; 5 to 14 days, early encapsulation, with early granulation tissue formation, takes place; 14 days and later, late encapsulation with well-developed capsule takes place. If abscess heals without surgical treatment, a fibrous cyst with scattered macrophages in the lumen may be all there is left. The surrounding granulation tissue with prominent neovascularization may complicate the picture, especially in small specimens and in IOC, potentially causing confusion with glioblastoma. *Caseating necrosis* is typically associated with infectious granulomas, especially *Mycobacterium tuberculosis*. Granulomatous diseases such as tuberculosis and sarcoidosis can diffusely involve leptomeninges and necrosis may be minimal, if at all present. Alternatively, a large intraparenchymal mass lesion can form by the coalescence of granulomas in tuberculous infections, that is, a tuberculoma, which may result in clinical and radiologic confusion with a neoplastic process in some cases. Again, the identification of macrophages is the key to appreciate the inflammatory nature of this process. Fungi that form hyphae, as opposed to yeast forms, tend to invade vessels. *Aspergillus* spp. and *Pseudallescheria boydii*[340] can also cause a hemorrhagic, necrotic mass lesion due to the invasion of the vessels and interference with the blood flow. Another fungal infection that is characterized by prominent necrosis is zygomycosis.[508] In both infections, fungal microorganisms can be extremely difficult to find and may be essentially invisible on routine sections **(Fig. 2-225)**, without the use of special stains, such as GMS; therefore, a high degree of suspicion becomes the key. Clinical history of immunosuppression and, especially for zygomycotic infections, a history of diabetes mellitus in a patient who presents with an infiltrative and necrotic upper respiratory tract mass are alerting features. Rheumatoid arthritis granulomas have necrobiotic collagen in the center and a palisading arrangement of histiocytes at the periphery, that is, palisading granulomas (see also "Cellular Enlargement and Multinucleation").[434] South American blastomycosis (paracoccidioidomycosis; *Paracoccidioides brasiliensis*)[509] has a tumefactive (pseudotumorous) form that is more commonly seen than the meningitis form of the disease. Up to several centimeters of nodules with necrotic centers

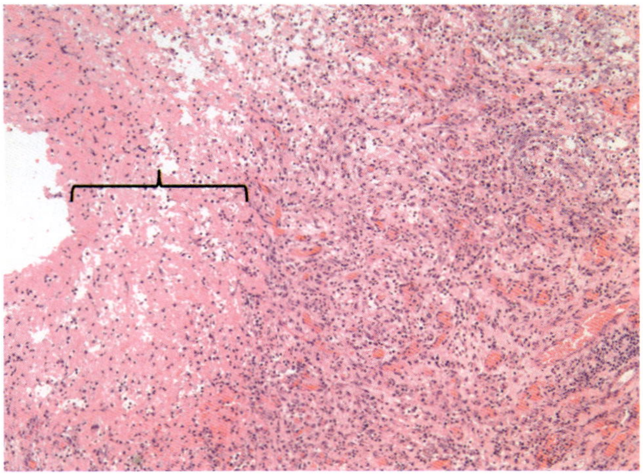

Figure 2-224. Abscess: Abscess cavity is filled with fibrinoid necrotic material (*bracket*) composed of inflammatory cells, fibrin, bacteria, and cellular breakdown products. The wall is composed of inflamed granulation tissue (**right side**) (H&E; original magnification: 100×).

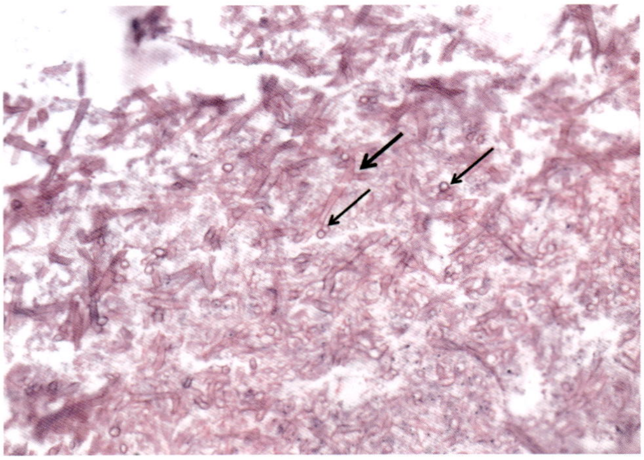

Figure 2-225. Zygomycosis: Necrotic material is filled with numerous fungal hyphae with no septation. Cross sections appear as round holes (*thin arrows*). Although the perfect example is difficult to find, right-angle branching (*thick arrow*) is also typical and is helpful in distinguishing this fungus from *Aspergillus* spp., which tend to have acute angle branching (H&E; original magnification: 400×).

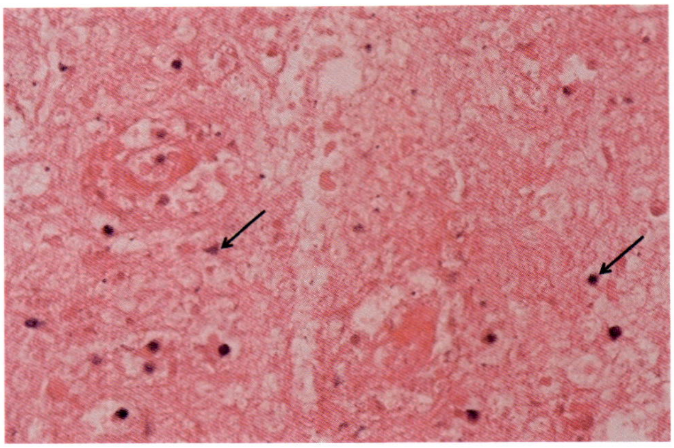

Figure 2-226. Toxoplasma cerebritis: This particular sample is entirely necrotic with scattered basophilic nuclear debris, some of which actually representing toxoplasma tachyzoites (*arrows*); however, they are difficult to identify without the use of immunohistochemistry, which in turn requires a high degree of suspicion and knowledge of clinical and radiologic features (H&E; original magnification: 400×).

are formed. They prefer cortex. Toxoplasmosis typically presents with multiple necrotic brain lesions in an immunocompromised patient. In this setting, the usual approach may be a stereotactic biopsy, resulting in a mostly necrotic small tissue. Again, attention to clinical information and a high degree of suspicion prevent a misdiagnosis of a high-grade malignancy. Identification of lymphocytes, plasma cells, and macrophages should also prompt a search for toxoplasma cysts and tachyzoites **(Fig. 2-226)**. The cyst forms are typically found at the periphery of the lesions and not in the necrotic center. Immunohistochemistry may be required in the identification and confirmation of tachyzoites, which may also be present in the macrophages.[510] The necrotic lesions may later cavitate. Another protozoan that involves the brain to create necrotic and hemorrhagic lesions is ameba.[511,512] Depending on the clinical presentation, *Naegleria fowleri, Acanthameba* and *Balamuthia spp*. are responsible for these lesions. Amebae are prominent in the leptomeninges and in the Virchow-Robin spaces, as well as within the neuroglial parenchyma, which is usually necrotic and hemorrhagic. Inflammation is variable and macrophages can cause difficulty in the identification of ameba. One or more amebic abscesses may occur as a result of hematogenous spread of *E. histolytica* from systemic sources such as liver.[513] They have hemorrhagic and necrotic contents and are otherwise similar in their wall structure to bacterial abscesses. Amebae may be identified in them. They may later cavitate in survivors. Parasites such as *A. cantonensis*[514] and *S. stercoralis*[352] can result in infarcts by occluding the vessels. The lesions may secondarily become infected, resulting in abscesses.[515] Toxocara canis (visceral larva migrans) causes lesions with necrotic center consisting of larvae, lymphocytes, macrophages, neutrophils, and eosinophil PMN leukocytes.[17] *Trypanosoma cruzi* (Chagas disease) can also cause cerebral infarction.[516]

Some diseases that are predominantly characterized by myelin loss can also eventually result in some degree of tissue necrosis and cavitation. For instance, Marchiafava-Bignami disease typically associated with chronic alcoholism, with or without malnourishment, involves mainly the genu and corpus of the corpus callosum and some lesions may cavitate.[517] Optic chiasm, anterior and posterior commissure, and middle cerebellar peduncle involvement can also be seen. Striatal necrosis is possible. There are histiocytic infiltrates, but lymphocytic inflammation is not seen. Devic disease (neuromyelitis optica) is the type that is most controversial to be an "MS variant." The lesions may be of necrotic nature and involve exclusively the optic nerves and spinal cord,[518] where they are typically central, involving both gray and white matter. Only occasional cases have typical MS lesions in other areas of the CNS parenchyma.[519] Acute necrotizing myelopathy[235] is characterized by an isolated necrotic lesion of the spinal cord and a relapsing clinical course.

Infarcts can be seen in association with neurodegenerative diseases or in isolation. Multiple infarcts of different stages of evolution are responsible for the stepwise deterioration in vascular dementia.[520] Chronic vascular insufficiency affecting the white matter over time results in the degeneration of parenchyma and a shrunken white matter with diffuse myelin and axon loss. This is typically the result of small vessel disease seen in the subcortical arteriosclerotic leukoencephalopathy (Binswanger disease).[521] PSP with brainstem and/or basal ganglionic infarcts is sometimes referred to as combined PSP. Arteriosclerotic or vascular pseudoparkinsonism[522] refers to parkinsonism that results from the cavitary infarcts in the substantia nigra and basal ganglia. Friedreich's ataxia can be associated with hypoxic–ischemic injury due to cardiomyopathy, especially in the cerebral and cerebellar cortex.

Apoptosis is the self-destruction of cells in a controlled manner through very complex mechanisms under various conditions. Some processes are characterized by a predominance of apoptosis rather than actual infarcts. Pontosubicular necrosis[274] is usually seen in association with other hypoxic–ischemic damage in other areas. Neuron loss and gliosis occur, but rather than an actual infarct, they are in the form of apoptotic debris. Internal granule layer neurons may undergo apoptosis in premature infants.[523] They are more vulnerable to hypoxic–ischemic damage in premature infants because Purkinje cells mature around 37 weeks and are not as vulnerable at that stage. In later life, Purkinje cells are easily recognized as red neurons. Apoptosis plays an important role in the development of the CNS. Trimethyltin causes neuron loss from the hippocampus, basal ganglia, entorhinal cortex, and amygdala. In addition, there is apoptotic destruction of neurons in the hippocampus and in other limbic structures.[524] In neoplasms, apoptosis is commonly seen in high-grade neoplasms with high cell turnover rate. There is also high mitotic activity in such situations. Some examples of this process are PNET, medulloblastoma, and small cell carcinoma **(Fig. 2-227)**.

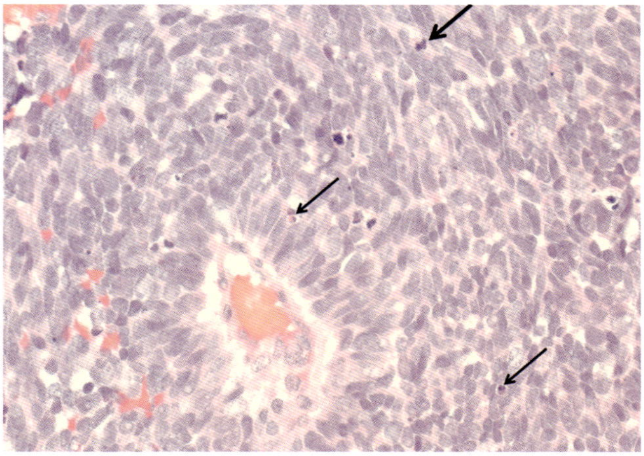

Figure 2-227. Apoptotic debris: Scattered apoptotic cells and debris (*thin arrows*) should not be mistaken for mitotic figures (*thick arrows*), and they altogether suggest a high-grade neoplasm with high turnover rate, as is the case in this metastatic small cell carcinoma (H&E; original magnification: 400×).

Cellular Arrangements

The way the cells are arranged, especially in neoplasms, provides clues to their diagnosis and differential diagnosis. Some of these, such as rosettes and peritheliomatous pattern, are discussed in

List of Findings/Checklist for Cellular Arrangements

AT A GLANCE

- Scherer's secondary structures
- Satellitosis
- Nuclear palisading
- Chordoid pattern
- Glandular/adenoid/ acinar pattern
- Nesting pattern
- Organoid pattern
- Neuropil-like islands
- Storiform pattern
- Cell-in-cell arrangement
- Whorl formation
- Swirling pattern
- Onion-bulb formation
- Pseudo-onion-bulb formation
- Sheet-like growth
- Cortical layering and neuronal arrangement abnormalities

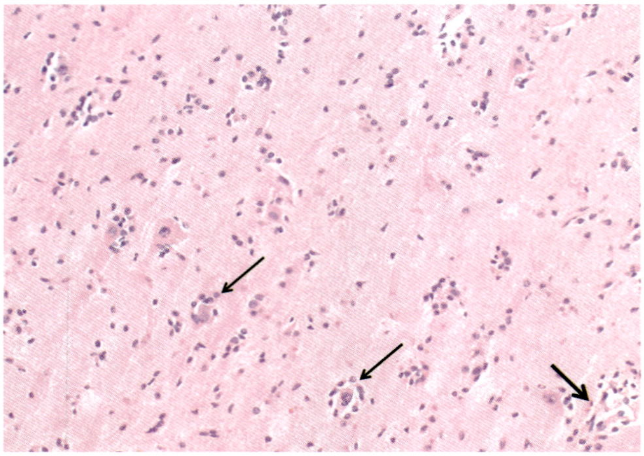

Figure 2-228. Satellitosis: Perineuronal (*thin arrows*) and perivascular (*thick arrow*) satelliting are secondary structures of Scherer commonly associated with glioma infiltration of the gray matter (H&E; original magnification: 100×).

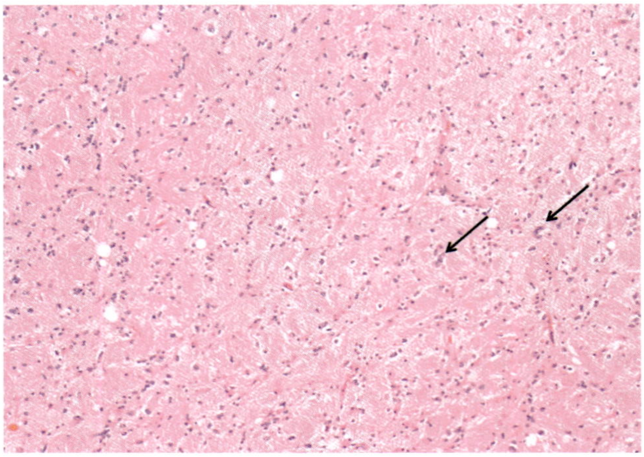

Figure 2-229. Glioma infiltrating along white matter fascicles appears in the form of cells in single files, may mimic gliomatosis, and can be difficult to identify. Atypical nuclei stand out (*arrows*) (H&E; original magnification: 100×).

"Perivascular Arrangements and Rosettes"; nodularity is discussed in "Nodular Arrangement."

Satellitosis **(Fig. 2-228)** is the perineuronal and perivascular aggregation of neoplastic glial cells infiltrating the gray matter. They constitute examples of *secondary structures of Scherer*[525,526] along with subpial and subependymal accumulation of glial neoplastic cells. Scherer's secondary structures are those arrangements that are formed through the interactions of neoplastic cells with the existing normal structures and include satellitosis, subpial accumulation of infiltrating glioma cells, and *interfascicular growth* **(Fig. 2-229)** in the form of neoplastic cells lined up among white matter tracts; however, the term is best known for satellitosis. These are seen more commonly in oligodendrogliomas and astrocytomas but are also present in some ependymal neoplasms, in spite of their relatively well-circumscribed nature.[527] *Subpial accumulation* of infiltrating neoplastic cells is a well-known feature of oligodendroglioma **(Fig. 2-230)**. Angiocentric glioma and medulloblastoma/PNET can also show this propensity to infiltrate through the cortex and accumulate under the pia. Germinoma growing on the basal surface of the brain may penetrate the pial surface to result in a superficially infiltrating process. Together with the reactive gliosis it may induce, arriving at the accurate diagnosis can become complicated in the small tissue samples. Scherer also described *primary and tertiary structures*.[525,526] Primary structures are those formed by the neoplastic cells, such as the ependymal canal formation by ependymomas and Wright rosettes in medulloblastoma. Tertiary structures are those formed as a result of interaction of neoplastic glial cells with the mesenchymal tissue, excluding vascular proliferation. This term applies typically to infiltration of the leptomeninges by the neoplasm and structures formed by the interaction of cellular and noncellular

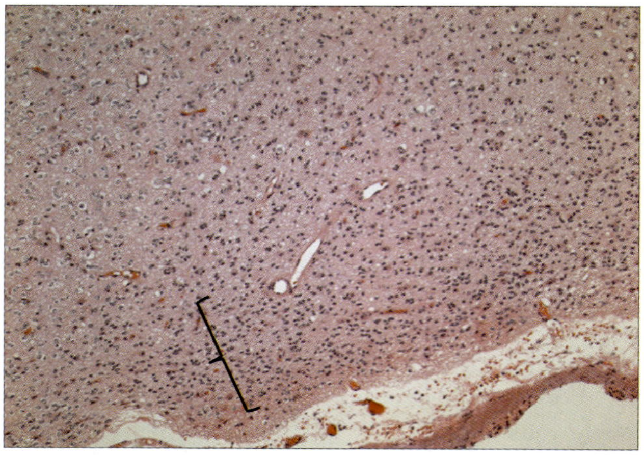

Figure 2-230. Subpial accumulation of neoplastic cells (*bracket*) is typical for some neoplasms, including oligodendroglioma, as in this case (H&E; original magnification: 100×).

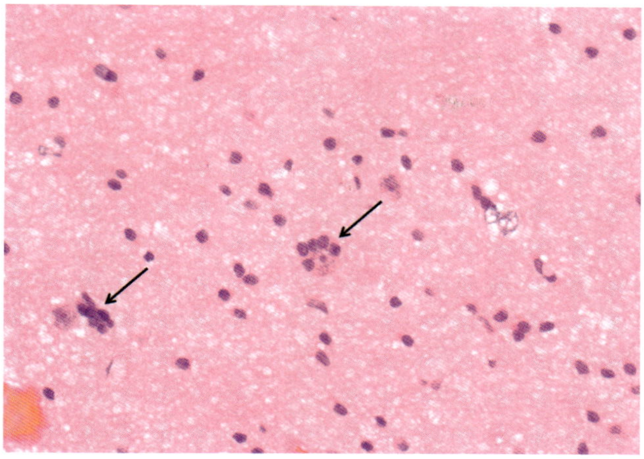

Figure 2-231. Satellitosis in nonneoplastic temporal lobe (*arrows*) is not uncommon and should not be mistaken for a neoplastic process, especially during intraoperative consultations (H&E; original magnification: 400×).

material, such as organization of necrosis. Primary and tertiary structures are not terms used as formal descriptions. Secondary structures have the practical diagnostic implication in that they help support the presence of an underlying glial neoplasm in a superficial biopsy that mainly shows cortical gray matter or help favor a glial neoplastic process in a mildly cellular specimen where the distinction between reactive gliosis and low-grade glial neoplasm is difficult. One caveat is that perineuronal satellitosis is a common finding in the temporal lobe in the absence of infiltrating glioma **(Fig. 2-231)**. Whether this finding is normal or is abnormal, but is with no apparent significance that it is considered normal, is not clear. It is sometimes considered as part of an ill-defined condition called microdysgenesis,[12,528] along with several other alterations, such as neurons in the white matter, which can be identified only by histologic evaluation. Although its definition and component findings are not consistent, it is considered to be a finding frequently associated with intractable epilepsy.[12,528,529] Nonetheless, it creates a pitfall in the interpretation of satellitosis. Therefore, knowledge of the location of a biopsy may be necessary, especially in small biopsy specimens and in IOC. In this type of temporal lobe satellitosis, the satelliting cells are bland and small cells, in contrast to glioma cells that tend to be larger and somewhat irregular, especially in the case of astrocytic neoplasms. This can be a difficult evaluation, however.

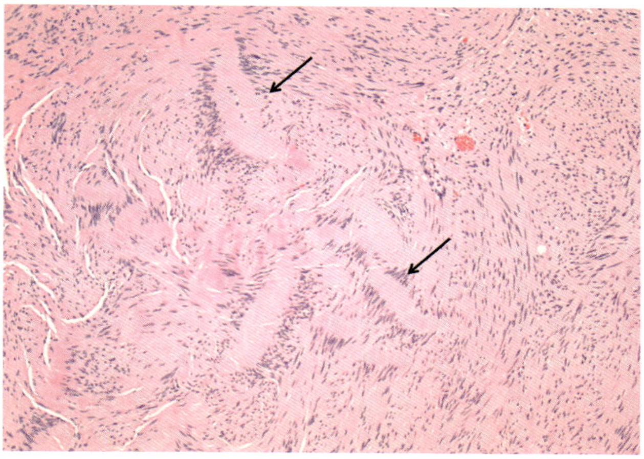

Figure 2-232. Schwannoma: Verocay bodies (*arrows*) are formed by a collagenous band between two strips of palisading nuclei in the cellular Antoni A areas of schwannoma. Nuclear palisading is not diagnostic of schwannoma and can occasionally be seen in a variety of other neoplasms (H&E; original magnification: 200×).

Another peculiar arrangement of neoplastic nuclei is *palisading*. Nuclear palisading is perhaps best known as a characteristic feature seen in Antoni A areas of schwannomas. The structure formed by the two layers of palisading nuclei with the eosinophilic anuclear strip in between, composed of cytoplasms of these cells and collagen, is called a *Verocay body* **(Fig. 2-232)**. Nuclear palisading is not pathognomonic for schwannoma and can be seen in several other neoplasms, though not as frequently. Palisaded encapsulated neuroma is composed of palisaded spindle cells and scattered axons. It is located in skin and superficial subcutaneous tissue, and in mucosae. It is surrounded by perineurium, except on the surface.[530] Oligodendroglioma, meningioma, and many other CNS neoplasms can occasionally have a focal palisading of their nuclei. A primary glial neoplasm with prominent nuclear palisading has been referred to as polar spongioblastoma; however, its existence as a distinct entity is doubtful, as this pattern is not specific. A *pseudopalisading* arrangement can be present surrounding the geographic areas of necrosis in glioblastoma due to the crowding of neoplastic cells. Nuclear palisading can be present focally in SFT and may result in confusion with schwannoma taken out of context. A low-grade neoplasm that combines subpial accumulation and palisading is angiocentric

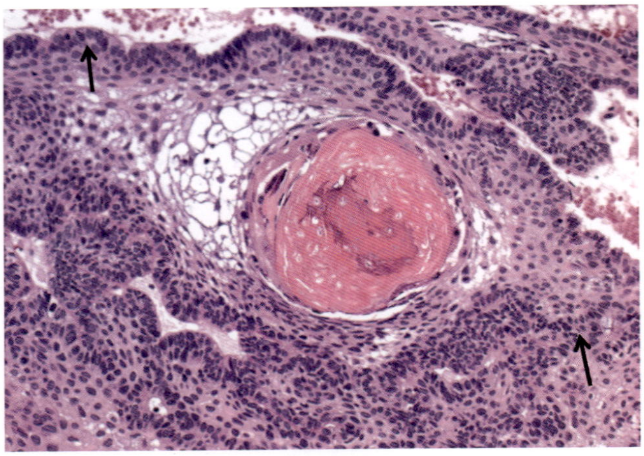

Figure 2-233. Craniopharyngioma: Adamantinomatous craniopharyngioma is characterized by squamoid islands with peripheral palisading of basaloid calls (*arrows*), loosely textured interior, and a central wet keratin, altogether called stellate reticulum (H&E; original magnification: 200×).

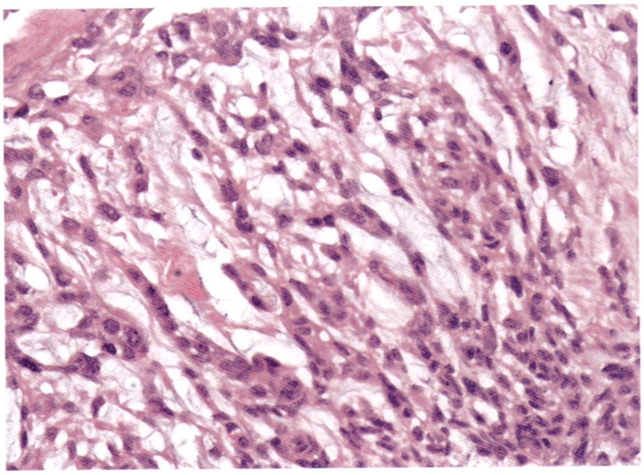

Figure 2-234. Chordoid meningioma: Neoplastic cells are arranged in files and trabeculae in a mucinous background, reminiscent of chordoma (H&E; original magnification: 400×).

glioma. One of its distinguishing features is a subpial accumulation of a thin layer of neoplastic cells with elongated nuclei aligned perpendicular to the surface, resulting in a palisading arrangement. In astroblastoma, elongated cells arranged perpendicular to thin hyalinized collagenous bands may also create a palisading or picket-fence appearance within these trabeculae. Palisading arrangement of basaloid cells at the periphery of anastomosing squamoid islands is characteristic for adamantinomatous craniopharyngioma **(Fig. 2-233)**. These squamous epithelial islands, rimmed by these palisading basaloid cells, have also a peculiar lacy arrangement of small squamoid cells in the center, called stellate reticulum. Within these solid islands, there may be pockets of obvious squamous cells with keratinization. Necrotizing granulomas with peripheral palisading of somewhat spindled histiocytes are referred to as palisading granuloma and are typically associated with lymphogranuloma venerium and rheumatoid nodule.[434]

Chordoid pattern refers to the arrangement of neoplastic cells in small groups or trabeculae in a myxoid background, as in chordomas, hence the descriptive term. In addition to chordomas, this pattern can be identified in chordoid meningioma **(Fig. 2-234)**, a histologic subtype of meningioma that places it in atypical (WHO grade II) meningioma. They are rarely associated with Castleman's disease.[126] Prominent inflammatory response and anemia may be present. The associated conditions respond to resection of the meningioma. The distinction of chordoma and chordoid meningioma on histologic grounds alone can be difficult; however, the midline skull base, especially clivus, and midline vertebral bone location of chordomas contrast with the eccentric dural-based presentation of meningiomas. Furthermore, the immunohistochemical characterization of chordoid meningiomas has been investigated and may be useful in difficult cases.[128] Chordoid glioma is a WHO grade II astrocytic neoplasm that typically occurs in the third ventricle and can also be distinguished by its glial immunohistochemical features in addition to its typical location.[531]

Glandular, adenoid, or acinar structure formation is a feature of adenocarcinomas. However, several primary neoplasms of the CNS can also have acinar architecture. Anterior pituitary gland is normally arranged in a nesting pattern of cells but can have a more obvious and larger acinar pattern, apparently as a reactive/reparative process. Some of them may have eosinophilic proteinaceous material in the lumen. While adenomas are typically composed of sheets of cells interrupted only by scattered vessels, the cells can form trabecular, organoid, perivascular pseudorosette-like or microcystic appearances. Secretory meningiomas have gland-like spaces with eosinophilic secretory material **(Fig. 2-235)**. They are not surrounded by an orderly layer of columnar or cuboidal cells as in a true gland, but rather by a few attenuated cells

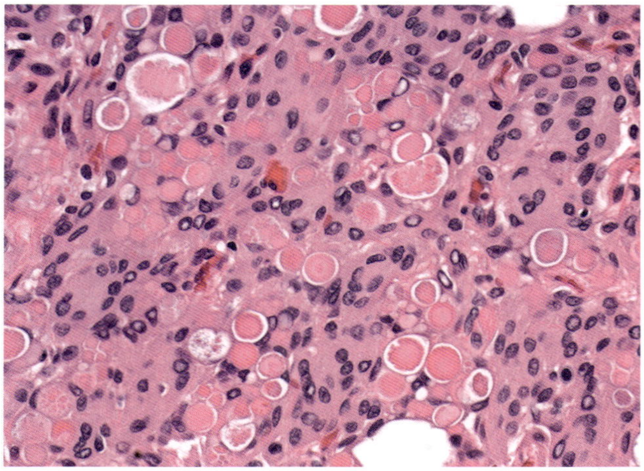

Figure 2-235. Secretory meningioma: Round eosinophilic material is present in the lumens of acinar structures formed by the meningioma cells (H&E; original magnification: 400×).

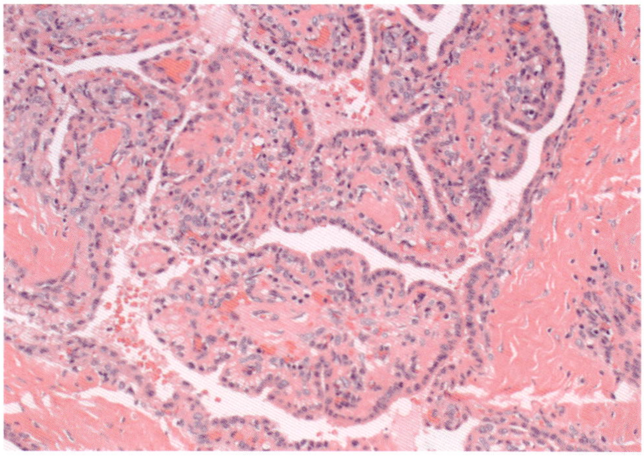

Figure 2-236. Endolymphatic sac tumor: Papillary structures are composed of fibrovascular cores lined by bland, low columnar, or cuboidal epithelial cells (H&E; original magnification: 200×).

encircling a round space. The secretory material is PAS positive and diastase resistant but is negative for mucin. They are, however, carcinoembryonic antigen (CEA) positive, although confusion with an adenocarcinoma is unlikely in the absence of cytologic atypia and the presence of typical meningioma morphology elsewhere. When small, they may appear like collagen bundles on H&E and are sometimes termed pseudopsammoma bodies.[532] In addition, the blood CEA levels may be associated with recurrences of secretory meningioma[533] and may also cause problems in the evaluation of patients with colorectal carcinoma. Focal glandular areas can rarely be seen in malignant meningiomas and show cytokeratin positivity. These areas should not be taken as evidence for the rare occasion of an adenocarcinoma metastasizing to a meningioma. Endolymphatic sac tumors, in addition to their papillary areas, may have glandular structures with variably microcystic appearance.[534] Their cells are typically cuboidal, uniform, and bland in contrast to a metastatic carcinoma **(Fig. 2-236)**. However, in some cases with eosinophilic proteinaceous material in the lumen and some nuclei with intranuclear cytoplasmic invaginations, metastatic thyroid carcinoma may become a concern. TTF-1, which is negative in endolymphatic sac tumor and positive in thyroid carcinomas, easily answers this question in difficult cases. Choroid plexus papillomas can be entirely or partially adenoid.[535] They are then termed choroid plexus adenoma. This feature does not have a prognostic implication; however, this may cause confusion in making the diagnosis. A small blue cell neoplasm with a dyscohesive pattern resulting in a layer of cells remaining attached to the collagenous bands and a subsequent pseudopapillary and *alveolar pattern* is typical for alveolar rhabdomyosarcoma. In this context, medulloblastoma with myogenic differentiation should be differentiated from embryonal rhabdomyosarcomas with admixed rhabdomyoblasts with bright eosinophilic fibrillary cytoplasm or strap cells with striations. Although typical cerebellar location is useful in the case of medulloblastoma, similar differentiation in an S-PNET may require immunohistochemistry and incorporation of clinical and radiologic information. A pattern that is referred to as alveolar but can also be described as organoid is seen in alveolar soft part sarcoma, which rarely can metastasize to CNS. *Organoid pattern* is characteristic of neuroendocrine neoplasms and is typically seen in paraganglioma and olfactory neuroblastoma **(Fig. 2-237)**. Some epithelioid melanomas can also have an organoid pattern. Specifically in paraganglioma, the clustering of the chief cells forming the organoid pattern is termed zellballen. They are surrounded by delicate elongated sustentacular cells. Sustentacular cells are not necessary for the diagnosis of paraganglioma, although their presence makes the diagnosis easier and helps avoid mistakes. It has been suggested that their disappearance may be associated with a

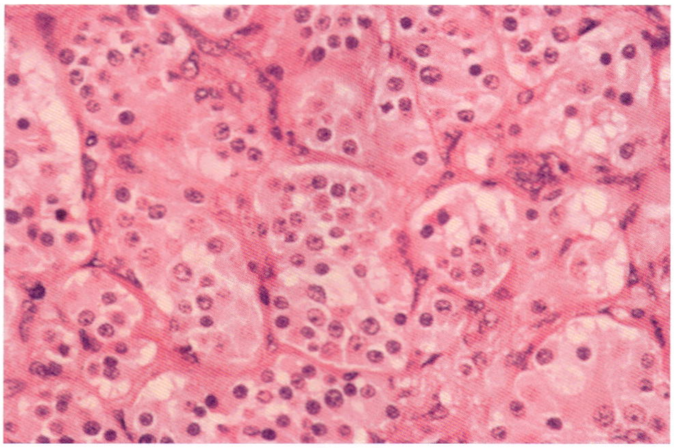

Figure 2-237. Paraganglioma: Uniform cells with bland nuclei form organoid arrangements. Their chromatin is finely granular, also called "salt and pepper," with small nucleoli (H&E; original magnification: 400×).

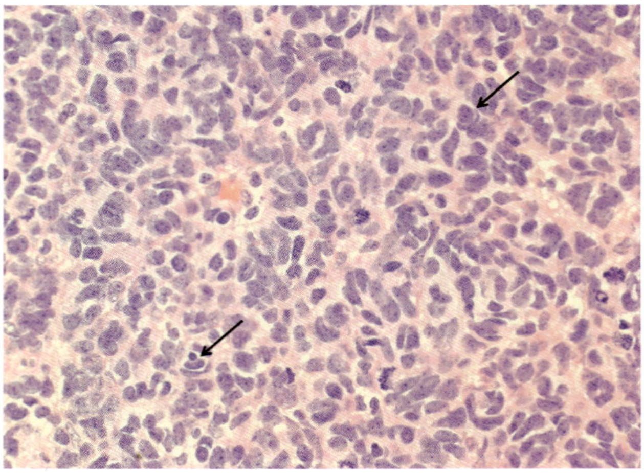

Figure 2-239. Anaplastic medulloblastoma: In addition to nuclear pleomorphism, there are cell-in-cell configurations (*arrows*) where one nucleus is wrapping around another, usually an apoptotic nucleus (H&E; original magnification: 400×).

more aggressive biologic behavior.[536,537] Some paragangliomas may have a trabecular arrangement of cells, separated by hyalinized vessels or myxoid matrix, mimicking a myxopapillary ependymoma. *Neuropil-like islands* refer to focal fibrillary areas reminiscent of neuropil. They are typically present in glioneuronal tumor with neuropil-like islands[538] **(Fig. 2-238)**, where they are admixed with oligodendroglial-like round cells, but can rarely be seen in other neoplasms, such as ependymoma[539] and choroid plexus papilloma.[540]

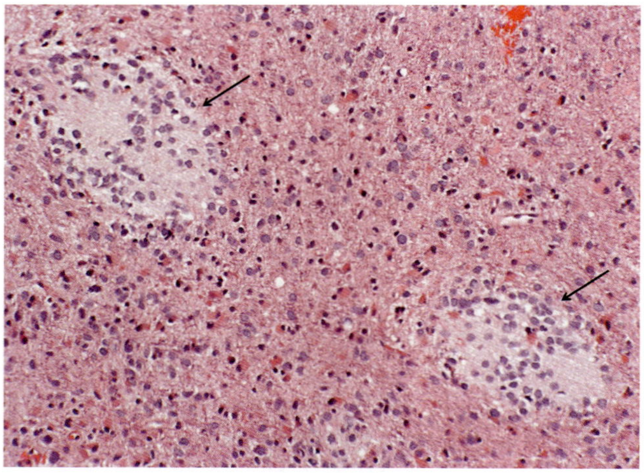

Figure 2-238. Neuropil islands: Pale foci with delicate fibrillary neuropil-like features (*arrows*) are present in an otherwise predominantly glial background with thick and bright eosinophilic fibrillarity in this glioneuronal tumor with neuropil-like islands (H&E; original magnification: 200×). (Courtesy of Marc K. Rosenblum, M.D., Department of Pathology, Memorial Sloan-Kettering Cancer Center, New York, NY.)

Storiform pattern is a peculiar arrangement of spindle cells typically associated with fibrohistiocytic neoplasms. It can rarely and focally be seen in fibroblastic meningiomas and the spindle cell population of PXA. *Cell-in-cell arrangement* or wrapping of one cell around another can be a feature of anaplastic medulloblastoma[541] **(Fig. 2-239)**. This is sometimes referred to as cannibalism or bird's eye appearance in the setting of other neoplasms such as metastatic carcinomas and in cytologic preparations. Other features of anaplastic medulloblastoma are pleomorphism, more prominent mitotic activity, apoptosis, and necrosis. These features, including cell-in-cell arrangement, can overlap with features of large cell medulloblastoma, where the nuclei are enlarged and rounded and have open chromatin pattern and prominent nucleoli, leading to difficulties in distinction of these two variants, hence, the combined term large cell/anaplastic medulloblastoma. Attempts to further stratify anaplastic medulloblastomas based on the degree of microscopic features have not yielded widely accepted results. Changes similar to those described for other medulloblastoma variants are sometimes seen in S-PNET, although these are not formally recognized as variants of S-PNET. A similar cell-in-cell arrangement,

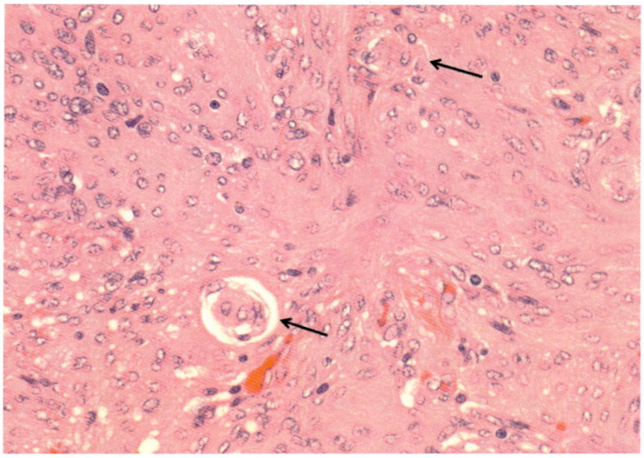

Figure 2-240. Meningioma: Meningioma cells are typically seen in a syncytial pattern where cytoplasmic borders cannot be easily identified due to the numerous interdigitations, creating a "sea" of cytoplasms. Whorl formation (*arrows*) is also a typical feature for meningioma and may resemble squamous eddies, although any confusion is unlikely in the absence of keratin formation and atypia (H&E; original magnification: 400×).

termed sickle-shaped embracing cell, has been identified in ATRT.[542] *Whorls* are typical features of meningiomas **(Fig. 2-240)**. They are formed by a peculiar formation of cells attempting to wrap around each other, forming a tangled cellular aggregate that usually stands out in the background of the usual cellularity of the meningioma. They are most frequent in transitional and psammomatous meningiomas but can be found in other histologic variants upon diligent search, aiding in the diagnosis. They are difficult to find and may be vague or completely absent in some histologic variants such as clear cell, chordoid and rhabdoid meningiomas. There may be a hyalinized or collagenized round center, which may later become calcified to form the psammoma bodies. They are also very useful on cytologic preparations (see Chapter 3). The identification of prominent meningothelial cell component, complete with whorls and intranuclear cytoplasmic invaginations, may represent meningothelial hyperplasia adjacent to other neoplasms, inflammatory processes, hemorrhages, and even meningiomas. This possibility should be kept in mind during the evaluation of small amounts of meningothelial cell groups. Since there is no magic amount or size for the diagnosis of meningioma, these cell groups should be interpreted in context, and the possibility of reactive proliferation should be considered, especially if there is some other pathologic process in the sample, such as a subdural hemorrhage. Rarely, meningioma may coexist together with a glioma or schwannoma as a composite neoplasm (see "Biphasic Pattern, Composite Lesions and Metaplastic Tissues"). A similar situation may arise even when dealing with a known meningioma. For instance, a thin strip of dura mater may be sent for IOC to evaluate the resection margin of a parasagittal meningioma to decide on the dural sinus intervention during surgery, or specimen from an actual dural sinus may be sent to confirm the involvement of the sinus by meningioma for further intervention. These evaluations are difficult as there is usually some degree of reactive meningothelial proliferation adjacent to meningioma and these specimens are typically cauterized. The knowledge of the histologic features of the actual meningioma may help in providing a comparison, but this approach will not be useful in meningothelial meningiomas, as meningothelial hyperplasia also has a meningothelial histology. Otherwise, the decision is one of judgment and communication with the surgeon to correlate with the intraoperative observations. *Sheet-like growth pattern* is a term used, along with other features, as a feature in the diagnosis of atypical (WHO grade II) meningioma and refers to the loss of usual

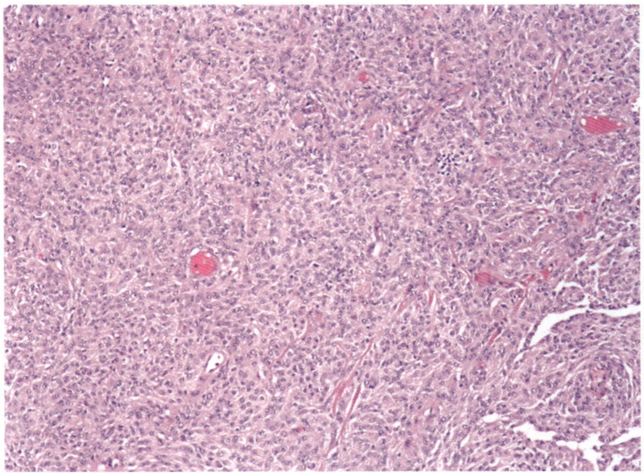

Figure 2-241. Meningioma: Monotonous sheet-like growth pattern is seen without any whorl formation or lobular, grouped arrangement of cells and is one of the features to take into consideration in grading these neoplasms (H&E; original magnification: 200×).

meningioma architecture with loss of whorls and fascicles[44] **(Fig. 2-241)**. A vaguely *swirling pattern* can be present in melanocytoma and melanoma. When melanin pigment is scarce or absent, they may be confused with meningioma, as all these lesions can have similar nuclear appearances, especially if cytologic atypia is not prominent in melanoma. A pattern similar to whorls, called *onion bulb,* is seen in the peripheral nerve. It is formed by the proliferation of Schwann cells creating multiple layers wrapped around each other and is seen in nerve biopsy specimens in medical disorders (see "Peripheral Nerve"). In intraneural perineurioma, they are formed by perineurial cell proliferation around individual or small groups of axons and are called *pseudo–onion bulbs* as they are not Schwann cells. They should not be confused with hereditary sensory motor neuropathies, which are diffuse systemic processes in contrast to the intraneural perineurioma, which results in localized thickening of the nerve.[543] Localized hypertrophic neuropathy is also a focal, likely reactive process. It has true onion bulbs consisting of Schwann cells and can easily be distinguished by being EMA-negative, while perineurial cells are EMA positive.

Cortical layering is altered in a variety of MCD. In the histologic picture corresponding to agyria/pachygyria, there is a *four-layer cortical ribbon*, comprised of three neuronal cell layers in addition to the molecular layer. Variable layering is seen in polymicrogyria, ranging from a two-layer cortex comprised of a thick and disorganized neuronal layer in addition to the molecular layer or a four-layer cortex as in agyria/pachygyria.[544] In addition, cortical ribbon, while winding up and down perpendicular to pial surface in an attempt to form gyration, is not separated by true sulci followed by leptomeninges, an appearance perfectly matching the gross description (see gross). *Band heterotopias*[545] are separated from the original cortical gray matter by a rim of white matter and have disorganized neuronal distribution, in contrast to normal cortex. The layering properties can be evaluated better when the neurons are highlighted by Neu-N. Presence of a *persistent subpial granule cell layer* is another abnormality associated with MCD[546] and should not be confused with a neoplastic infiltrate in the leptomeninges. *Dispersion of granular cell layer* in the dentate gyrus in the hippocampus is a finding that can be seen in hippocampal sclerosis and as a part of the so-called microdysgenesis in intractable epilepsy cases.[528,529] It may accompany MCD, although in that situation, it is without the hippocampal sclerosis. On the other hand, there are seizure cases with both hippocampal sclerosis and MCD or with both hippocampal sclerosis and neoplasms.

Papillary and Pseudopapillary Structures

A papilla is a fibrous or fibrovascular core covered by lining cells that separate it from a true lumen, as in choroid plexus. Pseudopapilla is a structure that is similar to papilla but does not have contact with a lumen or space. Pseudopapillae are so named because they superficially resemble papilla, such as in papillary ependymoma, or assume a papillary appearance due to secondary changes, such as necrosis leaving viable cells only around vessels, resulting in a pseudopapillary structure. These terms may be used interchangeably and not necessarily accurately in practice, and it is important to appreciate the biologic process underlying their

List of Findings/Checklist for Papillary and Pseudopapillary Structures

AT A GLANCE

Normal
- Choroid plexus
- Arachnoid granulations

Neoplastic
- Metastatic papillary carcinomas
    - Peritheliomatous pattern
- Choroid plexus neoplasms
- Papillary glioneuronal tumor
- Papillary tumor of the pineal region
- Papillary meningioma
- Papillary ependymoma
- Astroblastoma
- Papillary craniopharyngioma
- Pituitary adenoma
- Pilomyxoid astrocytoma
- Myxopapillary ependymoma
- Endolymphatic sac tumor

formation and the subsequent associations with specific pathologic processes.

Choroid plexus (see also "Choroid Plexus") is one of the only two papillary structures, along with arachnoid granulations, that are normally found in the nervous system. It is located in the ventricular system and is responsible for the production of cerebrospinal fluid. Its papillae are composed of a fibrovascular core surrounded by a layer of cuboidal epithelial cells resting on a basement membrane. It should be recognized as a normal structure in small tissue biopsies or resections, not to mistake it for a pathologic process, especially *choroid plexus neoplasm* or *metastatic papillary carcinoma*. This usually is not a problem given the bland appearance of *normal choroid plexus*. However, the problem may arise if the specimen is otherwise unremarkable and the choroid plexus fragment is interpreted as a choroid plexus neoplasm, usually a papilloma (WHO grade I).[547] In such situations, correlation with the radiologic and intraoperative findings is helpful, as choroid plexus papilloma is expected to show a mass-producing enlargement of choroid plexus, even though it is still cytologically and histologically bland. Papillomas are seen more commonly in the pediatric population with a second peak in adulthood, while the choroid plexus neoplasms in adults are relatively rare. Fortunately in terms of the differential diagnostic difficulty between choroid plexus carcinoma and metastatic carcinoma, choroid plexus carcinoma is predominantly seen in pediatric population.[548] In addition, the papillary pattern is no longer so prominent and is replaced by a solid growth pattern in choroid plexus carcinoma. Subtle microscopic differences can be identified between nonneoplastic choroid plexus and choroid plexus papilloma upon careful evaluation. Nonneoplastic choroid plexus epithelium has a cobblestone surface with individual cells' luminal surfaces bulging into the lumen, in that sense resembling a mesothelial surface **(Fig. 2-242)**. Epithelium of papilloma has still similar cuboidal cells but with a more straight linear surface **(Fig. 2-243)**. In addition, papillomas have more delicate, slender, elongated, and more branching papillae compared to the thicker and shorter, somewhat stocky papillae of nonneoplastic choroid plexus. When solid areas, necrosis, and more than an occasional mitotic figure are identified in a choroid plexus papilloma, the diagnosis of *atypical papilloma* (WHO grade II) should be considered **(Fig. 2-244)**. Papillary architecture is essentially absent or very limited, only to represent a possible lower-grade area, in *choroid plexus carcinoma* (WHO grade III). Due to their solid sheets of cytologically malignant cells, the differential diagnosis then includes a metastatic carcinoma. Rarely an isolated metastasis from an adenocarcinoma with papillary features may metastasize to choroid plexus, which can pose a serious problem, especially if it is a metastasis of unknown primary. Immunohistochemistry is frequently needed

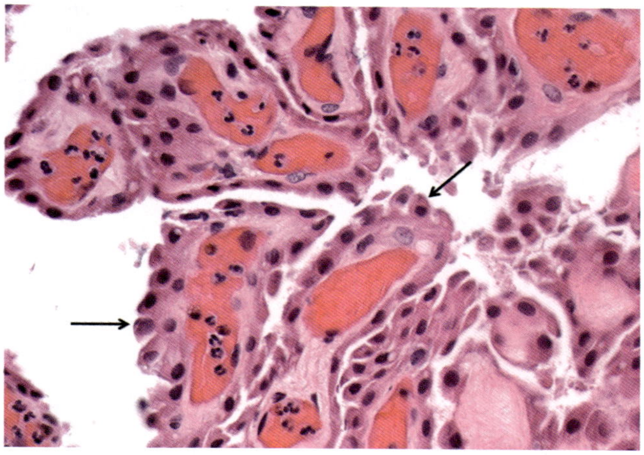

Figure 2-242. Choroid plexus: Epithelial cells normally show a hobnail arrangement (*arrows*), which is lost in papilloma (H&E; original magnification: 400×).

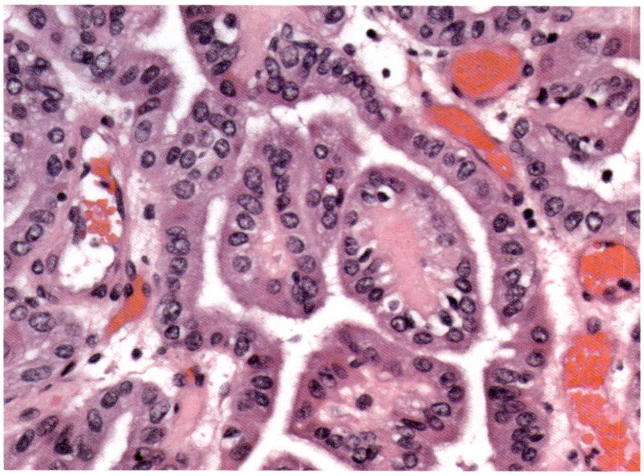

Figure 2-243. Choroid plexus papilloma: Compared to nonneoplastic choroid plexus, the papillary structures are somewhat more compact, the epithelial cells appear more crowded, and their surfaces are flat (H&E; original magnification: 400×).

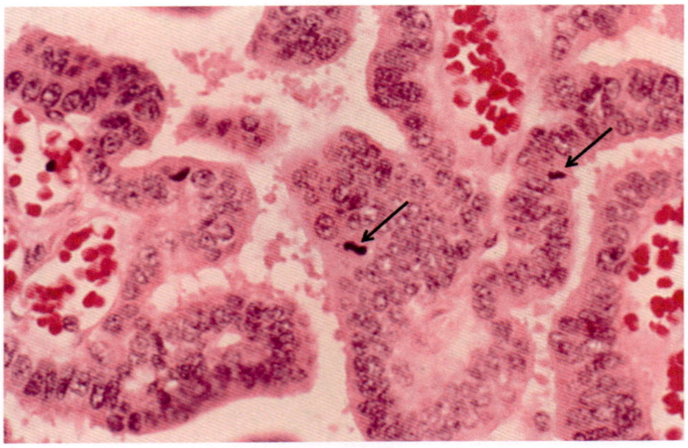

Figure 2-244. Atypical choroid plexus papilloma: There is more prominent cellular crowding with focal piling up of epithelial cells. Frequent mitotic figures (*arrows*) are present (H&E; original magnification: 400×).

in the differential diagnostic workup of papillary neoplasms, and transthyretin (prealbumin) is a highly sensitive and specific marker for choroid plexus neoplasms in this context[549,550] (see below) **(Table 2.23)**.[551] An unusual and surprising finding is the identification of loss of INI-1 expression in the nuclei of some choroid plexus papillomas and carcinomas, similar to ATRT and indicating that choroid plexus tumors may be seen in the setting of rhabdoid tumor predisposition syndrome.[552] This issue is further complicated by the presence of a rare choroid plexus carcinoma with rhabdoid features.[553]

Arachnoid granulations are broad and dense fibrous tissue cores lined by one or more, but with variable thickness of, meningothelial cells **(Fig. 2-245)**. These cells have features similar to those in other areas of leptomeninges, including formation of small multilayered piles, syncytial grouping, bland nuclear features, and intranuclear cytoplasmic invaginations, creating intranuclear pseudoinclusions. Although the microscopic appearance of arachnoid granulations is typical and they are easy to recognize, especially when one is aware of the dural sinus location of the submitted tissue, they can result in confusion if they are present unexpectedly. They can particularly be seen in dural margin specimens submitted to evaluate dural sinus invasion by meningioma during the resection of meningiomas that are close to dural sinuses. In fact, one potential problem in such specimens is the distinction of involvement by meningioma from reactive proliferation in meningothelial cells. Recognizing the arachnoid granulation architecture and being aware of the microscopic features of the particular meningioma should resolve this issue. Meningothelial cells, based on their microscopic features as described above, and arachnoid granulations are quite different from the cells and papillae of the papillary thyroid carcinoma, and this should not pose a problem in spite of the fibrous tissue cores and intranuclear cytoplasmic invaginations in both.

TABLE 2.23 Characteristic immunohistochemical features of the major papillary neoplasms of the CNS

Neoplasm	CK	EMA	CEA	GFAP	S-100	Syn.	Vim.	TTR	Pituitary Hormones
CPN	+	–	–	+/–	+/–	+/–	+	+	–
Carcinoma	+	+	+	–	–	–	+/–	–	–
PTPR	+[a]	–	N/A	+/–	+	+/–	+	–	–
PGNT	–	–	–	+	+	+	+	–	–
Ependymoma	–	+	–	+	+	–	+	–	–
Meningioma	+/–	+	–	–	–	–	+	–	–
Astroblastoma	–	+/–	–	+/–	+/–	–	+	–	–
Pituitary adenoma	+/–	–[b]	–	–[c]	–[c]	+	+/–	–	+

CNS, central nervous system; CK, cytokeratin; EMA, epithelial membrane antigen; CEA, carcinoembryonic antigen; GFAP, glial fibrillary acidic protein; Syn, synaptophysin; Vim., vimentin; TTR, transthyretin; CPN, choroid plexus neoplasm; PTPR, papillary tumor of the pineal region; PGNT, papillary glioneuronal tumor.

+, positive; –, negative; +/–, focal/variable; N/A, data not available.

[a]CK7-negative.

[b]Nonneoplastic pituitary is positive.[559]

[c]Folliculostellate cells are positive.[560]

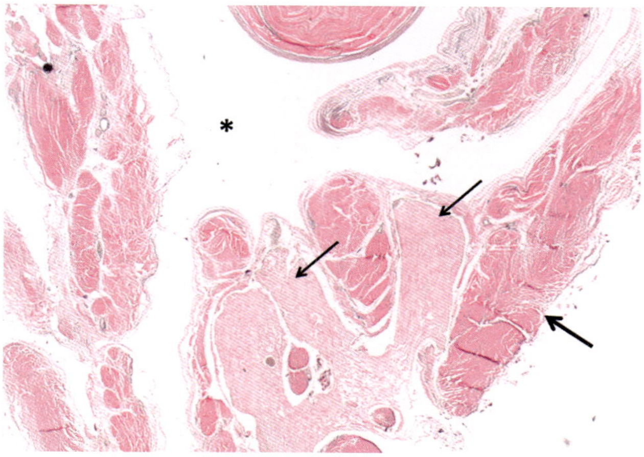

Figure 2-245. Arachnoid granulations: Papillary structures (*thin arrows*) lined by meningothelial cells protrude through the dura mater (*thick arrow*) into the dural sinus (*asterisk*). They are unlikely to be mistaken for any other significant pathologic process due to their peculiar appearance; however, they may catch the unwary by surprise if seen in fragments of surgical specimens (H&E; original magnification: 40×).

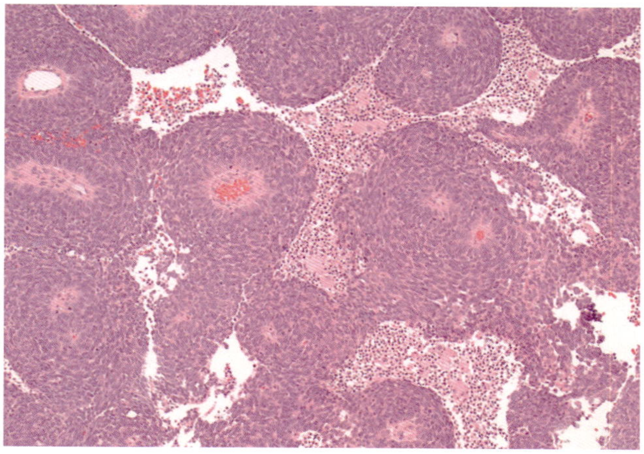

Figure 2-246. Metastatic carcinoma: A pseudopapillary architecture, termed peritheliomatous pattern, is formed due to necrosis leaving viable only those cells close to the vessels and is one of the features favoring metastatic carcinoma over a glial neoplasm, although this is by no means the rule (H&E; original magnification: 100×).

A wide variety of *carcinomas* of various organs, such as kidneys, ovaries, and thyroid gland, have papillary features and can metastasize to the CNS, presenting with papillary architecture. Serous and mucinous carcinomas of the ovary, urothelial carcinomas, and many other organ carcinomas can have predominantly papillary architecture. The main point in this context is to recognize them as of metastatic origin. The subsequent workup to identify their primary origin as needed is the same as the workup of any other metastatic malignancy. Their differential diagnosis from choroid plexus carcinoma is discussed above, under choroid plexus. Differentiating a metastatic carcinoma, especially when solid, from a glial neoplasm, such as glioblastoma with epithelioid cells, is important and can become a challenge in IOC. In general, metastatic carcinomas, solid or papillary, tend to be well-circumscribed from the surrounding reactive neuroglial tissue, while glial neoplasms have ill-defined borders due to their infiltrative nature. More readily appreciated on cytologic preparations, but are also seen on frozen and paraffin sections, carcinomas yield cell clusters with sharp borders and distinct cell boundaries, while glial neoplasms have glial processes protruding from the edges of the cellular fragments. In these fragments, cell borders are not clearly identified. Easily identified, uniformly prominent nucleoli, open chromatin pattern, and high mitotic rate also favor a metastatic carcinoma. As far as the role of papillary structures in this context, carcinomas tend to become extensively necrotic, resulting in pseudopapillary structures floating in this background of necrosis creating an appearance termed "peritheliomatous" **(Fig. 2-246)**. These pseudopapillae are formed by those few layers of cells closest to the vessels remaining viable. Even though it is possible for such pseudopapillary formations to be seen rarely in glioblastomas, the examination of the viable cells will also help with this distinction by the identification of other features described above.

Several *primary neoplasms* of the CNS, other than choroid plexus neoplasms, also have characteristic papillary/pseudopapillary architecture **(Table 2.23)**. As mentioned above, some glioblastomas may have pseudopapillary architecture within large areas of necrosis. *Papillary glioneuronal tumor*[388] is a WHO grade I neoplasm characterized by a loose architecture consisting of pseudopapillary structures formed by layers of small, uniform round cells. The layer immediately around the vessel is GFAP positive, while the outer layers forming the intervening cell population are neurocytic. Another neoplasm that has been recently incorporated in the WHO classification, though without a definitive

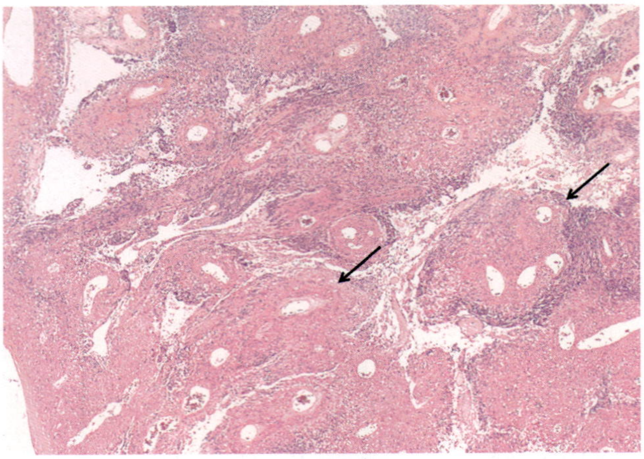

Figure 2-247. Papillary meningioma: A papillary pattern (*arrows*) is present in this meningioma, which also has rhabdoid features, a common coexistence, resulting in the bright eosinophilia of the papillae (H&E; original magnification: 40×).

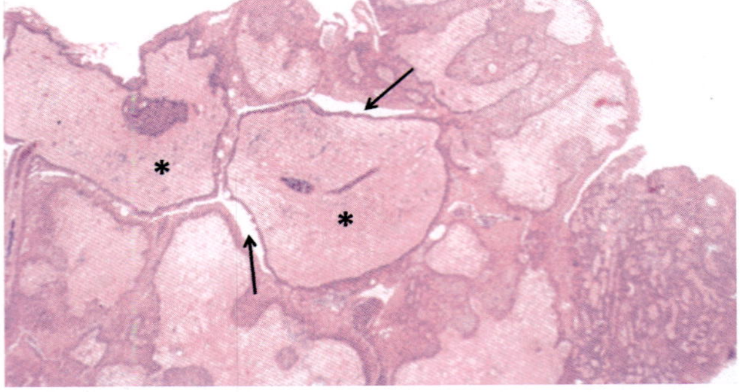

Figure 2-248. Papillary craniopharyngioma: Papillary architecture is due to the dehiscence (*arrows*) of the solid cellularity among the fibrovascular stroma (*asterisk*) (H&E; original magnification: 40×).

grade assignment, is *papillary tumor of the pineal region*.[554] Papillary structures lined by cytokeratin-positive cells can certainly create confusion with a metastatic carcinoma. They alternate with solid areas and can have true rosettes, also mimicking ependymoma, especially a papillary ependymoma; however, they are typically not EMA positive in contrast to ependymoma. EMA can sometimes be positive in a cytoplasmic dot-like pattern and GFAP can be focally positive. In addition, it shows neuroendocrine differentiation, as well as vimentin positivity. *Papillary meningioma*[555] is by definition a malignant (WHO grade III) meningioma. Its papillary nature can be quite subtle **(Fig. 2-247)**. The diagnostic feature is a peculiar reticulin network by a reticulin stain that shows extension of reticulin fibers radially away from the vessel wall among the neoplastic cells. *Papillary ependymoma* actually has pseudopapillary structures formed by the pseudorosettes standing out in the loose background cellularity. As such, instead of fibrovascular cores, their stroma is composed of glial processes and the central vessel that are forming the pseudorosettes. Immunohistochemistry may be needed in some cases to differentiate papillary ependymoma from papillary meningioma, using GFAP and S-100 protein positivity for ependymal differentiation, and to show the absence of glial processes in the pseudorosette-like areas of papillary meningioma. The presence of basement membrane, which can be highlighted by PAS, laminin, or collagen type IV, separating the epithelial cells of choroid plexus neoplasms from the stroma also helps distinguish it from papillary ependymoma. *Astroblastoma* can show a pseudopapillary architecture due to the pseudorosettes around hyalinized vessels and loose cellular background in other areas.

A pseudopapillary architecture forms as a result of dehiscence of the solid sheets of squamous cells in *papillary craniopharyngioma*.[556] The resulting loose pseudopapillae appear to float within the cystic cavity **(Fig. 2-248)**. They are formed by the cells still adherent to the fibrovascular cores of variable density and size. A pseudopapillary appearance can also form in some *pituitary adenomas* **(Fig. 2-249)** through a process similar to that in papillary craniopharyngioma. They are usually of gonadotroph type.[557] They may resemble the pseudorosettes of ependymoma and may cause confusion, especially in IOC. Noting the exact location of the lesion and communicating with the surgeon should clarify this situation in difficult cases. Another neoplasm common in the hypothalamic/suprasellar region is *pilomyxoid astrocytoma*.[390] One of its features is a peculiar radial arrangement of elongated neoplastic cells around vessels, altogether in a myxoid background. Although quite a distinct lesion in many other respects, a neoplasm with a superficial resemblance to PMA due to some overlapping histologic features is *myxopapillary ependymoma*. The perivascular arrangement of bland, round-to-oval cells and a myxoid background that is more prominent around the vessels result in the descriptive name of this neoplasm. *Endolymphatic sac tumor*[558]

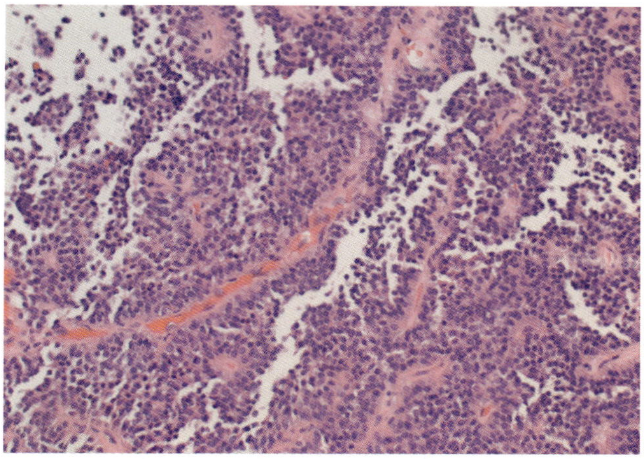

Figure 2-249. Pituitary adenoma: A pseudopapillary architecture is formed as a result of dehiscence of cellular areas and, together with the perivascular pseudorosette appearance, may resemble an ependymoma (H&E; original magnification: 200×).

develops within the temporal bone but may erode through the bone to present as a cerebellopontine angle tumor due to its destructive nature. It has a delicate, lacy papillary and glandular architecture with cuboidal epithelial cells and histologically can be easily distinguished from the more common spindle cell neoplasms in this region, that is, fibroblastic meningioma and schwannoma **(Fig. 2-250)**. It is positive for CK7, negative for CK20, and positive for EMA, S-100 protein, and GFAP. It is associated with von Hippel-Lindau (VHL) syndrome.

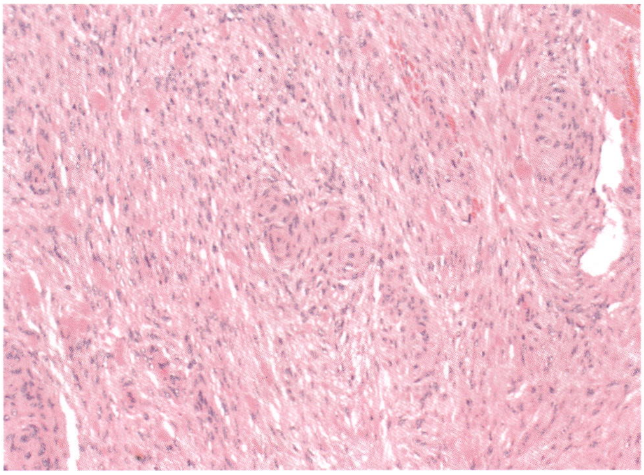

Figure 2-250. Fibroblastic meningioma: A spindle cell neoplasm is seen and might be difficult to recognize as meningioma in the absence of whorls (**center**) (H&E; original magnification: 200×).

Small Blue Cells

This discussion goes beyond the traditional description of small blue cell neoplasms such as PNET, lymphoma, and embryonal and alveolar rhabdomyosarcoma and, with a more descriptive approach, includes those variants with small blue cells of other neoplasms, such as small cell glioblastoma. The typical small blue cell neoplasm of the CNS is *PNET/medulloblastoma*. Medulloblastoma has traditionally been considered a PNET that occurs in the cerebellum; however, recent studies suggest that it may be a separate neoplasm of its own based on genetic differences.[561,562] They are histologically essentially identical neoplasms with primitive cells that may show variable degrees of differentiation along neuronal and/or glial lines. Typically, without any differentiation, the cells are small with minimal amount of cytoplasm that may not be readily visible. The nucleus is oval, is somewhat tapered, and

List of Findings/Checklist for Small Blue Cells

AT A GLANCE

- Primitive neuroectodermal tumor (PNET)/ medulloblastoma
- Medulloblastoma variants
- Supratentorial PNET
- Peripheral PNET
- Pineoblastoma
- Neoplasms with PNET-like areas
  - Atypical teratoid/rhabdoid tumor (ATRT)
  - Choroid plexus carcinoma
  - Glioblastoma multiforme (GBM) with PNET-like component
- Other small blue cell neoplasms
  - Lymphoma/leukemia
  - Rhabdomyosarcoma
  - Malignant peripheral nerve sheath tumor
  - Small cell carcinoma
- PNET mimickers
  - External granule layer
  - Internal granule layer
  - Germinal matrix
  - Small cell GBM
  - Anaplastic oligodendroglioma
  - Anaplastic ependymoma
  - Cellular ependymoma
  - Atypical meningioma
  - Treated prolactinoma
  - Crush artifact

is sometimes described as "carrot-shaped," with a course granular chromatin pattern with no obvious nucleoli. Mitotic figures are easily identified. Many apoptotic cells are present. Focal micronecroses can be present, but confluent areas of necroses are not typical. Vessels are not prominent, but vascular proliferation can be seen. The cellularity may be in the form of confluent sheets or may be arranged in a vague lobularity with areas of streaming of nuclei **(Fig. 2-251)**. Wright rosettes and true rosettes may be seen. It is common to find widespread immunohistochemical evidence of neuronal differentiation in medulloblastomas, even without obvious light microscopic features of such differentiation, but glial differentiation is less common and focal at best. Scattered GFAP-positive entrapped reactive astrocytes should not be taken as evidence of glial differentiation. PNETs are truly undifferentiated. Both PNETs and medulloblastomas can have variable degrees of neuronal differentiation with the development of neuropil-like background composed of neurites. These are usually seen in the form of pale nodules or elongated rounded areas standing out in the background of primitive cells. In these areas, nuclei become rounder and smaller, reminiscent of the internal granule cells of the cerebellum or those of central neurocytoma **(Fig. 2-252)**. Frank ganglion cell differentiation can be seen. In addition to the classical medulloblastoma with no further defining features, four medulloblastoma variants with prognostic implications have been recognized.[206] A medulloblastoma variant that is composed of such nodular structures surrounded by the small blue cells streaming around them is *desmoplastic/nodular medulloblastoma*.[563] The defining feature is the presence of dense reticulin network in the small cell areas surrounding the nodules **(Fig. 2-253)**. If the majority of the neoplasm is composed of nodules

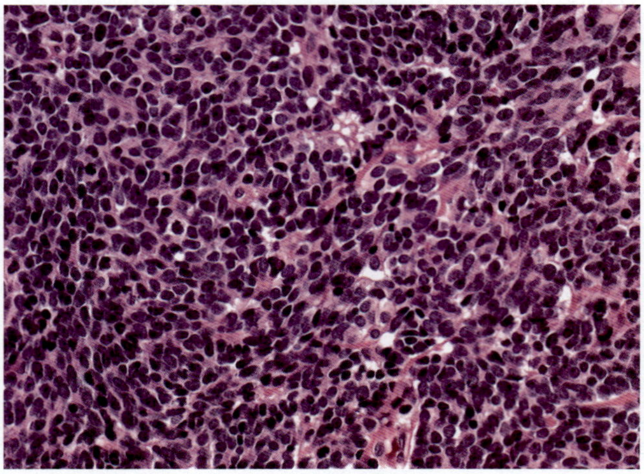

Figure 2-251. Medulloblastoma: Small, hyperchromatic cells with only minimal amount of cytoplasm are seen. Nuclei are oval to elongated and, in some areas, may form a streaming pattern (H&E; original magnification: 400×).

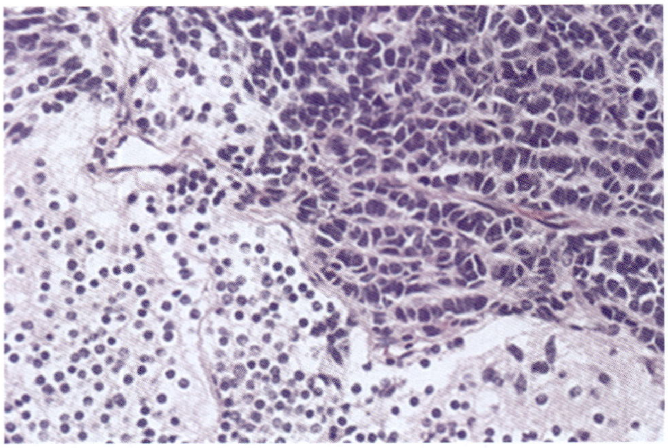

Figure 2-252. Medulloblastoma: The typical small blue cell morphology is seen at the top of the picture. Nuclear molding is prominent and may cause problems in distinguishing it from metastatic small cell carcinoma, fortunately a rare situation. The bottom part is more differentiated with round nuclei, a more uniform and finely granular chromatin pattern, and a neuropil-like background composed of the neuritic processes of these cells (H&E; original magnification: 400×).

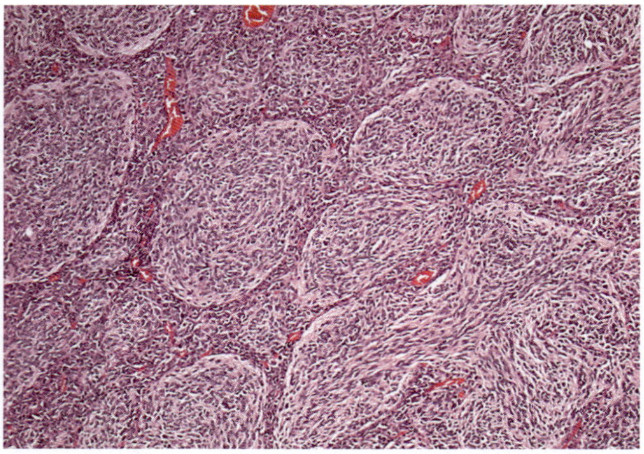

Figure 2-253. Desmoplastic medulloblastoma: Multiple better differentiated nodules with round nuclei and neuropil-like background are surrounded by the dense typical small blue cell areas. The latter is also rich in reticulin and can be highlighted by a reticulin stain (H&E; original magnification: 200×).

with neuronal differentiation without intervening primitive cell component, it is termed *medulloblastoma with extensive nodularity*.[564] In practice, because of overlapping features, it may be problematic to reliably distinguish *large cell and anaplastic medulloblastoma* variants, although described as separate variants, resulting in the diagnosis of large cell/anaplastic medulloblastoma. Synaptophysin shows a peculiar paranuclear dot-like positivity, especially in large cell medulloblastoma. While all medulloblastomas are WHO grade IV, large cell[565] and anaplastic variants imply a worse prognosis in this category. Medulloblastoma with extensive nodularity, while still WHO grade IV, has a better prognosis among medulloblastoma variants. The prognosis of desmoplastic/nodular medulloblastoma has been debatable; however, if strict criteria are followed, it has a better prognosis and nodularity in general seems to imply a better prognosis.[566] Large cell medulloblastoma has nuclei that are larger than the typical medulloblastoma. They are also round with open chromatin and prominent nucleoli, reminiscent of the nuclei of a large cell or immunoblastic lymphoma. Large, geographic areas of necrosis are common, as is brisk mitotic activity[567] **(Fig. 2-254)**. In anaplastic medulloblastoma, there are variable degrees of pleomorphism and cytologic atypia. Cell-in-cell configuration is common as is anaplasia defined by the presence of large, bizarre cells resulting in a striking pleomorphism.[541] Myogenic differentiation, formerly known as medullomyoblastoma, with rhabdomyoblastic differentiation can have additional rhabdomyoblastic cells and strap cells with cross striations. Medulloblastoma with melanotic differentiation, formerly known as melanotic medulloblastoma, has clusters, ribbons, or tubules of cells with melanin pigment. These histologic changes do not indicate a separate entity or distinct variant as these changes can be seen in any other variant or classical type of medulloblastoma and do not have prognostic significance. They also show respective immunohistochemical features for skeletal muscle and melanotic differentiation. Medulloblastoma/PNET-like small blue cell areas can be seen in *ATRT* and can be present to such an extent that the true nature of ATRT is obscured, resulting in a misdiagnosis in pediatric population. The loss of INI1 reactivity by immunohistochemistry will identify such neoplasms as ATRT, rather than PNET, an important prognostic and therapeutic distinction.[568]

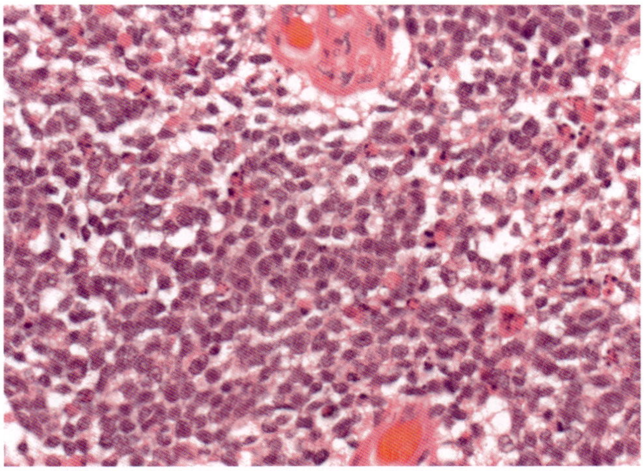

Figure 2-254. Large cell medulloblastoma: The nuclei are not the typical small blue cells of the classical medulloblastoma but rather have rounded contours with a more open chromatin and prominent nucleoli, resembling large B-cell lymphoma. Many apoptotic cells are also present and prominent necrosis is common (H&E; original magnification: 400×).

PNETs are given descriptive names based on their locations. In the cerebellum, they have been called medulloblastoma, which, as described above, may represent a separate category of neoplasms. In the pineal gland, they are called *pineoblastoma* and in the cerebral hemispheres, *cerebral or supratentorial PNET*. If they showed ependymal canal-like structures, they have traditionally then been called ependymoblastoma, a diagnosis the existence of which as an entity has been recently challenged, as similar structures can be seen in other entities. Pineoblastoma may be associated with bilateral retinoblastomas, referred to as trilateral retinoblastoma. *Peripheral PNET (pPNET/EWS)* can occur in the dura mater as a primary soft tissue neoplasm, can invade the dura mater from a primary focus in the surrounding bone, or can simply metastasize to the dura from an extracranial soft tissue site.[569,570] PNET can develop in association with peripheral/cranial nerves. Especially medulloblastoma and pineoblastoma, due to their proximity and propensity to infiltrate the ventricular system and leptomeninges, but all PNETs in general have a tendency to result in *CNS dissemination* by seeding the CSF.[571] Such small blue cells can then be identified by CSF cytology, which can be used in the follow-up of patients with these neoplasms. In surgical specimens, leptomeningeal

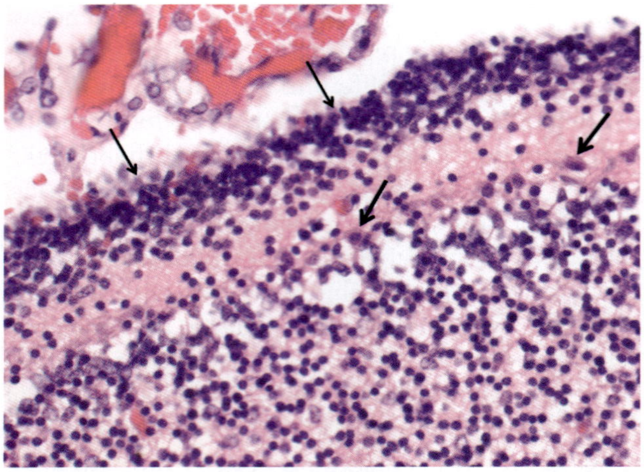

Figure 2-255. External granule layer: Also known as fetal layer of Obersteiner, this germinal layer (*thin arrows*) should not be mistaken for medulloblastoma infiltrating the leptomeninges. Immature Purkinje cells (*thick arrows*) and internal granule layer cells (**bottom**) are also seen (H&E; original magnification: 400×).

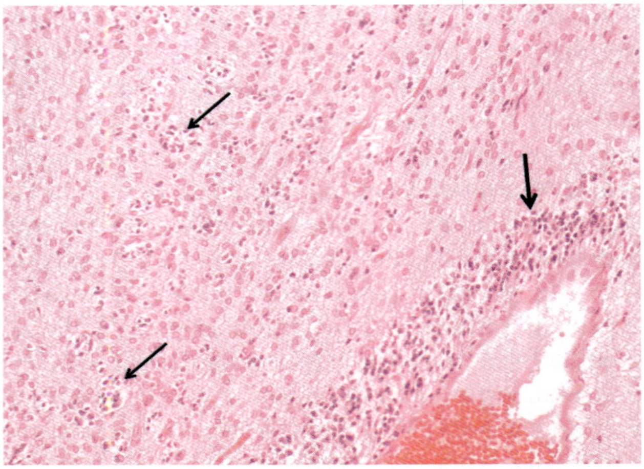

Figure 2-256. Germinal matrix cells: As the migration of the primitive cells of the germinal matrix continues, only small clusters are left behind scattered in the periventricular parenchyma (*thin arrows*) and around vessels (*thick arrow*), not to be confused with inflammation (H&E; original magnification: 200×).

infiltration of medulloblastoma can be identified. In pediatric patients who are younger than 1 year of age, the normally present *external granule layer (fetal layer of Obersteiner),* which gradually disappears by the age of one, may constitute a pitfall **(Fig. 2-255)**. Just like the cells of the periventricular germinal matrix in the brain, these cells in the cerebellum are the primitive cells that are destined to migrate and populate the cerebellum, and at this stage, they resemble the neoplastic primitive cells. They are smaller and their chromatin is not as coarse or nuclei as hyperchromatic. When admixed, the neoplastic cells may stand out as a different population. Likewise, the *periventricular germinal matrix* of the brain gradually starts thinning out at about 26 weeks of gestation, eventually down to small collections of cells around the vessels until term, and subsequently disappears with only the area between thalamus and caudate nucleus called ganglionic eminence persisting until the end of 1st year of life. Especially such perivascular residual cell groups may appear as inflammatory cells, collections of oligodendroglial cells resembling hamartomatous foci, or, if in larger sheets, PNET, especially in small specimens **(Fig. 2-256)**. Another similar trap in the diagnosis of medulloblastoma are the normal internal granule layer cells potentially misdiagnosed as neoplasm, especially in IOC (see Chapter 3). Attention to their small and round contours and the presence of large neurons representing Purkinje cells, being aware of the location and this pitfall are important to avoid this mistake. Adult cases are rare and usually occur in the third and fourth decades,[572] while cases in the fifth decade are extremely rare.[206] Nonetheless, sometimes in this age group, the differential diagnosis also includes *metastatic small cell carcinoma* **(Fig. 2-257)**. Large areas of confluent necrosis,

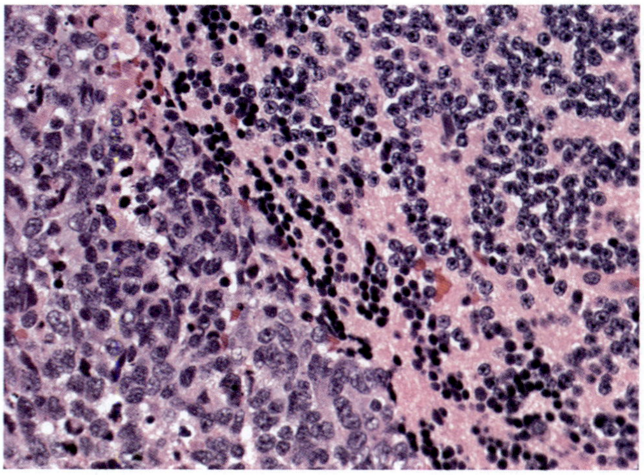

Figure 2-257. Metastatic small cell carcinoma (**bottom left**) cells may resemble medulloblastoma but are quite different than the round nuclei of the internal granule cells (**top right**) (H&E; original magnification: 400×).

resulting in peritheliomatous appearance due to groups of neoplastic cells remaining viable around the vessels, and an epithelial clustering if cytologic preparations are available favor a carcinoma. A history of previously diagnosed small cell carcinoma or the presence of a lung mass is also helpful, although these carcinomas can present with metastasis for the first time. In difficult cases, immunohistochemistry is useful in this differential diagnosis, with diffuse and strong cytokeratin positivity supporting the diagnosis of metastatic carcinoma. Some differentiating PNETs present as ganglioneuroblastoma, similar to their extra-CNS counterparts.[573] They may be mistaken for the more common ganglion cell neoplasms or gangliogliomas when neuroblastic component is not obvious.

Some of the *gliomas*, due to their increased cellularity and hyperchromasia, may mimic PNET. Especially anaplastic oligodendroglioma, anaplastic ependymoma, cellular ependymoma, and small cell glioblastoma[574] can occasionally cause differential diagnostic problems **(Fig. 2-258)**. The presence of Wright rosettes supports PNET/medulloblastoma. There are usually areas that yield clues to the true nature of the neoplasm elsewhere, if there is enough specimen to work with. In most cases, careful evaluation will reveal clues to the nature of the process. Immunohistochemistry may be needed in small tissue samples and in difficult cases. Glioblastoma with PNET-like areas[575] likely

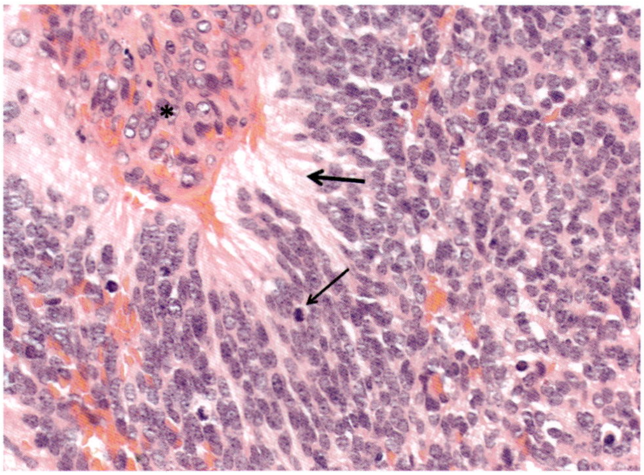

Figure 2-258. Anaplastic ependymoma: Hyperchromatic small cells with prominent mitotic activity (*thin arrow*) resemble PNET/medulloblastoma. Fibrillary zone of a pseudorosette (*thick arrow*) is seen around a proliferating vessel (*asterisk*) (H&E; original magnification: 400×).

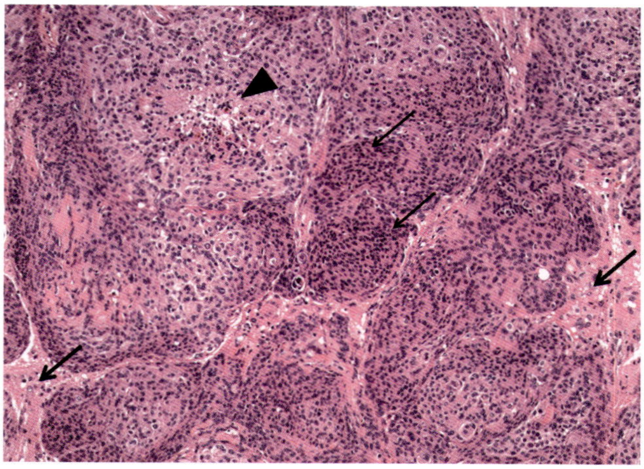

Figure 2-259. Atypical meningioma: Small cells with high nucleus-to-cytoplasm ratio are seen as darker cell groups (*thin arrows*) in the more eosinophilic background, and this is one of the features to take into consideration in the grading of meningiomas. In addition, this meningioma also invades and entraps the neuroglial parenchyma (*thick arrows*) and shows micronecrosis (*arrowhead*) (H&E; original magnification: 200×).

represents a metaplastic transformation of high-grade glioma; however, at least in some cases, it may overlap with the rare situation where an exuberant glial differentiation in a PNET takes place. Some *choroid plexus carcinomas* can have variable amounts of small cells, resembling PNET, and may represent choroid plexus–type differentiation in a PNET.[576] Groups of small cells with high nucleus-to-cytoplasm ratios can be found in some meningiomas, and this is one of the findings used in the diagnosis of *atypical (WHO grade II) meningioma*[577] **(Fig. 2-259)**. They stand out as groups of dark cells in the background of cells with more prominent cytoplasm. *Hematolymphoid neoplasms*, especially high-grade lymphoma such as Burkitt or diffuse large B-cell lymphoma, leukemic infiltrates especially acute lymphoblastic leukemia, or myeloid (granulocytic) sarcoma, can present as a small blue cell neoplasm. *Embryonal and alveolar rhabdomyosarcomas* also enter this differential diagnostic list but are rare in the CNS. Nonetheless, when faced with a small blue cell neoplasm, a broad differential diagnostic approach is needed, with an immunohistochemical panel covering these various possibilities. In some cases, cytogenetic and molecular diagnostic ancillary testing is also needed. Some highly cellular *MPNSTs* have a PNET-like appearance. In

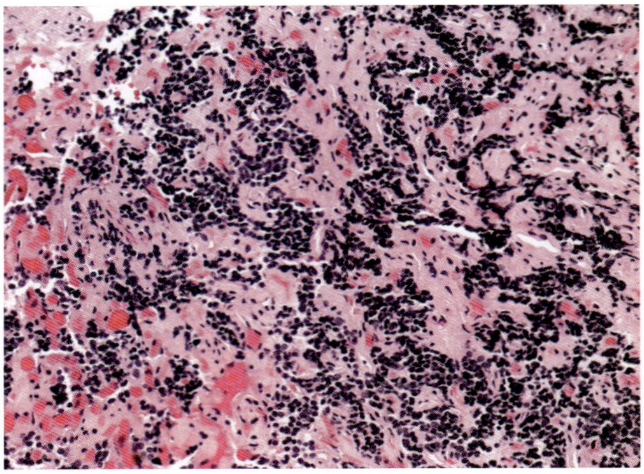

Figure 2-260. Treated prolactinoma: After bromocriptine treatment, prolactinoma can become atrophic, resulting in a small cell carcinoma–like or PNET–like appearance (H&E; original magnification: 400×).

addition, MPNST can also have areas resembling PNET.[578] The neuroblastoma-like schwannoma is a rare schwannoma variant that is composed of small cells and with a histology reminiscent of neuroblastoma, which may mimic PNET.[579]

Crush artifact results in a microscopic appearance of small cells with smudgy chromatin and, in extreme cases, a complete breakdown of nuclei, resulting in a sea of basophilic chromatin. This artifact can result in any cellular component to appear like a small blue cell neoplasm. Some cells are more prone to be affected by such an artifact. Cells of small cell carcinoma, lymphoma, and PNET are particularly prone. None of these diagnoses should be made based on the presence of crush artifact. In fact, no diagnosis should be made in areas with any artifact. A similar appearance can also occur in *prolactinoma after bromocryptin treatment*, when the cells become inactive with very small amount of cytoplasm remaining and the nuclei are shrunken **(Fig. 2-260)**.

Nodular and Nested Arrangement

In some lesions, the cellularity is interrupted by fibrovascular stroma to create large nodules or, in a smaller scale, an organoid/nested arrangement.

List of Findings/Checklist for Nodular and Nested Arrangement

AT A GLANCE

- Desmoplastic/nodular medulloblastoma
- Medulloblastoma with extensive nodularity
- Supratentorial primitive neuroectodermal tumor
- Germinoma
- Pineal parenchymal tumors
- Paraganglioma
- Melanoma
- Ganglion cell neoplasms
- Subependymal giant cell astrocytoma (SEGA)
- Dysembryoplastic neuroepithelial tumor
- Anaplastic oligodendroglioma
- Subependymoma
- Nonneoplastic anterior pituitary parenchyma
- Optic nerve
- Plexiform neurofibroma and schwannoma
- Chondrosarcoma
- Chordoma

This appearance is not specific or diagnostic for any particular entity but can narrow down the possibilities in a challenging case. Many lesions can have at least a partial nodular/nested architecture, while it is a common finding in some. In fact, some are named based on their nodular arrangement.

Desmoplastic/nodular medulloblastoma[563] is characterized by so-called pale islands in a background of primitive cells with more typical medulloblastoma features. These pale nodules represent better differentiated areas with more obvious neuronal features, neuropil-like fibrillary delicate eosinophilic background, and round, neurocytic nuclei, which show prominent Neu-N positivity in the background of negative primitive cells. This creates a negative image with the Ki-67 proliferative activity, which is prominent in the primitive cell population but is essentially absent within the nodules. The primitive cell areas among the nodules are rich in reticulin, resulting in the name. Nodular/desmoplastic medulloblastoma is the predominant histologic medulloblastoma variant seen in association with Gorlin syndrome. A medulloblastoma variant termed *medulloblastoma with extensive nodularity*[564] owing to the diffuse presence of nodular architecture without desmoplasia or primitive component also has a nodular

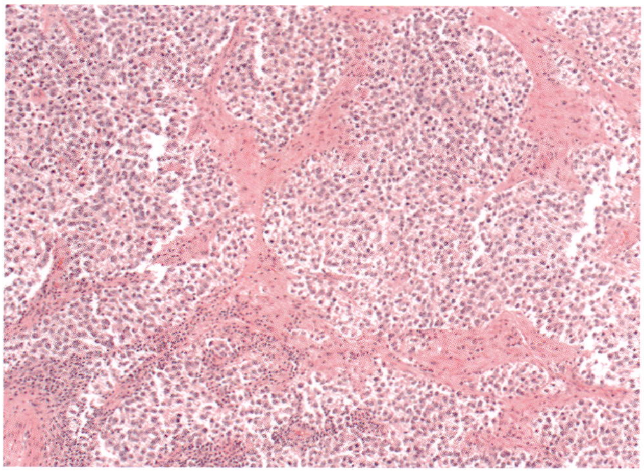

Figure 2-261. Germinoma: A nodular arrangement is created by the fibrous tissue bands that usually contain variable numbers of lymphocytes (**bottom**) (H&E; original magnification: 100×).

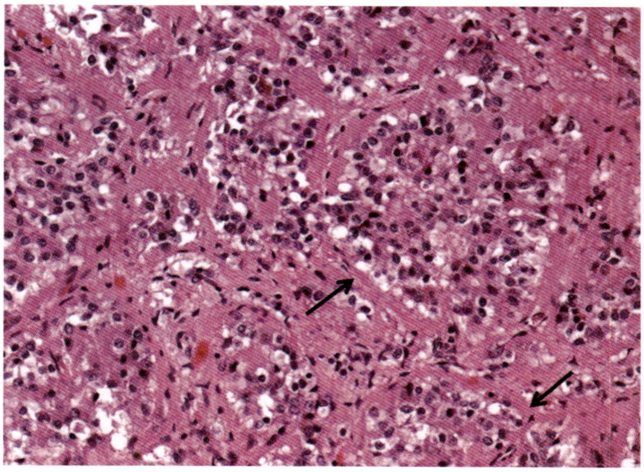

Figure 2-262. Pineal gland: Nonneoplastic pineal parenchyma has a nodular appearance (*arrows*) and should not be mistaken for a germinoma in small samples (H&E; original magnification: 200×).

architecture, as the name implies. The nodules are of irregular shapes and sizes and may appear as solid sheets in some areas where they are large or where they merge. Changes similar to what has been described for medulloblastoma variants can also be observed in *S-PNET*.

Germinoma is characterized in many cases by fibrovascular septae of variable thickness and prominence, dividing the neoplasm into cellular nodules. These septae are frequently associated with a lymphocytic infiltrate and sometimes granulomas, in some cases even obscuring the neoplasm **(Fig. 2-261)**. Given that the pineal region is the most common intracranial location for germinoma, *nonneoplastic pineal parenchyma* also has a nodular architecture, in some cases creating pitfalls and confusion for the unaware **(Fig. 2-262)**. Attention to the cellular detail and contrasting the back-to-back clear cells of the germinoma with the somewhat smaller and irregular cells of the pineal gland separated in a fibrillary background are helpful. The presence of calcifications should also alert one to the possibility of nonneoplastic pineal parenchyma. Some *pineal parenchymal tumors of intermediate differentiation* can be in a lobular pattern rather than diffuse sheets of cells and are divided by fibrovascular septae, referred to as pseudolobulated, as opposed to diffuse pattern.[398] This appearance may also create confusion with nonneoplastic pineal gland, which normally has a similar configuration, especially in small tissue samples. Furthermore, if the normal gland histology has been distorted by the commonly present cysts, calcifications, or hemorrhage, this distinction can become a problem. Unfortunately, the typically layered cyst wall may not be appreciated in such small tissues (see "Cystic Lesions").

Paraganglioma is characterized by an organoid pattern of solid sheets of uniform cells with neuroendocrine chromatin pattern and may look epithelioid. These sheets of cells are divided typically by a delicate fibrovascular, capillary network, creating the organoid pattern. This pattern is similar to that seen especially in many *epithelioid melanomas*; however, the large nuclei, open chromatin, and prominent nuclei of this type of melanoma should provide a stark contrast with paraganglioma. Diffuse S-100 protein positivity in melanoma contrasts with the S-100 protein positivity that is limited to variable numbers of sustentacular cells that are typically located at the periphery of the organoid groups in paraganglioma. In addition, MART-1, HMB-45, MiTF-1 positivity in melanoma and synaptophysin and chromogranin positivity in paraganglioma further clarify any confusion. It should be noted that some paragangliomas can have cytokeratin-positive cells and should not be interpreted as metastatic carcinoma.[124] *Metastatic carcinoma* can have a nodular appearance in some cases; however, the cytologic atypia, evidence of epithelial differentiation, such as squamous or glandular features, necrosis, peritheliomatous arrangement, and sharp border with the surrounding parenchyma all make it easy to avoid confusion. Occasionally, especially low-grade neuroendocrine carcinomas and prostate carcinomas can have a predominantly neuroendocrine appearance, obscuring their carcinoma origin. They only rarely metastasize to the CNS and any previous history should alert one to consider these possibilities. Nonetheless, surprises may occur. *Ganglion cell neoplasms* have a prominent thick vascular network that is further accentuated by the presence of variable numbers of perivascular lymphocytes, resulting in a somewhat nodular appearance of the parenchyma **(Fig. 2-263)**. Since some of the neoplasms may have low cellularity and may be difficult to assess, especially in small biopsy tissues, this vascular and nodular appearance can provide additional help in the differential diagnosis. *SEGA*, in addition to its syndromic association with tuberous sclerosis,[580] typical location, and cellular parenchyma containing large cells with abundant cytoplasm, also has a prominent vascular network resulting in a nodular architecture. These cells may be crowded around the vessels, creating a pseudorosette-like appearance. The cytohistomorphologic features, together with its clinical presentation, are quite characteristic for diagnosis.

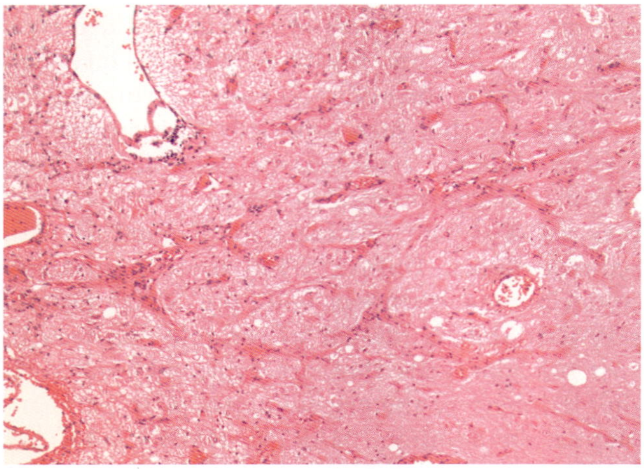

Figure 2-263. Ganglioglioma: A vague nodularity is created by the thick and branching vascular component and may draw attention to the abnormal nature of the tissue in subtle cases of ganglion cell neoplasms (H&E; original magnification: 100×).

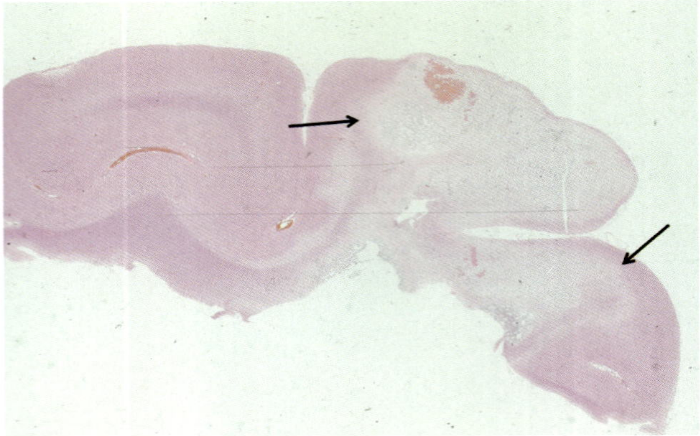

Figure 2-264. DNT is characterized by a primarily intracortical multinodularity (*arrows*) that can also be identified radiologically. The nodules are well-circumscribed (H&E; original magnification: 20×).

DNT[581] is characterized by multiple intracortical nodules **(Fig. 2-264)**, within which the more specific diagnostic features, such as oligodendroglial-like cells and floating neurons in a myxoid background, are seen. If adequate size of tissue is available, the identification of this superficial multinodular low-power appearance is very helpful in recognizing this entity. In other cases, referring to the radiologic features, which show the same finding, is useful. Otherwise, examining the nodules in high power may sometimes result in confusion with oligodendroglioma, especially if the floating neurons are not readily apparent. The borders of the nodules of DNT are sharply demarcated from the surrounding tissue and show no satellitosis in contrast to oligodendroglioma. Aside from this context, in general, *anaplastic oligodendroglioma* can assume a nodular appearance due to the division of cellular parenchyma by the proliferation of its vascular network **(Fig. 2-265)**. The high-grade nature of the neoplasm is readily obvious in such cases; however, its histologic typing may be difficult (see "Small Blue Cells"). *Subependymoma* is an incidental neoplasm in most cases.[582] It is a WHO grade I neoplasm typically located in the fourth ventricle and less so in the lateral ventricles. Sometimes, it comes to attention during a workup for another reason. Rarely, it may grow to a size or be located at a site to interfere with the CSF circulation,

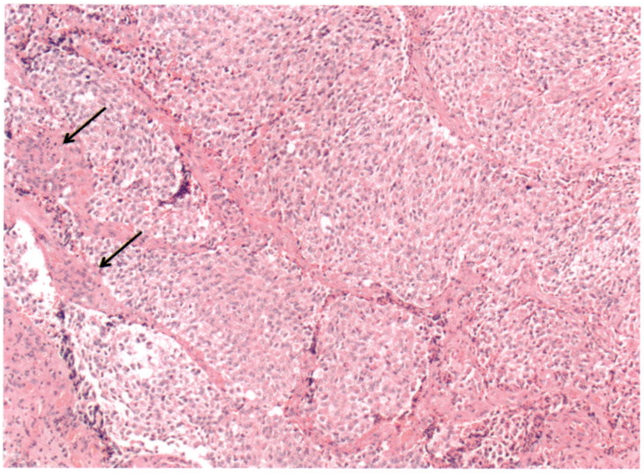

Figure 2-265. Anaplastic oligodendroglioma: Bundles of vascular proliferation (*arrows*) can divide the cellular parenchyma into nodules, a feature seen more commonly in anaplastic oligodendrogliomas than in astrocytic neoplasms (H&E; original magnification: 100×).

creating clinical findings. At any rate, an "intraventricular" or periventricular neoplasm may be sent for IOC and catch the pathologist by surprise. The typical grouped arrangement of its bland cells within the densely glial fibrillarity is an important clue. The cells may be associated with a myxoid background, resulting in small cellular and mucinous pools within the fibrillary background **(Fig. 2-266)**. Some superficial fragments may also represent the nodule bulging

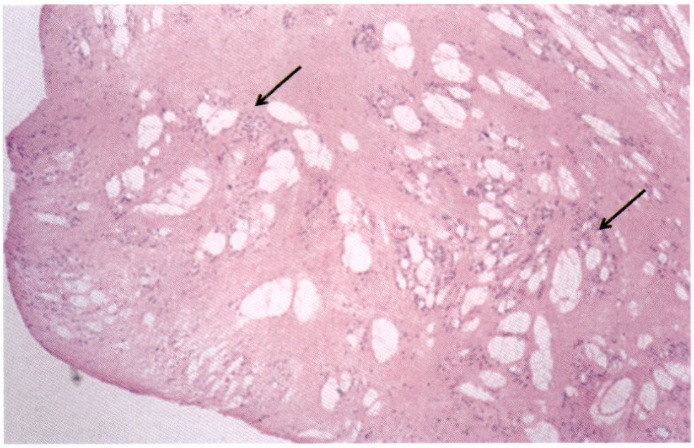

Figure 2-266. Subependymoma: Cellular groups and mucinous microcysts (*arrows*) are separated by dense glial tissue, resulting in an irregular nodularity in this mass protruding into the ventricle lumen (**left side**) (H&E; original magnification: 40×).

into the ventricular lumen and may be covered by ependymal cells. A significantly higher probability of recurrence has been attributed to the cellular variant, in contrast to reticular variant, of hemangioblastoma as an independent prognostic factor.[583] In the cellular variant, sheets of neoplastic cells are divided into groups that are devoid of reticulin by a reticulin rich stroma, in contrast to the classical pericellular reticulin network of the reticular variant.

A nested appearance is very useful in the sellar region to identify *nonneoplastic anterior pituitary parenchyma*. Its recognition becomes important in small tissues sent for IOC to distinguish it from hyperplastic or adenomatous pituitary tissue. Typically, the nesting pattern of nonneoplastic pituitary parenchyma is composed of cells forming groups of more or less similar sizes. They are composed of a mixture of cell types, that is, acidophil, basophil, and chromophobe, although one may predominate. In some cases, only one cell type can be identified, depending on the location of the sample in the gland, as the distribution of cells is not homogeneous in the parenchyma. For instance, the lateral parts of the parenchyma contain predominantly acidophilic cells that are growth hormone secreting, while the midportion is predominantly composed of basophilic ACTH-producing cells. However, attention to the nesting pattern avoids misinterpretation of such small, monotonous samples as adenoma. Another structure that normally has a compartmentalized structure is the *optic nerve* on cross section. While it may be easy to recognize it as a nerve when whole, it may appear unusual when seen in small fragments as part of a surgical specimen. In addition, one should be familiar with its appearance to further distinguish the presence of admixed cells representing a PA or other glioma, or neurofibroma, when the bulk of the neoplasm is not present but only infiltrating periphery is represented on the section. These conditions are typically seen as scattered larger and darker cells among the nerve fibers, and in the case of PA, identification of Rosenthal fibers should alert one to this possibility **(Fig. 2-267)**. *Plexiform neurofibroma and plexiform (multinodular) schwannoma*[584] are neoplasms characterized by their multinodular appearance due to involvement of multiple nerve fascicles **(Fig. 2-268)**. The nodules are therefore

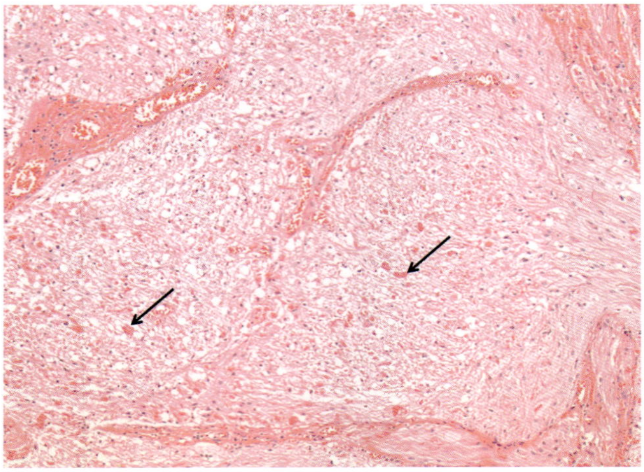

Figure 2-267. Optic nerve glioma: The usual septated nodularity of the optic nerve is still somewhat preserved, although distorted, and scattered Rosenthal fibers (*arrows*) draw attention to the presence of a PA infiltrating the nerve (H&E; original magnification: 100×).

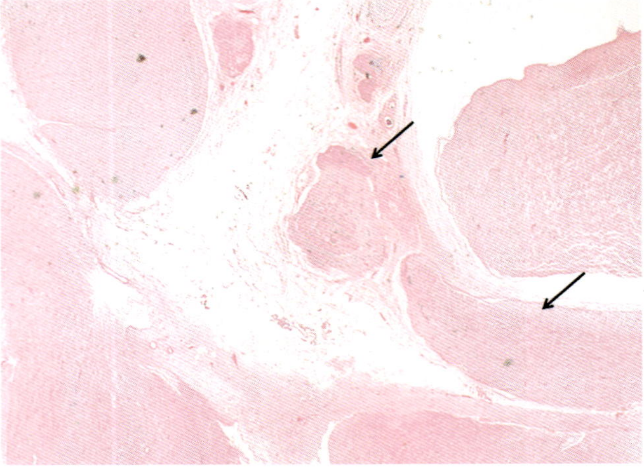

Figure 2-268. Plexiform neurofibroma: Expansion of individual nerve fascicles (*arrows*) by neurofibroma results in a multinodular appearance that is typical for plexiform neurofibroma (H&E; original magnification: 40×).

surrounded by perineurium, though in some fascicles, the neoplasm may "spill" into the surrounding tissues. There are frequent recurrences due to incomplete resections as a result of this irregular multinodularity. In the skin and superficial soft tissues, neurotropic desmoplastic melanoma[585] may also appear as a spindle cell process with admixed nerve fascicles and is only positive for S-100 protein and negative for the typical melanoma markers. Plexiform neurofibroma is, as a rule, associated with NF-1. Plexiform schwannoma is not associated with NF-1, but some cases may be seen in NF-2. Some are associated with schwannomatosis. *Neurothekeoma* is a multinodular, myxoid, variably cellular, well-circumscribed neoplasm that is composed of spindle and/or epithelioid cells and that may show some pleomorphism in some cases due to the presence of scattered larger and multinucleated cells. It should be distinguished from plexiform PNST as well as from plexiform fibrohistiocytic tumor. Neurothekeoma is S-100 protein negative and PGP 9.5 positive. It has been suggested that neurothekeoma and plexiform fibrohistiocytic tumors may be histogenetically related and may represent a spectrum based on their similar immunohistochemical features.[586]

Chondrosarcoma, mainly low-grade ones, has a lobular appearance to the chondroid matrix with variable cellularity **(Fig. 2-269)**, which can be lost as the grade increases. *Chordoma* on the other hand, which is the main differential diagnostic possibility in the skull base/clivus region, has a more compartmentalized appearance due to the thick fibrovascular septae dividing the myxoid areas of the neoplasm into irregular compartments or due to the separation of solid cellular groups by mucinous stroma **(Fig. 2-270)**.

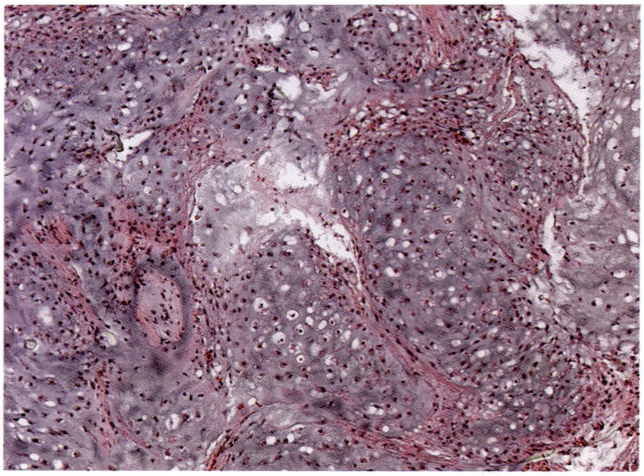

Figure 2-269. Chondrosarcoma: With or without the fibrous tissue septae, chondrosarcoma is typically arranged in a multinodular pattern (H&E; original magnification: 100×).

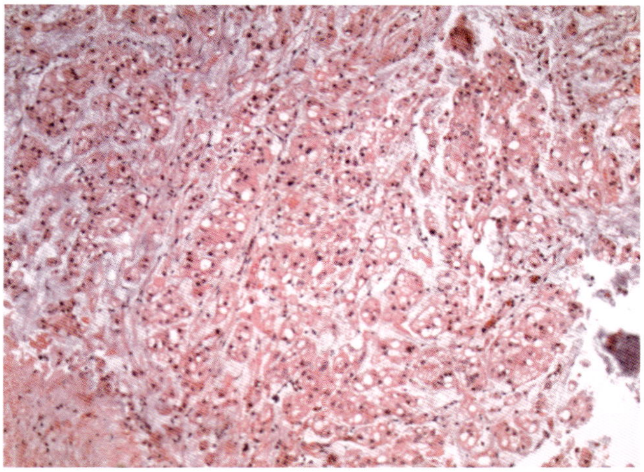

Figure 2-270. Chordoma: Cellular groups separated by mucinous stroma may assume a nodular appearance (H&E; original magnification: 200×).

Biphasic Pattern, Composite Lesions, and Metaplastic Tissues

Some neoplasms are characterized by a biphasic pattern that helps narrow down the differential diagnostic possibilities. Composite neoplasms are composed of two distinct, separately identified components, while some of those neoplasms are characterized by the admixture of two patterns that characterize them. Whether such associations of different histologic appearances, termed biphasic or composite, are a result of divergent differentiation from a single cell type or a metaplastic process that occurs in the cells of a neoplasm has been debated, and both arguments may be true in certain situations. In some of these lesions discussed below, defining them as biphasic or composite may become a philosophical point. The point is that these lesions have different histologic appearances in the same lesion, either separately or admixed with each other, metachronously (e.g., posttreatment changes in histologic type) or synchronously.

Of the nervous system neoplasms, *gliosarcoma* **(Fig. 2-271)** consists of a combination of glioblastoma and a sarcoma component. Rarely, the glial component may be an oligodendroglioma, resulting in an oligosarcoma.[587] The end result is a high-grade neoplasm with variable amounts of glial and sarcomatous areas. The resulting pattern is quite typical; however, in difficult situations, a reticulin stain highlights the differences between two patterns with rich pericellular reticulin network in the sarcomatous, spindle cell areas alternating with glial areas that are devoid of reticulin, except for vessel walls. A similar distinction can be made by GFAP immunohistochemistry, which provides a negative image of reticulin stain by highlighting the glial component. Gliosarcoma has historically been considered to have a slightly better prognosis compared to glioblastoma; other reports indicate a similar prognosis to glioblastoma.[588] Although a rare occurrence and has not been typically referred to as gliosarcoma, sarcomatous transformation of vascular elements,[589] as well as rhabdomyosarcomatous component,[590] has been reported in *subependymoma*. A conceptually similar alternating mesenchymal-appearing and neuroglial components are seen in *DIG/DIA*. The collagen-rich, spindle cell areas are quite sharply demarcated from the more cellular areas composed of a mixture of predominantly small cells and admixed ganglion cells. Ganglion cells and gemistocytic cells can be seen in both compartments. The biphasic pattern, although quite obvious in most cases on routine sections, can be further highlighted by reticulin and collagen stains. *Pilocytic astrocytoma (PA)* has loosely textured areas with bland round-to-oval nuclei sprinkled in a myxoid, edematous background alternating with piloid, less cellular glial areas in which the cells are relatively spindled and Rosenthal fibers can be present **(Fig. 2-272)**. While no prognostic significance is associated with this biphasic pattern, it can be useful to support the PA diagnosis along with other findings.

Ganglioglioma is composed of a ganglion cell component with an admixed glioma, which is typically a low-grade astrocytoma, although other gliomas can be present, such as pilocytic,[591] as well as features similar to gemistocytic astrocytoma or PXA-like areas. Ganglioglioma with tanycytic ependymoma[592] or oligodendroglioma[593] as its glial component has also been reported. The great majority of ganglioglioma is WHO grade I but can be anaplastic (WHO grade III).[594] Some cases with worrisome features beyond the typical ganglioglioma are termed atypical ganglioglioma, without a WHO grade designation. Ganglion cells resemble neurons with their nuclear and cytoplasmic features, but

List of Findings/Checklist for Biphasic Pattern, Composite Lesions, and Metaplastic Tissues

• AT A GLANCE

Biphasic Pattern

- Sarcomatous component in glial neoplasms
  - Gliosarcoma
  - Oligosarcoma
  - Subependymoma with sarcoma
- Desmoplastic infantile ganglioglioma/desmoplastic infantile astrocytoma
- Pilocytic astrocytoma
- Ganglioglioma
- Oligodendroglioma with ganglioglioma-like maturation
- Primitive neuroectodermal tumor (PNET) with extensive neuronal differentiation
- Papillary glioneuronal tumor
- Rosette-forming glioneuronal tumor
- Synovial sarcoma
- Solitary fibrous tumor
- Choriocarcinoma
- Peripheral nerve sheath neoplasms
  - Schwannoma
  - Psammomatous melanotic schwannoma
  - Schwannoma with meningothelial islands
  - Neurofibroma with schwannomatous nodules
  - Malignant peripheral nerve sheath tumor (MPNST) with divergent differentiation
  - Malignant perineurioma

Composite Pattern

- Oligoastrocytoma
- Glioblastoma with oligodendroglioma component
- Glioblastoma with PNET-like component
- Ependymal neoplasms
  - Subependymoma and ependymoma
  - Classical ependymoma and papillary or clear cell ependymoma

Ganglioglioma (GG)

  - GG with pleomorphic xanthoastrocytoma
  - GG with meningioma
  - GG with malformations of cortical development
- Complex dysembryoplastic neuroepithelial tumor
- Pineal neoplasms
  - Pineocytoma with pineoblastoma
  - Pineocytoma with pineal parenchymal tumor of intermediate differentiation
- Classical medulloblastoma with large cell/anaplastic component
- PNET/medulloblastoma with prominent glial differentiation
- Meningiomas
  - Papillary and rhabdoid meningioma
  - Meningioma and glioma
  - Meningioma and meningioangiomatosis
  - Meningioma and malignant meningioma with sarcomatous or carcinomatous areas
  - Meningioma with metastatic carcinoma
  - Meningioma and schwannoma
- Peripheral nerve sheath neoplasms
  - Schwannoma and perineurioma
  - Schwannoma and neurofibroma
  - MPNST arising from schwannoma, ganglioneuroma and ganglioneuroblastoma
- Pituitary adenoma and craniopharyngioma
- Pituitary adenoma and Rathke cleft cyst
- Germ cell neoplasms
  - Mixed germ cell neoplasms
  - Teratoma
  - Immature teratoma
  - Malignant teratoma
- Vascular malformation combinations
- Aneurysmal bone cyst and giant cell tumor of bone
- Metastases to neoplasms

Changes in Histology

- Posttreatment maturation in PNET and olfactory neuroblastoma
- Maturation in pilomyxoid astrocytoma
- Postradiation malignant transformation
- Secondary gliosarcoma
- Maturation in immature teratoma

Metaplastic Tissues

- Epithelial metaplasia
  - Glioblastoma
  - MPNST
- Osteocartilaginous metaplasia
  - Meningioma
  - Ependymoma
  - Choroid plexus papilloma
  - Medulloepithelioma
- Heterologous elements in MPNST

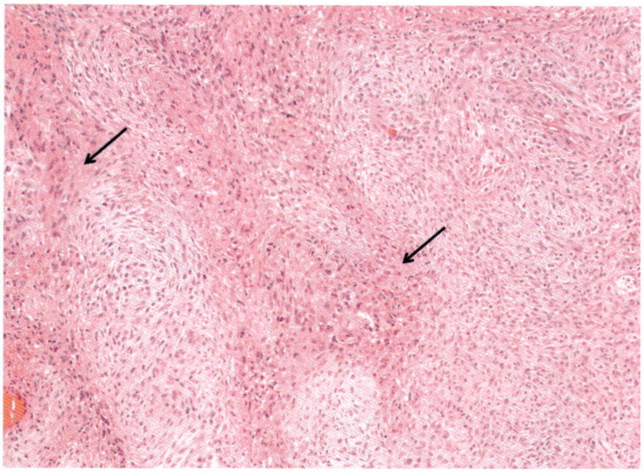

Figure 2-271. Gliosarcoma: A biphasic appearance is imparted by spindle cell sarcomatous areas alternating with the more eosinophilic glial areas (*arrows*). Their relative amounts may be variable, and sometimes, sarcomatous component may overrun the glial component (H&E; original magnification: 100×).

they show irregular grouping, dysmorphic features, binucleation, and cytoplasmic vacuolation and can be of variable sizes, from small cells that may be difficult to recognize as neurons to bizarre forms. In some cases, these changes are subtle and it may be difficult to appreciate the presence of a ganglion cell component in a glioma, as they appear like normal neurons. Diligent search eventually reveals abnormal forms. Such cases may also be difficult to distinguish from a glioma infiltrating a group of native neurons. The orderly distribution and uniform spacing of cytologically unremarkable and uniform neurons, as well as the presence of satellitosis, supports a glioma infiltrating a resident neuronal population. In addition, the presence of a thick vascular network, many times with variable numbers of perivascular small, round lymphocytes, preferentially temporal lobe location of a well-circumscribed mass with cyst and mural nodule formation, also supports the diagnosis of ganglioglioma. Plasma cells may be present admixed with this lymphocytic infiltrate. *Oligodendroglioma with ganglioglioma-like maturation*[595] may result in a misdiagnosis of oligodendroglioma as ganglioglioma with an oligodendroglial component. In this case, the ganglion cell component tends to be well-demarcated from the oligodendroglial areas, among several other defining features. *PNET* may show prominent and exclusively neuronal differentiation in some cases, and such cases may be termed cerebral neuroblastoma or ganglioneuroblastoma,[596] depending on the type of differentiation. *Papillary glioneuronal tumor*[597] is composed of an admixture of glial and neuronal populations. The GFAP-positive glial component is prominent around thick, hyalinized vessels, and the synaptophysin-positive neuronal component that has predominantly neurocytic features but may also show variable degrees of ganglion cell differentiation and can have cells with intermediate features is interspersed among these perivascular arrangements, creating a pseudopapillary appearance. *Rosette-forming glioneuronal tumor*[598] typically arises in the fourth ventricle or cerebellar vermis and is characterized by a peculiar arrangement of small, round neurocytic cells in single-layered rosettes with a central vessel or fibrillary neuropil-like neuritic processes, alternating with a glial component that has features resembling PA or oligodendroglioma **(Fig. 2-273)**. The rosettes are synaptophysin positive, while the admixed glial component is GFAP positive. A pituitary neoplasm with a pituitary adenoma-like secretory component and an admixed Rathke-like epithelial component has been described as pituitary blastoma.[599]

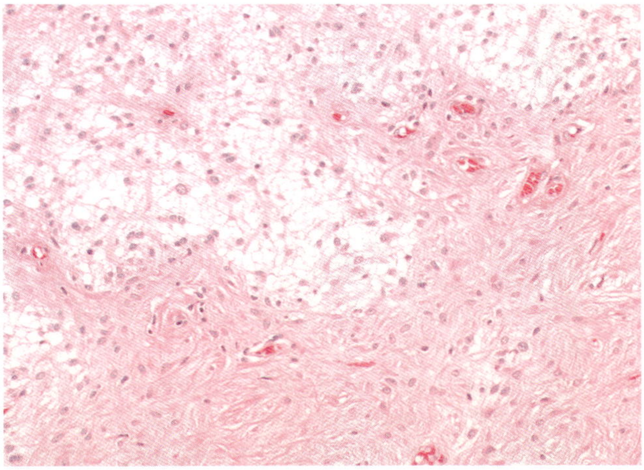

Figure 2-272. PA: Loosely textured areas with round nuclei (**top**) contrast with the dense piloid spindled areas (**bottom**) (H&E; original magnification: 200×).

Synovial sarcoma is the prototype of biphasic neoplasms in general pathology. It is a soft tissue neoplasm that can rarely metastasize from a distant site to the CNS or directly invade the CNS from the surrounding tissues.[600] In its biphasic

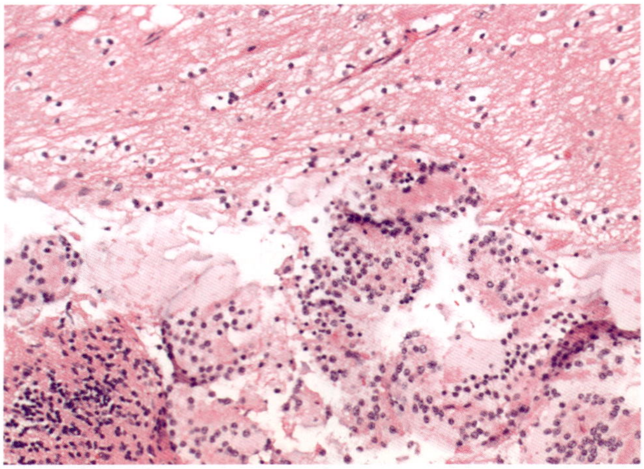

Figure 2-273. Rosette-forming glioneuronal tumor of the fourth ventricle: The mucinous areas with rosettes (**bottom**) alternate with the compact areas (**top**) that can have oligodendroglial or PA–like appearance (H&E; original magnification: 200×).

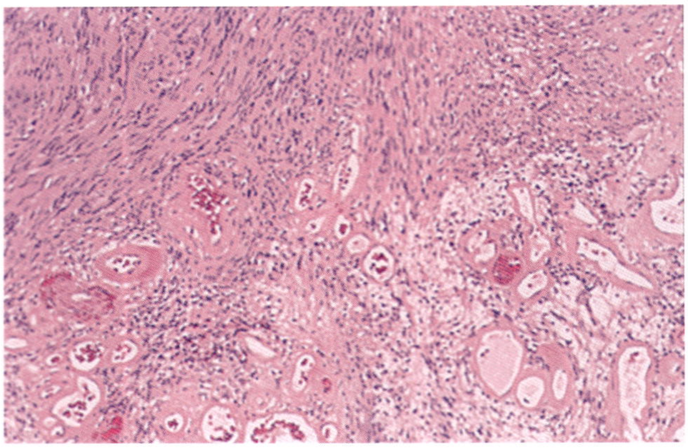

Figure 2-274. Schwannoma: Spindle cell compact Antoni A areas (**top**) and loosely textured Antoni B areas (**bottom**) with many hyalinized vessels, macrophages, and hemosiderin pigment are characteristic (H&E; original magnification: 200×).

form, variable amounts of spindle cell and epithelioid areas are admixed in a typical case, and monophasic synovial sarcomas composed exclusively of either component can also be seen. *Solitary fibrous tumor* has alternating cellular and collagenous areas that are imperceptibly merging with each other, creating what is described as a patternless pattern. *Choriocarcinoma* has syncytiotrophoblastic and cytotrophoblastic cell components. At low power, the former appears as a darker component due to more amphophilic and larger cytoplasm of the cells. Some embryonal carcinoma variants can have a somewhat darker cell population, creating a similar low-power appearance, and should not be confused with choriocarcinoma. In the so-called monophasic choriocarcinoma,[601] however, the syncytiotrophoblasts may be difficult to find and the neoplasm may not have the typical biphasic morphology. A similar picture can arise posttreatment. Choriocarcinoma is typically a highly hemorrhagic and necrotic malignant neoplasm that can even present with hemorrhage, and the cellular areas may prove to be difficult to find in the material.

Schwannoma is well-known for its biphasic pattern. The cellular spindle cell Antoni A areas alternate with loosely textured Antoni B areas where the neoplastic cells are round and are admixed with variable numbers of foamy macrophages, thick and hyalinized vessels, hemorrhage, cystic degeneration, and chronic inflammation **(Fig. 2-274)**. Although not so distinctly separated, in *psammomatous melanotic schwannoma*, a spindle cell and a somewhat epithelioid component can be identified. This picture is made more complicated by the presence of melanin pigment, lipid vacuoles, and psammomatous calcifications. These features are also reflected in the immunophenotype of the neoplasm. It is positive for melanocytic markers, such as HMB-45 and MART-1, while collagen type IV shows a pericellular pattern. Ordinary *schwannoma with meningothelial islands*[602] and *neurofibroma with schwannomatous nodules* are rare.[603] *MPNST with divergent differentiation*[604] can have, in addition, rhabdomyosarcomatous (also known as triton tumor), osteosarcomatous, chondrosarcomatous, angiosarcomatous, and epithelial (also known as glandular MPNST, typically containing benign glandular elements) component. These are frequently NF1-associated neoplasms and the prognosis is especially poor. *MPNST with perineurial differentiation* (also known as *malignant perineurioma*)[605] is a malignant neoplasm that is EMA positive and S-100 negative.

Composite neoplasms and lesions are composed of two separate histologically different components. They are different than the biphasic neoplasms discussed above, where the two components are admixed and constitute the characteristics of that particular neoplasm or lesion. The most common and well-known example of composite neoplasms in the CNS is *oligoastrocytoma*. It has two histologic varieties. The intermingled histology is characterized by one type of histologic appearance that is uniformly present throughout the neoplasm. Its hallmark is a histologic picture that is in between a typical oligodendroglioma and a typical astrocytoma. However, the less common and truly composite form of oligoastrocytoma suits better the discussion here. It is composed of separate and distinct areas of typical oligodendroglioma and typical astrocytoma histology. In general, the amount of a particular histologic component that is required to justify the diagnosis of a composite neoplasm is not well-defined. However, it has been suggested that the presence of as little as one 100× magnification field of oligodendroglioma component is significant enough for a diagnosis of oligoastrocytoma.[606] The subjectivity of the intermingled variant adds to the very low interobserver agreement rate and possibly to an artificially increased frequency of oligoastrocytoma diagnosis. Technically speaking, any combination of two of the three gliomas—astrocytic, oligodendroglial, and ependymal—can form a mixed glioma; however, the most common and essentially exclusive mixed glioma is oligoastrocytoma. Glioblastoma has variants with prognostic and therapeutic implications: *glioblastoma with primitive neuroectodermal tumor (PNET)–like component and glioblastoma with oligodendroglioma component*. They are both WHO grade IV neoplasms but with better prognoses than pure glioblastoma. The PNET component is histologically identical to the typical PNET and occurs together with an otherwise typical glioblastoma. The presence of PNET component allows the use of additional chemotherapeutic regimens in treatment.[575] Glioblastoma with oligodendroglioma component[607] is essentially an oligoastrocytoma with necrosis, with or without vascular proliferation, while an oligoastrocytoma with only vascular proliferation and increased mitotic activity (see "Mitotic Activity"), but without necrosis, constitutes an anaplastic oligoastrocytoma. For this reason, it can also be argued that glioblastoma with oligodendroglial component may also be considered hypothetically as a grade IV oligoastrocytoma.[379] The oligodendroglioma component puts this composite neoplasm prognostically between anaplastic oligoastrocytoma and pure glioblastoma. *Subependymoma with classical or anaplastic ependymoma component* can occasionally be encountered. The highest grade that can be identified should be assigned, but how much area is needed to upgrade is not clear. Likewise, *clear cell ependymoma and papillary ependymoma with classical ependymoma areas*, low or high grade, are also possible. A rare occurrence is the composite neoplasm composed of *rhabdoid meningioma with ganglioglioma*[608] and *PXA and ganglioglioma*.[609] It is not unusual for PXA to have neuronal features and immunohistochemical positivity for neuronal markers; in this case, there are clearly distinct components of PXA and ganglioglioma. *Ganglion cell neoplasms* can be present in association with other abnormalities, such as FCDs/MCD,[610] DNT,[611] and Rasmussen's encephalitis.[612] Spinal ganglion cell neoplasms may be associated with spinal deformities.[613] Some *DNTs* can be associated with a distinct glioma component and are termed "complex," as opposed to "simple" variant of DNT.[61] These nodules may be in the form of oligodendroglioma, oligoastrocytoma, or PA. A rare DNT can be associated with a ganglioglioma, and the presence of FCD in the adjacent cortex is also possible. Some angiocentric gliomas have been associated with MCD. *Pineoblastoma and pineocytoma* can rarely coexist in a pineal parenchymal neoplasm.[614] Pineocytoma component may be overlooked or confused with nonneoplastic pineal gland, especially if it is small. Likewise, pineocytomas and pineal parenchymal tumors of intermediate differentiation can show areas of transition to each other. Classic *medulloblastoma* may have variable foci of large cell, anaplastic, or nodular areas; however, diagnoses of such specific variants are made only when they predominate, although their presence in any degree should be documented. *Medulloepithelioma, medulloblastoma, and PNET* may show differentiation along neuronal and various glial lines, creating a picture with various appearances. Immature neuroepithelial component can be seen in *immature teratoma* and should be a consideration especially in the pineal region tumors in terms of differential diagnosis of pineoblastoma or an immature teratoma; the typical mature components may not be represented in the small biopsy tissues. In most situations, additional tissue with mature elements and/or typical features of one or more germ cell neoplasm types will be present to aid in this differential diagnosis. Rarely, the extensive glial differentiation in a PNET may obscure its true nature and may potentially lead to a diagnosis of a glial neoplasm. Hypothetically, a similar argument may be made for the glioblastoma with PNET-like component. Therefore, location, radiologic features, and intraoperative observations may prove to be extremely important in sorting through these possibilities in a given case. Papillary and rhabdoid histology may coexist in *malignant meningioma* with these histologic patterns.

Some of the other reported combinations are *meningioma and glioma*,[615,616] *meningioma and schwannoma*,[617] especially in the context of NF1, *meningioma and meningioangiomatosis*,[618] *schwannoma and perineurioma, neurofibroma and perineurioma*,[619] *schwannoma and neurofibroma*,[603] *craniopharyngioma and pituitary adenoma*,[620] which may also be in an intermingled form[621] **(Fig. 2-275)**, *pituitary adenoma and Rathke cleft cyst*,[620] and *mixed germ cell neoplasms*, with various combinations of teratomatous and non–teratomatous components. *Teratoma* has different types of tissues representing different germ layers. Teratoma with secondary malignant component, or *malignant teratoma*, is a mature or immature teratoma with a sarcoma or carcinoma arising in it, in contrast to an immature teratoma with immature elements. These malignant components are commonly undifferentiated spindle cell sarcoma, rhabdomyosarcoma, or

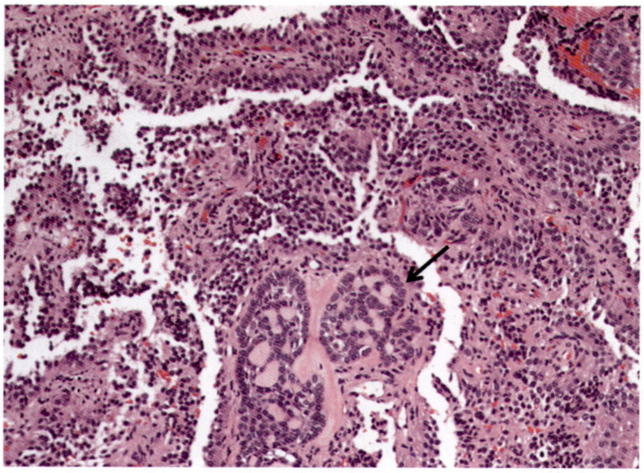

Figure 2-275. Pituitary adenoma and craniopharyngioma: Adamantinomatous craniopharyngioma islands (*arrow*) are present admixed with pituitary adenoma with pseudopapillary features (H&E; original magnification: 100×).

squamous cell carcinoma. Development of PNET also qualifies if it is at least the area of 40× magnification field in amount.[622] *MPNST* may develop from schwannoma, ganglioneuroma, and ganglioneuroblastoma. *Vascular malformations* of various types can coexist in the same lesion, such as cavernous angioma together with venous malformation or capillary telangiectasia.[623] *Aneurysmal bone cyst* can be associated with a variety of other neoplasms, most notably giant cell tumor of bone.

Metastases to other neoplasms can occur. Best known example in the CNS is metastasis to meningioma from especially lung and breast carcinoma, among others.[624,625] Usually, the metastasizing malignant neoplasm stands out in the background of low-grade meningioma; however, if the two neoplasms have somewhat similar histology, the diagnosis may be difficult and may require immunohistochemical workup. A malignant meningioma with a carcinoma-like histology should be ruled out. Typically, the clear distinction between the two components and, if necessary, immunohistochemical work-up should be helpful in this distinction. Metastasis to pituitary adenoma is rare but well-known.[626]

Different *posttreatment* histologic appearances can be seen in recurrences of some neoplasms. The new histology may be together with the original histology, creating a composite appearance, or the original histology may not be present anymore. Such changes in histology are best recognized in PNET and olfactory neuroblastoma. After treatment, a PNET may present as a ganglioneuroblastoma,[627] or an olfactory neuroblastoma may show differentiation into glandular elements mimicking adenocarcinoma or the nonneoplastic glandular elements of the upper respiratory system.[628] A similar process can be observed in the recurrences of PMA in the form of PA, with or without radiation treatment. This phenomenon is sometimes termed "maturation" and may lead to the identification of PA and PMA areas in the same neoplasm.[391] Whether focal perivascular arrangement of cells in PA represents a residual PMA or is an unremarkable histologic feature is not clear. In addition, malignant transformation in association with radiation treatment is also a well-recognized phenomenon. Postradiation sarcoma, such as MPNST in PA after radiation treatment, and postradiation meningioma are well-known.[629,630] Secondary gliosarcoma is the emergence of gliosarcoma after the initial diagnosis and treatment of a glioblastoma and is a rare occurrence.[631] Maturation of immature teratoma into mature teratoma in recurrences also occurs, likely related to treatment.[632,633] Confusion and misinterpretations can be avoided if this possibility is kept in mind, especially during IOC.

Metaplastic tissues can be present in some neoplasms. *Epithelial metaplasia* can rarely be present in glioblastoma.[634] Synonyms such as adenoid/epithelioid glioblastoma or adenoglioma are also used for this occurrence. These epithelial islands appear as distinct sheets, groups, or nests within the more obvious glial background and are positive for cytokeratin, contrasting with the GFAP-positive background. Similar epithelial metaplasias can also occur in malignant peripheral nerve sheath neoplasms, typically as a focal change, in the form of glandular, squamous, neuroendocrine, osseous, cartilaginous *metaplastic elements*.[604] *Osseous and/or cartilaginous metaplasia* can be seen in ependymoma,[635] meningioma, choroid plexus papilloma,[636] and medulloblastoma.[637] *Cartilage, bone, skeletal muscle, and irregular vessels* can be present in lipomas, supporting a hamartomatous origin.

Cellular Enlargement and Multinucleation

Cellular enlargement may have multiple implications. It may be infectious, such as viral infections; malformative, as in FCD; or neoplastic, as in giant cell glioblastoma. In general, enlarged cells are easy to spot in the background of other cells even if they are rare; however, their further characterization can be difficult in some cases. The following discussion should provide some guidance in the evaluation of lesions with large cells.

Giant cells can be multinucleated and being large with multiple nuclei leads to the term *multinucleated giant cell*. The first cell that comes to mind with multinucleated giant cell is a macrophage as seen in granulomatous inflammation. They are easy to identify in the context they are seen and do not pose a diagnostic problem. As in the case of general pathology, they are commonly associated with *granulomatous reactions*, such as in mycobacterial and fungal infections, as well as in sarcoidosis. They can have variable shapes and variable numbers of nuclei that are uniform among themselves. A typical giant cell is the Langhans-type giant cell in which the nuclei are arranged in a horseshoe pattern at the periphery of the cytoplasm. More commonly in the nonnecrotizing granulomas, they can have intracytoplasmic calcifications (Schaumann bodies) or asteroid bodies. They are not specific for any particular granulomatous process but have been usually described in association with the nonnecrotizing granulomas of sarcoidosis, which are also well-circumscribed with a thin peripheral small lymphocytic rim. Some of them can have a small, central fibrinoid necrosis, but necrosis is absent as a rule. Granulomas may not be present or prominent in immunocompromised patients. Parasitic infections can produce a prominent inflammatory reaction, including multinucleated giant cells in reaction to the parasite, sometimes as part of the infection and sometimes after the parasite is dead. Visceral larva migrans (*Toxocara canis*), cysticercus, angiostrongyliasis (*A. cantonensis*), and Schistosoma infections[638–641] are some examples of such situations. The remnants of the parasite can be identified within the inflammatory population and may help with its recognition. Granulomas, with or without multinucleated giant cells, can be seen as a prominent component of some neoplasms. Characteristically, germinomas can have granulomas,[435] which can be abundant enough to obscure the neoplastic cells, potentially resulting in misdiagnosis. Hodgkin lymphoma is another such neoplasm that can be complicated by granulomas.[436] In addition, Hodgkin lymphoma, which rarely involves the CNS,[642] depending on its histologic type, can have Reed-Sternberg cells with various appearances. Some of these cases may be extremely difficult to diagnose due to the paucity of the diagnostic Reed-Sternberg cells in the naturally reactive lymphoid population of Hodgkin lymphoma.[643] Some non-Hodgkin lymphomas, such as anaplastic large cell lymphoma, also come into this differential due to the presence of pleomorphic large cells. Multinucleated histiocytes are also seen in *foreign body giant cell* reaction, where their cytoplasm is shaped to accommodate the foreign material they are reacting to and their nuclei are grouped irregularly. In the CNS, they are commonly seen in reaction to embolization material within the vessels in

List of Findings/Checklist for Cellular Enlargement and Multinucleation

AT A GLANCE

Multinucleated Giant Cells

- Granulomatous reactions
  - Mycobacterial infections
  - Fungal infections
  - Parasitic infections
  - Viral infections
  - Sarcoidosis
  - Foreign body giant cell reaction
  - Xanthogranuloma
  - Vasculitis
  - Wegener's granulomatosis
  - Neoplasms
- HIV encephalitis
- Osteoclasts
- Touton giant cells
  - Xanthogranulomatous reactions
  - Juvenile xanthogranuloma
  - Pleomorphic xanthoastrocytoma
- Neoplasms
  - Giant cell glioblastoma
  - Glioblastoma
  - Ependymoma
  - Oligodendroglioma
  - Pilocytic astrocytoma
  - Ganglion cell neoplasms
  - Primitive neuroectodermal tumor/ medulloblastoma
  - Metastatic carcinoma and sarcoma
  - Neurothekeoma and plexiform fibrohistio-cytic tumor
  - Bone and soft tissue neoplasms
- Reactive
  - Giant cell reparative granuloma
  - Aneurysmal bone cyst
- Degenerative
  - "Ancient" change
  - Radiation change
- Syncytial trophoblasts
  - Choriocarcinoma
  - Germinoma and other germ cell neoplasms
- Astrocytic
  - Glial microhamartia
  - Giant axonal neuropathy

Large Cells

- Progressive multifocal leukoencephalopathy (PML)
- Balloon cells
  - Malformations of cortical development/ focal cortical dysplasia
  - Dysmorphic neurons
  - Neurodegenerative diseases
- Lhermitte-Duclos disease
- Subependymal giant cell astrocytome (SEGA)
- Subependymal nodules
- Prion diseases
- Inferior olivary hypertrophy
- Chromatolytic neurons
  - Spinal muscular atrophies
  - Niacin deficiency
- Storage diseases
- Ganglion cells
  - Ganglion cell neoplasms
  - Hamartomatous lesions
  - Differentiation in other neoplasms
  - Entrapment by infiltrating neoplasms

embolized neoplasms or vascular malformations. They are also common in reaction to surgical material in the previously operated patients. In addition, in *xanthogranulomas* of the choroid plexus, they are associated with cholesterol clefts resulting from hemorrhage and with keratin debris in craniopharyngiomas and in ruptured epidermoid/dermoid cysts **(Fig. 2-276)**. Xanthogranulomatous lesions[644] also occur in the pituitary/suprasellar region, in association with endolymphatic sac tumors, which, in the cerebellopontine angle, may be mistaken for xanthogranulomas or such reactions to a ruptured epidermoid cyst. Scattered multinucleated histiocytes in the white matter and especially around the blood vessels are seen in *HIV encephalitis*, but they may not necessarily be in the form of giant cells or multinucleated (see "White Matter and Myelin Disorders"). *Osteoclasts* are essentially specialized multinucleated histiocytes and are easy to recognize due to their association with bone trabeculae. They can increase in number and their nature may be obscured in cases of extensive bone destruction,

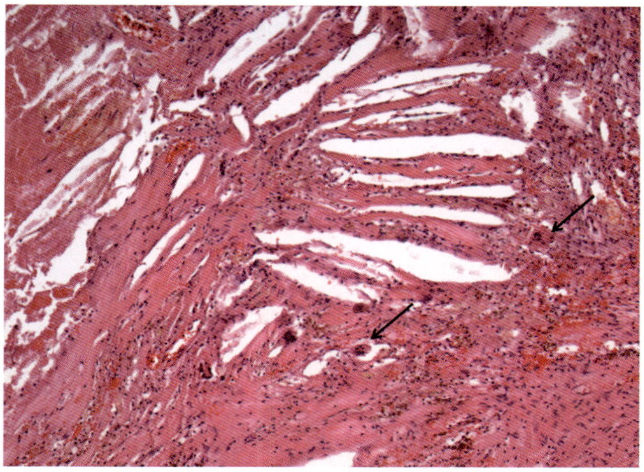

Figure 2-276. Xanthogranuloma: Many cholesterol clefts are seen in a hemorrhagic and inflammatory background with foamy histiocytes and multinucleated giant cells (*arrows*) (H&E; original magnification: 100×).

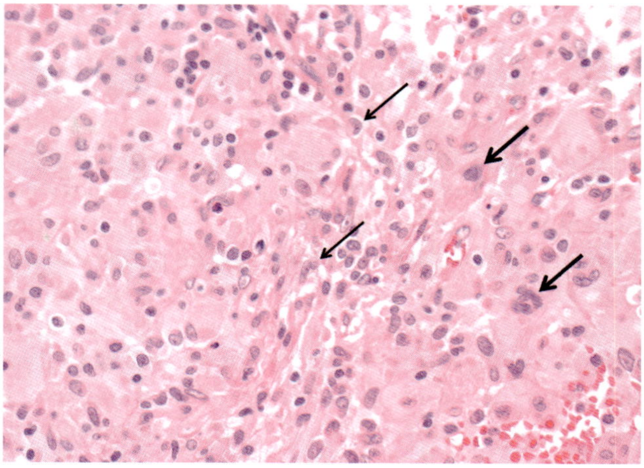

Figure 2-277. Juvenile xanthogranuloma: Many histiocytic cells with typical curved histiocyte nuclei (*thin arrows*), some of which are multinucleated giant cells (*thick arrows*), are present in a mixed inflammatory background (H&E; original magnification: 400×).

especially when the bone is overrun by an invasive/metastatic neoplasm or by a primary bone neoplasm. In such cases, the presence of these multinucleated giant cells should not be interpreted as part of the neoplasm. The same is true in the interpretation of immunohistochemical markers for histiocytes in the work-up of neoplasms. *Osteoclast-like giant cells* without atypia are seen in giant cell tumor of bone, in a background of small, spindle-to-oval cell population. They are typically quite regularly distributed in this background—one of the features helpful in distinguishing them from similar but nonneoplastic processes such as giant cell reparative granuloma[645] and aneurysmal bone cyst, which may be associated with other lesions.[646] Another type of multinucleated histiocyte is *Touton-type giant cell*. Its nuclei are grouped in the center of the cell and its cytoplasm usually has round-to-oval contours and a foamy or xanthomatous cytoplasm. It is typically associated with juvenile xanthogranuloma[647] and other histiocytic lesions that are usually seen in the soft tissues and dermis but can also occasionally occur in the CNS **(Fig. 2-277)**. Such lesions can occur as dural-based lesions, mimicking meningiomas, or as intraparenchymal mass lesions. A multinucleated giant cell with a similar appearance but neoplastic with atypical nuclei is seen in PXA, along with its mononuclear versions and prominent pleomorphism. The neoplastic nature of PXA is readily apparent and the differential diagnosis centers on distinguishing it from other neoplastic entities, such as glioblastoma. Glioblastoma commonly has mono- or multinucleated large cells but only occasionally with xanthomatous cytoplasms. Its giant cell variant can have abundant multinucleated giant cells that are obviously malignant and imply a better prognosis due to the better circumscription and, therefore, better resectability. This variant tends to be more common in BTPS type I cases.[41] A rare giant cell ependymoma has been described.[648] In regard to the xanthomatous quality of the cytoplasm, granular cell change seen in variable degrees in astrocytomas, including glioblastomas, can easily be recognized in the context of the astrocytic neoplasm, though their confusion with histiocytes may result in an erroneous diagnosis of a reactive process, as granular cell change is associated with a more aggressive biologic behavior. They are typically not in the form of giant cells or multinucleated, and immunohistochemical help may be needed. They are GFAP positive but may also show weak positivity with EMA and CD68,[428] as the latter is essentially a nonspecific lysosomal marker that can stain cells with an abundance of lysosomes. Experience with the more specific macrophage marker CD163[649] in this setting is needed. *Neoplastic multinucleated large cells* can be seen in various neoplasms but rarely cause diagnostic difficulty, as they remain scattered or remain as a focal change in the background of the otherwise typical neoplasm. Oligodendroglioma and PA can have such cells, sometimes described as "pennies on a plate" due to the peripheral circular arrangement of their nuclei. When seen in a background of otherwise typical WHO grade II astrocytoma, multinucleated giant cells may raise suspicion for the presence of a high-grade component elsewhere in the neoplasm. Ganglion cell neoplasms can have bizarre large ganglion cells, but their nuclei are usually not more than a few and they can easily be at least suspected of being neuronal origin due to their abundant cytoplasm with basophilic granularity and open chromatin with prominent nucleoli, resembling their nonneoplastic counterparts. They tend to form irregular groupings and are distributed in a disorganized manner **(Fig. 2-278)**. Rarely, a subtle case may cause diagnostic difficulty. The presence of rare abnormal forms, especially the identification of a binucleated ganglion cell, can help favor a neoplastic process. It should be remembered that very rarely, binucleated neurons can be seen in otherwise unremarkable brain; however, its nonneoplastic nature should be clear from the surrounding tissues. Metastatic carcinomas can have scattered multinucleated giant cells depending on their original histologic type. This may be in the form of occasional larger neoplastic cells with multiple atypical nuclei or more orderly distribution of

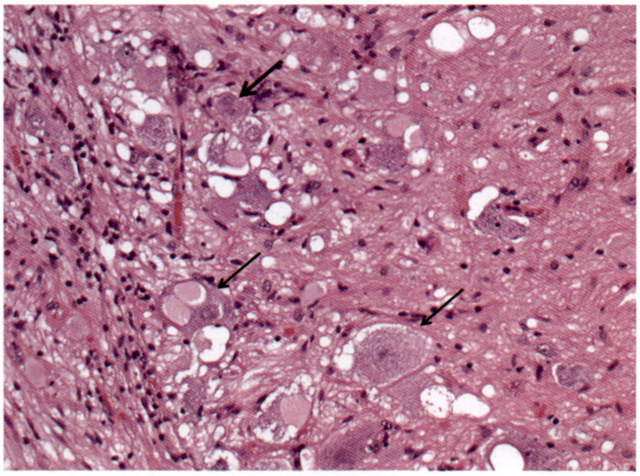

Figure 2-278. Ganglioglioma: Dysmorphic, giant ganglion cells (*thin arrows*) are present in an irregular distribution with grouping. Occasional binucleated forms (*thick arrow*) are also seen (H&E; original magnification: 400×).

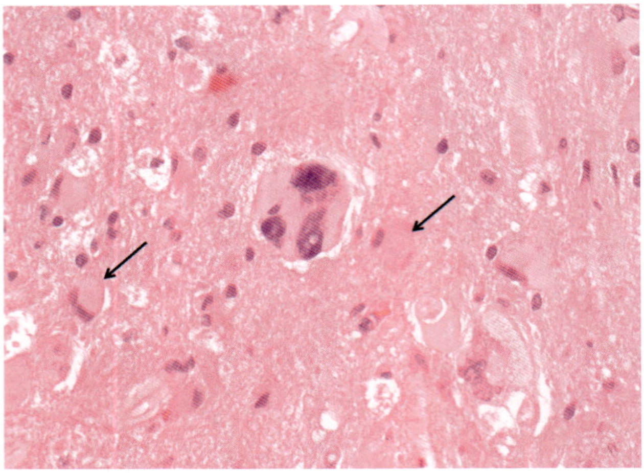

Figure 2-279. Radiation change: A bizarre cell with multinucleation, nuclear and cytoplasmic enlargement, and smudgy chromatin pattern is seen in the center, representing a neoplastic cell with radiation change. Other cells (*arrows*) may be difficult to identify as being neoplastic or reactive in isolation (H&E; original magnification: 400×).

osteoclast-like giant cells. Primary bone lesions, neoplastic such as giant cell tumor of bone or nonneoplastic such as aneurysmal bone cysts, can have osteoclastic giant cells. Various sarcomas, primary or metastatic, can also commonly have multinucleated giant cells, one prominent example being malignant fibrous histiocytoma. *Bizarre cellular changes,* often with multinucleation, occur in neoplastic and nonneoplastic cells as a result of radiation treatment **(Fig. 2-279)**. The knowledge of previous diagnosis and treatment, as well as the presence of other radiation-related changes, helps accurately identify such cellular enlargement. They typically have smudgy chromatin pattern and a proportionate enlargement of nucleus and cytoplasm. It is also important to be aware of and consider this type of change in the evaluation of recurrences of low-grade neoplasms that have been radiated after initial diagnosis so that they are not assigned a higher grade based on the cellular and vascular changes associated with radiation treatment. When there is obvious bulky neoplasm, it is easy to recognize a recurrence; however, when only scattered atypical cells are seen, it may be impossible to say anything more than "scattered atypical cells" with a comment describing the absence of a definitive neoplasm. Easily identified mitotic figures and increased proliferation index may help

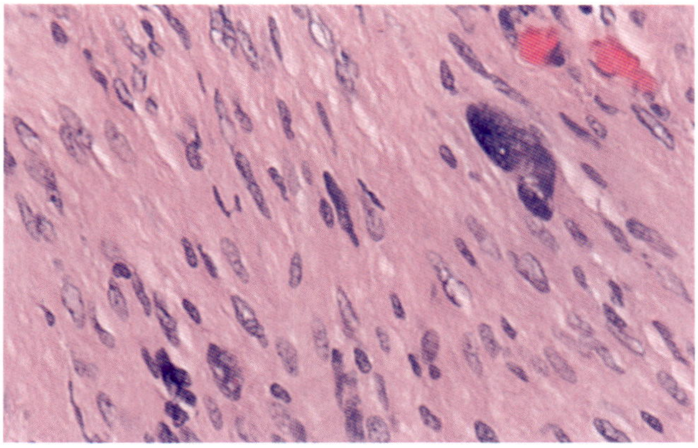

Figure 2-280. Schwannoma: So-called degenerative atypia, also known as ancient change, is characterized by nuclear enlargement and hyperchromasia and should not be interpreted as a sign of malignancy. Smudgy chromatin pattern and their isolated nature in a background of bland cells favor nonneoplastic origin (H&E; original magnification: 400×).

favor a neoplasm, though one should consider the presence of vascular changes and inflammatory cells and their contribution to these parameters. P53 overexpression in these scattered atypical cells supports their neoplastic, rather than reactive, nature. Scattered giant cells, usually with smudgy chromatin and irregular nuclear borders, can be seen in some neoplasms that are otherwise unremarkable benign examples of their kind. They represent a *degenerative change*, sometimes called "ancient" change, and are well-known in schwannomas **(Fig. 2-280)** but can also be present in other low-grade neoplasms, such as meningiomas, and more commonly in angiomatous and microcystic variants, subependymomas, and myxopapillary ependymomas. Scattered, large, hyperchromatic nuclei can be seen in an otherwise unremarkable pituitary adenoma without increased mitotic activity, proliferation index, or p53 overexpression. These cells have smudgy chromatin and also represent a degenerative change, with no prognostic significance. Adenomas should not be diagnosed as atypical adenoma based on these cells or other cytologic changes. The term atypical adenoma refers to increased mitotic activity, more than 3% proliferative index, and immunohistochemical p53 positivity, although this has not been consistently applied and the concept has not yet been settled.[650,651] Likewise, there is no significant correlation between the cytologic features and pituitary carcinoma, which is described as a pituitary neoplasm with distant metastasis and/or craniospinal dissemination. Scattered multinucleated giant cells can be present in the neoplastic cellular areas of germinomas and embryonal carcinomas and represent *syncytiotrophoblasts*.[652] The nuclei appear bunched up and have smudgy chromatin. The cytoplasm is amphophilic. They are positive for beta-HCG and may be responsible for elevated plasma beta-HCG levels. These findings should not prompt a diagnosis of choriocarcinoma. Scattered multinucleated giant cells can be seen in the atypical pineocytoma. Although they are not a predominant feature, they contribute to the "atypical" appearance along with the other cytologic changes. Neurothekeoma and plexiform fibrohistiocytic tumor also have variable numbers of multinucleated large neoplastic cells (see "Nodular Arrangement"). Viral infections such as Herpes virus and measles inclusion body encephalitis typically have multinucleation with intranuclear inclusions. Multinucleated giant cells associated with vessels, perivascular and/or intramural, are seen in giant cell arteritis and PACNS. They are closely associated with internal elastic lamina, and a Verhoeff-van Gieson stain can highlight the damage to the internal elastic lamina with ingested fragments of it within the cytoplasm of giant cells. Other inflammatory cells, such as lymphocytes, plasma cells, and macrophages are also present, as well as variable fibrous thickening of the vessel wall. Wegener's granulomatosis[653] also contains multinucleated giant cells associated with vague granulomas or floating in the necrosis. Glial microhamartoma[654] is a microscopic aggregate of mono- or *multinucleated dysplastic astrocytes*. They may form a quite pleomorphic population standing out in the background of an otherwise unremarkable parenchyma. They can be present adjacent to other malformative lesions, such as meningioangiomatosis typically associated with NF2. Due to the presence of quite atypical nuclei, they should not be confused with infiltrating high-grade glioma cells. Giant axonal neuropathy[655,656] results in deep white matter degeneration in the brain, cerebellum, and the long tracts of the spinal cord. It is associated with axonal swellings, especially in corticospinal tracts and posterior tracts, as well as peripheral nerves. Axonal spheroids are present also in the cerebral cortex and basal ganglia. Many Rosenthal fibers are present in the white matter and around vessels, resembling Alexander's disease. Occasional large, sometimes multinucleated astrocytes may be present and may resemble PML.

Aside from multinucleation, many of the *large cells* are similar to their normal counterparts with the exception of their larger size and some degree of dysmorphic features in some cases. PML also typically has enlarged and bizarre astrocytes as a result of viral cytopathic effect, sometimes potentially creating confusion with a neoplastic process. Some degree of enlargement and ballooning is usually present in anterior horn neurons of the spinal cord with increasing age. FCD/MCD[10] may have large cells with glassy eosinophilic, somewhat irregular cytoplasm devoid of Nissl substance. These are sometimes referred to as grotesque cells or *balloon cells*. They have mixed neuronal and glial features with a neuron-like nucleus and an astrocyte-like cytoplasm **(Fig. 2-281)**. They stain for both neuronal markers, such as synaptophysin, and GFAP. These may be together with large *dysmorphic neurons* that are easily recognized as of neuronal origin with their cytoplasmic features, including the presence of Nissl substance **(Fig. 2-282)**. Balloon cells qualify a FCD as Taylor type IIb. FCDs can be sporadic or may represent the tubers in the context

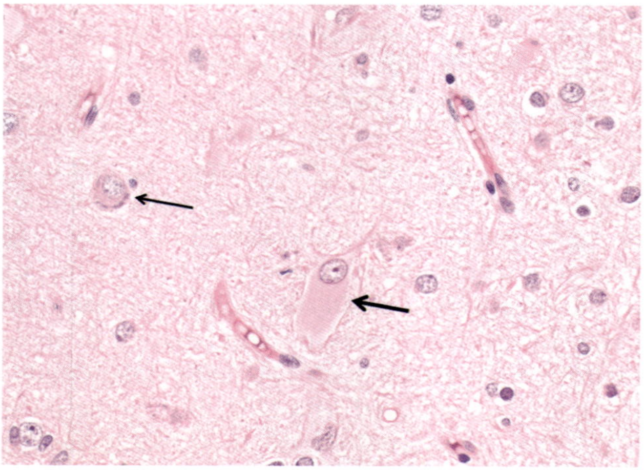

Figure 2-281. Balloon cell: A large cell (*thick arrow*), sometimes referred to as grotesque cell, is seen in this FCD and has a cytoplasm that is more consistent with astrocytic lineage, while its nucleus is similar to that of a neuron. A nearby neuron (*thin arrow*) is much smaller (H&E; original magnification: 400×).

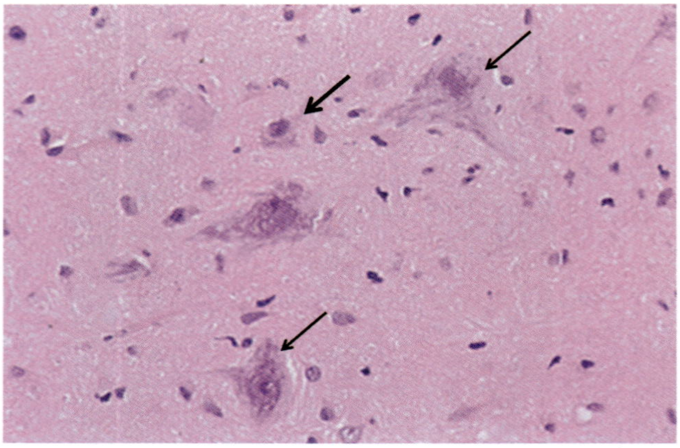

Figure 2-282. Dysmorphic neurons: Large, irregular neurons (*thin arrows*) with disorderly orientation are seen in this FCD. In contrast to the balloon cells, they can be easily recognized as neurons. A relatively normal nearby neuron (*thick arrow*) is also present (H&E; original magnification: 400×).

of tuberous sclerosis. In the latter case, they tend to be multiple and associated with other stigmata of tuberous sclerosis. Sometimes, a tuberous sclerosis patient may be recognized by the diagnosis of FCD, and such patients should be further investigated for the presence of other tuberous sclerosis features. FCD can be present next to other lesions, such as ganglion cell neoplasms. It has also been described in association with angiocentric glioma and other neoplasms.[610,657] Fetal mercury exposure can also result in heterotopias and cortical dysplasias in the brain and cerebellum. Changes in the cortex that are reminiscent of MCD due to a disorganized appearance of the neurons can be seen adjacent to destructive lesions, such as infarcts, that may have occurred during development. A histologic picture similar to that of the cortical dysplasia present in a more diffuse manner within the white matter, with large cells with glassy eosinophilic cytoplasms standing out in the background, likely represents radial glioneuronal heterotopias in the setting of tuberous sclerosis. In the cerebellum, complete replacement of internal granule layer neurons by ganglion cells, resulting in a diffuse but orderly expansion of the cerebellar foliar architecture, is diagnostic of Lhermitte-Duclos disease (dysplastic gangliocytoma of the cerebellum). Other possible findings in the CNS associated with Lhermitte-Duclos disease are neuronal heterotopias in the white matter, vascular malformations, syrinx formation, hydromyelia, and olivary hypertrophy. It can be a component of Cowden syndrome, as well.[658] SEGA is essentially entirely composed of large cells with neuron-like nuclei and astrocyte-like cytoplasm. These cells with abundant cytoplasm are densely packed and may impart an epithelioid look to the lesion. Close examination reveals a variable amount of fibrillary background. The cells have tapering cytoplasms and are arranged in groups or fascicles. They may be grouped around vessels rendering them prominent. SEGA is a WHO grade I neoplasm. It is well-circumscribed in spite of its cytologically atypical and worrisome appearance and contrasts with the infiltrative nature of high-grade glial neoplasms. Rare cases can have mitotic activity and foci of necrosis.[659] The histologic features of SEGA are the same as those of subependymal nodules and, although SEGA can measure from less than 1 cm to over several centimeters, there has been no definitive cutoff measurement. When a subependymal nodule becomes a SEGA is mainly dependent on when it results in clinical manifestations, which in turn is also associated with its location to some degree.[660–662] Sequential imaging follow-up demonstrates subependymal nodules to grow over time to become SEGA.[661]

Neuronal enlargement can also occur in diverse conditions.[17] Some swelling may occur in some cortical neurons in prion diseases. In niacin deficiency, cortical, spinal, and brainstem neurons are swollen. Inferior olivary hypertrophy is a form of degeneration associated with ipsilateral tegmental tract degeneration (see "Tract Degeneration"). It is hypertrophic with enlarged and vacuolated neurons. In general, chromatolytic neurons appear larger and they are typically grouped together in the nuclei that are affected by the process, rather than scattered individual cells. Some examples of chromatolytic neuronal changes are anterior horn neurons in spinal muscular atrophies; Betz cells, pontine nuclei, dentate nucleus, and anterior horn neurons in niacin deficiency; and spinal and brainstem neurons in porphyria. Storage diseases also result in enlargement of neurons, but usually in a diffuse manner, although some regions may be affected more prominently. GM1 and GM2 gangliosidoses, Niemann-Pick disease, fucosidosis, and Pompe disease are some examples. Vincristine can result in distention of spinal cord and brainstem neurons by neurofilament accumulation. Enlarged or ballooned neurons can be seen in association with neurodegenerative diseases. In CBD, scattered swollen cerebral cortical neurons that are positive for alpha–beta crystalline, neurofilament, and tau are seen. Such swollen neurons can rarely be seen in AD also and should be evaluated for CBD. Dementia with changes of CBD has CBD neuropathology without the clinical movement disorder but with the clinical features of frontotemporal dementia. Such swollen neurons can also be seen in the so-called frontal AD that has pathologic features of AD but has the clinical features of frontotemporal involvement. Scattered swollen neurons may be present in FTLD, including Pick's disease. Spinal motor neuron ballooning can be seen in ALS (see "Neuron Loss and Gliosis" for other features of these diseases).

Ganglion cell differentiation[42] can be seen mostly focally in neoplasms. The ganglion cells stand out and are easily identified in the background of a smaller neoplastic cell population. Medulloblastoma, PNET, neurocytoma (more common in extraventricular neurocytoma than in central neurocytoma), paraganglioma, pituitary adenoma, and even PA can have scattered ganglion cells. Especially in the latter, there is the possibility of entrapped resident neurons; however, the well circumscription of PA makes this possibility less likely. Nonetheless, this feature should not be interpreted as a ganglioglioma. Similar concern should be present for a neurofibroma infiltrating the dorsal root ganglia, entrapping the resident ganglion cells versus a ganglioneuroma. Truly neoplastic ganglion cells that do not have their surrounding satellite cells also tend to show irregular groupings and dysmorphic features. They are less likely to contain lipofuscin pigment that is so common and prominent in the nonneoplastic dorsal root ganglion cells, especially with advanced age. Especially medulloblastoma with extensive nodularity can undergo prominent and extensive ganglion cell differentiation, resembling a ganglion cell neoplasm or ganglioneuroblastoma. Similar differentiations in the form of maturation of a primitive neoplasm can also occur in olfactory neuroblastoma and PNET. This can be in the form of ganglion cell differentiation and, as in the case of olfactory neuroblastoma, also in the form of glandular/epithelial differentiation, reflecting the divergent differentiation potential of the primitive olfactory neuroepithelium. In pituitary adenoma, ganglion cell differentiation tends to occur more commonly in growth hormone cell adenomas.[663] There may be binucleated forms. They also express

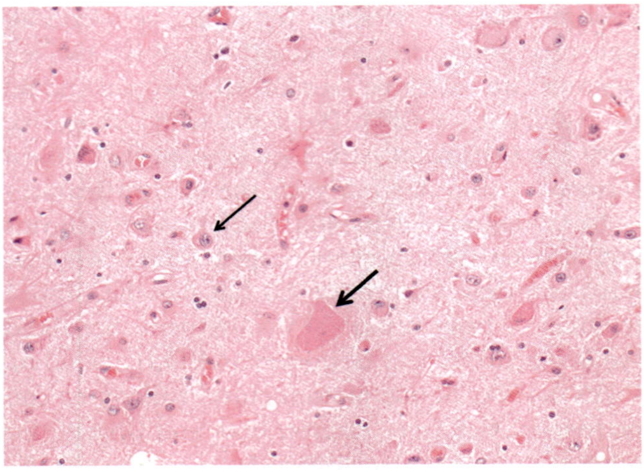

Figure 2-283. Neuronal gigantism: Enlargement of cerebral cortical neurons (*thick arrow*) can be seen after radiation treatment. A relatively unremarkable nearby neuron is also seen (*thin arrow*) (H&E; original magnification: 200×).

the pituitary hormone the adenoma cells secrete, as well as cytokeratin, supporting their metaplastic nature arising from the adenoma cells. They do not have any prognostic significance. Rarely, a pure ganglion cell neoplasm is present with or without the adenoma.[664,665] Whether this represents an entirely transformed pituitary adenoma or a gangliocytoma that happened to arise in the sella may be debatable. One of the rare complications of radiation therapy is a peculiar focal neuronal gigantism and cortical thickening[666] **(Fig. 2-283)**.

Nuclear Features

As in any microscopic evaluation, nuclear detail can provide valuable information, especially when the differential diagnostic possibilities have been reduced to a few with the help of clinical, radiologic, gross, and low-power microscopic pattern. Although there is much overlap, certain nuclear features are typically indicative of certain lesions or group of diseases. Unfortunately, the nuclear detail can vary significantly depending on the fixation and the quality of processing, sectioning, and staining, as well as the cytologic, frozen, or paraffin-embedded nature of the tissue. Therefore, as everything else, nuclear features should also be interpreted in the given context, together with other findings. Please also refer to Chapters 3 and 5 for additional details regarding the cytologic preparations.

List of Findings/Checklist for Nuclear Features

• AT A GLANCE

Nuclear Contours
- Spindled
- Wavy
- Round
- Raisinoid/cerebriform
- Irregular/thick nuclear membranes
- Nuclear grooves (coffee bean nuclei)
- Multilobation

Chromatin Pattern
- Salt and pepper chromatin
- Barr body
- Open chromatin pattern (with prominent nucleoli)
- Cartwheel chromatin
- Clumped chromatin
- Hyperchromasia
- Smudgy chromatin
- Coarse chromatin
- Ground-glass chromatin

Intranuclear Features
- Cytoplasmic invaginations (pseudoinclusion)
- Pseudo-pseudoinclusions
- Inclusions (see "Intranuclear Inclusions")
- Vacuolated nuclei

Nucleoli
- Chromocenters
- Micronucleoli
- Nucleoli/macronucleoli
- Irregular/bar-shaped nucleoli

Atypia/pleomorphism (See also "Cellular Enlargement and Multinucleation")

While the nuclei are usually round to oval and appear to be of no particular significance in terms of shape, there are some situations where a particular *nuclear contour* may be associated with a specific cell type or a group of lesions. In general, when the phrase *"spindle cell"* is attached to a description, it refers to the shape of the nucleus and it is implied that at least part of the differential diagnosis includes mesenchymal lesions. Sometimes, the inaccurate term "fibroblastic" may be erroneously used to refer to the general spindled appearance of the nuclei, since fibroblast is the prototype of spindle cells. In the CNS, mesenchymal lesions are typically dural based. Some prominent examples are hemangiopericytoma/SFT; metastatic or primary sarcomas, such as meningeal fibrosarcoma, leiomyosarcoma, and liposarcomas with dedifferentiated areas; and inflammatory myofibroblastic tumor. In the case of smooth muscle neoplasms, an association in some cases with immunosuppression, as in organ transplantation and AIDS, as well as with Epstein-Barr virus (EBV) has been noted. Smooth muscle neoplasms associated with EBV has been reported.[667,668] The histiocytic spindle cell lesion due to Mycobacterium avium-intracellulare infection, seen in immunocompromised patients, may be mistaken for a neoplastic process.[669] Cytologic preparations from these lesions show the negative images of the bacteria, especially if Romanowsky stain or a modification, is used.

Peripheral nerve sheath tumors, most notably schwannoma, neurofibroma, and MPNSTs, are also predominantly spindle cell neoplasms. In general, especially in the benign peripheral nerve sheath tumors, at least a subpopulation of nuclei have a *wavy contour* and typically one tip of the nucleus is pointy, in contrast to the other tip that tends to be blunt **(Fig. 2-284)**. These benign nuclei have uniform, homogeneous chromatin pattern. It is not unusual to have a smudgy dark chromatin in an occasional large, irregular nucleus, that is, ancient change, in these neoplasms and perineuriomas. They may be prominent and widespread.[670–672] Spindle or elongated nuclei are seen uniformly in a low-grade ependymoma variant, tanycytic ependymoma.[673] It is frequently seen in the spinal cord and can have a resemblance to schwannoma or PA, rather than the typical ependymoma. Perivascular pseudorosettes are rare and should be searched diligently in such cases, as true rosettes are not present. Even degenerative nuclear changes in the form of nuclear enlargement and pleomorphism can be present to cause further confusion with schwannoma, with no prognostic implications. Difficult cases may require immunohistochemical work-up with GFAP, S-100 protein, collagen type IV, and EMA. It is an intra-axial neoplasm with radiologic features similar to those of classical ependymoma. Spindle cell, sarcomatous areas may be a component of ATRT,[542] which should be considered as a possibility in young children, as actual spindle cell sarcomas are less likely in this age group.

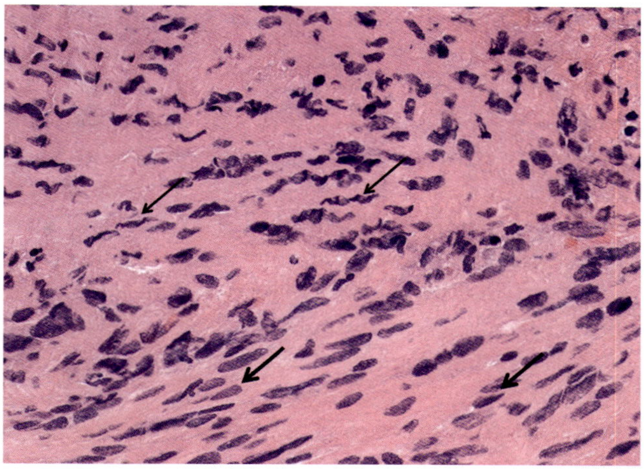

Figure 2-284. Schwannoma: As usually is the case with peripheral nerve sheath neoplasms, nuclei have a peculiar wavy appearance (*thin arrows*). One tip of many nuclei has a tendency to be more pointy than the other (*thick arrows*) (H&E; original magnification: 400×).

Meningiomas can be entirely spindle cell, termed fibroblastic meningioma. In cases with abundant collagen, the cells may be overtaken by the collagenous stroma and the spindle cells may become even blander. Cells of the fibroblastic meningioma tend to have plump, irregular, "fibroblastic," rather than typical, meningothelial nuclei. They have variably open chromatin and small nucleoli **(Fig. 2-285)**. The

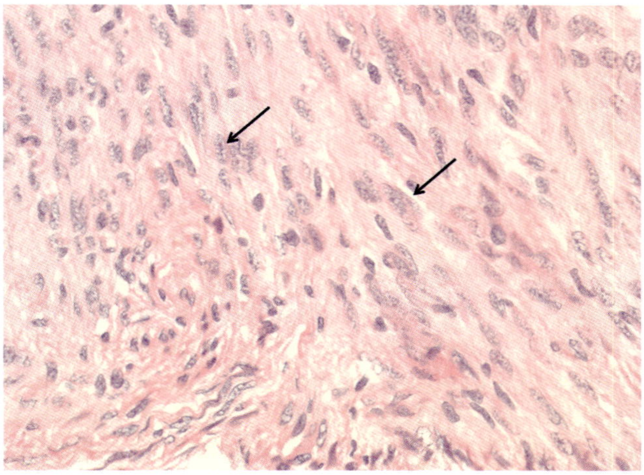

Figure 2-285. Fibroblastic meningioma: Nuclei resemble fibroblast nuclei in that they are plump with rounded tips, have open chromatin, and may have small nucleoli (*arrows*) (H&E; original magnification: 400×).

poles of the nuclei are usually blunt. Though harder to find, intranuclear cytoplasmic invaginations and occasional abortive whorls will usually clarify the lesion's meningothelial origin. In the malignant (WHO grade III; anaplastic) meningioma, a spindle cell component may be difficult to differentiate from a primary (or metastatic) meningeal sarcoma, or metastatic sarcomatoid carcinoma. Typically in malignant meningioma, there are other areas with more recognizable meningioma histology and usually a history of multiple resections with diagnosis of meningioma, supporting a malignant transformation in meningioma. The differential diagnosis of a spindle cell neoplasm in the cerebellopontine angle is fibroblastic meningioma and schwannoma. The typical cases are easy to distinguish with their characteristic histologic features; however, overlapping features are not uncommon, and composite form is possible (see "Biphasic Pattern, Composite Lesions and Metaplastic Tissues"). Fibroblastic meningiomas may have quite thin and wavy nuclei with pointy tips and may even show nuclear palisading, while schwannomas may not always have the biphasic appearance and may be composed only of cellular Antoni A areas. Rich, pericellular reticulin network, diffuse and strong S-100 protein positivity, and pericellular collagen type IV positivity with negative EMA favor schwannoma, while at least patchy EMA positivity is a feature of meningiomas. Fibroblastic meningiomas may have focal S-100 protein positivity, although not to the degree of the positivity seen in schwannomas. Reticulin tends to be more prominent in perivascular areas, and collagen type IV shows irregular focal positivity. A third and rare neoplasm that may present in the cerebellopontine angle (CPA) due to its bone-destructive nature and has a quite different, epithelioid papillary and glandular histology is endolymphatic sac tumor. Ingrowth of peripheral nerve fibers into the spinal cord parenchyma may be seen during the healing process of cord lesions, infarcts, hemorrhage, and traumatic lesions, resulting in a spindle cell proliferation that can range from small perivascular foci to larger areas **(Fig. 2-286)**. This process, called schwannosis, can be associated with neurofibromatosis, also.[402,674] Similar situations may also result in collagenous scarring of cord lesions in the long term. Melanocytoma, especially when amelanotic, can be confused with fibroblastic meningioma due to its bland cytologic features, frequent spindling, and

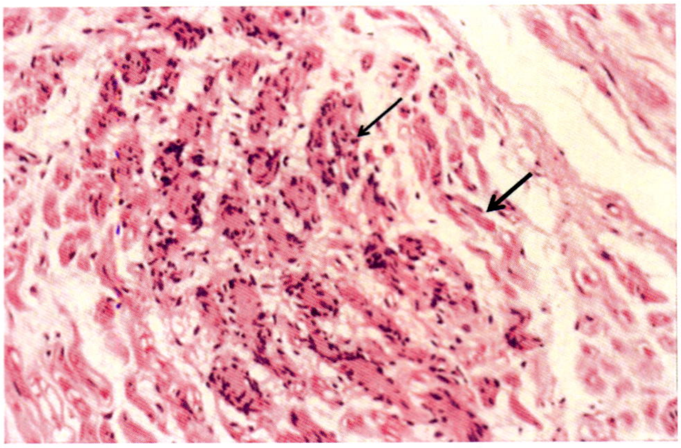

Figure 2-286. Schwannosis: This spinal nerve fascicle seen in a herniated nucleus pulposus excision specimen shows a peculiar schwannian proliferation (*thin arrow*) in some of its fibers, compared to the adjacent unremarkable ones (*thick arrow*). This process likely is reactive and occurred as a result of trauma due to herniated nucleus pulposus in this case (H&E; original magnification: 200×).

the presence of a vague swirling pattern of its cells. Melanocytoma tends to have more oval nuclear contours and a more prominent nucleolus compared to fibroblastic meningioma **(Fig. 2-287)**. In pigmented cases, melanotic schwannoma should be excluded.[675]

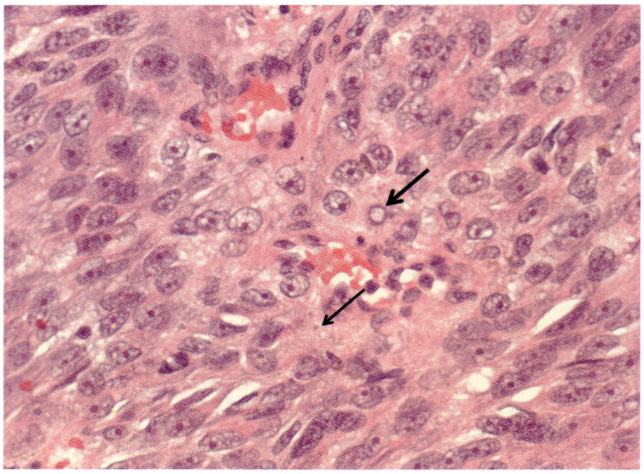

Figure 2-287. Melanocytoma: Striking resemblance of the nuclei to those of fibroblastic meningioma is further complicated by the intranuclear cytoplasmic invaginations (pseudoinclusions), which are also common in melanocytic cells (*thick arrow*). Although a very minimal finely granular pigment can be found after some search (*thin arrow*), obvious pigment is typically absent when most needed, as usual (H&E; original magnification: 400×).

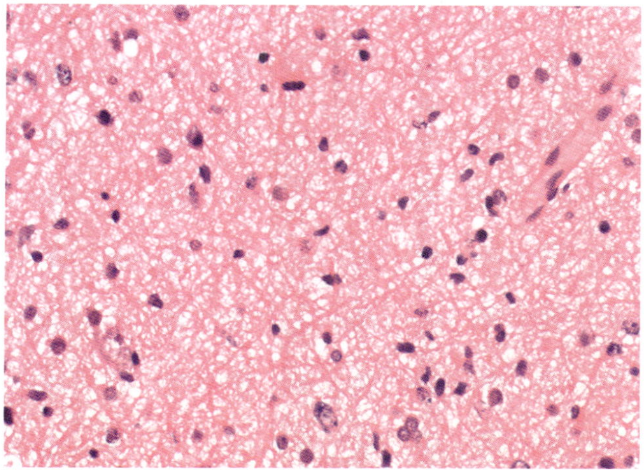

Figure 2-288. Astrocytoma: Hyperchromatic and irregular nuclei with only rare small nucleoli and with irregular distribution and orientation are characteristic for astrocytoma (H&E; original magnification: 400×).

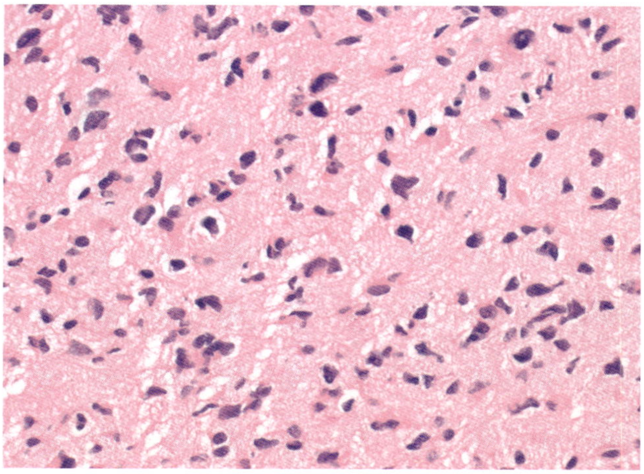

Figure 2-289. Oligodendroglioma: It is essentially impossible to make a diagnosis of oligodendroglioma based only on the paraffin sections of a previously frozen tissue, as it will look similar to an astrocytoma (compare to Fig. 2-288) (H&E; original magnification: 400×).

Cellular areas alternating with less cellular areas with thick collagen bundles, at least focally associated with a hemangiopericytomatous vascular pattern, are highly suggestive of a SFT in a dural-based spindle cell mass lesion. Hemangiopericytoma, on the other hand, has smaller and more round to oval, rather than elongated, spindle cells with a homogeneous cellularity and widespread branching, staghorn vascular pattern.

Spindle cells can be seen in glial neoplasms, especially in astrocytomas and especially in glioblastoma. In general, for glial neoplasms, nuclear spindling, irregularities, and angulated contours, especially combined with a coarse, hyperchromatic chromatin pattern, indicate astrocytic lineage **(Fig. 2-288)**. The spindling in glioblastoma can also be associated with sarcomatous component. Sarcomatous areas usually are perivascular, but this may be difficult to appreciate if these areas are widespread. They also stand out as more solid sheets or islands of compact cellularity in the fibrillary background of a relatively loosely textured glioblastoma component with spindled but smaller and darker nuclei. PXA typically has a spindled or elongated cell morphology to its astrocytic cells, sometimes resulting in a storiform pattern.

In surgical specimens, thermal artifact from cautery application creates an elongation of nuclei, typically in the same direction, giving them a false appearance of a spindle cell or an astrocytic appearance. The walls of any admixed vessels and any fibrous tissue fragments show a deep purple homogenization to provide a clue to the possibility of thermal artifact in such areas. In the fibrous tissue fragments, numerous irregular spaces are created as a result of retraction of tissue and cells. Such areas should not be included in the interpretation. Paraffin section of previously frozen oligodendroglioma shows the nuclei to appear angulated and spindled, resulting in an astrocytic appearance **(Fig. 2-289)**. This should be kept in mind while evaluating such previously frozen sections. Therefore, it is important to secure unfrozen tissue during intraoperative consultations, if no additional tissue can be provided for routine processing. A similar nuclear change can be seen in oligodendrogliomas after radiation treatment as a result of radiation effect, resulting in confusion, unnecessary upgrading, and possibly misdiagnosis as astrocytoma or glioblastoma in recurrent oligodendrogliomas. PNET, and especially S-PNET, can show frequent and considerable glial differentiation, as well as neuronal differentiation.[676] Glial areas tend to appear as more spindled areas within the primitive cell population. In some cases, recurrences of S-PNET may be predominantly in the form of a glioma. Among pituitary adenomas, especially TSH cell adenomas tend to have elongated cells with oval to spindled nuclei, creating a vague

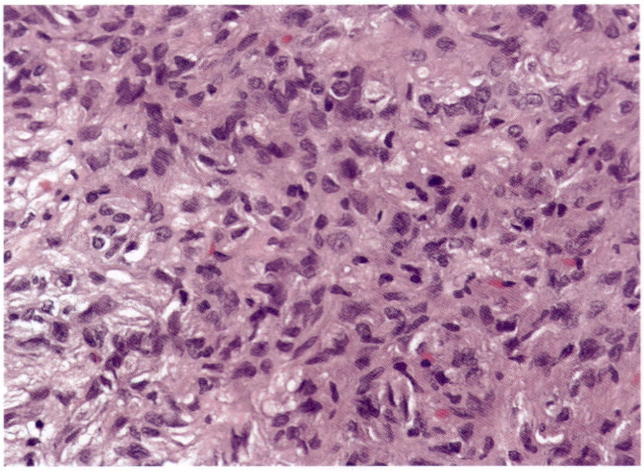

Figure 2-290. Pituicytoma: Due to the spindling and vague grouping of its cells, pituicytoma can easily be misdiagnosed as a fibroblastic meningioma or astrocytoma. Knowledge of its sellar/suprasellar location and awareness of its existence should help avoid such mishaps (H&E; original magnification: 400×).

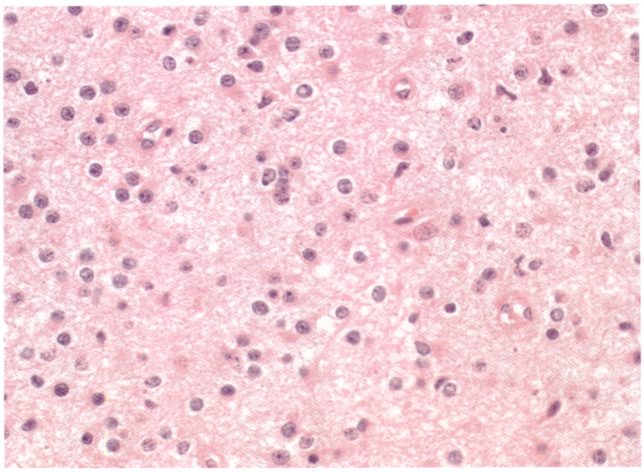

Figure 2-291. Oligodendroglioma: Almost perfectly and uniformly round nuclei with a finely granular chromatin and small nucleoli or chromocenters are characteristic of oligodendroglioma and constitute the main diagnostic feature for it among several other features mentioned elsewhere in this text (H&E; original magnification: 400×).

streaming or fascicular pattern. In the sellar region, the major neoplasms with a spindle cell morphology are spindle cell oncocytoma of the adenohypophysis, which has been suggested to originate from the folliculostellate cells[70,677] and pituicytoma[678] **(Fig. 2-290)**.

The *round nuclear contours* are typical for several neoplasms and cell types. In oligodendroglioma, round nuclei are considered to be the main diagnostic microscopic feature along with several other supportive features **(Fig. 2-291)**. Their presence is essential in the difficult distinction of pure oligodendroglioma from oligoastrocytoma, especially the intermingled type where clear and separate oligodendroglial and astrocytic components cannot be discerned but decision of whether the neoplasm is astrocytic or oligodendroglial is also a difficult one. Round nuclei are also important in the identification of an oligodendroglial component in other neoplasms, namely, glioblastoma with oligodendroglioma component. Other supportive features that can be present in oligodendroglioma in variable combinations and amounts are clear cytoplasm, microcalcifications, chicken-wire vasculature, finely granular chromatin, micronucleoli/chromocenters, and minigemistocytes. In general, the basophilic chromatin clump that is somewhat more prominent than the rest of the chromatin is referred to as chromocenter. When it is still small but assumes an eosinophilic or amphophilic quality, then it becomes a micronucleolus, and when it is obviously standing out as an eosinophilic structure in the nucleus in the background of the chromatin, then it is a nucleolus or macronucleolus. Nonneoplastic oligodendrogliocytes also have round nuclei. They are abundant in the white matter and can be seen lined up along the nerve fibers or in small groups. This appearance can be difficult to differentiate from a diffusely infiltrating low-grade oligodendroglioma that shows low cellularity. The nuclei of resting oligodendrogliocytes are smaller than their neoplastic counterparts and have a more condensed chromatin pattern that is more reminiscent of that of the small lymphocyte rather than the finely granular chromatin of the enlarged nucleus of the neoplastic oligodendrogliocytes with small nucleoli. When the nonneoplastic oligodendroglia group about the capillaries, they may resemble small lymphocytes around the vessels seen in inflammatory processes or sometimes with no particular explanation. Their perivascular tendencies should be apparent especially at low power, punctuating the monotonous cellularity of the white matter. Typical oligodendroglioma may rarely constitute the glioma component of a ganglioglioma.[593] In such cases, the differential diagnosis of this round cell component is between oligodendroglioma and a small, round neuronal/neurocytic population, which can be distinguished by the fibrillary background and by using immunohistochemistry. The expression of neuronal markers in oligodendrogliomas[679] and the ganglion cell like maturation in some oligodendrogliomas[595] may complicate this work-up. Another histologically very similar neoplasm especially in terms of round nuclei is central neurocytoma. It too has similar-sized round nuclei with finely granular chromatin pattern and micronucleoli/chromocenters. In some areas, its cells may even have clear cytoplasms and microcalcifications are frequently present to further mimic oligodendroglioma. Its background has a delicate, neuropil-like quality relative to the more glial background of oligodendroglioma. Noting its intraventricular location is also important, although extraventricular neurocytomas are also present, and helps avoid misdiagnosis as intraventricular oligodendroglioma.[680] It is possible, however, that some cases diagnosed as intraventricular oligodendroglioma before the description of central neurocytoma were in fact central neurocytomas.[681] Small, round cells of neurocytic nature, resembling those of central neurocytoma, can be seen in papillary glioneuronal tumor and rosette-forming glioneuronal tumor of the fourth ventricle but do not cause a diagnostic problem, as these neoplasms have distinct histologic features. Liponeurocytoma[682] is a peculiar neoplasm that arises only in adults, typically in the cerebellar vermis or hemispheres, occasionally in the cerebellopontine angle, and rarely in the supratentorial location within the ventricles. This neoplasm has cells similar to those of neurocytoma and, in addition, has a variably vacuolated cell population resembling mature adipose tissue. Pineal parenchymal tumors of intermediate differentiation can have sheets of uniform round cells that result in an oligodendroglioma- or neurocytoma-like appearance. Alternatively, they can be in a lobular arrangement, divided by fibrovascular septae. Only a few, if any, pineocytomatous rosettes can be seen. This roundness and uniformity are also seen in the smaller cells of pineocytomas, but they are punctuated by pineocytomatous rosettes and are easy to recognize as a pineal parenchymal tumor. The retention of the nuclear features, without reaching a small, blue cell or primitive neuroectodermal appearance, is important to note because vascular proliferation, necrosis, some degree of mitotic activity, and even leptomeningeal infiltration can be present in the high-grade variant of pineal parenchymal tumor of intermediate differentiation and should not be confused with pineoblastoma. This is especially true for the pleomorphic variant of low-grade PPTID, in which the pineocytomatous rosettes may be scant, if any.

Fetal stage neurons are usually very small and their nuclei may appear quite hyperchromatic and round. In brains of late fetal period where the germinal matrix cells have almost completed their migration, all there is left representing the residual portions of germinal matrix may be the small aggregates of perivascular cells with round nuclei. These small groups usually have a skewed or polarized appearance around the vessel. Another cell type with round nuclei that can be extremely devastating for the unwary is the small neurons of the cerebellar internal granule layer. They present a particular challenge in the cytologic preparations of the cerebellar tissue in intraoperative consultations. Their identification on frozen sections is easier due to the recognition of the cerebellar cortical architecture. They have round, hyperchromatic nuclei with condensed chromatin and a central chromocenter. They are similar to the cells of the central neurocytoma. Their darker and condensed chromatin is useful in telling them apart from oligodendrogliomas, while the presence of easily identified chromocenter helps in differentiating them from nonneoplastic oligodendrogliocytes and lymphocytes.

The great majority of lymphomas in the brain are of diffuse large B-cell type, and as such, especially in cellular specimens where they present as sheets of cells, they may be difficult to distinguish from carcinomas or high-grade gliomas. This confusion is more likely in diffusely infiltrating pattern of lymphomas, rather than those forming sheet-like growth and/or angiocentric pattern **(Fig. 2-292)**. Nuclear features are especially useful in at least suspecting the possibility of a high-grade lymphoma in a diffusely infiltrating process in small samples. Close examination of the nuclei reveals a finely granular to *open chromatin pattern with multiple nucleoli that tend to be located closer to the nuclear membrane*. The nuclear membrane is typically irregular with convolutions. In follicular lymphomas with a

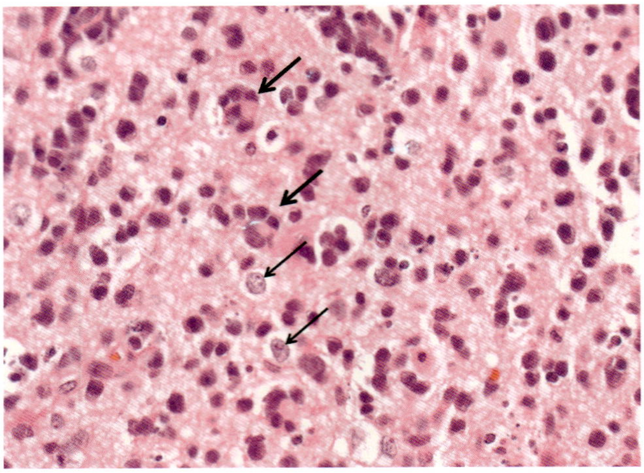

Figure 2-292. Lymphoma: When it diffusely infiltrates the parenchyma, lymphoma can be difficult to recognize. Small groupings (*thick arrows*) may further mimic a glial neoplasm. Since the great majority of CNS lymphomas are diffuse large B-cell type, at least some large nuclei with open chromatin pattern, one or more eccentric nucleoli, and irregular nuclear membranes (*thin arrows*) should help raise the suspicion to initiate appropriate workup for diagnosis (H&E; original magnification: 400×).

variable mixture of small and large cells, the small cell population shows a darker, denser chromatin with a *raisinoid nucleus*, that is, small cleaved cell, with no nucleoli. In T-cell lymphomas, the nuclei tend to have a prominent convoluted *cerebriform pattern*.[683] *Nuclear grooves*, resulting in coffee bean or cleaved nuclei, are characteristic for Langerhans cell histiocytosis[684] **(Fig. 2-293)**. They are also seen as a characteristic feature of papillary thyroid carcinoma, which only rarely metastasizes to the CNS[685] and which also comes into the differential diagnosis of cytoplasmic intranuclear invaginations (pseudoinclusions) (see below).

Multilobated nucleus is typical for Creutzfeldt astrocyte, a type of reactive astrocyte that is nonspecific but is commonly associated with inflammatory processes and especially inflammatory demyelinating conditions **(Fig. 2-294)**. Another cell with similar but larger and more hyperchromatic nucleus is megakaryocyte, which can be identified in the circulation, usually stuck in a capillary in autopsy tissue, as well as occasionally in extramedullary hematopoietic foci.

A good example of an association of a diagnosis with a particular *chromatin pattern* is the *salt and pepper chromatin* pattern seen in neuroendocrine

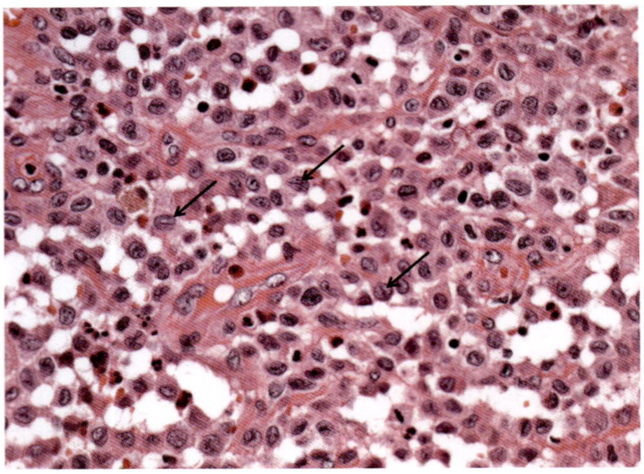

Figure 2-293. Langerhans cell histiocytosis: Nuclei of many neoplastic cells have grooves (*arrows*) that should be sought for in a mixed inflammatory population, especially when eosinophil PMN leukocytes are present, not to overlook this process (H&E; original magnification: 400×).

cell nuclei **(Fig. 2-295)**. In the CNS, this chromatin pattern is seen in pituitary neoplasms and paraganglioma. Neuroendocrine neoplasms of other sites that may metastasize to the CNS also have salt and pepper chromatin pattern, and they should be

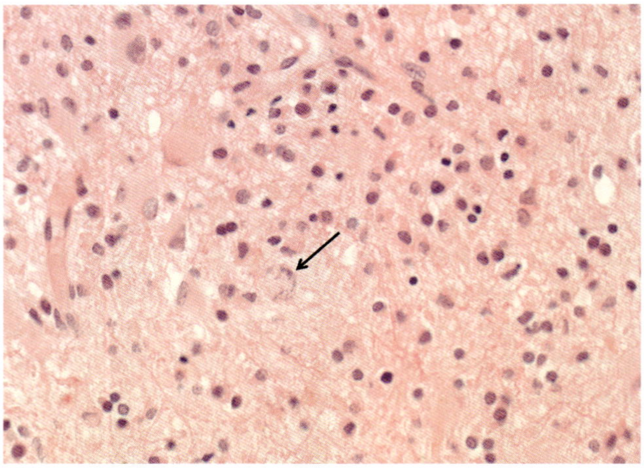

Figure 2-294. Creutzfeldt astrocyte: A fragmented, granular, or multilobated nucleus (*arrow*) is seen in a cell that is usually larger than the surrounding population, except for the reactive astrocytes. They may be difficult to identify without a search due to their fragmented nuclei and pale appearance. Creutzfeldt astrocytes are not diagnostic for, but are usually seen in association with, demyelinating processes and are different than mitotic cells in metaphase (H&E; original magnification: 400×).

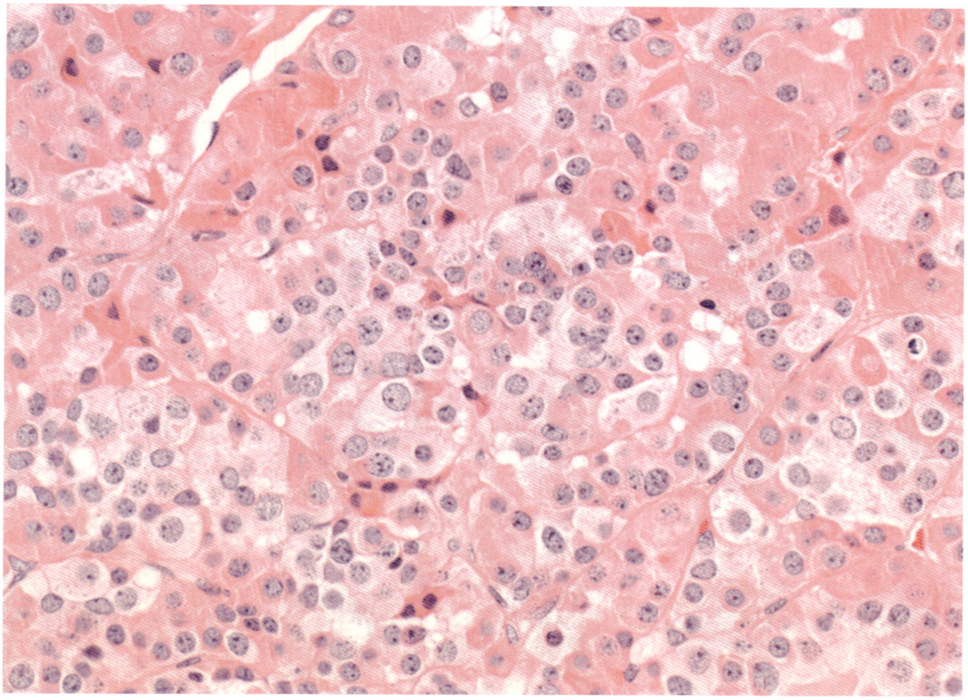

Figure 2-295.
Neuroendocrine chromatin pattern: Also commonly referred to as "salt and pepper" chromatin due to its finely granular quality, this chromatin pattern is considered typical for neuroendocrine cells, as seen in this nonneoplastic anterior pituitary parenchyma, and their neoplasms. Small nucleoli or chromocenters are also commonly present (H&E; original magnification: 400×).

considered in the context of metastatic neoplasms just like any other general pathologic feature. Pituitary adenoma diagnosis is usually straightforward given the location of the lesion. However, in IOC and small biopsies, or in ectopic sites such as in sphenoid sinus mucosa, bone, brain, or other organs as in the cases of invasive adenoma or pituitary carcinoma, pituitary gland origin may not be thought of as a top possibility. In pituitary adenoma with perivascular arrangement of cells (see perivascular arrangements), together with the frozen artifact, one may get a pseudorosette impression of an ependymoma. The finely granular chromatin pattern then helps support "pituitary adenoma" over ependymoma, which has a relatively coarse, not so crisp chromatin and may also have chromocenters or micronucleoli. Meningiomas that grow into the sella may rarely present as "pituitary adenomas." Their pale chromatin pattern and intranuclear cytoplasmic invaginations (pseudoinclusions) and optically clear nuclei (Orphan Annie eye nuclei)[686] are useful in favoring meningioma (see below). Another peculiar finding in meningioma, especially identified on cytologic preparations due to better preservation of nuclear detail, is the presence of *Barr body* in some female cases.[42,687] Especially on smear preparations, pituitary adenoma cytoplasms tend to strip off of the nucleus, leaving many naked nuclei in a granular eosinophilic background. This appearance, in the right context, is also highly suggestive of pituitary adenoma; however, sometimes, the question of lymphoid population, inflammatory with small, round lymphocytes or neoplastic with features of a low-grade lymphoma, may arise. Again, the finely granular, uniform chromatin pattern, along with the monomorphic population of cells, favors pituitary adenoma over lymphocytes in inflammation, which have dark, condensed chromatin and form a polymorphic population. In cases of low-grade lymphoma that is composed of small lymphoid cells, the uniformity is also expected; however, the nuclear membranes tend to be irregular with somewhat raisinoid contours. Similar picture can be seen in plasma cell lesions, especially plasma cell myeloma. Even if the cytoplasms of the pituitary adenoma cells are intact to some extent, they may also accentuate the eccentric nucleus, creating a plasmacytoid appearance. However, the cytoplasms of pituitary adenoma cells are not amphophilic nor do they have a paranuclear huff. In addition, the typical *"cartwheel" chromatin pattern*, sometimes referred to as "clockface" or plasmacytoid, should be obvious in plasma cells. In high-grade or plasmablastic plasma cell myeloma, this typical chromatin may not be identified. Instead, it may be replaced by an immunoblast-like open chromatin with large nucleolus, an appearance that is still not compatible with pituitary adenoma. In essentially all cases, the nature of the process becomes obvious on tissue sections. In cases where any uncertainty exists, immunohistochemical studies should easily clarify the issue.

Round nuclei with similar chromatin pattern can be seen in neurocytoma. Neurocytoma nuclei tend to have a chromatin pattern that is reminiscent of the internal granule layer cells of the cerebellum, in that they have more *clumped chromatin with a chromocenter*, although they are slightly larger. That way, they can also be distinguished from small lymphocytes. In the neuroglial parenchyma, such round cell neoplasms as neurocytoma need to be distinguished from oligodendroglioma. The latter also has a finely granular chromatin but is more open and uniform rather than crisp and with a chromocenter or a small nucleolus.

Large nucleus with open chromatin pattern and prominent nucleolus is typically considered to be associated with malignant processes. However, in the CNS, neuron nuclei match this definition, also. Fortunately, their neuronal nature is usually very clear on sections due to their cytoplasmic features, distribution, and location. Sometimes, these large pyramidal neurons can become a source of misdiagnosis in cytologic preparations, especially in CSF cytology, resulting in confusion with melanoma (supported by granular cytoplasmic lipofuscin pigment) or metastatic carcinoma. In general, this kind of chromatin pattern is considered typical for metastatic carcinomas. In fact, one has to be careful with making a glial neoplasm diagnosis, no matter how high grade, in the abundance of such nuclei, and consider the possibility of a metastatic carcinoma when faced with a clearly neoplastic process **(Fig. 2-296)**. There are exceptions both ways, however. Especially squamous cell carcinomas may have a coarse and condensed chromatin with no prominent nucleoli, unless they are high grade **(Fig. 2-297)**. This in turn is a chromatin pattern seen in high-grade glial neoplasms, especially anaplastic astrocytoma and glioblastoma. Both neoplasms can have abundant cytoplasm and show spindling, creating more overlap between them. The presence of adenoid/epithelioid areas in glioblastomas may further complicate the issue. On the other hand, some neoplasms with neuronal/ganglion cell differentiation can have such cells with only a small amount of cytoplasm but with nuclear features suggesting a neuronal origin. Usually in gangliogliomas, scattered dysplastic or immature ganglion cells may stand out only due to their open chromatin pattern and prominent

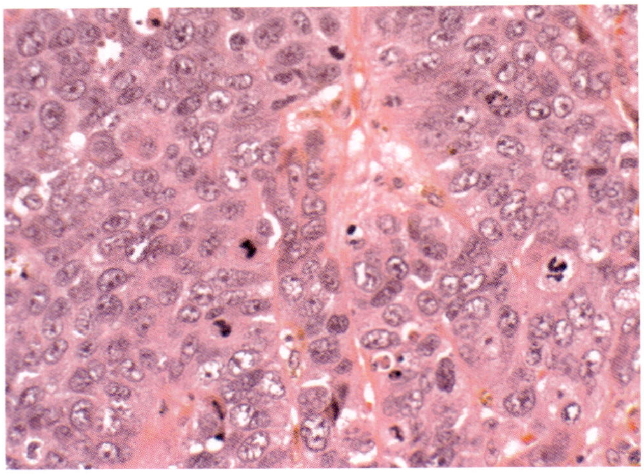

Figure 2-296. Metastatic carcinoma: Open chromatin, uniformly prominent one or more nucleoli, and a brisk mitotic rate that is higher than that of a typical high-grade glial neoplasm should make one to suspect a metastatic carcinoma in the differential diagnosis of difficult cases (H&E; original magnification: 400×).

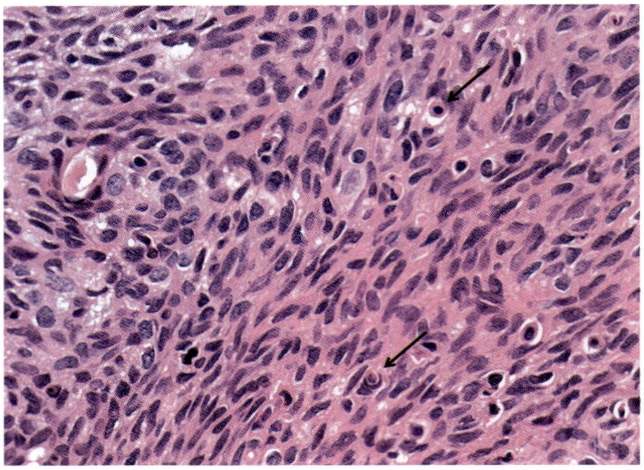

Figure 2-297. Metastatic squamous cell carcinoma: The nuclear features described in Figure 2-296 may not apply to squamous cell carcinomas, which tend to have a more condensed chromatin. Nucleoli are not readily identified. Scattered dyskeratotic cells (*arrows*) and a streaming quality to the cells are features suggesting a squamous cell carcinoma (H&E; original magnification: 400×).

nucleoli. In reactive astrocytes, nuclei can be so active that they assume an open chromatin pattern with a prominent nucleolus. In general, however, in an average specimen, there are usually areas that are typical enough to reveal the true nature of the neoplasm. In more difficult cases, immunohistochemistry and electron microscopy can be utilized. Typically in Alzheimer type II glia, which may have little or no GFAP positivity, the nuclei may resemble those of a neuron. They may have irregular and lobulated nuclei in globus pallidus, where they are especially prominent. Alzheimer type II astrocytes are associated with hyperammonemia states, such as in hepatic encephalopathy and Wilson's disease. They are also seen in AIDS without liver failure, Morel's laminar sclerosis, and mitochondrial DNA depletion syndrome and in Canavan's disease, a leukodystrophy also involving the U-fibers.

Ground-glass or hazy, homogeneous chromatin pattern suggests the possibility of viral inclusion. Usually there is a very thin, speckled chromatin pushed against the nuclear membrane, making it look thicker than normal. Such nuclei can be seen in JC virus–infected oligodendrogliocytes in PML, typically at the periphery of the demyelinating foci, and in HSV infections in the neuronal nuclei. Ground-glass appearance of the nucleus can sometimes be used interchangeably in general pathology to refer to the optically clear nuclei as seen in papillary thyroid carcinomas. In spite of the jargon in terminology, the important point is to note that the nuclei may assume a ground-glass appearance because of viral inclusions or optic clearing (Orphan Annie eye nuclei) **(Fig. 2-298)**, which is different from intranuclear cytoplasmic invaginations (pseudoinclusions) **(Fig. 2-299)**. More details and various substance accumulations from a general surgical pathologic standpoint have been discussed extensively.[688] See also "Intranuclear Inclusions."

Intranuclear pseudoinclusions are invaginations of cytoplasm into the nucleus due to the nuclear irregularities or convolutions. When seen in the perfect angle, they appear like round vacuoles filled with cytoplasm. As such, they are of the same quality as the cytoplasm. They are surrounded by nuclear membrane and then the circular remaining nucleus around them. When seen from the side, the cytoplasm is seen protruding into the C-shaped nucleus. The nuclear irregularity

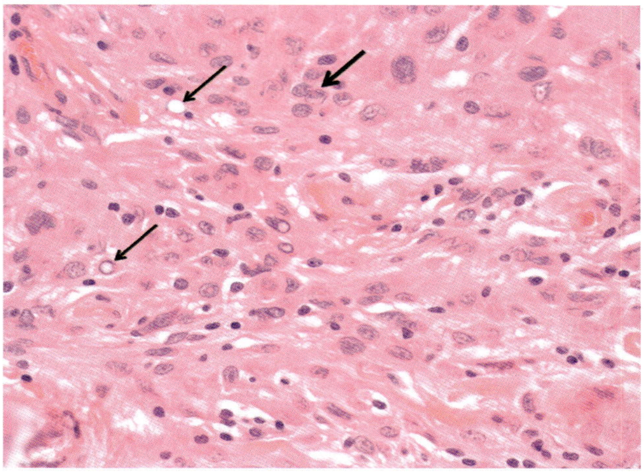

Figure 2-298. Meningioma: A ground-glass or optically clear quality to some nuclei (*thin arrows*) is also known as "Orphan Annie eye" nuclei and is different than intranuclear cytoplasmic invaginations (pseudoinclusions) (*thick arrow*) (H&E; original magnification: 400×).

mentioned here is not necessarily associated with malignancy, although malignant cells typically have nuclear membrane irregularities. In the CNS, intranuclear cytoplasmic invagination or pseudoinclusion is most notably associated with meningioma. In general, it is also a well-known

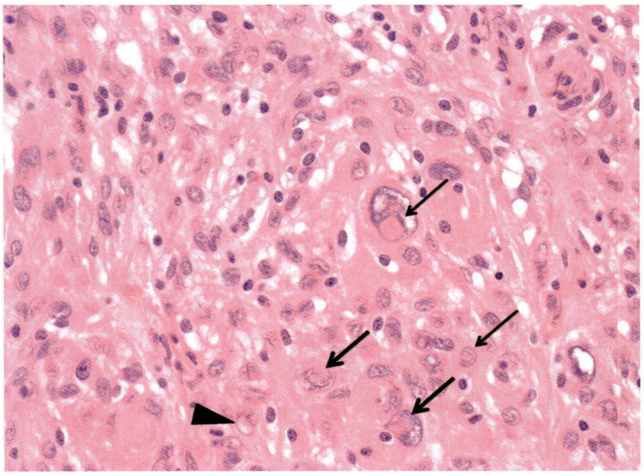

Figure 2-299. Meningioma: Intranuclear cytoplasmic invaginations or pseudoinclusions have a quality similar to the cytoplasm (*thin arrows*), and they are due to the irregularities of the nuclear membrane as seen when nuclei are appropriately oriented (*thick arrows*). A clear nucleus is also present (*arrowhead*) (H&E; original magnification: 400×).

cytologic feature of melanoma and papillary thyroid carcinoma. However, the latter two malignancies are otherwise remarkably different from meningioma, and together with all the other features taken into account, this distinction should not become a problem. One exception is melanocytoma, which can have several overlapping features with meningioma, including intranuclear cytoplasmic invaginations. Melanocytomas are typically spindle cell neoplasms with a swirling pattern of cells mimicking whorls and may cause diagnostic problems when melanin pigment is scarce or absent. Such intranuclear pseudoinclusions can sometimes be seen in schwannoma, ganglion cell component of ganglioglioma, and PXA. Otherwise, it is not uncommon to find a rare pseudoinclusion in many other lesions, if searched diligently. Potential pitfalls are to confuse them with a true inclusion of some sort, or, with immunohistochemical stains, to interpret them as nuclear staining. Cells of endolymphatic sac tumor may have intranuclear pseudoinclusions, which may add to the confusion with metastatic thyroid carcinoma in cases with glandular and/or papillary architecture, especially if the glandular areas have eosinophilic proteinaceous material in the lumen, resembling colloid. Immunohistochemical studies resolve any confusion. Pseudo-pseudoinclusions, which are artifactual bubbly appearance of the nucleus, should not be mistaken for pseudoinclusions.[688] Ferritinopathy is associated with peculiar vacuolated neuronal and glial nuclei with globular eosinophilic intranuclear inclusions.[121]

The involvement of the nucleolus in neoplasia is a complex process detailed elsewhere.[689] In general, the *prominence of nucleolus* in a cell is linked with the nuclear activity and, in the case of neoplasia, with increasing malignancy. Many cells normally can have prominent nucleoli in their baseline state, however. In the brain, the most notable example is the pyramidal neuron. Due to its high activity in protein synthesis, it normally has a "malignant-looking" nucleus, with open chromatin, corresponding to euchromatin, and a prominent nucleolus. Due to this appearance, the pitfall is to confuse them with melanoma cells, especially together with the cytoplasmic lipofuscin pigment mimicking melanin, or adenocarcinoma, usually in cytology setting (see above). In general, nucleolus prominence is an alarming feature for malignancy, and in borderline cases, it can help one be concerned for malignancy. In the CNS, the ganglion cell component of gangliogliomas has prominent nucleoli just like nonneoplastic neurons. However, even in highly malignant neoplasms such as glioblastoma, they are not uniformly present, in accord with the general rule that prominent nucleoli are not a feature of most primary CNS neoplasms (see above). As for metastatic carcinomas, a small cell carcinoma (i.e., poorly differentiated neuroendocrine carcinoma) typically does not show nucleoli. In that sense, it is similar to cells of medulloblastoma or PNET. This absence of nucleoli favors a small cell carcinoma (or, medulloblastoma/PNET, depending on the situation) over a lymphoma, based on the nuclear and nucleolar features. Large cell medulloblastoma has nuclear, chromatin, and nucleolar appearance similar to a diffuse large B-cell lymphoma, possibly with the exception of a more rounder and regular nuclear border. Prominence of nucleolus is typical in adenocarcinoma. Prominent nucleolus is one of the features used, along with other features, to diagnose atypical (WHO grade II) meningioma.[44] Diffuse large B-cell lymphomas, the most common type of lymphoma seen in the CNS, have cells with nuclei with typical features (see above "nuclear contours"). They typically have one or more nucleoli that are placed closer to or attached to the nuclear membrane, rather than central. Open chromatin pattern and prominent nucleoli in an epithelioid neoplasm with high mitotic activity, that is, resembling a carcinoma, should also bring to mind nonteratomatous germ cell neoplasm, especially in pineal and suprasellar regions. In germinoma, the prominent nucleoli can assume irregular contours with a somewhat spindled or bar-shaped appearance.[42] Among pituitary adenomas, prominent nucleoli, along with chromatin clearing, nuclear enlargement, and pleomorphism, is a uniform feature of silent subtype III adenoma, many of which show aggressive biologic behavior with invasion and recurrences. They are nonfunctional adenomas, even though some degree of immunohistochemical positivity for a combination of hormones is seen. Scattered larger cells with prominent nucleoli and an open chromatin pattern may represent ganglion cell differentiation in a pituitary adenoma, and they can be relatively easily identified by their overall neuronal features. *Micronucleoli* or even *chromocenters* (see above) are useful in distinguishing oligodendroglial nuclei from astrocytic nuclei. Among other features, their presence favors an oligodendroglial lineage. Central neurocytoma also has chromocenters or small central nucleoli.

The definition of, or lack thereof, the terms interchangeably used as *nuclear and/or cytologic atypia or anaplasia* is a very subjective one; hence, "atypia is in the eye of the beholder."[690] Depending on the particular context, one or more of nuclear enlargement, increasing nucleus-to-cytoplasm ratio, hyperchromasia, nuclear membrane irregularities, open chromatin pattern, coarse chromatin pattern, prominence of nuclear membrane (due to margination of heterochromatin), and enlargement and/or prominence of nucleoli are used as features to look for. As such, it is associated with increasing degree of malignancy and decreasing differentiation. This concept is also dependent on the type of lesion at hand. For instance, the atypia seen in a glioblastoma is not the same and does not fulfill the same criteria as the one seen in pituitary adenoma. As such, as discussed above, normal neuron can easily qualify as an atypical cell, when taken out of context. Whatever its definition may be, there are a few caveats in its interpretation. Some neoplasms, especially neuroendocrine neoplasms such as pituitary adenoma and paraganglioma, can have cytologic atypia with no influence on their biologic behavior. It is also common to have large cells in some low-grade neoplasms such as PA and schwannoma, among others, and should not be interpreted as a sign of more aggressive behavior. Therefore, "atypia" should be interpreted in context. For instance, the so-called ancient change or degenerative atypia can be seen in neurofibroma, with no diagnostic or prognostic significance. Cellular neurofibromas do not typically have atypical cells, but if atypical cells are seen and p53 overexpression is identified, a malignant change should be suspected. Mitotic figures may not be useful in this differential, as a few mitotic figures can be seen in both lesions.[691]

Pleomorphism is usually regarded as an atypical feature associated with neoplastic processes. In general, it is used for nuclei and refers to the variable shapes and sizes of the component cells relative to each other, hence nuclear pleomorphism, even though the definition is true for the entirety of the cell. It can be seen in malignant, benign, or nonneoplastic conditions; can be the identifying features of some lesions; may constitute a pitfall when seen in reactive conditions; or may simply be an insignificant finding in some cases. In malignant neoplasms, the degree of pleomorphism tends to increase as the grade increases. In contrast to some neoplasms such as Wilms' tumor, where favorable or unfavorable prognostic information can be obtained based on the degree of pleomorphism,[692] there are no such lesions in the CNS where pleomorphism can be used in this manner, with the possible exception of anaplastic medulloblastoma.[541]

Aside from the usual malignancy-related pleomorphism, for example, as seen in glioblastoma, among others, one particular glial neoplasm that made a name based on pleomorphism is PXA. In addition to the prominent pleomorphism, the neoplastic cells also have xanthomatous cytoplasms. Overall, this highly atypical appearance creates the pitfall of mistaking this WHO grade II neoplasm for a high-grade one, such as glioblastoma. However, noticing the difficulty in finding mitotic figures, the presence of EGBs, the absence of necrosis, and vascular proliferation help avoid this mistake.[42] In addition, PXA is usually a superficial, well-circumscribed neoplasm with cyst and mural nodule formation in a young adult. Even when anaplastic features such as increased mitotic activity, necrosis, and vascular proliferation are seen, appreciating the true nature of the neoplasm avoids the diagnosis of glioblastoma. Another CNS neoplasm that can have significant pleomorphism to result in misinterpretation is hemangioblastoma. Typically presenting in the cerebellum of a young adult as cyst and mural nodule formation, in the setting of von Hippel-Lindau syndrome or as a sporadic lesion, hemangioblastoma is composed of clear cells and prominent vascular component. While a straightforward diagnosis in its typical presentation, especially in the setting of IOC and without the knowledge of clinical and radiologic features, its nuclear pleomorphism, combined with rich vascular component, can result in an appearance of high-grade glial neoplasm. The clear cytoplasms may not be appreciated on frozen sections and on cytologic preparations, as they are fragile and are destroyed during preparation. The absence of glial processes in the background and the hemorrhagic nature of the material should alert one to consider a diagnostic alternative to glial neoplasm. In endocrine neoplasms in general, and specifically in pituitary adenoma in the CNS, nuclear pleomorphism is common and does not have any diagnostic or prognostic implications. However, it can be quite prominent in some cases and should not prompt consideration of a more aggressive biologic behavior, such as invasive adenoma and atypical adenoma, or impending metastasis to imply pituitary carcinoma.

Variable numbers of larger cells or giant cells can be seen in many contexts (see "Cellular Enlargement and Multinucleation" for more details).

Nuclear Inclusions

Accumulations within the nucleus of different cell types can be seen in a broad spectrum of diseases including neurodegenerative and viral or can be of yet unknown significance. In some situations, the intranuclear inclusions and nucleoli can have overlapping microscopic features, leading to confusion. For nucleoli, please see "Nuclear Features." It is also useful to see "Cytoplasmic Inclusions" and "Neuron Loss and Gliosis" to identify additional features, and tissue involvement patterns further distinguish those disorders with similar intranuclear inclusions.

Marinesco body is a round eosinophilic inclusions with a vague halo and a faint orange hue **(Fig. 2-300)**. They are seen in substantia nigra neurons and can be of variable size but are typically about the size of the nucleolus or slightly larger. They have historically been of no clinical significance; however, recent studies have suggested that they may be linked to and represent the early stages of some neurodegenerative diseases.[693] Immunohistochemically, they are positive for ubiquitin. The inclusions of *neuronal intranuclear inclusion disease (NIID)*[694] are similar to Marinesco bodies, though they are more eosinophilic. Similar inclusions are also seen in *fragile-X tremor/ataxia syndrome (FXTAS)* in diverse areas of the CNS and PNS, as well as in pituitary gland, adrenal medulla, and testis[695,696] **(Fig. 2-301)**. In *multiple system atrophy (MSA)*,[697] neuronal and glial intranuclear accumulations can be seen by alpha-synuclein immunohistochemistry and by silver impregnation techniques. They are mainly in basis pontis and putamen and can be seen as delicate fibrillary structures lined up against the nuclear membrane or as rod-like structures. There may also be motor neuron–type inclusions. *Dentatorubropallidoluysial atrophy*[698] can have neuronal intranuclear inclusions that are ubiquitin-positive immunohistochemically and may be as diffuse accumulation within the nucleus or as distinct inclusions in the affected regions. Somewhat irregular neuronal intranuclear ubiquitin-positive inclusions are also present in *Huntington disease*. Inclusions are more common and easier to

List of Findings/Checklist for Nuclear Inclusions

AT A GLANCE

Nonviral Inclusions
- Marinesco body
- Neuronal intranuclear inclusion disease
- Fragile-X tremor/ataxia syndrome
- Multiple system atrophy
- Dentatorubropallidoluysian atrophy
- Huntington disease
- Frontotemporal lobar degeneration with ubiquitin-immunoreactive inclusions
- Kennedy's disease
- Neurofilament inclusion body disease
- SCA1
- SCA3
- SCA7
- Ferritinopathy

Viral Inclusions
- Herpes simplex virus
- Cytomegalovirus
- Progressive multifocal leukoencephalopathy
- Measles
  - Subacute sclerosing panencephalitis
  - Measles inclusion body encephalitis
- Varicella-zoster virus (VZV)

Pseudoinclusions
- Meningioma
- Melanocytic neoplasms
- Metastatic thyroid papillary carcinoma
- Metastatic adenocarcinoma of the lung
- Dutcher bodies

Pseudo-pseudoinclusions
- Artifact

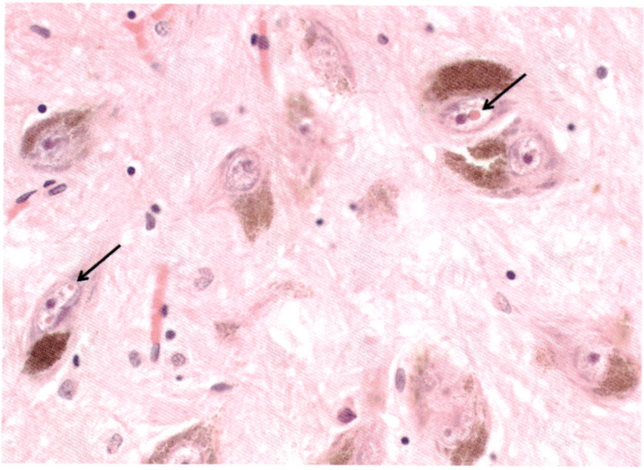

Figure 2-300. Marinesco bodies: Round, eosinophilic one or more intranuclear structures of variable sizes, but typically about the size of the nucleolus, are usually present with increasing age in the pigmented neurons of the substantia nigra (*arrows*). They can have a thin halo when near condensed areas of the chromatin and should not be mistaken for viral inclusions (H&E; original magnification: 400×).

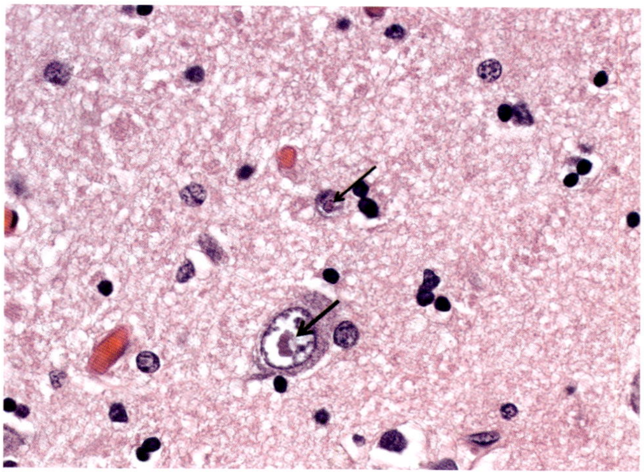

Figure 2-301. Fragile-X ataxia tremor syndrome (FXTAS): Similar to Marinesco bodies, but with a pale and dull eosinophilic quality, these intranuclear inclusions can be seen in different cell types in the body and mainly in neurons and glial cells in the CNS. Multiple neuronal (*thick arrow*) inclusions and an astrocytic (*thin arrow*) inclusion are present in this picture (H&E; original magnification: 600×).

find in younger cases as they correlate with the number of triplet repeats. Ubiquitin and huntingtin immunostains are positive in neuron nuclei and axons.[699] *Frontotemporal lobar degeneration with ubiquitin-only immunoreactive changes (FTLD-U)*[700] can occasionally have neuronal intranuclear ubiquitin-positive inclusions in the dentate gyrus, amygdala, and cerebral cortex. Neuronal cytoplasmic inclusions are also seen in the dentate gyrus, amygdala, and cortex. *Spinobulbar muscular atrophy (Kennedy's disease)*[701] is a CAG repeat expansion disorder with facial, hypoglossal, and spinal motor neuron degeneration, sparing the third, fourth, and sixth cranial nerve nuclei. Nuclear ubiquitin-positive inclusions in neurons of affected regions, as well as in other tissues such as skin, heart, kidney, and testis, are present. *Neurofilament inclusion body disease*, currently also referred to as FTLD with intermediate filament inclusions (FTLD-IF),[702] predominantly has cytoplasmic but sometimes neuronal intranuclear inclusions.[122] *SCA1*[698] is associated with atrophy of the cerebellum, pons, and inferior olives, as well as spinal cord. Mutant ataxin-1 and ubiquitin positivity by immunohistochemistry is seen in neuron nuclei. *SCA3 (Machado-Joseph disease)* has cerebello-olivary sparing but neuron loss in dentate nucleus and superior cerebellar peduncle, along with spinocerebellar tract degeneration. Clarke's column, substantia nigra, and anterior horn neurons are also involved. Ataxin-3 and ubiquitin-positive intranuclear neuronal inclusions are identified.[703] *SCA7*[698] is associated with cerebellar cortical atrophy, spinocerebellar and olivocerebellar tract degeneration, as well as degeneration of motor neurons of the brainstem and spinal cord. Substantia nigra and subthalamic nucleus are also involved. Neuronal intranuclear inclusions with expanded polyglutamine repeats are present in inferior olives. Essentially all polyglutamine expansion disorders also have variable neuronal intranuclear inclusions.[698] *Ferritinopathy* has peculiar vacuolated neuronal and glial nuclei with globular eosinophilic intranuclear inclusions reminiscent of NIID. Some are positive for ubiquitin and neurofilament.[121]

Intranuclear viral inclusions are typical for several viral infections. In *HSV*, the intranuclear inclusions are large enough to fill the entire nucleus, pushing the chromatin to the nuclear membrane and creating a pale, hazy eosinophilic ground-glass appearance to the nucleus.

Multinucleation with nuclear molding can be seen. HSV infection typically involves the medial temporal lobe by a hemorrhagic, necroinflammatory process, and inclusions may be difficult to find as they may resemble disintegrating nuclei. In *CMV*, intranuclear inclusions are also eosinophilic and large, surrounded by a halo, creating the "owl-eye" appearance. The cells are enlarged and can also have eosinophilic granular intracytoplasmic inclusions. CMV infection can be seen as an opportunistic infection in immunocompromised individuals or in the newborn in periventricular regions and ventricular surfaces as part of TORCH group of infections, resulting in ventriculitis and destructive encephalitis. *JC virus* inclusions in *progressive multifocal leukoencephalopathy (PML)* result in enlargement of oligodendroglial nuclei by a diffuse ground-glass plum-colored inclusion **(Fig. 2-302)**. They are typically prominent toward the periphery of the demyelinating lesions. *SSPE*, which occurs many years after the initial measles infection, has inclusions that are somewhat similar to PML inclusions in that they are also seen in enlarged oligodendroglial nuclei, are dark eosinophilic, and result in ground-glass appearance in the nuclei **(Fig. 2-303)**. There is demyelination due to oligodendroglial involvement, as well as neuron loss due to the involvement of neurons. *Measles inclusion body encephalitis* and the autoimmune acute measles encephalomyelitis are other pathologic

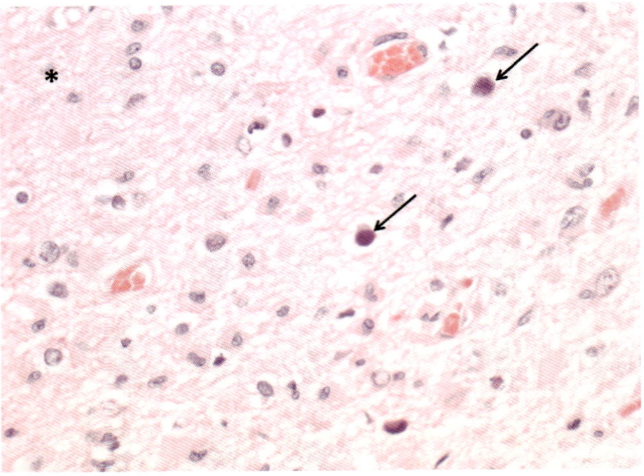

Figure 2-302. PML: Enlarged oligodendroglial nuclei have a plum-colored ground-glass quality (*arrows*) due to viral inclusions. The background is pale and gliotic due to myelin loss, and the lesion has a relatively well-defined border with the more eosinophilic, that is, in this case better myelinated, surrounding tissues (*asterisk*), emphasizing that the diagnostic inclusions are more likely to be found at the periphery of the lesion (H&E; original magnification: 400×).

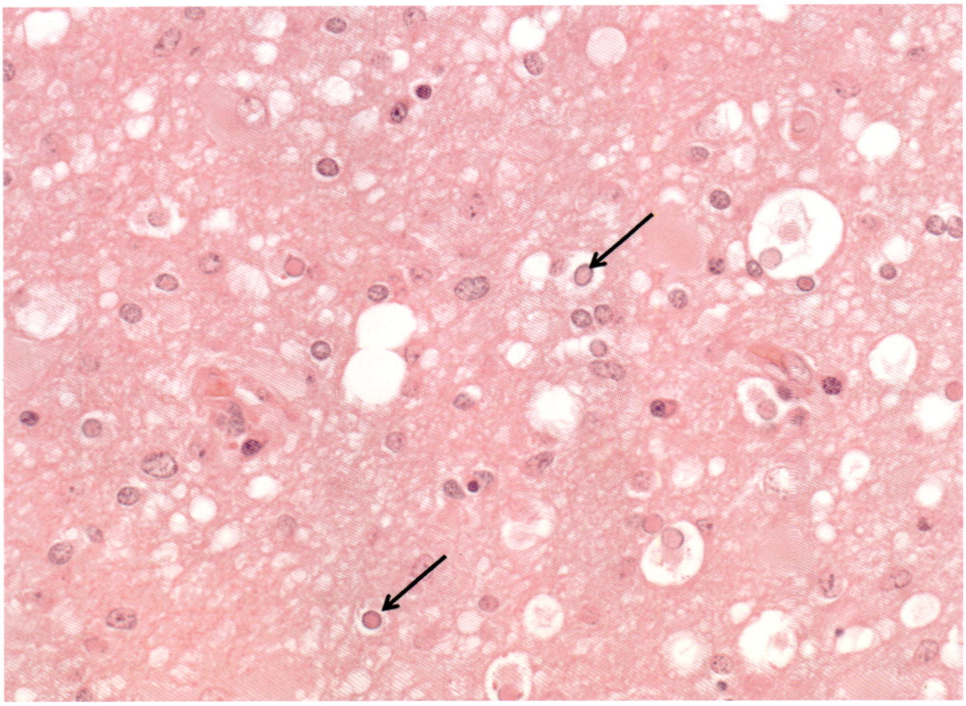

Figure 2-303. SSPE: Many nuclei have a homogeneous pale eosinophilic quality (*arrows*) (H&E; original magnification: 400×).

processes associated with measles infection.[704] The former occurs within a year of the initial infection in immunocompromised hosts and also has intranuclear inclusions. Multinucleated cells with intranuclear inclusions in oligodendroglia, astrocytes, and neurons, as well as less well-defined cytoplasmic inclusions, can be seen. In *VZV* ventriculitis, viral inclusions are seen in ependymal cell nuclei.

Various intranuclear accumulations may appear as ground-glass nuclei (see also "Nuclear Features"), *optically clear nuclei*, inclusions, *pseudoinclusions*, and *pseudo-pseudoinclusions*.[688] Aside from viral inclusions, substances such as surfactant may accumulate in the nucleus, creating a pseudoinclusion, and may be useful in the identification of lung origin of a metastatic carcinoma when detected by surfactant immunohistochemistry. Intranuclear cytoplasmic invaginations (pseudoinclusions) are, while nonspecific, highly characteristic for meningioma, although they can be seen in metastatic thyroid papillary carcinoma, in melanocytic neoplasms, and occasionally in several other neoplasms in the CNS, as well as in the form of Dutcher bodies in plasma cell myeloma. Pseudo-pseudoinclusions occur as an artifact and appear as multiple ill-defined bubbles within the nucleus and should not be confused with more significant inclusions **(Fig. 2-304)**. Needless to say, with the exception of cytoplasmic intranuclear invaginations, accurate evaluation of inclusions in frozen tissue is essentially impossible. An in-depth and extensive review of various intranuclear inclusions, especially from a general pathology standpoint, is available.[688]

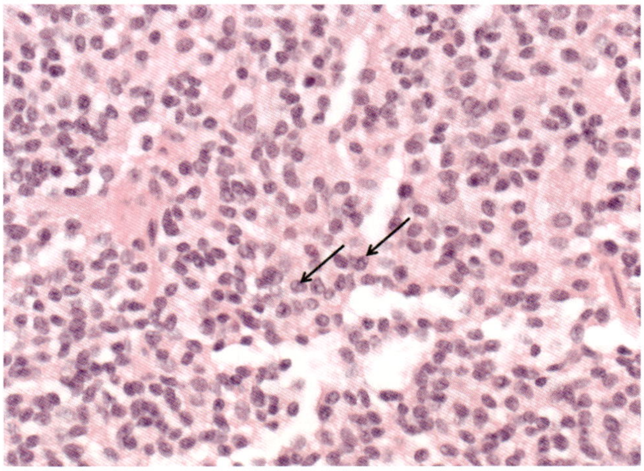

Figure 2-304. Pseudo-pseudoinclusions: Nuclei have an artifactual bubbly appearance due to multiple vacuoles (*arrows*), which should not be mistaken for a more significant finding (H&E; original magnification: 400×).

Mitotic Activity

Mitotic activity is usually used in the grading of neoplasms and its presence can become useful in subtle situations by allowing one to favor a neoplasm, although this situation is not without pitfalls. The presence of mitotic activity is no surprise, as the cells forming the neoplasm should be coming from somewhere, and that would be the division of the cells. That is why a certain level of mitotic activity is meaningful in certain situations. However, some neoplasms by nature are

List of Findings/Checklist for Mitotic Activity

AT A GLANCE

- Mitotic counts
- Meningioma
- Oligodendroglioma
- Fibrillary astrocytoma
- Oligoastrocytoma
- Pilocytic astrocytoma
- Ependymoma
- Pleomorphic xanthoastrocytoma
- Metastatic versus primary neoplasms
- Reactive versus neoplastic processes
- Astroblastoma
- Choroid plexus neoplasms
- Neurocytoma
- Pineal parenchymal tumors
- desmoplastic infantile ganglioglioma/ desmoplastic infantile astrocytoma
- SEGA
- Mesenchymal neoplasms
- Hemangiopericytoma
- Melanocytic neoplasms
- Peripheral nerve sheath tumors
    - Cellular schwannoma
    - Plexiform schwannoma
    - Cellular neurofibroma
    - MPNST
- Granular cell tumor
- Pituitary adenoma

so slow-growing that identification of only a few mitotic figures may be significant in a given context. In addition, the presence of "atypical mitotic figures," that is, bizarre forms resulting in tripolar or multipolar mitotic spindles, is in general more significant for malignancy. In regard to the nervous system neoplasms, in many situations, an "increased mitotic activity" is significant regardless of whether mitotic figures are typical or atypical, while a definitive mitotic count has been determined in the grading of some of the primary neoplasms. Otherwise, what constitutes an increased mitotic activity is highly subjective; however, in general, if mitotic figures can easily be identified by checking several areas on the tissue, without the need to spend minutes on high power, it is considered increased. Further evaluation can be pursued once a mitotic figure is identified and additional ones may or may not be found. Eventually, other factors, such as the type of the lesion and the size of the tissue, should also be incorporated in the final interpretation (see below). Mitotic counts are traditionally performed using 10 consecutive "high power fields" (HPFs), which means a standard 40× objective and 10× ocular, resulting in a 400× magnification. Other definitions of HPF also exist.[705] Several different areas with a likelihood of mitotic activity, such as an area where a mitotic figure has already been identified, or areas with other atypical features, that is, hypercellularity and cytologic atypia are selected, and multiple counts are performed to find the maximum number of mitotic figures per 10 HPFs. It should be noted that based on studies done in other organ lesions, the surface area that one HPF covers may vary depending on the technical specifications of the optic system, that is, from microscope to microscope,[706] even though different systems may result in 400× magnification, with wide variations in the final mitotic count.[707] Some investigators used surface area represented as mm^2.[577] The details and variables of mitosis counting have been investigated and discussed previously in other organ neoplasms.[708–711] To circumvent these potential problems, using a mitotic index expressing the number of mitotic figures as a percentage of the total number of neoplastic cells has been found useful.[707] In current practice, however, such details are not taken into account, and a "mitotic count per 10 HPFs" is used without further qualifications. In addition to the HPF surface area, the thickness of the section and the strict criteria to identify mitotic figures and not mistake apoptotic cells with mitotic figures are also important factors. Relatively recently, an immunohistochemical stain, phosphohistone-H protein, has been used to aid in the identification and counting of cells in mitosis[712,713] and showed correlation with WHO grading system.[714] The time until the fixation of the tissue and whether the tissue has been previously frozen may also interfere with mitotic counts.[715,716] Some bizarre mitotic figures may mimic Creutzfeldt astrocyte, although the confusion would me more worrisome the other way around.

In *meningioma*, identification of four or more mitotic figures per 10 HPFs indicates a diagnosis of atypical (WHO grade II) meningioma.[717] Mitotic counts high enough to qualify a meningioma as WHO grade II may be present in otherwise histologically unremarkable meningiomas. Therefore, a diligent evaluation for mitotic activity should be carried out in any meningioma, since this is a crucial feature for grading. In preoperatively *embolized meningioma*, mitotic figures may be present around the infarcted areas as part of the reactive activity and can create an illusion of increased mitotic count.[718,719] Noting that the meningioma has been embolized and the location of mitotic figures limited to around the infarct and searching for mitotic activity away from these areas for grading purposes should avoid misinterpretation. One of the definitions of anaplastic (WHO grade III; malignant) meningioma is a 20 or more mitotic figures per 10 HPFs.[717]

In *oligodendroglioma*, although a definitive number has not been mentioned in the WHO classification,[720] a mitotic count of six or more per 10 HPFs was found to be significant to indicate a diagnosis of anaplastic (WHO grade III) oligodendroglioma,[380] even if vascular proliferation and/or necrosis is not present. Mitotic count is also important in the grading of *astrocytoma*, although definitive rules are not present. In fibrillary astrocytomas, increased mitotic activity is "judged" by correlating the frequency of mitotic figures with the amount of material examined. For instance, in a fibrillary astrocytoma of low grade (WHO grade II), a few mitotic figures found after a laborious search in a material with several sections are not significant enough to upgrade it to anaplastic (WHO grade III) astrocytoma, while a single mitotic figure in a small fragment of tissue, such as a stereotactic biopsy material, is significant enough to at least raise this suspicion. How to handle mitotic activity in *oligoastrocytoma* is not clear; however, using 6 or more mitotic figures per 10 HPFs has sometimes been used, as in oligodendrogliomas.[721] In *PAs*, a mitotic figure per 250× microscopic field has been reported to be concerning for a more aggressive behavior.[504] *Anaplastic ependymoma* is designated by an increased mitotic count, although other features such as vascular proliferation, increased cellularity, and pseudopalisading necrosis are also usually present. Again, a definitive number for mitotic count has not been identified; however, various studies suggested variable numbers, that is, 5 to 10 mitotic figures per 10 HPFs. In fact, grading of especially posterior fossa ependymomas in childhood is not well-defined and can be problematic. It is not uncommon to find confluent and prominent areas of necrosis in these neoplasms, which should not be taken as a sign of anaplasia in isolation, and mitotic activity should be evaluated.[506,507] The presence of five or more mitotic figures per 10 HPFs in a *pleomorphic xanthoastrocytoma (PXA)*, a WHO grade II astrocytic neoplasm, indicates a more aggressive biologic behavior. These cases may also show necrosis, with or without pseudopalisading. Such PXAs are termed PXA with anaplastic features; however, an official grade (e.g., WHO grade III) has not been assigned to them.[505] Mitotic figures are naturally easier to find in high-grade neoplasms, such as *glioblastoma, PNET*, and *medulloblastoma*. They are also very frequent in *metastatic carcinoma*. In fact, as a general guideline, in a high-grade neoplasm with epithelioid features, the abundance of mitotic figures, among other features, should raise suspicion for metastatic carcinoma over glioblastoma.

In glial neoplasms or in reactive, inflammatory, or infectious processes, mitotic figures can be present in the *vascular component*, especially endothelial cells, even without the presence of definitive vascular proliferation, which can potentially result in misinterpretation as high grade. Obviously, in the presence of definitive vascular proliferation, the issue of mitotic figures will not become a problem. They can also be seen in the reactive *lymphohistiocytic population* present around the vessels in neoplastic as well as nonneoplastic conditions. The mitotic activity in reactive/inflammatory conditions should not be mistaken as an indication of malignancy, especially in pseudoneoplastic lesions such as demyelinating lesions and infarcts. Similar comments are in order for the interpretation of proliferative activity by Ki-67 immunohistochemistry. The presence of mitotic figures is one of the several features to evaluate in the differential diagnosis of *reactive gliosis* versus a neoplastic glial process (see "Hypercellularity"). The term granular mitosis has been used variably to refer to mitotic cells apparently in prophase and other times to erroneously refer to the multilobated nucleus of, *Creutzfeldt astrocyte* **(Fig. 2-294)**. It is not diagnostic for, but is frequently seen in, demyelinating conditions.

Although a formal WHO grading is not present for *astroblastoma*, it can be divided into well-differentiated and anaplastic (malignant) groups based on general features, such as vascular proliferation and necrosis, applicable to grading of other neoplasms. Mitotic count is usually around 1 per 10 HPFs in well-differentiated and more than five in anaplastic version.[722] *Choroid plexus papilloma* (WHO grade I) with 2 or more mitotic figures per 10 HPFs is designated as atypical choroid plexus papilloma (WHO grade II), although additional atypical features are also present, such as fusion of papillary structures to form cribriforming, solid sheets, hypercellularity, nuclear pleomorphism, and necrosis. In choroid plexus carcinomas, brisk mitotic activity, which is usually more than 5 per 10 HPFs, is one of the five features to be evaluated along with increased cellularity, nuclear pleomorphism, blurring of papillary pattern and sheet formation, and necrosis. Four of these five features are needed to make a diagnosis of malignancy in a choroid plexus neoplasm.[547] Some *neurocytomas*, central or extraventricular, can have more than an occasional mitotic figure, are associated with vascular proliferation and necrosis, and have been designated as atypical neurocytomas,[499,500] without a WHO grade. They also tend to have a Ki-67 proliferation index of more than 2%. An anaplastic version of neurocytoma has not been designated and is debatable; however, atypical neurocytoma tends to behave more aggressively than the usual neurocytoma, with recurrences. It has been suggested that mitotic counts correlate with the grading of *pineal parenchymal tumors*,[398] with zero mitotic figures per 10 HPFs in pineocytoma and less than 6 per 10 HPFs for low-grade pineal parenchymal tumor of intermediate differentiation. Variable numbers of mitotic figures, that is, less than, equal to, or more than 6 per 10 HPFs, depending on other factors in conjunction with the degree of neurofilament expression, can be seen in high-grade pineal parenchymal tumor of intermediate differentiation. Mitotic count is variable in pineoblastoma, although their typical PNET morphology provides adequate grading information in and of itself. A WHO grade I neoplasm that can rarely have an increased mitotic activity is *DIG/DIA*, with no prognostic implications. A similar situation can be seen in *SEGA*.

In general, mitotic activity is also important in the diagnosis and grading of *mesenchymal neoplasms*. *Hemangiopericytoma* (WHO grade II) can have scattered mitotic figures, but a mitotic count of more than 5 per 10 HPFs and/or necrosis is a feature of anaplastic (WHO grade III) hemangiopericytoma, associated with two of hypercellularity, cytologic atypia, and hemorrhage.[501] In rare cases of soft tissue sarcomas that can be seen in the nervous system, their respective rules should be applied, as outlines in soft tissue texts and literature.

In *melanocytic neoplasms*, the differentiation of melanocytoma from melanoma can sometimes be difficult if melanoma is not clearly malignant and has bland features. This distinction then is based on a constellation of features, one of which is mitotic activity, along with proliferation index, necrosis, and cytologic features. There is considerable overlap between the mitotic counts between grades, but typically, melanocytomas have 0-1 mitotic figures per 10 HPFs and a proliferation index of 2% or less, while melanomas have higher counts and indices, both up to 15. These figures are somewhat in between for intermediate grade lesions and a lot higher in metastatic melanomas.[47]

Cellular schwannoma[178] may be difficult to distinguish from MPNST. While necrosis is not a feature, small foci may be present but are without pseudopalisading. The presence of pseudopalisading is suspicious for MPNST. The neoplasm is composed only of cellular Antoni A areas of the schwannoma. Cellular whorls may be seen. In this context, mitotic activity provides an important feature. Mitotic count is typically less than 4 in 10 HPFs. Cellular schwannoma may rarely be associated with NF1 or another MPNST; therefore, identification of an MPNST at another site when multiple neoplasms are present should not bias one. *Plexiform (multinodular) schwannoma*[178] can have mitotic activity. It has a multinodular arrangement, mostly composed of Antoni A areas, and may be associated with NF1 or schwannomatosis in some cases. The nodules are surrounded by perineurium. Local recurrence due to irregular borders and multinodularity can be seen. These features can result in consideration of malignancy in some cases, especially if mitotic activity is present. Especially in the cutaneous and subcutaneous soft tissues, desmoplastic neurotropic melanoma is also a consideration (see "Nodular Arrangement"). Another differential diagnostic concern is distinguishing a *low-grade MPNST* or the nerve margin of an MPNST from localized intraneural neurofibroma in a somewhat cellular intraneural proliferation when mitotic figures are identified. MPNST is typically a deep-seated mass lesion, associated with large nerve trunks as in retroperitoneum or posterior mediastinum. Close communication with the surgeon and awareness of the clinical situation usually resolve any confusion. *Cellular neurofibroma*[691,723] can also add to the confusion, as well as the presence of enlarged nuclei as an ancient degenerative change that can commonly be seen in PNSTs. Among other features, the presence of strong and prominent p53 positivity is also useful by favoring malignancy. *Malignant granular cell tumors*[503] may be well-circumscribed or have infiltrative borders. Mitotic activity is one of the many features to evaluate in diagnosing a malignant granular cell tumor. Three of the marked cellularity, pleomorphism, high nucleus-to-cytoplasm ratio, the presence of nucleoli, brisk mitotic activity (most show mitotic counts of more than 5 per 10 HPFs), spindle cells, and necrosis are needed for this diagnosis, although most cases are readily obvious. Lymphovascular invasion and destructive behavior may be seen. Melan-A and microphthalmia transcription factor-1 can be positive. It has been reported that the usually incidental granular cell tumor of the neurohypophysis may have atypical features.[724]

Pituitary adenoma can further be qualified as "atypical adenoma" based on multiple parameters, including increased mitotic activity, a Ki-67 proliferation index of more than 3%, and p53 overexpression; however, these criteria do not appear to be well-settled or uniformly applied.[650,725]

Ependymal Surfaces

Ependymal lining is a layer of columnar ependymal cells with stereocilia, resting on subependymal glial tissue with no basement membrane. It is not unusual to have foci of ependymal denudation on the ependymal surfaces. The glial tissue reacts and proliferates to form small nodules protruding into the ventricular lumen. They are called *granular ependymitis* or, more accurately, since they are not necessarily inflammatory, *ependymal granulations*[726] **(Fig. 2-305)**. In the more exuberant versions of this process, simultaneously proliferating ependymal cells can be entrapped within the glial proliferation to result in a more complicated appearance with an admixture of ependymal cell groups or rosettes and prominent gliosis. In pediatric cases, they can be associated with evidence of previous hemorrhage, such as hemosiderin pigment, suggesting a germinal matrix hemorrhage or irritation by intraventricular hemorrhage as the initiator. In most cases, no definitive cause can be identified, even though they are common findings in autopsies. In others, they can be associated with obvious hemorrhagic or inflammatory/infectious processes involving the ventricles. Ependymal granulations are different from normal ependymal surface folding and nodulations that are uniformly covered by ependymal cells with no evidence of tissue injury or proliferation. In the brain and especially in the occipital horns of the lateral ventricles, the ependymal surfaces are pinched during development and can result in irregular acinar structures or small *groups of ependymal cells entrapped within the parenchyma*.[727] These should not be interpreted as ependymoma or confused with metastatic adenocarcinoma in small biopsy specimens or during IOC. In the spinal cord, the *central canal* is patent in the newborn and gradually becomes obliterated in time to result in an irregular aggregate of ependymal cells in its place. As in the brain, these ependymal cell aggregates may be a source of confusion in small samples. Also, developmental abnormalities, such as *duplication or hydromyelia*, that is, cystic dilation of the central canal filled with CSF and lined by ependymal cells, in contrast to *syrinx*, where ependymal lining is not present, can be identified. A pair of normal, symmetrical structures protruding into the fourth ventricle in the medulla oblongata represent *area postrema* **(Fig. 2-306)**. When seen as a whole on an autopsy section, it is easy to recognize this structure; however, for the unwary, they may look like microscopic gangliogliomas due to their ganglion cells in a fibrillary, loose, or edematous background. *Biondi bodies or rings* are mainly identified in

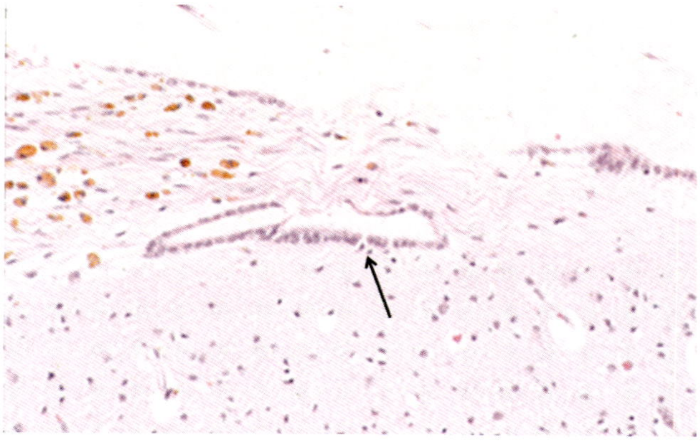

Figure 2-305. Ependymal granulation: Ependymal lining is denuded as a result of irritation and injury, in this case apparently due to intraventricular hemorrhage based on the hemosiderin pigment (**left side**). Underlying parenchyma shows reactive glial and ependymal proliferation, entrapping ependymal cells (*arrow*). The whole process may form multiple small nodules bulging into the ventricle lumen (H&E; original magnification: 200×).

List of Findings/Checklist for Ependymal Surfaces

AT A GLANCE

- Ependymal granulations
- Entrapped ependymal cells
- Central canal
- Hydromyelia-syrinx
- Area postrema
- Biondi bodies
- CMV infection
- VZV infection
- Bacterial infections
- Shunt infections
- Fungal infections
- Chemical/aseptic ventriculitis
- Hamartomas-candle guttering
- SEGA
- Subependymoma

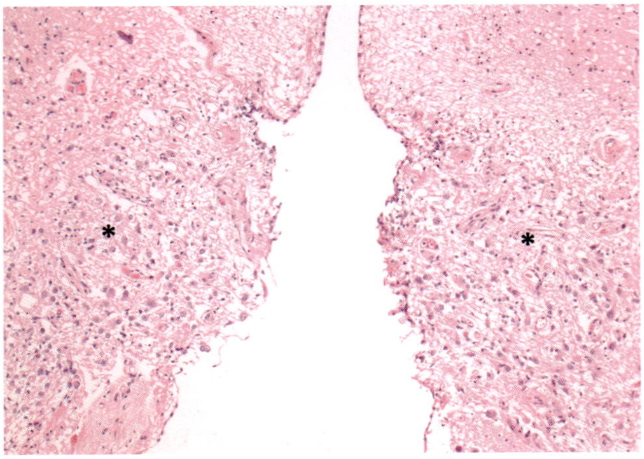

Figure 2-306. Area postrema: In the medulla oblongata and on the surfaces of the caudal fourth ventricle are symmetrical structures bulging into the ventricle (*asterisk*) composed of groups of neurons in a loose background. They are easily identified in autopsies due to better orientation and represent an example of many normal structures in the CNS, which can have unusual histologic features (H&E; original magnification: 100×).

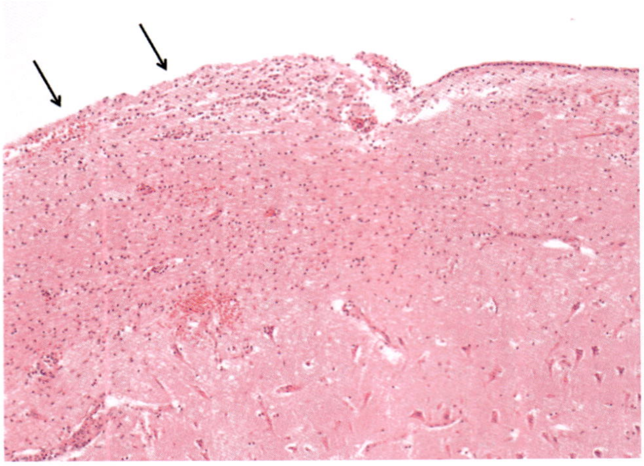

Figure 2-307. Ependymitis: Ependymal lining is denuded and the subependymal tissues are infiltrated by PMN leukocytes (*arrows*) (H&E; original magnification: 100×).

choroid plexus cells but can also be seen in ependymal cells. They are age-related changes in the form of fibrillary or ring-like structures that are positive for amyloid by thioflavin-S, Congo red, and beta-amyloid. They are also increased in AD.[728]

CMV infection[729] favors the ventricular surfaces and periventricular tissues. Ependymal cells may harbor viral inclusions and should be evaluated carefully, especially in immunocompromised cases. Especially congenital infections are characterized predominantly by ventricular and periventricular involvement with tissue destruction and dystrophic calcifications. *VZV* also has a predilection to cause ventriculitis, and viral inclusions can be seen in ependymal cell nuclei.[730] Especially *bacterial meningitis*[731] can spread in a retrograde manner to the ventricular system and can cause ventriculitis, ependymitis, and choroid plexitis **(Fig. 2-307)**. Ventriculitis, rather than meningitis, is predominant in the primary infections of the ventricular surfaces, as seen in *shunt infections*.[732] Essentially any intracranial infection can make its way into the ventricles, including fungal infections, resulting in changes in the choroid plexus and ependyma, such as *granulomas* in these locations in some cases of histoplasmosis. *Chemical or aseptic ventriculitis* may occur as a result of chemical irritation by ruptured cyst contents or can occur as a side effect of medications.[733,734]

Small nodules of hamartomatous nature can protrude into the ventricular surface in tuberous sclerosis and are termed *subependymal nodule or candle guttering*. *SEGA*[580] is also seen in the context of tuberous sclerosis and, taken out of context, can result in confusion due to its large, bizarre cells. The typical groupings of these overall uniform cells with tapered cytoplasms, usually packed close to each other in a fibrillary background, especially with a history of tuberous sclerosis are characteristic for this WHO grade I neoplasm. *Subependymoma*[582] is a WHO grade I ependymal neoplasm that is found on the ependymal surfaces, usually protruding into the lumen, typically in the fourth ventricle, although this is not the rule. It is usually seen as an incidental finding at autopsy but may come to clinical attention due to obstruction to CSF circulation, resulting in syncope or headache. It has a characteristic lobulated pattern with small groups of cells in a partially mucinous, fibrillary background. It is covered for the most part by ependymal cells on the surface.

There are many conditions that involve the ventricular system; however, they typically constitute gross structural abnormalities, such as hydrocephalus, and do not provide material for microscopic evaluation. In addition, there are several intraventricular neoplastic processes arising from particular locations; however, they are typically small tissue samples or resection material from surgical procedures, and any relevant specific location information, if needed, is obtained from radiologic findings. For instance, chordoid glioma is thought to arise from organum vasculosum in the anterior aspect of the third ventricle,[735] while PTPR is thought to arise from specialized ependyma of the subcommissural organ in the posterior aspect of the third ventricle.[554]

Choroid Plexus

Choroid plexus is composed of branching fibrovascular cores lined by a cuboidal epithelium resting on a basement membrane. The epithelial cells form a hobnail appearance on their surface and have eosinophilic, finely granular cytoplasm and a central to slightly basally located round, bland nucleus. A cytoplasmic pale area or sometimes even a vague vacuole can be present in the cytoplasm, an age-related change. *Biondi bodies or rings* are delicate ring or arc-shaped age-related accumulations in the cytoplasm. They are positive for amyloid by Thioflavin-S, Congo red, and beta-amyloid immunohistochemistry, as well as by PAS and silver stains. They are also increased in AD.[728] Another age-related change is inclusion bodies that are positive by iron stains, indicating iron accumulation.[736,737]

Choroid plexus papilloma (see also "Papillary and Pseudopapillary Structures") also consists of complex fibrovascular cores lined by cuboidal or somewhat columnar epithelium, forming a mass lesion. Otherwise, in small biopsies, it may be difficult to distinguish from nonneoplastic choroid plexus. One subtle difference is that in choroid plexus papilloma, the surface hobnailing arrangement of epithelial cells is lost, resulting in a flat surface. Areas of coalescence and solid sheet formation, necrosis, and increased mitotic activity should be sought, as these features indicate *choroid plexus carcinoma*. Although a superficial invasion of the neuroglial tissue can be seen in choroid plexus papillomas, extensive invasion is a feature of carcinomas. There is also an associated increase in cytologic atypia and Ki-67 proliferation index in carcinomas. When there are some atypical features, but they are not widespread and prominent enough to justify a diagnosis of choroid plexus carcinoma, *atypical papilloma* is diagnosed.[547] Some choroid plexus papillomas may be a component of Aicardi syndrome, associated with corpus callosum agenesis, infantile spasms, and retinal abnormalities.[738] Rare cases of choroid plexus neoplasms may be multiple with or without an association with Aicardi syndrome.[739–741] Whether what is described as villous hypertrophy of the choroid plexus, which involves multiple ventricles and results in hydrocephalus,[742,743] actually represents multiple choroid plexus papillomas is debatable. They may also be a component of von Hippel-Lindau syndrome[744] and Down syndrome.[745] Choroid plexus carcinomas can be a component of familial tumor syndromes.[746] Choroid plexus neoplasms in general may be multiple, involving more than one ventricle, and may also be seen rarely outside the ventricles. The differential diagnosis of choroid plexus carcinoma includes *metastatic carcinoma*. This may become a difficult differential diagnosis and may require immunohistochemistry. Papillary ependymoma enters into the differential diagnosis of the papillary choroid plexus neoplasms. It has glial stroma and the lining cells do not rest on a basement membrane as choroid plexus cells do. Choroid plexus stroma can have remnants of *meningeal cell groups and glial tissue*, which can be a source for intraventricular meningiomas[747] and gliomas,[748] respectively. Other rare neoplasms that can be seen in the choroid plexus include hemangiopericytoma,[749] SFT,[750] lymphoma,[751] and metastatic carcinoma,[752] among which renal cell carcinoma has a particular propensity.[752,753] An even rarer neoplasm is the *choroid plexus adenoma* that is characterized

List of Findings/Checklist for Choroid Plexus

AT A GLANCE

- Choroid plexus neoplasms
  - Papilloma
  - Atypical papilloma
  - Carcinoma
  - Adenoma
- Metastatic carcinoma
- Meningioma
- Glioma
- Edematous stroma
- Choroid plexus cyst
- Hemorrhage
- Choroid plexitis
- Xanthogranuloma/cholesterol granuloma
- Accumulations
  - Biondi bodies/rings
  - Argyrophilic material
  - Calcium oxalate

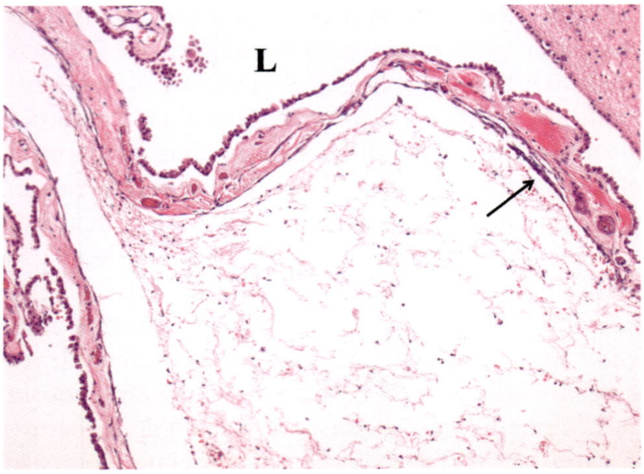

Figure 2-308. Choroid plexus cyst: Identified as an incidental finding in an autopsy of an adult, the cyst is lined by attenuated choroid plexus epithelium (*arrow*) (L: ventricle lumen) (H&E; original magnification: 100×).

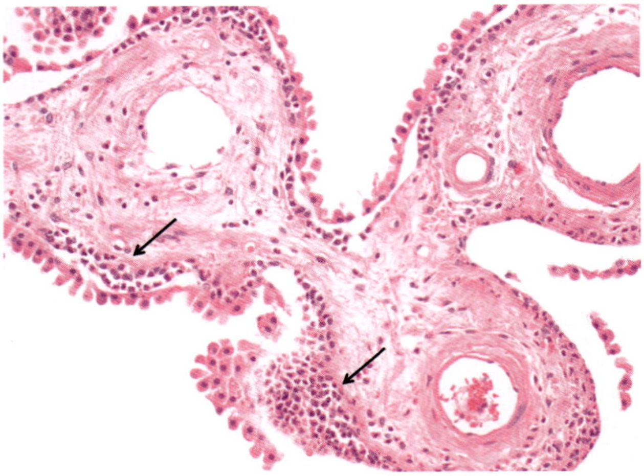

Figure 2-309. Choroid plexitis: Similar to ependymitis, the lining epithelium is sloughing off and many PMN leukocytes are present in the underlying stroma (*arrows*) (H&E; original magnification: 400×).

by adenoid structures instead of papillary architecture, also mimicking metastatic carcinoma in spite of its relatively bland appearance.[534]

Choroid plexus stroma tends to become edematous and develop cystic dilatations. *True cysts* that are lined by choroid plexus epithelium are common in adults **(Fig. 2-308)** but may be associated with trisomies in pediatric population.[754] In intrauterine life and in neonates, choroid plexus may be a source of hemorrhage as part of the hypoxic–ischemic injury that can present as *hemorrhage* in various parts of the intracranial structures, including dura mater. Infections within the ventricles, resulting in ventriculitis/ependymitis, such as those seen in the retrograde extension of acute inflammation in cases of meningitis, can also involve the choroid plexus, resulting in *choroid plexitis* **(Fig. 2-309)**, including the lymphocytic infiltrate of aseptic meningitis that can also be present in choroid plexus. Essentially any infection involving the brain can make its way into the ventricular system and involve choroid plexus. These include fungal infections such as histoplasmosis, which can present with granulomas in the choroid plexus (see also "Ependymal Surfaces"). *Xanthoma and xanthogranuloma*[755] are usually incidental findings, typically in the lateral ventricles and sometimes bilaterally. Xanthoma is composed of sheets of lipid-laden macrophages **(Fig. 2-310)**, while xanthogranuloma results from a reaction to the lipid content with cholesterol clefts, foreign body giant cell reaction to cholesterol crystals, lipid-laden macrophages, hemorrhage, and inflammation, forming a well-circumscribed reactive nodular lesion that can be calcified.

Rarely, *argyrophilic material accumulation* can be seen in the choroid plexus epithelial cells in aluminum intoxication and in dialysis encephalopathy.[756] Birefringent *calcium oxalate crystals* can be

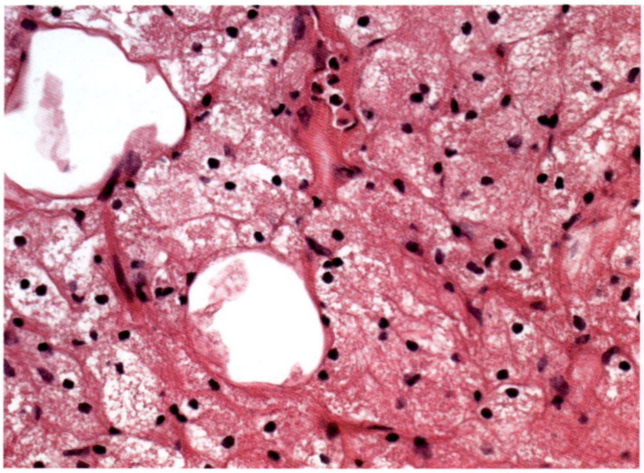

Figure 2-310. Xanthoma: Compact sheets of foamy histiocytes are seen and may occasionally need to be distinguished from metastatic clear cell carcinomas, such as clear cell renal cell carcinoma (H&E; original magnification: 400×).

present in vessel walls and perivascular areas in parenchyma, meninges, and choroid plexus in ethylene glycol intoxication.[310]

Cystic Lesions

The contents and lining of a cyst help identify its nature. In surgical specimens, it is not unusual to receive only unoriented fragments of cyst wall and, depending on its nature, the cyst contents may have been washed away during surgery or in fixative. Still, minute amount of cyst contents may be attached to the surface of the cyst lining. Nonetheless, it is the lining that determines the nature of the cyst. Many are nonneoplastic, developmental cysts, while some are pseudocysts.

List of Findings/Checklist for Cystic Lesions

AT A GLANCE

Squamous Lining
- Epidermoid cyst
- Dermoid cyst
- Pilonidal cyst
- Teratoma
- Craniopharyngioma
  - Adamantinomatous
  - Papillary
- Rathke cleft cyst (squamous metaplasia)

Columnar, Cuboidal, and Mucinous Lining
- Colloid cyst
- Endodermal cyst
- Rathke cleft cyst

Others
- Arachnoid cyst
- Dural cyst
- Choroid plexus cyst
- Glioependymal (ependymal) cyst
- Nerve root (Tarlov) cyst
- Periventricular matrix cyst
- Pineal cyst
- Synovial cyst

Other Cyst-like Lesions
- Parasites
  - Cysticercosis
  - Echinococcosis
  - Sparganosis
- Tuberculosis
- Abscess
- Neoplasms
  - Glioblastoma
  - Metastatic carcinoma
  - Low-grade neoplasms with cyst and mural nodule

Relatively limited types of cysts are seen in the CNS. More common and clinically significant ones are lined by *stratified squamous epithelium* or *columnar/cuboidal epithelium* with some component of mucinous cells. *Colloid cyst of the third ventricle* and *endodermal (neuroenteric, enterogenous) cyst* **(Fig. 2-311)** are similar lesions in different locations, though both tend to be midline. Both are lined by a single or multiple layers of columnar, mucinous epithelium.[757] *Rathke cleft cyst* also has a similar lining,[758] but it may commonly have variable amount of squamous metaplasia[759] **(Fig. 2-312)**. In some cases, the squamous metaplasia may be extensive and occupy the entire cyst lining, resulting in a squamous cyst. Usually, a mucicarmine or other mucin stain will highlight a few residual mucinous cells entrapped within this squamous metaplasia. Together with the sellar/suprasellar location and the smooth lining, this finding supports Rathke cyst. Occasionally, samples from repeated resections for craniopharyngioma (see below) after radiation treatment may have a stratified squamous epithelial lining without the typical stellate reticulum or palisading basaloid cells. Such cases may be difficult to differentiate from Rathke cleft cyst based only on microscopic examination; however, the previous diagnosis and history are very useful, as well as the identification of very small more typical adamantinomatous epithelium and wet keratin upon diligent search. Nuclear beta-catenin positivity in adamantinomatous craniopharyngioma remnants also supports the diagnosis.[760]

Cysts that are lined by stratified squamous epithelium are *epidermoid and dermoid cysts*.[761] The difference is that the latter also has skin adnexa, such as hair follicles and sebaceous glands, in its wall. Epidermoid cysts are typically in the temporal lobe and cerebellopontine angle, while the dermoid cysts are midline on the convexities, may even be intraosseous or in the scalp, and may be completely disconnected from the brain. The lining epithelium may be extremely

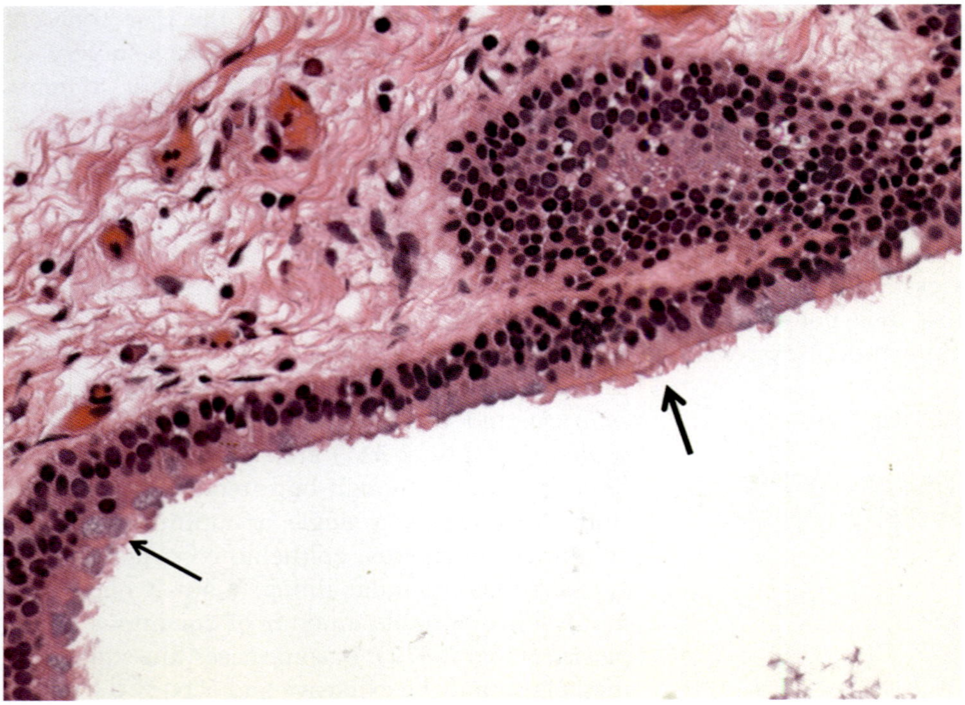

Figure 2-311. Enterogenous cyst: Thin connective tissue cyst wall and a columnar or cuboidal epithelial lining are seen. Goblet cells with mucin (*thin arrow*), as well as ciliated cells (*thick arrow*), are present, mimicking various endodermal epithelial tissues (H&E; original magnification: 400×).

attenuated and rests on a thin, fibrous collagen tissue wall. If the cyst has ruptured and a foreign body giant cell reaction has occurred against the

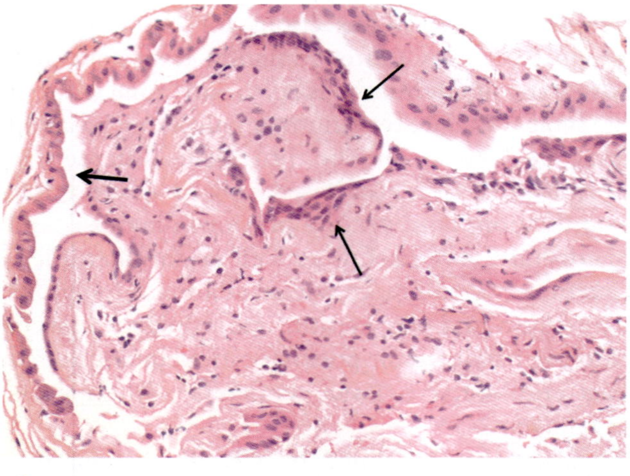

Figure 2-312. Rathke cleft cyst: Wrinkled cyst lining after excision shows areas lined by columnar or cuboidal epithelium (*thick arrow*) that focally shows squamous metaplasia (*thin arrows*). The latter is useful in distinguishing Rathke cleft cyst from cysts with similar lining epithelia, such as colloid cyst and enterogenous cyst; however, the typical locations and presentations of these cysts rarely leave room for any confusion (H&E; original magnification: 200×).

keratinous contents, lining epithelium may not be identified in those areas. No matter how attenuated the lining squamous epithelium might be, diligent search reveals keratohyalin granules in the superficial cells and intercellular junctions between the keratinocytes **(Fig. 2-313)**. Rarely, the development of squamous cell carcinoma has been reported in these cysts.[762,763] A cystic neoplasm with keratinization is *craniopharyngioma*.[764,765] The squamoid epithelium of adamantinomatous craniopharyngioma has a peculiar appearance in solid areas. These islands form interconnected trabecular arrangements with peripheral palisading of the basaloid neoplastic cells and a central loosely textured arrangement called stellate reticulum. Areas of keratinization are frequently present in the center of these epithelial islands. Keratinization is not flaky but is in the form of tightly packed cell groups sometimes seen as squamous ghosts and is referred to as wet keratin due to its waxy appearance. When the neoplasm is extremely cystic, the lining squamous epithelium may be attenuated to only a few layers but usually retains its palisading arrangement at the periphery. Cells are uniform and bland. Rare squamous cell carcinomas may arise in craniopharyngioma, possibly in association

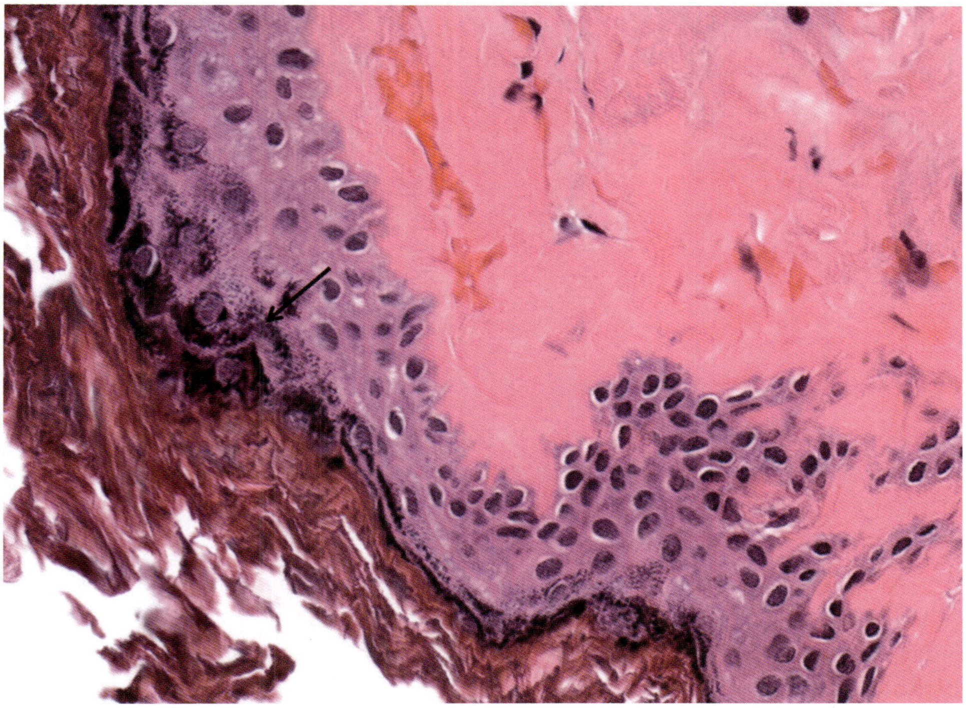

Figure 2-313. Epidermoid cyst: Keratinizing stratified squamous epithelial lining is similar to epidermis with flaky (as opposed to "wet") keratin and a granular layer (*arrow*), both of which are helpful in distinguishing epidermoid cyst from adamantinomatous and papillary craniopharyngiomas (H&E; original magnification: 400×).

with radiation treatment.[766] *Papillary craniopharyngioma*[556,765] is actually a solid neoplasm but becomes variably cystic as it grows due to loosening and separation of squamous epithelial component, leaving fibrovascular cores of tissue covered by this epithelium floating in the cystic space. The squamous epithelium of papillary craniopharyngioma does not have keratohyalin granules and does not keratinize. Especially the *teratomatous component of germ cell neoplasms* can have variable amount of cystic component. It is usually associated with the epidermoid or endodermal components and is lined by their corresponding epithelia.

Arachnoid cyst[764] is a developmental cyst that is formed between the layers of arachnoid membrane and may be lined by a simple arachnoid cell layer. The cyst wall can have a thin collagenous layer, but the lining epithelium may be extremely attenuated or denuded **(Fig. 2-314)**. In some situations, this term may inaccurately be used to refer to a compensatory expansion of the subarachnoid space due to a parenchymal loss, such as an underlying infarct. A similar situation is the posterior fossa cyst of *Dandy-Walker malformation*, in which a large cystic cavity filled with CSF is in continuity with the subarachnoid space and fourth ventricle due to the absence of vermis. Its wall is composed of fibrous leptomeninges on the outside and an inner glioependymal layer, which sometimes may contain residual cerebellar tissue. This condition should be distinguished from large arachnoid and glioependymal cysts in that region, which may distort and hide the developed

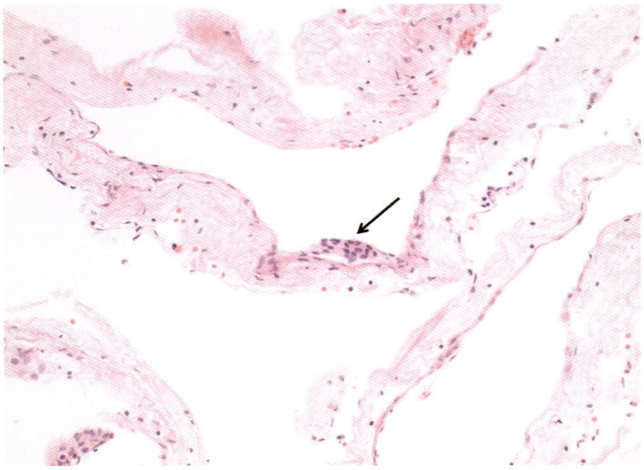

Figure 2-314. Arachnoid cyst: Delicate thin cyst wall is lined by an extremely attenuated arachnoid cell layer with occasional meningothelial cell groups (*arrow*) (H&E; original magnification: 200×).

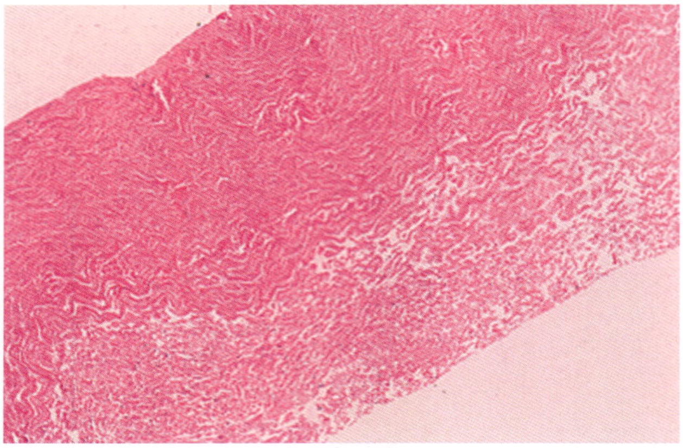

Figure 2-315. Dural cyst: The wall of this rare cyst is composed of thick collagenous connective tissue similar to dura mater, with no epithelial lining (H&E; original magnification: 100×).

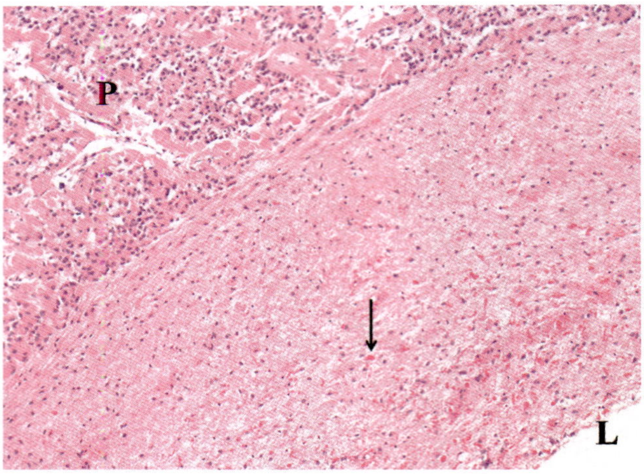

Figure 2-316. Pineal cyst: Cyst has no lining epithelium but a layer of gliotic tissue, usually with many Rosenthal fibers (*arrow*) separating the pineal parenchyma (*P*) from the cyst lumen (*L*) (H&E; original magnification: 100×).

vermis.[767] *Dural cyst* is a very rare condition that develops within the layers of dura mater, and its wall consists of fibrous tissue like the dura mater **(Fig. 2-315)**. It can grow to very large size to produce mass effect or may be small and within the dural sinus to cause occlusion of the sinus.[768,769] *Choroid plexus cyst* has been discussed in "Choroid Plexus." *Glioependymal, or ependymal, cysts*[770,771] are septated cysts of variable size, lined by ependymal cells, which may be extremely attenuated or denuded especially in large cysts under pressure. The lining cells have no basement membrane and are in direct contact with the underlying glial tissue. *Pineal cyst*[772] is very common and occurs as a degenerative change in the pineal gland. Its lining is composed of gliotic tissue that also contains Rosenthal fibers and sometimes evidence of previous hemorrhage. Variable amount of pineal parenchyma may be present in the outer layer of the cyst and may resemble a neoplasm due to its distorted architecture **(Fig. 2-316)**. Fibrotic meninges can be seen as an outermost layer, though not always present. Due to cystic nature and the presence of Rosenthal fibers, which are also commonly present in the pineal region regardless of the presence of a cyst, it should be distinguished from PA. Typically, awareness of this situation, correlation with radiologic findings, and close communication with the surgeon to identify where exactly the sample is originating from should resolve this problem in difficult cases. In addition, neuronal markers help identify the surrounding cells as pineal parenchyma. *Periventricular matrix cysts*, or subependymal matrix cysts or simply periventricular cysts, are probably related to ependymal cysts and develop as a result of resolution of previous destructive lesions, such as hemorrhage, and usually indicate a previous hypoxic–ischemic injury in perinatal period. Residual germinal matrix cell groups can be present in its lining **(Fig. 2-317)**.

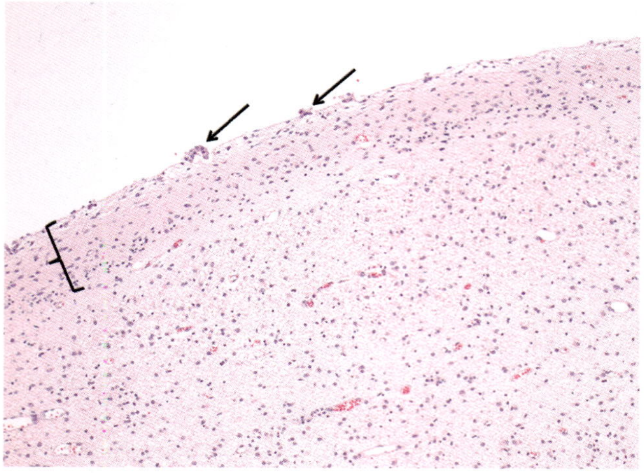

Figure 2-317. Subependymal matrix cyst: These cysts are typically periventricular and have a gliotic lining (*bracket*), separating the neuroglial parenchyma from the cyst lumen. There may be small groups of ependymal cells on the surface (*arrows*) (H&E; original magnification: 100×).

Hydromyelia refers to the expansion of the central canal of the spinal cord. It is lined by ependymal cells. Larger examples may appear like a cyst; however, they are not true cysts by definition and the process is similar to the dilation of the cerebral ventricles for various reasons. *Syringomyelia* on the other hand is a cavity in the spinal cord parenchyma and is not lined by any cells. In that sense, syrinx is similar to the periventricular matrix cyst in the brain. Syringomyelia and hydromyelia can coexist and can be connected. They may be associated with other anomalies in the CNS. A cyst that occurs in association with spinal nerve roots is *Tarlov cyst, or spinal nerve root cyst*. It is devoid of a lining layer and the wall contains the nerve fascicles **(Fig. 2-318)**. It typically arises in the lumbosacral region and may interfere with urinary bladder function or result in radiculopathy.[773] *Synovial cyst*, also known as ganglion cyst and sometimes referred to as spinal extradural cyst, commonly occurs in association with facet joints of the spine, typically in the lumbar region, but may be unassociated with the joints, as well. Its lining commonly consists of fibrous tissue without a cell layer but may also have synovial cells **(Fig. 2-319)**. Rarely, a *pilonidal cyst or sinus* in the sacral skin may be surgically removed and may histologically resemble epidermoid or dermoid cyst with its keratin content and keratinizing stratified squamous epithelium, that is, skin. Frequently, it has a prominent foreign body and inflammatory reaction against the hair it contains.

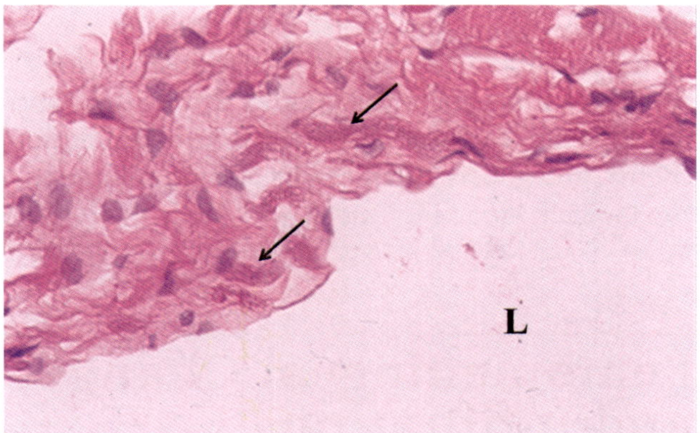

Figure 2-318. Tarlov cyst: Also referred to as nerve root cyst, its wall consists of spinal nerve fascicles with otherwise unremarkable nerve fibers (*arrows*) and no lining epithelium (L: lumen) (H&E; original magnification: 400×).

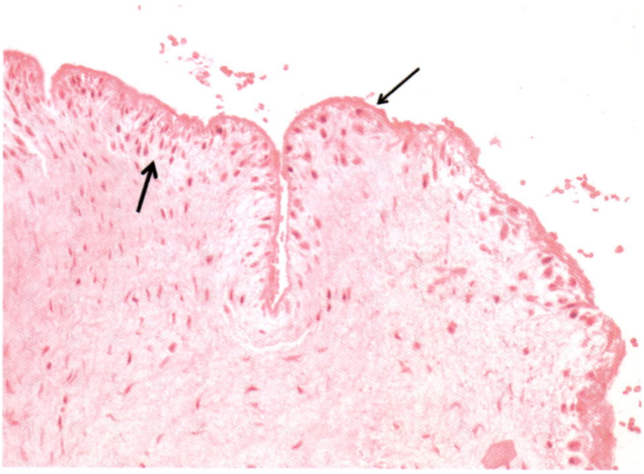

Figure 2-319. Synovial cyst: The lining is usually fibrous tissue with no epithelial lining. Fibrin and hemorrhage can be present (*thin arrow*). A synovial cell proliferation may be present on the surface (*thick arrow*) (H&E; original magnification: 200×).

Based on the above description of various cysts, the *cyst contents* may be variable. *Mucinous material* is seen in those cysts lined by a mucin-secreting epithelium, such as colloid cyst, endodermal cyst, and Rathke cleft cyst, as well as the cystic endodermal component of germ cell neoplasms. Condensed mucinous and proteinaceous contents may sometimes be a source of confusion. For instance, in colloid cyst, there may be linear structures in aggregates, mimicking fungal hyphae or the sulfur granules of Actinomyces,[774] while in some other cysts, the proteinaceous/fibrinous material may actually form a membrane, mimicking a cyst wall or parasite grossly and microscopically. Synovial cyst typically contains mucinous material. *Keratinous contents* are associated with those cysts lined by squamous epithelium, such as epidermoid and dermoid cysts, craniopharyngiomas, and the cystic epidermoid components of germ cell neoplasms. Craniopharyngioma contents are usually thick, hemorrhagic, dark brown with admixed keratinous debris and are described as "machinery oil." Other cysts such as arachnoid cyst, Tarlov cyst, and glioependymal cyst have clear or blood-tinged *CSF or extracellular fluid*.

There are many *other conditions* that present with a cystic lesion and most are malformative, such as meningocele, meningomyelocele, hydrocephalus, and hydranencephaly, and others may be destructive, such as multicystic leukomalacia and remote infarcts. Their identification and interpretation mainly require gross evaluation, and microscopic evaluation may be needed for confirmation. Several other lesions can have cystic components. For instance, neoplasms like glioblastoma or metastatic carcinoma with extensive necrosis or hemorrhage may assume a cystic nature filled with necrotic material and are described as such on imaging. Likewise, large necrotic lesions of tuberculosis, that is, tuberculoma, may resemble cystic mass lesions. Remote infarcts also become cystic once the necrotic debris is cleared away and is replaced by CSF and glial tissue. Low-grade neoplasms such as ganglioglioma, PA, PXA, and hemangioblastoma have a cyst and mural nodule configuration. Their cystic component is filled with clear or blood-tinged fluid, and the mural nodule represents the solid neoplastic area, although their cystic nature cannot be appreciated in fragmented surgical specimens. These lesions are not lined by a particular layer, but their walls are formed by malignant cells in the case of metastatic carcinoma and glioblastoma, and reactive neuroglial parenchyma in infarcts and in the cystic component of low-grade neoplasms. One needs to be familiar with their nature to avoid confusion after reading the details of their radiologic descriptions. Schwannoma can frequently show variable degrees of cystic degeneration and, in some cases, become completely cystic. Similarly, abscesses are filled with pus and are surrounded by granulation tissue wall with acute and chronic inflammatory component. Encapsulation starts with granulation tissue in 1 to 2 weeks and, after 2 weeks, gradually better developed outer fibrous abscess wall forms. If abscess heals without surgical treatment, a fibrous cyst with scattered macrophages in the lumen may be all there is left. Parasitic infections such as cysticercosis and echinococcosis also form cystic lesions containing the parasites and are readily identified by their typical features. Cysticercosis[775] has clear cysts that may float in the subarachnoid space and in the ventricular system. Cyst wall is undulated and has an outer surface hairy layer composed of microtrichia rather than cilia, a cellular layer, and an inner reticular loose fibrillary layer **(Fig. 2-320)**. Hydatid cyst is rare in the CNS; however, it also has a characteristic appearance. Echinococcosis[776] is caused by *Echinococcus granulosus*, which is unilocular, and *Echinococcus multilocularis* (alveolaris), which is in the form of multiple smaller cysts. The outer fibrous layer comes from the host, while the middle cuticular layer and inner germinal layer belong to the parasite. There may be mild gliosis and a few lymphocytes as a reaction. When these parasites die, granulation tissue and giant cell reaction occur, together with many neutrophil and eosinophil PMN leukocytes, eventually resulting in fibrosis and calcification. The appearance of cyst contents at this stage may mimic an abscess if the parasite components are not appreciated. Sparganosis lesions[777] consist of a degenerating central worm, surrounding fibrous capsule, lymphocytic inflammation, edema, and gliosis. Cavities lined by granulation tissue indicate larva migration.

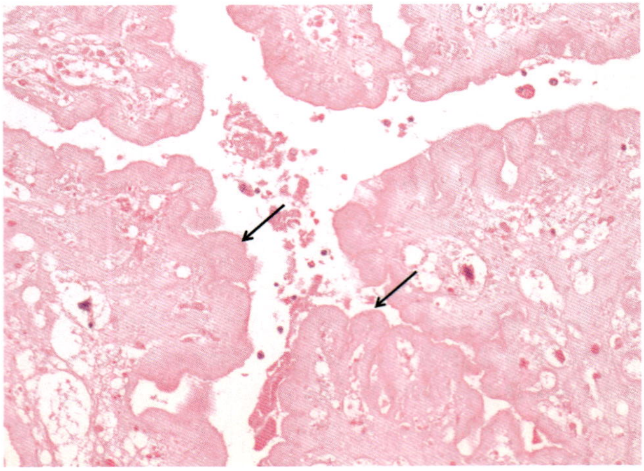

Figure 2-320. Cysticercus: Undulated cyst wall forms projections and has microvillus layer (*arrows*). The organism can be recognized easily because of its distinct morphology even after it is dead; however, if its fragments are seen in a surgical material, it may be difficult to distinguish from condensed fibrin or other proteinaceous material, or vice versa (H&E; original magnification: 200×).

Leptomeningeal Changes and Infiltrations

This discussion excludes the processes that arise in association with the meninges, such as meningioma, soft tissue lesions, meningitis, and malignant or reactive hematolymphoid processes that

List of Findings/Checklist for Leptomeningeal Changes and Infiltrations

• AT A GLANCE

- Neoplastic infiltration
- Craniospinal dissemination
- Glioneuronal heterotopias
- Meningeal gliomatosis
- Fibrosis

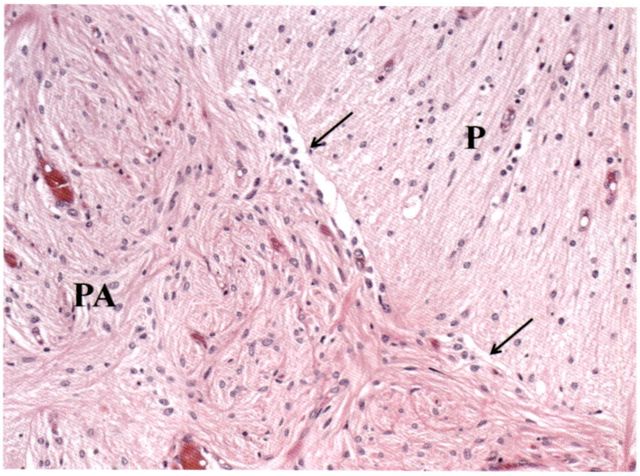

Figure 2-321. PA: Infiltration of leptomeninges and an exophytic growth are common for PA, especially in the brainstem and cerebellum. A sharp distinction (*arrows*) is present between the neuroglial parenchyma (*P*) and the overlying neoplasm (PA). The latter has piloid histology (H&E; original magnification: 200×).

typically involve the meninges, which are mentioned in their respective discussions. Instead, it focuses mainly on the neoplasms that arise in the brain parenchyma and have a tendency to infiltrate the meninges.

Many *neoplasms* can infiltrate the leptomeninges. *Leptomeningeal carcinomatosis*,[778,779] instead of the pathologically inaccurate term carcinomatous meningitis, is more common than the involvement of subarachnoid space by primary neoplasms. It refers to the subarachnoid spread of any malignancy but, in practice and more commonly, is used to refer to a metastatic malignancy, the great majority of which consists of carcinomas. Clinical suspicion and leptomeningeal enhancement lead to cytologic evaluation of CSF, in some cases multiple times to make the diagnosis, and open biopsy may occasionally be needed. Some of the primary neoplasms remain localized but some progress to widespread *craniospinal seeding*. Medulloblastoma, PNET, and especially pineoblastoma due to its proximity to the ventricular system are particularly prone to seed the CSF (see "Small Blue Cells"). Another intraventricular neoplasm with a tendency to seed the CSF is choroid plexus carcinoma. Other *choroid plexus neoplasms* can also result in such dissemination, though less frequently. Of the *glial neoplasms, oligodendroglioma* has a particular tendency to infiltrate the cortical gray matter and form a subpial accumulation of cells, eventually infiltrating the subarachnoid space. *Pilocytic astrocytoma* tends to grow on the surface of the cerebellum and brainstem, where it is densely piloid with many Rosenthal fibers **(Fig. 2-321)**. PMA demonstrates a similar behavior and owes its more aggressive nature at least in part to its tendency to produce craniospinal seeding. Glioblastoma, fibrillary astrocytoma, and ependymoma are also capable of leptomeningeal infiltration. ATRT can grow in an exophytic manner and commonly results in craniospinal seeding, commonly at the time of initial presentation.[780]

Several low-grade glial neoplasms are typically located superficially and may be naturally in touch with overlying leptomeninges. PXA, ganglioglioma, and DIG/DIA, actually a dural-based neoplasm, commonly involve the leptomeninges. PXA can extend along the vessels through the Virchow-Robin spaces deeper into the neuroglial parenchyma.[42] Gliofibroma is a biphasic neoplasm with a glial component and a fibroblastic component that is bland in contrast to gliosarcoma, where the spindle cell component is sarcomatous. SEGA has also been reported to result in craniospinal seeding.[781] Meningioma, due to its location, may result in craniospinal seeding; however, this is a relatively infrequent occurrence compared to those neoplasms mentioned above. In general, it may not be readily obvious that the neoplasm is infiltrating the subarachnoid space, especially if there is a large amount of neoplasm in large sheets, overrunning the normal tissues. In such cases, presence of large-caliber vessels entrapped within the neoplasm represents the subarachnoid vessels and indicates the subarachnoid space involvement by the neoplasm.

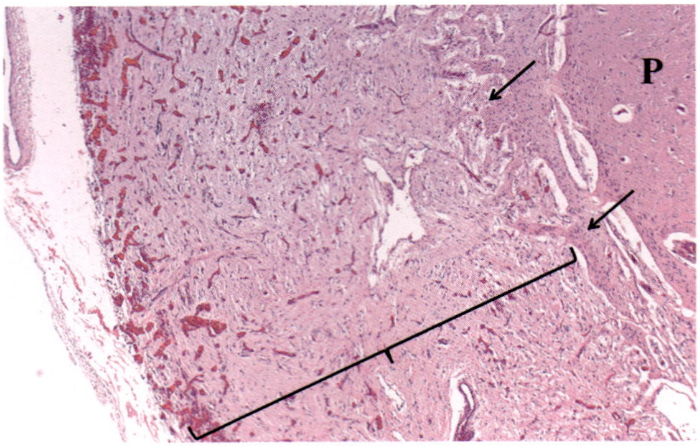

Figure 2-322. Leptomeningeal glioneuronal heterotopia: Abundant neuroglial tissue is present in the leptomeninges, forming a distinct layer (*bracket*) that can be easily distinguished from the parenchyma (*P*) by a clear border (*arrows*) in spite of some surface irregularities (H&E; original magnification: 40×).

Leptomeningeal glioneuronal heterotopias **(Fig. 2-322)**[782] are common in association with malformations, but especially common in some of them, such as MCD, holoprosencephaly, migration defects, atelencephaly, and cerebro-ocular dysplasia. Glial neoplasms located in the meninges with no parenchymal component are thought to arise from such heterotopic tissue. *Diffuse leptomeningeal gliomatosis*[783] is a glial neoplasm that diffusely involves the leptomeninges, without an intraparenchymal component. Clinically and radiologically, it may be confused with meningitis. *Leptomeningeal fibrosis* is an age-related change seen with increasing age especially in the parasagittal convexities. Focal fibrosis may be seen in specimens resected during seizure surgery and is a result of preoperative work-up with electrodes. These can be associated with chronic inflammation and small infarcts with linear or rounded contours due to electrode placement.

References

1. Zulch KJ, ed. *Histological Typing of Tumours of the Central Nervous System, International Histological Classification of Tumours, No. 21*. Geneva, Switzerland: World Health Organization; 1979.
2. Louis DN, Ohgaki H, Wiestler OD, et al., eds. *WHO Classification of Tumours of the Central Nervous System*. Lyon, France: IARC Press; 2007.
3. Fuller GN, Kros JM. Gliomatosis cerebri. In: Louis DN, Ohgaki H, Wiestler OD, et al., eds. WHO *Classification of Tumours of the Central Nervous System*. Lyon, France: IARC Press; 2007:50–52.
4. Rollins KE, Kleinschmidt-DeMasters BK, Corboy JR, et al. Lymphomatosis cerebri as a cause of white matter dementia. *Hum Pathol*. 2005;36:282–290.
5. Niess C, Grauel U, Toennes SW. Incidence of axonal injury in human brain tissue. *Acta Neuropathol*. 2002;104:79–84.
6. Markesbery WR, Jicha GA, Liu H, et al. Lewy body pathology in normal elderly subjects. *J Neuropathol Exp Neurol*. 2009;68:816–822.
7. Nishio S, Fujiwara S, Aiko Y, et al. Hypothalamic hamartoma. Report of two cases. *J Neurosurg*. 1989;70:640–645.
8. Squires LA, Constantini S, Miller DC, et al. Hypothalamic hamartoma and the Pallister-Hall syndrome. *Pediatr Neurosurg*. 1995;22:303–308.
9. Prayson RA. Diagnostic challenges in the evaluation of chronic epilepsy-related surgical neuropathology. *Am J Surg Pathol*. 2010;34:e1–e13.
10. Palmini A, Najm I, Avanzini G, et al. Terminology and classifications of the cortical dysplasia. *Neurology*. 2004;62:S2–S8.
11. Hardiman O, Burke T, Phillips J, et al. Microdysgenesis in resected temporal neocortex: incidence and clinical significance in focal epilepsy. *Neurology*. 1988:38:1041–1047.
12. Kasper BS, Chang BS, Kasper EM. Microdysgenesis: Historical roots of an important concept in epilepsy. *Epilepsy Behav*. 2009;15:146–153.
13. Goto N, Kaneko M. Olivary enlargement: chronological and morphometric analyses. *Acta Neuropathol*. 1981;54: 275–282.
14. Ho KL, Chang CH, Yang SS, et al. Neuropathologic findings in thanatophoric dysplasia. *Acta Neuropathol*. 1984;63:218–228.
15. ten Donkelaar HJ, Hoevenaars F, Wesseling P. A case of Joubert's syndrome with extensive cerebral malformations. *Clin Neuropathol*. 2000;19:85–93.
16. Powers JM, Moser HW, Moser AB, et al. Fetal cerebrohepatorenal (Zellweger) syndrome: dysmorphic, radiologic, biochemical, and pathologic findings in four affected fetuses. *Hum Pathol*. 1985;16:610–620.
17. Ellison D, Love S, Chimelli L, et al. *Neuropathology. A Reference Text of CNS Pathology*. Philadelphia, PA: Elsevier; 2004.
18. Barth PG, Aronica E, de Vries L, et al. Pontocerebellar hypoplasia type 2: a neuropathological update. *Acta Neuropathol*. 2007;114:373–386.
19. Bertrand I, Gruner J. The status verrucosus of the cerebral cortex. *J Neuropathol Exp Neurol*. 1955;14:331–347.
20. Gilbert LA, Dudley AW Jr, Meisner L, et al. New neurological findings in trisomy 13. *Archiv Pathol Lab Med*. 1977;101:540–544.
21. Soto Ares G, Deries B, Delmaire C, et al. Cerebellar cortical dysplasia: MRI aspects and significance. *J Radiol*. 2004;85:729–740.
22. Hanaway J, Netsky MG. Heterotopias of the inferior olive. Relation to Dandy-Walker malformation and correlation with experimental data. *J Neuropathol Exp Neurol*. 1971;30:380–389.
23. Halliday J, Chow CW, Wallace D, et al. X linked hydrocephalus: a survey of a 20 year period in Victoria, Australia. *J Med Genet*. 1986;23:23–31.
24. Michotte A, De Meirleir L, Lissens W, et al. Neuropathological findings of a patient with pyruvate dehydrogenase E1 alpha deficiency presenting as a cerebral lactic acidosis. *Acta Neuropathol*. 1993;85:674–678.
25. Panayi M, Gokhale D, Mansour S, et al. Prenatal diagnosis in a family with X-linked hydrocephalus. *Prenat Diagn*. 2005;25:930–933.
26. Ogata H, Oka K, Mitsudome A. Hydrocephalus due to acute aqueductal stenosis following mumps infection: report of a case and review of the literature. *Brain Develop*. 1992;14: 417–419.
27. Jellinger G. Anatomopathology of non-tumoral aqueductal stenosis. *J Neurosurg Sci*. 1986;30:1–16.

28. Horvath E, Kovacs K, Scheithauer BW. Pituitary hyperplasia. *Pituitary*. 1999;1:169–179.

29. Burger PC, Scheithauer BW, Vogel FS. *Surgical Pathology of the Nervous System and Its Coverings*. 4th edition, New York. Churchill–Livingstone. 2002.

30. Bruner JM, Saya H, Moser RP. Immunocytochemical detection of p53 in human gliomas. *Mod Pathol*. 1991;4:671–674.

31. Yaziji H, Massarani-Wafai R, Gujrati M, et al. Role of p53 immunohistochemistry in differentiating reactive gliosis from malignant astrocytic lesions. *Am J Surg Pathol*. 1996;20:1086–1090.

32. Schittenhelm J, Mittelbronn M, Nguyen TD, et al. WT1 Expression distinguishes astrocytic tumor cells from normal and reactive astrocytes. *Brain Pathol*. 2008;18:344–353.

33. Camelo-Piragua S, Jansen M, Ganguly A, et al. A sensitive and specific diagnostic panel to distinguish diffuse astrocytoma from astrocytosis: chromosome 7 gain with mutant isocitrate dehydrogenase 1 and p53. *J Neuropathol Exp Neurol*. 2011;70:110–115.

34. Colodner KJ, Montana RA, Anthony DC, et al. Proliferative potential of human astrocytes. *J Neuropathol Exp Neurol*. 2005;64:163–169.

35. Burger PC, Shibata T, Kleihues P. The use of the monoclonal antibody Ki-67 in the identification of proliferating cells: application to surgical neuropathology. *Am J Surg Pathol*. 1986;10:611–617.

36. Deckert M, Reifenberger G, Wechsler W. Determination of the proliferative potential of human brain tumors using the monoclonal antibody Ki-67. *J Cancer Res Clin Oncol*. 1989;115:179–188.

37. Lombardi D, Scheithauer BW, Piepgras D, et al. "Angioglioma" and the arteriovenous malformation-glioma association. *J Neurosurg*. 1991;75:589–566.

38. Nazek M, Mandybur TI, Kashiwagi S. Oligodendroglial proliferative abnormality associated with arteriovenous malformation: report of three cases with review of the literature. *Neurosurgery*. 1988;23:781–785.

39. Raore B, Schniederjan M, Prabhu R, et al. Metastasis infiltration: an investigation of the postoperative brain-tumor interface. *Int J Radiat Obcol Biol Phys*. 2011;81:1075–1080.

40. Burger PC, Vollmet RT. Histologic factors of prognostic significance in the glioblastoma multiforme. *Cancer*. 1980;46:1179–1186.

41. Lusis EA, Travers S, Jost SC, et al. Glioblastomas with giant cell and sarcomatous features in patients with Turcot syndrome type 1: a clinicopathological study of 3 cases. *Neurosurgery*. 2010;67:811–817.

42. Burger PC, Scheithauer BW. *Tumors of the Central Nervous System. AFIP Atlas of Tumor Pathology*. Washington, DC: American Registry of Pathology; 2007.

43. Wang M, Tihan T, Rojiani AM, et al. Monomorphous angiocentric glioma: a distinctive epileptogenic neoplasm with features of infiltrating astrocytoma and ependymoma. *J Neuropathol Exp Neurol*. 2005;64:875–881.

44. Perry A, Louis DN, Scheithauer BW, et al. *Meningiomas*. In: Louis DN, Ohgaki H, Wiestler OD, et al., eds. *WHO Classification of Tumours of the Central Nervous System*. Lyon, France: IARC Press; 2007:163–172.

45. Kim NR, Choe G, Shin SH, et al. Childhood meningiomas associated with meningioangiomatosis: report of five cases and literature review. *Neuropathol Appl Neurobiol*. 2002;28:48–56.

46. Giangaspero F, Guiducci A, Lenz FA, et al. Meningioma with meningioangiomatosis: a condition mimicking invasive meningiomas in children and young adults: report of two cases and review of the literature. *Am J Surg Pathol*. 1999;23: 872–875.

47. Brat DJ, Giannini C, Scheithauer BW, et al. Primary melanocytic neoplasms of the central nervous systems. *Am J Surg Pathol*. 1999;23:745–754.

48. Asa SL. Practical pituitary pathology, what does the pathologist need to know? *Arch Pathol Lab Med*. 2008;132: 1231–1240.

49. Scheithauer BW, Woodruff JM, Erlandson RA. *Tumores of the Peripheral Nervous System. Atlas of Tumor Pathology*. Washington, DC: Armed Forces Institute of Pathology; 1999.

50. Von Diemling A, Burger PC, Nakazato Y, et al. Diffuse astrocytoma. In: Louis DN, Ohgaki H, Wiestler OD, et al., eds. WHO *Classification of Tumors of the Central Nervous System*. Lyon, France: IARC Press; 2007:25–29.

51. Peraud A, Ansari H, Bise K, et al. Clinical outcome of supratentorial astrocytoma WHO grade II. *Acta Neurochir*. 1998;140:1213–1222.

52. Tihan T, Vohra P, Berger MS, et al. Definition and diagnostic implications of gemistocytic astrocytomas: a pathological perspective. *J Neurooncol*. 2006;76:175–183.

53. Meenakshi-Sundaram S, Mahadevan A, Taly AB, et al. Wilson's disease: a clinico-neuropathological autopsy study. *J Clin Neurosci*. 2008;15:409–417.

54. Mossakowski MJ. Some remarks on the morphology and histochemistry of the so-called Opalski cells. *Acta Neuropathol*. 1965;4:659–668.

55. Takashima S, Becker LE. Developmental changes of glial fibrillary acidic protein in cerebral white matter. *Arch Neurol*. 1983;40:14–18.

56. Perry A, Fuller CE, Judkins AR, et al. INI1 expression is retained in composite rhabdoid tumors, including rhabdoid meningiomas. *Mod Pathol*. 2005;18:951–958.

57. Stevens EA, Stanton CA, Nichols K, et al. Rare intraparenchymal choroid plexus carcinoma resembling atypical teratoid/rhabdoid tumor diagnosed by immunostaining for INI1 protein. *J Neurosurg*. 2009;4:368–371.

58. Fruhwald MC, Hasselblatt M, Wirth S, et al. Nonlinkage of familial rhabdoid tumors to SMARCB1 implies a second locus for the rhabdoid tumor predisposition syndrome. *Pediatr Blood Cancer*. 2006;47:273–278.

59. Kleinschmidt-DeMasters BK, Alassiri AH, Birks DK, et al. Epithelioid versus rhabdoid glioblastomas are distinguished by monosomy 22 and immunohistochemical expression of INI-1 but not claudin 6. *Am J Surg Pathol*. 2010;34:341–354.

60. Gokden M, Roth KA, Carroll SL, et al. Clear cell neoplasms and pseudoneoplastic lesions of the central nervous system. *Semin Diagn Pathol*. 1997;14:253–269.

61. Daumas-Duport C, Varlet P, Bacha S, et al. Dysembryoplastic neuroepithelial tumors: nonspecific histological forms—a study of 40 cases. *J Neurooncol*. 1999;41:267–280.

62. Almefty K, Pravdenkova S, Colli BO, et al. Chordoma and chondrosarcoma: similar, but quite different, skull base tumors. *Cancer*. 2007;110:2457–2467.

63. Hoch BL, Nielsen GP, Liebsch NJ, et al. Base of skull chordomas in children and adolescents: a clinicopathologic study of 73 cases. *Am J Surg Pathol*. 2006;30:811–818.

64. Mobley BC, McKenney JK, Bangs CD, et al. Loss of SMARCB1/INI1 expression in poorly differentiated chordomas. *Acta Neuropathol*. 2010;120:745–753.

65. Horvath E, Kovacs K, Singer W, et al. Acidophil stem cell adenoma of the human pituitary: clinicopathologic analysis of 15 cases. *Cancer*. 1981;47:761–771.

66. Brat DJ, Scheithauer BW, Medina-Flores R, et al. Infiltrative astrocytomas with granular cell features (granular cell astrocytomas) a study of histopathologic features, grading, and outcome. *Am J Surg Pathol*. 2002;26:750–757.

67. Cohen-Gadol AA, Pichelmann MA, Link MJ, et al. Granular cell tumor of the sellar and suprasellar region: clinicopathologic study of 11 cases and literature review. *Mayo Clin Proc*. 2003;78:567–573.

68. Carstens PH, Yacoub O. Importance of angulate bodies in the diagnosis of granular cell tumors (schwannomas). *Ultrastruct Pathol*. 1993;17:271–278.

69. Giangaspero F, Cenacchi G. Oncocytic and granular cell neoplasms of the central nervous system and pituitary gland. *Semin Diagn Pathol*. 1999;16:91–97.

70. Roncaroli F, Scheithauer BW, Cenacchi G, et al. 'Spindle cell oncocytoma' of the adenohypophysis: a tumor of folliculostellate cells? *Am J Surg Pathol*. 2002;26:1048–1055.

71. Vajtai I, von Gunten M, Fung C, et al. Oncocytic ependymoma: a new morphological variant of high-grade ependymal neoplasm composed of mitochondrion-rich epithelioid cells. *Pathol Res Pract*. 2011;207:49–54.

72. Zunarelli E, Tallarico E, Valentini A, et al. Oncocytic meningioma: study of eight new cases and analysis of 13 reported cases. *Pathology*. 2010;42:587–589.

73. Connor DH, Neafie RC, Dooley JR. African trypanosomiasis. In: Binford CH, Connor DH, ed. *Pathology of Tropical and Extraordinary Diseases:* An Atlas. Washington, DC: AFIP; 1976:252–257.

74. Sanno N, Teramoto A, Osamura RY, et al. Pathology of pituitary tumors. *Neurosurg Clin N Am*. 2003;14:25–39.

75. George DH, Scheithauer BW, Kovacs K, et al. Crooke's cell adenoma of the pituitary:an aggressive variant of corticotroph adenoma. *Am J Surg Pathol*. 2003;27:1330–1336.

76. Rodriguez D, Gauthier F, Bertini E, et al. Infantile Alexander disease: spectrum of GFAP mutations and genotype-phenotype correlation. *Am J Hum Genet*. 2001;69:1134–1140.

77. Harding BN, Surtees RA. *Metabolic and Neurodegenerative Diseases of Childhood. Greenfield's Neuropathology*. London, UK: Edward Arnold; 2008:482–514.

78. Rubinstein LJ. Tumors of the central nervous system. In: *Atlas of Tumor Pathology*. Fascicle 6, 2nd. series, Washington, DC: AFIP; 1972.

79. Walkley SU. Cellular pathology of lysosomal storage disorders. *Brain Pathol*. 1998;8:175–193.

80. Tellez I, Cabello A, Franch O, et al. Chromatolytic changes in the central nervous system of patients with the toxic oil syndrome. *Acta Neuropathol*. 1987;74:354–361.

81. Kotaki H, Nakajima K, Tanimura Y, et al. Appearance of intoxication in rats by intraperitoneal administration of clioquinol. *J Pharmacobiodyn*. 1983;6:773–783.

82. Marker SC, Howard RJ, Groth KE, et al. A trial of vidarabine for cytomegalovirus infection in renal transplant patients. *Arch Intern Med*. 1980;140:1441–1444.

83. Oehmichen M, Auer RN, Konig HG. *Forensic Neuropathology and Associated Neurology*. Berlin, Germany: Springer; 2009.

84. Vinters HV, Kleinschmidt-DeMasters BK. General pathology of the central nervous system. In: Love S, Louis DN, Ellison DW, ed. *Greenfield's Neuropathology.* 8th ed. vol. 1. London, UK: Edward Arnold; 2008:1–62.

85. Frank S, Tolnay M. Frontotemporal lobar degeneration: toward the end of confusion. *Acta Neuropathol*. 2009;118:629–631.

86. Kovacs GG, Botond G, Budka H. Protein coding of neurodegenerative dementias: the neuropathological basis of biomarker diagnostics. *Acta Neuropathol*. 2010;119:389–408.

87. Dickson DW. Neuropathology of non-Alzheimer degenerative disorders. *Int J Clin Exp Pathol*. 2009;3:1–23.

88. Gibb WR, Scott T, Lees AJ. Neuronal inclusions of Parkinson's disease. *Mov Disord*. 1991;6:2–11.

89. Jellinger KA. Formation and development of Lewy pathology: a critical update. *J Neurol*. 2009;256:270–279.

90. Ikemura M, Saito Y, Sengoku R, et al. Lewy body pathology involves cutaneous nerves. *J Neuropathol Exp Neurol*. 2008;67:945–953.

91. Jellinger KA. A critical reappraisal of current staging of Lewy-related pathology in human brain. *Acta Neuropathol*. 2008;116:1–16.

92. Cummings JL. Reconsidering diagnostic criteria for dementia with lewy bodies. *Rev Neurol Dis*. 2004;1:31–34.

93. Hayashida K, Oyanagi S, Mizutani Y, et al. An early cytoplasmic change before Lewy body maturation: an ultrastructural study of the substantia nigra from an autopsy case of juvenile parkinsonism. *Acta Neuropathol*. 1993;85:445–448.

94. Okamoto K, Mizuno Y, Fujita Y. Bunina bodies in amyotrophic lateral sclerosis. *Neuropathology*. 2008;28:109–115.

95. Brunnstrom H, Englund E. Comparison of four neuropathological scales for Alzheimer's disease. *Clin Neuropathol*. 2011;30:56–69.

96. Newell KL, Hyman BT, Growdon JH, et al. Application of the National Institute on Aging (NIA)-Reagan Institute criteria for the neuropathological diagnosis of Alzheimer disease. *J Neuropathol Exp Neurol*. 1999;58:1147–1155.

97. Braak H, Braak E. Neuropathological staging of Alzheimer-related changes. *Acta Neuropathol*. 1991;82:239–259.

98. Litvan I, Hauw JJ, Bartko JJ, et al. Validity and reliability of the preliminary NINDS neuropathologic criteria for progressive supranuclear palsy and related disorders. *J Neuropathol Exp Neurol*. 1996;55:97–105.

99. Morris HR, Lees AJ, Wood NW. Neurofibrillary tangle parkinsonian disorders—tau pathology and tau genetics. *Movement Disord*. 1999;14:731–736.

100. McKee AC, Cantu RC, Nowinski CJ, et al. Chronic traumatic encephalopathy in athletes: progressive tauopathy after repetitive head injury. *J Neuropathol Exp Neurol*. 2009;68:709–735.

101. Habuchi C, Iritani S, Sekiguchi H, et al. Clinicopathological study of diffuse neurofibrillary tangles with calcification. With special reference to TDP-43 proteinopathy and alpha-synucleinopathy. *J Neurol Sci*. 2011;301:77–85.

102. Ferrer I, Santpere G, van Leeuwen FW. Argyrophilic grain disease. *Brain*. 2008;131:1416–1432.

103. Goldman JE. The association of actin with Hirano bodies. *J Neuropathol Exp Neurol*. 1983;42:146–152.

104. Cairns NJ, Bigio EH, Mackenzie IR, et al. Neuropathologic diagnostic and nosologic criteria for frontotemporal lobar degeneration: consensus of the Consortium for Frontotemporal Lobar Degeneration. *Acta Neuropathol*. 2007;114:5–22.

105. Yokota O, Tsuchiya K, Terada S, et al. Basophilic inclusion body disease and neuronal intermediate filament inclusion disease: a comparative clinicopathological study. *Acta Neuropathol*. 2008;115:561–575.

106. Ikeda K, Tsuchiya K. Motor neuron disease group accompanied by inclusions of unidentified protein signaled by ubiquitin. *Neuropathology*. 2004;24:117–1124.

107. Przedborski S, Jackson-Lewis V. Mechanisms of MPTP toxicity. *Movement Disord*. 1998;13:35–38.

108. Josephs KA, Petersen RC, Knopman DS, et al. Clinicopathologic analysis of frontotemporal and corticobasal degenerations and PSP. *Neurology*. 2006;66:41–48.

109. Davis RL, Holohan PD, Shrimpton AE, et al. Familial encephalopathy with neuroserpin inclusion bodies. *Am J Pathol*. 1999;155:1901–1913.

110. Jellinger KA, Lantos PL. Papp-Lantos inclusions and the pathogenesis of multiple system atrophy: an update. *Acta Neuropathol*. 2010;119:657–667.

111. Wakabayashi K, Takahashi H. Cellular pathology in multiple system atrophy. *Neuropathology*. 2006;26:338–345.

112. Keith-Rokosh J, Ang LC. Progressive supranuclear palsy: a review of co-existing neurodegeneration. *Can J Neurol Sci*. 2008;35:602–608.

113. Vogel H, Horoupian DS. Filamentous degeneration of neurons. A possible feature of cytosine arabinoside neurotoxicity. *Cancer*. 1993;71:1303–1308.

114. Dahl D, Bignami A, Bich NT, et al. Immunohistochemical characterization of neurofibrillary tangles induced by mitotic spindle inhibitors. *Acta Neuropathol*. 1980;51:165–168.

115. Wakabayashi K, Hayashi S, Yoshimoto M, et al. NACP/alpha-synuclein-positive filamentous inclusions in astrocytes and oligodendrocytes of Parkinson's disease brains. *Acta Neuropathol*. 2000;99:14–20.

116. Kawashima T, Furuta A, Doh-ura K, et al. Ubiquitin-immunoreactive skein-like inclusions in the neostriatum are not restricted to amyotrophic lateral sclerosis, but are rather aging-related structures. *Acta Neuropathol*. 2000;100:43–49.

117. Takei Y, Mirra SS. Intracytoplasmic hyaline inclusion bodies in the nerve cells of the hypoglossal nucleus in human autopsy material. *Acta Neuropathol*. 1971;17:14–23.

118. Wen GY, Wisniewski HM, Kascsak RJ. Biondi ring tangles in the choroid plexus of Alzheimer's disease and normal aging brains: a quantitative study. *Brain Res*. 1999;832:40–46.

119. Obari A, Sano T, Ohyama K, et al. Clinicopathological features of growth hormone-producing pituitary adenomas: difference among various types defined by cytokeratin distribution pattern including a transitional form. *Endocr Pathol.* 2008;19:82–91.

120. Harding BN, Ramani P, Thurley P. The familial syndrome of proliferative vasculopathy and hydranencephaly-hydrocephaly: immunocytochemical and ultrastructural evidence for endothelial proliferation. *Neuropathol Appl Neurobiol.* 1995;21:61–67.

121. Mancuso M. Davidzon G. Kurlan RM, et al. Hereditary ferritinopathy: a novel mutation, its cellular pathology, and pathogenetic insights. *J Neuropathol Exp Neurol.* 2005;64:280–294.

122. Josephs KA. Holton JL. Rossor MN, et al. Neurofilament inclusion body disease: a new proteinopathy?. *Brain.* 2003;126:2291–2303.

123. Langer CJ, Besse B, Gualberto A, et al. The evolving role of histology in the management of advanced non-small-cell lung cancer. *J Clin Oncol.* 2010;28:5311–5320.

124. Moran CA, Rush W, Mena H. Primary spinal paragangliomas: a clinicopathological and immunohistochemical study of 30 cases. *Histopathology.* 1997;31:167–173.

125. Berho M, Suster S. Mucinous meningioma: report of an unusual variant of meningioma that may mimic metastatic mucin-producing carcinoma. *Am J Surg Pathol.* 1994;18:100–106.

126. Kepes JJ, Chen WY-K, Conners MH, et al. Chordoid meningeal tumors in young individuals with peritumoral lymphoplasmacellular infiltrates causing systemic manifestations of the Castleman syndrome. *Cancer.* 1988;62:391–406.

127. Couce ME, Aker FV, Scheithauer BW. Chordoid meningioma: a clinicopathologic study of 42 cases. *Am J Surg Pathol.* 2000;24:899–905.

128. Sangoi AR, Dulai MS, Beck AH, et al. Distinguishing chordoid meningiomas from their histologic mimics an immunohistochemical evaluation. *Am J Surg Pathol.* 2009;33:669–681.

129. Oakley GJ, Fuhrer K, Seethala RR. Brachyury, SOX-9, and podoplanin, new markers in the skull base chordoma vs chondrosarcoma differential: a tissue microarray-based comparative analysis. *Mod Pathol.* 2008;21:1461–1469.

130. Wang WL, Abramson JH, Ganguly A, et al. The surgical pathology of notochordal remnants in adult intervertebral disks a report of 3 cases. *Am J Surg Pathol.* 2008;32:1123–1129.

131. Yamaguchi T, Suzuki S, Ishiiwa H, et al. Benign notochordal cell tumors a comparative histological study of benign notochordal cell tumors, classic chordomas, and notochordal vestiges of fetal intervertebral discs. *Am J Surg Pathol.* 2004;28:756–761.

132. Yamaguchi T, Watanabe-Ishiiwa H, Suzuki S, et al. Incipient chordoma: a report of two cases of early-stage chordoma arising from benign notochordal cell tumors. *Mod Pathol.* 2005;18:1005–1010.

133. Tosi L, Rigoli G, Beltramello A. Fibrocartilaginous embolism of the spinal cord: a clinical and pathogenetic reconsideration. *J Neurol Neurosurg Psychiatry.* 1996;60:55–60.

134. Hoch B, Hermann G. Migrated herniated disc mimicking a neoplasm. *Skelet Radiol.* 2010;39:1245–1249.

135. Lin CS, Schwartz IS, Chapman I. Calcification of mitral annulus fibrosus with systemic embolization: a clinicopathologic study of 16 cases. *Arch Pathol Lab Med.* 1987;111:411–414.

136. Fuller GN. Intraoperative consultation and optimal processing. In: Perry A, Brat DJ, eds. *Practical Surgical Neuropathology*, Philadelphia, PA: Churchill Livingstone; 2010:35–46.

137. Neumann MA, Cohn R. Progressive subcortical gliosis, a rare form of presenile dementia. *Brain.* 1967;90:405–418.

138. Gambetti P, Dong Z, Yuan J, et al. A novel human disease with abnormal prion protein sensitive to protease. *Ann Neurol.* 2008;63:697–708.

139. Matsusue E, Kinoshita T, Sugihara S, et al. White matter lesions in panencephalopathic type of Creutzfeldt-Jakob disease: MR imaging and pathologic correlations. *AJNR Am J Neuroradiol.* 2004;25:910–918.

140. Jansen C, Head MW, Rozemuller AJ, et al. Panencephalopathic Creutzfeldt-Jakob disease in the Netherlands and the UK: clinical and pathological characteristics of nine patients. *Neuropathol Appl Neurobiol.* 2009;35:272–282.

141. Collins S, McLean CA, Masters CL. Gerstmann-Straussler-Scheinker syndrome, fatal familial insomnia, and kuru: a review of these less common human transmissible spongiform encephalopathies. *J Clin Neurosci.* 2001;8:387–397.

142. Ironside JW, Head MW. Neuropathology and molecular biology of variant Creutzfeldt-Jakob disease. *Curr Top Microbiol Immunol.* 2004;284:133–159.

143. Harding BN. Progressive neuronal degeneration of childhood with liver disease (Alpers-Huttenlocher syndrome): a personal review. *J Child Neurol.* 1990;5:273–287.

144. Kishi M, Yamamura Y, Kurihara T, et al. An autopsy case of mitochondrial encephalomyopathy: biochemical and electron microscopic studies of the brain. *J Neurol Sci.* 1988;86:31–40.

145. Brockington M, Alsanjari N, Sweeney MG, et al. Kearns-Sayre syndrome associated with mitochondrial DNA deletion or duplication: a molecular genetic and pathological study. *J Neurol Sci.* 1995;131:78–87.

146. Chang LW. The neurotoxicology and pathology of organomercury, organolead, and organotin. *J Toxicol Sci.* 1990;15:125–151.

147. Kobayashi Z, Tsuchiya K, Takahashi M, et al. Morel's laminar sclerosis showing apraxia of speech: distribution of cortical lesions in an autopsy case. *Neuropathology.* 2010;30:76–83.

148. Tobias SM, Robitaille Y, Hickey WF, et al. Bilateral Rasmussen encephalitis: postmortem documentation in a five-year-old. *Epilepsia.* 2003;44:127–130.

149. Miller D, MuzinichM, Tacazon M, et al. Histopathology of an unidentified bright object in the brain of an adult patient with neurofibromatosis type 1. *J Neuropathol Exp Neurol.* 2009;68:592–593.

150. Bell JE. The neuropathology of adult HIV infection. *Rev Neurol.* 1998;154:816–829.

151. Mirra SS, Heyman A, McKeel D, et al. The Consortium to Establish a Registry for Alzheimer's Disease (CERAD). Part II. Standardization of the neuropathologic assessment of Alzheimer's disease. *Neurology.* 1991;41:479–486.

152. Mizusawa H, Yen S-H, Llena JF. Pathology of the dentate nucleus in progressive supranuclear palsy: a histological, immunohistochemical and ultrastructural study. *Acta Neuropathol.* 1989;78:419–428.

153. Su M, Yoshida Y, Hirata Y, et al. Degeneration of the cerebellar dentate nucleus in corticobasal degeneration: neuropathological and morphometric investigations. *Acta Neuropathol.* 2000;99:365–370.

154. Yamanouchi H, Yokoo H, Yuhara Y, et al. An autopsy case of ornithine transcarbamylase deficiency. *Brain Dev.* 2002;24:91–94.

155. Kumada S, Hayashi M, Mizuguchi M, et al. Cerebellar degeneration in hereditary dentatorubral-pallidoluysian atrophy and Machado-Joseph disease. *Acta Neuropathol.* 2000;99:48–54.

156. Kobayashi K, Morikawa K, Fukutani Y, et al. Ramsay Hunt syndrome: progressive mental deterioration in association with unusual cerebral white matter change. *Clin Neuropathol.* 1994;13:88–96.

157. Ishikawa A, Oyanagi K, Tanaka K, et al. A non-familial Huntington's disease patient with grumose degeneration in the dentate nucleus. *Acta Neurol Scand.* 1999;99:322–326.

158. Iijima M, Ishino H, Seno H, et al. An autopsy case of Alzheimer disease with myoclonus and periodic spikes on EEG. *Jpn J Psychiatry Neurol.* 1994;48:615–621.

159. Cavanagh JB. Corpora-amylacea and the family of polyglucosan diseases. *Brain Res Rev.* 1999;29:265–295.

160. Hazrati LN, Kleinschmidt-DeMasters BK, Handler MH, et al Astrocytic inclusions in epilepsy: expanding the spectrum of filaminopathies. *J Neuropathol Exp Neurol.* 2008;67:669–676.

161. Hayashi T, Ago K, Ago M, et al.Two patterns of beta-amyloid precursor protein (APP) immunoreactivity in cases of blunt head injury. *Legal Med*. 2009;11:171–173.

162. Grahama DI, Smith C, Reicharda R, et al. Trials and tribulations of using b-amyloid precursor protein immunohistochemistry to evaluate traumatic brain injury in adults. *Forensic Sci Int*. 2004;146:89–96.

163. Posthumus J, Mohila C, Richards V, et al. β-Amyloid precursor protein immunoreactivity in infant brains: a detailed look at pattern of injury. *J Neuropathol Exp Neurol*. 2011;70:523.

164. Kruer M, Hiken M, Gregory A, et al. Novel histopathologic findings in molecularly-confirmed pantothenate kinase-associated neurodegeneration. *Brain*. 2011;134:947–958.

165. Sung JH, Mastri AR, Park SH. Axonal dystrophy in the gracile nucleus in children and young adults. Reappraisal of the incidence and associated diseases. *J Neuropathol Exp Neurol*. 1981;40:37–45.

166. Graham DG. Neurotoxicants and the cytoskeleton. *Curr Opin Neurol*. 1999;12:733–737.

167. Aoki N, Tsuchiya K, Togo T, et al. Gray matter lesions in Nasu-Hakola disease: a report on three autopsy cases. *Neuropathology*. 2011;31:135–143.

168. Walterfang M, Fahey M, Desmond P, et al. White and gray matter alterations in adults with Niemann-Pick disease type C: a cross-sectional study. *Neurology*. 2010;75:49–56.

169. Powers JM, Moser HW. Peroxisomal disorders: genotype, phenotype, major neuropathologic lesions, and pathogenesis. *Brain Pathol*. 1998;8:101–120.

170. Steward CG. Neurological aspects of osteopetrosis. *Neuropathol Appl Neurobiol*. 2003;29:87–97.

171. Takahashi T, Arai N, Shimamura M, et al. Autopsy case of acute encephalopathy linked to familial hemiplegic migraine with cerebellar atrophy and mental retardation. *Neuropathology*. 2005;25:228–234.

172. Schmidt RE, Dorsey D, Parvin CA, et al. Dystrophic axonal swellings develop as a function of age and diabetes in human dorsal root ganglia. *J Neuropathol Exp Neurol* 1997;56:1028–1043.

173. Bang OY, Kim DI, Yoon SR, et al. Idiopathic hypertrophic pachymeningeal lesions: correlation between clinical patterns and neuroimaging characteristics. *Eur Neurol*. 1998;39:49–56.

174. Vedam-Mai V, Ullman M, Okun M, et al. Collagenous fibrosis: a rare tissue reaction of deep brain stimulation (DBS). *J Neuropathol Exp Neurol*. 2011;70:549.

175. Foschini MP, D'adda T, Bordi C, et al. Amyloid stroma in meningiomas. *Virchows Arch A Pathol Anat Histopathol*. 1993;422:53–59.

176. Foreid H, Barroso C, Evangelista T, et al. Intracerebral amyloidoma: case report and review of the literature. *Clin Neuropathol*. 2010;29:217–222.

177. Stavrou T, Dubovsky EC, Reaman GH, et al. Intracranial calcifications in childhood medulloblastoma: relation to nevoid basal cell carcinoma syndrome. *AJNR Am J Neuroradiol*. 2000;21:790–794.

178. Kurtkaya-Yapicier O, Scheithauer B, Woodruff JM. The pathobiologic spectrum of Schwannomas. *Histol Histopathol*. 2003;18:925–934.

179. Moskowitz MA, Winickoff RN, Heinz ER. Familial calcification of the basal ganglions: a metabolic and genetic study. *N Engl J Med*. 1971;285:72–77.

180. Morgante L, Vita G, Meduri M, et al. Fahr's syndrome: local inflammatory factors in the pathogenesis of calcification. *J Neurol*. 1986;233:19–22.

181. Malat J, Virapongse C. Brain calcification in Kallman's syndrome. Computed tomographic appearance. *Pediatr Neurosci*. 1985–1986;12:257–259.

182. Patel PJ. Some rare causes of intracranial calcification in childhood: computed tomographic findings. *Eur J Pediatr*. 1987;146:177–180.

183. Avrahami E, Katz A, Bornstein N, et al. Computed tomographic findings of brain and skull in myotonic dystrophy. *J Neurol Neurosurg Psychiatry*. 1987;50:435–438.

184. Andres RH, Schroth G, Remonda L. Neurological picture. Extensive cerebral calcification in a patient with systemic lupus erythematosus. *J Neurol Neurosurg Psychiatry*. 2008;79:365.

185. Chung SH, Chen SC, Chen WJ, et al. Symmetric basal ganglia calcification in a 9-year-old child with MELAS. *Neurology*. 2005;65:19.

186. Fitzsimons RB. The mitochondrial myopathies: 9 case reports and a literature review. *Clin Exp Neurol*. 1981;17:185–210.

187. Verma A, Moraes CT, Shebert RT, et al. A MERRF/PEO overlap syndrome associated with the mitochondrial DNA 3243 mutation. *Neurology*. 1996;46:1334–1336.

188. Klunemann HH, Ridha BH, Magy L, et al. The genetic causes of basal ganglia calcification, dementia, and bone cysts: DAP12 and TREM2. *Neurology*. 2005;64:1502–1507.

189. Valdivieso EM, Scholtz CL. Diffuse meningocerebral angiodysplasia and renal agenesis: a case report. *Pediatr Pathol*. 1986;6:119–126.

190. Marques-Dias MJ, Gonzalez CH, Rosemberg S. Mobius sequence in children exposed in utero to misoprostol: neuropathological study of three cases. *Birth Defects Res*. 2003;67:1002–1007.

191. Lanzi G, D'Arrigo S, Drumbl G, et al. Aicardi-Goutieres syndrome: differential diagnosis and aetiopathogenesis. *Funct Neurol*. 2003;18:71–75.

192. Rapin I, Weidenheim K, Lindenbaum Y, et al. Cockayne syndrome in adults: review with clinical and pathologic study of a new case. *J Child Neurol*. 2006;21:991–1006.

193. Williams D, Patel C, Fallet-Bianco C, et al. Fowler syndrome-a clinical, radiological, and pathological study of 14 cases. *Am J Med Genet*. 2010;152:153–160.

194. Pfaender M, D'Souza WJ, Trost N, et al. Visual disturbances representing occipital lobe epilepsy in patients with cerebral calcifications and coeliac disease: a case series. *J Neurol Neurosurg Psychiatry*. 2004;75:1623–1625.

195. Epps RE, Pittelkow MR, Su WP. TORCH syndrome. *Semin Dermatol*. 1995;14:179–186.

196. Kulkarni AM, Baskar S, Kulkarni ML, et al. Fetal intracranial calcification: pseudo-TORCH phenotype and discussion of related phenotypes. *Am J Med Genet*. 2010;152:930–937.

197. Dickson DW, Belman AL, Park YD, et al. Central nervous system pathology in pediatric AIDS: an autopsy study. *APMIS*. 1989;8:40–57.

198. Remsen LG, McCormick CI, Sexton G, et al. Long-term toxicity and neuropathology associated with the sequencing of cranial irradiation and enhanced chemotherapy delivery. *Neurosurgery*. 1997;40:1034–1040.

199. Mahaley MS Jr, Whaley RA, Blue M, et al. Central neurotoxicity following intracarotid BCNU chemotherapy for malignant gliomas. *J Neurooncol*. 1986;3:297–314.

200. Sakamaki H, Onozawa Y, Yano Y, et al. Disseminated necrotizing leukoencephalopathy following irradiation and methotrexate therapy for central nervous system infiltration of leukemia and lymphoma. *Radiat Med*. 1993;11:146–153.

201. Anders KH, Becker PS, Holden JK, et al. Multifocal necrotizing leukoencephalopathy with pontine predilection in immunosuppressed patients: a clinicopathologic review of 16 cases. *Hum Pathol*. 1993;24:897–904.

202. Liubinas SV, Maartens N, Drummond KJ. Primary melanocytic neoplasms of the central nervous system. *J Clin Neurosci*. 2010;17:1227–1232.

203. Gempt J, Buchmann N, Grams AE, et al. Black brain: transformation of a melanocytoma with diffuse melanocytosis into a primary cerebral melanoma. *J Neuro-Oncol*. 2011;102:323–328.

204. Smith AB, Rushing EJ, Smirniotopoulos JG. Pigmented lesions of the central nervous system: radiologic-pathologic correlation. *Radiographics*. 2009;29:1503–1524.

205. Rosenblum MK, Erlandson RA, Aleksic SN, et al. Melanotic ependymoma and subependymoma. *Am J Surg Pathol*. 1990;14:729–736.

206. Giangaspero F, Eberhart CG, Haapasalo H, et al. Medulloblastoma. In: Louis DN, Ohgaki H, Wiestler OD, et al., eds. *WHO Classification of Tumours of the Central Nervous System*. Lyon, France: IARC Press; 2007:132–140.
207. Kapadia SB, Frisman DM, Hitchcock CL, et al. Melanotic neuroectodermal tumor of infancy. Clinicopathological, immunohistochemical, and flow cytometric study. *Am J Surg Pathol*. 1993;17:566–573.
208. Schmidbauer M, Budka H, Pilz P. Neuroepithelial and ectomesenchymal differentiation in a primitive pineal tumor ("pineal anlage tumor"). *Clin Neuropathol*. 1989;8:7–10.
209. Sharma MC, Mahapatra AK, Gaikwad S, et al. Pigmented medulloepithelioma: report of a case and review of the literature. *Childs Nerv Syst*. 1998;14:74–78.
210. Vajtai I, Yonekawa Y, Schauble B, et al. Melanotic astrocytoma. *Acta Neuropathol*. 1996;91:549–553.
211. Soffer D, Lach B, Constantini S. Melanotic cerebral ganglioglioma: evidence for melanogenesis in neoplastic astrocytes. *Acta Neuropathol*. 1992;83:315–323.
212. Watanabe K, Ando Y, Iwanaga H, et al. Choroid plexus papilloma containing melanin pigment. *Clin Neuropathol*. 1995;14:159–161.
213. Fenichel GM, Bazelon M. Studies on neuromelanin. II. Melanin in the brainstems of infants and children. *Neurology*. 1968;18:817–820.
214. Rudow G, O'Brien R, Savonenko AV, et al. Morphometry of the human substantia nigra in ageing and Parkinson's disease. *Acta Neuropathol*. 2008;115:461–470.
215. Beach TG, Sue LI, Walker DG, et al. Marked microglial reaction in normal aging human substantia nigra: correlation with extraneuronal neuromelanin pigment deposits. *Acta Neuropathol*. 2007;114:419–424.
216. Keller JN. Age-related neuropathology, cognitive decline, and Alzheimer's disease. *Ageing Res Rev*. 2006;5:1–13.
217. Jolly RD, Dalefield RR, Palmer DN. Ceroid, lipofuscin and the ceroid-lipofuscinoses (Batten disease). *J Inherit Metab Dis*. 1993;16:280–283.
218. March PA, Wurzelmann S, Walkley SU. Morphological alterations in neocortical and cerebellar GABAergic neurons in a canine model of juvenile Batten disease. *Am J Med Genet*. 1995;57:204–212.
219. Shannon P, Wherrett JR, Nag S. A rare form of adult onset leukodystrophy: orthochromatic leukodystrophy with pigmented glia. *Can J Neurol Sci*. 1997;24:146–150.
220. Monji A, Morimoto N, Okuyama I, et al. Effect of dietary vitamin E on lipofuscin accumulation with age in the rat brain. *Brain Res*. 1994;634:62–68.
221. Gaytan-Garcia S, Kaufmann JC, Young GB. Adult onset Hallervorden-Spatz syndrome or Seitelberger's disease with late onset: variants of the same entity? A clinicopathological study. *Clin Neuropathol*. 1990;9:136–142.
222. Cordonnier C. Brain microbleeds. *Pract Neurol*. 2010;10:94–100.
223. Kleinschmidt-Demasters BK. Gamna-Gandy bodies in surgical neuropathology specimens: observations and a historical note. *J Neuropathol Exp Neurol*. 2004;63:106–112.
224. Vogel FS. Studies on the pathogenesis of kernicterus, with special reference to the nature of kernicteric pigment and its deposition under natural and experimental conditions. *J Exp Med*. 1953;98:509–520.
225. Sherwood AJ, Smith JF. Bilirubin encephalopathy. *Neuropathol Appl Neurobiol*. 1983;9:271–285.
226. Barnes S, Hurst W. A further note on hepatolenticular degeneration. *Brain*. 1926;49:36–60.
227. Gomez BL, Nosanchuk JD. Melanin and fungi. *Curr Opin Infect Dis*. 2003;16:91–96.
228. Takei H, Goodman JC, Powell SZ. Cerebral phaeohyphomycosis caused by ladophialophora bantiana and Fonsecaea monophora: report of three cases. *Clin Neuropathol*. 007;26:21–27.
229. Churukian JC. *Pigments and Minerals*. In: Bancroft JD, Gamble M, eds. *Theory and Practice of Histological Techniques*. 5th ed. Edinburgh, UK: Churchill Livingstone; 2002:243–268.
230. Dolinak D, Matshes E. *Medicolegal Neuropathology: A Color Atlas*. Boca Raton, FL: CRC Press; 2002.
231. Daikha-Dahmane F, Dommergues M, Narcy F, et al. Congenital erythropoietic porphyria: prenatal diagnosis and autopsy findings in two sibling fetuses. *Pediatr Dev Pathol*. 2001;4:180–184.
232. Hu W, Lucchinetti CF. The pathological spectrum of CNS inflammatory demyelinating diseases. *Semin Immunopathol*. 2009;31:439–453.
233. Kepes JJ. Large focal tumor-like demyelinating lesions of the brain: intermediate entity between multiple sclerosis and acute disseminated encephalomyelitis? A study of 31 patients. *Ann Neurol*. 1993;33:18–27.
234. Grcevic N. Concentric lacunar leukoencephalopathy. *Archiv Neurol*. 1960;2:266–273.
235. Katz JD, Ropper AH. Progressive necrotic myelopathy: clinical course in 9 patients. *Archiv Neurol*. 2000;57:355–361.
236. Fazio R, Radaelli M, Furlan R. Neuromyelitis optica: concepts in evolution. *J Neuroimmunol*. 2011;231:100–104.
237. Del Valle L, Pina-Oviedo S. HIV disorders of the brain: pathology and pathogenesis. *Front Biosci*. 2006;11:718–732.
238. Souraud JB, Faivre A, Waku-Kouomou D, et al. Adult fulminant subacute sclerosing panencephalitis: pathological and molecular studies—a case report. *Clin Neuropathol*. 2009; 28:213–218.
239. Adams JM. Severe demyelinating diseases in childhood: a clinicopathological study. *J Natl Med Assoc*. 1978;70:171–178.
240. Kleinschmidt-DeMasters BK, Amlie-Lefond C, Gilden DH. The patterns of varicella zoster virus encephalitis. *Hum Pathol*. 1996;27:927–938.
241. Alderson L, Fetell MR, Sisti M, et al. Sentinel lesions of primary CNS lymphoma. *J Neurol Neurosurg Psychiatry*. 1996;60:102–105.
242. Kleinschmidt-Demasters BK, Rojiani AM, Filley CM. Central and extrapontine myelinolysis: then…and now. *J Neuropathol Exp Neurol*. 2006;65:1–11.
243. Serdaru M. Hausser-Hauw C. Laplane D, et al. The clinical spectrum of alcoholic pellagra encephalopathy. A retrospective analysis of 22 cases studied pathologically. *Brain*. 1988;111:829–842.
244. Johkura K, Naito M, Naka T. Cortical involvement in Marchiafava-Bignami disease. *AJNR Am J Neuroradiol*. 2005;26:670–673.
245. Sato Y, Tabira T, Tateishi J. Marchiafava-Bignami disease, striatal degeneration, and other neurological complications of chronic alcoholism in a Japanese. *Acta Neuropathol*. 1981;53:15–20.
246. Poe LB, Dubowy RL, Hochhauser L, et al. Demyelinating and gliotic cerebellar lesions in Langerhans cell histiocytosis. *AJNR Am J Neuroradiol*. 1994;15:1921–1928.
247. Grois N, Prayer D. Prosch H, et al. Neuropathology of CNS disease in Langerhans cell histiocytosis. *Brain*. 2005;128:829–838.
248. Lindzen E, Jewells V, Bouldin T, et al. Progressive tumefactive inflammatory central nervous system demyelinating disease in an acquired immunodeficiency syndrome patient treated with highly active antiretroviral therapy. *J Neurovirol*. 2008;14:569–573.
249. Berciano J, Berciano MT, Polo JM, et al. Creutzfeldt-Jakob disease with severe involvement of cerebral white matter and cerebellum. *Virchows Arch A Pathol Anat Histopathol*. 1990;417:533–538.
250. Moore-Maxwell CA, Datto MB, Hulette CM. Chemotherapy-induced toxic leukoencephalopathy causes a wide range of symptoms: a series of four autopsies. *Mod Pathol*. 2004;17:241–247.
251. Filley CM. Toxic leukoencephalopathy. *Clin Neuropharmacol*. 1999:22:249–260.
252. Matsubayashi J, Tsuchiya K, Matsunaga T, et al. Methotrexate-related leukoencephalopathy without radiation therapy: distribution of brain lesions and pathological heterogeneity on two autopsy cases. *Neuropathology*. 2009;29:105–115.

253. Suzuki K, Takemura T, Okeda R, et al. Vascular changes of methotrexate-related disseminated necrotizing leukoencephalopathy. *Acta Neuropathol*. 1984;65:145–149.

254. Minagawa M, Maeshiro H, Kato K, et al. A rare form of leucodystrophy. Neuroaxonal leucodystrophy (Seitelberger). *Psychol Neurol Jpn*. 1980;82:488–503.

255. Tanaka J. Nasu-Hakola disease: a review of its leukoencephalopathic and membranolipodystrophic features. *Neuropathology*. 2000;20:25–29.

256. Schiff D, Lopes MB. Neuropathological correlates of reversible posterior leukoencephalopathy. *Neurocrit Care*. 2005;2:303–305.

257. Jayawant S, Halpin S, Wallace S. Menkes kinky hair disease: an unusual case. *Eur J Paediatr Neurol*. 2000;4:131–134.

258. Volpe JJ. Brain injury in premature infants: a complex amalgam of destructive and developmental disturbances. *Lancet Neurol*. 2009;8:110–124.

259. Leviton A, Gilles FH. Morphologic correlates of age at death of infants with perinatal telencephalic leukoencephalopathy. *Am J Pathol*. 1971;65:303–309.

260. Mehta PS, Bruccoleri A, Brown HW, et al. Increase in brain stem cytokine mRNA levels as an early response to chemical-induced myelin edema. *J Neuroimmunol*. 1998;88:154–164.

261. Adityanjee, Munshi KR, Thampy A. The syndrome of irreversible lithium-effectuated neurotoxicity. *Clin Neuropharmacol*. 2005;28:38–49.

262. Haller L, Adams H, Merouze F, et al. Clinical and pathological aspects of human African trypanosomiasis (T. B. gambiense) with particular reference to reactive arsenical encephalopathy. *Am J Trop Med Hyg*. 1986;35:94–99.

263. Besser R, Kramer G, Thumler R, et al. Acute trimethyltin limbic-cerebellar syndrome. *Neurology*. 1987;37:945–950.

264. Mullick FG. Hexachlorophene toxicity—human experience at the Armed Forces Institute of Pathology. *Pediatrics*. 1973; 51:395–399.

265. Pascual LL, Merino VC, Estruch CB. Demyelinization and occipital atrophy due to cyclosporin A. *Neurologia*. 1999;14:459.

266. Bech RA, Waldemar G, Gjerris F, et al. Shunting effects in patients with idiopathic normal pressure hydrocephalus: correlation with cerebral and leptomeningeal biopsy findings. *Acta Neurochir*. 1999;141:633–639.

267. Hamlat A, And M, Sid-ahmed S, et al. Theoretical considerations on the pathophysiology of normal pressure hydrocephalus (NPH) and NPH-related dementia. *Med Hypotheses*. 2006;67:115–123.

268. Casseb J, Penalva-de-Oliveira AC. The pathogenesis of tropical spastic paraparesis/human T-cell leukemia type I-associated myelopathy. *Braz J Med Biol Res*. 2000;33:1395–1401.

269. Powers JM, DeCiero DP, Ito M, et al. Adrenomyeloneuropathy: a neuropathologic review featuring its noninflammatory myelopathy. *J Neuropathol Exp Neurol*. 2000;59:89–102.

270. Platt B, Fiddler G, Riedel G, et al. Aluminium toxicity in the rat brain: histochemical and immunocytochemical evidence. *Brain Res Bull*. 2001;55:257–267.

271. McLaughlin AIG, Kazantzis G, King E, et al. Pulmonary fibrosis and encephalopathy associated with the inhalation of aluminium dust. *Br J Ind Med*. 1962;19:253–263.

272. Reusche E, Seydel U. Dialysis-associated encephalopathy. Light and electron microscopic morphology and topography with evidence of aluminum by laser microprobe mass analysis. *Acta Neuropathol*. 1993;86:249–258.

273. Davis LE, Kornfeld M, Mooney HS, et al. Methylmercury poisoning: long-term clinical, radiological, toxicological, and pathological studies of an affected family. *Ann Neurol*. 1994;35:680–688.

274. Takizawa Y, Takashima S, Itoh M. A histopathological study of premature and mature infants with pontosubicular neuron necrosis: neuronal cell death in perinatal brain damage. *Brain Res*. 2006;1095:200–206.

275. Gogus S, Yalaz K, Gucsavas M, et al. Subacute necrotizing encephalopathy (Leigh syndrome): report of two juvenile cases with fatal outcome. *Turk J Pediatr*. 1994;36:57–65.

276. Pal PK, Samil A, Caine DB. Manganese neurotoxicity: a review of clinical features, imaging and pathology. *Neurotoxicology*. 1999;20:227–238.

277. Walker RH, Jung HH, Danek A. Neuroacanthocytosis. *Handb Clin Neurol*. 2011;100:141–151.

278. Rafalowska J, Drac H, Jamrozik Z. Neuroacanthocytosis. Review of literature and case report. *Folia Neuropathol*. 1996;34:178–183.

279. Danek A, Rubio JP, Rampoldi L, et al. McLeod neuroacanthocytosis: genotype and phenotype. *Ann Neurol*. 2001;50:755–764.

280. Aizawa H, Kwak S, Shimizu T, et al. A case of adult onset pure pallidal degeneration. I. Clinical manifestations and neuropathological observations. *J Neurol Sci*. 1991;102:76–82.

281. Miyazu K, Kobayashi K, Fukutani Y, et al. Membranous lipodystrophy (Nasu-Hakola disease) with thalamic degeneration: report of an autopsied case. *Acta Neuropathol*. 1991;82:414–419.

282. Schmidtke K. Wernicke-Korsakoff syndrome following attempted hanging. *Rev Neurol*. 1993;149:213–216.

283. Mizusawa H, Ohkoshi N, Sasaki H, et al. Degeneration of the thalamus and inferior olives associated with spongiform encephalopathy of the cerebral cortex. *Clin Neuropathol*. 1988;7:81–86.

284. Martin JJ, Leroy JG. Thalamic lesions in a patient with Menkes kinky-hair disease. *Clin Neuropathol*. 1985;4:206–209.

285. Nagayama M, Shinohara Y, Furukawa H, et al. Fatal familial insomnia with a mutation at codon 178 of the prion protein gene: first report from Japan. *Neurology*. 1996;47:1313–1316.

286. Pittella JE, Nogueira AM. Pontoneocerebellar hypoplasia: report of a case in a newborn and review of the literature. *Clin Neuropathol*. 1990;9:33–38.

287. Koeppen AH. The pathogenesis of spinocerebellar ataxia. *Cerebellum*. 2005;4:62–73.

288. Williams RS, Marshall PC, Lott IT, et al. The cellular pathology of Menkes steely hair syndrome. *Neurology*. 1978;28:575–583.

289. Kamiya M, Yamanouchi H, Yoshida T, et al. Ataxia telangiectasia with vascular abnormalities in the brain parenchyma: report of an autopsy case and literature review. *Pathol Int*. 2001;51:271–276.

290. Gordon N. Carbohydrate-deficient glycoprotein syndromes. *Postgrad Med J*. 2000;76:145–149.

291. Ishikawa K, Mizusawa H. On autosomal dominant cerebellar ataxia (ADCA) other than polyglutamine diseases, with special reference to chromosome 16q22.1-linked ADCA. *Neuropathology*. 2006;26:352–360.

292. Bolla L, Palmer RM. Paraneoplastic cerebellar degeneration. Case report and literature review. *Archiv Intern Med*. 1997;157:1258–1262.

293. Shannon P, Pennacchio LA, Houseweart MK, et al. Neuropathological changes in a mouse model of progressive myoclonus epilepsy: cystatin B deficiency and Unverricht-Lundborg disease. *J Neuropathol Exp Neurol*. 2002;61:1085–1091.

294. Hadjivassiliou M, Grunewald RA, Sharrack B, et al. Gluten ataxia in perspective: epidemiology, genetic susceptibility and clinical characteristics. *Brain*. 2003;126:682–691.

295. Crawley AC, Walkley SU. Developmental analysis of CNS pathology in the lysosomal storage disease alpha-mannosidosis. *J Neuropathol Exp Neurol*. 2007;66:687–697.

296. Fukuhara N. Fukuhara disease. *Brain Nerve/Shinkei Kenkyu no Shinpo*. 2008;60:53–58.

297. Mangano WE, Montine TJ, Hulette CM. Pathologic assessment of cerebellar atrophy following acute lithium intoxication. *Clin Neuropathol*. 1997;16:30–33.

298. Crooks R, Mitchell T, Thom M. Patterns of cerebellar atrophy in patients with chronic epilepsy: a quantitative neuropathological study. *Epilepsy Res*. 2000;41:63–73.

299. Feki M, Souissi M, Mebazaa A. Vitamin E deficiency. Etiopathogenesis, clinical, histopathologic, and electrical features, and main etiologies. *Ann Med Interne*. 2001;152:392–397.

300. Dooley JM, Stewart WA, Hayden JD, et al. Brainstem calcification in Mobius syndrome. *Pediatr Neurol*. 2004;30:39–41.

301. Dierick I, Baets J, Irobi J, et al. Relative contribution of mutations in genes for autosomal dominant distal hereditary motor neuropathies: a genotype-phenotype correlation study. *Brain*. 2008;131:1217–1227.

302. Baker AB. The nervous system in trichloroethylene intoxication; an experimental study. *J Neuropathol Exp Neurol* 1958;17:649–655.

303. Dipti S, Childs AM, Livingston JH, et al. Brown-Vialetto-Van Laere syndrome: variability in age at onset and disease progression highlighting the phenotypic overlap with Fazio-Londe disease. *Brain Dev*. 2005;27:443–446.

304. Guidetti D, Vescovini E, Motti L, et al. X-linked bulbar and spinal muscular atrophy or Kennedy disease: clinical, neurophysiological, neuropathological, neuropsychological and molecular study of a large family. *J Neurol Sci*. 1996;135: 140–148.

305. Wenning GK, Geser F. Multiple system atrophy. *Rev Neurol*. 2003;159:3S31–3S38.

306. Tateishi J. Subacute myelo-optico-neuropathy: clioquinol intoxication in humans and animals. *Neuropathology*. 2000;20:S20–S24.

307. Brown P, Marsden CD. The stiff man and stiff man plus syndromes. *J Neurol*. 1999;246:648–652.

308. Gazic B, Pisem J, Dolenc-Groselj L, et al. Paraneoplastic encephalomyelitis/sensory motor peripheral neuropathy—an autopsy case study. *Folia Neuropathol*. 2005;43:113–117.

309. Di Rocco A, Simpson DM. AIDS-associated vacuolar myelopathy. *AIDS Patient Care STDS*. 1998;12:457–461.

310. Schochet SS Jr, Nelson J. Exogenous toxic-metabolic diseases including vitamin deficiency. In: Davis RL, Robertson DM, eds. *Textbook of Neuropathology*. 3rd ed. Baltimore, MD: Williams & Wilkins; 1997:511–546.

311. Anheim M, Tranchant C. Peripheral neuropathies associated with hereditary cerebellar ataxias. *Rev Neurol*. 2011;167: 72–76.

312. Eto K, Tokunaga H, Nagashima K, et al. An autopsy case of minamata disease (methylmercury poisoning)—pathological viewpoints of peripheral nerves. *Toxicol Pathol*. 2002;30:714–722.

313. Kennedy P, Cavanagh JB. Spinal changes in the neuropathy of thallium poisoning. A case with neuropathological studies. *J Neurol Sci*. 1976;29:295–301.

314. Walther PJ, Rossitch E Jr, Bullard DE. The development of Lhermitte's sign during cisplatin chemotherapy. Possible drug-induced toxicity causing spinal cord demyelination. *Cancer*. 1987;60:2170–2172.

315. Spriggs DR, Stopa E, Mayer RJ, et al. Fludarabine phosphate (NSC 312878) infusions for the treatment of acute leukemia: phase I and neuropathological study. *Cancer Res*. 1986;46:5953–5958.

316. Striefler M, Cohn DF, Hirano A, et al. The central nervous system in a case of neurolathyrism. *Neurology*. 1977;27:1176–1178.

317. Boyes WK, Cooper GP. Acrylamide neurotoxicity: effects on far-field somatosensory evoked potentials in rats. *Neurobehav Toxicol Teratol*. 1981;3:487–490.

318. Alpers BJ, Lewy FH. Changes in the nervous system following carbon disulfide poisoning in animals and in man. *Arch Neurol Psychiatry*. 1940;44:725–739.

319. Altenkirch H, Wagner HM, Stoltenburg G, et al. Nervous system responses of rats to subchronic inhalation of *N*-hexane and *N*-hexane + methyl-ethyl-ketone mixtures. *J Neurol Sci*. 1982;57:209–219.

320. Jokanovic M, Kosanovic M, Brkic D, et al. Organophosphate induced delayed polyneuropathy in man: an overview. *Clin Neurol Neurosurg*. 2011;113:7–10.

321. Tsuchiya K, Ozawa E, Haga C, et al. Constant involvement of the Betz cells and pyramidal tract in multiple system atrophy: a clinicopathological study of seven autopsy cases. *Acta Neuropathol*. 2000;99:628–636.

322. Eusebio A, Azulay JP, Witjas T, et al. Assessment of cortico-spinal tract impairment in multiple system atrophy using transcranial magnetic stimulation. *Clin Neurophysiol*. 2007;118:815–823.

323. Boelmans K, Kaufmann J, Bodammer N, et al. Corticospinal tract atrophy in corticobasal degeneration. *Arch Neurol*. 2006;63:462–463.

324. Josephs KA, Katsuse O, Beccano-Kelly DA, et al. Atypical progressive supranuclear palsy with corticospinal tract degeneration. *J Neuropathol Exp Neurol*. 2006;65:396–405.

325. Pandolfo M. Friedreich ataxia. *Archiv Neurol*. 2008;65: 1296–1303.

326. Riess O, Rub U, Pastore A, et al. SCA3: neurological features, pathogenesis and animal models. *Cerebellum*. 2008;7: 125–137.

327. Garden GA, La Spada AR. Molecular pathogenesis and cellular pathology of spinocerebellar ataxia type 7 neurodegeneration. *Cerebellum*. 2008;7:138–149.

328. Robitaille Y, Lopes-Cendes I, Becher M, et al. The neuropathology of CAG repeat diseases: review and update of genetic and molecular features. *Brain Pathol*. 1997;7:901–926.

329. Iwabuchi K, Yagishita S. An autopsied case of idiopathic late cortical cerebellar atrophy—comparison with other cortical cerebellar atrophy. *Clin Neurol*. 1990;30: 1190–1196.

330. Scheithauer BW, Forno LS, Dorfman LJ, et al. Neuroaxonal dystrophy (Seitelberger's disease) with late onset, protracted course and myoclonic epilepsy. *J Neurol Sci*. 1978;36: 247–258.

331. Landi G, Vulani F, Anzalone N. Variable angiographic findings in patients with stroke and neurosyphilis. *Stroke*. 1990;21:333–338.

332. Kirkpatrick JB. Neurologic infections due to bacteria, fungi, and parasites. In: Davis RL, Robertson DM, eds. *Textbook of Neuropathology*. 3rd ed. Baltimore, MD: Williams & Wilkins; 1997:823–926.

333. Topakian R, Stieglbauer K, Nussbaumer K, et al. Cerebral vasculitis and stroke in Lyme neuroborreliosis. Two case reports and review of current knowledge. *Cerebrovasc Dis*. 2008;26:455–461.

334. Koh SB, Kim BJ, Park MH, et al. Clinical and laboratory characteristics of cerebral infarction in tuberculous meningitis: a comparative study. *J Clin Neurosci*. 2007;14: 1073–1077.

335. Mousseaux E, Plouin PF, Touze E, et al. Fibromuscular dysplasia of cervical and intracranial arteries. *Int J Stroke*. 2010;5:296–305.

336. Suzuki J, Takaku A. Cerebrovascular "moyamoya" disease: disease showing abnormal net-like vessels in base of brain. *Arch Neurol*. 1969;20:288–299.

337. Dubrovsky T, Curless R, Scott G, et al. Cerebral aneurysmal arteriopathy in childhood AIDS. *Neurology*. 1998;51: 560–565.

338. Peters G, du Plessis DG, Humphrey PR. Cerebral Whipple's disease with a stroke-like presentation and cerebrovascular pathology. *J Neurol Neurosurg Psychiatry*. 2002;73: 336–339.

339. Cairns AG, North KN. Cerebrovascular dysplasia in neurofibromatosis type 1. *J Neurol Neurosurg Psychiatry*. 2008;79:1165–1170.

340. Kleinschmidt-DeMasters BK. Central nervous system aspergillosis: a 20-year retrospective series. *Hum Pathol*. 2002;33:116–124.

341. Frater JL, Hall GS, Procop GW. Histologic features of zygomycosis: emphasis on perineural invasion and fungal morphology. *Arch Pathol Lab Med*. 2001;125:375–378.

342. Chen M, Caplan L. Intracranial dissections. *Front Neurol Neurosci*. 2005;20:160–173.

343. Day AL, Gaposchkin CG, Yu CJ, et al. Spontaneous fusiform middle cerebral artery aneurysms: characteristics and a proposed mechanism of formation. *J Neurosurg*. 2003;99: 228–240.

344. Aarabi B. Management of traumatic aneurysms caused by high-velocity missile head wounds. *Neurosurg Clin N Am*. 1995;6:775–797.

345. Parkinson D, West M. Traumatic intracranial aneurysms. *J Neurosurgery*. 1980;52:11–20.

346. Rosenblum WI. Fibrinoid necrosis of small brain arteries and arterioles and miliary aneurysms as causes of hypertensive hemorrhage: a critical reappraisal. *Acta Neuropathol*. 2008;116:361–369.

347. Fukutake T. Cerebral autosomal recessive arteriopathy with subcortical infarcts and leukoencephalopathy (CARASIL): from discovery to gene identification. *J Stroke Cerebrovasc Dis*. 2011;20:85–93.

348. Kabins S, Keller R, Naragi S, et al. Viral ascending radiculomyelitis with severe hypoglycorrachia. *Arch Intern Med*. 1976;136:933–935.

349. Franchini M, Zaffanello M, Veneri D. Advances in the pathogenesis, diagnosis and treatment of thrombotic thrombocytopenic purpura and hemolytic uremic syndrome. *Thromb Res*. 2006;118:177–184.

350. Erbetta A, Salmaggi A, Sghirlanzoni A, et al. Clinical and radiological features of brain neurotoxicity caused by antitumor and immunosuppressant treatments. *Neurol Sci*. 2008;29:131–137.

351. Walker DH, Parks FM, Betz TG, et al. Histopathology and immunohistologic demonstration of the distribution of *Rickettsia typhi* in fatal murine typhus. *Am J Clin Pathol*. 1989;91:720–724.

352. Neefe LI, Pinilla O, Garagusi VF, et al. Disseminated strongyloidiasis with cerebral involvement: a complication of corticosteroid therapy. *Am J Med*. 1973;55:832–838.

353. Wachter RM, Burke AM, MacGregor RR. *Strongyloides stercoralis* hyperinfection masquerading as cerebral vasculitis. *Arch Neurol*. 1984;41:1213–1216.

354. Ghatak NR. Pathology of cerebral embolization caused by nonthrombotic agents. *Hum Pathol*. 1975;6:599–610.

355. Mehta RI, Mehta RI, Solis OE, et al. Hydrophilic polymer emboli: an under-recognized iatrogenic cause of ischemia and infarct. *Mod Pathol*. 2010;23:921–930.

356. Uppal S, Dash S, Sharer L, et al. Spinal cord infarction secondary to nucleus pulposus embolization in pregnancy. *Mod Pathol*. 2004;17:121–124.

357. Tehrani M, Friedman TM, Olson JJ, et al. Intravascular thrombosis in central nervous system malignancies: a potential role in astrocytoma progression to glioblastoma. *Brain Pathol*. 2008;18:164–171.

358. Miller DV, Salvarani C, Hunder GG, et al. Biopsy findings in primary angiitis of the central nervous system. *Am J Surg Pathol*. 2009;33:35–43.

359. Hotchi M. Pathological studies on Takayasu arteritis. *Heart Vessels*. 1992;7:11–17.

360. Amano S, Hazama F. Neural involvement in kawasaki disease. *Acta Pathol Jpn*. 1980;30:365–373.

361. Cordonnier C. Brain microbleeds: more evidence, but still a clinical dilemma. *Curr Opin Neurol*. 2011;24:69–74.

362. Ferro JM. Vasculitis of the central nervous system. *J Neurol*. 1998;245:766–776.

363. Myung J, Kim B, Yoon BW, et al. B-cell dominant lymphocytic primary angiitis of the central nervous system: four biopsy-proven cases. *Neuropathology*. 2010;30:123–130.

364. Kleinschmidt-DeMasters BK, Geier JM. Pathology of high-dose intraarterial BCNU. *Surg Neurol*. 1989;31:435–443.

365. Citron B, Halpern M, McCarron M, et al. Necrotizing angiitis associated with drug abuse. *N Engl J Med*. 1970;283:1003–1011.

366. Fredericks R, Lefkowitz D, Challa V, et al. Cerebral vasculitis associated with cocaine abuse. *Stroke*. 1991;22:1437–1439.

367. Daras M, Koppel B, Atos-Radizon E. Cocaine-induced choreoathetoid movements ("crack dancing"). *Neurology*. 1994;44:751–752.

368. Garcia JH, Ho KL. Pathology of hypertensive arteriopathy. *Neurosurg Clin N Am*. 1992;3:497–507.

369. Weller RO, Boche D, Nicoll JA. Microvasculature changes and cerebral amyloid angiopathy in Alzheimer's disease and their potential impact on therapy. *Acta Neuropathol*. 2009;118:87–102.

370. Okeda R, Nisihara M. An autopsy case of Fabry disease with neuropathological investigation of the pathogenesis of associated dementia. *Neuropathology*. 2008;28:532–540.

371. Kretzschmar HA, Wagner H, Hubner G, et al. Aneurysms and vacuolar degeneration of cerebral arteries in late-onset acid maltase deficiency. *J Neurol Sci*. 1990;98:169–183.

372. Froberg K, Dorion RP, McMartin KE. The role of calcium oxalate crystal deposition in cerebral vessels during ethylene glycol poisoning. *Clin Toxicol*. 2006;44:315–318.

373. Judice DJ, LeBlanch HJ, McGarry PA. Spinal cord vasculitis presenting as a spinal cord tumor in a heroin addict. Case report. *J Neurosurg*. 1978;48:131–134.

374. Burger PC, Mahley MS Jr, Dudka L, et al. The morphologic effects of radiation administered therapeutically for intracranial gliomas: a postmortem study of 25 cases. *Cancer*. 1979;44:1256–1272.

375. Uematsu Y, Fujita K, Tanaka Y, et al. Gamma knife radiosurgery for neuroepithelial tumors: radiological and histological changes. *Neuropathology*. 2001;21:298–306.

376. Horowitz MB, Jungreis CA, Quisling RG, et al. Vein of Galen aneurysms: a review and current perspective. Ajnr: *Am J Neuroradiol*. 1994;15:1486–1496.

377. Kimura A, Tan CF, Wakida K, et al. Venous congestive myelopathy of the cervical spinal cord: an autopsy case showing a rapidly progressive clinical course. *Neuropathology*. 2007;27:284–289.

378. Haddad SF, Moore SA, Schelper RL, et al. Vascular smooth muscle hyperplasia underlies the formation of glomeruloid vascular structures of glioblastoma multiforme. *J Neuropath Exp Neurol*. 1992;51:488–492.

379. Scheithauer BW, Fuller GN, VandenBerg SR. The 2007 WHO classification of tumors of the nervous system: controversies in surgical neuropathology. *Brain Pathol*. 2008;18: 307–316.

380. Giannini C,Scheithauer BW, Weaver AL, et al. Oligodendrogliomas: reproducibility and prognostic value of histologic diagnosis and grading. *J Neuropathol Exp Neurol*. 2001;60: 248–262.

381. Tihan T, Burger PC, Pomper M, et al. Subacute diencephalic angioencephalopathy: biopsy diagnosis and radiological features of a rare entity. *Clin Neurol Neurosurg*. 2001;103:160–167.

382. Kristof RA, Van Roost D, Wolf HK, et al.Intravascular papillary endothelial hyperplasia of the sellar region. Report of three cases and review of the literature. *J Neurosurg*. 1997;86: 558–563.

383. Guillou L, Fletcher JA, Fletcher CDM, et al. Extrapleural solitary fibrous tumor and haemangiopericytoma. In: Fletcher CDM, Unni K, Mertens F, eds. *Pathology and Genetics: Tumours of Soft Tissue and Bone*. Lyon, France: IARC Press; 2002:86–90.

384. Connor DH, Neafie RC, Hockmeyer WT. Malaria. In: Binford CH, Connor DH, eds. *Pathology of Tropical and Extraordinary Diseases: An Atlas*. Washington, DC: AFIP; 1976:273–283.

385. Ponzoni M, Ferreri AJ. Intravascular lymphoma: a neoplasm of 'homeless' lymphocytes? *Hematol Oncol*. 2006;24: 105–112.

386. Russell DS. The pathology of intracranial tumours. *Postgrad Med J*. 1950;26:109–125.

387. Rubinstein LJ. *Tumors of the Central Nervous System. Second Series, Fascicle 6*. Washington, DC: AFIP; 1972.

388. Komori T, Scheithauer BW, Anthony DC, et al. Papillary glioneuronal tumor: a new variant of mixed neuronal-glial neoplasm. *Am J Surg Pathol*. 1998;22:1171–1183.

389. Lellouch-Tubiana A, Boddaert N, Bourgeois M, et al. Angiocentric neuroepithelial tumor (ANET): a new epilepsy-related clinicopathological entity with distinctive MRI. *Brain Pathol*. 2005;15:281–286.

390. Tihan T, Fisher PG, Kepner JL, et al. Pediatric astrocytomas with monomorphous pilomyxoid features and a less favorable outcome. *J Neuropathol Exp Neurol*. 1999;58: 1061–1068.

391. Ceppa EP, Bouffet E, Griebel R, et al. The pilomyxoid astrocytoma and its relationship to pilocytic astrocytoma: report of a case and a critical review of the entity. *J Neurooncol*. 2007;81:191–196.

392. Perry A, Brat DJ. Astrocytic and Oligodendroglial Tumors. In: Perry A, Brat DJ, eds. *Practical Surgical Neuropathology*. Philadelphia, PA: Churchill Livingtsone; 2011:63–102.

393. Judkins AR, Ellison DW. Ependymoblastoma: Dear, Damned, Distracting Diagnosis, Farewell! *Brain Pathol*. 2010;20: 133–139.

394. Eberhart CG, Brat DJ, Cohen KJ, et al. Pediatric neuroblastic brain tumors containing abundant neuropil and true rosettes. *Pediatr Dev Pathol*. 2000;3:346–352.

395. Sato K, Kubota T. Pathology of pineal parenchymal tumors. *Prog Neurol Surg*. 2009;23:12–25.

396. McLean IW, Burnier MN, Zimmerman LE, et al. *Tumors of the Eye and Ocular Adnexa. Atlas of Tumor Pathology*. Washington, DC: Armed Forces Institute of Pathology; 1994.

397. Fevre-Montange M, Szathmari A, Champier J, et al. Pineocytoma and pineal parenchymal tumors of intermediate differentiation presenting cytologic pleomorphism: a multicenter study. *Brain Pathol*. 2008;18:354–359.

398. Jouvet A, Saint-Pierre G, Fauchon F, et al. Pineal parenchymal tumors: a correlation of histological features with prognosis in 66 cases. *Brain Pathol*. 2000;10:49–60.

399. Komori T, Scheithauer BW, Hirose T. A rosette-forming glioneuronal tumor of the fourth ventricle: infratentorial form of dysembryoplastic neuroepithelial tumor? *Am J Surg Pathol*. 2002;26:582–591.

400. Stemmer-Rachmamimov AO, Wiestler OD, Louis DN. *Neurofibromatosis Type 2. WHO Classification of Tumours of the Central Nervous System*. Lyon, France: IARC Press; 2007:210–214.

401. Ishihara M, Miyagawa-Hayashino A, Nakashima Y, et al. Intracerebral schwannoma in a child with infiltration along perivascular spaces resembling meningioangiomatosis. *Pathol Int*. 2009;59:583–587.

402. Norenberg MD, Smith J, Marcillo A. The pathology of human spinal cord injury: defining the problems. *J Neurotrauma*. 2004;21:429–440.

403. Jallo GI, Kothbauer K, Mehta V, et al. Meningioangiomatosis without neurofibromatosis: a clinical analysis. *J Neurosurg*. 2005;103:319–324.

404. Omeis I, Hillard VH, Braun A, et al. Meningioangiomatosis associated with neurofibromatosis: report of 2 cases in a single family and review of the literature. *Surg Neurol*. 2006;65:595–603.

405. Kim SU, de Vellis J. Microglia in health and disease. *J Neurosci Res*. 2005;81:302–313.

406. Garden GA, Moller T. Microglia biology in health and disease. *J Neuroimmune Pharmacol*. 2006;1:127–137.

407. Treml A, Bannykh S, Fan X. CD68 vs. CD163, Which Is More Sensitive and Specific in Various Brain Lesions? *Mod Pathol*. 2009;22:335A.

408. Merrill JE, Chen IS. HIV-1, macrophages, glial cells, and cytokines in AIDS nervous system disease. *FASEB J*. 1991;5: 2391–2397.

409. Arribas JR, Storch GA, Clifford DB, et al. Cytomegalovirus encephalitis. *Ann Intern Med*. 1996;125:577–587.

410. Levi ME, Quan D, Ho JT, et al. Impact of rituximab-associated B-cell defects on West Nile virus meningoencephalitis in solid organ transplant recipients. *Clin Transplant*. 2010;24:223–228.

411. Chen-Plotkin AS, Christopoulos KA, Venna N. Demyelinating polyneuropathy and herpes simplex lumbosacral radiculitis in a patient with chronic HIV infection. *AIDS*. 2007;21:1663–1664.

412. Dutta MK, Saha V, Sarkar P. Detection of rabies virus in different tissues of experimentally infected mice at preclinical and postclinical stages of the disease. *Indian J Exp Biol*. 1992;30:877–880.

413. Trask TW, Trask RP, Aguilar-Cordova E, et al. Phase I study of adenoviral delivery of the HSV-tk gene and ganciclovir administration in patients with current malignant brain tumors. *Mol Ther*. 2000;1:195–203.

414. Tremont-Lukats IW, Fuller GN, Ribalta T, et al. Paraneoplastic chorea: case study with autopsy confirmation. *Neuro Oncol*. 2002;4:192–195.

415. Storstein A, Krossnes B, Vedeler CA. Autopsy findings in the nervous system and ovarian tumour of two patients with paraneoplastic cerebellar degeneration. *Acta Neurol Scand*. 2006;183:69–70.

416. Takei H, Wilfong A, Malphrus A, et al. Dual pathology in Rasmussen's encephalitis: a study of seven cases and review of the literature. *Neuropathology*. 2010;30:381–391.

417. Dewil M, Van Den Bosch L, Robberecht W. Microglia in amyotrophic lateral sclerosis. *Acta Neurolog Belg*. 2007;107:63–70.

418. Nag S. Cerebral changes in chronic hypertension: combined permeability and immunohistochemical studies. *Acta Neuropathol*. 1984;62:178–184.

419. Imaizumi T, Nishizaka S, Ayabe M, et al. Probable chronic viral encephalitis with microglial nodules in the entire brain: a case report with necropsy. *Med Sci Monit*. 2005;11:23–26.

420. Porta J, Carota A, Pizzolato GP, et al. Immunopathological changes in human cerebral malaria. *Clin Neuropathol*. 1993;12:142–146.

421. Bertrand E, Szpak GM, Pilkowska E, et al. Central nervous system infection caused by Borrelia burgdorferi. Clinico-pathological correlation of three post-mortem cases. *Folia Neuropathol*. 1999;37:43–51.

422. Kleinschmidt-Demasters BK. Disseminated Fusarium infection with brain abscesses in a lung transplant recipient. *Clin Neuropathol*. 2009;28:417–421.

423. Watters JJ, Schartner JM, Badie B. Microglia function in brain tumors. *J Neurosci Res*. 2005;81:447–455.

424. Hulette CM. Microglioma, a histiocytic neoplasm of the central nervous system. *Mod Pathol*. 1996;9:316–319.

425. Phowthongkum P, Puengchitprapai A, Udomsantisook N, et al. Spindle cell pseudotumor of the brain associated with *Mycobacterium haemophilum* and *Mycobacterium simiae* mixed infection in a patient with AIDS: the first case report. *Int J Infect Dis*. 2008;12:421–424.

426. Matthiessen L, Marche C, Labrousse F, et al. Neuropathology of the brain in 174 patients who died of AIDS in a Paris hospital 1982–1988. *Ann Med Intern*. 1992;143:43–49–.

427. Kobayashi Z, Tsuchiya K, Takahashi M, et al. An autopsy case of chronic active Epstein-Barr virus infection (CAEBV): distribution of central nervous system (CNS) lesions. *J Neurol Sci*. 2008;275:170–177.

428. Shi Y. Morgenstern N. Granular cell astrocytoma. *Arch Pathol Lab Med*. 2008;132:1946–1950.

429. Alfieri A, Gazzeri R, Galarza M, et al. Surgical treatment of intracranial Erdheim-Chester disease. *J Clin Neurosci*. 2010;17:1489–1492.

430. Sun W, Nordberg ML, Fowler MR. Histiocytic sarcoma involving the central nervous system: clinical, immunohistochemical, and molecular genetic studies of a case with review of the literature. *Am J Surg Pathol*. 2003;27:258–265.

431. Darwish BS, Fowler A, Ong M, et al. Intracranial syphilitic gumma resembling malignant brain tumour. *J Clin Neurosci*. 2008;15:308–310.

432. Strickland-Marmol LB, Fessler RG, Rojiani AM. Necrotizing sarcoid granulomatosis mimicking an intracranial neoplasm: clinicopathologic features and review of the literature. *Mod Pathol*. 2000;13:909–913.

433. Urich H. Neurosarcoidosis or granulomatous angiitis: a problem of definition. *Mt Sinai J Med*. 1977;44:718–725.

434. Kim RC, Collins GH. The neuropathology of rheumatoid disease. *Hum Pathol*. 1981;12:5–15.
435. Utsuki S, Oka H, Tanizaki Y, et al. Pathological features of intracranial germinomas with reference to fibrous tissue and granulomatous change. *Brain Tumor Pathol*. 2005;22: 9–13.
436. Sacks EL, Donaldson SS, Gordon J, et al. Epithelioid granulomas associated with Hodgkin's disease: clinical correlations in 55 previously untreated patients. *Cancer*. 1978;41:562–567.
437. Carpinteri R, Patelli I, Casanueva FF, et al. Pituitary tumours: inflammatory and granulomatous expansive lesions of the pituitary. *Best Pract Res Clin Endocrinol Metab*. 2009;23: 639–650.
438. Leporati P, Landek-Salgado MA, Lupi I, et al. IgG4-related hypophysitis: a new addition to the hypophysitis spectrum. *J Clin Endocrinol Metab*. 2011;96:1971–1980.
439. Roy K, Bhattacharyya AK, Tripathy P, et al. Intracranial epidermoid—a 10-year study. *J Indian Med Assoc*. 2008;106:450–453.
440. Tateno F, Sakakibara R, Kishi M, et al. Bupivacaine-induced chemical meningitis. *J Neurol*. 2010;257:1327–1329.
441. Pearce JM. Mollaret's meningitis. European Neurology. 2008;60:316–317.
442. Teot LA, Sexton CW. Mollaret's meningitis: case report with immunocytochemical and polymerase chain reaction amplification studies. *Diagn Cytopathol*. 1996;15:345–348.
443. Ribalta T, McCutcheon IE, Neto AG, et al. Textiloma (gossypiboma) mimicking recurrent intracranial tumor. *Arch Pathol Lab Med*. 2004;128:749–758.
444. Lana-Peixoto MA. Devic's neuromyelitis optica: a critical review. *Arq Neuropsiquiat*. 2008;66:120–138.
445. Louis DN, Frosch MP, Mena H, et al. *Non-Neoplastic Diseases of the Central Nervous System. Atlas of Nontumor Pathology*. Washington, DC: American Registry of Pathology; 2008.
446. Gray F, Bazille C, Adle-Biassette H, et al. Central nervous system immune reconstitution disease in acquired immunodeficiency syndrome patients receiving highly active antiretroviral treatment. *J Neurovirol*. 2005;11:16–22.
447. Best T, Finlayson M. Two forms of encephalitis in opportunistic toxoplasmosis. *Arch Pathol Lab Med*. 1979;103: 693–696.
448. Johnson MD, Powell SZ, Boyer PJ, et al. Dural lesions mimicking meningiomas. *Hum Pathol*. 2002;33:1211–1226.
449. Tyler LN, Joseph L, Waldron JA, et al. Central nervous system findings in 65 multiple myeloma autopsies. *Mod Pathol*. 2002;15:9A.
450. Bruno MC, Ginguene C, Santangelo M, et al. Lymphoplasmacyte rich meningioma. A case report and review of the literature. *J Neurosurg Sci*. 2004;48:117–124.
451. Swain RS, Tihan T, Horvai AE, et al. Inflammatory myofibroblastic tumor of the central nervous system and its relationship to inflammatory pseudotumor. *Hum Pathol*. 2008;39:410–419.
452. Brat DJ, Scheithauer BW, Staugaitis SM, et al. Third ventricular chordoid glioma: a distinct clinicopathologic entity. *J Neuropathol Exp Neurol*. 1998;57:283–290.
453. Brown JA, Gomez-Leon G. Subdural hemorrhage secondary to extramedullary hematopoiesis in postpolycythemic myeloid metaplasia. *Neurosurgery*. 1984;14:588–591.
454. Slater JP. Extramedullary hematopoiesis in a subdural hematoma. Case report. *J Neurosurg*. 1966;25:211–214.
455. Zec N, Cera P, Towfighi J. Extramedullary hematopoiesis in cerebellar hemangioblastoma. *Neurosurgery*. 1991;29:34–37.
456. O'Brien CE, Saratsis AM, Voyadzis JM. Granulocytic sarcoma in a patient with blast crisis mimicking a chronic subdural hematoma. *J Clin Oncol*. 2011;29:569–571.
457. Stevenson VL, Hardie RJ. Acanthocytosis and neurological disorders. *J Neurol*. 2001;248:87–94.
458. Challa VR, Moody DM, Bell MA. The Charcot-Bouchard aneurysm controversy: impact of a new histologic technique. *J Neuropathol Exp Neurol*. 1992;51:264–271.
459. Sutherland GR, Auer RN. Primary intracerebral hemorrhage. *J Clin Neurosci*. 2006;13:511–517.
460. Karayel F, Turan AA, Sav A, et al. Methanol intoxication: pathological changes of central nervous system (17 cases). *Am J Forensic Med Pathol*. 2010;31:34–36.
461. Prockop LD, Chichkova RI. Carbon monoxide intoxication: an updated review. *J Neurol Sci*. 2007;262:122–130.
462. Zimmerman RA, Bilaniuk LT. Pediatric head trauma. *Neuroimaging Clin N Am*. 1994;4:349–366.
463. Bonnier C, Nassogne MC, Evrard P. Outcome and prognosis of whiplash shaken infant syndrome: late consequences after a symptom-free interval. *Develop Med Child Neurol*. 1995;37:943–956.
464. Sganzerla EP, Tomei G, Rampini P, et al. A peculiar intracerebral hemorrhage: the gliding contusion, its relationship to diffuse brain damage. *Neurosurg Rev*. 1989;12:215–218.
465. Love S. Autopsy approach to stroke. *Histopathology*. 2011;58:333–351.
466. Chan C, Fryer J, Herkes G, et al. Fatal brain stem event complicating acute pancreatitis. *J Clin Neurosci*. 2003;10: 351–358.
467. Rachinger J, Fellner FA, Stieglbauer K, et al. MR changes after acute cyanide intoxication. *AJNR Am J Neuroradiol*. 2002;23:1398–1401.
468. Sato Y, Kondo T, Ohshima T. Traumatic tear of the basilar artery associated with vertebral column injuries. *Am J Forensic Med Pathol*. 1997;18:129–134.
469. Cohen MC, Scheimberg I. Evidence of occurrence of intradural and subdural hemorrhage in the perinatal and neonatal period in the context of hypoxic ischemic encephalopathy: an observational study from two referral institutions in the United Kingdom. *Pediatr Dev Pathol*. 2009;12:169–176.
470. Kuhn E, Dorji T, Rodriguez J, et al. Extramedullary erythropoiesis in chronic subdural hematoma simulating metastatic small round cell tumor. *Int J Surg Pathol*. 2007;15: 288–291.
471. Ferrer I, Kaste M, Kalimo H. *Vascular Diseases. Greenfield's Neuropathology*. London, UK: Hodder Arnold; 2008: 121–240.
472. Brown AW, Brierley JB. The earliest alterations in rat neurons and astrocytes after anoxia-ischaemia. *Acta Neuropathol*. 1973;23:9–22.
473. Mohr JP. Lacunes. *Neurol Clin*. 1983;1:201–221,
474. Bargallo N, Burrel M, Berenguer J, et al. Cortical laminar necrosis caused by immunosuppresive therapy and chemotherapy. *AJNR Am J Neuroradiol*. 2000;21:479–484.
475. Bladin CF, Chambers BR. Frequency and pathogenesis of hemodynamic stroke. *Stroke*. 1994;25:2179–2182.
476. Moulin T. Crepin-Leblond T. Chopard JL, et al. Hemorrhagic infarcts. *Eur Neurol*. 1994;34:64–77.
477. Gates PC. Cerebral venous thrombosis: a retrospective review. *Aust NZ J Med*. 1986;16:766–770.
478. Milhorat TH. Capocelli AL Jr. Anzil AP, et al. Pathological basis of spinal cord cavitation in syringomyelia: analysis of 105 autopsy cases. *J Neurosurg*. 1995;82:802–812.
479. Meschia JF. Brott TG. Brown RD Jr. Genetics of cerebrovascular disorders. *Mayo Clin Proc*. 2005;80:122–132.
480. Fukuhara N. Strokelike episodes in MERRF. *Ann Neurol*. 1985;18:368.
481. Hutchinson M. O'Riordan J. Javed M, et al. Familial hemiplegic migraine and autosomal dominant arteriopathy with leukoencephalopathy (CADASIL). *Ann Neurol*. 1995;38:817–824.
482. Scott RM. Smith ER. Moyamoya disease and moyamoya syndrome. *N Engl J Med*. 2009;360:1226–1237.
483. Vinters HV, Anders KH, Barach P. Focal pontine leukoencephalopathy in immunosuppressed patients. *Arch Pathol Lab Med*. 1987;111:192–196.

484. Park YD, Belman AL, Kim TS, et al. Stroke in pediatric acquired immunodeficiency syndrome. *Ann Neurol.* 1990;28:303–311.

485. Leeuwis JW, Wolfs TF, Braun KP. A child with HIV-associated transient cerebral arteriopathy. *AIDS.* 2007;21:1383–1384.

486. Robb J. Chalmers L. Rojiani A, et al. Multifocal necrotizing leukoencephalopathy: an unusual complication of acute leukemia. *Arch Neurol.* 2006;63:1028–1029.

487. Bruck W, Heise E, Friede RL. Leukoencephalopathy after cisplatin therapy. *Clin Neuropathol.* 1989;8:263–265.

488. Baker WJ, Royer GL Jr, Weiss RB. Cytarabine and neurologic toxicity. *J Clin Oncol.* 1991;9:679–693.

489. Blaes AH, Santa-Cruz KS, Lee CK, et al. Necrotizing leukoencephalopathy following CHOP chemotherapy. *Leukemia Res.* 2008;32:1611–1614.

490. Miyoshi K, Matsuoka T, Mizushima S. Familial holotopistic striatal necrosis. *Acta Neuropathol.* 1969;13:240–249.

491. Kovacs GG, Hoftberger R, Majtenyi K, et al. Neuropathology of white matter disease in Leber's hereditary optic neuropathy. *Brain.* 2005;128:35–41.

492. Al-Shammari NE, El-Beltagi AH, Al-Far SA, et al. Syphilitic arteritis involving the origin of the cervical internal carotid artery. *Neurosciences.* 2010;15:122–125.

493. de Carvalho CA, Allen JN, Zafranis A, et al. Coccidioidal meningitis complicated by cerebral arteritis and infarction. *Hum Pathol.* 1980;11:293–296.

494. Parker JC Jr, McCloskey JJ, Lee RS. The emergence of candidosis. The dominant postmortem cerebral mycosis. *Am J Clin Pathol.* 1978;70:31–36.

495. Hideyama T, Aono G, Uesaka Y, et al. A 95-year-old female with autopsy-proven cerebral necrosis due to candidiasis who developed stroke-like manifestations. *Clin Neurol.* 2005;45:230–234.

496. Kikumoto Y, Kai Y, Morinaga H, et al. Fabry disease exhibiting recurrent stroke and persistent inflammation. *Intern Med.* 2010;49:2247–2252.

497. Kleihues P, Burger PC, Aldape KD, et al. Glioblastoma. In: Louis DN, Ohgaki H, Wiestler OD, et al., eds. *WHO Classification of Tumours of the Central Nervous System.* Lyon, France: IARC Press; 2007:33–49.

498. Rong Y, Durden DL, Van Meir EG, et al. 'Pseudopalisading' necrosis in glioblastoma: a familiar morphologic feature that links vascular pathology, hypoxia, and angiogenesis. *J Neuropathol Exp Neurol.* 2006;65:529–539.

499. Sharma MC, Deb P, Sharma S, et al. Neurocytoma: a comprehensive review. *Neurosurg Rev.* 2006;29:270–285.

500. Lenzi J, Salvati M, Raco A, et al. Central neurocytoma: a novel appraisal of a polymorphic pathology. Our experience and a review of the literature. *Neurosurg Rev.* 2006;29:286–292.

501. Giannini C, Rushing EJ, Hainfellner JA. Haemangiopericytoma. In: Louis DN, Ohgaki H, Wiestler OD, et al., eds. WHO *Classification of Tumours of the Central Nervous System.* Lyon, France: IARC Press; 2007:178–180.

502. Judkins AR, Montone KT, LiVolsi VA, et al. Sensitivity and specificity of antibodies on necrotic tumor tissue. *Am J Clin Pathol.* 1998;110:641–646.

503. Fanburg-Smith JC, Meis-Kindblom JM, Fante R, et al. Malignant granular cell tumor of soft tissue: diagnostic criteria and clinicopathologic correlation. *Am J Surg Pathol.* 1998;22:779–794.

504. Tomlinson FH, Scheithauer BW, Hayostek CJ, et al. The significance of atypia and histologic malignancy in pilocytic astrocytoma of the cerebellum: a clinicopathologic and flow cytometric study. *J Child Neurol.* 1994;9:301–310.

505. Giannini C, Scheithauer BW, Burger PC, et al. Pleomorphic xanthoastrocytoma: what do we really know about it? *Cancer.* 1999;85:2033–2045.

506. Figarella-Branger D, Civatte M, Bouvier-Labit C, et al. Prognostic factors in intracranial ependymomas in children. *J Neurosurg.* 2000;93:605–613.

507. Tihan T, Zhou T, Holmes E, et al. The prognostic value of histological grading of posterior fossa ependymomas in children: a Children's Oncology Group study and a review of prognostic factors. *Mod Pathol.* 2008;21:165–177.

508. Goel A, Kini U, Shetty S. Role of histopathology as an aid to prognosis in rhino-orbito-cerebral zygomycosis. *Indian J Pathol Microbiol.* 2010;53:253–257.

509. Paniago AM, de Oliveira PA, Aguiar ES, et al. Neuroparacoccidioidomycosis: analysis of 13 cases observed in an endemic area in Brazil. *Trans R Soc Trop Med Hygiene.* 2007;101:414–420.

510. Khoury H, Adkins D, Brown R, et al. Successful treatment of cerebral toxoplasmosis in a marrow transplant recipient: contribution of a PCR test in diagnosis and early detection. *Bone Marrow Transplant.* 1999;23:409–411.

511. Recavarren-Arce S, Velarde C, Gotuzzo E, et al. Amoeba angeitic lesions of the central nervous system in Balamuthia mandrilaris amoebiasis. *Hum Pathol.* 1999;30:269–273.

512. Singh P, Kochhar R, Vashishta RK, et al. Amebic meningoencephalitis: spectrum of imaging findings. *AJNR Am J Neuroradiol.* 2006;27:1217–1221.

513. Sundaram C, Prasad BC, Bhaskar G, et al. Brain abscess due to Entamoeba histolytica. *J Assoc Physicians India.* 2004;52:251–252.

514. Bourque AC, Conboy G, Miller LM, et al. Pathological findings in dogs naturally infected with Angiostrongylus vasorum in Newfoundland and Labrador, Canada. *J Vet Diagn Invest.* 2008;20:11–20.

515. Masdeu JC, Tantulavanich S, Gorelick PP, et al. Brain abscess caused by *Strongyloides stercoralis*. *Arch Neurol.* 1982;39:62–63.

516. Carod-Artal FJ. Tropical causes of epilepsy. *Revista de Neurologia.* 2009;49:475–482.

517. Nicoli F, Vion-Dury J, Chave B, et al. Marchiafava-Bignami disease: interhemispheric disconnection, Balint syndrome, spontaneously favourable outcome. *Rev Neuro.* 1994;150:157–161.

518. Baudoin D, Gambarelli D, Gayraud D, et al. Devic's neuromyelitis optica: a clinicopathological review of the literature in connection with a case showing fatal dysautonomia. *Clin Neuropathol.* 1998;17:175–183.

519. Nakamura M, Endo M, Murakami K, et al. An autopsied case of neuromyelitis optica with a large cavitary cerebral lesion. *Mult Scler.* 2005;11:735–738.

520. Jellinger KA. The enigma of vascular cognitive disorder and vascular dementia. *Acta Neuropathol.* 2007;113:349–388.

521. Roman GC. Senile dementia of the Binswanger type. A vascular form of dementia in the elderly. *JAMA.* 1987;258:1782–1788.

522. Sibon I, Fenelon G, Quinn NP, et al. Vascular parkinsonism. *J Neurol.* 2004;251:513–524.

523. Allais A, Burel D, Roy V, et al. Balanced effect of PACAP and FasL on granule cell death during cerebellar development: a morphological, functional and behavioural characterization. *J Neurochem.* 2010;113:329–340.

524. Lefebvre d'Hellencourt C, Harry GJ. Molecular profiles of mRNA levels in laser capture microdissected murine hippocampal regions differentially responsive to TMT-induced cell death. *J Neurochem.* 2005;93:206–220.

525. Scherer HJ. Structural development in gliomas. *Am J Cancer.* 1938;34:333–351.

526. Peiffer J, Kleihues P. Hans-Joachim Scherer (1906–1945), pioneer in glioma research. *Brain Pathol.* 1999;9:241–245.

527. Lehman NL. Patterns of brain infiltration and secondary structure formation in supratentorial ependymal tumors. *J Neuropathol Exp Neurol.* 2008;67:900–910.

528. Arai N, Takahashi T, Komori T, et al. Diagnostic surgical neuropathology of intractable epilepsy. *Neuropathology.* 2007;27:594–600.

529. Kaufmann WE, Galaburda AM. Cerebrocortical microdysgenesis in neurologically normal subjects: a histopathologic study. *Neurology.* 1989;39:238–244.

530. Jokinen CH, Ragsdale BD, Argenyi ZB. Expanding the clinicopathologic spectrum of palisaded encapsulated neuroma. *J Cutan Pathol* 2010;37:43–48.

531. Wilson JL, Ellis TL, Mott RT. Chordoid meningioma of the third ventricle: a case report and review of the literature. *Clin Neuropathol.* 2011;30:70–74.

532. Kepes JJ. The fine structure of hyaline inclusions (pseudopsammoma bodies) in meningiomas. *J Neuropathol Exp Neurol*. 1975;34:282–294.

533. Louis DN, Hamilton AJ, Sobel RA, et al. Pseudopsammomatous meningioma with elevated serum carcinoembryonic antigen: a true secretory meningioma. Case report. *J Neurosurg*. 1991;74:129–132.

534. Folker RJ, Meyerhoff WL, Rushing EJ. Aggressive papillary adenoma of the cerebellopontine angle: case report of an endolymphatic sac tumor. *Am J Otolaryngol*. 1997;18: 135–139.

535. Aquilina K, Nanra JS, Allcutt DA, et al. Choroid plexus adenoma: case report and review of the literature. *Childs Nerv Syst*. 2005;21:410–415.

536. Kliewer KE, Wen DR, Cancilla PA, et al. Paragangliomas: assessment of prognosis by histologic, immunohistochemical, and ultrastructural techniques. *Hum Pathol*. 1989;20:29–39.

537. Achilles E, Padberg BC, Holl K, et al. Immunocytochemistry of paragangliomas—value of staining for S-100 protein and glial fibrillary acid protein in diagnosis and prognosis. *Histopathology*. 1991;18:453–458.

538. Teo JG, Gultekin SH, Bilsky M, et al. A distinctive glioneuronal tumor of the adult cerebrum with neuropil-like (including "rosetted") islands: report of 4 cases. *Am J Surg Pathol*. 1999;23:502–510.

539. Gessi M, Marani C, Geddes J, et al. Ependymoma with neuropil-like islands: a case report with diagnostic and histogenetic implications. *Acta Neuropathol*. 2005;109:231–234.

540. Hasselblatt M, Jeibmann A, Guerry M, et al. Choroid plexus papilloma with neuropil-like islands. *Am J Surg Pathol*. 2008;32:162–166.

541. Eberhart CG, Kepner JL, Goldthwaite PT, et al. Histopathologic grading of medulloblastomas. *Cancer*. 2002;94: 552–560.

542. Ho DM, Hsu CY, Wong TT, et al. Atypical teratoid/rhabdoid tumor of the central nervous system: a comparative study with primitive neuroectodermal tumor/medulloblastoma. *Acta Neuropathol* 2000;99:482–488.

543. Boyanton BL Jr, Jones JK, Shenaq SM, et al. Intraneural perineurioma: a systematic review with illustrative cases. *Arch Pathol Lab Med*. 2007;131:1382–1392.

544. Fabregues I, Ferrer I, Cusi MV, et al. Fine structure based on the Golgi method of the abnormal cortex and heterotopic nodules in pachygyria. *Brain Dev*. 1984;6:317–322.

545. Pilz D, Stoodley N, Golden JA. Neuronal migration, cerebral cortical development, and cerebral cortical anomalies. *J Neuropathol Exp Neurol*. 2002;61:1–11.

546. Rickert CH. Cortical dysplasia: neuropathological aspects. *Childs Nerv Syst*. 2006;22:821–826.

547. Paulus W, Brandner S. Choroid plexus tumours. In: Louis DN, Ohgaki H, Wiestler OD, et al., eds. *WHO Classification of Tumours of the Central Nervous System*. Lyon, France: IARC Press; 2007:81–86.

548. Geerts Y, Gabreels F, Lippens R, et al. Choroid plexus carcinoma: A report of two cases and review of the literature. *Neuropaediatrics*. 1996;27:143–148.

549. Paulus W, Janisch W. Clinicopathologic correlations in epithelial choroid plexus neoplasms: a study of 52 cases. *Acta Neuropathol*. 1990;80:635–641.

550. Herbert J, Cavallaro T, Dwork AJ. A marker for primary choroid plexus neoplasms. *Am J Pathol*. 1990;136:1317–1325.

551. Ang LC, Taylor AR, Bergin D, et al. An immunohistochemical study of papillary tumors in the central nervous system. *Cancer*. 1990;65:2712–2719.

552. Gessi M, Giangaspero F, Pietsch T. Atypical teratoid/rhabdoid tumors and choroid plexus tumors: when genetics "surprise" pathology. *Brain Pathol*. 2003;13:409–414.

553. Tena-Suck ML, Gomez-Amador JL, Ortiz-Plata A, et al. Rhabdoid choroid plexus carcinoma: a rare histological type. *Arquivos de Neuro-Psiquiatria*. 2007;65:705–709.

554. Jouvet A, Fauchon F, Liberski P, et al. Papillary tumor of the pineal region. *Am J Surg Pathol*. 2003;27:505–512.

555. Samuel K, Juwin L, Lucie JN, et al. Papillary meningioma: a malignant variant of meningioma. *Cancer*. 1975;36:1363–1373.

556. Giangaspero F, Burger PC, Osborne DR, et al. Suprasellar papillary squamous epithelioma ("papillary craniopharyngioma"). *Am J Surg Pathol*. 1984;8:57–64.

557. Sano T, Yamada S. Histologic and immunohistochemical study of clinically non-functioning pituitary adenomas: special reference to gonadotropin-positive adenomas. *Pathol Int*. 1994;44:697–703.

558. Luff DA, Simmons M, Malik T, et al. Endolymphatic sac tumours. *J Laryngol Otol*. 2002;116:398–401.

559. Kasper M, Kasper M, Kern F, et al. Immunohistochemical studies on human pituitary gland and adenomas. *J Hirnforsch*. 1991;32:725–734.

560. Giometto B, Miotto D, Botteri M, et al. Folliculo-stellate cells of human pituitary adenomas: immunohistochemical study of the monocyte/macrophage phenotype expression. *Neuroendocrinology*. 1997;65:47–52.

561. Burnett ME, White EC, Sih S, et al. Chromosome arm 17p deletion analysis reveals molecular genetic heterogeneity in supratentorial and infratentorial primitive neuroectodermal tumors of the central nervous system. *Cancer Genet Cytogenet*. 1997;97:25–31.

562. Behdad A, Perry A. Central Nervous System Primitive Neuroectodermal Tumors: A Clinicopathologic and Genetic Study of 33 Cases. *Brain Pathol*. 2010;20:441–450.

563. Katsetos CD, Herman MM, Frankfurter A, et al. Cerebellar desmoplastic medulloblastomas. A further immunohistochemical characterization of the reticulin-feee pale islands. *Arch Pathol Lab Med*. 1989;113:1019–1029.

564. Giangaspero F, Perilongo G, Fondelli MP, et al. Medulloblastoma with extensive nodularity: a variant with favorable prognosis. *J Neurosurg*. 1999;91:971–977.

565. Giangaspero F, Rigobello L, Badiali M, et al. Large-cell medulloblastomas. A distinct variant with highly aggressive behavior. *Am J Surg Pathol*. 1992;16:687–693.

566. McManamy CS, Pears J, Weston CL, et al. Nodule formation and desmoplasia in medulloblastomas-defining the nodular/desmoplastic variant and its biological behavior. *Brain Pathol*. 2007;17:151–164.

567. Brown HG, Kepner JL, Perlman EJ, et al. "Large cell/anaplastic" medulloblastomas: a Pediatric Oncology Group Study. *J Neuropathol Exp Neurol*. 2000;59:857–865.

568. Dang T, Vassilyadi M, Michaud J, et al. Atypical teratoid/rhabdoid tumors. *Childs Nerv Syst*. 2003;19:244–248.

569. Mobley BC, Roulston D, Shah GV, et al. Peripheral primitive neuroectodermal tumor/Ewing's sarcoma of the craniospinal vault: case reports and review. *Hum Pathol*. 2006;37:845–853.

570. Dedeurwaerdere F, Giannini C, Sciot R, et al. Primary peripheral PNET/Ewing's sarcoma of the dura: a clinicopathologic entity distinct from central PNET. *Mod Pathol*. 2002;15: 673–678.

571. Fouladi M, Gajjar A, Boyett JM, et al. Comparison of CSF cytology and spinal magnetic resonance imaging in the detection of leptomeningeal disease in pediatric medulloblastoma or primitive neuroectodermal tumor. *J Clin Oncol*. 1999;17:3234–3237.

572. Lai R. Survival of patients with adult medulloblastoma: a population-based study. *Cancer*. 2008;112:1568–1574.

573. Sabatino G, Lauriola L, Sioletic S, et al. Occipital ganglio-neuroblastoma in an adult. *Acta Neurochir*. 2009;151: 495–496.

574. Perry A, Aldape KD, George DH, et al. Small cell astrocytoma: an aggressive variant that is clinicopathologically and genetically distinct from anaplastic oligodendroglioma. *Cancer*. 2004;101:2318–2326.

575. Perry A, Miller CR, Gujrati M, et al. Malignant gliomas with primitive neuroectodermal tumor-like components: a clinicopathologic and genetic study of 53 cases. *Brain Pathol*. 2009;19:81–90.

576. Janzer RC, Kleihues P. Primitive neuroectodermal tumor with choroid plexus differentiation. *Clin Neuropathol*. 1985;4:93–98.

577. Perry A, Stafford SL, Scheithauer BW, et al. Meningioma grading: an analysis of histologic parameters. *Am J Surg Pathol*. 1997;21:1455–1465.

578. Shintaku M, Nakade M, Hirose T. Malignant peripheral nerve sheath tumor of small round cell type with pleomorphic spindle cell sarcomatous areas. *Pathol Int*. 2003;53:478–482.

579. Suchak R. Luzar B. Bacchi CE, et al. Cutaneous neuroblastoma-like schwannoma: a report of two cases, one with a plexiform pattern, and a review of the literature. *J Cutan Pathol*. 2010;37:997–1001.

580. Roach ES, DiMario FJ, Kandt RS, et al. Tuberous Sclerosis Consensus Conference recommendations for diagnostic evaluation. National Tuberous Sclerosis Association. *J Child Neurol*. 1999;14:401–407.

581. Daumas-Duport C, Scheithauer BW, Chodkiewitz JP, et al. Dysembryoplastic neuroepithelial tumor: a surgically curable tumor of young patients with intractable partial seizures. Report of thirty-nine cases. *Neurosurgery*. 1987;23:545–556.

582. Maiuri F, Gangemi M, Iaconetta G, et al. Symptomatic subependymomas of the lateral ventricles. Report of eight cases. *Clin Neurol Neurosurg*. 1997;99:17–22.

583. Hasselblatt M, Jeibmann A, Gerß J, et al. Cellular and reticular variants of haemangioblastoma revisited: a clinicopathologic study of 88 cases. *Neuropathol Appl Neurobiol*. 2005;31:618–622.

584. Berg JC, Scheithauer BW, Spinner RJ, et al. Plexiform schwannoma: a clinicopathologic overview with emphasis on the head and neck region. *Hum Pathol*. 2008;39:633–640.

585. Newlin HE, Morris CG, Amdur RJ, et al. Neurotropic Melanoma of the Head and Neck With Clinical Perineural Invasion. *Am J Clin Oncol*. 2005;28:399–402.

586. Jaffer S. Ambrosini-Spaltro A. Mancini AM, et al. Neurothekeoma and plexiform fibrohistiocytic tumor: mere histologic resemblance or histogenetic relationship? *Am J Surg Pathol* 2009;33:905–913.

587. Rodriguez FJ. Scheithauer BW. Jenkins R, et al. Gliosarcoma arising in oligodendroglial tumors ("oligosarcoma"): a clinicopathologic study. *Am J Surg Pathol*. 2007;31:351–362.

588. Han SJ, Yang I, Tihan T, et al. Primary gliosarcoma: key clinical and pathologic distinctions from glioblastoma with implications as a unique oncologic entity. *J Neurooncol*. 2010;96:313–320.

589. Louis DN, Hedley-Whyte ET, Martuza RL. Sarcomatous proliferation of the vasculature in a subependymoma. *Acta Neuropathol*. 1989;78:332–335.

590. Tomlinson FH, Scheithauer BW, Kelly PJ, et al. Subependymoma with rhabdomyosarcomatous differentiation: report of a case and literature review. *Neurosurgery*. 1991;28:761–768.

591. Hirose T, Scheithauer BW, Lopes MB, et al. Ganglioglioma: an ultrastructural and immunohistochemical study. *Cancer*. 1997;79:989–1003.

592. Hayashi S, Kameyama S, Fukuda M, et al. Ganglioglioma with a tanycytic ependymoma as the glial component. *Acta Neuropathol*. 2000;99:310–316.

593. Johnson MD, Jennings MT, Toms ST. Oligodendroglial ganglioglioma with anaplastic features arising from the thalamus. *Pediatr Neurosurg*. 2001;34:301–305.

594. Becker AJ, Wiestler OD, Figarella-Branger D, et al. Ganglioglioma and gangliocytoma. In: Louis DN, Ohgaki H, Wiestler OD, et al., eds. *WHO Classification of Tumours of the Central Nervous System*. Lyon, France: IARC Press; 2007:103–105.

595. Perry A, Burton SS, Fuller GN, et al. Oligodendroglial neoplasms with ganglioglioma-like maturation: a diagnostic pitfall. *Acta Neuropathol*. 2010;120:237–252.

596. Tanaka M, Shibui S, Nomaru K, et al. Pineal ganglioneuroblastoma in an adult. *J Neurooncol*. 1999;44:169–173.

597. Govindan A, Mahadevan A, Bhat DI, et al. Papillary glioneuronal tumor-evidence of stem cell origin with biphenotypic differentiation. *J Neurooncol*. 2009;95:71–80.

598. Solis OE, Mehta RI, Lai A, et al. Rosette-forming glioneuronal tumor: a pineal region case with IDH1 and IDH2 mutation analyses and literature review of 43 cases. *J Neurooncol*. 2011;102:477–484.

599. Scheithauer BW, Kovacs K, Horvath E, et al. Pituitary blastoma. *Acta Neuropathol* 2008;116:657–666.

600. Siegel HJ, Dunahm WH, Lopez-Ben R, et al. Intracranial metastasis from synovial sarcoma. *Orthopedics*. 2008;31:405.

601. Ulbright TM, Young RH, Scully RE. Trophoblastic tumors of the testis other than classic choriocarcinoma: "monophasic" choriocarcinoma and placental site trophoblastic tumor: a report of two cases. *Am J Surg Pathol*. 1997;21:282–288.

602. Ludemann W, Stan AC, Tatagiba M, et al. Sporadic unilateral vestibular schwannoma with islets of meningioma: case report. *Neurosurgery*. 2000;47:451–452.

603. Feany MB, Anthony DC, Fletcher CD. Nerve sheath tumours with hybrid features of neurofibroma and schwannoma: a conceptual challenge. *Histopathology*. 1998;32:405–410.

604. Ducatman BS, Scheithauer BW, Piepgras DG, et al. Malignant peripheral nerve sheath tumors. A clinicopathologic study of 120 cases. *Cancer*. 1986;57:2006–2021.

605. Rosenberg AS, Langee CL, Stevens GL, et al. Malignant peripheral nerve sheath tumor with perineurial differentiation: "malignant perineurioma". *J Cutan Pathol*. 2002;29:362–367.

606. Coons SW, Johnson PC, Scheithauer BW, et al. Improving diagnostic accuracy and interobserver concordance in the classification and grading of primary gliomas. *Cancer*. 1997;79:1381–1393.

607. He J, Mokhtari K, Sanson M, et al. Glioblastoma with an oligodendroglioma component: a pathological and molecular study. *J Neuropathol Exp Neurol*. 2001;60:863–871.

608. Bannykh SI, Perry A, Powell HC, et al. Malignant rhabdoid meningioma arising in the setting of preexisting ganglioglioma: a diagnosis supported by fluorescence in situ hybridization. Case report. *J Neurosurg*. 2002;97:1450–1455.

609. Hattab EM, Martin SE, Shapiro SA, et al. Pleomorphic xanthoastrocytoma and oligodendroglioma: collision of 2 morphologically and genetically distinct anaplastic components. *J Neurosurg*. 2011;114:1648–1653.

610. Prayson RA, Fong J, Najm I. Coexistent pathology in chronic epilepsy patients with neoplasms. *Mod Pathol*. 2010;23:1097–1103.

611. Piao YS, Lu DH, Chen L, et al. Neuropathological findings in intractable epilepsy: 435 Chinese cases. *Brain Pathol*. 2010;20:902–908.

612. Firlik KS, Adelson PD, Hamilton RL. Coexistence of a ganglioglioma and Rasmussen's encephalitis. *Pediatr Neurosurg*. 1999;30:278–282.

613. Park SH, Chi JG, Cho BK, et al. Spinal cord ganglioglioma in childhood. *Pathol Res Pract*. 1993;189:189–196.

614. Schild SE, Scheithauer BW, Schomberg PJ, et al. Pineal parenchymal tumors: clinical, pathologic, and therapeutic aspects. *Cancer*. 1993;72:870–880.

615. Matyja E, Kuchna I, Kroh H, et al. Meningiomas and gliomas in juxtaposition: casual or causal coexistence? Report of two cases. *Am J Surg Pathol*. 1995;19:37–41.

616. Suzuki K, Momota H, Tonooka A, et al. Glioblastoma simultaneously present with adjacent meningioma: case report and review of the literature. *Neurooncol*. 2010;99:147–153.

617. Izci Y, Secer HI, Gonul E, et al. Simultaneously occurring vestibular schwannoma and meningioma in the cerebellopontine angle: case report and literature review. *Clin Neuropathol*. 2007;26:219–223.

618. Deb P, Gupta A, Sharma MC, et al. Meningioangiomatosis with meningioma: an uncommon association of a rare entity—report of a case and review of the literature. *Childs Nerv Syst*. 2006;22:78–83.

619. Kazakov DV, Pitha J, Sima R, et al. Hybrid peripheral nerve sheath tumors: schwannoma-perineurioma and neurofibroma-perineurioma. A report of three cases in extradigital locations. *Ann Diagn Pathol*. 2005;9:16–23.

620. Karavitaki N, Scheithauer BW, Watt J, et al. Collision lesions of the sella: co-existence of craniopharyngioma with gonadotroph adenoma and of Rathke's cleft cyst with corticotroph adenoma. *Pituitary*. 2008;11:317–323.

621. Gokden M, Mrak RE. Pituitary adenoma with craniopharyngioma component. *Hum Pathol*. 2009;40:1189–1193.

622. Hattab EM. Germ cell tumors. In: *Practical Surgical Neuropathology*. Philadelphia, PA: Churchill Livingstone; 2007:333–352.

623. Challa VR, Moody DM, Brown WR. Vascular malformations of the central nervous system. *J Neuropathol Exp Neurol*. 1995;54:609–621.

624. Pamphlett R. Carcinoma metastasis to meningioma. *J Neurol Neurosurg Psychiatry*. 1984;47:561–563.

625. Baratelli GM, Ciccaglioni B, Dainese E, et al. Metastasis of breast carcinoma to intracranial meningioma. *J Neurosurg Sci*. 2004;48:71–73.

626. Hoellig A, Niehusmann P, Flacke S, et al. Metastasis to pituitary adenoma: case report and review of the literature. *Cent Eur Neurosurg*. 2009;70:149–153.

627. Collini P, Mezzelani A, Modena P, et al. Evidence of neural differentiation in a case of post-therapy primitive neuroectodermal tumor/ewing sarcoma of bone. *Am J Surg Pathol*. 2003;27:1161–1166.

628. Miura K, Mineta H, Yokota N, et al. Olfactory neuroblastoma with epithelial and endocrine differentiation transformed into ganglioneuroma after chemoradiotherapy. *Pathol Int*. 2001;51:942–947.

629. Al-Mefty O, Topsakal C, Pravdenkova S, et al. Radiation-induced meningiomas: clinical, pathological, cytokinetic, and cytogenetic characteristics. *J Neurosurg*. 2004;100:1002–1013.

630. Scheithauer BW, Erdogan S, Rodriguez FJ, et al. Malignant peripheral nerve sheath tumors of cranial nerves and intracranial contents a clinicopathologic study of 17 Cases. *Am J Surg Pathol*. 2009;33:325–338.

631. Han SJ, Yang I, Otero JJ, et al. Secondary gliosarcoma after diagnosis of glioblastoma: clinical experience with 30 consecutive patients. *J Neurosurg*. 2010;112:990–996.

632. Shaffrey ME, Lanzino G, Lopes MB, et al. Maturation of intracranial immature teratomas. Report of two cases. *J Neurosurg*. 1996;85:672–676.

633. Yu L, Krishnamurthy S, Chang H, et al. Congenital maturing immature intraventricular teratoma. *Clin Imaging*. 2010;34:222–225.

634. Rodriguez FJ, Scheithauer BW, Giannini C, et al. Epithelial and pseudoepithelial differentiation in glioblastoma and gliosarcoma: a comparative morphologic and molecular genetic study. *Cancer*. 2008;113:2779–2789.

635. Jain A, Rishi A, Suri V, et al. Recurrent ependymoma with cartilaginous metaplasia in an adult: report of a rare case and review of literature. *Clin Neuropathol*. 2009;28:101–104.

636. Corcoran GM, Frazier SR, Prayson RA. Choroid plexus papilloma with osseous and adipose metaplasia. *Ann Diagn Pathol*. 2001;5:43–47.

637. Anwer UE, Smith TW, DeGirolami U, et al. Medulloblastoma with cartilaginous differentiation. *Arch Pathol Lab Med*. 1989;113:84–88.

638. Chandy MJ, Rajshekhar V, Ghosh S, et al. Single small enhancing CT lesions in Indian patients with epilepsy: clinical, radiological and pathological considerations. *J Neurol Neurosurg Psychiatry*. 1991;54:702–705.

639. Hughes AJ, Biggs BA. Parasitic worms of the central nervous system: an Australian perspective. *Intern Med J*. 2002;32:541–553.

640. Saleem S, Belal AI, el-Ghandour NM. Spinal cord schistosomiasis: MR imaging appearance with surgical and pathologic correlation. *AJNR Am J Neuroradiol*. 2005;26:1646–1654.

641. Musso C, Castelo JS, Tsanaclis AM, et al. Visceral larva migrans granulomas in liver and central nervous system of children who died of bacterial or viral meningitis. *Clin Neuropathol*. 2006;25:288–290.

642. Foo WC, Desjardins A, Cummings TJ. Primary intracerebral Hodgkin lymphoma with recurrence. *Clin Neuropathol*. 2011;30:75–79.

643. Schnitzer B. Hodgkin lymphoma. *Hematol Oncol Clin North Am*. 2009;23:747–768.

644. Hicks MJ, Albrecht S, Trask T, et al. Symptomatic choroid plexus xanthogranuloma of the lateral ventricle. Case report and brief critical review of xanthogranulomatous lesions of the brain. *Clin Neuropathol*. 1993;12:92–96.

645. Saw S, Thomas N, Gleeson MJ, et al. Giant cell tumour and central giant cell reparative granuloma of the skull: do these represent ends of a spectrum? A case report and literature review. *Pathol Oncol Res*. 2009;15:291–295.

646. Haddad GF, Hambali F, Mufarrij A, et al. Concomitant fibrous dysplasia and aneurysmal bone cyst of the skull base. Case report and review of the literature. *Pediatr Neurosurg*. 1998;28:147–153.

647. Fulkerson DH, Luerssen TG, Hattab EM, et al. Long-term follow-up of solitary intracerebral juvenile xanthogranuloma. Case report and review of the literature. *Pediatr Neurosurg*. 2008;44:480–485.

648. Barbagallo GM, Caltabiano R, Parisi G, et al. Giant cell ependymoma of the cervical spinal cord: case report and review of the literature. *Eur Spine J*. 2009;18:186–190.

649. Lau SK, Chu PG, Weiss LM. CD163: a specific marker of macrophages in paraffin-embedded tissue samples. *Am J Clin Pathol*. 2004;122:794–801.

650. Scheithauer BW, Gaffey TA, Lloyd RV, et al. Pathobiology Of Pituitary Adenomas And Carcinomas. *Neurosurgery*. 2006;59:341–353.

651. Perry A, Scheithauer BW. Commentary: Classification and grading of pituitary tumors. Observations of two working neuropathologists. *Acta Neuropathol*. 2006;111:68–70.

652. Utsuki S, Oka H, Tanaka S, et al. Long-term outcome of intracranial germinoma with hCG elevation in cerebrospinal fluid but not in serum. *Acta Neurochir*. 2002;144:1151–1154.

653. Nordmark G, Boquist L, Ronnblom L. Limited Wegener's granulomatosis with central nervous system involvement and fatal outcome. *J Intern Med*. 1997;242:433–436.

654. Teruo S, Yasuto H. A 25-year-old woman with multiple brain tumors who died after a course of 1 year and 6 months. *Neuropathology*. 2003;23:364–366.

655. Thomas C, Love S, Powell HC, et al. Giant axonal neuropathy: correlation of clinical findings with postmortem neuropathology. *Ann Neurol*. 1987;22:79–84.

656. Kretzschmar HA, Berg BO, Davis RL. Giant axonal neuropathy. A neuropathological study. *Acta Neuropathol*. 1987;73:138–144.

657. Marburger TB, Prayson RA. Angiocentric glioma: a clinicopathologic review of five tumors with identification of associated cortical dysplasia. *Mod Pathol* 2010;23:378A.

658. Perez-Nunez A, Lagares A, Benitez J, et al. Lhermitte-Duclos disease and Cowden disease: clinical and genetic study in five patients with Lhermitte-Duclos disease and literature review. *Acta Neurochir*. 2004;146:679–690.

659. Shepherd CW, Scheithauer BW, Gomez MR, et al. Subependymal giant cell astrocytoma: a clinical, pathological, and flow cytometric study. *Neurosurgery*. 1991;28:864–868.

660. Kingsley DP, Kendall BE, Fitz CR. Tuberous sclerosis: a clinicoradiological evaluation of 110 cases with particular reference to atypical presentation. *Neuroradiology*. 1986;28:38–46.

661. Kim SK, Wang KC, Cho BK, et al. Biological behavior and tumorigenesis of subependymal giant cell astrocytomas. *J Neurooncol*. 2001;52:217–225.

662. Perry A. Familial tumor syndromes. In: Perry A, Brat DJ, eds. *Practical Surgical Neuropathology*. Philadelphia, PA: Churchill Livingstone; 2007:427–454.

663. Isidro ML, Iglesias Diaz P, Matias-Guiu X, et al. Acromegaly due to a growth hormone-releasing hormone-secreting intracranial gangliocytoma. *J Endocrinol Invest*. 2005;28:162–165.

664. Scheithauer BW, Silva AI, Parisi JE, et al. Ganglioglioma of the neurohypophysis. *Endocrine Pathol*. 2008;19:112–116.

665. Serri O, Berthelet F, Belair M, et al. An unusual association of a sellar gangliocytoma with a prolactinoma. *Pituitary*. 2008;11:85–87.

666. Gaughen JR, Bourne TD, Aregawi D, et al. Focal neuronal gigantism: a rare complication of therapeutic radiation. *Am J Neuroradiol*. 2009;30:1933–1935.

667. Kleinschmidt-DeMasters BK, Mierau GW, Sze CI, et al. Unusual dural and skull-based mesenchymal neoplasms: a report of four cases. *Hum Pathol*. 1998;29:240–245.

668. Sivendran S, Vidal CI, Barginear MF. Primary intracranial leiomyosarcoma in an HIV-infected patient. *Int J Clin Oncol*. 2011;16:63–66.

669. Morrison A, Gyure KA, Stone J, et al. Mycobacterial spindle cell pseudotumor of the brain: a case report and review of the literature. *Am J Surg Pathol*. 1999;23:1294–1299.

670. Darwish BS, Balakrishnan V, Maitra R. Intramedullary ancient schwannoma of the cervical spinal cord: case report and review of literature. *J Clin Neurosci*. 2002;9:321–323.

671. Ugokwe K, Nathoo N, Prayson R, et al. Trigeminal nerve schwannoma with ancient change. Case report and review of the literature. *J Neurosurg*. 2005;102:1163–1165.

672. Hornick JL, Fletcher CD. Soft tissue perineurioma: clinicopathologic analysis of 81 cases including those with atypical histologic features. *Am J Surg Pathol*. 2005;29:845–858.

673. Ishihama H, Nakamura M, Funao H, et al. A rare case of spinal dumbbell tanycytic ependymoma. *Spine*. 2011;36:E612–E614.

674. Louis DN, Ramesh V, Gusella JF. Neuropathology and molecular genetics of neurofibromatosis 2 and related tumors. *Brain Pathol*. 1995;5:163–172.

675. Azarpira N, Torabineghad S, Sepidbakht S, et al. Cytologic findings in pigmented melanotic schwannoma: a case report. *Acta Cytol*. 2009;53:113–115.

676. Janss AJ, Yachnis AT, Silber JH, et al. Glial differentiation predicts poor clinical outcome in primitive neuroectodermal brain tumors. *Ann Neurol*. 1996;39:481–489.

677. Borota OC, Scheithauer BW, Fougner SL, et al. Spindle cell oncocytoma of the adenohypophysis: report of a case with marked cellular atypia and recurrence despite adjuvant treatment. *Clin Neuropathol*. 2009;28:91–95.

678. Phillips JJ, Misra A, Feuerstein BG, et al. Pituicytoma: characterization of a unique neoplasm by histology, immunohistochemistry, ultrastructure, and array-based comparative genomic hybridization. *Arch Pathol Lab Med*. 2010;134:1063–1069.

679. Perry A, Scheithauer BW, Macaulay RJ, et al. Oligodendrogliomas with neurocytic differentiation. A report of 4 cases with diagnostic and histogenetic implications. *J Neuropathol Exp Neurol*. 2002;61:947–955.

680. Yuen ST, Fung CF, Ng TH, et al. Central neurocytoma: its differentiation from intraventricular oligodendroglioma. *Childs Nerv Syst*. 1992;8:383–388.

681. Nishio S, Tashima T, Takeshita I, et al. Intraventricular neurocytoma: clinicopathological features of six cases. *J Neurosurg*. 1988;68:665–670.

682. Chakraborti S, Mahadevan A, Govindan A, et al. Supratentorial and cerebellar liponeurocytomas: report of four cases with review of literature. *J Neurooncol*. 2011;103:121–127.

683. Zonenshayn M, Sharma S, Hymes K, et al. Mycosis fungoides metastasizing to the brain parenchyma: case report. *Neurosurgery*. 1998;42:933–937.

684. Ghosal N, Kapila K, Kakkar S, et al. Langerhans cell histiocytosis infiltration in cerebrospinal fluid: a case report. *Diagn Cytopathol*. 2001;24:123–125.

685. Angeles-Angeles A, Chable-Montero F, Martinez-Benitez B, et al. Unusual metastases of papillary thyroid carcinoma: report of 2 cases. *Ann Diagn Pathol*. 2009;13:189–196.

686. DeLellis RA. Orphan annie eye nuclei: a historical note. *Am J Surg Pathol*. 1993;17:1067.

687. Zankl H, Seidel H, Zang KD. Cytological and cytogenetical studies on brain tumors. V. Preferential loss of sex chromosomes in human meningiomas. *Humangenetik*. 1975;27:119–128.

688. Ip YT, Dias Filho MA, Chan JK. Nuclear inclusions and pseudoinclusions: friends or foes of the surgical pathologist? *Int J Surg Pathol*. 2010;18:465–481.

689. Derenzini M, Montanaro L, Trere´ D. What the nucleolus says to a tumour pathologist. *Histopathology*. 2009;54:753–762.

690. Volk EE, Prayson RA. Hamartomas in the setting of chronic epilepsy: a clinicopathologic study of 13 cases. *Hum Pathol*. 1997;28:227–232.

691. Lin BT, Weiss LM, Medeiros LJ. Neurofibroma and cellular neurofibroma with atypia: a report of 14 tumors. *Am J Surg Pathol*. 1997;21:1443–1449.

692. Zuppan CW, Beckwith JB, Luckey DW. Anaplasia in unilateral Wilms' tumor: a report from the National Wilms' Tumor Study Pathology Center. *Hum Pathol*. 1988;19:1199–1209.

693. Beach TG, Walker DG, Sue LI, et al. Substantia nigra Marinesco bodies are associated with decreased striatal expression of dopaminergic markers. *J Neuropathol Exp Neurol*. 2004;63:329–337.

694. Kimber TE, Blumbergs PC, Rice JP, et al. Familial neuronal intranuclear inclusion disease with ubiquitin positive inclusions. *J Neurol Sci*. 1998;160:33–40.

695. Greco CM, Hagerman RJ, Tassone F et al. Neuronal intranuclear inclusions in a new cerebellar tremor/ataxia syndrome among fragile X carriers. *Brain*. 2002;125:1760–1771.

696. Gokden M, Al-Hinti JT, Harik SI. Peripheral nervous system pathology in fragile X tremor/ataxia syndrome (FXTAS). *Neuropathology*. 2009;29:280–284.

697. Nishie M, Mori F, Yoshimoto M, et al. A quantitative investigation of neuronal cytoplasmic and intranuclear inclusions in the pontine and inferior olivary nuclei in multiple system atrophy. *Neuropathol Appl Neurobiol*. 2004;30:546–554.

698. Yamada M, Sato T, Tsuji S, et al. CAG repeat disorder models and human neuropathology: similarities and differences. *Acta Neuropathol*. 2008;115:71–86.

699. DiFiglia M, Sapp E, Chase KO, et al. Aggregation of huntingtin in neuronal intranuclear inclusions and dystrophic neurites in brain. *Science*. 1997;277:1990–1993.

700. Snowden J, Neary D, Mann D. Frontotemporal lobar degeneration: clinical and pathological relationships. *Acta Neuropathol*. 2007;114:31–38.

701. Adachi H, Katsuno M, Minamiyama M, et al.Widespread nuclear and cytoplasmic accumulation of mutant androgen receptor in SBMA patients. *Brain*. 2005;128:659–670.

702. Woulfe J, Gray DA, Mackenzie IR. FUS-immunoreactive intranuclear inclusions in neurodegenerative disease. *Brain Pathol*. 2010;20:589–597.

703. Fujigasaki H, Uchihara T, Koyano S, et al. Ataxin-3 is translocated into the nucleus for the formation of intranuclear inclusions in normal and Machado-Joseph disease brains. *Exp Neurol*. 2000;165:248–256.

704. Liebert UG. Measles virus infections of the central nervous system. *Intervirology*. 1997;40:176–184.

705. Rosai J. *Ackerman's Surgical Pathology*. Vol. 2, St. Louis, MO: Mosby; 2004:1609–1612.

706. Ellis PSJ, Whitehead R. Mitosis counting—a need for reappraisal. *Hum Pathol*. 1981;12:3–4.

707. Quinn CM, Wright NA. The clinical assessment of proliferation and growth in human tumours: evaluation of methods and application as prognostic variables. *J Pathol*. 1990;160:93–102.

708. Silverberg SG. Reproducibility of the mitosis count in the histologic diagnosis of smooth muscle tumors of the uterus. *Hum Pathol*. 1976;7:451–454.

709. Scully RE. Mitosis counting—I. *Hum Pathol*. 1976;7:481–482.

710. Kempson RL. Mitosis counting—II. *Hum Pathol*. 1976;7:482–483.

711. Norris HJ. Mitosis counting—III. *Hum Pathol*. 1976;7: 483–484.

712. Fukushima S, Terasaki M, Sakata K, et al Sensitivity and usefulness of anti-phosphohistone-H3 antibody immunostaining for counting mitotic figures in meningioma cases. *Brain Tumor Pathol*. 2009;26:51–57.

713. Habberstad AH, Gulati S, Torp SH. Evaluation of the proliferation markers Ki-67/MIB-1, mitosin, survivin, pHH3, and DNA topoisomerase IIalpha in human anaplastic astrocytomas—an immunohistochemical study. *Diagn Pathol*. 2011;6:43.

714. Ribalta T, McCutcheon IE, Aldape KD, et al. The mitosis-specific antibody anti-phosphohistone-H3 (PHH3) facilitates rapid reliable grading of meningiomas according to WHO 2000 criteria. *Am J Surg Pathol*. 2004;28:1532–1536.

715. Graem NN, Helweg-Larsen E. Mitotic activity and delay in fixation of tumour tissue. *Acta Pathol Microbial Stand*. 1979;87:375–378.

716. Kronqvist P, Kuopio T, Collan Y. Quantitative thresholds for mitotic counts in histologic grading: confirmation in nonfrozen samples of invasive ductal breast cancer. *Ann Diagn Pathol*. 2000;4:65–70.

717. Perry A, Louis DN, Scheithauer BW, et al. Meningiomas. In: Louis DN, Ohgaki H, Wiestler OD, et al., eds. *WHO Classification of Tumours of the Central Nervous System*. Lyon, France: IARC Press; 2007:164–172.

718. Ng HK, Poon WS, Goh K, et al. Histopathology of post-embolized meningiomas. *Am J Surg Pathol*. 1996;20:1224–1230.

719. Perry A, Chicoine MR, Filiput E, et al. Clinicopathologic assessment and grading of embolized meningiomas: a correlative study of 64 patients. *Cancer*. 2001;92:701–711.

720. Reifenberger G, Kros JM, Louis DN, et al. Anaplastic oligodendroglioma. In: Louis DN, Ohgaki H, Wiestler OD, et al., eds. WHO *Classification of Tumours of the Central Nervous System*. Lyon, France: IARC Press; 2007:60–62.

721. Brat DJ, Perry A. Astrocytic and oligodendroglial tumors. In: *Practical Surgical Neuropathology*. Perry A, Brat DJ, eds. Philadelphia, PA: Churchill Livingstone; 2007:63–102.

722. Aldape KD, Rosenblum MK. Astroblastoma. In: Louis DN, Ohgaki H, Wiestler OD, et al., eds. *WHO Classification of Tumours of the Central Nervous System*. Lyon, France: IARC Press; 2007:88–89.

723. Liapis H, Dehner LP, Gutmann DH. Neurofibroma and cellular neurofibroma with atypia: a report of 14 tumors. *Am J Surg Pathol*. 1999;23:1156–1158.

724. Kasashima S, Oda Y, Nozaki J, et al. A case of atypical granular cell tumor of the neurohypophysis. *Pathol Int*. 2000;50:568–573.

725. Perry A. Scheithauer BW. Commentary: Classification and grading of pituitary tumors. Observations of two working neuropathologists. *Acta Neuropathol*. 2006;111:68–70.

726. Gray F, Gherardi R, Keohane C, et al. Pathology of the central nervous system in 40 cases of acquired immune deficiency syndrome (AIDS). *Neuropathol Appl Neurobiol*. 1988;14: 365–380.

727. Alvarez LA, Kato T, Llena JF, et al. Ependymal foldings and other related ependymal structures in the cerebral aqueduct and fourth ventricle of man. *Acta Anat*. 1987;129: 305–309.

728. Wolburg H, Paulus W. Choroid plexus: biology and pathology. *Acta Neuropathol*. 2010;119:75–88.

729. Kleinschmidt-DeMasters BK, Gilden DH. The expanding spectrum of herpesvirus infections of the nervous system. *Brain Pathol*. 2001;11:440–451.

730. Kleinschmidt-DeMasters BK, Gilden DH. Varicella-Zoster virus infections of the nervous system: clinical and pathologic correlates. *Arch Pathol Lab Med*. 2001;125:770–780.

731. Hughes DC, Raghavan A, Mordekar SR, et al. Role of imaging in the diagnosis of acute bacterial meningitis and its complications. *Postgr Med J*. 2010;86:478–485.

732. Beer R, Lackner P, Pfausler B, et al. Nosocomial ventriculitis and meningitis in neurocritical care patients. *J Neurol*. 2008;255:1617–1624.

733. Kulkarni V, Daniel RT, Pranatartiharan R. Spontaneous intraventricular rupture of craniopharyngioma cyst. *Surg Neurol*. 2000;54:249–253.

734. Al Ferayan A, Russell NA, Al Wohaibi M, et al. Cerebrospinal fluid lavage in the treatment of inadvertent intrathecal vincristine injection. *Childs Nerv Syst*. 1999;15:87–89.

735. Leeds NE, Lang FF, Ribalta T, et al. Origin of chordoid glioma of the third ventricle. *Arch Pathol Lab Med*. 2006;130:460–464.

736. Moos T. Brain iron homeostasis. *Danish Med Bull*. 2002;49:279–301.

737. Benkovic SA, Connor JR. Ferritin, transferrin, and iron in selected regions of the adult and aged rat brain. *J Comp Neurol*. 1993;338:97–113.

738. Aicardi J. Aicardi syndrome. *Brain Dev*. 2005;27:164–171.

739. Rovit RL, Schechter MM, Chodroff P. Choroid plexus papillomas: observations on radiographic diagnosis. *AJR Am J Roentgenol*. 1970;110:608–617.

740. Yoshino A, Katayama Y, Watanabe T, et al. Multiple choroid plexus papillomas of the lateral ventricle distinct from villous hypertrophy. Case report. *J Neurosurg*. 1998;88:581–585.

741. Taggard DA, Menezes AH. Three choroid plexus papillomas in a patient with Aicardi syndrome. A case report. *Pediatr Neurosurg*. 2000;33:219–223.

742. Hirano H, Hirahara K, Asakura T, et al. Hydrocephalus due to villous hypertrophy of the choroid plexus in the lateral ventricles. Case report. *J Neurosurg*. 1994;80:321–323.

743. Davis LE. A physio-pathologic study of the choroid plexus with the report of a case of villous hypertrophy. *J Med Res*. 1924;44:521–534.

744. Blamires TL, Maher ER. Choroid plexus papilloma. A new presentation of von Hippel-Lindau (VHL) disease. *Eye*. 1992;6:90–92.

745. Hori A, Walter GF, Haas J, et al. Down syndrome complicated by brain tumors: case report and review of the literature. *Brain Dev*. 1992;14:396–400.

746. Gonzalez KD, Noltner KA, Buzin CH, et al. Beyond Li Fraumeni Syndrome: clinical characteristics of families with p53 germline mutations. *J Clin Oncol*. 2009;27:1250–1256.

747. Liu M, Wei Y, Liu Y, et al. Intraventricular meningiomas: a report of 25 cases. *Neurosurg Rev*. 2006;29:36–40.

748. Dumont AS, Farace E, Schiff D, et al. Intraventricular gliomas. *Neurosurg Clin N Am*. 2003;14:571–591.

749. Bunai Y, Akaza K, Tsujinaka M, et al. Sudden death due to undiagnosed intracranial hemangiopericytoma. *Am J Forensic Med Pathol*. 2008;29:170–172.

750. Surendrababu NR, Chacko G, Daniel RT, et al. Solitary fibrous tumor of the lateral ventricle: CT appearances and pathologic correlation with follow-up. *AJNR Am J Neuroradiol*. 2006;27:2135–2136.

751. Rumana M, Kirmani A, Khursheed N, et al. Primary B-cell lymphoma of choroid plexus in a 30-year-old immunocompetent male. *Clin Neuropathol*. 2011;30:152–154.

752. Siomin V, Lin JL, Marko NF, et al. Stereotactic radiosurgical treatment of brain metastases to the choroid plexus. *Int J Radiat Oncol Biol Physics*. 2011;80:1134–1142.

753. Vecil GG, Lang FF. Surgical resection of metastatic intraventricular tumors. *Neurosurg Clin N Am*. 2003;14:593–606.

754. Denis E, Dufour P, Valat AS, et al. Choroid plexus cysts and risks of chromosome anomalies. Review of the literature and proposed management. *J Gynecol Obstet Biol Reprod*. 1998;27:144–149.

755. Muenchau A, Laas R. Xanthogranuloma and xanthoma of the choroid plexus: evidence for different etiology and pathogenesis. *Clin Neuropathol*. 1997;16:72–76.

756. Reusche E. Argyrophilic inclusions distinct from Alzheimer neurofibrillary changes in one case of dialysis-associated encephalopathy. *Acta Neuropathol*. 1997;94:612–616.

757. Lach B, Scheithauer BW. Colloid cyst of the third ventricle: a comparative ultrastructural study of neuraxis cysts and choroid plexus epithelium. *Ultrastruct Pathol*. 1992;16: 331–3349.

758. Graziani N, Dufour H, Figarella-Branger D, et al. Do the suprasellar neurenteric cyst, the Rathke cleft cyst and the colloid cyst constitute a same entity? *Acta Neurochir*. 1995;133:174–180.

759. Zada G, Lin N, Ojerholm E, et al. Craniopharyngioma and other cystic epithelial lesions of the sellar region: a review of clinical, imaging, and histopathological relationships. *Neurosurg Focus*. 2010;28:E4.

760. Cao J, Lin JP, Yang LX, et al. Expression of aberrant beta-catenin and impaired p63 in craniopharyngiomas. *Br J Neurosurg*. 2010;24:249–256.

761. Guidetti B, Gagliardi FM. Epidermoid and dermoid cysts. Clinical evaluation and late surgical results. *J Neurosurg*. 1977;47:12–18.

762. Agarwal S, Rishi A, Suri V, et al. Primary intracranial squamous cell carcinoma arising in an epidermoid cyst—a case report and review of literature. *Clin Neurol Neurosurg*. 2007;109:888–891.

763. Nishio S, Takeshita I, Morioka T, et al. Primary intracranial squamous cell carcinomas: report of two cases. *Neurosurgery*. 1995;37:329–332.

764. Shin JL, Asa SL, Woodhouse LJ, et al. Cystic lesions of the pituitary: clinicopathological features distinguishing craniopharyngioma, Rathke's cleft cyst, and arachnoid cyst. *J Clin Endocrinol Metab*. 1999;84:3972–3982.

765. Pekmezci M, Louie J, Gupta N, et al. Clinicopathological characteristics of adamantinomatous and papillary craniopharyngiomas: University of California, San Francisco experience 1985–2005. *Neurosurgery*. 2010;67:1341–1349.

766. Aquilina K, Merchant TE, Rodriguez-Galindo C, et al. Malignant transformation of irradiated craniopharyngioma in children: report of 2 cases. *J Neurosurg*. 2010;5:155–161.

767. Kollias SS, Ball WS Jr, Prenger EC. Cystic malformations of the posterior fossa: differential diagnosis clarified through embryologic analysis. *Radiographics*. 1993;13:1211–1231.

768. Inagaki T. Yamanouchi Y. Nishimura T, et al. Intracranial dural cyst. *Childs Nerv Syst*. 1998;14:69–73.

769. Ojemann JG, Moran CJ, Gokden M, et al. Sagittal sinus occlusion by intraluminal dural cysts. Report of two cases. *J Neurosurg*. 1999;91:867–870.

770. Boockvar JA, Shafa R, Forman MS, et al. Symptomatic lateral ventricular ependymal cysts: criteria for distinguishing these rare cysts from other symptomatic cysts of the ventricles—case report. *Neurosurgery*. 2000;46:1229–1233.

771. Gherardi R, Lacombe MJ, Porer J, et al. Asymptomatic encephalic intraparenchymatous neuroepithelial cysts. *Acta Neuropathol*. 1984;63:264.

772. Engel U, Gottschalk S, Niehaus L, et al. Cystic lesions of the pineal region: MRI and pathology. *Neuroradiology*. 2000;42:399–402.

773. Voyadzis JM, Bhargava P, Henderson FC. Tarlov cysts: a study of 10 cases with review of the literature. *J Neurosurg*. 2001;95:25–32.

774. Powers JM, Dodds HM. Primary actinomycoma of the third ventricle—the colloid cyst. *Acta Neuropathol*. 1977;37:21–26.

775. Oeberst JL, Barnard JJ, Bigio EH, et al. Neurocysticercosis. *Am J Forensic Med Pathol*. 2002;23:31–35.

776. Taratuto AL, Venturiello SM. Echinococcosis. *Brain Pathol*. 1997;7:663–672.

777. Rengarajan S, Nanjegowda N, Bhat D, et al. Cerebral sparganosis: a diagnostic challenge. *Br J Neurosurg*. 2008;22:784–786.

778. Shapiro WR, Posner JB, Ushio Y, et al. Treatment of meningeal neoplasms. *Cancer Treat Rep*. 1977;61:733–743.

779. Wasserstrom WR, Glass JP, Posner JB. Diagnosis and treatment of leptomeningeal metastases from solid tumors: experience with 90 patients. *Cancer*. 1982;49:759–772.

780. Hilden JM, Meerbaum S, Burger P, et al. Central nervous system atypical teratoid/rhabdoid tumor: results of therapy in children enrolled in a registry. *J Clin Oncol* 2004;22:2877–2884.

781. Telfeian AE, Judkins A, Younkin D, et al. Subependymal giant cell astrocytoma with cranial and spinal metastases in a patient with tuberous sclerosis. Case report. *J Neurosurg*. 2004;100:498–500.

782. Lammens M. Neuronal migration disorders in man. *Eur J Morphol*. 2000;38:327–333.

783. Keith T, Llewellyn R, Harvie M, et al. A report of the natural history of leptomeningeal gliomatosis. *J Clin Neurosci*. 2011;18:582–585.

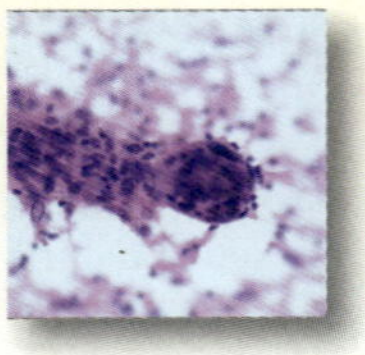
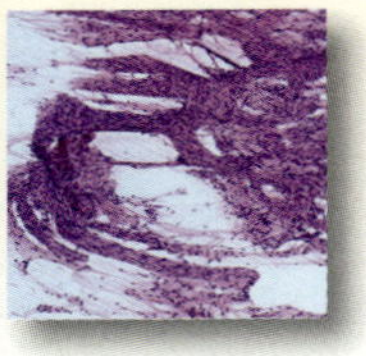
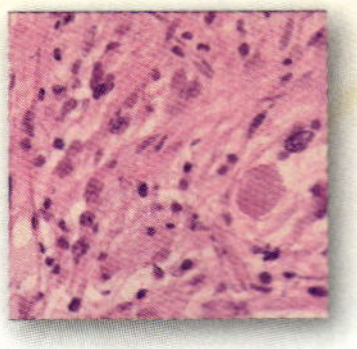

CHAPTER 3

Intraoperative Consultations

Introduction

Intraoperative consultation (IOC) is a very crucial component of surgical neuropathology. Its intimidating nature is at least in part due to the unfamiliarity with it of surgical pathologists and cytopathologists, who may not have adequate experience with the interpretation of neuropathologic samples. IOC is preferred over the common daily and admittedly more practical term "frozen," which represents only the frozen section component of this apparently simple but paradoxically extremely complex process. Multiple modalities are involved in IOC. Gross examination of the tissue; selection of the fragments for further microscopic examination; preparation and evaluation of cytologic slides and frozen sections; review of clinical, intraoperative, and radiologic findings (see Chapter 4); discussion with the surgeon; allocation of tissue for ancillary tests, such as electron microscopy, microbiology, flow cytometry, and cytogenetics, as needed; and additional recommendations to the surgeon are all part of this process.[1] As such, this process is much more involved than simply glancing at a slide and is therefore more appropriately referred to as IOC. Tissue selection for cytologic examination and frozen sections is especially important, so that various different areas of the tissue with different qualities can be sampled, keeping in mind the heterogeneity of the neoplasms of the central nervous system (CNS). This also assures that some tissue is saved for formalin fixation and routine processing without subjecting to freezing and associated artifacts. Orientation of larger fragments for frozen sections is another consideration that can be addressed by gross examination of the fresh tissue. Bone and extensively calcified portions can be separated and saved for decalcification, as forceful smearing or frozen sectioning will not be productive. See Chapter 1 for general descriptions of specimen types encountered in neuropathology.

The systematical discussions of IOC on individual entities have been provided in detail elsewhere.[1,2] In accord with the approach taken in this text, the discussion in this chapter, as in the previous chapters discussing gross and microscopic features, centers on the pathologic findings, their differential diagnoses and analyses. However, this will not be a mere repetition of the previous section on microscopic features but will add to them mainly by emphasizing those features that are relevant to the cytologic evaluation and frozen tissue sections in the context of IOC, as the individual findings and their differential diagnoses, especially as they relate to tissue sections (in this case, frozen sections), are essentially the same and have already been discussed in Chapter 2. As such, the differential diagnosis of a lesion with giant cells still includes those discussed in Chapter 2 under "Cellular Enlargement and Multinucleation." Therefore, this chapter is intended to complement Chapter 2 in terms of description of cytologic features that can be identified in various lesions, rather than a repetition of the entire subject. While this text starts from the pathologic features and works its way toward a specific diagnosis, which is what really happens in real life, it is important to note that a final check to make sure the pathologic interpretation is in accord with the general clinical and radiologic features is essential mainly to avoid pitfalls and mistakes, which are discussed as appropriate mainly in Chapter 2 in regard to various situations. Otherwise, the pathologist should of course make, or at least suggest, the diagnosis that is dictated by the findings in the tissue examined. After all, that is why the IOC is being obtained from pathology, that is, to learn what the pathologic findings are, and not simply for the pathologist to agree with the interpretations of the surgeon and/or the radiologist. One way to assure this is to approach the pathologic evaluation without any other bias from the clinical, radiologic, and other laboratory findings, or any previous diagnoses. It is only after a preliminary impression and a working diagnosis are formed that the entire circumstances should be put in context. This allows the pathologist to keep an open mind. Having at least one alternative diagnosis, preferably a short list of differential diagnostic possibilities, even when the diagnosis appears most obvious is the best insurance against complications. This same approach is certainly advisable for any type of pathologic evaluation but is most important in the IOC setting, where resources, such as consultation, further reading, and special stains, are limited and time is of essence. Knowledge of any previous diagnoses, and if available, reviewing those slides, can be of tremendous help with the interpretation of the findings and providing a more meaningful evaluation of the current situation. That being said, there are and will be difficult cases, for which even a general classification of the lesion may not be possible. The pathologist should not hesitate to defer such diagnoses, and these cases should be discussed with the surgeon. Most neurosurgeons are very open to this type of communication. Especially those with a solid understanding of pathology and its importance for their patients' management do not see this as a "nuisance from an incompetent pathologist" but, instead, welcome the opportunity to even review the slides together while discussing the findings, possibilities, and limitations. This also provides the pathologist with an understanding of the surgeon's plans and the reason for this IOC. This way, even if a specific diagnostic line may not be provided, a mutual understanding of the situation and a plan that is in the best interest of the patient can be established, and adequate tissue for further workup, including special studies, can be secured.

Cytologic Evaluation

Cytologic examination of the tissue is a crucial component of IOC in neuropathology. It can be performed by using conventional smear techniques, crush/squash preparations, touch/imprint preparations, scrape preparations, or a combination of these. Crush or touch preparations (TPs) may have the added advantage of preserving the architectural histologic features without distorting them with smearing. For instance, the microcysts of subependymoma may also be observed on crush preparations.[3] An actual needle aspiration method using an 18-gauge spinal tap needle with subsequent smear preparations has also been studied[4]; however, it did not enjoy much popularity in practice, likely due to the development of stereotactic biopsy method, which offered solid tissue cores with the added advantage of histologic evaluation. Fine needle aspiration can actually be used efficiently[5] at least in selected situations with great degree of accuracy and allow the application of ancillary techniques such as electron microscopy.[6] Either way by avoiding artifacts associated with freezing and cutting the tissue, it allows one to examine the cellular detail. In addition, it is possible to evaluate patterns on cytologic preparations in many situations as on tissue sections. It also allows minimal use of tissue and saving as much of it as possible for routine sections and ancillary tests. Becoming familiar with the cytologic evaluation of tissue allows one to examine even the smallest amount of tissue from which obtaining frozen sections would have been essentially impossible due to the risk of cutting through a miniscule fragment. This can especially be very important in stereotactic biopsy specimens.[7] In some cases, one may not even have to use tissue fragments to prepare smears. Touch or imprint preparations, obtained simply by touching the slide to the tissue, can provide invaluable information in some situations.[8] Most institutions use cytologic preparations together with frozen section evaluation,[9] taking advantage of both modalities, although some studies showed a higher sensitivity, positive and negative predictive values, as well as greater overall diagnostic efficiency for cytologic techniques over frozen sections.[10] Variable success has been reported for the cytologic evaluations, however,[11,12] which further provides comfort in using combined cytologic and histologic methods. Admittedly, both techniques have advantages and limitations and what works for the pathologist and institution, for the given situation, and eventually for the patient should be considered the best method. While evaluating the results of a study, or one's own success rate, the criteria used for diagnostic accuracy should also be kept in mind. The more specific diagnoses demanded, in contrast to broad ones such as low-grade glioma, the more likely that a lower concordance rate with the final diagnosis will be obtained. Another factor is certainly the experience of the pathologist. Cytologic evaluation can be used for nonneoplastic/infectious lesions, as well, with the added advantage of avoiding the contamination of the cryostat with potentially infectious specimens; however, the diagnostic accuracy for nonneoplastic lesions is not as good as it is for neoplastic lesions.[13]

In contrast to the usual cytologic techniques employing Papanicolaou and/or Romanowsky type of stains, cytologic preparations in neuropathology IOC are stained with the usual H&E, and the characteristics described in this chapter and other neuropathology texts are based on H&E staining. However, the use of other stains depends on personal preferences. The features of the major CNS neoplasms and cells based on routine cytologic stains have been described,[14] and many cases are described based on cytologic staining methods in the cytology literature. There are several variables that need to be taken into consideration while evaluating a cytologic preparation. For instance, cellularity is also dependent on factors other than the absolute cellularity of the tissue. The larger the tissue used to prepare the smear, the more cellular the preparation will be. Therefore, it is best that the smears are prepared by the pathologist who will evaluate them. This will also provide information on ease of smearing, consistency, and nature of the tissue, which may be relevant to interpretation in some cases. The thickness of the smear and how much tissue is used are also related, which in turn affect cellularity. If the smears will be prepared by someone other than who will interpret them, it is preferable that the preparation be done by the same person as much as possible. This ensures some degree of consistency for the procedure and for subsequent evaluation. Typically, a 1- to 2-mm^3 tissue fragment is sufficient for an adequate smear.[15] Sampling and evaluating different areas of the tissue on the same glass slide are also possible by placing the pieces side by side on the slide and smearing them parallel to each other.[16]

All in all, cytology is another way of looking at the same cells and lesions that are dealt with on a routine basis by histologic approach. A thorough knowledge of these lesions and familiarity with their histologic features, as well as the cytologic features as they apply to tissue sections, should put the findings identified on cytologic preparations in perspective **(Fig. 3-1)**.

Background Features

It has to be remembered that, while cytology refers to the examination of the cells and is traditionally mainly concerned with the nuclear features, the interpretation of cytologic preparations is no different than the approach to a tissue section in principle. In neuropathology, evaluation of background helps narrow down the differential diagnostic possibilities rapidly.

The smears from nonlesional neuroglial tissue produce a *homogeneous smear pattern* on the slide. This can even be seen with naked eye. Microscopically, the background is homogeneous with finely granular neuropil components in which delicate capillaries and nuclei are scattered. Upon close examination, axons can be seen as delicate lines running in different directions. Naked nuclei are variable in size. The larger ones, representing neurons whose cytoplasms have been stripped off during smearing, are round to oval and have a relatively finely granular and lighter chromatin. A prominent nucleolus is also present. Smaller nuclei are mainly in two forms. They are both round. Some have dark chromatin and appear pyknotic. They are almost perfectly round. These nuclei represent oligodendroglial cells. Also round but somewhat more irregular and larger compared to these are astrocytes. Their chromatin can be seen easier than that of oligodendroglia. They do not have visible nucleoli. No cytoplasms or processes emanating from these cells can be appreciated **(Fig. 3-2)**.

In a lesion of neuroglial nature, neoplastic or reactive, the appearance of the slide to the naked

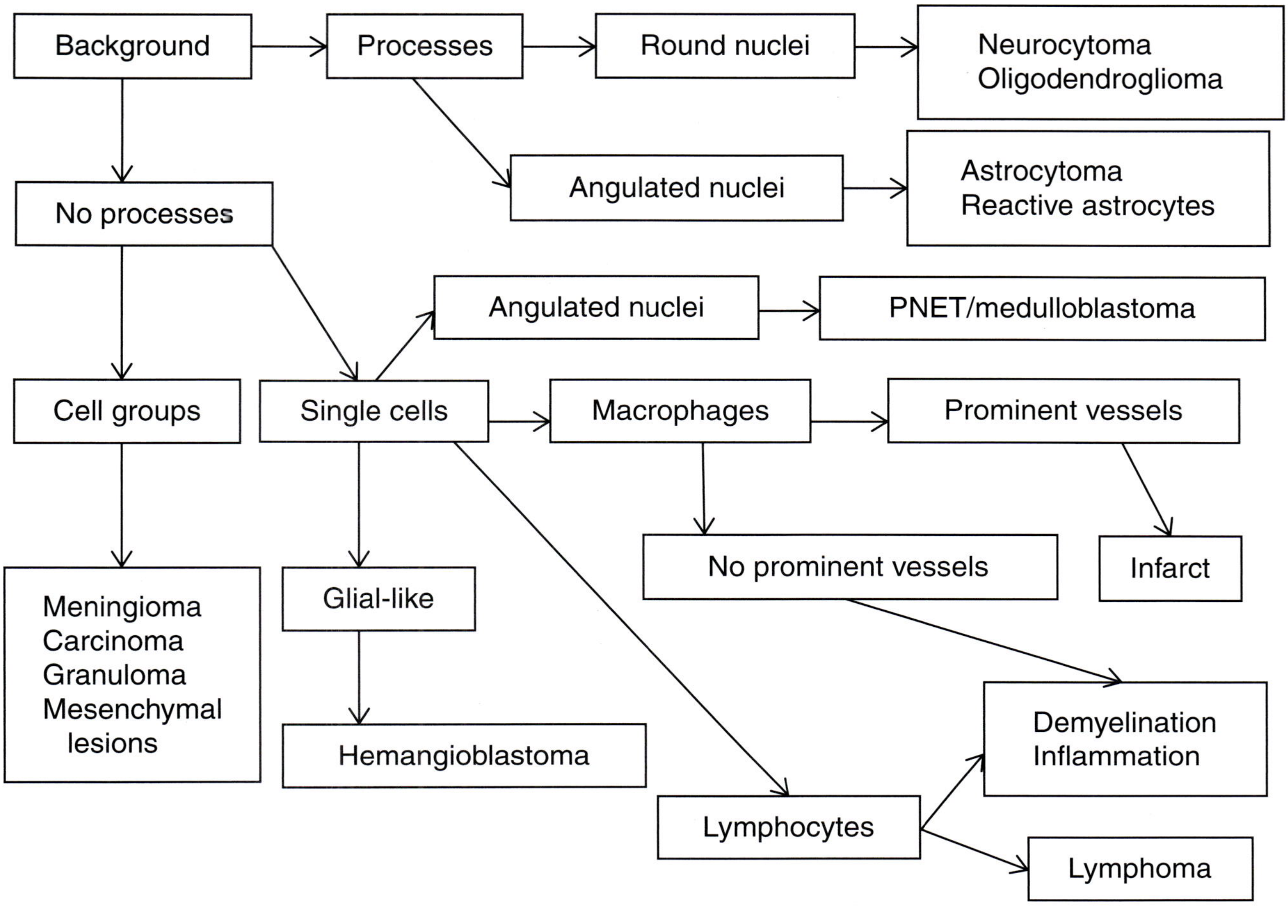

Figure 3-1. Algorithm for evaluation of smear preparations. (PNET, primitive neuroectodermal tumor.)

eye is one of *heterogeneous smear pattern* speckled with thicker tissue fragments alternating with open areas. Microscopic examination shows an abundance of prominent processes in the background, creating a *fibrillary background*, among other variable features depending on the nature of the pathologic process. These processes are predominantly astrocytic, whether neoplastic or reactive.

List of Findings/Checklist for Background Features

AT A GLANCE

- Smear pattern
  - Homogeneous
  - Heterogeneous
- Background
  - Fibrillary
    - Glial (reactive or neoplastic)
    - Neural
    - Glial mimickers (schwannoma and meningioma)
  - Mucinous/basophilic
    - Low-grade glioma
    - Metastatic adenocarcinoma
    - Cysts
    - Contaminants (paranasal sinus mucosa)
  - Necrotic
    - Neoplastic
    - Nonneoplastic
    - Pseudonecrosis
  - Hemorrhagic
  - Granular
    - Lymphoglandular bodies
  - Clean
  - Keratinous debris
  - Calcifications

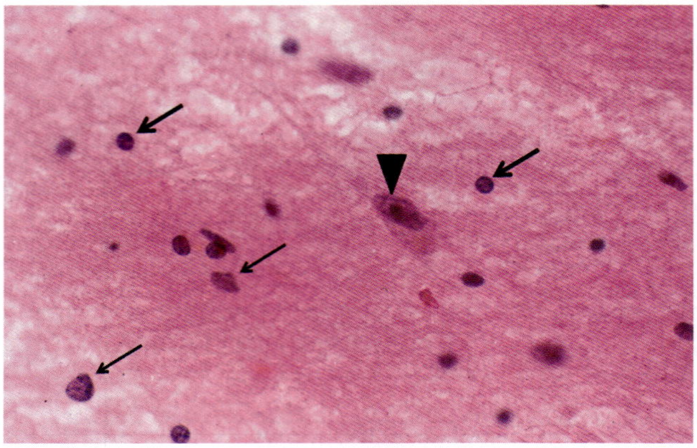

Figure 3-2. Nonlesional brain smear: A finely granular, homogeneous background is formed by the neuropil components. Nuclei appear naked. A neuron (*arrowhead*) has prominent cytoplasm with a light yellow-brown hue due to lipofuscin pigment, but when striped off of its cytoplasm, neuron nucleus can easily be recognized with its large size and prominent nucleolus. Other smaller nuclei are mainly of astrocytes (*thin arrows*), which are somewhat irregular and have a relatively open chromatin, and oligodendrogliocytes (*thick arrows*), which are similar to those of a small, round lymphocyte (H&E; original magnification: 400×).

Therefore, upon initial low-power examination, in an abnormal smear, that is, one without the homogeneous granular and nonfibrillary background as described above for nonlesional neuroglial tissue, whether the background is fibrillary helps classify the process broadly as glial or nonglial **(Fig. 3-3)**. As in routine paraffin sections, background fibrillarity can also be seen in central neurocytoma, but the processes are very delicate compared to thick and glassy eosinophilic astrocytic processes. They are thin, lacey, and not as straight or smoothly curved as and as brightly eosinophilic as the astrocytic processes **(Fig. 3-4)**. In astrocytic neoplasms, the processes appear to come out of the edges of the tissue fragments. These fragments have a syncytial internal structure in which the nuclei are sprinkled. In reactive astrocytosis, astrocytes tend to be identified individually and have prominent cytoplasms from which the processes come out, and this feature can be seen in essentially all astrocytes available for review **(Fig. 3-5)**. Depending on the cause of this reactive process, the background may have admixed inflammatory cells and/or macrophages. In contrast, astrocytic neoplasms have a prominent

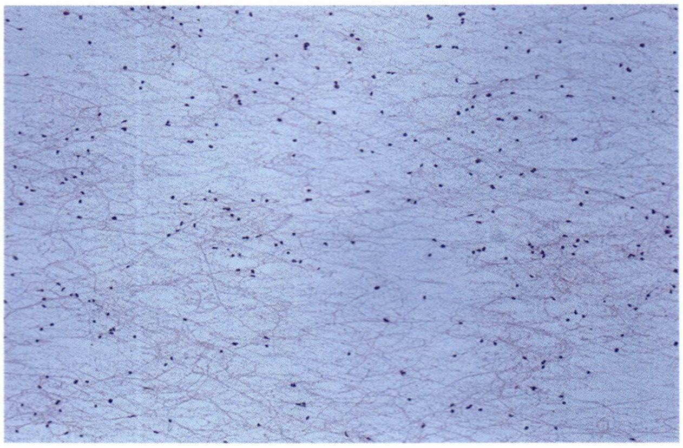

Figure 3-3. Abnormal brain smear background: No matter how hypocellular the smear may be, the prominent fibrillarity in the background indicates a glial lesion, though not necessarily neoplastic (H&E; original magnification: 100×).

fibrillary background in which the cells appear to be entangled **(Fig. 3-6)**. Pilocytic astrocytoma (PA) has astrocytic processes that are thinner than the fibrillary astrocytoma but extremely long, that is, piloid, that can sometimes extend across an entire low-power microscope field. At some point along these processes, a somewhat oval nucleus lies parallel to it, and the processes are seen to come out of both ends of this nucleus **(Fig. 3-7)**. Other features such as Rosenthal fibers and thick vessels can also be identified by cytologic evaluation.[17] Tanycytic

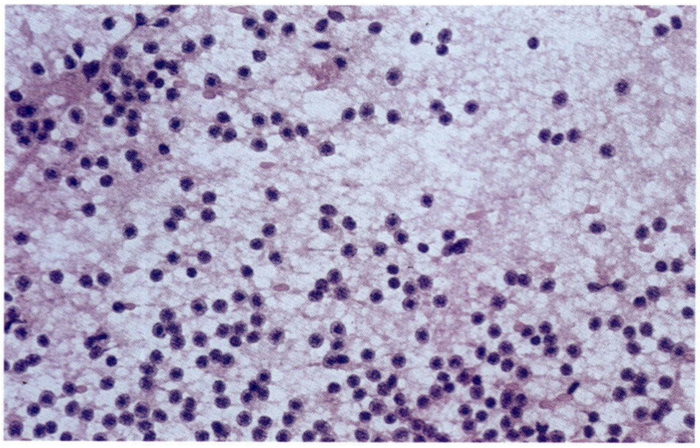

Figure 3-4. Central neurocytoma: The background fibrillarity is due to the neuritic processes and is therefore composed of delicate, lacy, and short processes. Neurocytic nuclei are similar to oligodendroglial nuclei with round contours, uniform chromatin, and small nucleolus or chromocenter (H&E; original magnification: 400×).

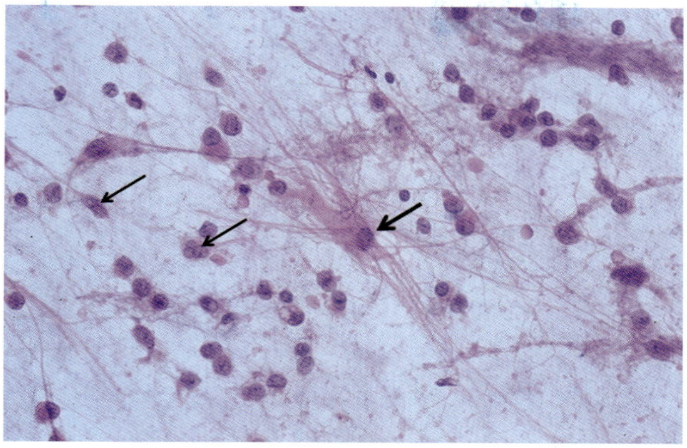

Figure 3-5. Reactive process: Reactive astrocyte (*thick arrow*) with abundant cytoplasm and many prominent processes is easily identified individually. Although not necessarily present in all reactive conditions, a mixed inflammatory background is seen in this case. The segmented nuclei of many PMN leukocytes can clump up to look like lymphocytes (*thin arrows*) in cytologic preparations (H&E; original magnification: 400×).

ependymoma lacks the usual ependymal features and may resemble PA or schwannoma with its tapered long processes, elongated nuclei, and lack of perivascular pseudorosettes.[18] Another common feature is a thin, *mucinous, basophilic background*. This type of mucinous background is also common in oligodendroglioma. Oligodendroglioma is not as rich in the number of processes as an astrocytoma.

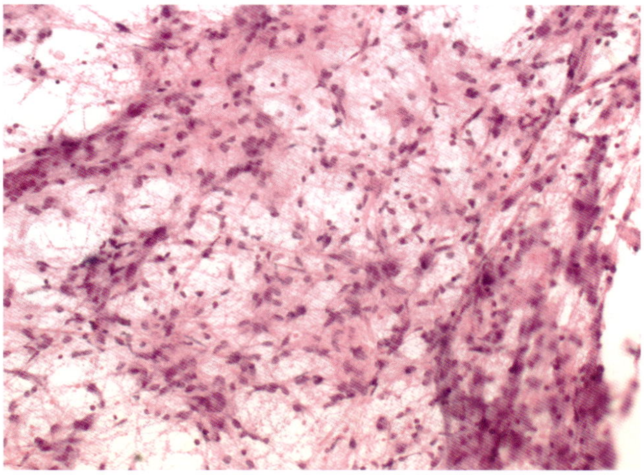

Figure 3-6. Glial neoplasm: In contrast to reactive astrocytosis, glial neoplasms have a rich fibrillary background within which the nuclei are entangled and form a monomorphous population (H&E; original magnification: 200×).

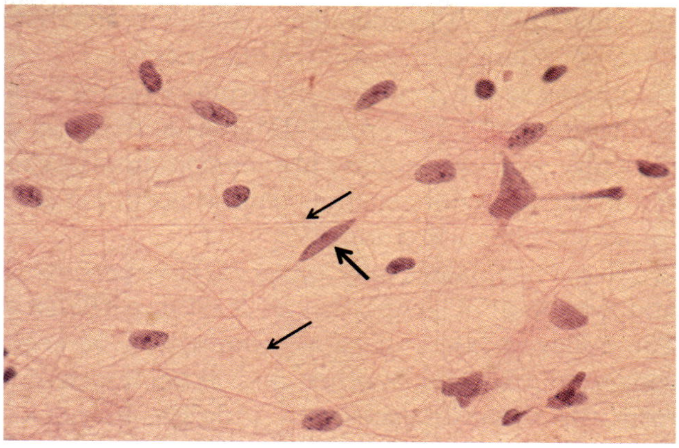

Figure 3-7. Pilocytic astrocytoma: The glial processes of PA are thin and extremely long (*thin arrows*). Some are clearly associated with elongated nuclei (*thick arrow*). The nuclei may be pleomorphic but have a finely granular and uniform chromatin with or without chromocenters or nucleoli (H&E; original magnification: 400×).

Its processes are also thinner than the fibrillary astrocytoma and can be difficult to identify in the mucinous background. Tanycytic ependymomas can also have elongated, piloid cell processes and may cause significant confusion with PA. In addition, since they have a paucity of perivascular pseudorosettes and an absence of true rosettes, the mucinous background, Rosenthal fibers, and eosinophilic granular bodies (EGB) should be searched for to support a diagnosis of PA, keeping in mind that they are not necessarily present in every PA or in every specimen. Mucinous background should alert one to the possibility of metastatic adenocarcinoma, especially in the presence of highly atypical cells. It is not specific for a metastatic adenocarcinoma and can also be seen in low-grade glial neoplasms, as described above. The contents of colloid cyst, Rathke cleft cyst and endodermal cyst, and mucinous components of germ cell neoplasms can also have mucinous background. One pitfall that is applicable to transsphenoidal resections for pituitary lesions is the sphenoid sinus mucosa or mucinous sinus contents admixed with the actual lesion, creating an impression that one is dealing with a Rathke cleft cyst. In general, when mucin is identified, epithelial cells should be searched for in an attempt to identify the source of the mucin. Enteric and colloid cysts have mucinous background with admixed columnar/cuboidal cells, which can contain intracellular mucin or can be ciliated.[19,20] Myxopapillary ependymoma can have abundant mucin and mimic metastatic carcinoma or other neoplasms.[21] It may present as a soft tissue mass and create differential diagnostic difficulty with other mass lesions commonly seen in the sacral region, such as chondrosarcoma and mucinous adenocarcinoma.[22]

Some neoplasms may appear to have processes and mimic glial neoplasms at least superficially. The collagen fibers of schwannoma can be seen separated from each other and extending away from the tissue fragment. In addition, its nuclei also are sprinkled in a syncytial tissue fragment. However, the commonly cerebellopontine angle location, the difficulty in smearing the tissue due to its collagen content, and the spindled, somewhat wavy nuclei with pointy tips raise the possibility of schwannoma as a diagnosis **(Fig. 3-8)**. As for cerebellopontine angle location, it should be remembered that rare gliomas can occur in association with cranial nerve VIII as an extraaxial neoplasm due to the presence of Obersteiner-Redlich zone away from the brainstem. In fact, a rare intraosseous presentation can also be seen in the temporal bone. The other neoplasm that may falsely appear to have processes is meningioma. Fibrillary appearance in meningioma is usually

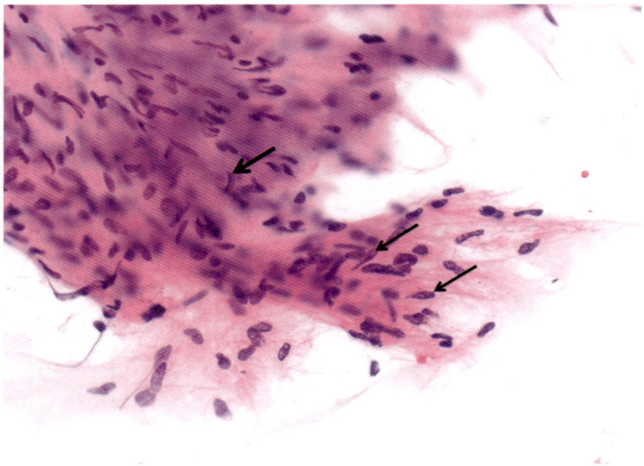

Figure 3-8. Schwannoma: The edge of a fragment that was resistant to smearing shows a somewhat fibrillary appearance, but these "processes" are wispy rather that crisp and are formed by matrix and cytoplasms that fade and disappear. The cytoplasmic borders cannot be identified. Many nuclei have typical pointy tips (*thin arrows*), while some are wavy or curved (*thick arrow*) (H&E; original magnification: 400×).

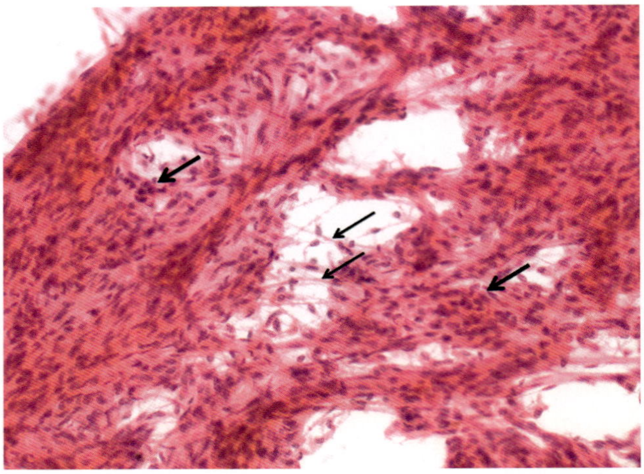

Figure 3-9. Meningioma: This predominantly fibroblastic meningioma cells show elongation of their cytoplasms (*thin arrows*) both as an artifact of smearing, as well as separation of tissue, and may mimic a glial lesion. In spite of the predominantly spindled nuclei and apparent resistance to smearing, as the tissue remained as a thick fragment, this fibroblastic meningioma still shows clues in the form of vague whorl formation (*thick arrows*) to reveal its nature (H&E; original magnification: 200×).

the result of elongation of cytoplasms as a smear artifact **(Fig. 3-9)**.

As alarming as it may seem, a *necrotic background* does not necessarily imply a high-grade neoplasm, although that possibility certainly should be considered **(Fig. 3-10)**. Necrosis can be

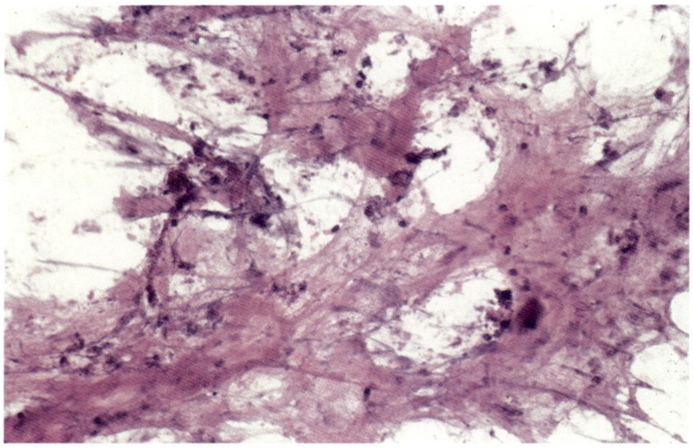

Figure 3-10. Necrosis: A mixture of amorphous eosinophilic debris and nuclear debris is seen. No further information can be obtained based only on this finding without any viable component, except for the presence of a lesion (H&E; original magnification: 400×).

seen in high-grade neoplasms, glial or metastatic, in infectious processes, and in infarcts. When necrosis is identified, other features should be searched for to further support or reject these possibilities **(Table 3.1)**. Usually, there are viable areas that can provide additional clues to the nature of the pathologic process, for example, inflammatory cells or multinucleated giant cells in infectious processes such as toxoplasmosis or necrotizing granulomas, respectively, or foamy macrophages with

TABLE 3.1 Differential diagnosis and typical features of necrotic lesions

Features	GBM	Metastatic Carcinoma	Lymphoma	Tumefactive Infectious Granuloma	Toxoplasmosis
Cells	Glial, entangled with processes	Epithelial groups	Lymphoid, single cells	Macrophages/multinucleated giant cells and lymphocytes	Mixed inflammatory macrophages, small lymphocytes, plasma cells, PMNL
Background	Necrotic, fibrillary	Necrotic, mucin, keratin	Necrotic, lymphoglandular bodies	Necrotic, granulomas	Necrotic, basophilic granular debris
Nuclei	Spindled, angulated, hyperchromatic, pleomorphic, rare nucleoli	Open chromatin, prominent nucleoli	Open chromatin, one or more prominent nucleoli	Bland, spindled or round, bean-shaped eccentric	Bland, round or bean-shaped
Cytoplasms	Processes are variably prominent	Abundant; thin, vacuolated, or dyskeratotic; sharp borders	Inconspicuous	Foamy, variable amount	Variable according to inflammatory cells
Mitotic activity	Present	Prominent	Prominent	Rare	Rare
Vessels	Proliferating, lacy reticulin	May be thick	May be thick, with perivascular cuffs; multiple layers of circular reticulin	May be thick, with surrounding inflammatory cells	May be thick, with surrounding inflammatory cells
Histologic features	Infiltrative borders, pseudopalisading necrosis	Sharp borders, peritheliomatous pattern, acinar formations, keratinization	May be solid, infiltrating, perivascular; with or without sharp borders	Sharp borders, granulomas at the edge	Cyst forms and tachyzoites can be seen
Radiologic features	Ring-enhancing mass, irregular borders	Ring-enhancing mass, may be multifocal, well-circumscribed, peritumoral edema and mass effect common	Ring-enhancing mass, may be multifocal, well-circumscribed, peritumoral edema and mass effect common, restricted diffusion common	Ring-enhancing mass, may be multifocal; perilesional edema; mass effect	Multiple ring-enhancing lesions, perilesional edema
Location	Anywhere, may cross corpus callosum (butterfly lesion)	Anywhere, may cross corpus callosum (butterfly lesion)	Anywhere, may cross corpus callosum (butterfly lesion)	Anywhere	Periventricular white matter

GBM, glioblastoma multiforme; PMNL, polymorphonuclear leukocytes.

intracytoplasmic debris in infarcts. One should be careful with a diagnosis of high-grade neoplasm in the presence of inflammation and especially macrophages. Other necrotic lesions may represent infectious processes that present as a mass lesion mimicking a neoplasm, such as toxoplasmosis[13] or mucormycosis.[23] Infectious nature of the lesion and the microorganisms may be easier to identify on cytologic preparations and should be sought in necrotic/inflammatory/reactive specimens. Smears may appear necrotic as a result of crush artifact due to aggressive smearing. Alternatively, an obviously inflammatory/infectious process may masquerade as another, such as toxoplasmosis that can present as a brain abscess, even on cytologic examination,[24] underscoring the importance of nonbiased approach and detailed evaluation of the material. Sometimes, the nuclei can appear smudged and cytoplasms fall apart to create a debris-like appearance in the background, that is, *pseudonecrosis*. It is more likely to occur with those tissue fragments that are somewhat resistant to smearing, necessitating the use of excessive force by the inexperienced.

The presence of erythrocytes in the background is not unusual for any surgical material; however, it is usually in the form of fresh blood and is not the dominant feature. A *hemorrhagic background* with lysed erythrocytes and fibrin can be seen in hemorrhagic/vascular lesions. One particular neoplasm is hemangioblastoma,[25,26] where in such a background, tissue fragments are scattered. The fragments are difficult to break apart by smearing and have distinct borders. The nuclei can show considerable pleomorphism and irregularity in a syncytial arrangement in these fragments. The presence of hemorrhagic background and the absence of processes should alert one to the possibility of hemangioblastoma, rather than glioma **(Fig. 3-11)**. Cells with intact foamy cytoplasms can be identified especially at the edges of the tissue fragments.

An eosinophilic *granular background* can be produced by the fragmentation of delicate cytoplasms of pituitary adenoma cells as a smear artifact. The naked nuclei are seen floating in this kind of background, mimicking a small blue cell neoplasm or a lymphoid process **(Fig. 3-12)**. Close examination reveals the relatively bland, round nuclei with smooth nuclear membranes, finely granular chromatin pattern, and an absence of mitotic activity and apoptotic debris, in contrast to the small blue cell neoplasms that are typically high-grade malignancies. Nuclear pleomorphism can be present, as usual for endocrine neoplasms, and should not be taken as a sign of malignancy

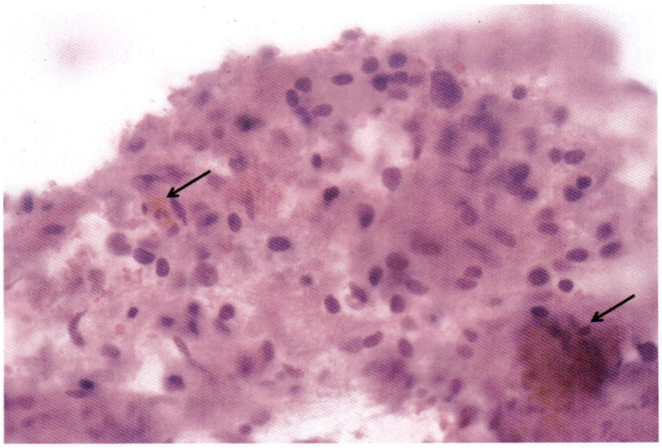

Figure 3-11. Hemangioblastoma: Typically in fragments with a granular eosinophilic background are pleomorphic irregular nuclei, creating a glial appearance due to the destruction of the fragile cytoplasms of the neoplastic cells; however, no processes are present. Evidence of blood or lysed erythrocytes (*arrows*) is commonly present. Scattered spindled nuclei in the fragment likely represent endothelial cells of the vascular network. A few intact stromal cells with microvesicular or foamy cytoplasm can rarely be seen at the edges of these fragments in some cases (H&E; original magnification: 400×).

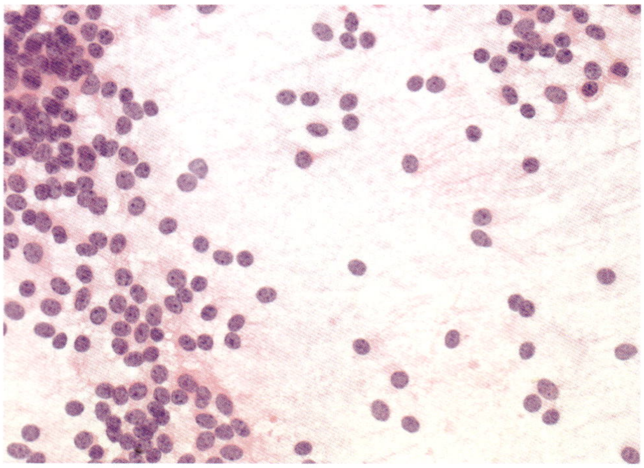

Figure 3-12. Pituitary adenoma: Granular background is formed by the fragile cytoplasms destroyed by smearing, leaving naked uniform round-to-oval nuclei with finely granular chromatin pattern (H&E; original magnification: 400×).

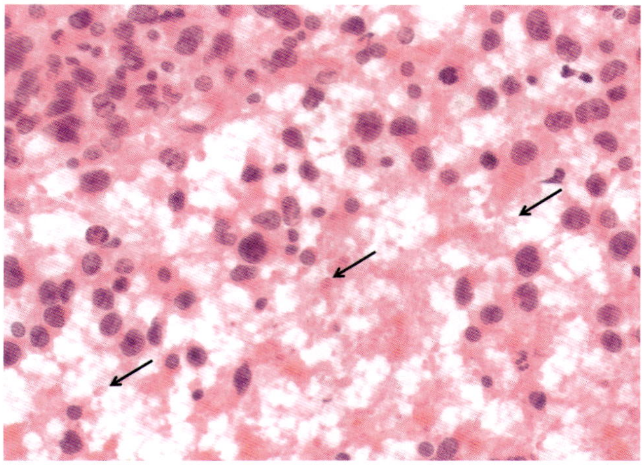

Figure 3-13. Lymphoma: Many large lymphoid cells with irregular nuclear membrane, open chromatin, and one or more prominent, usually eccentric nucleoli are seen individually distributed in a granular, necrotic background that contains small eosinophilic blebs called lymphoglandular bodies (*arrows*) representing cytoplasmic fragments and supporting the lymphoid nature of this population (H&E; original magnification: 400×).

or aggressive biologic behavior. The so-called *lymphoglandular bodies* are small, variable-sized cytoplasmic fragments and are characteristic of a lymphoid process. They represent the fragments of fragile cytoplasms that fall apart during smearing **(Fig. 3-13)**. They are not always but frequently present in association with lymphoid lesions. They should not be taken as a diagnostic feature for lymphoma; however, they indicate that one is dealing with a lymphoid population, reactive or neoplastic. For instance, in a high-grade neoplasm with individually scattered pleomorphic cells, their identification allows one to favor a lymphoma over melanoma, sarcoma, or an undifferentiated malignant neoplasm. Their absence does not rule out, but their presence support the presence of a lymphoid population.

A predominantly *clean background* does not rule out a malignant process. For instance, primitive neuroectodermal tumor (PNET)/medulloblastoma can have a clean background with no identifying features, such as necrosis, mucin or processes, and the small blue cells with essentially no visible cytoplasm scattered throughout the slide. This appearance may resemble a lymphoid process, although nuclear morphology is quite different. Cells with neuritic differentiation may have delicate polar processes attached to them, giving them a comet-like appearance. This does not reach to the level to create a fibrillary background, however. Meningiomas, soft tissue lesions such as hemangiopericytoma and solitary fibrous tumor, and schwannomas are other neoplasms that tend to have an overall clean background. Reactive inflammatory and demyelinating conditions also tend to have a clean background in spite of their abundant cellularity, including the presence of macrophages. Specifically, no necrosis is present.

The background of dermoid or epidermoid cysts can have abundant *keratinous debris*. In fact, the entire specimen that is available for review may consist of this type of material. When in thick clusters, these anucleated keratinous cells and keratin flakes do not take up eosin and remain as thick, clear chunks of material mimicking a foreign material or artifact **(Fig. 3-14)**.

Calcifications are commonly seen, and their differential diagnosis is similar to those seen on tissue sections, more specifically related to mostly low-grade, long-standing neoplasms and bone dust artifact. In some rare situations, what appear to be calcifications may turn out to be the calcareous corpuscles of cysticercus, allowing cytologic diagnosis while also causing potential mistakes.[27]

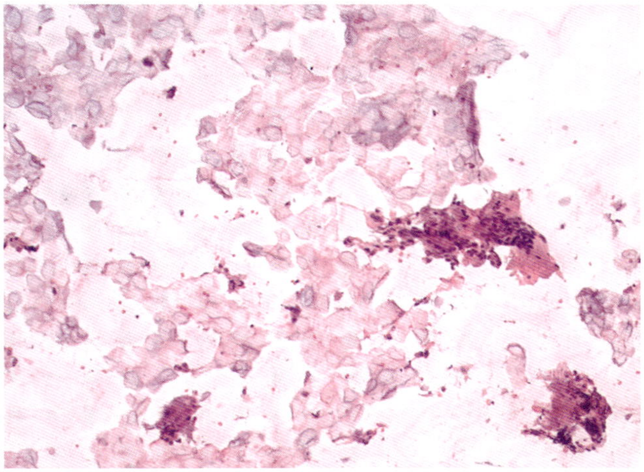

Figure 3-14. Keratinous debris: Numerous anuclear flaky keratinized cells are seen piled up in large groups. They do not stain well and may easily be missed as artifact when there are only a few. Occasional cellular groups consist of foreign body giant cell reaction (H&E; original magnification: 100×).

Tissue Fragments and Cell Groups

The smeared tissue tends to stay together in small clusters on the slide. The background may have any of the features described above in "Background Features," and it may or may not have individually scattered cells. The characteristics of the small tissue islands that could not be completely broken by smearing can provide clues to the nature of the process.

The tissue tends to remain in large, *thick fragments* in mesenchymal neoplasms and schwannoma. The inspection of the slide by naked eye shows one or two thick chunks and air bubbles under the coverslip due to the thickness of tissue fragments **(Fig. 3-15)**. In general, the cytologic detail is difficult to evaluate in such fragments due to their thickness and suboptimal staining. Evaluation of the edges of such fragments can provide valuable information. Nuclear detail can be seen in the thin edges. The edges of the fragments are irregular and reveal the spindle nuclei with no distinct cytoplasmic borders, within the collagenous stroma.

The presence of speckled smear pattern due to the tissue fragments on the slide, in contrast to a homogeneous smear pattern, implies lesional tissue **(Fig. 3-16)**. The glial fragments have a tangled appearance due to glial processes, especially at their edges. Their interior is thicker, and it may be difficult to trace individual processes in these areas, resulting in a *syncytial appearance*, in which nuclei are scattered.

Metastatic carcinoma and meningioma, most notably meningothelial meningioma, appear as *epithelioid clusters* with distinct borders. The component cells are tightly packed and have prominent cytoplasms in most cases. The whorls and nuclear pseudoinclusions of meningioma are distinctive on smears, also **(Fig. 3-17)**, and are essentially diagnostic of meningioma in this setting.[28] Rarely, special histologic types of meningioma can also be recognized. Chordoid meningioma can have cords of uniform cells with round nuclei but surprisingly without significant mucinous background.[29] Secretory meningioma can show the round eosinophilic so-called pseudopsammoma bodies.[2] Even

List of Findings/Checklist for Tissue Fragments and Cell Groups

AT A GLANCE

- Thick fragments resistant to smearing
- Syncytial fragments
- Epithelioid fragments
- Vessels and perivascular arrangements
- Papillae

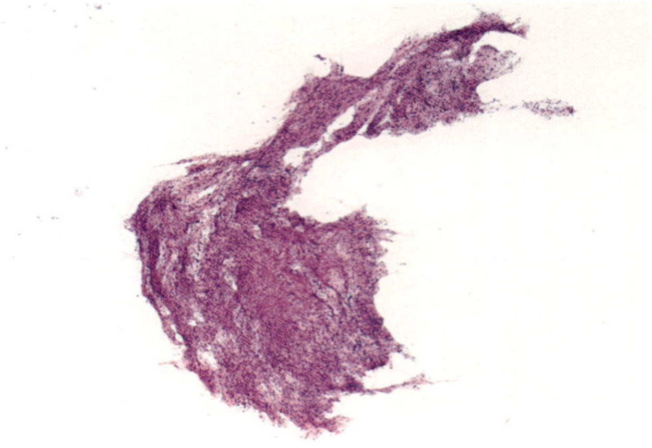

Figure 3-15. Mesenchymal fragment: Mesenchymal fragments, typically from neoplasms such as schwannoma, as in this case, are resistant to smearing resulting in this type of thick chunks of tissue but can still be evaluated for details at their edges. Trying to forcefully smear such lesions usually results in crush artifact and causes difficulty in interpretation (H&E; original magnification: 40×).

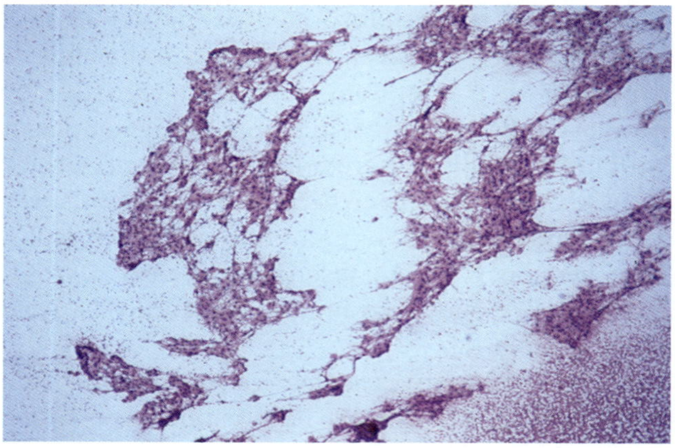

Figure 3-16. Speckled pattern of abnormal smear: The fragments can be smeared easily and have many smaller fragments and even individual cells, in contrast to the homogeneous pattern of nonlesional neuroglial tissue. These patterns can also be seen with naked eye on the glass slide (H&E; original magnification: 100×).

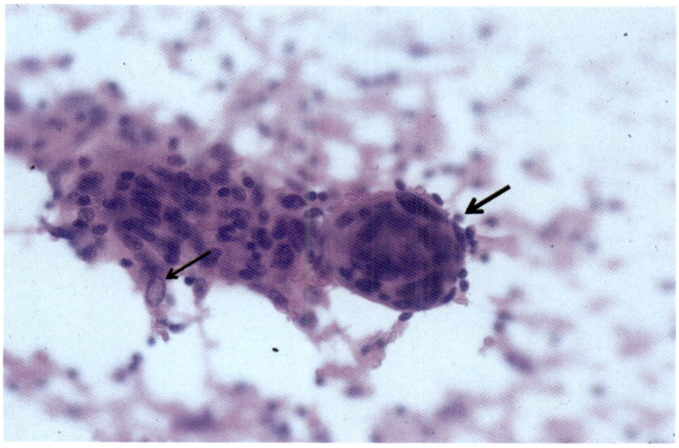

Figure 3-17. Meningioma: Syncytial group of cells, in which cytoplasmic borders cannot usually be identified, is seen. A whorl formation (*thick arrow*) is present and a nucleus has a pseudoinclusion (*thin arrow*) (H&E; original magnification: 400×).

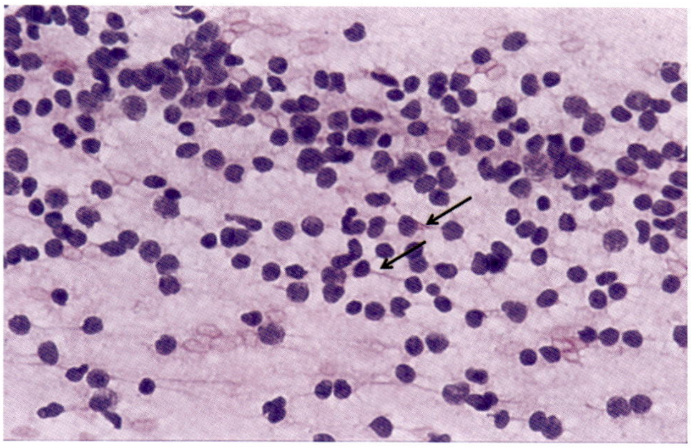

Figure 3-19. Medulloblastoma: The cells tend to be distributed individually. Some cells have neuritic processes (*arrows*), indicating neuronal differentiation. The nuclei of such cells may have a more open chromatin pattern and even a small nucleolus (H&E; original magnification: 400×).

in poorly differentiated or undifferentiated carcinomas, such as small cell carcinoma, in which the cohesiveness is expected to be impaired, it is still possible to see this type of epithelial clustering in a smaller scale, in the background of more prominent single-cell population **(Fig. 3-18)**. In the case of a small blue cell neoplasm where the differential diagnosis is small cell carcinoma and medulloblastoma (or, PNET) **(Fig. 3-19)**, this epithelial clustering favors carcinoma. Otherwise, both can have rosette formation, nuclear molding, high mitotic activity and apoptotic debris, high nucleus-to-cytoplasm ratios, and generally absent nucleoli. In addition, medulloblastomas can show subtle features suggesting neuronal differentiation in the form of delicate neurites emanating from the cell, or rarely, glial differentiation in the form of glial processes, supporting the diagnosis.

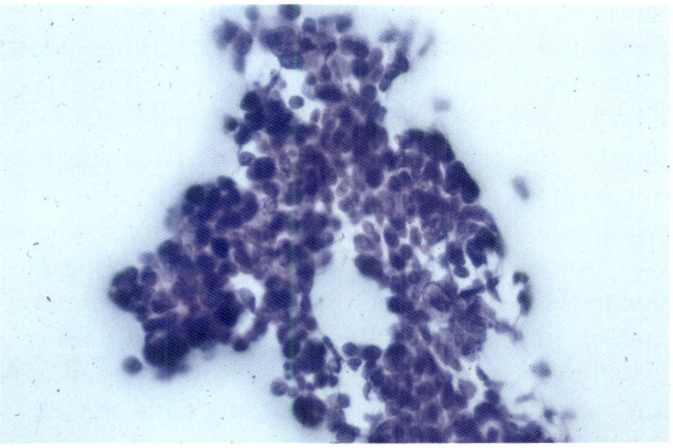

Figure 3-18. Small cell carcinoma: Small cells with cytoplasms that are too small in amount to be readily identified form an epithelial group. The nuclei are variable in shape, from round to oval to even spindled. They have a coarse chromatin pattern and no nucleoli. While the cells may also be spread individually, and there is considerable overlap with medulloblastoma/PNET, this type of epithelial grouping favors carcinoma (H&E; original magnification: 400×).

Pretty much any lesion, including cysts with epithelial lining, can have epithelial clusters with sharp borders and distinct cytoplasmic outlines. In nonneoplastic epithelia, the orderly arrangement of cells creates a honeycomb appearance in the monolayered sheets. In carcinomas, they form three-dimensional, disorderly clusters with nuclear pleomorphism, in addition to chromatin changes. Craniopharyngiomas have sheets or clusters of small, basaloid squamoid cells in a background where ghost-like wet keratin can be identified.[30,31] Papillary craniopharyngioma[32] also has squamoid cells that are in between fully developed squamous cells of the epidermoid cyst and the small basaloid cells of the craniopharyngioma and does not contain keratin. If there is keratin and/or better differentiated squamous cells, other entities such as epidermoid cyst,[33] dermoid cyst, or squamous cell carcinoma should be considered. In the sellar/suprasellar region, squamous component of germ

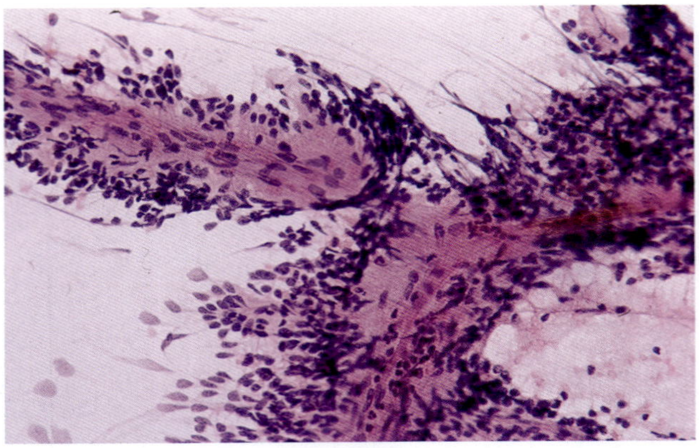

Figure 3-20. Ependymoma: Two pseudorosettes, formed by the perivascular arrangement of neoplastic cells, are seen. Glial fibrillarity is not prominent elsewhere but can be identified at the periphery of the pseudorosettes, along with other cellular details (H&E; original magnification: 400×).

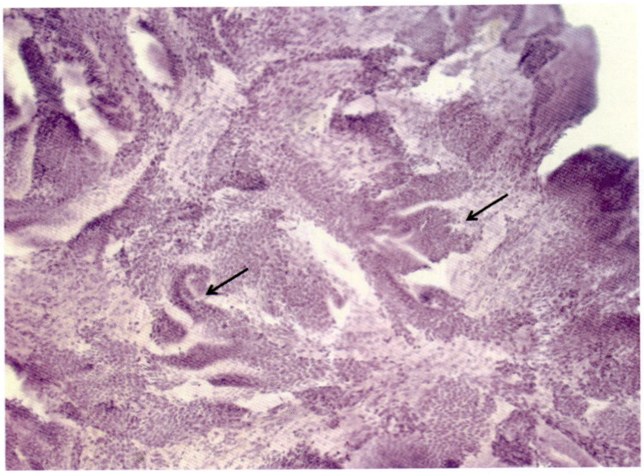

Figure 3-21. Choroid plexus papilloma: Even though a thick fragment has formed on this crush preparation, the outlines of papillary structures (*arrows*) can be seen. In many other areas, a honeycomb effect is created from the top view due to the orderly arrangement of epithelial cells in this low-grade neoplasm (H&E; original magnification: 100×).

cell neoplasms, as well as Rathke cleft cyst,[31] which can have considerable squamous component in addition to columnar cells, should also be remembered. In addition, while dealing with any kind of squamous lesion, contamination of the slide with the anuclear squames from the bare hands during preparation should be kept in mind as a pitfall. They are easily identified as artifacts on frozen sections since they are just randomly scattered on a different plane of focus but may become potentially confusing on cytologic preparations.

In some lesions, tissue fragments are composed mainly of a vessel with a population of cells surrounding it. The edges of such fragments are ragged due to irregular cellular distribution. The glial processes are not prominent at the edges, even if they are present in some of these lesions. The *pseudorosettes* of ependymoma[34] can be seen longitudinally, with a prominent vessel, surrounding anuclear zone composed of fibrillary material representing the processes of the ependymal cells, and the crowded nuclei at a uniform distance from the vessel wall **(Fig. 3-20)**. The fragment's outer edge is irregular with crowded nuclei, and even though these too are glial cells, the processes are not a prominent feature of the fragment edges. Intracytoplasmic lumina may be identified and should not be mistaken for metastatic signet ring cell carcinoma.[35] A similar tendency for perivascular crowding of cells but without such orderly pseudorosette formation can also be seen in reactive astrocytosis. The cellularity is less prominent, not as tightly packed as in ependymoma and tends to spread out from the vessels in a thin layer rather than the three-dimensional configurations in ependymoma. Lymphoid cells, inflammatory or neoplastic, also can form perivascular arrangements, imitating their distribution on tissue sections. They tend to be loosely arranged and individually scattered in the background. A *papillary pattern* can be apparent in choroid plexus neoplasms, especially papillomas[36,37] **(Fig. 3-21)**, while choroid plexus carcinomas look more similar to other carcinomas, due to their solid sheet formation and loss of papillary architecture. Endolymphatic sac tumors can also have papillary fragments.[38] Both fragments and papillary architecture, along with the characteristic cytoplasmic accumulations, have been observed in atypical teratoid rhabdoid tumor.[39]

Nuclear Features

Nuclear features identified on cytologic preparations and the implications of various cytologic features are similar to those described in Chapter 2,

List of Findings/Checklist for Nuclear Features

AT A GLANCE

- Irregular
- Round
- Enlarged/pleomorphic/bizarre
- Binucleation/multinucleation
- Without cytoplasm
- Nuclear molding
- Nuclear grooves
- Spindled
- Pseudoinclusions

"Microscopic Features." Cytologic preparations show the nuclei as three-dimensional objects with a depth and provide more detail due to rapid fixation and paucity of artifacts if prepared appropriately. Tissue sections on the other hand provide an essentially two-dimensional cross section of the nucleus and only at a given level. Therefore, the appearances may differ, although general rules of interpretation remain the same.

The general architectural, cytoplasmic, and background features provide ample information to classify the lesion for the purposes of IOC. However, nuclear detail can provide crucial information in many situations. The oval, somewhat spindled, *irregular nuclei* of fibrillary astrocytoma may also have angular contours with sharp corners. They are hyperchromatic with no nucleoli, at least in low-grade astrocytoma. In contrast, oligodendroglial nuclei are almost perfectly *round* with smooth nuclear membrane, relatively open chromatin pattern, and a small nucleolus or chromocenter. In fact, if other features of the smear are not taken into account, these nuclei may resemble lymphoid nuclei, mainly due to the round contours. Another neoplasm with uniform nuclei is neurocytoma.[40] Its nuclei also have small, indistinct nucleoli but are more hyperchromatic compared to oligodendroglioma. It is difficult to distinguish anaplastic from low-grade gliomas solely based on the nuclear features. Mitotic figures are usually difficult to find on smears and many cases can be difficult even in the presence of large amount of tissue on histologic examination. Therefore, cytologic atypia becomes important and should be evaluated carefully. The degree of cytologic atypia, hyperchromasia, and the coarseness of chromatin can also aid in the cytologic diagnosis of atypical (WHO Grade II) meningioma,[2,41] although it is found to be easier to diagnose malignant (WHO Grade III) meningioma than distinguishing Grades I and II.[42] Medulloblastomas can be diagnosed as large cell/anaplastic or other variants using cytologic features, which are essentially the cytologic versions of the histologic features, such as cell wrapping, apoptosis/necrosis, and nuclear enlargement.[43,44] In the context of round nuclei and small blue cells, internal granule cells of the cerebellum should be kept in mind as a pitfall. They resemble small round lymphocytes but may also be mistaken for medulloblastoma due to cerebellar origin of the specimen **(Fig. 3-22)**. The typical neuropil-like fibrillary background and the presence of a scattered Purkinje cell should help identify this tissue as nonlesional cerebellum. Pituitary adenoma can be seen in the form of many round, naked nuclei when the cytoplasms of the cells are fragmented to form the granular background seen in some cases. The nuclei are round to oval with smooth nuclear membranes and finely granular chromatin pattern. Small nucleoli can be present.

Dark, angulated but monomorphic nuclei of small cells with small amount of cytoplasm that may superficially resemble an astrocytoma can be seen in hemangiopericytoma. The glial background is not present. The cells tend to disperse

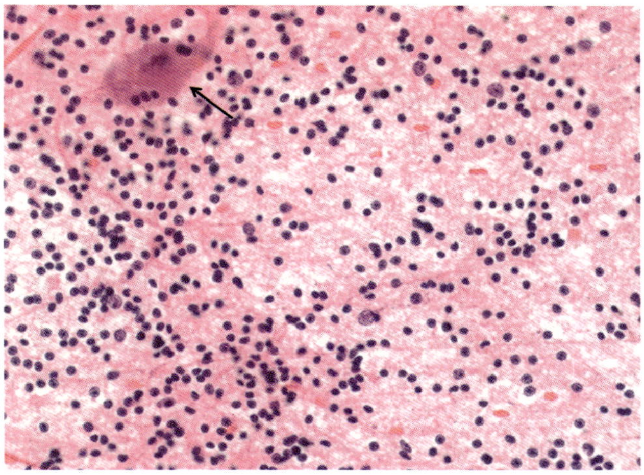

Figure 3-22. Nonlesional cerebellum: Unless this possibility is considered and the presence of a Purkinje cell (*arrow*) noticed, small, round internal granule cells may mimic inflammation or a small blue cell neoplasm (H&E; original magnification: 400×).

TABLE 3.2 Differential diagnosis and typical features of neoplasms with giant cells and pleomorphism

Features	PXA[45,46]	SEGA[47,48]	GBM
Cells	Large, pleomorphic, xanthomatous; multinucleation; spindling	Large, uniform, tapering; may have binuclear cells	Large, pleomorphic; may have bizarre, multinucleated cells; spindling
Mitotic activity	Rare, if any	Rare, if any	Present, may be prominent and atypical
Background on cytologic preparations	Clean (necrosis rare), fibrillarity not prominent	Clean, processes with polar tendency, fibrillarity may be prominent	Necrotic, fibrillarity prominent
Vessels	May be prominent, perivascular lymphocytes	Vague and rare perivascular pseudorosettes	Proliferating (perivascular lymphocytes rare)
Other findings	Nuclear pseudoinclusions, EGB, rich pericellular reticulin	Vague grouping of cells	Pseudopalisading necrosis
Radiologic features	Enhancing cyst and mural nodule, well-circumscription, calcifications	Diffuse enhancement, well-circumscription, calcifications	Ring-enhancing mass, irregular borders
Location	Superficial temporal lobe	Subependymal/ intraventricular	Anywhere, may cross corpus callosum (butterfly lesion)

PXA, pleomorphic xanthoastrocytoma; SEGA, subependymal giant cell astrocytoma; GBM, glioblastoma multiforme; EGB, eosinophilic granular bodies.

individually and do not form the syncytial arrangements or whirling seen in meningioma, nor do they have the nuclear pseudoinclusions that are commonly seen in meningioma.

Glioblastoma also has astrocytic nuclei, but their appearance is variable, ranging from uniform dark, small nuclei to pleomorphic *large nuclei* with prominent nucleoli to even include multinucleated giant cells **(Table 3.2)**. Its nuclear features can overlap with those of carcinomas, especially due to the presence of prominent nuclei that may be present in many cells. In general, a widespread prominence of nucleoli should be an alerting sign to consider the possibility of metastatic carcinoma. Large, round *naked nuclei* with prominent nucleoli stripped off of their cytoplasm can represent ganglion cell nuclei in a ganglion cell neoplasm, such as ganglioglioma. Intact ganglion cells can also be seen if the material is smeared gently, avoiding fragmentation of cytoplasms, in which case binucleated or dysplastic forms can be easily identified. Otherwise, the presence of such nuclei can raise the suspicion in a background that is typical of a low-grade glial neoplasm. Nuclear changes of radiation treatment can result in bizarre mono- or multinuclear cells with smudgy chromatin, with or without nucleoli. In cytology context, they may be difficult to distinguish from the nuclei of a recurrent glioblastoma with bizarre cells.

The main differential diagnosis of small nuclei with a coarse chromatin pattern, no nucleoli, with very small amount of or invisible cytoplasm is metastatic small cell carcinoma and PNET/medulloblastoma. *Nuclear molding*, high mitotic activity, rosette formation, and frequent apoptotic bodies are common features; however, small cell carcinoma tends to show epithelial clustering, as discussed in "Tissue Fragments." In terms of pineal parenchymal tumors, one tricky point in regard to their cytologic features is that higher-grade tumors, while appearing more PNET-like, tend to be more uniform, while the pleomorphic variant of pineocytoma can appear more worrisome for a malignant neoplasm due to its pleomorphism. *Nuclear grooves* have been described in ependymoma and can be a useful feature to distinguish it from other glial neoplasms.[49] They are also well-recognized features of Langerhans cell histiocytosis and papillary thyroid carcinoma.

Of the *spindle cell lesions*, peripheral nerve sheath tumors stand out with their peculiar nuclear features. Both schwannoma and neurofibroma have spindled and wavy nuclei with pointy tips. They lie parallel to the collagen bundles in the tissue fragments. This nuclear appearance, along with other

TABLE 3.3 Differential diagnosis and typical features of common neoplasms in the cerebellopontine angle

Features	Fibroblastic Meningioma	Schwannoma
Cells	Spindled	Spindled
Nuclei	"Fibroblast"-like, round tips (some may be pointy), small nucleoli	Wavy contours, dark chromatin, one tip pointy: nucleoli rare
Cytoplasm	Indistinct, elongated, syncytial	Indistinct, elongated, syncytial
Cytologic preparations	Grouped or dyscohesive cells, cytoplasms may resemble glial processes, rare whorls and nuclear pseudoinclusions	Thick fragments, resistant to smearing, collagenous background
Histologic features	Rare whorls and pseudoinclusions	Biphasic, nuclear palisading, admixed or adjacent nerve/axons
Vessels	Unremarkable	Thick, hyalinized
Other findings	Calcifications	Hemorrhage/hemosiderin
Radiologic features	Extraaxial, dura-based, well-circumscribed enhancing mass; calcifications possible	Extraaxial, well-circumscribed, enhancing mass; temporal bone erosion, internal auditory meatus expansion

features, is very helpful in distinguishing schwannoma from fibroblastic meningioma in a cerebellopontine angle tumor **(Table 3.3)**.[50] Ancient change in schwannoma results in large, irregular nuclei. They should not be alarming for a malignant process. They are usually few in number and have a smudgy, not crisp, chromatin pattern.

Intranuclear cytoplasmic invaginations, also referred to as *intranuclear pseudoinclusions*, are useful in the diagnosis of meningioma. In fact, among the CNS neoplasms, meningioma is the only one to show prominent and widespread intranuclear cytoplasmic invaginations that can be easily identified. In the context of poorly differentiated malignant neoplasms, intranuclear cytoplasmic invaginations are typically associated with melanoma. Along with binucleation, creating the so-called double mirror image nuclei, plasmacytoid cytology with eccentric nuclei, single-cell distribution, and, if one is fortunate, melanin pigment, this nuclear feature supports the diagnosis, or can raise the suspicion for melanoma in obscure cases. Intranuclear cytoplasmic invaginations are also one of the diagnostic features of papillary thyroid carcinoma, although it rarely metastasizes to the CNS. They can also be present in many cells with nuclei that are irregular enough to create such an appearance. However, they rarely are a prominent feature of neoplasms other than those mentioned so far. Some examples are ganglion cells of ganglion cell neoplasms, hemangioblastoma, schwannoma, metastatic carcinoma, sarcoma, and plasma cell myeloma, known as the Dutcher bodies in the latter. Viral inclusions can be identified in selected cases to even allow difficult diagnoses, such as measles encephalitis.[6] In progressive multifocal leukoencephalopathy, nuclear changes similar to those identified on tissue sections such as atypical changes in astrocyte nuclei and viral inclusions in oligodendroglial nuclei can also be identified by cytologic examination of smears prepared from needle biopsy.[51]

Biphasic Pattern

As in tissue sections, it is possible to see on cytologic preparations the tissue fragments representing different components of a lesion. The most common situation is the presence of nonneoplastic or reactive neuroglial fragments admixed with the actual lesional tissue fragments, such as a metastatic carcinoma. Depending on how prominent or well-represented each component is, this biphasic appearance

List of Findings/Checklist for Biphasic Pattern

AT A GLANCE

- Nonglial neoplasm with reactive glial tissue
- Heterogeneous glial neoplasm
- Germinoma
- Others

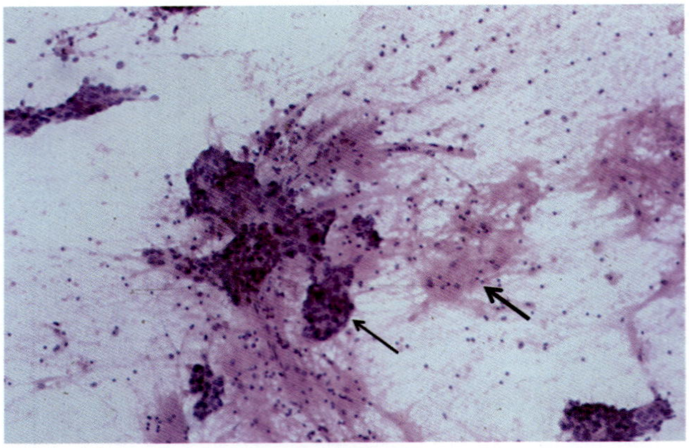

Figure 3-23. Biphasic appearance: The hyperchromatic cellular epithelial groups of metastatic carcinoma (*thin arrow*) alternate with the admixed neuroglial fragments (*thick arrow*) (H&E; original magnification: 200×).

can potentially lead to misdiagnosis as a reactive or nonlesional tissue, or even as a low-grade glial neoplasm. It is important to see the gross specimen and try to sample the areas with different gross appearances. In addition, the frozen sections will also help identify an obscure area of interest. This biphasic appearance also underscores the importance of evaluating the entire slide, which may be difficult to do in the rush and pressure of the IOC. However, low-power scanning of the slide should easily highlight the presence of more than one component on the smear **(Fig. 3-23)**. While the possibilities are many as outlined in Chapter 2, "Microscopic Features," a few of the more common ones in the cytologic context will be mentioned here.

Neuroglial tissue fragments may accompany meningioma on the same slide and should prompt to look for brain invasion on tissue sections. Normally, meningiomas are easily detached and removed from the brain surface, but brain tissue is more likely to remain attached to the meningioma if there is invasion, a feature that is typically first noticed by the surgeon. A similar appearance where neuroglial fragments alternate with cellular clusters is also possible in metastatic carcinoma. As expected, gliosarcoma has mesenchymal and glial components,[52] and complicated appearances may occur due to divergent differentiation, such as PNET-like areas.[53]

Sometimes, even though the material is not composed of different components, the nature of the lesion can make the smear look as though there are different components. This usually occurs in poorly differentiated or high-grade neoplasms where they are somewhat dyscohesive to result in easily detached cells creating a single-cell distribution in the background in addition to tissue fragments. This appearance may also be caused by the thicker areas of the smear alternating with less cellular areas, or parts of the cellular component remaining attached with stromal or vascular components. For instance, granulomatous processes and other inflammatory processes can result in this picture.

Germ cell neoplasms, depending on the amount of lymphocytic infiltrate they may have, can appear like an inflammatory process, especially if the neoplastic cells are obscured. On the other hand, with their large nuclei, clear chromatin pattern, and prominent nucleoli, the individually distributed neoplastic cells may appear like large lymphoid cells, mimicking a lymphoma **(Fig. 3-24)**. Considering germinoma as a possibility and the knowledge of the lesion's location and radiologic features usually clarify this question. The presence of a lymphocytic population is also helpful in directing the attention to other possibilities in pituitary lesions, such as lymphocytic hypophysitis.

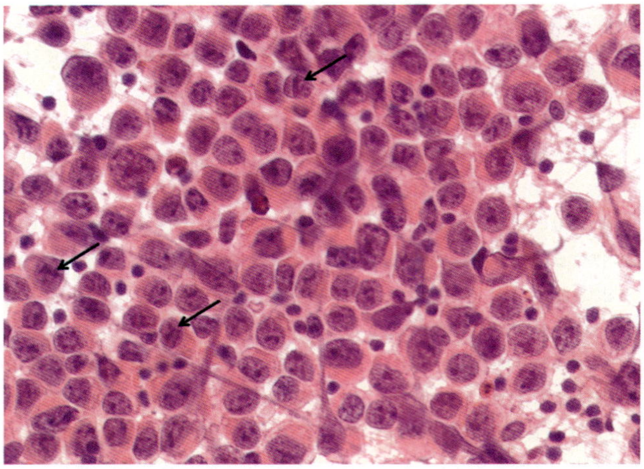

Figure 3-24. Germinoma: Crowded large neoplastic cells may mimic carcinoma, but close evaluation reveals their individual distribution due to small distances among them. Their nuclei may be reminiscent of large B-cell lymphoma although they tend to be rounder, and their cytoplasm is more abundant. Their nucleoli are typically pleomorphic with various shapes, including elongated ones (*arrows*), or several may be lined up together (H&E; original magnification: 400×).

Myxopapillary ependymomas can result in papillary, mesenchymal-like component and a cellular myxoid component, creating a biphasic appearance.[21]

Diffuse Cellularity without Tissue Fragments

It is not uncommon to have a homogeneous smear pattern with no tissue fragments or cellular aggregates. The smear of *nonlesional neuroglial parenchyma* has been described above in "Background Features." It is typically paucicellular with scattered naked nuclei, including the large ones with nucleoli, representing neuronal nuclei. Diffuse and homogeneous cellularity on a smear indicates the presence of a cellular lesion with not much stroma, vessels, or epithelial clustering, although such lesions, for example, lymphoma, may be deceiving when admixed with and entangled in fibrillary neuroglial tissue (see above "Biphasic Pattern"). *Low-grade glial neoplasms*, especially PA and oligodendroglioma, as well as central neurocytoma and pituitary adenoma, can have a uniform distribution of cells and can further be identified based on the nuclear, background, and cytoplasmic features described in other sections. Rarely, a smear can be *acellular*. This is usually because the fragment selected for cytologic evaluation may be resistant to smearing as is the case in schwannomas, mesenchymal neoplasms, fibrous tissue, and extremely gliotic tissue. This fragment remains as a thick tissue on the slide.

Pituitary adenoma, even though an epithelial neoplasm, smears in a diffusely cellular pattern with only small clusters,[54] making it easier to differentiate from metastatic carcinoma. Nuclei of pituitary adenoma rarely show the obvious atypia associated with malignancy. They have a finely granular and uniform chromatin pattern, described as salt and pepper chromatin that is characteristic for neuroendocrine cells. Pituitary adenoma cells have a plasmacytoid appearance due to their eccentric nuclei in many cases. However, their cytoplasm, except maybe for basophilic adenomas, does not show the prominent paranuclear huff and the amphophilia of the plasma cell cytoplasm. In addition, the cartwheel chromatin pattern is not present in pituitary adenoma nuclei. It should be remembered however that plasma cell myeloma cells may become atypical and lose their typical nuclear features, making their recognition difficult. Nonetheless, there are usually scattered more typical cells in the population allowing recognition of the population as plasmacytic. Nonneoplastic pituitary tissue may also be confused with adenoma. Adenomas are monomorphous while the nonneoplastic pituitary tissue consists of a mixture of more than one cell type, that is, acidophilic, basophilic, and chromophobic. It should be remembered that the acidophilic cells are more frequent in the lateral aspects of the gland and may yield a relatively monomorphous population for this reason, mimicking adenoma. Tissue sections should highlight their nesting pattern, supporting nonneoplastic origin. In the IOC setting, good quality frozen sections and a sample that is devoid of various tissue artifacts, such as crush artifact, are most helpful for this evaluation. TPs are also more cellular in adenomatous tissue due to the effacement of the reticulin network, resulting in higher cellular yield in adenomas, compared to nonneoplastic pituitary tissue, where cells are in contact with the reticulin framework, making the TPs less cellular or even essentially acellular. Due to the monotony of a round nuclear population, oligodendroglioma may be a consideration; however, the complete absence of glial processes and the uniform presence of plasmacytoid cytoplasms make this differential a relatively easy one. In addition, sellar location together with the cytologic picture described here is virtually diagnostic of pituitary adenoma.

Lymphoma consists of individual cells with large nuclei with irregular nuclear membranes, that is, for the most part large cleaved cells as the great majority of CNS lymphomas are diffuse large B-cell lymphomas, and prominent one or more nucleoli.[55]

List of Findings/Checklist for Diffuse Cellularity without Tissue Fragments

AT A GLANCE

- Nonlesional neuroglial tissue
- Low-grade glioma
- Clean background
- Pituitary adenoma

Cytoplasmic Features

As is the case with nuclei, cytoplasms may appear quite different on cytologic preparations because of their three-dimensional nature without the effects of formalin fixation and paraffin embedding. However, the general principles remain the same. In fact, as with the nuclei, cytoplasmic detail can be seen better due to relative lack of artifacts and the ability to evaluate three-dimensional structures on cytologic preparations.

In carcinomas, cytoplasmic borders are distinct and individual *cell borders* can be identified even in the thick cellular groups **(Fig. 3-25)**. Adenocarcinoma cells typically have thin and microvesicular or foamy appearing cytoplasm due to mucin content, or a small intracytoplasmic vacuole representing *lumen formation*. A small dot-like inspissated mucin can be present within this vacuole. Those carcinomas with no mucin but with other *accumulations* in the cytoplasm, such as lipid or glycogen, resulting in clear cytoplasm on routine sections, show thin and delicate cytoplasms on cytologic preparations. Multiple microvesicle formation is also typically associated with adenocarcinomas, regardless of their type. In contrast, squamous cell carcinomas tend to have thick eosinophilic cytoplasms. In cellular groups, their desmosomes can be seen as intercellular bridges, supporting a squamous nature in cases in which keratinization is not readily apparent. Squamous cell carcinomas can be recognized easily due to abundant bright eosinophilic keratin formation, but keratin is usually limited to small ill-defined eddies or even single cells that stand out among other cells because of their bright eosinophilic, thick appearance, that is, dyskeratotic cells.

Prominent eosinophilic cytoplasm is also present in gemistocytes. They are thick glassy and eosinophilic. These astrocytes are usually seen as individual cells, even when they are in tissue fragments, and can be identified by their processes. Mini- or microgemistocytes are smaller versions of gemistocytes, are seen in oligodendrogliomas, and are of oligodendroglial origin with nuclei similar to those of oligodendrogliomas but with no or few processes **(Fig. 3-26)**. In some meningothelial

List of Findings/Checklist for Cytoplasmic Features

AT A GLANCE

- Distinct cell borders
- Lumen/vacuole formation
- Cytoplasmic accumulations
- Eosinophilic cytoplasm
- Foamy cytoplasm
- Granular cytoplasm
- Plasmacytoid cells
- Indistinct cytoplasm

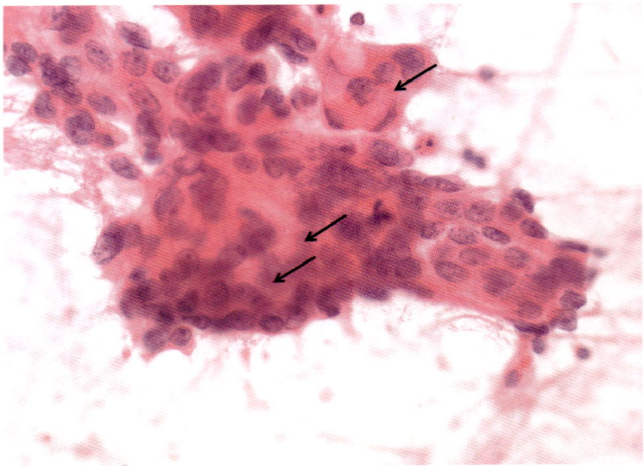

Figure 3-25. Metastatic carcinoma: In contrast to low-grade neoplastic or nonneoplastic epithelia, the honeycomb arrangement of cells is lost and they are piled up irregularly. The group has sharp borders with no processes. Distinct cytoplasmic borders can be identified (*arrows*) better by focusing up and down. Many cells have prominent nucleoli (H&E; original magnification: 400×).

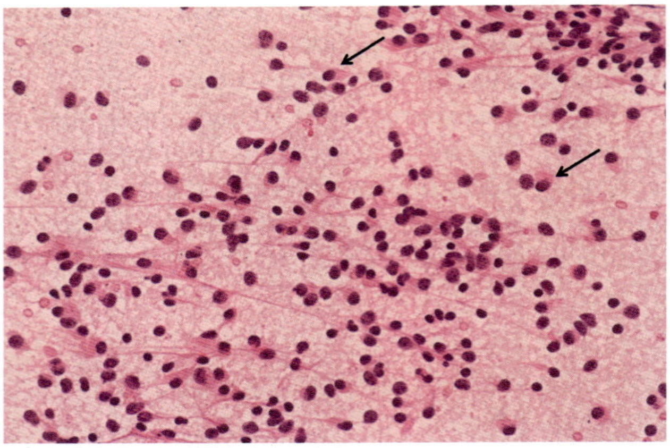

Figure 3-26. Oligodendroglioma: The nuclei are uniform and round and the background is fibrillary, though not as prominently as in an astrocytic neoplasm. Many minigemistocytes (*arrows*) with small amount of eosinophilic eccentric cytoplasm are also present (H&E; original magnification: 200×).

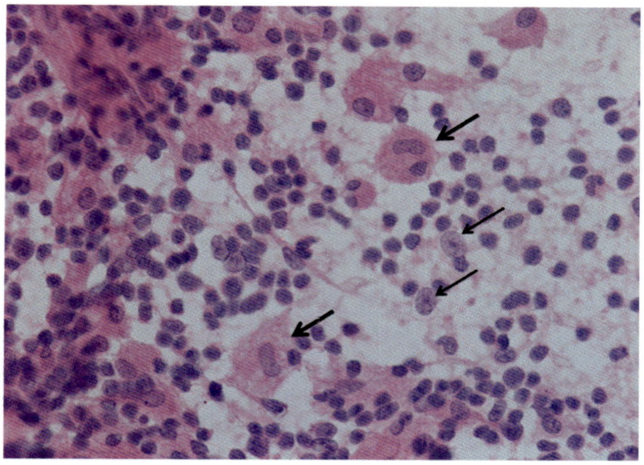

Figure 3-27. Demyelinating process: Many small lymphocytes and macrophages (*thick arrows*) with their curved, kidney-shaped eccentric nuclei and foamy cytoplasms are present. A few large lymphoid cells (*thin arrows*) are also present and should not be mistaken for a large cell lymphoma. The background is clean and not necrotic (H&E; original magnification: 400×).

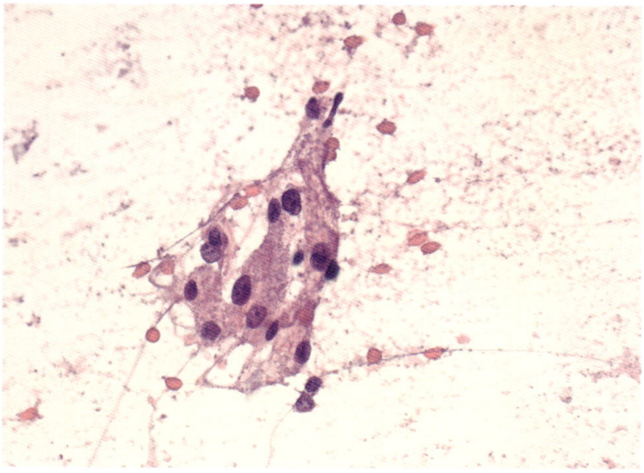

Figure 3-28. Granular cell astrocytoma: Granular cells mimic macrophages. They may be associated with a few processes and do not have the typical macrophage nuclei, and the background is devoid of inflammatory cells (H&E; original magnification: 400×).

meningiomas, cells of the syncytial groups can be separated as a result of the stretching of the group, allowing the cytoplasmic borders to be seen. The interdigitating cytoplasmic borders then may appear as processes, resulting in cells reminiscent of gemistocytes. Their cytoplasms are not as thick, glassy, and brightly eosinophilic as gemistocytes but are thin and somewhat amphophilic. When the overall features are taken into account, the distinction is not problematic.

Foamy, bubbly, or microvesicular cytoplasm is seen in macrophages, usually together with some debris or pigment. Hemangioblastomas and cells with xanthomatous features, such as seen in pleomorphic xanthoastrocytomas, can also have such cytoplasms. Macrophages should be recognized **(Fig. 3-27)** and the lesion should be further evaluated for the possibility of a reactive/inflammatory process. Cells of granular cell astrocytoma can be a great mimicker of macrophages **(Fig. 3-28)**.

Occasional cells with bright eosinophilic *granular cytoplasm* can be seen in oligodendrogliomas. In leukemic infiltrates and granulocytic (myeloid) sarcoma, eosinophil precursors also stand out among other cells and may provide a clue to the hematologic nature of the infiltrate. Acidophilic cells of the pituitary gland and adenomas also have a finely, but not so brightly eosinophilic cytoplasm. Their presence admixed with other cell types in a pituitary smear suggests that one is likely dealing with a nonadenomatous tissue, based on the mixture of cell types. Granular cell tumors are well-recognized for their granular cytoplasm. Hurthle cell neoplasms of the thyroid gland rarely if ever metastasize to the CNS but present as cells with eosinophilic granular cytoplasms. *Plasmacytoid cells* with eccentric nucleus are so named descriptively due to their resemblance to plasma cells, and some lesions may consist predominantly of plasmacytoid cells, creating a short list of differential diagnostic possibilities **(Table 3.4)**. While typical cells are easily recognized as part of an inflammatory process, plasma cell myeloma, melanoma, paraganglioma, and pituitary adenoma cells can be plasmacytoid.

Some cells do not have any visible cytoplasm to discuss, other than their small amount, resulting in high nucleus-to-cytoplasm ratios. Small cell carcinoma, lymphoma, and PNET/medulloblastoma are the typical examples.

Vessels

The vascular structures, whether prominent or not, can provide important clues to the diagnosis. *Vascular proliferation* **(Table 3.5)** is a high-grade

TABLE 3.4 Differential diagnosis and typical features of lesions with plasmacytoid cells

Features	Plasma Cell Myeloma	Melanoma	Paraganglioma	Pituitary Adenoma
Cytoplasm	Amphophilic, paranuclear huff	Amphophilic or eosinophilic, thin, pigment	Eosinophilic, granular	Basophilic-to-eosinophilic, granular
Nuclei	Hyperchromatic, binucleated forms, Dutcher bodies, cartwheel chromatin in low-grade lesions, pleomorphism in high-grade lesions	Hyperchromatic, variably round or spindled, binucleated forms, pseudoinclusions, prominent nucleoli, pleomorphism, frequent mitoses	Salt and pepper chromatin, chromocenters or small nucleoli, uniform	Salt and pepper chromatin, chromocenters or small nucleoli, uniform
Cytologic preparations	Single cells, clean or proteinaceous background	Single cells and small groups, hemorrhagic and/or necrotic background	Single cells and small groups, clean background	Single cells and small groups, naked nuclei, clean or granular background
Histologic features	Sheets of cells	Sheets of cells, organoid pattern	Organoid pattern	Sheets of cells punctuated by vessels
Location	Anywhere	Anywhere	Cauda equina	Sella turcica

feature in glial neoplasms and results in a diagnosis of glioblastoma in astrocytic neoplasms. Its identification is relatively easy with branching thick vessels standing out in the cellular background **(Fig. 3-29)**. Usually, high cellularity and atypia, as well as the presence of necrosis, also support the diagnosis of high-grade glioma. One pitfall to this appearance is PA in which vessels can be prominent. This

TABLE 3.5 Differential diagnosis and typical features of lesions with prominent vessels

Features	GBM	PA	Abscess
Cells	Glial, atypical, entangled with processes	Oval to elongated, piloid processes, bland nuclei	Fibroblastic, enlarged, atypical, many mixed inflammatory cells
Background	Necrotic	Clean, may be mucinous	Necroinflammatory
Cytologic preparations	Necrotic, fibrillarity prominent	Cellular, fibrillarity prominent	May have granulation tissue fragments resistant to smearing
Vessels	Proliferating	Prominent, thick, hyalinized, or multichannel	Prominent, cuffed by inflammatory cells
Histologic features	Pseudopalisading necrosis, hypercellular glial neoplasm	Low cellularity paradoxical to vascular prominence; dense and loose areas, myxoid background	Layered abscess wall may be seen
Others	Thrombosed vessels, infiltrative borders	Rosenthal fibers, EGB, leptomeningeal infiltration, well-defined borders	Reactive astrocytes, microorganisms may be seen, well-defined borders
Radiologic features	Ring-enhancing mass, irregular borders	Enhancing cyst and mural nodule, well-circumscribed	Ring-enhancing mass, uniform-regular borders, well-circumscribed, peritumoral edema, may be multifocal
Location	Anywhere, may cross corpus callosum (butterfly lesion)	Cerebellum, optic pathway, hypothalamus, brainstem preferred	Anywhere

GBM, glioblastoma multiforme; PA, pilocytic astrocytoma; EGB, eosinophilic granular bodies.

List of Findings/Checklist for Vessels

AT A GLANCE

- Normal thick vessels
- Vascular proliferation
- Capillaries

prominence, however, is paradoxical to the low cellularity and bland cellular features **(Fig. 3-30)**. Granulation tissue also has prominent vessels as part of its vascular and fibroblastic proliferation. This is usually associated with a prominent inflammatory infiltrate of variable acute and chronic nature, creating a cellular background. Especially if it is rich in macrophages, their variably and sometimes spindled nuclei can resemble a neoplastic process. The vessels of ependymoma become prominent due to the pseudorosettes, but they are not necessarily proliferating when the actual vascular components are examined. Proliferating vessels are typically cellular and branching, but some normal thick vessels can have a deceiving appearance due to their cellular walls. The spindled nuclei in the walls of such thick normal vessels are arranged very orderly and parallel to each other. In larger vessels with two layers of smooth muscle (circular and longitudinal), the two sets of such nuclei can be observed aligned perpendicular to each other. In contrast, the nuclei of proliferating vessels are irregular and pleomorphic. Such normal vessels should not be interpreted as vascular proliferation. Nonlesional neuroglial tissue and low-grade glial neoplasms have thin vasculature, and especially low-grade oligodendrogliomas are known for their network of delicate capillaries, creating the chickenwire vasculature as seen on the tissue sections.

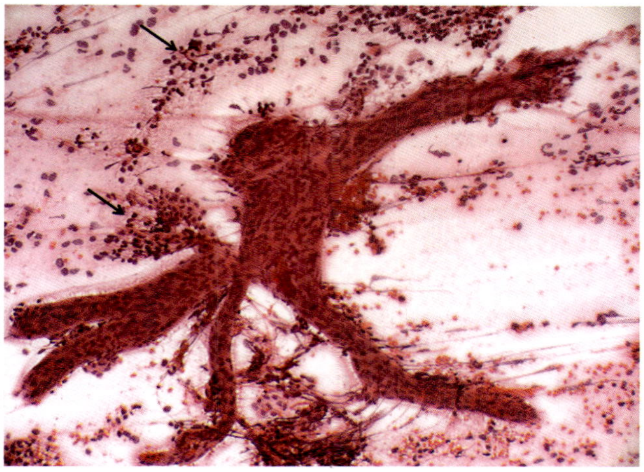

Figure 3-29. Glioblastoma: Prominent thick and branching vessels are seen in a necrotic background with many hyperchromatic cells (*arrows*) (H&E; original magnification: 200×).

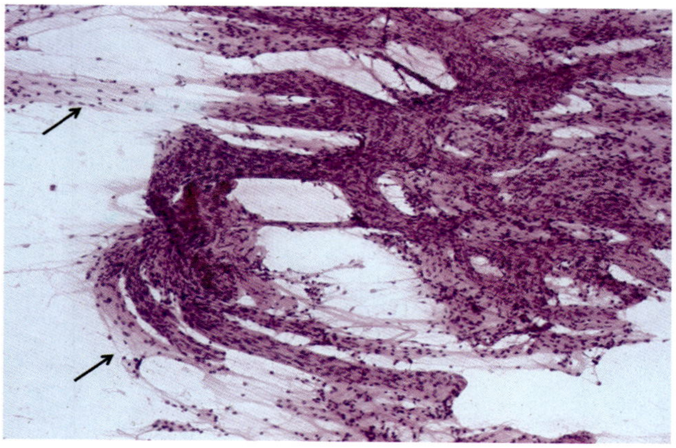

Figure 3-30. Pilocytic astrocytoma: Thick, branching vessels, reminiscent of those seen in glioblastoma, create a paradox with the low cellularity and bland cells (*arrows*) in a clean background (H&E; original magnification: 200×).

Touch Preparations

The utility of TPs in neuropathology has not been well-settled, while it continues to have a relatively limited place. The main limitation for TP stems from the nature of the neuroglial tissue. Due to the presence of a meshwork of cellular processes in glial lesions, the cell yield is usually too low for optimal evaluation. In cellular lesions, poorly differentiated carcinomas and undifferentiated neoplasms, cell yield is better due to the

List of Findings/Checklist for Touch Preparations

AT A GLANCE

- Cellular yield
- Quality and artifacts
- Preservation of architecture
- Preservation of cytoplasm
- Pituitary tissue

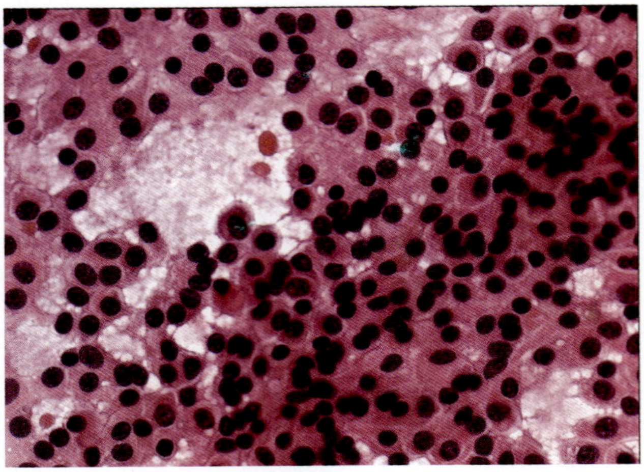

Figure 3-31. Pituitary adenoma: Touch preparation is less prone to creating artifacts, leaving the cytoplasms intact and preserving the sheet-like arrangement of the epithelial cells. Evaluation of cytoplasms shows that the population is monomorphic. Taken out of context, this picture may be impossible to distinguish from paraganglioma, especially without help from the frozen sections, which may show the organoid architecture of paraganglioma (H&E; original magnification: 400×).

dyscohesive nature of these neoplasms. Likewise, in neoplasms with no intercellular junctions, such as melanoma and lymphoma, TP is also useful. Traditionally, perhaps the best-known use of TP in neuropathology is the evaluation of *pituitary tissue*.[56,57] Due to the nesting architecture of nonneoplastic anterior pituitary gland and the close association of pituitary cells with the reticulin network, only occasional cells fall onto the slide; however, adenomas yield many cells due to the disruption of reticulin network and formation of sheets of cells **(Fig. 3-31)**.

In contrast to smear preparations, TPs tend to be less cellular in neuropathology practice because the processes of the neuroglial cells prevent the cells from falling onto the slide. On the other hand, TP allows one to see the cells and tissue fragments in a more natural state in contrast to smear preparations, because the former does not create artifactual distortions of the cells since there is no squashing and pulling involved.

A *cellular TP* is an indirect evidence of the cellular nature of the lesion and likely of its nonglial nature, too, since many cells can fall onto the slide. Another advantage of TP is the relative preservation of fragile cytoplasms of some cell types that otherwise have a tendency to break apart during smearing. Prominent examples are macrophages, stromal cells of hemangioblastoma, and neurons. Macrophages are important to recognize to appreciate the infarct and the reactive or inflammatory nature of the process. Stromal cells of hemangioblastoma allow mistaking the lesion for a glial neoplasm. Without their cytoplasms, neuronal nuclei may appear quite atypical and may at least result in some confusion.

Bone specimens that may be submitted for IOC are good candidates for TP evaluation. That way, any hematolymphoid process or metastatic malignancy can be identified in many cases. Larger bone fragments, however, as well as densely fibrous tissue fragments may need to be scraped and the scraped material smeared in an attempt to dislodge cells that may be stuck in dense fibrous tissue.

The general cytologic features for the recognition of various lesions remain similar to those described in other sections of this chapter.

Frozen Section

It should be clear from various discussions that in many situations, the cytologic detail can be evaluated a lot better on cytologic preparations, and it is highly recommended that frozen sections are used in conjunction with cytologic preparations.

The distinction of oligodendroglial from astrocytic neoplasms is not necessary, and a diagnosis such as low-grade glial neoplasm should suffice for all practical purposes. Given the difficulties associated with distinction of many of these neoplasms, as well as the subjectivity with mixed oligoastrocytomas, forcing a more specific diagnosis during IOC is likely to lead to many discrepancies with no meaningful intraoperative impact. Evaluation of cytologic preparations will reveal better nuclear detail to aid in this differential diagnosis, as needed. Nonneoplastic lesions of inflammatory, reactive, infectious, or hemorrhagic nature also pose a particular problem in IOC and seem to be more prone to discrepancies due to misdiagnosis as neoplasms.[58]

Freezing may create extensive chromatin distortion, resulting in changes reminiscent of pseudoinclusions or the clear nuclei. Such features should be evaluated on cytologic preparations to avoid misinterpretations. Likewise, cytoplasm of ganglion cells can become glassy eosinophilic and may appear like gemistocytes or reactive astrocytes, or may allow them to bland into the eosinophilic background, resulting in a diagnosis of glioma for a ganglioglioma. In a neoplasm with a prominent vascular network with perivascular lymphocytes and a nodular appearance, such dysplastic ganglion cells should be searched for. Ice crystal artifact is common in frozen sections and especially in neuroglial tissue and can interfere with the interpretations in several ways. Obviously, the tissue distortion will alter the architectural features. In addition, because the cells in the residual solid areas of the sections are squeezed together, those areas may artificially appear more cellular than they are, resulting in a neoplastic appearance of an otherwise unremarkable or gliotic tissue. Alternatively, many small vacuolations in the tissue may create the illusion that an otherwise very cellular tissue is hypocellular at low-power evaluation **(Fig. 3-32)**. This also occurs commonly in lesions with an edematous or mucinous, loose background, such as low-grade gliomas or PA. The spaces of the ice crystal artifact may contain stain residue and mimic microcysts with faint mucinous material, creating the false impression of a low-grade glial neoplasm in a gliotic or otherwise nonneoplastic tissue.

As a side effect of freezing, nuclei of the cells of lymphoma can appear darker and more irregular, mimicking astrocytoma. This is a problem especially in the diffusely infiltrating lymphomas. Nonetheless, since the great majority of lymphomas in the CNS are of diffuse large B-cell type, close attention to the chromatin pattern and the presence of prominent, one or more nucleoli, as well as at least a focal tendency to form perivascular cuffs, should alert one to the possibility of a lymphoid process. As is the case with metastatic carcinoma versus glial neoplasm, lymphomas too tend to have a higher mitotic activity compared to glial neoplasms, although this may be highly variable in a given case. Likewise, a similar change can occur in the round and bland nuclei of neurocytoma and result in their shrunken and dark appearance, which may potentially be confused with that of astrocytoma or PNET.

Iatrogenic foreign material used for hemostatic and embolization purposes is commonly present in the tissue sent for IOC and can create unusual appearances, confusing the unwary[59] **(Fig. 3-33)**. These, and other artifacts, which have been discussed

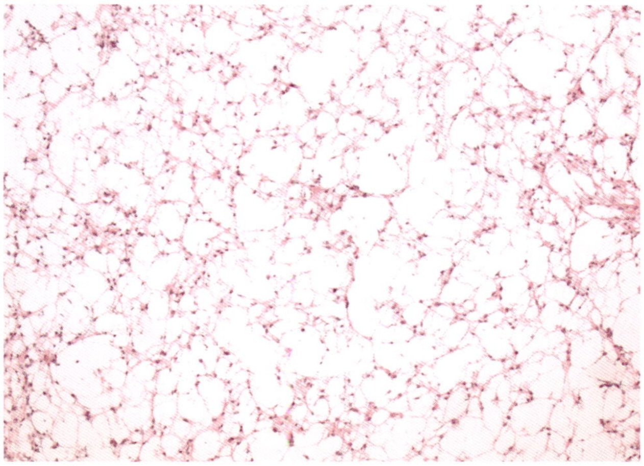

Figure 3-32. Ice crystal artifact: This common artifact more commonly forms in low-grade neoplasms with a myxoid background or edematous tissues. It distorts the architecture and alters the appearance of cellularity (H&E; original magnification: 100×).

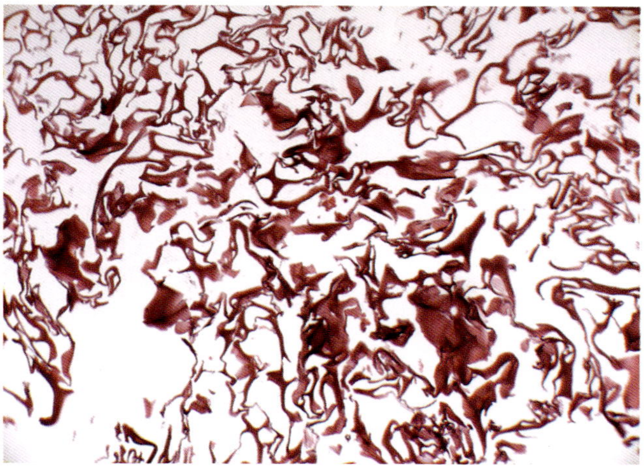

Figure 3-33. Iatrogenic material: Absorbable gelatin sponge, also known as Gelfoam®, may grossly mimic tissue and fungal microorganisms microscopically (H&E; original magnification: 100×).

TABLE 3.6 Other common pitfalls especially problematic during IOC[a]

Finding	Differential Diagnosis
Small blue cells (posterior fossa)	- Cerebellar internal granule layer - Medulloblastoma - Cerebellar external granule layer - Medulloblastoma infiltration of leptomeninges - Metastatic small cell carcinoma - Inflammation - Lymphoma
Small blue cells (cerebrum)	- PNET - Germinal matrix - Inflammation - Lymphoma - Olfactory bulb small neurons - Olfactory neuroblastoma infiltration through cribriform plate (orbital surfaces of frontal lobes)
Mildly increased cellularity	- "Atypical glial proliferation" - Reactive gliosis - Low–grade glial neoplasm - Infiltrating periphery of glial neoplasm - Tissue submitted as "margin" of a glioma - Microglial proliferation - Infiltrating lymphoma - Infiltrating germinoma (on hypothalamic or pineal region surfaces)
Clear cells in cerebellum	- Hemangioblastoma - Metastatic clear cell renal cell carcinoma - Glial neoplasm - Macrophage–rich lesions
Macrophages and macrophage-like cells	- Inflammation/infection - Demyelination - Infarct - Ameba - Granular cell astrocytoma - Lymphoma - Glial neoplasm - Hemangioblastoma - Xanthoma/xanthogranuloma
Hematolymphoid population	- Inflammation/infection - Reactive lesions (inflammatory pseudotumor, IHP) - Demyelination - Leukemic infiltrate - Lymphoma - Langerhans cell histiocytosis - Lymphoplasmacyte–rich meningioma - Extramedullary hematopoiesis
Round cells (oligodendroglial-like cells)	- Oligodendroglioma - DNT - Neurocytoma - PA - Clear cell ependymoma - Clear cell meningioma - RFGNT - Collapsed white matter

[a]Also see the detailed discussions in Chapter 2 and additional differential diagnostic situations in Chapter 4 "Radiologic Features."
IOC, intraoperative consultation; PNET, primitive neuroectodermal tumor; IHP, idiopathic hypertrophic pachymeningitis; DNT, dysembryoplastic neuroepithelial tumor; RFGNT, rosette-forming glioneuronal tumor of the fourth ventricle; PA, pilocytic astrocytoma.

TABLE 3.7 Other common situations that need to be kept in mind and addressed during IOC[a]

Normal/nonlesional tissue vs. lesional/neoplastic tissue with special emphasis on:
- Nonneoplastic/hyperplastic anterior pituitary parenchyma vs. pituitary adenoma
- Nonneoplastic posterior pituitary/pituitary stalk vs. PA
- Nonneoplastic pineal gland vs. pineal parenchymal neoplasm vs. germinoma
- Nonneoplastic pineal gland/cyst vs. PA
- Cerebellum (see Table 3.6)
- Temporal lobe with satellitosis vs. infiltrating glioma

Reactive process vs. glial neoplasm
Piloid astrocytosis next to another lesion vs. PA
Recurrent glioma vs. radiation changes
High–grade vs. low–grade neoplasm
Oligodendroglioma vs. DNT
Infiltrating vs. well–circumscribed neoplasm
Primary vs. metastatic neoplasm
Ganglion cell neoplasm vs. malformation of cortical development
Ganglion cells as part of the neoplasm vs. native ganglion cells infiltrated by the neoplasm
Malformative vs. neoplastic process
Squamous epithelium–lined nonneoplastic cyst vs. craniopharyngioma
Artifact vs. diagnostically significant change with special emphasis on:
- Thermal artifact in vessels vs. high–grade neoplasm
- Thermal artifact in nuclei vs. spindle cell neoplasm vs. astrocytoma
- Tissue vacuolation due to thermal artifact vs. vascular lesion
- Ice crystal artifact vs. microcysts
- Ice crystal artifact vs. truly hypocellular or hypercellular tissue
- Collapsed/retracted vessels vs. vascular malformation
- Necrosis vs. pseudonecrosis
- Bone dust vs. calcification
- Capillaries vs. fungal hyphae
- Foreign/iatrogenic material and changes against it vs. other pathologically significant change

[a]Also see the detailed discussions in Chapter 2 and additional differential diagnostic situations in Chapter 4 "Radiologic Features."
IOC, intraoperative consultation; PA, pilocytic astrocytoma; DNT, dysembryoplastic neuroepithelial tumor.

in Chapter 2, have also been explained in detail elsewhere.[60,61]

In general, an awareness of the pitfalls and potentially problematic areas **(Tables 3.6 and 3.7)** should help avoid the great majority of the problems, such as diagnosing a high-grade glial neoplasm in the presence of features that are typically associated with low-grade glial neoplasms **(Fig. 3-34)**. Using frozen sections in conjunction with cytologic preparations also increases the accuracy of interpretation especially in selected situations **(Fig. 3-35)**. In addition, an awareness of the purpose of IOC and a final check **(Table 3.8)** should become a habit and eliminate any unnecessary distress associated with uncertainty and should still allow valuable contributions to the management of the patient.

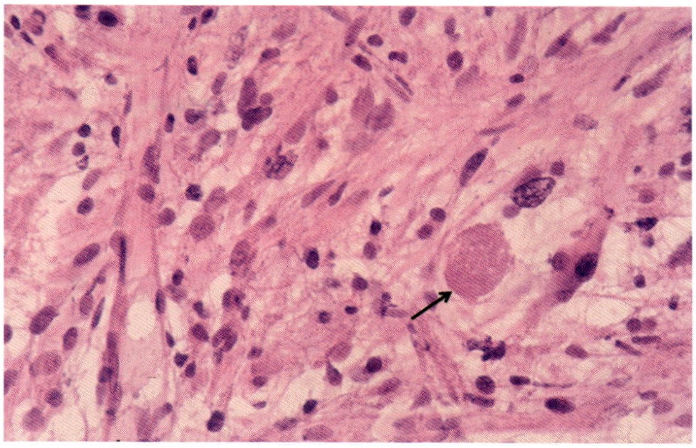

Figure 3-34. Pleomorphic xanthoastrocytoma: In spite of the worrisome cytologic features, the presence of EGB (*arrow*) should alert one to the possibility of a low-grade neoplasm (H&E; original magnification: 400×).

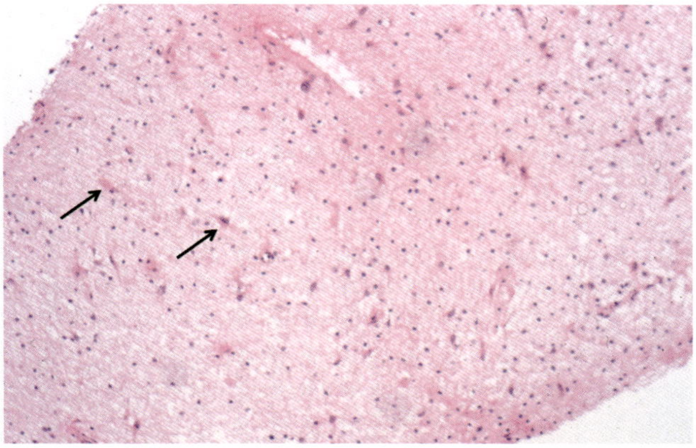

Figure 3-35. Gliosis: Frozen sections can be very useful in evaluating the tissue architecture and cellularity. In this case of reactive astrocytosis, diagnosis on cytologic preparations may be difficult due to variable cellularity. On frozen section, the cellularity is mildly increased, and the astrocytic proliferation shows an orderly distribution (*arrows*), favoring a reactive process (H&E; original magnification: 200×).

TABLE 3.8 Final crucial questions

- Is the tissue representative of the lesion based on the pathologic, clinical, radiologic findings and discussion with the surgeon?
- What is the pathologic diagnosis?
- What are the alternative differential diagnostic possibilities?
- Is there a previous diagnosis, history of treatment, or other relevant history?
- Is the pathologic diagnosis in accord with the clinical scenario and radiologic findings?
- Would it be helpful to obtain consultation from another neuropathologist or other pathologist colleague?
- Will the IOC diagnosis be confirmed after reviewing paraffin sections and final workup?
- If a specific/definitive diagnosis cannot be made, what other information can be useful to the pathologist?
- If a specific/definitive diagnosis cannot be made, what other useful information (such as reactive, primary, or metastatic neoplasm; high-grade or low-grade glial neoplasm; well-circumscribed or infiltrative glial neoplasm; etc.) can be provided to the surgeon?
- Is additional tissue available or needed for definitive diagnosis, and which, if any, recommendations (such as tissue from borders of the lesion, tissue from non-necrotic areas, submitting for cultures, etc.) can be given to the surgeon?
- Is additional tissue needed to triage for additional studies (microbiology, flow cytometry, cytogenetics, biochemical testing, electron microscopy, etc.)?

References

1. Burger PC. *Smears and Frozen Sections in Surgical Neuropathology. A Manual*. Baltimore, MD: PB Medical Publishing; 2009.
2. Burger PC, Scheithauer BW. *Tumors of the Central Nervous System, AFIP Atlas of Tumor Pathology*. Washington, DC: American Registry of Pathology; 2007.
3. Inayama Y, Nishio Y, Ishii M, et al. Crush and imprint cytology of subependymoma: a case report. *Acta Cytol*. 2001;45:636–640.
4. Liwnicz BH, Henderson KS, Masukawa T, et al. Needle aspiration cytology of intracranial lesions: a review of 84 cases. *Acta Cytol*. 1982;26:779–786.
5. Seliem RM, Assaad MW, Gorombey SJ, et al. Fine-needle aspiration biopsy of the central nervous system performed freehand under computed tomography guidance without stereotactic instrumentation. *Cancer*. 2003;99:277–284.
6. Poon TP, Tchertkoff V, Win H. Subacute measles encephalitis with AIDS diagnosed by fine needle aspiration biopsy. A case report. *Acta Cytol*. 1998;42:729–733.
7. Chandrasoma PT, Apuzzo MLJ. *Stereotactic Brain Biopsy*. New York: Igaku-Shoin; 1989.
8. Martinez AJ, Pollack I, Hall WA, et al. Touch preparations in the rapid intraoperative diagnosis of central nervous system lesions: a comparison with frozen sections and paraffin-embedded sections. *Mod Pathol*. 1988;1:378–384.
9. Firlik KS, Martinez AJ, Lunsford LD. Use of cytological preparations for the intraoperative diagnosis of stereotactically obtained brain biopsies: a 19-year experience and survey of neuropathologists. *J Neurosurg*. 1999;91:454–458.
10. Hayden R, Cajulis RS, Frias-Hidvegi D, et al. Intraoperative diagnostic techniques for stereotactic brain biopsy: cytology versus frozen section histopathology. *Stereotact Funct Neurosurg*. 1995;65:187–193.
11. Marshall LF, Adams H, Doyle D, et al. The histological accuracy of the smear technique for neurosurgical biopsies. *J Neurosurg*. 1973;39:82–88.
12. Mennel HD, Rossberg C, Lorenz H, et al. Reliability of simple cytological methods in brain tumour biopsy diagnosis. *Neurochirurgia*. 1989;32:129–134.
13. Cajulis RS, Hayden R, Frias-Hidvegi D, et al. Role of cytology in the intraoperative diagnosis of HIV-positive patients undergoing stereotactic brain biopsy. *Acta Cytol*. 1997;41:481–486.
14. Cetin N, Gokden M. Evaluation of Papanicolaou (PAP), Diff-Quik (DQ) and Hematoxylin-Eosin (H&E) Staining Methods in Cytopathology of the Central Nervous System (CNS). *Cancer Cytopathol*. 2005;105:339–340.
15. Ironside JW, Moss TH, Louis DN, et al. *Diagnostic Pathology of Nervous System Tumours*. London, UK: Churchill-Livingstone; 2002.
16. Joseph JT. *Diagnostic Neuropathology Smears*. Philadelphia, PA: Lippincott Williams & Wilkins; 2007.
17. Teo JG, Ng HK. Cytodiagnosis of pilocytic astrocytoma in smear preparations. *Acta Cytol*. 1998;42:673–678.
18. Dvoracek MA, Kirby PA. Intraoperative diagnosis of tanycytic ependymoma: pitfalls and differential diagnosis. *Diagn Cytopathol*. 2001;24:289–292.
19. Ballesteros E, Greenebaum E, Merriam JC. Fine-needle aspiration diagnosis of enterogenous cyst of the orbit: a case report. *Diagn Cytopathol*. 1997;16:450–453.
20. Parwani AV, Fatani IY, Burger PC, et al. Colloid cyst of the third ventricle: cytomorphologic features on stereotactic fine-needle aspiration. *Diagn Cytopathol*. 2002;27:27–31.
21. Bradly DP, Reddy VB, Cochran E, et al. Comparison of cytological features of myxopapillary ependymomas on crush preparations. *Diagn Cytopathol*. 2009;37:607–612.
22. Layfield LJ. Cytologic differential diagnosis of myxoid and mucinous neoplasms of the sacrum and parasacral soft tissues. *Diagn Cytopathol*. 2003;28:264–271.
23. Deshpande AH, Munshi MM. Rhinocerebral mucormycosis diagnosis by aspiration cytology. *Diagn Cytopathol*. 2000;23:97–100.
24. McLeod R, Berry PF, Marshall WH Jr, et al. Toxoplasmosis presenting as brain abscesses. Diagnosis by computerized tomography and cytology of aspirated purulent material. *Am J Med*. 1979;67:711–714.
25. Commins DL, Hinton DR. Cytologic features of hemangioblastoma: comparison with meningioma, anaplastic astrocytoma and renal cell carcinoma. *Acta Cytol*. 1998;42:1104–1110.
26. Ortega L, Jimenez-Heffernan JA, Perna C. Squash cytology of cerebellar haemangioblastoma. *Cytopathology*. 2002;13:184–185.
27. Kaw YT. Cytologic diagnosis of neurocysticercosis. A case report. *Acta Cytol*. 1994;38:87–89.
28. Mukunyadzi P, Palmer HE, Husain M, et al. Cytologic features of central nervous system tumors. *Acta Cytol*. 2000;44:922.
29. Lui PC, Chau TK, Wong SS, et al. Cytology of chordoid meningioma: a series of five cases with emphasis on differential diagnoses. *J Clin Pathol*. 2007;60:1024–1028.
30. Smith AR, Elsheikh TM, Silverman JF. Intraoperative cytologic diagnosis of suprasellar and sellar cystic lesions. *Diagn Cytopathol*. 1999;20:137–147.
31. Daneshbod Y, Monabati A, Kumar PV, et al. Intraoperative cytologic crush preparation findings in craniopharyngioma: a study of 72 cases. *Acta Cytol*. 2005;49:7–10.

32. Madhavan M, P JG, Abdullah Jafri J, et al. Intraventricular squamous papillary craniopharyngioma: report of a case with intraoperative imprint cytology. *Acta Cytol.* 2005;49:431–434.

33. Silverman JF, Timmons R, Harris LS. Fine needle aspiration cytology of primary epidermoid cyst of the brain. *Acta Cytol.* 1985;29:989–993.

34. Ng HK. Cytologic features of ependymomas in smear preparations. *Acta Cytol.* 1994;38:331–334.

35. Otani M, Fujita K, Yokoyama A, et al. Imprint cytologic features of intracytoplasmic lumina in ependymoma. A report of two cases. *Acta Cytol.* 2001;45:430–434.

36. Buchino JJ, Mason KG. Choroid plexus papilloma. Report of a case with cytologic differential diagnosis. *Acta Cytol.* 1992;36:95–97.

37. Pai RR, Kini H, Rao VS, et al. Choroid plexus papilloma diagnosed by crush cytology. *Diagn Cytopathol.* 2001;25:165–167.

38. Murphy BA, Geisinger KR, Bergman S. Cytology of endolymphatic sac tumor. *Mod Pathol.* 2001;14:920–924.

39. Parwani AV, Stelow EB, Pambuccian SE, et al. Atypical teratoid/rhabdoid tumor of the brain: cytopathologic characteristics and differential diagnosis. *Cancer.* 2005;105:65–70.

40. Klysik M, Gavito J, Boman D, et al. Intraoperative imprint cytology of central neurocytoma: the great oligodendroglioma mimicker. *Diagn Cytopathol.* 2010;38:202–207.

41. Vogelsang PJ, Nguyen GK, Mielke BW. Cytology of atypical and malignant meningiomas in intraoperative crush preparations. *Acta Cytol.* 1993;37:884–888.

42. Ali S, Nassar A, Siddiqui MT. Crush preparations of meningiomas: can grading be accomplished? *Diagn Cytopathol.* 2008;36:827–831.

43. Kumar PV, Hosseinzadeh M, Bedayat GR. Cytologic findings of medulloblastoma in crush smears. *Acta Cytol.* 2001;45:542–546.

44. Takei H, Dauser RC, Adesina AM. Cytomorphologic characteristics, differential diagnosis and utility during intraoperative consultation for medulloblastoma. *Acta Cytol.* 2007;51:183–192.

45. Kobayashi S, Hirakawa E, Haba R. Squash cytology of pleomorphic xanthoastrocytoma mimicking glioblastoma. A case report. *Acta Cytol.* 1999;43:652–658.

46. Bleggi-Torres LF, Gasparetto EL, Faoro LN, et al. Pleomorphic xanthoastrocytoma: report of a case diagnosed by intraoperative cytopathological examination. *Diagn Cytopathol.* 2001;24:120–122.

47. Altermatt HJ, Scheithauer BW. Cytomorphology of subependymal giant cell astrocytoma. *Acta Cytol.* 1992;36:171–175.

48. Takei H, Florez L, Bhattacharjee MB. Cytologic features of subependymal giant cell astrocytom: a review of 7 cases. *Acta Cytol.* 2008;52:445–450.

49. Kumar PV. Nuclear grooves in ependymoma. Cytologic study of 21 cases. *Acta Cytol.* 1997;41:1726–1731.

50. Kobayashi S. Meningioma, neurilemmoma and astrocytoma specimens obtained with the squash method for cytodiagnosis. A cytologic and immunochemical study. *Acta Cytol.* 1993;37:913–922.

51. Suhrland MJ, Koslow M, Perchick A, et al. Cytologic findings in progressive multifocal leukoencephalopathy. Report of two cases. *Acta Cytol.* 1987;31:505–511.

52. Parwani AV, Berman D, Burger PC, et al. Gliosarcoma: cytopathologic characteristics on fine-needle aspiration (FNA) and intraoperative touch imprint. *Diagn Cytopathol.* 2004;30:77–81.

53. Hayashi T, Kushida Y, Kadota K, et al. Cytopathologic features of gliosarcoma with areas of primitive neuroepithelial differentiation of the brain in squash smears. *Diagn Cytopathol.* 2009;37:906–909.

54. Ng HK. Smears in the diagnosis of pituitary adenomas. *Acta Cytol.* 1998;42:614–618.

55. Yu GH, Montone KT, Frias-Hidvegi D, et al. Cytomorphology of primary CNS lymphoma: review of 23 cases and evidence for the role of EBV. *Diagn Cytopathol.* 1996;14:114–120.

56. Martinez AJ, Moossy J. Pituitary adenoma: diagnosis by intraoperative imprints. *J Neuropathol Exp Neurol.* 1983;42:307.

57. Powell SZ. Intraoperative consultation. Cytologic preparations, and frozen section in the central nervous system. *Arch Pathol Lab Med.* 2005;129:1635–1652.

58. Plesec TP, Prayson RA. Frozen section discrepancy in the evaluation of central nervous system tumors. *Arch Pathol Lab Med.* 2007;131:1532–1540.

59. Barbolt TA, Odin M, Leger M, et al. Pre-clinical subdural tissue reaction and absorption study of absorbable hemostatic devices. *Neurol Res.* 2001;23:537–542.

60. Ribalta T, McCutcheon IE, Neto AG, et al. Textiloma (gossypiboma) mimicking recurrent intracranial tumor. *Arch Pathol Lab Med.* 2004;128:749–758.

61. Fuller GN. Intraoperative consultation and optimal processing. In: *Practical Surgical Neuropathology.* Perry A, Brat DJ, editors, Philadelphia, PA: Churchill Livingstone; 2011:35–45.

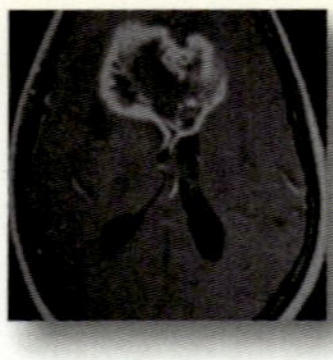

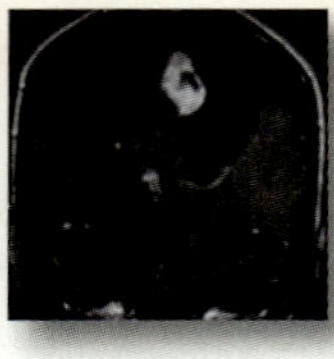

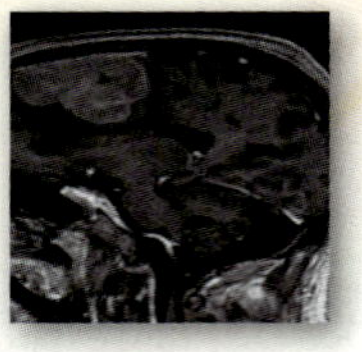

CHAPTER 4

Radiologic Features

Introduction

This chapter is not intended to be a comprehensive text on neuroradiology. It is not even intended to be a neuroradiologic source for any level of professional in that field or in other specialties who work with neuroradiology on a routine basis as part of their practice and who order and interpret neuroradiologic studies, such as neurology and neurosurgery. Instead, this chapter is intended to be a source to complement the studies of the pathologist in understanding the basic radiologic patterns and differential diagnoses, without getting too involved in radiology as a specialty and without getting too technical. In many cases, the pathologic process may be obvious. In others, the situation may not be as clear, and any additional help from clinical, intraoperative, and radiologic findings may provide a big help to the neuropathologist in interpreting the pathologic findings. In still others, correlating the pathologic findings with clinical and/or radiologic findings helps avoid misinterpretations of the case as a whole. For instance, a small biopsy sample that shows only a low-grade fibrillary astrocytoma but has areas of enhancement on imaging should alert one to refrain from definitive grading and include a comment on the possibility of sampling variation and histologic heterogeneity of the glial neoplasms. This knowledge in intraoperative consultation should prompt the pathologist to alert the surgeon and request a more representative tissue. In an era of smaller tissue samples available for pathologic evaluation, neuroradiology provides a means for understanding the exact location and any peculiar structural specifics of the lesion. Using the high resolution and the ability to generate thin slices, identification of the exact location of a given lesion allows the pathologist to approach the autopsy examination in a more targeted way. In a small biopsy tissue with a myxoid background, oligodendroglial-like cells result in a long differential diagnostic list. On the other hand, correlating these findings with the neuroradiologic findings of intracortical multinodularity and erosion of the internal table will direct the neuropathologist to consider a long-standing lesion, likely associated with intractable seizures, and bring dysembryoplastic neuroepithelial tumor to the top of the list. The pattern of a subtle atrophy can be identified on radiologic imaging, providing guidance for autopsy evaluation of neurodegenerative diseases. Fetal ultrasound can identify malformations and can be of invaluable help in pediatric neuropathologic autopsy evaluation, especially considering the artifacts associated with pediatric brains. In other words, neuroradiology can serve as gross pathology to the neuropathologist, when actual gross pathology is not available or is suboptimal. Similar to the various techniques and special stains in pathology, neuroradiologic evaluation utilizes multiple modalities and techniques and is a constantly evolving field; however, the pathologist should be familiar with at least the basic radiologic patterns and be able to understand the major descriptions used in the neuroradiology report. This information is particularly useful during intraoperative consultations,[1] when there is not enough time for further workup, investigation, and, in many cases, opportunities for consultation. The pathologist is primarily responsible for the interpretation of the gross and microscopic findings. Any other information should only be used to aid in the interpretation of the tissue by the pathologist and should not be used to replace it. In critical situations, discussion of all findings in a conference or directly with the neurosurgeon, neurologist, or neuroradiologist as appropriate may be both educational and more helpful. Neuroradiology texts,[2] chapters in neuropathology texts,[3] descriptions of

List of Findings/Checklist for Radiologic Features

AT A GLANCE

Using neuroradiologic information in neuropathologic evaluation
- Direct X-ray film
  - Calcifications
  - Bone lesions
- Computerized tomography (CT)
  - Calcifications
  - Bone lesions
    - Erosion, thinning, scalloping
    - Hyperostosis
  - Density/attenuation (iso-, hypo-, hyper-)
- Magnetic resonance (MR) imaging
  - Intensity (iso-, hypo-, hyper-)
  - T1-weighted images
  - T2-weighted images
  - Fluid attenuated nversion recovery (FLAIR)

Contrast enhancement
- Non-enhancement
- Homogeneous enhancement
- Heretogeneous enhancement
- Rim/ring enhancement
- Cyst and enhancing mural nodule pattern
- Multifocal enhancement
- Enhancement along ependymal surfaces
- Meningeal enhancement

Mass effect

Edema
- Peritumoral
- Periventricular/subependymal

Cystic lesions

Syrinx formation

Intraaxial lesions

Extraaxial lesions

Dural-based lesions

Lesions with dural tail

Intramedullary lesions

Intraduralextramedullary lesions

Extradural lesions

Pineal region

Sellar-suprasellar region

Cerebellopontine angle

Intraventricular

Posterior fossa

Butterfly lesions

Lesion borders
- Well-circumscribed lesions

Multifocal lesions

Multilobular-multinodular lesions

White matter involvement
- Diffuse
- Multifocal

Other radiologic techniques
- Angiography
  - Conventional
  - CT-angiography (CTA)
  - MR-angiography (MRA)
- Diffusion-weighted imaging (DWI)
  - Restricted diffusion
  - Unrestricted diffusion
- Diffusion tensor imaging-Tractography
- MR spectroscopy (MRS)
- Functional MRI
- Positron emission tomography (PET)

radiologic features of specific entities in neuropathology texts, especially in regard to surgical neuropathology,[4,5] as well as review papers[6,7] provide opportunities for more detailed study of the subject. The tables in this chapter provide a quick overview of lesions with a particular radiologic feature; however, many lesions may present with different patterns and therefore may be mentioned in more than one table. The tables included in this chapter summarize the differential diagnoses of common lesions with particular findings. Some other features, for instance, calcifications, hemorrhage, and cystic lesions, are in Chapter 2 and are not repeated here unless they have significant radiologic identifying findings. Lesions that are more likely to be seen in certain anatomical locations are also discussed in Chapter 1 and are briefly reviewed here to emphasize the role of radiology in the identification of location and in subsequent diagnosis when that information may not be readily available.

Routine Radiologic Techniques

Direct x-ray film is the basic technique and is best for the evaluation of bones as well as identification of

TABLE 4.1 Common translucent/lytic lesions of bones

Dermoid cyst/dermal sinus
Meningocele/encephalocele
Hemangioma
Osteomyelitis
Lytic metastases
Lymphoma/leukemia
Plasma cell myeloma/multiple myeloma
Langerhans cell histiocytosis
Chordoma
Aneurysmal bone cyst
Erosion of bone due to underlying lesion (dysembryoplastic neuroepithelial tumor, cortical malformation, low-grade glial neoplasm, arachnoid cyst, etc.)
Invasion of bone by intracranial or extracranial neoplasm (meningioma, soft tissue neoplasms, squamous cell carcinoma of the skin, etc.)

calcifications. Fractures and sclerotic or lytic lesions can be seen. It can be practically and conveniently performed in the morgue for the evaluation of the body before autopsy, especially in cases of suspected congenital skeletal malformations and trauma. *Computerized tomography (CT)* is also a good technique for the evaluation of bones. Fractures, skull base lesions, erosions, and whether the lesion is lytic, sclerotic, or expansile can be demonstrated[8] **(Tables 4.1 and 4.2)**. Calcifications are also well visualized, but the changes in soft tissue structures are not seen as good. *Erosion or scalloping* of the bone surfaces overlying a lesion is typically associated with longstanding, and therefore low-grade neoplasms such as dysembryoplastic neuroepithelial tumor,[9] and ganglioglioma,[10] cortical malformations, and nonneoplastic cysts[11] can result in this change. In addition, meningiomas can result in *hyperostotic reactive changes* in the adjacent bone, typically when they infiltrate the bone, but sometimes without any infiltration[12,13] **(Fig. 4-1)**. *Density* or *attenuation* refers to the differences among the absorption of the x-rays by the tissues.[3,6–8] The attenuation of cerebrospinal fluid is taken as a baseline, with tissues such as bone and blood, as well as normal parenchyma absorbing more x-rays and therefore are also referred to as hyperattenuating, resulting in *hyperdense* images that are brighter relative to the adjacent parenchyma, while adipose tissue and fluid such as edema and cerebrospinal fluid are hypoattenuating, that is, allowing

TABLE 4.2 Common sclerotic/osteoblastic lesions of bone

Hyperostosis frontalis interna
Osteopetrosis
Paget's disease
Chronic osteomyelitis
Meningioma
Osteoblastic metastases
Fibrous dysplasia
Osteoma
Osteoid osteoma
Osteoblastoma
Osteosarcoma
Chordoma
Chondrosarcoma

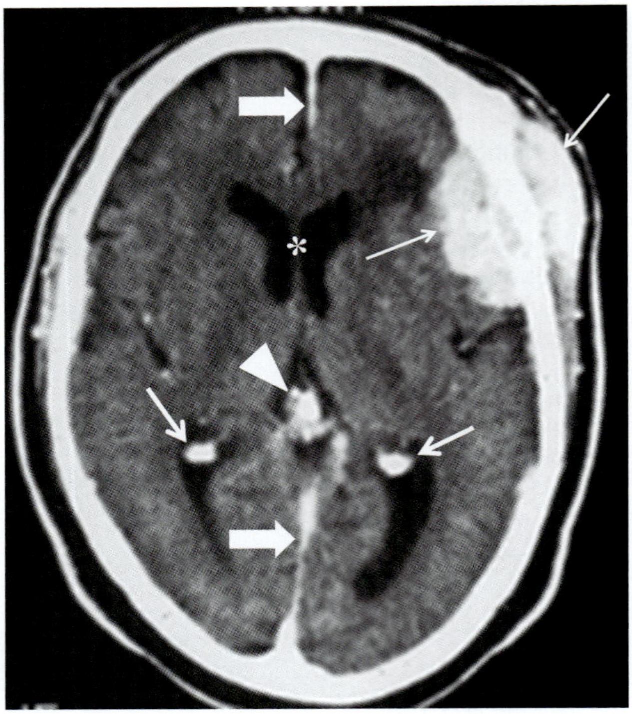

Figure 4-1. Hyperostosis and normal structures: A meningioma in the left frontal lobe infiltrating the overlying bone caused extensive hyperostosis and thickening of bone admixed with enhancing infiltrating meningioma (*thin arrows*). In addition to bone, CT shows other calcified structures, such as choroid plexus (*thick arrows*) and pineal gland (*arrowhead*), which are also highlighted as enhancing structures. Falx cerebri is also enhanced (*block arrows*), providing a reference point for septum pellucidum (*asterisk*) for the evaluation of midline shift. In this case, a mild midline shift to the right is present (axial postcontrast CT).

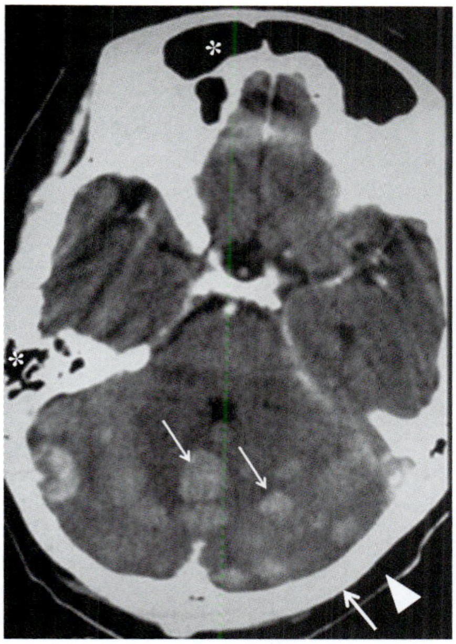

Figure 4-2. Multifocal lesion and normal structures: Many contrast-enhancing lesions (*thin arrows*) are present in the cerebellum, which proved to be metastatic endometrial adenocarcinoma after biopsy. Bone (*thick arrow*) can be seen as a hyperdense structure, while subcutaneous adipose tissue (*arrowhead*) is hypodense. Air in the frontal sinuses and mastoid air cells (*asterisk*) is also hypodense (axial postcontrast CT).

more x-rays to pass through, resulting in *hypodense* areas that are darker on the image, and are toward the other end of the attenuation spectrum. Tissues with more density and cellularity or acute hemorrhage are hyperdense, while those that contain fluid, air, or adipose tissue are hypodense **(Fig. 4-2)**. *Magnetic resonance (MR) imaging* is a technique that uses magnetic field and not x-rays or ionizing radiation. Based on the time from excitation and the collection of emitted waves, as well as the time until the protons return to their resting state after excitation, the generated images are referred to as *T1 or T2 weighted*. In addition, the intensities of the tissues and lesions are referred to as *isointense*, *hypointense*, or *hyperintense* typically relative to a normal structure, such as white matter. T1-weighted images are better for the evaluation of anatomical details of the lesion, while T2-weighted images provide information of its water content. For instance, edema and infectious processes as well as high water content of a neoplasm or cyst generally result in hypointensity on T1- **(Fig. 4-3)** and hyperintensity on T2-weighted images

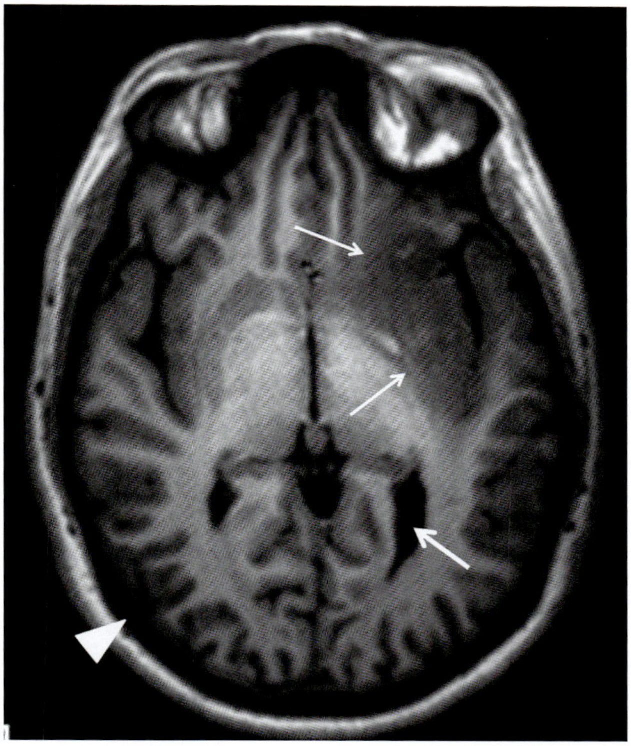

Figure 4-3. Low-grade fibrillary astrocytoma and normal structures: An irregular lesion is present in the left anterior insula and basal ganglia (*thin arrows*). It is hypointense compared to white matter in this T1-weighted image. Cerebrospinal fluid (*thick arrow*) and bone (*arrowhead*) normally appear *black* with essentially no signal, while the subcutaneous adipose tissue overlying the bone is bright, in contrast to CT seen in Figure 4-2 (axial T1-weighted MRI).

(Fig. 4-4), helping further characterize them. Although many pathologic processes tend to be hyperintense on T2-weighted images, those lesions with a dense fibrous connective tissue component, for example, meningioangiomatosis, fibroblastic meningioma, and desmoplastic infantile ganglioglioma, as well as dura mater, tend to be hypointense.[6] White matter foci that are hyperintense on T2-weighted images, referred to as T2-hyperintense foci or unidentified bright objects, can be seen in a wide variety of conditions,[14] including dilated Virchow-Robin spaces. An association with neurofibromatosis type 1 has been proposed in children.[15] *Fluid-attenuated inversion recovery (FLAIR)* also highlights water content and is especially good for this purpose to highlight peritumoral edema **(Fig. 4-5)**. In contrast to CT, MR is not a good technique for the evaluation of bones, but is superior for soft tissues **(Fig. 4-6)**.

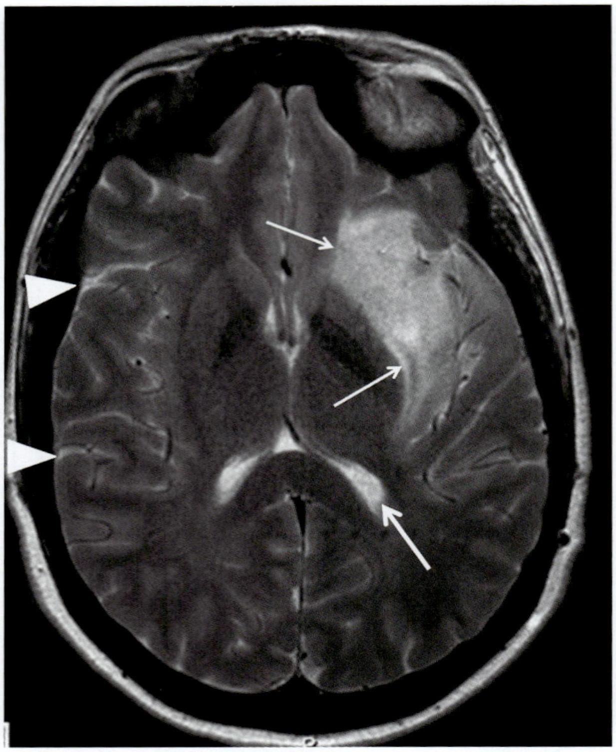

Figure 4-4. Low-grade fibrillary astrocytoma and CSF: The same lesion seen in Figure 4-3 (*thin arrows*) and the CSF in the ventricular system (*thick arrow*) and subarachnoid space (*arrowheads*) are hyperintense (axial T2-weighted MRI).

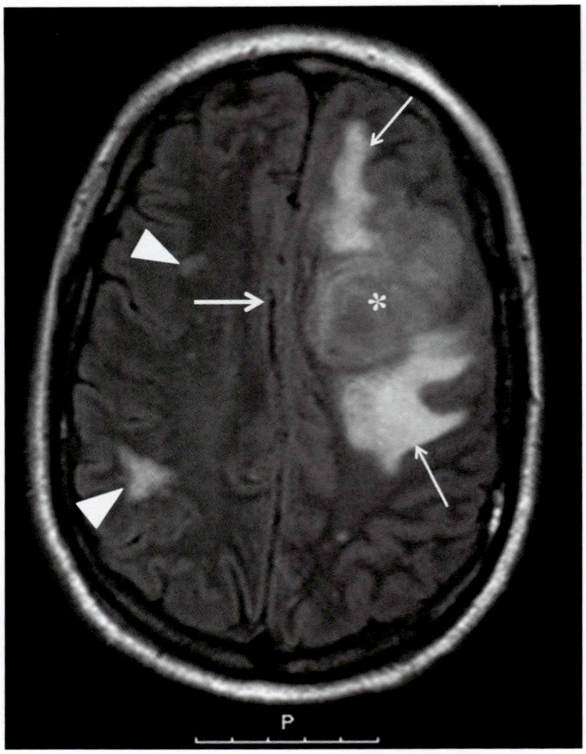

Figure 4-5. Peritumoral edema and midline shift: The metastatic carcinoma (*asterisk*) and the peritumoral edema (*thin arrows*) that are seen as hyperintensities in this FLAIR image result in a mass effect with a midline shift to the right (*thick arrow*). Several foci of apparent ischemic white matter foci (*arrowheads*) are also present in the right hemisphere (axial FLAIR MRI).

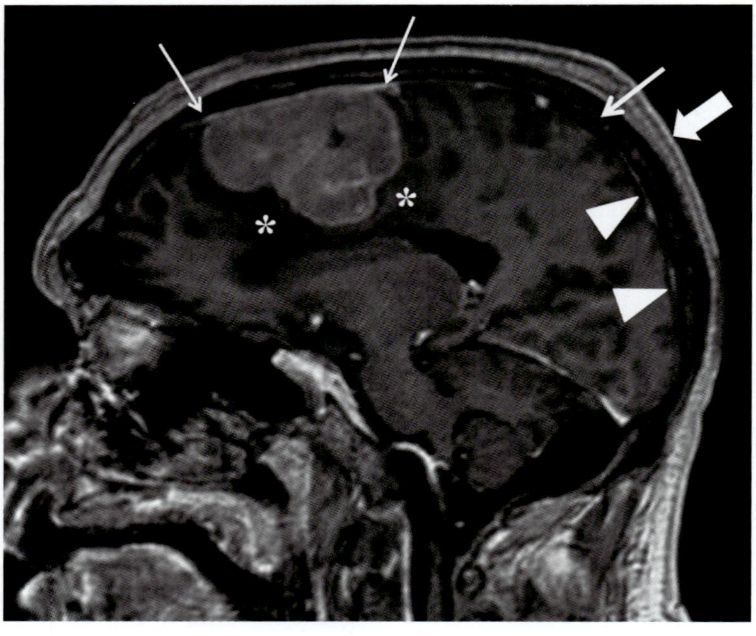

Figure 4-6. Dural-based mass and dural tail: This heterogeneously enhancing meningioma has a broad dural base with enhancing elongated dural tails (*thin arrows*) at the periphery of the dural attachment. The heterogeneity of enhancement, in contrast to the usual homogeneous enhancement of meningiomas, is due to necrosis and variations in internal structure in this atypical meningioma. Adjacent brain parenchyma is edematous (*asterisk*), which is hypointense on T1-weighted image. In MR images, subcutaneous adipose tissue has bright signal (*block arrow*). Diploe (*thick arrow*) is relatively prominent and is bordered by dark signal of the inner and outer tables on both sides. Dura mater is seen as a bright line next to the brain parenchyma (*arrowheads*) (sagittal postcontrast T1-weighted MRI).

Contrast Enhancement

Both CT and MR can be performed after administering a contrast medium, which is typically an iodine-containing material for CT and gadolinium for MR. These substances leak into the tissues where there is disruption of blood–brain barrier and cannot be cleared from those areas as in the rest of the neuroglial tissue, resulting in their identification in the subsequent images. This is called *enhancement* and provides very useful clues. Blood vessels naturally enhance due to the presence of contrast medium in their lumens **(Fig. 4-7)**, but the blood–brain barrier will not allow this material to pass into the tissues, except where it is normally absent, such as in the choroid plexus, pineal gland, pituitary gland, and falx cerebri **(Fig. 4-1)**. Extraaxial lesions, such as meningiomas, tend to enhance as there is normally no blood–brain barrier in that location **(Fig. 4-6)**. Enhancement in intraaxial lesions may or may not be an indication of a high-grade neoplasm, depending on other features and the pattern of enhancement. Glioblastoma shows *ring enhancement*[16–23] **(Table 4.3)** due to central necrosis and the proliferation of abnormal vessels in the viable tissue in its periphery **(Fig. 4-7)**. On the other hand, pilocytic astrocytoma, along with several other low-grade and well-circumscribed neoplasms, shows a *cyst and enhancing mural nodule* pattern[24–29] **(Table 4.4; Fig. 4-8)**. In other cases, enhancement may be *heterogeneous* **(Table 4.5; Fig. 4-6)**, *homogeneous* **(Table 4.6)**, or absent, that is, *nonenhancing* **(Table 4.7)** lesions.[30–32] The presence of cysts, hemorrhage, calcifications, and necrosis results in a heterogeneous enhancement **(Fig. 4-9)**. High-grade

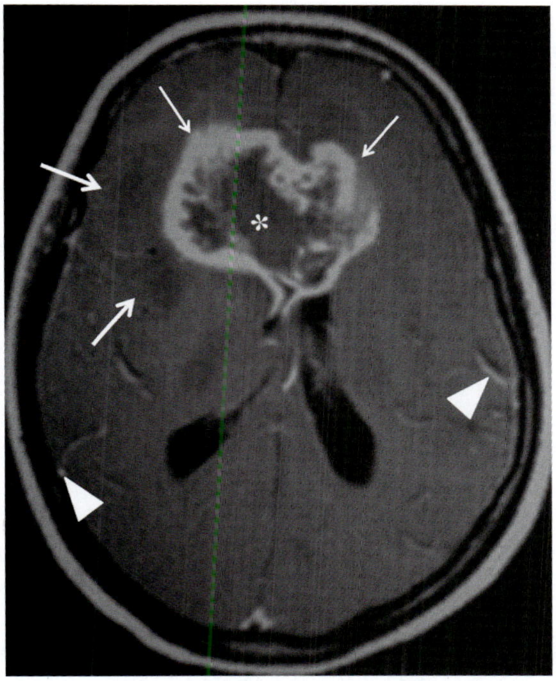

Figure 4-7. Ring-enhancing and butterfly lesion: A lesion (*thin arrows*) is situated straddling the corpus callosum, creating a "butterfly" appearance. The enhancement is at its periphery, completely surrounding the central area (*asterisk*), which is nonenhancing due to necrosis. Peritumoral edema is present in the right hemisphere as a hypointense region in this T1-weighted image (*thick arrows*). Normal vessels are highlighted in other areas due to the presence of contrast material in them (*arrowheads*) (axial postcontrast T1-weighted MRI).

TABLE 4.3 Common lesions typically presenting with ring/rim or peripheral enhancement

Subacute and chronic/resolving hematomas
Subacute infarction
Abscess
Necrotic granuloma
Toxoplasmosis
Cystic neoplasms (see table 4.4)
Glioblastoma
Metastatic carcinoma with central necrosis
Lymphoma
Rosette-forming glioneuronal tumor
Radiation necrosis
Necrotizing leukoencephalopathy
Infarct (rare)
Tumefactive demyelination (demyelinating pseudotumor; incomplete ring, C-shaped or horseshoe-shaped enhancement)

TABLE 4.4 Main neoplasms typically presenting with cyst and mural nodule formation

Pilocytic astrocytoma
Ganglioglioma
Desmoplastic infantile ganglioglioma/desmoplastic infantile astrocytoma (cyst may be multilocular)
Hemangioblastoma
Pleomorphic xanthoastrocytoma
Extraventricular neurocytoma
Papillary glioneuronal tumor

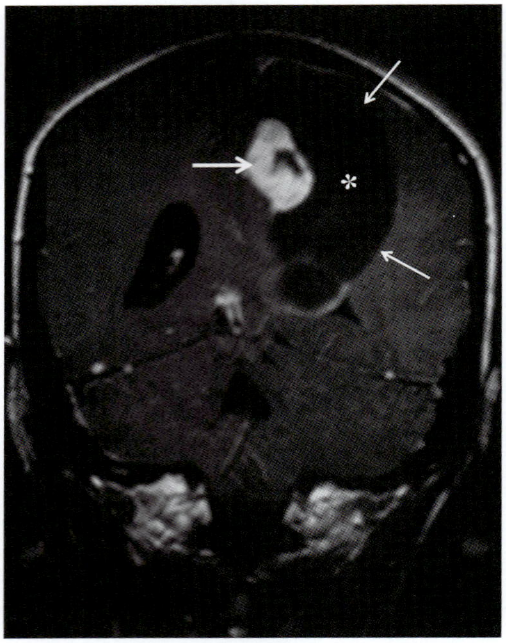

Figure 4-8. Cyst and mural nodule formation: A lesion representing a pilocytic astrocytoma with well-defined smooth borders (*thin arrows*) is present in the left hemisphere. The cyst contents (*asterisk*) are isointense to CSF seen within the occipital horn of the right lateral ventricle, in which parts of normally enhancing choroid plexus can be seen. An enhancing mural nodule (*thick arrow*) is present attached to the wall of the cyst (coronal postcontrast T1-weighted MRI).

gliomas, metastatic neoplasms, infarcts, and cerebritis tend to have heterogeneous enhancement. Meningioma, lymphoma, and anaplastic glial neoplasms such as anaplastic oligodendroglioma, but not anaplastic astrocytoma,[33] tend to enhance homogeneously. The absence of enhancement indicates an intact blood–brain barrier and is therefore associated with low-grade gliomas, anaplastic astrocytomas, and nonneoplastic cysts, such as arachnoid cyst. *Multifocal enhancement* within a lesion can be seen in the presence of multiple enhancing lesions or in multiple foci of high-grade progression in a low-grade infiltrating glioma. *Enhancement along the ependymal surfaces* is indicative of involvement of these surfaces by a pathologic process through cerebrospinal fluid (CSF) dissemination or by direct infiltration through the parenchyma[34–37] **(Table 4.8; Fig. 4-10)**. It may be accompanied by leptomeningeal/subarachnoid involvement by neoplastic or inflammatory processes that starts with the involvement of one and progresses to involve the other compartment. Either way, dissemination of a neoplastic

TABLE 4.5 Commonly heterogeneously enhancing lesions
Ependymoma
Subependymoma (if multiple cyst formation and calcification are present)
Subependymal giant cell astrocytoma
Anaplastic oligodendroglioma
Primitive neuroectodermal tumor
Central neurocytoma
Papillary tumor of the pineal region
Papillary glioneuronal tumor
Craniopharyngioma
Germ cell neoplasms other than germinoma
Radiation necrosis (with a "soap bubble" appearance)
Chemotherapy-induced leukoencephalopathy (in foci of demyelination and necrosis)

TABLE 4.6 Commonly homogeneously enhancing lesions
Vascular malformation
Infarction
Aneurysm
Granulomatous inflammation
Ependymoma (including subependymoma and myxopapillary ependymoma)
Chordoid glioma
Pilomyxoid astrocytoma
Meningioma
Melanocytoma
Lymphoma
Primitive neuroectodermal tumor
Pineocytoma
Paraganglioma
Choroid plexus neoplasms
Germinoma
Active/acute multiple sclerosis lesions

TABLE 4.7 Commonly nonenhancing lesions
Remote/chronic/cystic infarction
Arachnoid cyst
Epidermoid/dermoid cyst
Parasitic cyst
Low-grade and anaplastic fibrillary astrocytoma
Low-grade oligodendroglioma
Chronic multiple sclerosis lesions
Progressive multifocal leukoencephalopathy
Gliomatosis cerebri

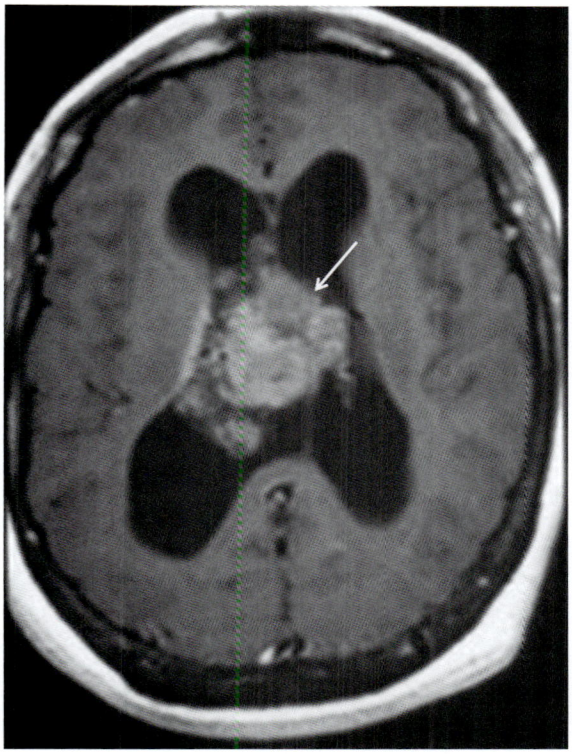

Figure 4-9. Intraventricular heterogeneously enhancing lesion: This central neurocytoma forms an intraventricular mass (*arrow*) with a multilobular and heterogeneously enhancing interior. Lateral ventricles are dilated due to the obstruction of the foramen of Monro that occurs commonly in intraventricular lesions producing a ball and valve effect (axial postcontrast T1-weighted MRI).

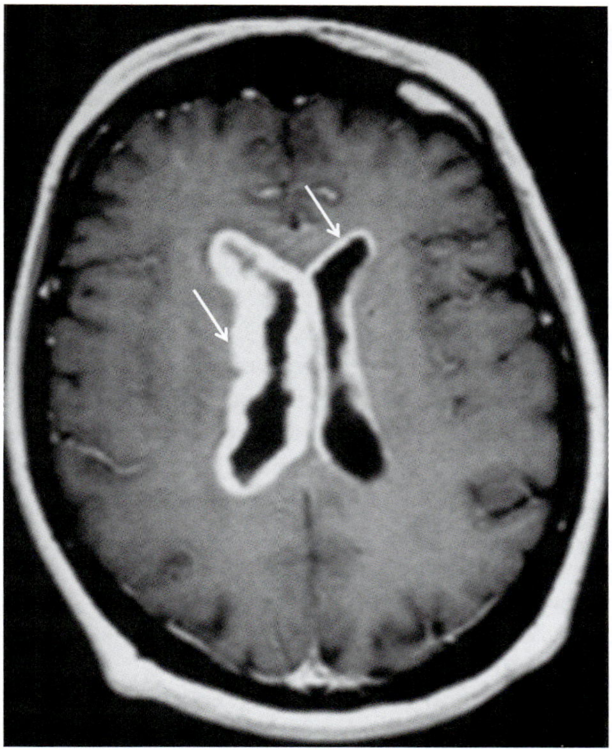

Figure 4-10. Ependymal lining enhancement: Pathologic processes that involve the ventricular surfaces, including neoplasms that seed the CSF, in this case a glioblastoma that is not seen in this particular image, result in the enhancement of ventricular surfaces (*arrows*) (axial postcontrast T1-weighted MRI).

or inflammatory process through the CSF is a bad prognostic sign and is associated with eventual craniospinal dissemination. *Meningeal enhancement*, with or without involvement of ependymal surfaces, can also be seen in a variety of inflammatory or neoplastic processes[38–43] **(Table 4.9)**.

TABLE 4.8 Lesions that can result in enhancement of ependymal surfaces

Ventriculitis
Retrograde infiltration by metastatic carcinomas from meningeal carcinomatosis
Germ cell neoplasms
Primitive neuroectodermal tumor/pineoblastoma
Infiltration by primary parenchymal neoplasms (e.g., glioblastoma)
Lymphoma/leukemia infiltration

TABLE 4.9 Common lesions resulting in diffuse or patchy meningeal enhancement without mass formation

Meningeal fibrosis
Meningitis
Sarcoidosis
Meningeal inflammation
Pachymeningitis
Dural sinus thrombosis
Meningioma en plaque
Lymphomatous involvement
Leukemic involvement
Meningeal carcinomatosis
Infiltration by primary malignancies and craniospinal seeding (choroid plexus neoplasms, pineoblastoma, ependymoma, germ cell neoplasms, oligodendroglioma, medulloblastoma)
Intracranial hypotension

Mass Effect and Edema

Mass effect refers to the changes that occur as a result of space-occupying lesions and is usually associated with high-grade neoplasms and rapidly enlarging processes such as edema with or without accompanying mass lesions. In addition, highly infiltrative neoplasms may not produce mass effect as they result in only minimal displacement of the tissues. Midline shift **(Figs. 4-1 and 4-5)**, compression of the ventricles, effacement of sulci, and various herniations are signs of mass effect. Therefore, encephalitis, abscess, metastatic carcinomas, large acute demyelinating lesions, intraparenchymal hemorrhage, glioblastoma, supratentorial primitive neuroectodermal tumors, and radiation necrosis are more likely to result in mass effect. *Peritumoral edema* may occur with or without mass effect, but certainly contributes to any mass effect. It is also seen typically around rapidly growing lesions such as cerebritis, abscess, and metastatic carcinomas. High-grade meningiomas and those with brain invasion also tend to have peritumoral edema in the surrounding brain tissue. In addition, angiomatous, microcystic, and secretory meningiomas can be associated with peritumoral edema. Edema is seen especially well in FLAIR images **(Fig. 4-5)**. A peculiar *periventricular/subependymal edema* can be seen in hydrocephalus cases with increased intraventricular pressure.[44]

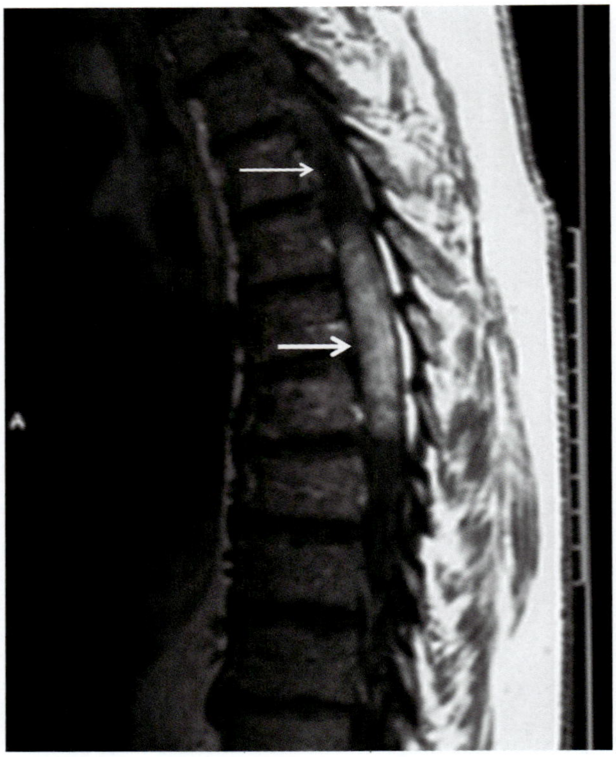

Figure 4-11. Syrinx formation: This ependymoma with heterogeneous interior results in this intramedullary enhancing mass (*thick arrow*) with iso- or hypointense, roughly triangular cystic areas at one or both poles, more prominent in the upper pole (*thin arrow*) in this case (sagittal postcontrast T1-weighted MRI).

Lesion Characteristics and Location

Various *cysts*, including those in the lesions with cyst and mural nodule formation, usually have contents that are isointense to CSF **(Fig. 4-8)**, but they can be hyperintense if they have a high protein content and/or hemorrhage. In the spinal cord, some neoplasms are especially associated with *syrinx* formation,[45,46] which is similar to the cyst in the cyst and mural nodule formation and is seen in the parenchyma corresponding to the upper and lower poles of the neoplasm. Pilocytic astrocytoma and ependymoma are prominent examples **(Fig. 4-11)**.

Radiologic images provide detailed information about the exact location of the lesion, its borders, multiplicity, and other features that may not be otherwise available to the neuropathologist or may not be readily discerned from the examination of the tissue sample. Lesions are broadly classified as being *intraaxial* or *extraaxial*, depending on whether they are within the neuroglial parenchyma or outside it, respectively. In superficially located lesions, this distinction helps narrow down the differential diagnosis. Intraaxial lesions directly arise from the parenchyma and are located within it. They are mainly glial neoplasms, infectious and inflammatory lesions, and malformative lesions, while extraaxial lesions are somewhat more limited **(Table 4.10)**. Some extraaxial lesions are closely associated with dura mater and are said to be *dural based*[47] **(Fig. 4-6)**. Meningioma is the classical example, among others, such as reactive or neoplastic lymphoid proliferations as well as histiocytic proliferations such as Rosai-Dorfman disease that typically mimic meningioma clinically and radiologically. Likewise, by virtue of their tendency to infiltrate the dura, some intraaxial neoplasms such as gliosarcoma, desmoplastic infantile ganglioglioma, and pleomorphic

TABLE 4.10 Common extraaxial mass lesions

Meningioma
Metastatic neoplasms
Hematolymphoid malignancies
Lymphoid/histiocytic proliferations
Hemangiopericytoma/solitary fibrous tumor
Inflammatory myofibroblastic tumor
Inflammatory pseudotumor
Peripheral nerve sheath neoplasms
Bone and soft tissue neoplasms
Sarcoidosis
Fungal or mycobacterial infections
Abscess

xanthoastrocytoma may also appear dural based. In addition, some of these dural-based lesions are associated with a characteristic elongated, tapering tail-like structure along the dura mater next to the lesion, which usually enhances similar to the lesion and is referred to as *dural tail* **(Fig. 4-6)**. While it is most typically associated with meningiomas, several other lesions can also have dural tails[2,48–56] **(Table 4.11)**. In the spinal cord, locations are referred to as *intramedullary* or *extramedullary*, with the latter further classified as *intradural* or *extradural*. These locations help classify the lesions and narrow down the differential diagnosis **(Tables 4.12 through 4.14)**. Other characteristic locations that are particularly helpful in a similar manner are *pineal region* **(Table 4.15)**, *sellar–suprasellar region* **(Table 4.16)**, *cerebellopontine angle* **(Table 4.17)**, and *intraventricular* **(Fig. 4-9)**. *Posterior fossa* is also associated more prominently with a limited number of neoplasms, especially

TABLE 4.11 Lesions that may be associated with enhancing dural tail

Meningioma
Dural metastatic disease
Dural sarcomas
Lymphomatous/leukemic involvement
Intraaxial neoplasm infiltrating leptomeninges
Bone neoplasms involving dura mater
Subacute subdural and epidural hematomas
Postoperative dural reaction
Subdural or epidural abscess
Infectious or noninfectious pachymeningitis

TABLE 4.12 Common intramedullary spinal cord focal lesions

Ependymoma (including myxopapillary ependymoma)
Astrocytic neoplasms (including pilocytic astrocytoma)
Paraganglioma
Demyelinating process
Vascular malformation

TABLE 4.13 Common intradural–extramedullary spinal cord focal lesions

Meningioma
Schwannoma
Neurofibroma
Hemangiopericytoma/solitary fibrous tumor
Lymphoma/leukemia and other hematolymphoid processes
Drop metastases
Metastases
Vascular malformation
Nonneoplastic cysts
Granulomatous inflammatory processes

TABLE 4.14 Common spinal extradural focal lesions

Soft tissue neoplasms
Bone neoplasms
Osteomyelitis extension
Bacterial infection/epidural abscess
Lymphoma/leukemia
Plasma cell myeloma
Metastases

TABLE 4.15 Common pineal region lesions

Germ cell neoplasms
Pineal parenchymal neoplasms
Pineal cyst
Glial neoplasms
Papillary tumor of the pineal region

TABLE 4.16 Common sellar–suprasellar lesions

Pituitary adenoma
Rathke cleft cyst
Spindle cell oncocytoma of the adenohypophysis
Pituicytoma
Granular cell tumor
Lymphocytic hypophysitis
Granulomatous hypophysitis
Langerhans cell histiocytosis
Pituitary apoplexy/infarct
Pilocytic astrocytoma
Pilomyxoid astrocytoma
Craniopharyngioma
Meningioma
Germ cell neoplasms
Hypothalamic hamartoma

TABLE 4.17 Common cerebellopontine angle lesions

Schwannoma
Meningioma
Epidermoid cyst
Choroid plexus neoplasm (extending from the fourth ventricle)
Exophytic brainstem glioma
Paraganglioma
Endolymphatic sac tumor

TABLE 4.18 Typically well-circumscribed lesions

Pilocytic astrocytoma
Pilomyxoid astrocytoma
Subependymal giant cell astrocytoma
Pleomorphic xanthoastrocytoma
Ependymoma
Subependymoma
Myxopapillary ependymoma
Chordoid glioma
Astroblastoma
Hemangioblastoma
Ganglion cell neoplasms
Dysembryoplastic neuroepithelial tumor
Papillary glioneuronal tumor
Primitive neuroectodermal tumor/medulloblastoma
Pineal parenchymal neoplasms
Atypical teratoid rhabdoid tumor
Choroid plexus papilloma
Meningioma
Mesenchymal neoplasms
Melanocytoma
Metastatic neoplasms
Abscess

in the pediatric population. These include medulloblastoma, pilocytic astrocytoma, ependymoma, and choroid plexus neoplasms. A peculiar intraaxial location, creating a peculiar radiologic appearance, is the so-called *butterfly lesion* involving the corpus callosum to cross the midline and involve both cerebral hemispheres **(Fig. 4-7)**. These are typically glioblastoma, lymphoma, or, less commonly, metastatic carcinoma and show a ring-enhancing pattern, although other rare processes such as demyelinating and infectious diseases are also possible.[57,58] *Borders of the lesion*, especially of neoplasms, can be very useful in difficult cases. Unfortunately, they are not readily available for microscopical evaluation in small tissue samples. In such situations, radiologic images can provide this information **(Table 4.18)**. Well circumscription is a finding that is typically associated with low-grade neoplasms amenable to complete or near-complete resection **(Figs. 4-8 and 4-12)**. *Multifocality* is a feature that is characteristically associated with a hematogenously spreading processes, mainly metastatic neoplasms **(Fig. 4-2)** and hematogenous abscesses; however, many other processes of diverse etiologies

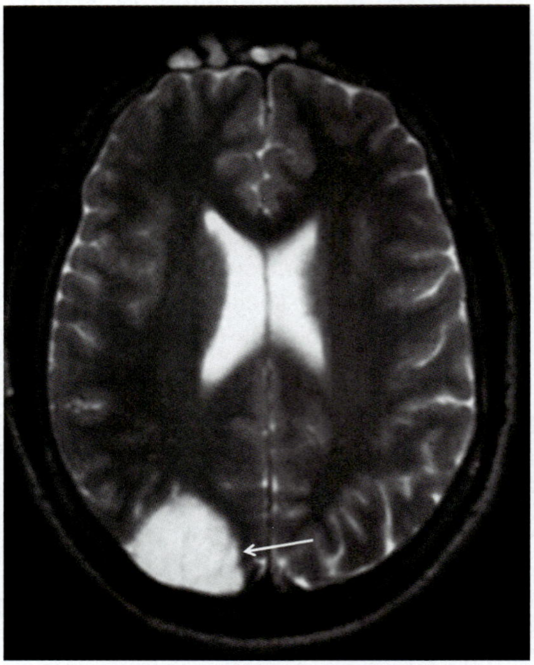

Figure 4-12. Multinodular well-circumscribed lesion: This dysembryoplastic neuroepithelial tumor is well circumscribed and has a multinodular interior that is also reflected in its borders (*arrow*). The outlines of gyri can be seen within it because of the intracortical location of this hyperintense lesion (axial T2-weighted MRI).

TABLE 4.19 Common multifocal lesions

Metastatic carcinoma
Metastatic melanoma
Lymphoma
Glioblastoma
Hemangioblastoma (especially those associated with von Hippel-Lindau syndrome)
Hematogenous abscesses
Granulomatous infections
Toxoplasmosis
Cysticercosis
Multiple sclerosis
Progressive multifocal leukoencephalopathy
Atypical teratoid rhabdoid tumor
Intraparenchymal hemorrhage (especially due to cerebral amyloid angiopathy)
Meningioma
Germ cell neoplasms (especially metastatic ones)

can be multifocal **(Table 4.19; Fig. 4-13)**. A *multilobular–multinodular* internal structure, while nonspecific, is associated more commonly with particular neoplasms of various grades, histologic

TABLE 4.20 Commonly multilobular/multinodular lesions

Central neurocytoma
Choroid plexus neoplasms
Dysembryoplastic neuroepithelial tumor
Pineoblastoma
Medulloblastoma with extensive nodularity
Astroblastoma

types, and locations **(Table 4.20; Fig. 4-12)**. *White matter abnormalities* can be diffuse or multifocal and are similar to their respective diseases described in Chapter 1, "Gross Features." For instance, leukodystrophies result in diffuse involvement, while demyelinating diseases such as multiple sclerosis result in multifocal involvement. In general, white matter lesions tend to be hyperintense on T2-weighted images and iso- or hypointense on T1-weighted images.[59] Gliomatosis cerebri also shows diffuse involvement with increased signal; however, it tends to be more prominent in one hemisphere[60] **(Fig. 4-14)**.

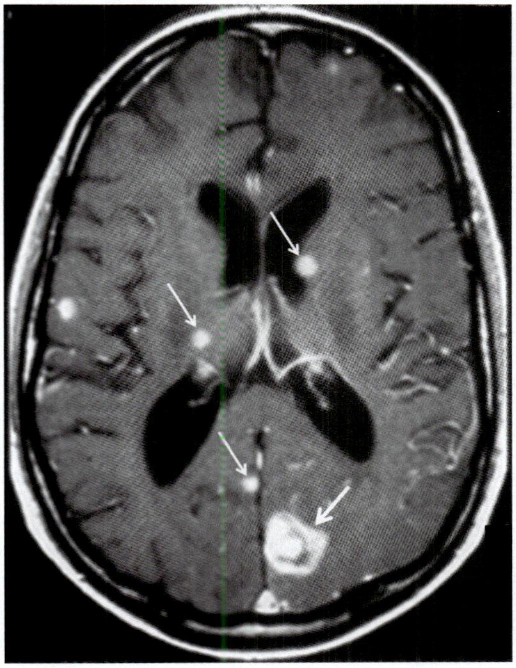

Figure 4-13. Multifocal lesions: Toxoplasmosis, in this case in the setting of acquired immunodeficiency syndrome, is seen as multiple lesions randomly scattered within the brain parenchyma (*thin arrows*). A larger lesion is assuming a ring-enhancing appearance due to central necrosis (*thick arrow*) (axial postcontrast T1-weighted image).

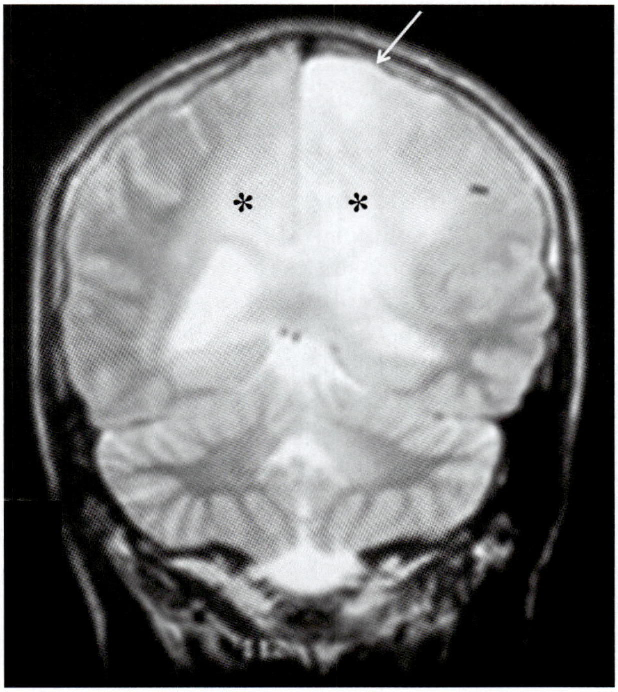

Figure 4-14. Diffuse white matter abnormality: Many processes that diffusely involve the white matter, as in this case of gliomatosis cerebri, result in widespread signal abnormalities (*asterisk*). The hyperintensity is more prominent in the left hemisphere (coronal T2-weighted image).

Advanced Radiologic Techniques

Angiographic methods, using conventional angiography, CT angiography (CTA), or MR angiography (MRA), help evaluate the vascular lesions such as aneurysms and vascular malformations, the vascularity of neoplasms, and the displacement and location of the vessels relative to a neoplasm, aiding in the surgical planning. MRA can be performed without a contrast agent. Several other advanced techniques provide additional information that is critical not only for diagnosis but also for planning of treatment, especially surgical approach.[61] *Diffusion-weighted MR imaging (diffusion-weighted image, DWI)*[62] provides information on random motion of water molecules. If that motion is restricted, as in cytotoxic edema, where water is entrapped within the cell, there will be hyperintense DWI (a.k.a., *restricted diffusion*). Abscesses and epidermoid cysts, as well as high-grade and therefore relatively hypercellular neoplasms, tend to have restricted diffusion, in contrast to necrosis, which shows *unrestricted diffusion* and is hypointense on DWI. Restricted diffusion has been identified as a constant finding in lymphomas,[63] although it can be seen in other highly cellular neoplasms such as glioblastoma and primitive neuroectodermal tumor. DWI can also give information in cases of edema that is not associated with cellularity. For instance, vasogenic edema around metastatic carcinoma or abscess shows high or unrestricted diffusion. Infiltrating tumors, due to the infiltrating cells, tend to have restricted diffusion. Postoperative injury also tends to have restricted diffusion. *Diffusion tensor imaging* and *tractography* are useful in the evaluation of white matter tracts. The directions of the tracts in the three-dimensional space can be highlighted in different colors. That way, whether the tracts are infiltrated or displaced by neoplasms and which tracts are affected can be identified.[64] *MR spectroscopy*[62] measures tissue metabolites. Choline peak gives information on cell membrane. Increased choline peak shows increased cell turnover and therefore suggests a neoplastic process. *N*-acetylaspartate is a neuronal marker and is decreased in neoplasms. Lactate peak provides information about necrotic component. *Functional magnetic resonance imaging*[59] is used to evaluate the status of critical areas such as motor areas relative to the neoplasm and provides useful information for surgical planning. Nuclear medicine techniques such as *positron emission tomography (PET) scan* are used to evaluate the metabolic activity in the tissues using a radioactive material called tracer and identifying its utilization in the tissues. Among other uses, PET scans are useful in the identification of highly active neoplasms and especially helpful in the differential diagnosis of delayed radiation necrosis versus recurrent high-grade glial neoplasm, such as glioblastoma, by detecting the high metabolic activity in the latter.[65]

References

1. Burger PC. *Smears and Frozen Sections in Surgical Neuropathology*. Baltimore, MD: PB Publishing; 2009.
2. Jinkins JR, Leite CDC. *Neurodiagnostic Imaging: Pattern Analysis and Differential Diagnosis*. Philadelphia, PA: Lippincott-Raven; 1998.
3. Wippold FJ II. Neuroradiology: the surrogate of gross neuropathology. In: *Practical Surgical Neuropathology*. Perry A, Brat DJ, ed. Philadelphia, PA: Churchill Livingstone; 2010: 47–62.
4. Burger PC, Scheithauer BW. *Tumors of the Central Nervous System, AFIP Atlas of Tumor Pathology*. Washington, DC: American Registry of Pathology; 2007.
5. Louis DN, Ohgaki H, Wiestler OD, et al. *World Health Organization Classification of Tumours of the Central Nervous System*. 4th ed. Lyon, France: IARC Press; 2007.
6. Burger PC, Nelson JS, Boyko OB. Diagnostic synergy in radiology and surgical neuropathology: neuroimaging techniques and general interpretive guidelines. *Arch Pathol Lab Med*. 1998;122:609–619.
7. Burger PC, Nelson JS, Boyko OB. Diagnostic synergy in radiology and surgical neuropathology: radiographic findings of specific pathologic entities. *Arch Pathol Lab Med*. 1998;122:620–632.
8. Woodruff WW. *Fundamentals of Neuroimaging*. Philadelphia, PA: W.B. Saunders Company; 1993.
9. Stanescu Cosson R, Varlet P, Beuvon F, et al. Dysembryoplastic neuroepithelial tumors: CT, MR findings and imaging follow-up: a study of 53 cases. *J Neuroradiol*. 2001;28:230–240.
10. Zhang D, Henning TD, Zou LG, et al. Intracranial ganglioglioma: clinicopathological and MRI findings in 16 patients. *Clin Radiol*. 2008;63:80–91.
11. Ibarra R, Kesava PP. Role of MR imaging in the diagnosis of complicated arachnoid cyst. *Pediatr Radiol*. 2000;30:329–331.
12. Terstegge K, Schorner W, Henkes H, et al. Hyperostosis in meningiomas: MR findings in patients with recurrent meningioma of the sphenoid wings. *AJNR Am J Neuroradiol*. 1994;15:555–560.
13. Min JH, Kang SH, Lee JB, et al. Hyperostotic meningioma with minimal tumor invasion into the skull. *Neurol Med Chir*. 2005;45:480–483.
14. Bekiesinska-Figatowska M. T2-hyperintense foci on brain MR imaging. *Med Sci Monit*. 2004;10:80–87.
15. DeBella K, Poskitt K, Szudek J, et al. Use of "unidentified bright objects" on MRI for diagnosis of neurofibromatosis 1 in children. *Neurology*. 2000;54:1646–1651.

16. Remick SC, Diamond C, Migliozzi JA, et al. Primary central nervous system lymphoma in patients with and without the acquired immune deficiency syndrome. A retrospective analysis and review of the literature. *Medicine*. 1990;69:345–360.

17. Vidal JE, Cimerman S, da Silva PR, et al. Tuberculous brain abscess in a patient with AIDS: case report and literature review. *Rev Inst Med Trop Sao Paulo*. 2003;45:111–114.

18. Anzalone N, Scotti R, Riva R. Neuroradiologic differential diagnosis of cerebral intraparenchymal hemorrhage. *Neurol Sci*. 2004;25:S3–S5.

19. Xia L, Lin S, Wang ZC, et al. Tumefactive demyelinating lesions: nine cases and a review of the literature. *Neurosurg Rev*. 2009;32:171–179.

20. Reiche W, Schuchardt V, Hagen T, et al. Differential diagnosis of intracranial ring enhancing cystic mass lesions—role of diffusion-weighted imaging (DWI) and diffusion-tensor imaging (DTI). *Clin Neurol Neurosurg*. 2010;112:218–225.

21. Garg RK, Sinha MK. Multiple ring-enhancing lesions of the brain. *J Postgrad Med*. 2010;56:307–316.

22. Aiken AH. Central nervous system infection. *Neuroimaging Clin N Am*. 2010;20:557–580.

23. Toh CH, Wei KC, Ng SH, et al. Differentiation of brain abscesses from necrotic glioblastomas and cystic metastatic brain tumors with diffusion tensor imaging. *AJNR Am J Neuroradiol*. 2011;32:1646–1651.

24. Palma L, Guidetti B. Cystic pilocytic astrocytomas of the cerebral hemispheres. Surgical experience with 51 cases and long-term results. *J Neurosurg*. 1985;62:811–815.

25. Wilms G, Raaijmakers C, Goffin J, et al. MR features of intracranial hemangioblastomas. *J Belge Radiol*. 1992;75:469–475.

26. Rippe DJ, Boyko OB, Radi M, et al. MRI of temporal lobe pleomorphic xanthoastrocytoma. *J Comput Assist Tomogr*. 1992;16:856–859.

27. Bouvier-Labit C, Daniel L, Dufour H, et al. Papillary glioneuronal tumour: clinicopathological and biochemical study of one case with 7-year follow up. *Acta Neuropathologica*. 2000;99:321–326.

28. Shin JH, Lee HK, Khang SK, et al. Neuronal tumors of the central nervous system: radiologic findings and pathologic correlation. *Radiographics*. 2002;22:1177–1189.

29. Alexiou GA, Stefanaki K, Sfakianos G, et al. Desmoplastic infantile ganglioglioma: a report of 2 cases and a review of the literature. *Pediatr Neurosurg*. 2008;44:422–425.

30. Reeder MM, Bradley WG. *Gamuts in Neuroradiology*. New York: Springer-Verlag; 1993.

31. Al-Okaili RN, Krejza J, Woo JH, et al. Intraaxial brain masses: MR imaging-based diagnostic strategy—initial experience. *Radiology*. 2007;243:539–550.

32. Castillo M. *Neuroradiology Companion: Methods, Guidelines, and Imaging Fundamentals*. 4th ed. Philadelphia, PA. Lippincott Williams & Wilkins; 2012.

33. Matar E, Cook RJ, Fowler AR, et al. Post-contrast enhancement as a clinical indicator of prognosis in patients with anaplastic astrocytoma. *J Clin Neurosci*. 2010;17:993–996.

34. Dubois PJ, Martinez AJ, Myerowitz RL, et al. Subependymal and leptomeningeal spread of systemic malignant lymphoma demonstrated by cranial computed tomography. *J Comput Assist Tomogr*. 1978;2:218–221.

35. Awad I, Bay JW, Rogers L. Leptomeningeal metastasis from supratentorial malignant gliomas. *Neurosurgery*. 1986;19:247–251.

36. Shima H, Nishizaki T, Ishihara H, et al. Recurrent intracranial germinoma with dissemination along the ventricular catheter: a case report. *J Clin Neurosci*. 2002;9:708–710.

37. Guerini H, Helie O, Leveque C, et al. Diagnosis of periventricular ependymal enhancement in MRI in adults. *J Neuroradiol*. 2003;30:46–56.

38. River Y, Schwartz A, Gomori JM, et al. Clinical significance of diffuse dural enhancement detected by magnetic resonance imaging. *J Neurosurg*. 1996;85:777–783.

39. Sakamoto S, Kitagaki H, Ishii K, et al. Gadolinium enhancement of the cerebrospinal fluid in a patient with meningeal fibrosis and cryptococcal infection. *Neuroradiology*. 1997;39:504–505.

40. Grossman SA, Krabak MJ. Leptomeningeal carcinomatosis. *Cancer Treat Rev*. 1999;25:103–119.

41. Mokri B. Spontaneous intracranial hypotension. *Curr Neurol Neurosci Rep*. 2001;1:109–117.

42. Joseph FG, Scolding NJ. Neurosarcoidosis: a study of 30 new cases. *J Neurol Neurosurg Psychiatry*. 2009;80:297–304.

43. Ruiz-Ares G, Collantes-Bellido E, Rodriguez de Rivera F, et al. Primary diffuse leptomeningeal gliomatosis mimicking meningeal tuberculosis. *Neurologist*. 2011;17:160–163.

44. Bydder GM, Pennock JM, Steiner RE, et al. The NMR diagnosis of cerebral tumors. *Magn Reson Med*. 1984;1:5–29.

45. Goy AMC, Pinto RS, Raghavendra BN, et al. Intramedullary spinal cord tumors: MR imaging, with emphasis on associated cysts. *Radiology*. 1986;161:381–386.

46. Do-Dai DD, Brooks MK, Goldkamp A, et al. Magnetic resonance imaging of intramedullary spinal cord lesions: a pictorial review. *Curr Probl Diagn Radiol*. 2010;39:160–185.

47. Johnson MD, Powell SZ, Boyer PJ, et al. Dural lesions mimicking meningiomas. *Hum Pathol*. 2002;33:1211–1226.

48. Rokni-Yazdi H, Sotoudeh H. Prevalence of "dural tail sign" in patients with different intracranial pathologies. *Eur J Radiol*. 2006;60:42–45.

49. Sahin F, Saydam G, Ertan Y, et al. Dural plasmacytoma mimicking meningioma in a patient with multiple myeloma. *J Clin Neurosci*. 2006;13:259–261.

50. Zeidman LA, Ankenbrandt WJ, Du H, et al. Growth rate of non-operated meningiomas. *J Neurol*. 2008;255:891–895.

51. Rokni-Yazdi H, Azmoudeh Ardalan F, Asadzandi Z, et al. Pathologic significance of the "dural tail sign". *Eur J Radiol*. 2009;70:10–16.

52. Peltier J, Fichten A, Lefranc M, et al. Follicular dural lymphoma. Case report. *Neurochirurgie*. 2009;55:345–349.

53. Furtado SV, Venkatesh PK, Dadlani R, et al. Adult medulloblastoma and the "dural-tail" sign: rare mimic of a posterior petrous meningioma. *Clin Neurol Neurosurg*. 2009;111:540–543.

54. Nayak L, Abrey LE, Iwamoto FM. Intracranial dural metastases. *Cancer*. 2009;115:1947–1953.

55. Ghosal N, Dadlani R, Furtado SV, et al. Dural based primary osteosarcoma in right fronto-temporal region with review of literature. *Neurol India*. 2010;58:128–130.

56. Wu B, Liu W, Zhu H, et al. Primary glioblastoma of the cerebellopontine angle in adults. Case report. *J Neurosurg*. 2011;114:1288–1293.

57. Rieth KG, Di Chiro G, Cromwell LD, et al. Primary demyelinating disease simulating glioma of the corpus callosum: report of three cases. *J Neurosurg*. 1981;55:620–624.

58. Lee HJ, Williams R, Kalnin A, et al. Toxoplasmosis of the corpus callosum: another butterfly. *AJR Am J Roentgenol*. 1996;166:1280–1281.

59. Zee CS. *Neuroradiology*. New York: McGraw-Hill; 1996.

60. Vates GE, Chang S, Lamborn KR, et al. Gliomatosis cerebri: a review of 22 cases. *Neurosurgery*. 2003;53:261–271.

61. Sherman JH, Hoes K, Marcus J, et al. Neurosurgery for brain tumors: update on recent technical advances. *Curr Neurol Neurosci Rep*. 2011;11:313–319.

62. Al-Okaili RN, Krejza J, Wang S, et al. Advanced MR imaging techniques in the diagnosis of intraaxial brain tumors in adults. *Radiographics*. 2006;26:S173–S189.

63. Zacharia TT, Law M, Naidich TP, et al. Central nervous system lymphoma characterization by diffusion-weighted imaging and MR spectroscopy. *J Neuroimaging*. 2008;18:411–417.

64. Field AS, Wu YC, Alexander AL. Principal diffusion direction in peritumoral fiber tracts: color map patterns and directional statistics. *Ann N Y Acad Sci*. 2005;1064:193–201.

65. Heiss WD, Raab P, Lanfermann H. Multimodality assessment of brain tumors and tumor recurrence. *J Nucl Med*. 2011;52:1585–1600.

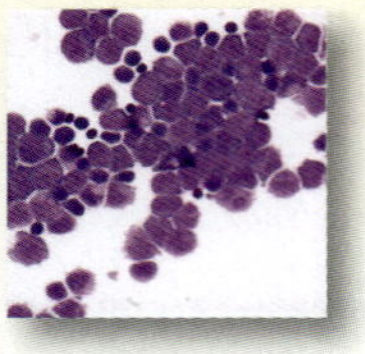
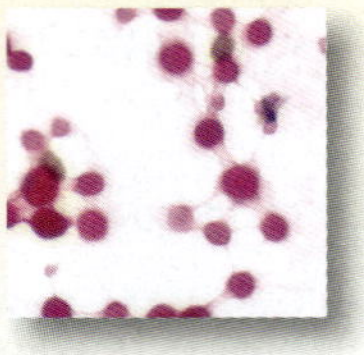
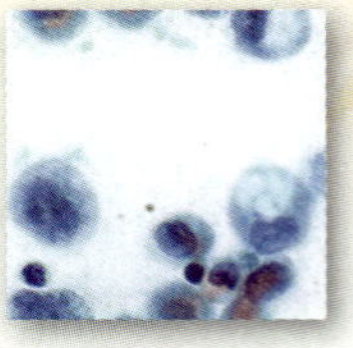

CHAPTER 5

Cerebrospinal Fluid

Introduction

Cytologic examination of cerebrospinal fluid (CSF) is an important tool in the evaluation of central nervous system (CNS) pathology. While the cytologic evaluation of smear preparations in the context of intraoperative consultation (IOC) is a practice that is essentially limited to neuropathology practice for all practical intents and purposes even though chapters are present in cytopathology texts and papers in cytopathology literature, the opposite is true for CSF cytology. Therefore, this chapter is not intended to be a comprehensive CSF cytology text, which is discussed in depth elsewhere in prominent cytopathology textbooks.[1–3] Nonetheless, it provides an area of considerable overlap between cytopathology and neuropathology knowledge and certainly requires a great deal of insight on the pathologic processes of the CNS. The air-dried slides are typically stained with a Romanowsky stain or one of its variations, while alcohol-fixed slides are stained with Papanicolaou stain. Romanowsky is especially useful in the evaluation of hematolymphoid cells and extracellular material, while Papanicolaou stain provides better nuclear detail. Their interpretation requires familiarity with their specifics, especially for the neuropathologist who is used to working with hematoxylin-eosin on smear preparations.

CSF cytology provides a window into the CNS, albeit limited, that is less invasive than the biopsy procedures. Compared to its relatively simple nature, it has a wide use in the diagnosis and follow-up of a number of diseases, with the potential of providing very useful information. It should be remembered that its use is limited to the processes that involve the CSF and the structures involved in its circulation. In that context, and with the knowledge of the potential processes that can be evaluated by CSF cytology, its advantages are maximized. The main areas where CSF cytology is utilized are (1) diagnosis of metastatic neoplasms, such as metastatic carcinoma, melanoma, and involvement by hematolymphoid malignancies; (2) identification of infectious agents, typically opportunistic, in the setting of immunosuppression, most notably human immunodeficiency virus (HIV) positivity; (3) inflammatory processes; (4) diagnosis of primary CNS neoplasms such as pineal region neoplasms, medulloblastoma, and choroid plexus neoplasms; and (5) follow-up of neoplasms, such as hematolymphoid neoplasms, germinoma, and medulloblastoma.

CSF can be obtained by several different methods, the most common being the usual lumbar puncture. Ommaya reservoir, ventriculoperitoneal shunt aspiration, and cisterna magna aspirations are other examples. The method used to obtain the specimen can affect its quality, especially its cellularity, and may result in some pitfalls in its interpretation. Therefore, knowledge of the source of the specimen may be important in its evaluation.

Gross Features

Normal CSF is a clear, colorless fluid, just like water. Any deviation from this appearance indicates some type of abnormality.[4] A *thick consistency* or *increased viscosity* can be due to mucinous material. *Mucin* may be due to the presence of actual mucin as a result of metastatic adenocarcinoma or due to the mucinous capsules of Cryptococcus infection. A rare source of mucinous material is ruptured nucleus pulposus. In rare

List of Findings/Checklist for Gross Features

AT A GLANCE

- Normal
- Thick/viscous fluid
  - Mucin
    - Adenocarcinoma
    - Cryptococcus infection
    - Ruptured nucleus pulposus
- Thick/cloudy appearance
  - Increased cellularity
  - Increased protein
  - Microorganisms
  - Pus (green-yellow)
  - Fat embolism (oily)
  - Contrast material
- Hardening
  - Abundant blood
  - Pus
  - Increased protein
- Tissue fragments
  - Ruptured nucleus pulposus
  - Infarct
  - Neoplasms
- Color
  - Hemorrhage (pink-red)
    - Aneurysm
    - Dissection of parenchymal hemorrhage
    - Germinal matrix hemorrhage
    - Traumatic tap
  - Xanthochromia (clear yellow-green)
    - Pigments
    - Very high protein

traumatic ruptures, fragments of intervertebral disc/nucleus pulposus can detach and make their way into the subarachnoid space. In this context, these fragments may travel to other levels of the spinal cord and present with cord compression. In some cases, they may even be sent as a specimen for IOC. A *thick and cloudy appearance* may be due to abundant cellularity of the fluid; usually, more than 500 cells/μL is needed for this type of cloudy appearance to occur. Increased cells also impart a sparkling quality to the specimen, called Tyndall effect.[5] Increased protein and microorganisms are other causes for cloudy appearance. If, in addition to being thick and cloudy, it also has a yellow-green color, it is purulent due to the presence of pus, as seen in cases of purulent (suppurative, bacterial, acute) meningitis. The thick appearance can have an "oily" quality to it in fat embolism due to the presence of fat globules or due to the presence of contrast material in postmyelogram specimens.

An obvious *hardening* of the specimen can be seen in actual clotting if there is abundant blood, which is also accompanied by a red color, or suppurative meningitis or in cases of increased protein as in Froin's syndrome. Actual *tissue fragments* can be seen in cases of infarcts, where necrotic tissue fragments may detach to fall into the CSF. This is especially possible in cases of cerebellar tonsillar herniation, where the herniated tonsillar tissue becomes ischemic and friable. Traumatic rupture of nucleus pulposus can also result in tissue fragments. Neoplastic tissue fragments from choroid plexus neoplasms or ependymomas may fall into the CSF.

A *color change* to pink-red without actual thickening of the fluid indicates the presence of blood, which can be due to actual hemorrhage or traumatic tap. The hemorrhage in the subarachnoid space is commonly due to an aneurysm rupture or dissection of an intracerebral hemorrhage into the subarachnoid spec through the brain parenchyma. In premature infants, germinal matrix hemorrhage is another reason for hemorrhagic CSF. If the specimen is collected in multiple consecutive tubes, in traumatic taps, the color of the fluid will get lighter and closer to normal in the later tubes, whereas in actual hemorrhage, all tubes will show similar color. Somewhat yellow-brown discoloration is called xanthochromia and indicates the presence of pigment that may be bilirubin due to jaundice, hemorrhage, or melanin pigment from melanocytic lesions including metastatic melanoma, or in cases of hypercarotenemia. Very high protein content can also result in xanthochromia.

Background Features

Due to the naturally low cellularity and small amount of the great majority of the CSF specimens, they are processed by concentrating techniques such as centrifuged or monolayer preparations, which tend to homogenize the fluid and eliminate any background features. Therefore, the background is essentially clean in CSF cytology, but rarely a mucinous or proteinaceous material in the background can be seen in prominent cases of metastatic adenocarcinoma or hemorrhage, respectively. In rare cases where necrotic tissue fragments fall into the CSF, a granular necrotic background can be present. In general, however, the clues that can be gained from the noncellular background material is limited in CSF cytology.

Hematolymphoid Cells

Normal CSF is essentially acellular with a rare lymphocyte and erythrocyte. Any more cellularity than that is abnormal. The presence of *bone marrow elements* is certainly concerning in terms of involvement by a leukemic infiltrate, especially if there is a history of one. In lumbar puncture procedure, the needle may scrape the vertebral arches to contaminate the sample with bone marrow elements.[6] The recognition and diagnosis principle is similar to the situation with extramedullary hematopoiesis on tissue sections, except that there may not be many cells to work with in the CSF. Nonetheless, the representation of at least two lineages with a range of maturation should alert one to this possibility. Leukemias on the other hand are monomorphous, and the acute leukemias are the ones that most commonly involve the CNS, resulting in a blastic population. In fact, in most cases, the difficulty is with recognizing the leukemic nature of this population, which may be quite scant. Chronic myelogenous leukemia, due to the maturation, can appear like an acute inflammatory infiltrate; however, close evaluation of the cells actually reveal admixed immature cells. Together with the previous history of leukemia, the diagnosis becomes easier. On the other hand, meningeal involvement by leukemia is not necessarily associated with neurologic findings.[7]

Another condition that may mimic bone marrow contamination or even a maturing leukemic infiltrate is acute *inflammation*. In acute meningitis, the infiltrate is predominantly composed of mature polymorphonuclear (PMN) leukocytes **(Fig. 5-1)**. A few small, round lymphocytes can be present. The latter can be more prominent in cases of partially treated bacterial meningitis and should not be

List of Findings/Checklist for Hematolymphoid Cells

AT A GLANCE

- Bone marrow elements
  - Contamination
  - Leukemic involvement
  - Peripheral blood contamination with leukemic cells
- Inflammation
  - Polymorphonuclear leukocytes
  - Mononuclear cells
  - Mixed
    - Treated bacterial meningitis
    - Early stage viral meningitis
    - Tuberculosis
    - Lyme disease
    - Mollaret meningitis
    - Chemical meningitis
    - Multiple sclerosis (PMN leukocytes absent)
- Erythrocytes
  - Traumatic tap
  - Hemorrhage
- Lymphocytes
  - Viral/aseptic meningitis
  - Lymphoma
  - Germinoma
- Plasma cells
  - Inflammatory
  - Neoplastic
- Macrophages/multinucleated giant cells
  - Granulomatous infection
  - Multiple sclerosis
  - Chronic inflammation
- Pigment
  - Hemosiderin
  - Radio-opaque material

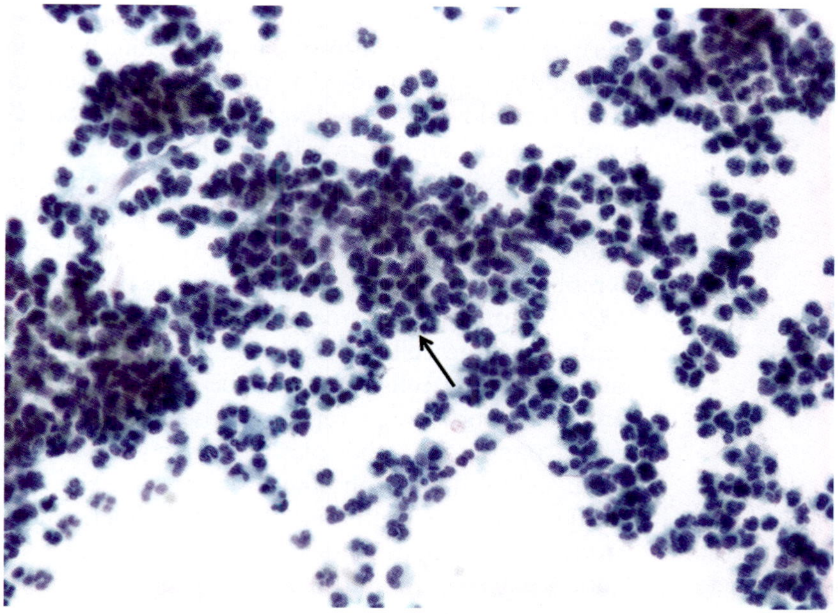

Figure 5-1. Bacterial meningitis: Abundant polymorphonuclear leukocytes are present. Careful search may reveal intracytoplasmic bacteria (*arrow*), in this case, cocci (Papanicolaou; original magnification: 400×).

confused with viral (aseptic) meningitis **(Fig. 5-2)**. In viral meningitis, the inflammatory population is essentially entirely composed of small, round lymphocytes. It too has a very early PMN leukocyte-predominant phase that lasts a day or two, before becoming exclusively lymphocytic. Admixed activated lymphocytes and plasma cells are also present. Monocytes appear in the later stages. In bacterial meningitis, careful search can reveal *bacteria* in the cytoplasms of PMN leukocytes. The background bacteria are not as dependable in general as the cytology sample is not processed under sterile conditions. However, in the appropriate clinical context and with the presence of PMN leukocytes, they support the diagnosis of bacterial meningitis. Prominence of eosinophil PMN leukocytes has been identified as an indication of parasitic infection in the right clinical context, even if the organism cannot be directly detected.[8]

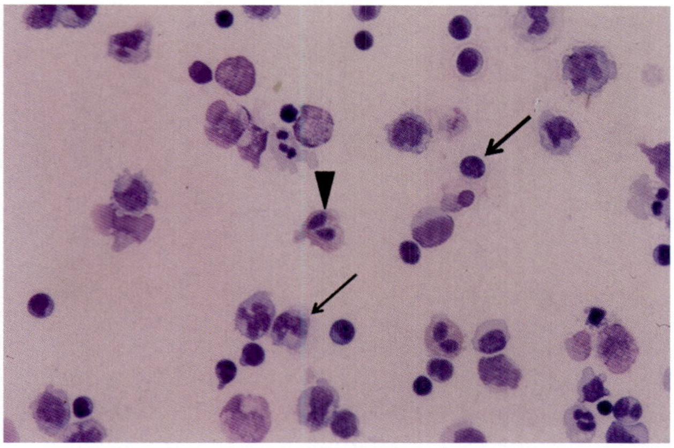

Figure 5-2. Treated bacterial meningitis: There is a mixed inflammatory population. Neutrophil polymorphonuclear leukocytes (*thin arrow*) are still abundant, with admixed lymphocytes (*thick arrow*). Scattered eosinophil polymorphonuclear leukocytes (*arrowhead*) are also present (Romanowsky; original magnification: 400×).

Peripheral blood contamination can occur as a result of traumatic procedure. It is usually not a problem to recognize the presence of peripheral blood contamination with occasional small, round lymphocytes and PMN leukocytes in a background of abundant erythrocytes. If the leukocytes tend to aggregate, they may create an inflammatory appearance, but noticing their proportionally few numbers relative to abundant erythrocytes should prevent this problem. Another problem with peripheral blood contamination is in actual leukemia cases in which the CSF examination is performed to diagnose CNS involvement.[7] In such cases of peripheral blood contamination and the presence of leukemic cells, before making a diagnosis of involvement of the CNS by leukemia, the peripheral blood blast count should be checked **(Fig. 5-3)**. Suspicion may be raised and the procedure may be repeated, but a definitive diagnosis should be avoided in cases in which the leukemia is not in remission and there is peripheral blood contamination of the specimen, showing leukemic

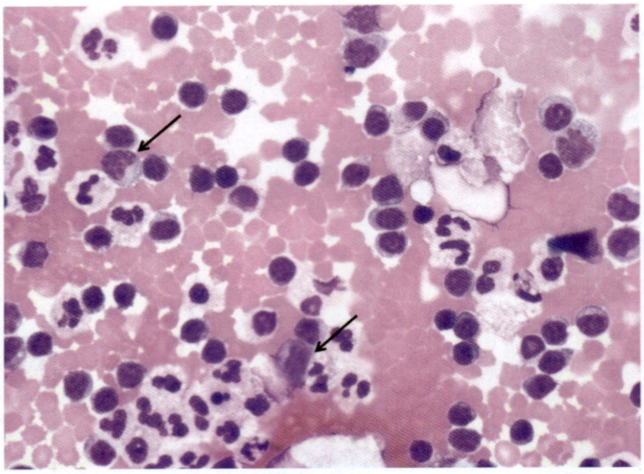

Figure 5-3. Peripheral blood contamination: Numerous erythrocytes, along with polymorphonuclear leukocytes and lymphocytes are present. In addition, there are blastic cells (*arrows*) in this leukemic patient. A diagnosis of leukemic involvement of the CSF should not be made in the presence of peripheral blood contamination, and peripheral blood counts should be checked (Romanowsky; original magnification: 400×).

cells. Such a diagnosis should only be made without peripheral blood contamination **(Fig. 5-4)**.

The *lymphocytic population* of viral meningitis can mimic lymphoma. The polymorphous population seen in reactive/inflammatory processes consisting of small round lymphocytes, activated lymphocytes, plasma cells, and, depending on the stage of the disease, PMN leukocytes or monocytes favors a reactive/inflammatory population; however, this feature may not be as obvious as one would like,[9] and cytologic atypia may be present in the lymphoid cells. Besides, lymphomas of follicle center origin can have a mixture of small and large lymphoid cells **(Fig. 5-5)**. In general, the lymphomas involving the CNS are more likely to be of predominantly large cell type, that is, diffuse large B-cell lymphomas **(Fig. 5-6)**. However, this is not always true. An admixture of small round lymphocytes and scattered large cells can also be seen in germinomas. The large cells represent the malignant cells, and the lymphocytes represent the reactive lymphoid population. This picture can potentially be confused with a lymphoma, as is the case even on tissue sections. Therefore, immunohistochemical studies on additional slides, or flow cytometric evaluation may be required. Unless the sample is very cellular, these additional techniques may not be performed, necessitating requesting additional sample solely for this purpose. Depending on the set up in the individual institution, communication with the clinical team may be needed to ensure that the sample is not further divided for clinical laboratory tests that have already been performed in the initial

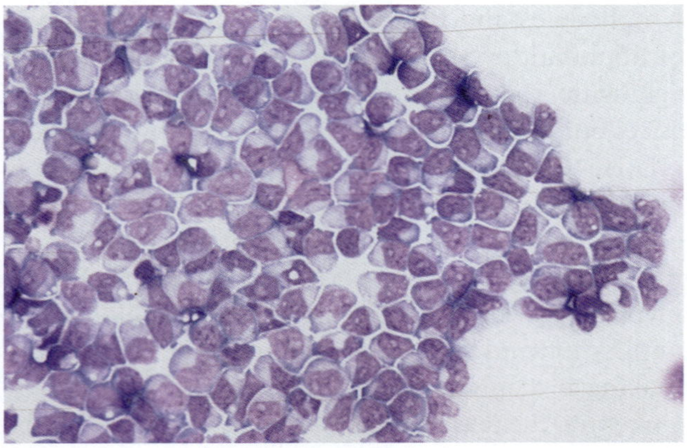

Figure 5-4. Leukemic involvement: Numerous blastic cells are present in this CSF from a patient with acute lymphoblastic leukemia. No blood components are seen (Romanowsky; original magnification: 400×).

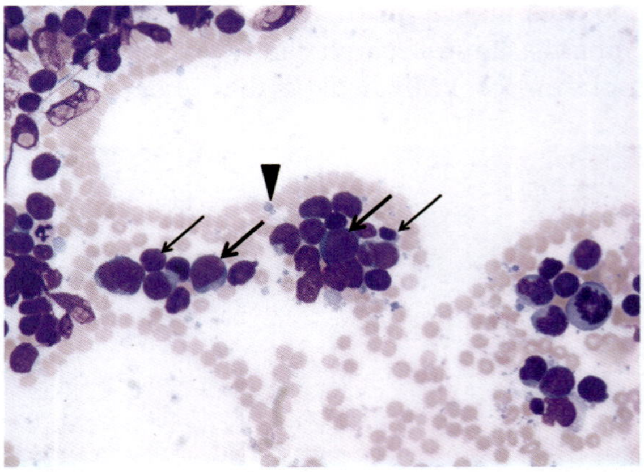

Figure 5-5. Follicle center lymphoma: A spectrum of lymphoid cells, from small cleaved centrocytes (*thin arrows*) to large centroblastic cells (*thick arrows*) are seen. Rare small, round mature lymphocytes may be present. Macrophages or polymorphonuclear leukocytes are not seen. Lymphoglandular bodies are also present (*arrowhead*) to support the lymphoid, but not necessarily malignant, nature of the population and help distinguish it from other small blue cell populations (Romanowsky; original magnification: 400×).

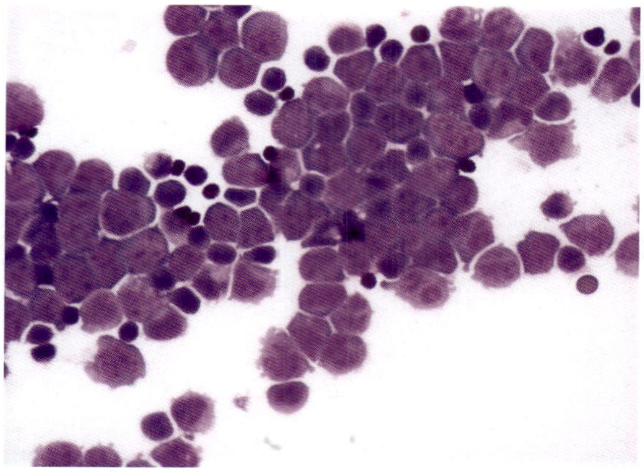

Figure 5-6. Diffuse large B-cell lymphoma: The lymphoid population is almost exclusively composed of large lymphoid cells with irregular nuclei and multiple nucleoli. They appear to form compact groups due to crowding, but the cells are still identified separate from others. Especially in a patient with a previously established diagnosis, this diagnosis can at least be suggested even in the presence of only a few cells (Romanowsky; original magnification: 400×).

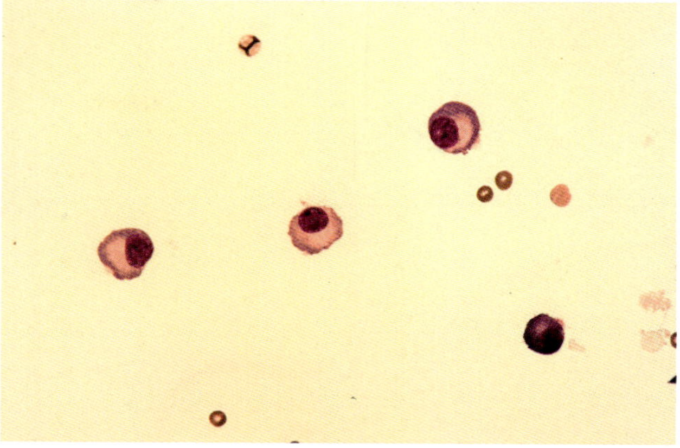

Figure 5-7. Plasma cell myeloma: Scattered atypical plasma cells have lost their typical cartwheel or clockface chromatin pattern but can still be recognized as plasma cells. No other inflammatory cell is present. In a patient with a previous diagnosis of plasma cell myeloma, these findings at least suggest CSF involvement (Romanowsky; original magnification: 400×).

sample, and directly sent for flow cytometry. It is possible to see cells with viral inclusions especially in infections that typically cause encephalitis, such as herpes encephalitis; however, this is a very rare occurrence.

Tuberculosis also produces a cellular population similar to viral meningitis,[10] starting with PMN leukocytes and becoming mononuclear with the appearance of lymphocytes, plasma cells, and macrophages,[11] or such a brief temporary picture may develop in the course of treatment for tuberculosis.[12] A similar picture is also present in Lyme disease[13] and Mollaret meningitis[14,15]; the latter is a rare, apparently aseptic condition that is recurrent. It too starts with an acute phase of PMN leukocyte population, gradually phasing into a mixed lymphoplasmacytic and monocytic population. The monocytes have nuclei described as "footprints in the sand."

An exclusively *plasmacytic population* is seen in the involvement of leptomeninges by plasma cell myeloma.[16] In many cases, this population is easily recognized as being composed of plasma cells, while in others, the cells may be difficult to recognize as plasma cells **(Fig. 5-7)**. They may resemble immunoblasts and even melanoma cells due to their eccentric large nuclei with prominent nucleoli. Prominent nucleoli indicate plasmablastic/immunoblastic transformation in plasma cell myeloma. Usually, admixed typical plasma cells and a morphologic spectrum in between these extremes help identify the process as plasmacytic. This distinction and the suspicion of the diagnosis of plasma cell myeloma, of course, are possible when there are large numbers of cells to evaluate. Typically, however, whether in plasma cell lesions or in other hematolymphoid populations, there are only a few cells to evaluate and one has to incorporate the clinical information and other laboratory findings in the interpretation. Atypical appearance of lymphoid[11] and plasmacytoid[17] cells is not unusual in a variety of infections and reactive conditions and should not be taken as a malignant process.

Chemical meningitides due to intrathecal chemotherapy or epidermoid cyst contents coming in contact with leptomeninges can result in a variable acute and/or chronic inflammatory reaction.[18] In multiple sclerosis,[19] the inflammatory reaction is mainly of lymphocytic and monocytic with an absence of PMN leukocytes. Macrophages may be in the form of foam cells and contain myelin debris. Plasma cells may be present.

Multinucleated giant cells are also rare to see but can be seen in tuberculosis, in sarcoidosis, or as a foreign body giant cell reaction after surgical procedures. Macrophages with *hemosiderin*

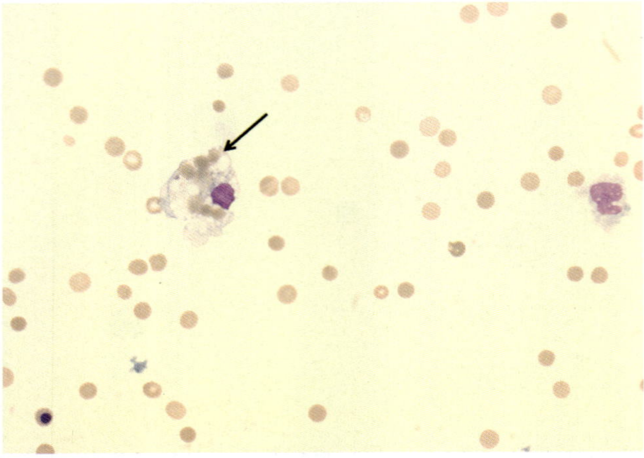

Figure 5-8. Subarachnoid hemorrhage: There are many erythrocytes. A macrophage shows erythrophagocytosis (*arrow*). A monocyte is also seen on the far right (Romanowsky; original magnification: 400×).

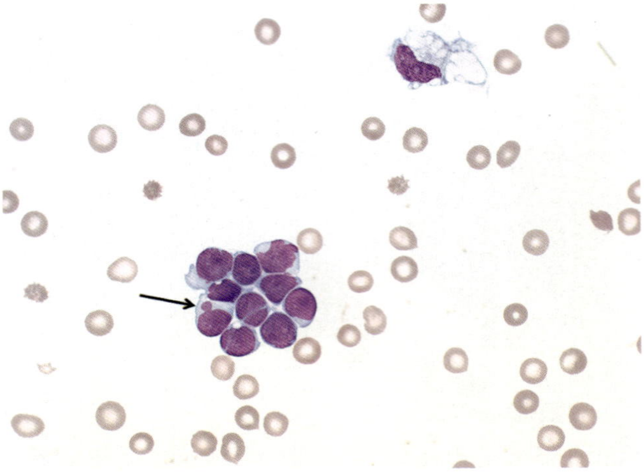

Figure 5-9. Small blue cells of presumed germinal matrix origin in a premature infant with intraventricular hemorrhage: They appear blastic, mimicking a PNET/medulloblastoma. In addition, a nuclear bleb (*arrow*) is present. A macrophage is present in the upper right (Romanowsky: original magnification: 600×).

pigment can be seen in subarachnoid hemorrhage. Erythrophagocytosis and hemosiderin pigment are the definitive diagnostic cytologic features for true subarachnoid hemorrhage[20] **(Fig. 5-8)**. Cytologic diagnosis of subarachnoid hemorrhage cannot be made simply based on the presence of blood since contamination cannot be ruled out. One way to distinguish between blood contamination as a result of traumatic tap and actual subarachnoid hemorrhage is the multiple tube collection method (see "Gross Features" above). In addition, it rarely becomes a problem left for the pathologist to figure out because significant subarachnoid hemorrhage is typically obvious by clinical presentation and radiologic imaging. In premature infants, germinal matrix hemorrhage is another situation where hemorrhagic CSF is seen with similar findings.[21] The presence of small groups of atypical cells that may be worrisome for a malignant process due to their small amount of cytoplasm, nucleoli, and nuclear molding, imitating a small blue cell neoplasm, can be confusing in this context or later in life in association with ventriculoperitoneal shunt placement for hydrocephalus **(Fig. 5-9)**. They have been identified as being of germinal matrix origin.[22] A pigment that is pale yellow and is lighter in color than hemosiderin can be seen in the cytoplasm of macrophages and may represent the *radiopaque material* used in myelography.[2]

Microorganisms

Cytologic examination of CSF is a useful tool to investigate the involvement of CNS by infectious agents. Especially in the era of HIV infection, the opportunistic infections involving CNS have increased dramatically. Regardless of the immune status and its effects on the formation of inflammatory response, it is not unusual to find microorganisms in a noninflammatory background. In addition, only a few microorganisms may be present in the entire set of slides, making their identification quite tricky. Especially in the case of immunosuppression

List of Findings/Checklist for Microorganisms

AT A GLANCE

- Bacteria
- Fungi
- Viral inclusions
- Parasites
- Artifacts
  - Air bubbles
  - Talc powder
  - Plane of focus

and opportunistic infections, identification of one microorganism does not exclude the possibility that others may be present.

Identification of *bacteria* in the cytoplasms of PMN leukocytes or in the background in acute meningitis is possible but is not crucial. Part of the specimen has been already submitted for microbiologic evaluation, and the clinical and microscopical features (see "Hematolymphoid Cells") support the diagnosis. Since cytologic specimens are not processed under sterile conditions, only the intracytoplasmic bacteria are considered evidence for the intravital presence of bacteria and of true infection, although the presence of abundant bacteria in the background of an acute inflammatory infiltrate in the right clinical context is also significant.

Cytologic evaluation of CSF is frequently utilized in search for opportunistic *fungal infections* in the setting of HIV positivity. However, especially in acellular appearing specimens, only rare fungal yeast forms may be present. In such apparently "blank" slides, the potential danger is to easily lose the correct plane of focus during screening since there are no prominent reference points to focus on. This issue can be addressed by using a noncellular material, a rare erythrocyte or even an artifact as a point of reference, or the focusing can be made using another cellular slide with the same thickness. The other end of the spectrum is to have a slide that is overcrowded by microorganisms that they may be overlooked as inflammatory cells or blood at low power. Otherwise, the general diagnostic principles apply to the recognition of specific fungi as in tissue pathology. The cell walls of all fungi stain black with GMS and are PAS positive. Histoplasma species are 2 to 5 μm round-to-oval yeast forms typically found in the cytoplasm of macrophages. They have a thin halo around them, representing their capsule. From the perfect angle, they may have a safety pin-like appearance due to a pale area in the center **(Fig. 5-10)**. Cryptococcosis is the most common fungal infection of the CNS diagnosed very accurately and easily by cytologic examination of the CSF.[23] The yeast forms are 4 to 10 μm, almost perfectly round and may show narrow-based budding **(Fig. 5-11)**. They have a thick, clear capsule that is positive for mucin stains such as mucicarmine, Alcian blue, and PAS, a distinguishing feature from other fungal yeast forms **(Fig. 5-12)**. Cytologic evaluation of India ink-treated preparations help highlight the cryptococcal yeast forms as negative images since they do not absorb the ink due to their capsules. This method is not superior or necessary, however,[24] as careful routine cytologic evaluation and modern laboratory tests are also efficient. In addition, Cryptococcus yeast forms are extremely pleomorphic with variable sizes

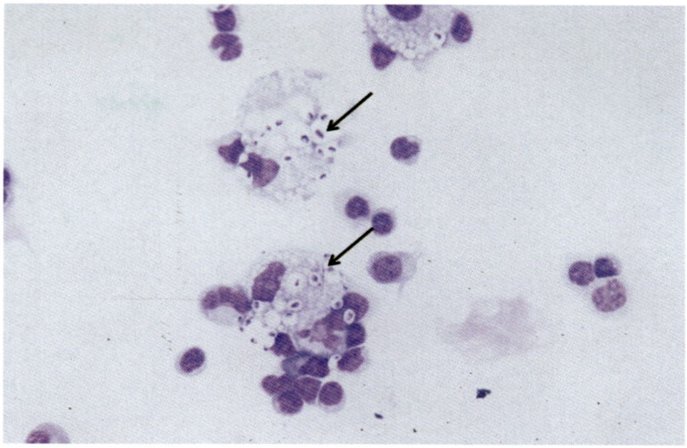

Figure 5-10. Histoplasmosis: There are many fungal yeast forms within the cytoplasm of macrophages (*arrows*). They are only several micrometers when compared to small lymphocytes in the field and appear to be within a vacuole (Romanowsky; original magnification: 400×).

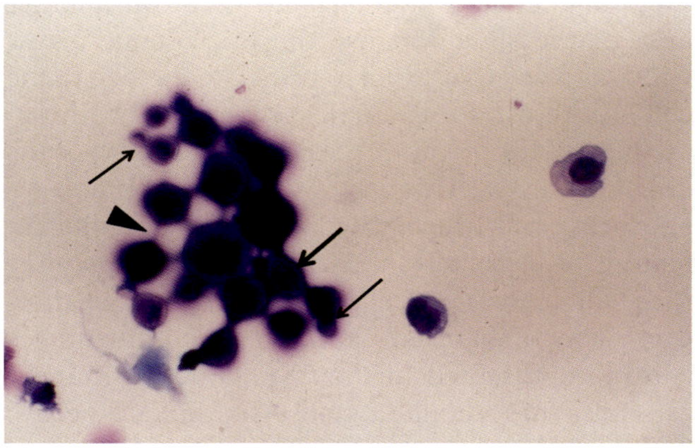

Figure 5-11. Cryptococcosis: Many fungal yeast forms are packed together, mimicking lymphocytes at low power magnification. Some of them are actually larger than macrophages (**far right**), have cell walls (*thick arrow*), and show narrow-based budding (*thin arrows*). They remain at a distance from each other (*arrowhead*) due to their capsules (Romanowsky; original magnification: 400×).

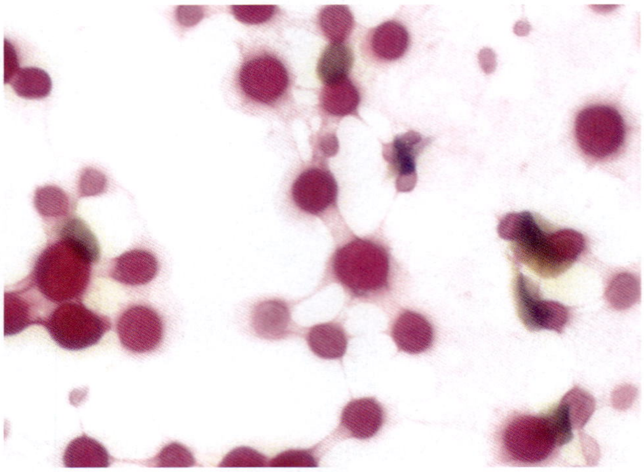

Figure 5-12. Cryptococcosis: The presence of mucinous capsule helps distinguish them from other yeast forms (Mucicarmine; original magnification: 400×).

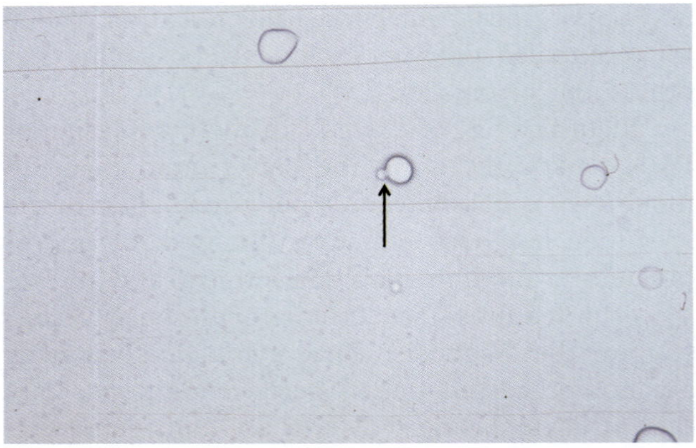

Figure 5-13. Air bubbles: Clear round structures may mimic fungal yeast forms, complete with budding appearance (*arrow*) (unstained areas of the slide; original magnification: 400×).

in contrast to Histoplasma, which is uniformly small at 1 to 5 μm and Blastomyces yeast forms, which are uniformly large around 10 to 12 μm. Cryptococcus shows narrow-based budding, while Blastomyces shows broad-based budding. In terms of the judgment of size of a cell or structure in general in cytology, especially in hypocellular specimens, comparison with an erythrocyte, which measures about 7 μm, or a small lymphocyte, which measures about 7 to 8 μm, is very useful. Even when there are no erythrocytes or lymphocytes in the field, one can find them on another area of the slide and use the microscope arrow width as a reference tool to translate the size to the cell of interest, for example, one-half the width of the base of the arrow or the size of the width of the tail of the arrow. This way, a surprisingly innocent-appearing cell in isolation, which is a significant feature of especially metastatic carcinomas, may turn out to be very large relative to an erythrocyte. Any fungus that can involve leptomeninges can be represented in the CSF. Other prominent examples are Candida and Aspergillus species, and Zygomycosis, which present as hyphae, or as pseudohyphae in the case of Candida. Rarely, fungi commonly known for their yeast forms may present with hyphae.[25] Microscopic air bubbles under the coverslip and talc powder are artifacts that may appear as fungal yeast forms. Both are clear and show no staining. The sharp refractile borders of air bubbles and absence of any internal structure help them identified as such and not as fungal yeast forms **(Fig. 5-13)**. Talc powder has a thick crystalloid appearance **(Fig. 5-14)** with a maltese cross birefringence in the center when examined under polarized light. Corpora amylacea[26] constitute another source of misdiagnosis for fungal yeast forms. They can fall into the CSF from the

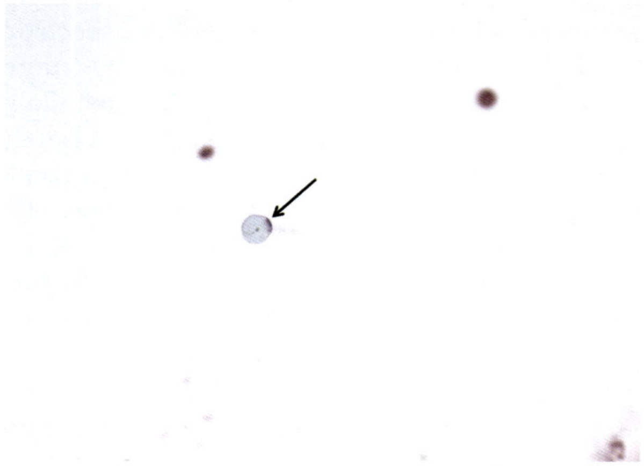

Figure 5-14. Talc powder: Refractile, roughly round structure that does not pick up any stain (*arrow*) can be suspected as an artifact. It appears on a different plane of focus when compared to two blurry cells in the field since it is thicker, and has a dot in the center. Polarized light examination confirms its nature, although it is not needed in most cases (Papanicolaou; original magnification: 400×).

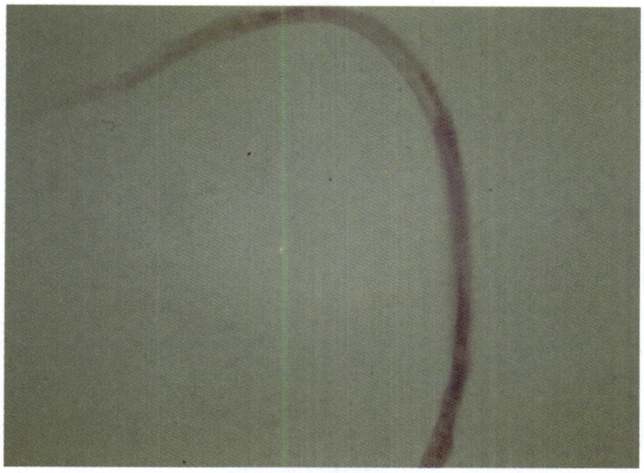

Figure 5-15. *Strongyloides stercoralis*: A thin, hair-like eosinophilic organism with an internal architecture is seen and may be mistaken for an artifact (Romanowsky; original magnification: 400×). (Courtesy of Neriman Gokden, M.D., Department of Pathology, University of Arkansas for Medical Sciences, Little Rock, AR.)

ventricular surfaces and are more likely to be identified in the shunt aspiration fluids.

Rarely, *viral inclusions*, such as herpes simplex virus,[27] or *parasites*, such as Strongyloides **(Fig. 5-15)**, ameba[28,29] **(Fig. 5-16)**, and hydatidosis,[30] can be identified.

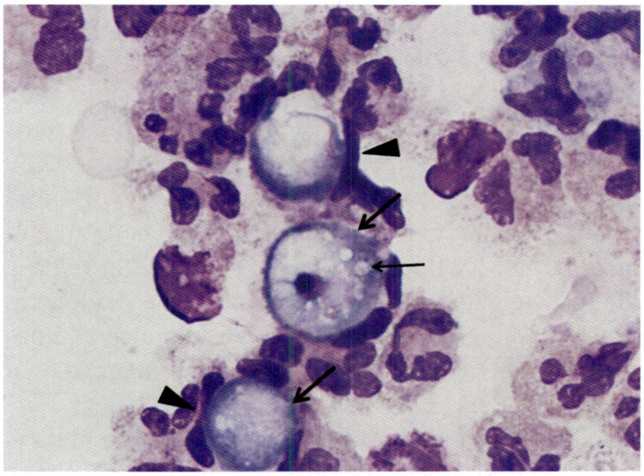

Figure 5-16. Amebic meningoencephalitis: Large, foamy organisms (*thick arrows*) resemble macrophages with their abundant, round cytoplasms, as well as with their erythrophagocytosis (*thin arrow*). Many polymorphonuclear leukocytes are present, some attacking the amebae (*arrowheads*) (Romanowsky; original magnification: 400×.) (Courtesy of Neslihan Cetin, M.D., Department of Pathology, Arkansas Children's Hospital, Little Rock, AR.)

Metastatic Malignancies

Hematolymphoid malignancies involving the leptomeninges and seeding the CSF are discussed under "Hematolymphoid Cells" above. Here, nonhematolymphoid neoplasms will be mentioned. Diffuse involvement of leptomeninges by a metastatic neoplasm, usually a carcinoma, is referred to as *meningeal carcinomatosis*, a term more accurate than carcinomatous meningitis for the obvious reason that it is not an inflammatory process.

In CSF cytology, the general cytology rule of *carcinomas* presenting in tightly packed groups of cells rarely holds true. In fact, there may only be a few cells to work with in most cases and they are in the form of individual cells **(Fig. 5-17)**. In addition, detached from their intercellular connections with other cells, they round up in the fluid, regardless of their original shape. This may make them difficult to recognize as carcinoma and differentiate from other malignancies, such as melanoma and even high-grade lymphoma. Again, because of the limitation with the number of cells, the possibility of preparing additional slides for immunohistochemical work up may not be possible in many cases. Therefore, the most important point is to be able to recognize the presence of malignant neoplastic cells and use all available information in history, especially previous diagnoses, if any. The presence of a tightly packed group or cell-in-cell configuration, which is also referred to as cannibalism or bird's eye appearance, is helpful to support an epithelial origin **(Fig. 5-18)**. The cell-in-cell architecture should not be mistaken for the whorl of meningioma. The nuclear atypia helps favor carcinoma. Since the carcinomas that most commonly metastasize to the brain are lung and

List of Findings/Checklist for Metastatic Malignancies

AT A GLANCE

- Hematolymphoid neoplasms
- Carcinomas
- Melanoma
- Small cell carcinoma
- Pitfalls
    - Choroid plexus cells
    - Chondrocytes

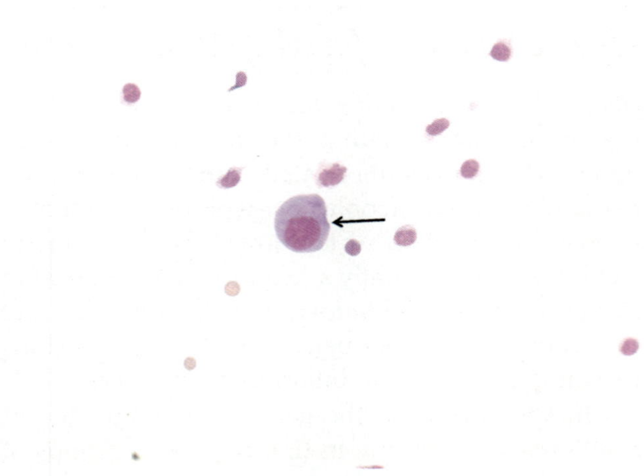

Figure 5-17. Metastatic carcinoma: A cell with eccentric nucleus and prominent nucleolus is present (*arrow*). Although its size may not be appreciated in isolation, this cell is huge when compared to the nearby lymphocytes and monocytes. It assumed, as many metastatic individual malignant cells do, a round contour floating in the fluid, free from its anchors with other cells. The patient had a previous diagnosis of non–small cell carcinoma of the lung (Romanowsky; original magnification: 400×).

breast carcinomas,[31] with the exception of small cell lung carcinoma (see below), they typically have the large cells with abundant cytoplasm and an eccentric large nucleus with a prominent nucleolus. In some adenocarcinomas, a cytoplasmic

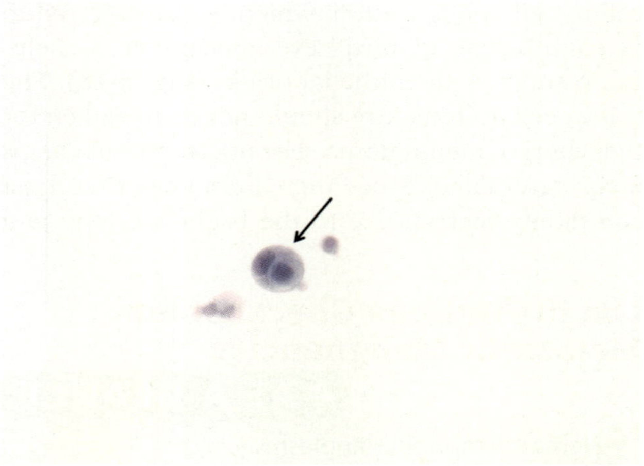

Figure 5-18. Cell-in-cell configuration: One atypical cell is hugging another with similar features (*arrow*), supporting an epithelial origin. The cells are very large when compared to nearby cells (Papanicolaou; original magnification: 400×).

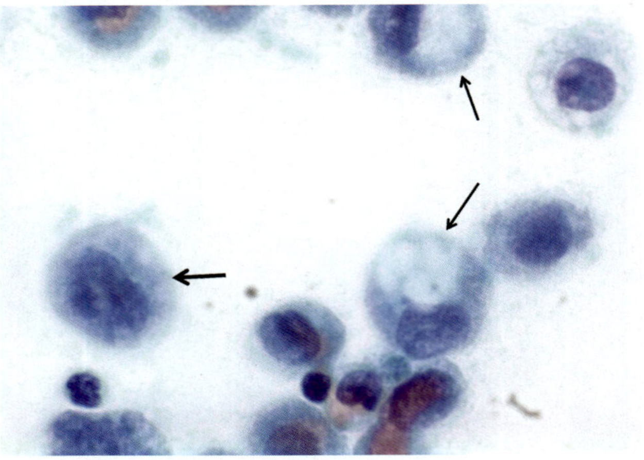

Figure 5-19. Metastatic adenocarcinoma: Large cells with large eccentric nuclei (*thick arrow*) are present. Many have multiple vacuoles in their cytoplasms, some pushing and indenting the nucleus (*thin arrows*) (Papanicolaou; original magnification: 400×).

vacuole containing mucin may be present. The entire cytoplasm may be distorted by multiple variable-sized vacuoles, pushing the nucleus to the side and indenting it **(Fig. 5-19)**. The differential diagnosis of a carcinoma cell with no such obvious features is melanoma. Unfortunately, melanin pigment is not always present to help with this differential diagnosis. If present, binucleation and intranuclear cytoplasmic invaginations favor melanoma **(Fig. 5-20)**. *Melanoma* cells have a denser and darker eosinophilic cytoplasm and may even have a peripheral amphophilic rim creating a plasmacytoid appearance in a larger scale **(Fig. 5-21)**. Instead, carcinoma cells usually have thin and lightly staining cytoplasm. Intracytoplasmic melanin pigment, while certainly helpful, can create a diagnostic trap when absorbed into the cytoplasm of macrophages. Siderophages should also be considered as a possible pitfall for the diagnosis of melanoma.

The differential diagnosis of epithelial cells is normal *choroid plexus cells*,[32] which can be present as small groups consisting of a few cells. They cannot be always distinguished from ependymal cells and are usually referred to as choroid plexus/ependymal cells. The cells are smaller than carcinoma cells. They have round nuclei; small, inconspicuous nucleoli; and small amount of cytoplasm. They can be more prominent in shunt aspirations and may actually appear as small tissue fragments

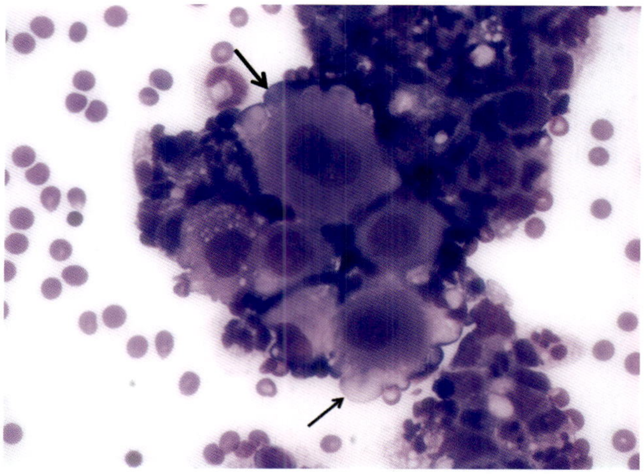

Figure 5-20. Metastatic melanoma: Large cells with abundant cytoplasm are essentially impossible to distinguish from metastatic carcinoma, especially when they cluster as in this field, without the help of clinical information and special stains. Melanin pigment is usually not present, especially when it is desperately needed, as in this case. Prominent single central nucleoli and binucleation (*thick arrow*) help favor melanoma. The irregular blebbing of cytoplasmic borders (*thin arrow*) is an artifact of centrifuge procedure, produced when cells hit the slide (Romanowsky; original magnification: 400×).

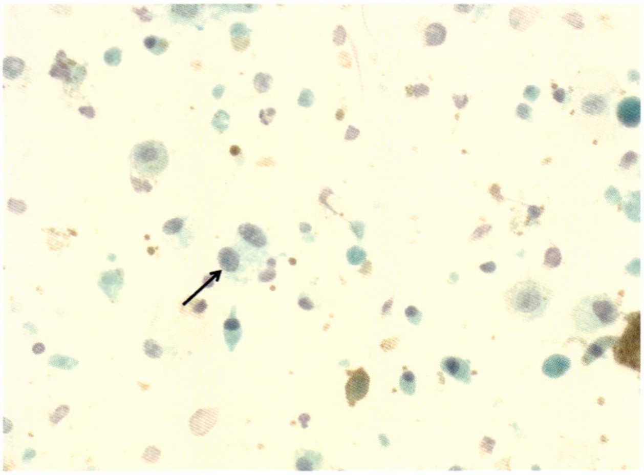

Figure 5-21. Metastatic melanoma: Abundant dusty, finely granular, brown-green pigment is present. Melanoma cells have prominent nucleoli (*arrow*), as well as eccentric nuclei creating a plasmacytoid appearance. Background is necrotic with nuclear and cytoplasmic debris (Papanicolaou; original magnification: 400×).

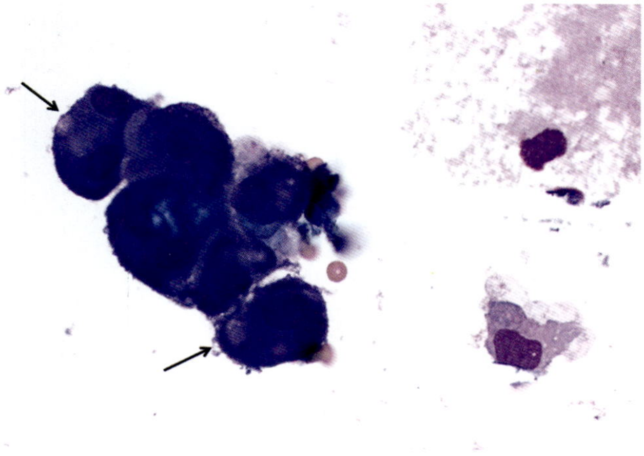

Figure 5-22. Choroid plexus cells: A group of several epithelioid cells are present in this shunt aspiration fluid. Although all cells appear somewhat larger on air-dried smears due to spreading, they are only slightly larger than a nearby monocyte (**right lower corner**). Their surfaces create a hobnail configuration, and well-defined vacuoles (*arrows*) are present in the cytoplasm, as in tissue sections (Romanowsky; original magnification: 400×).

(Fig. 5-22). They may also be more prominent in number in cases of choroid plexus neoplasms, especially of the fourth ventricle.

Chondrocytes can be present as individual cells or in groups of a few cells. They are present as a result of contamination from the lumbar puncture if the needle scrapes a facet joint or penetrates the intervertebral disc.[33] They create a pitfall by imitating carcinoma cells due to their grouping and especially adenocarcinoma due to the basophilic chondroid matrix around them, which appears like mucin. Their nuclei appear atypical due to their small, shrunken and hyperchromatic nature. However, this appearance contrasts with the nuclei of adenocarcinoma, which are large with prominent nucleoli. Perinuclear clear spaces in chondrocytes represent their lacunae and also provide a clue to their nature **(Fig. 5-23)**. The knowledge that chondrocytes can be present and cause such a problem is the most important way to avoid this pitfall, as is the case in many other situations in pathology.

Metastatic small cell carcinoma cells can look exactly like medulloblastoma/PNET cells, and special stains and clinical correlation are required to interpret them **(Fig. 5-24)**. This situation is mainly a problem in middle age and older adults who may have small cell carcinoma of the lung. They do not

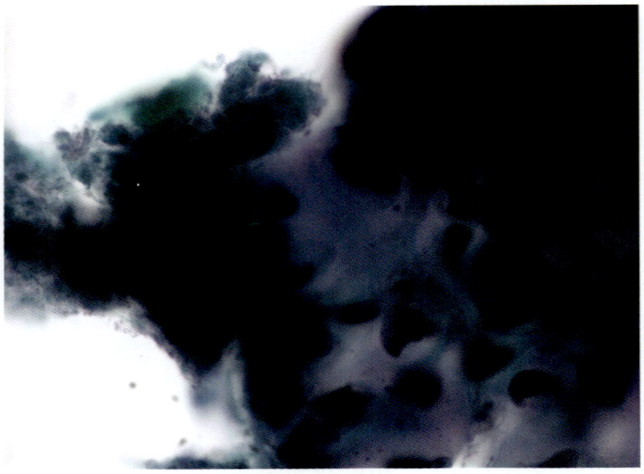

Figure 5-23. Chondrocytes: A group of chondrocytes with dark and angular nuclei are seen within their basophilic chondroid matrix, which altogether may be mistaken for metastatic adenocarcinoma with mucin (Papanicolaou; original magnification: 400×).

pose a problem in the pediatric population due to the absence of small cell carcinoma in this age group, although other solid small blue cell neoplasms, such as neuroblastoma can rarely be seen in the CSF. These cells in general have small hyperchromatic elongated or angular nuclei with coarse chromatin pattern and inconspicuous or small nucleoli. They have very small amount of barely visible cytoplasm, resulting in a high nucleus-to-cytoplasm ratio. They may form small groups composed of a few cells, in which nuclear molding can be identified. Mitotic figures and apoptotic debris may be seen.

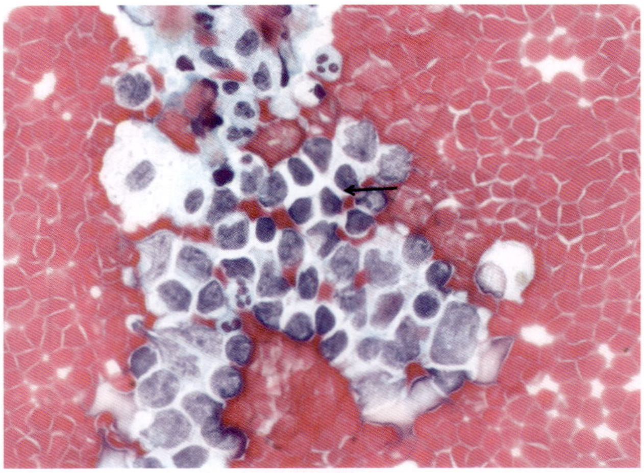

Figure 5-24. Metastatic small cell carcinoma: Malignant cells are only about twice the size of erythrocytes and leukocytes and have inconspicuous nucleoli, if any, and small amount of cytoplasm based on the narrow distance among the nuclei, many of which show nuclear molding (*arrow*). Although this is a large epithelioid group, identical cells can be seen in PNET/medulloblastoma (Papanicolaou; original magnification: 400×).

Primary CNS Neoplasms

Even though the idea of diagnosing primary CNS neoplasms by CSF cytology sounds very logical and it is possible to find several studies in the literature evaluating the use of CSF cytology in this context, in practice, it does not go much beyond wishful thinking with the exception of a few specific situations where CSF cytology is useful. The main context where primary CNS neoplasms are identified in the CSF is the follow-up cytologic evaluation for the assessment of CNS seeding, effectiveness of treatment, and identification of recurrences in previously diagnosed neoplasms that are well known for CSF spread. These are mainly medulloblastoma and germinoma.

Small blue cells with angulated nuclei, coarse chromatin pattern, inconspicuous nucleoli, and inconspicuous cytoplasm, resulting in high nucleus-to-cytoplasm ratios, indicate *medulloblastoma* in a pediatric patient with previous history or a cerebellar mass, *pineoblastoma* if there is a pineal mass, or *retinoblastoma* if there is an intraocular mass **(Fig. 5-25)**. The latter can infiltrate the optic nerve and make its way to the subarachnoid space around the optic nerve. On the other hand, in an older adult, metastatic small cell carcinoma, which has essentially the same cytologic appearance, should be ruled out. Clinical history and radiologic findings, as well as the presence of a lung mass or a previous

List of Findings/Checklist for Primary CNS Neoplasms

AT A GLANCE

- Medulloblastoma
- Pineoblastoma
- Retinoblastoma
- Germinoma
- Others

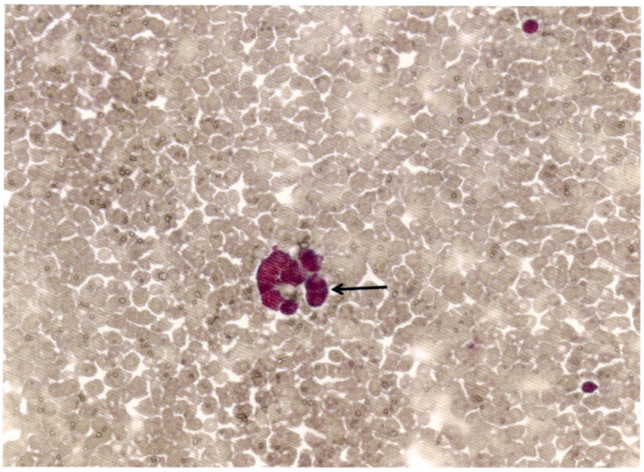

Figure 5-25. Medulloblastoma: Cells similar to those shown in Figure 5-24, that is, slightly larger than erythrocytes, with high nucleus-to-cytoplasm ratios, small amount of cytoplasm and inconspicuous nucleoli, are seen. They are somewhat dyscohesive relative to those of small cell carcinoma in Figure 5-24. They also show nuclear molding (*arrow*) (Romanowsky; original magnification: 400×).

diagnosis, should help favor the metastasis. In addition, for a metastatic small cell carcinoma to present in the CSF, it has to present as meningeal carcinomatosis or as a mass lesion that infiltrates the leptomeninges. Likewise, medulloblastoma has a tendency to infiltrate the leptomeninges and result in CSF and craniospinal seeding. If additional unstained slides with enough cells are present, cytokeratin immunohistochemistry can be performed to identify the carcinomatous nature of these cells. Synaptophysin may not be useful in this context as medulloblastoma is largely positive for synaptophysin, like the small cell carcinoma. In children, metastatic embryonal rhabdomyosarcoma and primitive neuroectodermal tumor/Ewing sarcoma are other considerations with similar cytologic features.[34]

Germinoma[35,36] may imitate a lymphoid process due to the presence of a reactive lymphoid infiltrate and admixed individual large cells, which represent the malignant cells. The large cells can also mimic carcinoma cells due to their round nuclei and prominent nucleoli. The immunohistochemistry for OCT4 or SALL-4 should be positive for germinoma cells, but experience is limited, if any, on their application in cytology. The best approach is a comprehensive one that takes into account all the clinical and radiologic findings, along with pathologic features.

In most cases of CSF cytology with significant findings, especially with malignant cells, there is usually a previous history or diagnosis, allowing a targeted approach with the knowledge of what is being looked for. This makes the interpretation of the findings easier.

Other primary neoplasms that can be identified in the CSF, but relatively rarely, are glial neoplasms,[35–37] including ependymoma,[38,39] pilocytic astrocytoma,[40] pleomorphic xanthoastrocytoma,[41] and oligodendroglioma[35] **(Fig. 5-26)**, as well as choroid plexus neoplasms,[42] meningioma,[37] and melanocytic lesions.[43] Intraoperative CSF sampling has been used to perform staging as part of surgery for primary neoplasms to identify medulloblastoma/PNET, ependymoma, and pilocytic astrocytoma.[44] As in the case of tissue diagnosis, the presence of a few meningothelial cells should not be considered diagnostic of meningioma, as nonneoplastic meningothelial cells can be present as contaminants **(Fig. 5-27)**. Likewise, if the needle enters the neuroglial parenchyma during the procedure, neurons and glial cells may be seen[32] and

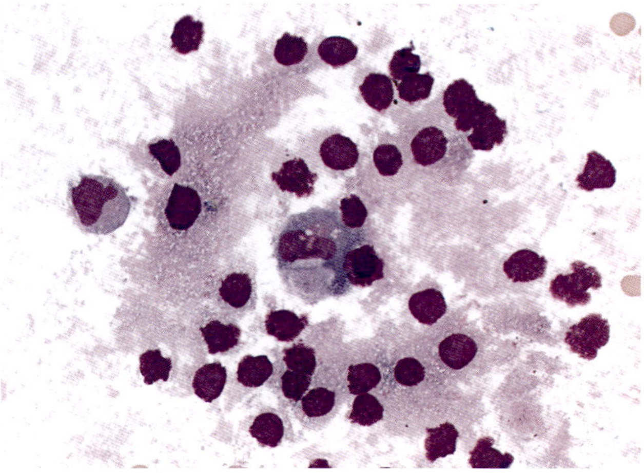

Figure 5-26. Oligodendroglioma: A loose group of round nuclei are seen in a granular background formed by their disintegrating cytoplasms. They are slightly larger than mature lymphocytes based on the comparison with the erythrocytes on the right and their chromatin pattern is not as clumped as in mature lymphocytes. The patient had a previous diagnosis of oligodendroglioma with extensive leptomeningeal infiltration (Romanowsky; original magnification: 400×).

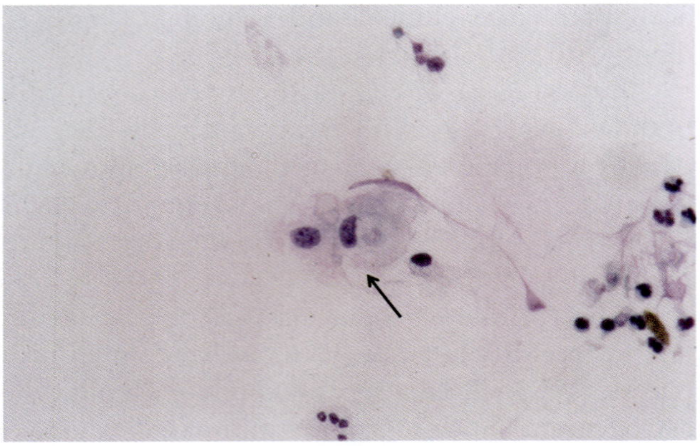

Figure 5-27. Meningothelial cells: A loose whorl formation attempt is present by two large epithelioid cells (*arrow*) and may mimic cell-in-cell configuration of metastatic carcinoma. They have finely granular and uniform chromatin. There was no history or clinical/radiologic evidence of mass lesions in other organs, though this does not necessarily exclude the possibility of metastatic carcinoma (Papanicolaou; original magnification: 400×).

should not be interpreted as evidence of a primary neoplasm **(Fig. 5-28)**. Neurons, due to their prominent nucleoli and cytoplasmic lipofuscin pigment, can be mistaken for melanoma cells. They are usually associated with a small amount of surrounding

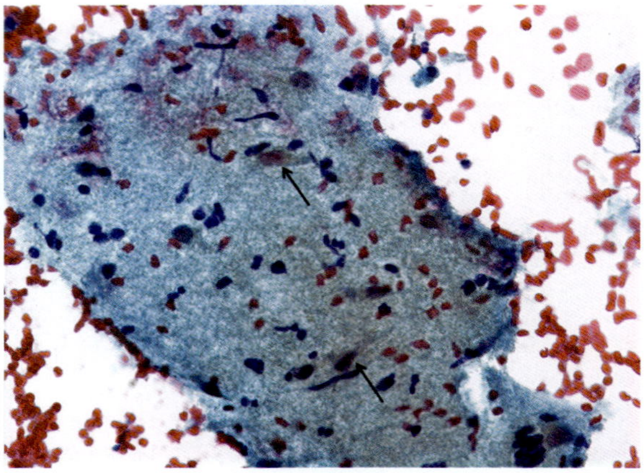

Figure 5-28. Neuroglial tissue fragment: A fragment of neuroglial tissue is seen in this shunt aspiration fluid. Neuropil is loosely textured and fibrillary, mimicking fibrin. Close evaluation shows different types of nuclei, representing glial cells. Neurons (*arrows*) are also present with their somewhat triangular cytoplasms and dusty brown lipofuscin pigment, and should not be mistaken for malignant cells, such as melanoma (Papanicolaou; original magnification: 200×).

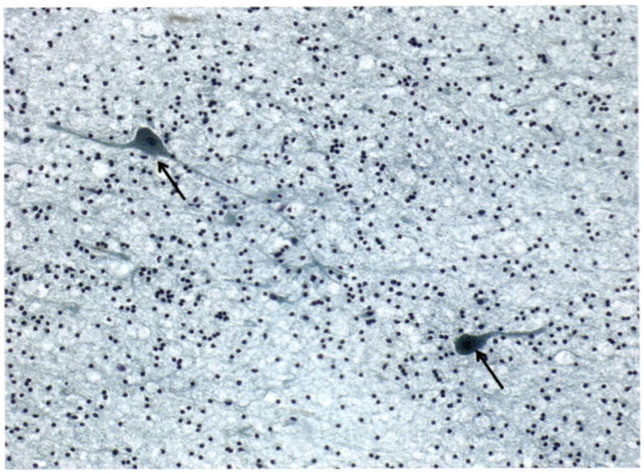

Figure 5-29. Cerebellar tissue: This CSF from a patient with cerebellar tonsillar herniation contains abundant small round cells representing the internal granule cells and should not be mistaken for inflammation, lymphoma, or a small blue cell neoplasm. Two Purkinje cells (*arrows*) are also present. The field is reminiscent of a smear preparation due to high cellularity. The fine, lacy fibrillarity in the background represents neuropil (Papanicolaou; original magnification: 100×).

neuropil. Neuropil may be difficult to recognize, as its fine fibrillarity and dispersed appearance may mimic proteinaceous or fibrinous material. Neuropil and neuroglial cells can be present and can be abundant in cases of infarct. Especially in cerebellar tonsillar herniation, the ischemic friable tonsillar tissue may fall into the spinal subarachnoid space to present in the CSF **(Fig. 5-29)**. They should not be mistaken for a glial neoplasm.

References

1. Bigner SH, Johnston WW. *Cytopathology of the Central Nervous System*. Chicago, IL: ASCP Press; 1994.
2. Koss LG, Melamed MR. *Koss' Diagnostic Cytopathology and Its Histopathologic Bases*. Baltimore, MD: Lippincott Williams & Wilkins; 2006.
3. DeMay RM. *The Art and Science of Cytopathology*. Chicago, IL: ASCP Press; 2011.
4. Walts AE. Cerebrospinal fluid cytology: selected issues. *Diagn Cytopathol*. 1992;8:394–408.
5. Simon RP, Abele JS. Spinal-fluid pleocytosis estimated by the Tyndall effect. *Ann Intern Med*. 1978;89:75–76.
6. Spriggs AI, Boddington MM. Leukaemic cells in cerebrospinal fluid. *Br J Haematol* 1959;5:83–91.
7. Nies BA, Malmgren RA, Chu EW, et al. Cerebrospinal fluid cytology in patients with acute leukemia. *Cancer*. 1965;18: 1385–1391.
8. Kuberski T. Eosinophils in the cerebrospinal fluid. *Ann Intern Med*. 1979;91:70–75.
9. Ross JS, Magro C, Szyfelbein W, et al. Cerebrospinal fluid pleocytosis in aseptic meningitis: cytomorphic and immunocytochemical features. *Diagn Cytopathol*. 1991;7:532–535.

10. Pelc S, De Maertelaere E, Denolin-Reubens R. CSF cytology of acute viral meningitis and meningoencephalitis. *Eur Neurol*. 1981;20:95–102.

11. Jeren T, Beus I. Characteristics of cerebrospinal fluid in tuberculous meningitis. *Acta Cytol*. 1982;26:678–680.

12. Teoh R, O'Mahony G, Yeung VT. Polymorphonuclear pleocytosis in the cerebrospinal fluid during chemotherapy for tuberculous meningitis. *J Neurol*. 1986;233:237–241.

13. Razavi-Encha F, Fleury-Feith J, Gherardi R, et al. Cytologic features of cerebrospinal fluid in Lyme disease. *Acta Cytol*. 1987;31:439–440.

14. Evans H. Cytology of Mollaret meningitis. *Diagn Cytopathol*. 1993;9:373–376.

15. Teot LA, Sexton CW. Mollaret's meningitis: case report with immunocytochemical and polymerase chain reaction amplification studies. *Diagn Cytopathol*. 1996;15:345–348.

16. Schluterman KO, Fassas AB, Van Hemert RL, et al. Multiple myeloma invasion of the central nervous system. *Arch Neurol*. 2004;61:1423–1429.

17. Kraft R, Altermatt HJ, Nguyen-Tran Q. Differential diagnosis of atypical plasma cells in the cerebrospinal fluid. *Deutsche Medizinische Wochenschrift*. 1989;114:1729–1733.

18. Fukushima T, Sumazaki R, Koike K, et al. A magnetic resonance abnormality correlating with permeability of the blood-brain barrier in a child with chemical meningitis during central nervous system prophylaxis for acute leukemia. *Ann Hematol*. 1999;78:564–567.

19. Zeman D, Adam P, Kalistova H, et al. Cerebrospinal fluid cytologic findings in multiple sclerosis. A comparison between patient subgroups. *Acta Cytol*. 2001;45:51–59.

20. Buruma OJ, Janson HL, Den Bergh FA, et al. Blood-stained cerebrospinal fluid: traumatic puncture or haemorrhage? *J Neurol Neurosurg Psychiatr*. 1981;44:144–147.

21. Craver RD. The cytology of cerebrospinal fluid associated with neonatal intraventricular hemorrhage. *Pediatr Pathol Lab Med*. 1996;16:713–719.

22. Fernandes SP, Penchansky L. Tumorlike clusters of immature cells in cerebrospinal fluid of infants. *Pediatr Pathol Lab Med*. 1996;16:721–729.

23. Bernad PG, Szyfelbein WM, Weiss HD, et al. Diagnosis of cryptococcal meningitis by cytologic methods: an old technique revisited. *Neurology*. 1980;30:102–105.

24. Cohen J. Comparison of the sensitivity of three methods for the rapid identification of *Cryptococcus neoformans*. *J Clin Pathol*. 1984;37:332–334.

25. Williamson JD, Silverman JF, Mallak CT, et al. Atypical cytomorphologic appearance of *Cryptococcus neoformans*: a report of five cases. *Acta Cytol*. 1996;40:363–370.

26. Preissig SH, Buhaug J. Corpora amylacea in cerebrospinal fluid. A source of possible diagnostic error. *Acta Cytol*. 1978;22:511–514.

27. Gupta PK, Gupta PC, Roy S, et al. Herpes simplex encephalitis, cerebrospinal fluid cytology studies. Two case reports. *Acta Cytol*. 1972;16:563–565.

28. Petry F, Torzewski M, Bohl J, et al. Early diagnosis of Acanthamoeba infection during routine cytological examination of cerebrospinal fluid. *J Clin Microbiol*. 2006;44:1903–1904.

29. Cetin N, Blackall D. *Naegleria fowleri* Meningoencephalitis. *Blood*. 2012;119:3658

30. Sherwani RK, Abrari A, Jayrajpuri ZS, et al. Intracranial hydatidosis. Report of a case diagnosed on cerebrospinal fluid cytology. *Acta Cytol*. 2003;47:506–508.

31. Bigner SH, Johnston WW. The diagnostic challenge of tumors manifested initially by the shedding of cells into cerebrospinal fluid. *Acta Cytol*. 1984;28:29–36.

32. Mathios AJ, Nielsen SL, Barrett D, et al. Cerebrospinal fluid cytomorphology identification of benign cells originating in the central nervous system. *Acta Cytol*. 1977;21:403–412.

33. Leiman G, Klein C, Berry AV. Cells of nucleus pulposus in cerebrospinal fluid: a case report. *Acta Cytol*. 1980;24:347–349.

34. Geisinger KR, Hajdu SI, Helson L. Exfoliative cytology of nonlymphoreticular neoplasms in children. *Acta Cytol*. 1984;28:16–28.

35. Naylor B. The cytologic diagnosis of cerebrospinal fluid. *Acta Cytol*. 1964;8:141–149.

36. Chhieng DC, Elgert P, Cohen JM, et al. Cytology of primary central nervous system neoplasms in cerebrospinal fluid specimens. *Diagn Cytopathol*. 2002;26:209–12,

37. Kline TS. Cytologic examination of the cerebrospinal fluid. *Cancer*. 1962;15:591–597.

38. Qian X, Goumnerova LC, De Girolami U, et al. Cerebrospinal fluid cytology in patients with ependymoma: a bi-institutional retrospective study. *Cancer*. 2008;114:307–314.

39. Moreno L, Pollack IF, Duffner PK, et al. Utility of cerebrospinal fluid cytology in newly diagnosed childhood ependymoma. *J Pediatr Hematol/Oncol*. 2010;32:515–518.

40. Browne TJ, Goumnerova LC, De Girolami U, et al. Cytologic features of pilocytic astrocytoma in cerebrospinal fluid specimens. *Acta Cytol*. 2004;48:3–8.

41. Lacoste-Collin L, d'Aure D, Aziza J, et al. Cerebrospinal fluid cytologic findings of a pleomorphic xanthoastrocytoma: a case report. *Acta Cytol*. 2010;54:871–874.

42. Kim K, Greenblatt SH, Robinson MG. Choroid plexus carcinoma. Report of a case with cytopathologic differential diagnosis. *Acta Cytol*. 1985;29:846–849.

43. Zunarelli E, Bettelli S, Reggiani-Bonetti L, et al. Cerebrospinal fluid cytology in a case of primary diffuse leptomeningeal and pineal melanocytic lesion, with histological confirmation. *Pathology*. 2010;42:292–295.

44. Souweidane MM, Morgenstern PF, Christos PJ, et al. Intraoperative arachnoid and cerebrospinal fluid sampling in children with posterior fossa brain tumors. *Neurosurgery*. 2009;65:72–78.

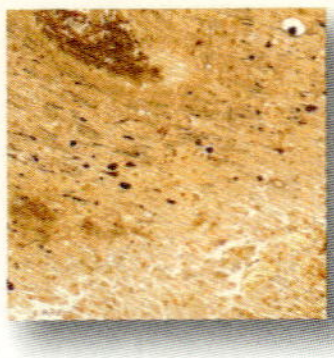
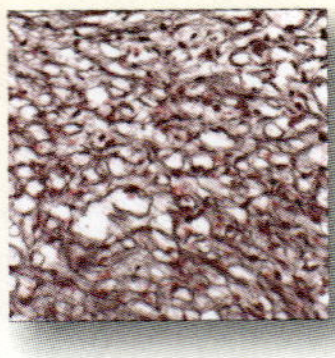
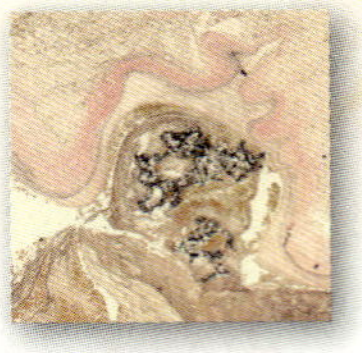

C H A P T E R 6

Histochemistry

Introduction

Together with the advances in immunohistochemistry (IHC), the need for and the use of classical histochemistry have diminished considerably. For instance, glial fibrillary acidic protein (GFAP) IHC has replaced phosphotungstic acid hematoxylin (PTAH) for the demonstration of astrocytic processes, and neurofilament IHC is being widely used instead of Bielschowsky silver stain for the evaluation of axons especially in surgical material such as the interpretation of biopsy tissue in demyelinating disease. Still, there are many traditional basic histochemical stains that are both practical and cost-efficient and that also provide important useful information in many lesions and supportive evidence for others. The following discussion provides the practical aspects of histochemistry as it applies to diagnostic use in neuropathology. While there are many staining methods for various components in tissues, only the most commonly used ones in daily practice are discussed here, with the understanding that different institutions and pathologists may prefer some over the others. More details and technical aspects are available in specialized texts.[1,2] Techniques used in muscle and nerve biopsy evaluation are discussed in their respective chapters. The details and meanings of the findings identified by these methods have been discussed in Chapter 2 "Microscopic Features" and will not be repeated here.

Bielschowsky and Other Silver Methods

Many silver impregnation methods are available, including Bielschowsky silver stain, Gallyas, and Palmgren methods.[3] Bielschowsky method is the most commonly used stain for the demonstration of axons and various accumulations and inclusions in the neuron, all of which stain black. It provides a means for assessing the axon structure and density. As such, it has a variety of uses. It helps identify and confirm *axonal spheroids*, irregularities, and swellings in diseases characterized by them, such as diffuse axonal injury, the periphery of infarcts **(Fig. 6-1)**, neuroaxonal dystrophy, and chemotherapy-induced leukoencephalopathy. It can be used to assess the presence and *density of axons* in demyelinating disorders, where there is relative preservation of axons, or in cases of subacute arteriosclerotic leukoencephalopathy, where the axonal density is also decreased. *Dystrophic neurites* with irregular swellings and distortions rather than actual axonal spheroids can be seen in the background in various neurodegenerative diseases such as Alzheimer's disease and Lewy body pathology and can be highlighted by Bielschowsky stain. However, they are better evaluated using more specific immunohistochemical markers such as tau and synuclein, depending on the disease process. In addition, many *cytoplasmic inclusions* are highlighted by Bielschowsky stain in neurodegenerative diseases (see Chapter 2). These range from neurofibrillary tangles to Pick bodies in neurons to glial cytoplasmic inclusions in corticobasal degeneration. Plaque pathology and plaque stages can be seen in detail **(Figs. 6-2 and 6-3)** with this stain, and it is a requirement for the neuropathologic diagnostic criteria, which are mainly based on the identification of neuritic plaques, used by Consortium to Establish a Registry for Alzheimer's Disease (CERAD),[4] while the evaluation of neurofibrillary tangle frequency and distribution is required for Braak staging[5] **(Fig. 6-3)**. Argyrophilic

List of Findings/Checklist for Silver Methods

AT A GLANCE

- Axons
  - Spheroids
  - Dystrophic axons
  - Density
  - Plaque pathology
- Accumulations/inclusions
  - Neurodegenerative diseases
  - Neuronal accumulations
  - Glial plaques
  - Glial inclusions
- Artifacts
- Pineal gland
- Cerebellum
  - Torpedoes
  - Empty baskets
  - Purkinje cell arborization
  - Grumose degeneration
  - Asteroids

grain disease diagnosis, as the name implies, is also made by the use of a silver stain to show the coils or grains of argyrophilic material. Similar to neuritic plaques, *astrocytic plaques* can form in corticobasal degeneration and are identified by silver methods. Other *glial accumulations* described as coils or thorns can also be highlighted in corticobasal

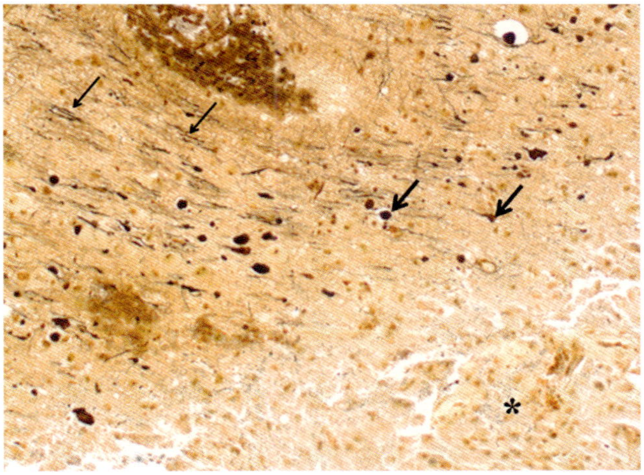

Figure 6-1. Axonal spheroids: The accumulation of axonal transport material in the axons (*thin arrows*) resulted in the formation of axonal spheroids (*thick arrows*) at the border of an infarct (*asterisk*) (Bielschowsky; original magnification: 200×).

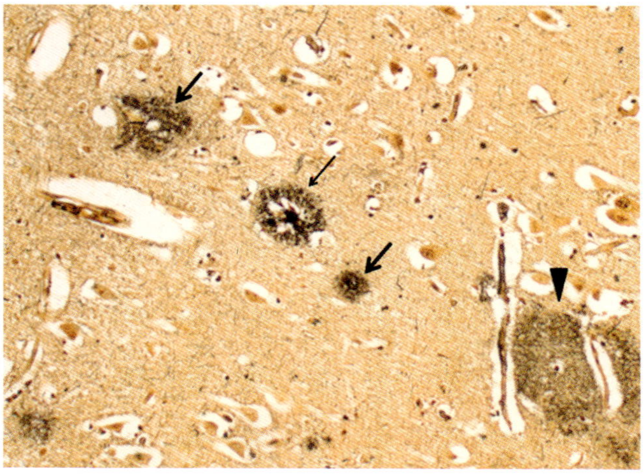

Figure 6-2. Plaques in Alzheimer's disease: Various stages of development are highlighted. The most typical mature neuritic plaque (*thin arrow*) has a central densely staining core corresponding to amyloid accumulation, sometimes with a halo formation around it, separating it from the dystrophic neurites at its periphery. Other neuritic plaques (*thick arrows*) are without the dense core but still contain irregular thickened dystrophic neurites. A diffuse plaque (*arrow head*) is also seen and has a more homogeneous staining pattern without the irregularities and thickenings of the dystrophic neurites (Bielschowsky; original magnification: 200×).

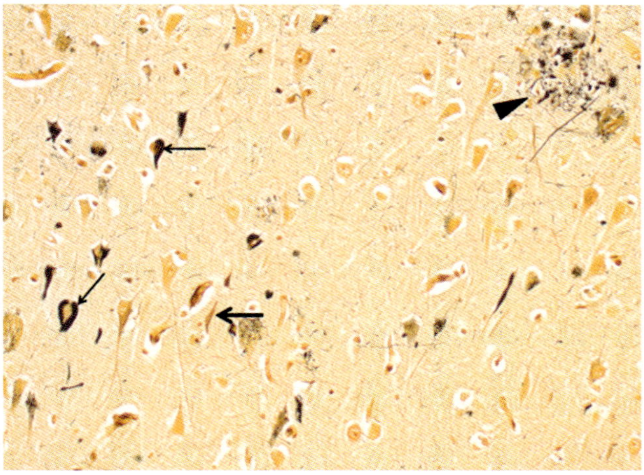

Figure 6-3. Neurofibrillary tangles: Cytoplasmic elongated black-staining structures next to neuron nuclei (*thin arrows*) represent neurofibrillary tangles. Some may be relatively pale and free in the neuropil (*thick arrow*). They represent the burnt-out tangles after the death of the neuron. A neuritic plaque is also seen (*arrow head*) (Bielschowsky; original magnification: 200×).

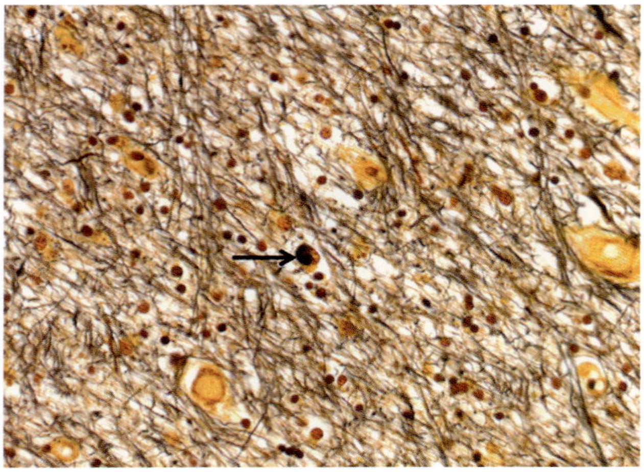

Figure 6-4. Glial cytoplasmic inclusion (*arrow*): The inclusion is seen in variable numbers in the cytoplasm of glial cells, as seen in an oligodendroglial cell in the white matter in this case of corticobasal degeneration (Bielschowsky; original magnification: 400×).

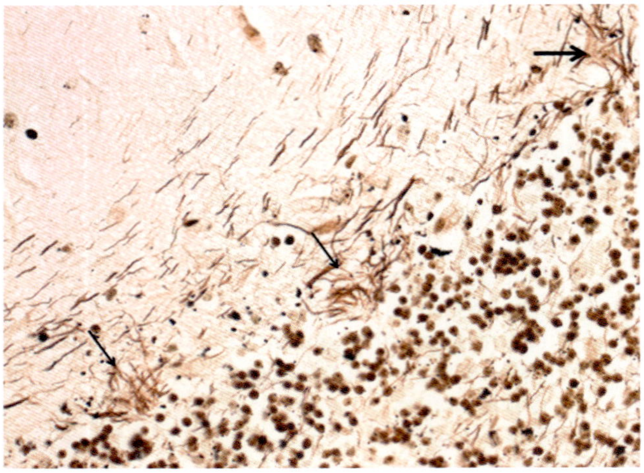

Figure 6-5. "Empty baskets": In disorders associated with the degeneration of Purkinje cell, the basket cells are seen without a Purkinje cell (*thin arrows*), indicating the drop-out of Purkinje cells. An intact Purkinje cell is seen together with its basket cell (*thick arrow*). Internal granule layer is in the bottom right; molecular layer is in the upper left (Bielschowsky; original magnification: 400×).

degeneration and in many other neurodegenerative diseases[6] **(Fig. 6-4)**.

Bielschowsky stain, in spite of its great help with many findings, can be difficult to appropriately perform with a high degree of consistency and requires experience. The differentiation can be very variable, from very faint staining to very dark staining with precipitates and *artifacts*, especially if it is not performed frequently enough to keep experience level high. The nuclei and vessel walls can stain and may cause confusion in interpretation. Especially, nuclei may appear as inclusions, or if the counterstaining is too pale, inclusions may be mistaken for nuclei. Therefore, careful evaluation and search are required. Standard Bielschowsky method can be modified, or Gallyas stain, another silver impregnation method, can be used to show the neurofibrillary tangles and plaque pathology better. Axonal staining tends to become less prominent in such modifications.

In the *pineal gland*, club-shaped terminal processes of pinocytes and pineocytomas are highlighted by Bielschowsky although this finding is of limited use in the light of location and good clinical and radiologic information. In cerebellum, evaluation of *cerebellar degeneration* and Purkinje cell loss can be facilitated by the identification of the so-called empty basket cells devoid of Purkinje cells **(Fig. 6-5)**. Torpedoes are also highlighted, just like axonal swellings in the white matter. The prominent arborization of Purkinje cell dendrites can be highlighted when needed, as in the case of Menkes' disease. The grumose degeneration in the dentate nucleus is better identified with a silver stain showing the perineuronal granular swellings. Asteroid-like structures may be seen by Bielschowsky stain in the cerebellum of patients with Pelizaeus-Merzbacher disease.[7]

Myelin Stains

The most commonly used stain for myelin is Luxol fast blue (LFB). Since staining only myelin may be difficult to interpret in terms of orientation to the particular areas on the section without contrast with the background and to facilitate identification of neurons and other accumulations, it can be combined with PAS and cresyl violet (LFB/PAS/CV), or with PAS, Nissl stain, and hematoxylin.

Myelin stains are used to evaluate the presence or loss of myelin especially in the pale areas in the white matter that may be suspected of having demyelination on routine H&E stain. Many lesions that are associated with myelin loss will be highlighted

List of Findings/Checklist for Myelin Stains

AT A GLANCE

- Myelin loss
  - Pattern
  - Location
- Demyelinating disease
- Infarct
- Tract degeneration
- Periventricular leukomalacia
- Perinatal telencephalic leukoencephalopathy/ Periventricular leukomalacia
- Leukodystrophy/dysmyelination
- Hypothalamic hamartoma
- Dysplastic gangliocytoma of the cerebellum
- Hypermyelination
- Malformations of inferior olivary and dentate nuclei
- Central and peripheral myelin

as pale areas by these stains. These range from classical multiple sclerosis plaques to progressive multifocal leukoencephalopathy (PML) lesions to carbon monoxide poisoning. The *location* and *pattern* of myelin loss are important and should be correlated with the clinical and radiologic information for the maximum yield to be obtained from the interpretation (see "White Matter Changes and Myelin Disorders" in Chapter 2). Whether myelin loss is focal, diffuse, multifocal, perivascular, or in some other pattern such as concentric or targetoid are important to note and can certainly be better evaluated with myelin stains. There are also methods to selectively show the degenerating myelin, for example, Marchi method; however, they are relatively difficult to perform on a routine basis and are usually not necessary for the evaluation of tissues and disorders encountered in daily practice.

One important use of myelin stains in especially small biopsy tissue is the evaluation of an apparently nonneoplastic lesion with many macrophages, with or without other inflammatory cells. The differential diagnosis of infarct versus myelin loss requires a myelin stain coupled with an axon stain, such as Bielschowsky silver stain or neurofilament IHC, to show the preferential loss of myelin with a relative preservation of axons in *demyelinating lesions* and loss of both myelin and axons in *infarcts*. The myelin debris ingested by macrophages can be seen with its blue color in earlier stages (gitter cells) but assumes a PAS-positive quality in later stages with further breakdown. One of the more common uses of myelin stains is the evaluation of spinal cord cross sections to better identify *tract degenerations* (see "Tract Degeneration" in Chapter 2).

LFB/PAS/CV stain can be used to outline the lesions of *periventricular leukomalacia* better as a pale center due to myelin loss and increased PAS staining at its edges, due to PAS-positive debris in the macrophages around the lesion or as a patch if there are many macrophages. *Perinatal telencephalic leukoencephalopathy*, sometimes used interchangeably with periventricular leukomalacia, but refers more to lesions without cavitation or tissue destruction, and with diffuse gliosis, myelin pallor, and mulberries, can also be better highlighted by an LFB/PAS/CV. Identification of myelin loss and myelin components in macrophages is facilitated by myelin stains in *leukodystrophies/dysmyelinating disorders* and disorders associated with *myelin breakdown*, such as GM1 and 2 gangliosidoses and neuronal ceroid lipofuscinosis (Batten's disease).

Evaluation of myelinated axons can provide interesting and useful findings in some other situations. For instance, in *hypothalamic hamartoma*, myelin stains show the absence of the usual thick myelinated bundles of normal hypothalamus in the hamartoma, helping with the differential diagnosis from normal hypothalamic tissue, as hypothalamic hamartomas can appear notoriously unremarkable.[8] In *dysplastic gangliocytoma of the cerebellum* (Lhermitte-Duclos disease), while the typical radiologic, gross, and histopathologic features are characteristic, myelin stains can also highlight additional features by showing the abnormal orientation of the myelinated axons in the molecular layer,[9] where they are aligned perpendicular to the pial surface in the superficial layers and parallel to it in the deeper layers. *Hypermyelination* in cerebral cortex (etat fibromyelinique) and status marmoratus (marbling) in thalamus and basal ganglia are better highlighted.[10] Abnormalities in the myelinated fibers associated with the *malformations* of the brain stem nuclei, especially inferior olivary nuclei as well as dentate nuclei, can be highlighted by a myelin stain and support the abnormal development in these structures.[7]

The staining characteristics of *central myelin* produced by oligodendroglia and of *peripheral myelin* produced by Schwann cells are different, with the latter staining darker blue with LFB/PAS/CV stain. This difference is best seen in spinal cord and brainstem sections that also include spinal and cranial nerves, respectively, and therefore showing the Obersteiner-Redlich zone that is the transition zone between the central and peripheral myelination.[11] The disorders involving the peripheral myelin are discussed in Chapter 9.

Lipids

The most important consideration in the identification of lipids in tissues is advance planning and securing frozen tissue. Working with frozen tissue is a routine part of skeletal muscle biopsy processing, but it may easily be overlooked in surgical specimens and even in autopsies. The diagnosis and classification of many metabolic inherited disorders, such as leukodystrophies, are now made by genetic and biochemical testing, and reliance on lipid stains has decreased. Nonetheless, in some cases, demonstration of lipid may be useful for diagnosis, such as fat embolism or identification of myelin breakdown products. Especially in autopsy cases, the tissue saved in formalin can be rinsed in water and samples can be frozen to perform lipid stains. This is not possible in paraffin-embedded tissues as the lipids dissolve in the solvent solutions during processing.

List of Findings/Checklist for Lipids

AT A GLANCE

- Lipids
  - Oil Red O
    - Neutral lipids
    - Tissue damage
    - Myelin degeneration
    - Fat embolism
    - Hemangioblastoma
    - Clear cell renal cell carcinoma
  - Sudan Black B
    - Neutral and complex lipids
    - Normal and degenerating myelin
    - Leukodystrophies
    - Others
    - Lipofuscin

Very briefly, *lipids* are broadly divided into two groups[12,13]: simple (neutral or nonpolar) lipids and complex (polar) lipids. Simple lipids, or *neutral lipids* as they are more commonly known, contain fatty acids, cholesterol, cholesteryl esters, and glycerides, such as triglycerides. *Complex lipids* are further divided into two broad groups as phospholipids (or glycerophospholipids) including sphingomyelin and glycolipids, which include cerebrosides, sulfatides, and gangliosides.

Mainly two lipid stains are used in routine diagnostic practice. More commonly used *oil red O* (ORO) is a general practical stain for neutral lipids and stains them bright red. It provides a good tool to evaluate the lipids that are released when there is *tissue damage* **(Fig. 6-6)** or the lipids that are stored in mature adipose tissue or skeletal muscle (see Chapter 9). As such, the neutral lipids that are formed after *myelin degeneration* can be highlighted, providing a means of identifying areas of myelin degeneration. The foamy cells of *hemangioblastoma*[14] and the cells of *renal cell carcinoma*[15] contain neutral lipids and can be stained by ORO. This may provide an additional tool to distinguish these neoplasms from glial neoplasms and other carcinomas; however, there are immunohistochemical markers that can be used as part of an

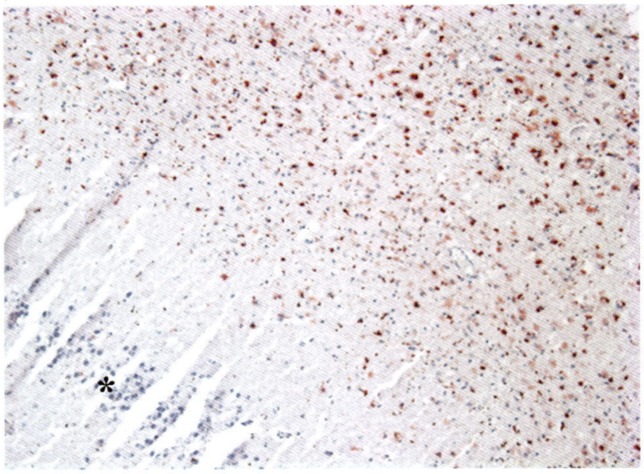

Figure 6-6. Neutral lipids: Pyramidal cell layer of hippocampus shows extensive degeneration and lipid accumulation, seen as bright red globules, in this case of Alpers-Huttenlocher syndrome (Alpers' disease; progressive neuronal degeneration of childhood with liver disease). Dentate gyrus is seen in bottom left (*asterisk*) (Oil red O; original magnification: 100×).

immunohistochemical panel to provide more specific results. On the other hand, the use of ORO during intraoperative consultation has been suggested as a rapid and practical tool in appropriate cases of clear cell neoplasms.[16]

Sudan Black B stains both the neutral lipids and complex lipids. As such, it stains both the *degenerating and normal myelin*. As such, it can also provide a means of evaluating the myelin and myelin loss. Various components that it stains show differences in color and staining quality, though it may be difficult to distinguish these details. While neutral lipids stain blue-black, phospholipids may be gray, and myelin components may appear bronze if examined under polarized light. A group of *leukodystrophies* has been historically referred to as orthochromatic leukodystrophies based on their sudanophilic staining (although ORO can also be used for this purpose), including adrenoleukodystrophy, Pelizaeus-Merzbacher disease, and Cockayne disease, as well as others, while some others have been characterized by the presence of more characteristic features, such as globoid cell leukodystrophy and metachromatic leukodystrophy.[7] GM1 and GM2 gangliosidoses, neuronal ceroid lipofuscinosis (Batten's disease),[17] as it also stains *lipofuscin*, Niemann-Pick disease,[18] mucopolysaccharidoses, Fabry disease, and Farber disease, among many others, are characterized by sudanophilic material.[7]

Periodic Acid-Schiff (PAS) Stain

Periodic acid-Schiff (PAS) stains glycoproteins and glycogen. It is performed before (PAS without diastase) and after (PAS with diastase; PAS/D) diastase treatment. If the staining is present without diastase but does not occur after diastase reaction, this confirms that the staining substance is glycogen. In addition, many other intracellular and extracellular accumulations, as well as tissue components, can be identified with PAS. Glycogen is diastase-sensitive, while other PAS-positive substances, mainly glycoproteins, are diastase-resistant. Therefore, *glycogen accumulation* in metabolic hereditary diseases, such as Pompe disease (type II glycogenosis), can be suspected with this method. Abundant cytoplasmic glycogen is a characteristic feature of several neoplasms that have clear cells. *Clear cell meningioma,*[19] *germinoma,*[20] and *primitive neuroectodermal tumor (PNET)/Ewing sarcoma* (peripheral PNET)[21] that can metastasize to the central nervous system (CNS), directly infiltrate it arising from

List of Findings/Checklist for PAS Stain

AT A GLANCE

PAS Positive Diastase Sensitive

- Glycogen
  - Glycogen storage diseases
  - Neoplasms
    - Clear cell meningioma
    - Germinoma
    - PNET/Ewing sarcoma
  - Amebae

PAS Positive Diastase Resistant

- Predominantly extracellular accumulations
  - Secretory meningioma
  - Yolk sac tumor
  - Eosinophilic granular bodies
  - Myxopapillary ependymoma
  - Papillary tumor of the pineal region
  - CADASIL
  - Basement membranes
- Predominantly cytoplasmic accumulations
  - Alveolar soft part sarcoma
  - Pituitary adenoma
  - Granular cell tumor
  - Lafora bodies
  - Acute lead poisoning
  - Neuroserpin inclusions
- Macrophages
  - Whipple disease
  - Amebae
  - Dysmyelinations/leukodystrophies
  - Infantile osteopetrosis
  - Demyelination
- Others
  - Mucin
  - Fungi
  - Mycobacteria
  - Parasites

skull bones, or may arise as a primary neoplasm in the dura mater are characterized by cytoplasmic glycogen, a feature that can be used to support the diagnosis in the appropriate context. In reality, however, each of these neoplasms has more specific and diagnostic immunohistochemical phenotypes, and PAS is only rarely needed at best.

Several accumulations are PAS-positive and diastase-resistant and constitute characteristic features for some other neoplasms. The eosinophilic material (also called pseudopsammoma bodies) in *secretory meningioma*[22] is one of them. PAS after diastase treatment helps identify easier the intra- and extracytoplasmic globules in *yolk sac tumor*.[23] Likewise, *eosinophilic granular bodies* seen in various low-grade CNS neoplasms, such as ganglioglioma and pleomorphic xanthoastrocytoma, are also highlighted by PAS, and they are diastase-resistant. In addition, in hemangioblastomas, cytoplasmic hyaline inclusions can be identified.[16] Collagen balloons of *myxopapillary ependymoma* are also PAS-positive and diastase-resistant. Many examples of *papillary tumor of the pineal region* have cytoplasmic PAS-positive, diastase-resistant granules.[24] Granular PAS-positive, diastase-resistant extracellular accumulations in the vessel walls are seen in cerebral autosomal dominant arteriopathy with subcortical infarcts and leukoencephalopathy (*CADASIL*).[25] They are associated with the basement membranes and smooth muscle layer. PAS is a simple method to reveal the presence of *basement membranes*. It can make the vascular endothelial basement membranes and its reduplications more prominent, allowing the evaluation of vessel wall infiltration by inflammatory cells. It provides a simple way to show the presence of basement membrane in papillary choroid plexus neoplasms, in contrast to papillary ependymomas, contributing to their differential diagnosis.

Intracytoplasmic crystalloid inclusions in *alveolar soft part sarcoma* can be highlighted by PAS and are diastase-resistant.[26] PAS-positive, diastase-resistant cytoplasmic granules in *thyrotroph and corticotroph adenomas* of the anterior pituitary represent lysosomes.[27] They are a characteristic feature of these adenomas, although they may not be very obvious and may be difficult to identify even with PAS stain. *Granular cell tumor* in posterior pituitary is characterized by cytoplasms packed with lysosomes, which are made more prominent by a PAS stain. They are diastase resistant. The so-called angulate bodies that can be identified in the stroma of these neoplasms also have similar staining features. *Lafora body* is PAS positive and diastase resistant,[28] with fragmented edges. In *lead poisoning*,[29] PAS may highlight globular diastase-resistant material within the perivascular proteinaceous material and in the cytoplasm of astrocytes. Neuronal inclusion bodies (Collins bodies) seen in *dementia with neuroserpin accumulation* (familial encephalopathy with neuroserpin inclusion bodies) are also PAS positive and diastase resistant, in addition to being neuroserpin positive by IHC.[30]

Small groups of macrophages within the parenchyma may represent *Whipple disease*. These macrophages contain cytoplasmic PAS-positive granular material representing the degenerating bacteria,[31] which may also be Grocott (Gomori) methenamine silver (GMS) positive and gram-positive, although the latter may not be useful due to bacterial degeneration.[7] It may be difficult to distinguish *amebic microorganisms* from these macrophages, as well as from other *macrophages* with cytoplasmic debris. The PAS positivity in amebae is due at least in part to glycogen accumulation[7] and is therefore diastase sensitive, and they are negative for macrophage markers by IHC. Their perivascular location, necrotic and hemorrhagic background, and clinicopathologic context are helpful. *Gaucher cells*[32] and macrophages in *Krabbe's disease*[33] can be highlighted by PAS due to the cytoplasmic accumulations. *Infantile osteopetrosis* can have neuronal cytoplasmic lipofuscin-like pigment accumulation that is PAS positive and diastase resistant and is seen as eosinophilic round ill-defined inclusions.[34]

PAS is commonly combined with LFB, a myelin stain that stains myelin blue. Macrophages in the acute stages of a *demyelinating process* contain myelin debris that stains blue with LFB. In the later stages, PAS-positive, diastase-resistant debris representing degraded myelin predominates. LFB/PAS stain can be additionally useful in subtle cases of *periventricular leukomalacia* by outlining these areas better as a pale center and increased staining at the edges, due to PAS-positive debris in the macrophages around the lesion or as a patch if there are many macrophages. The mulberries can be identified easier by PAS in *telencephalic leukoencephalopathy*, where the lesions are typically without cavitation and tissue destruction but with diffuse gliosis.

Other common PAS-positive, diastase-resistant materials are mucin and cell walls of fungal microorganisms, which are identified by more specific stains. When they are abundant, mycobacteria can be seen as PAS-positive bacteria and should not be confused with other bacilli in cases of *Mycobacterium* avium intracellulare infections, where microorganisms tend to be abundant in macrophages. Parasites such as Schistosoma and Echinococcus are also PAS positive, and especially the degenerating fragments of the former can be highlighted in the inflammatory background.

Reticulin Stain

Reticulin stain uses argyrophil silver techniques for the demonstration of these fine fibers associated with type I and III collagens.[35] In general, reticulin fibers tend to surround groups of cells in *epithelial neoplasms* and highlight the acinar/glandular structures in adenocarcinomas, while they are mainly pericellular in *mesenchymal neoplasms*, surrounding individual cells or small groups of cells. Therefore, a rich reticulin network is seen in sarcomas, while it is sparse in carcinomas and limited to vascular structures in many glial neoplasms. It is useful in identifying the sarcomatous component in *gliosarcoma*, resulting in a biphasic pattern, that is, reticulin-rich sarcomatous areas admixed and alternating with reticulin-poor glial areas. Some mainly low-grade glial neoplasms are characterized by a rich reticulin network, which is useful in supporting their diagnoses, even though it is a result of their superficial location and close association with and infiltration of the overlying leptomeninges, creating this reticulin-rich reaction. *Desmoplastic infantile ganglioglioma/astrocytoma,*[36] *pleomorphic xanthoastrocytoma,* and giant cell glioblastoma are characterized by areas of rich pericellular reticulin fibers.[37] Collagen balloons of *myxopapillary ependymoma* can be highlighted by reticulin stain, although they are usually obvious on H&E, and this staining does not provide additional crucial diagnostic information. *Desmoplastic/nodular medulloblastoma* has a rich reticulin network among the pale islands that are devoid of reticulin fibers.[38] It is a diagnostic feature of this medulloblastoma variant **(Fig. 6-7)**.

In *schwannoma*, reticulin is seen as pericellular staining, similar to collagen type IV. A similar feature

List of Findings/Checklist for Reticulin Stain

AT A GLANCE

- Carcinoma
- Sarcoma
- Gliosarcoma
- Desmoplastic infantile ganglioglioma/astrocytoma
- Pleomorphic xanthoastrocytoma
- Myxopapillary ependymoma
- Desmoplastic/nodular medulloblastoma
- Schwannoma
- Fibroblastic meningioma
- Melanocytoma
- Hemangiopericytoma/solitary fibrous tumor
- Hemangioblastoma
- Pituitary adenoma/hyperplasia/infarct
- Lymphoma
- Abscess
- Glioblastoma multiforme
- Gumma
- Necrotizing granuloma/tuberculosis

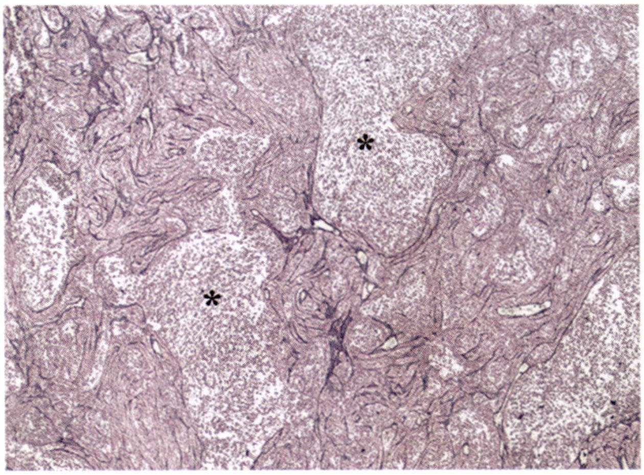

Figure 6-7. Desmoplastic medulloblastoma: More differentiated, reticulin-poor nodular islands (*asterisks*) are surrounded by reticulin-rich areas composed of cells with primitive neuroectodermal cytologic features (Reticulin; original magnification: 100×).

can be seen to some degree in *fibroblastic meningioma* but typically as a focal finding. It is probably more important in the differential diagnosis of schwannoma from melanocytoma, another spindle cell neoplasm that can mimic schwannoma and fibroblastic meningioma. In *melanocytoma*, reticulin is limited for the most part to perivascular areas. Papillary meningioma is characterized by papillary structures formed by perivascular neoplastic cells, mimicking pseudopapillae. They may in fact be formed artifactually as a result of separation of the loose tissue. The presence of rich perivascular reticulin and its radial extension into the cellular parenchyma surrounding the vessel is considered highly characteristic and is useful in distinguishing truly papillary meningiomas from otherwise artifactual pseudopapillary formations that may be seen in other types of meningioma.[39,40] This distinction is important as papillary meningiomas are malignant, that is, WHO grade III neoplasms.[41] In the evaluation of *hemangiopericytoma* (HPC)/*solitary fibrous tumor* (SFT), to distinguish HPC from SFT, the pericellular reticulin network favors HPC, while less prominent and mainly perivascular reticulin pattern favors SFT.[42] Many such neoplasms have hybrid or overlapping features, and reticulin also helps highlight their respective features in such neoplasms. *Hemangioblastoma* is typically associated with a prominent pericellular reticulin pattern **(Fig. 6-8)**, which can be used to support this diagnosis in small, distorted tissues. However, in addition to this reticular pattern, it also has a cellular variant in which reticulin fibers surround groups of cells **(Fig. 6-9)**. The latter can be associated with a higher likelihood of recurrence.[43]

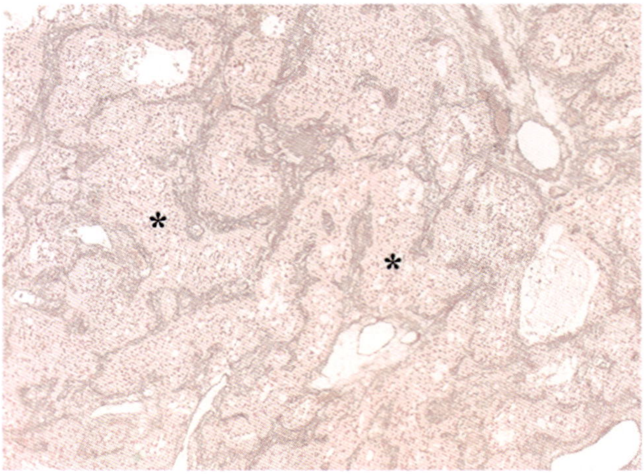

Figure 6-9. Hemangioblastoma: In contrast to the more typical reticular variant shown in Figure 6-8, cellular hemangioblastomas have a reticulin network that surrounds groups of cells (*asterisk*), mimicking an epithelial neoplasm (Reticulin; original magnification: 100×).

Evaluation of reticulin network is crucial in the diagnosis of *pituitary lesions*.[44] The normal nesting pattern of the anterior pituitary parenchyma **(Fig. 6-10)** is expanded and distorted in pituitary

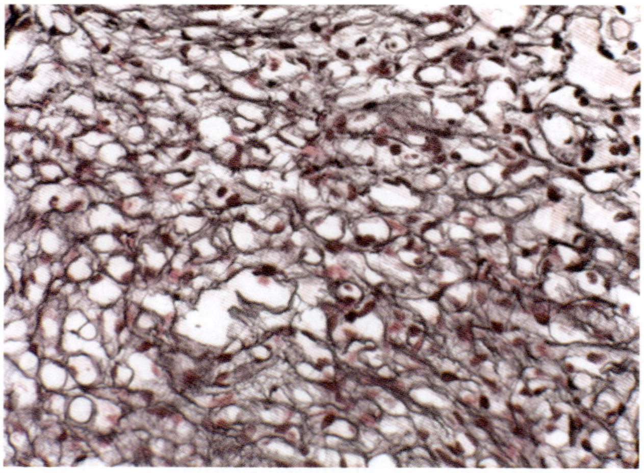

Figure 6-8. Hemangioblastoma: Pericellular reticulin pattern is typical of hemangioblastoma and is useful in the differential diagnosis of difficult cases (Reticulin; original magnification: 400×).

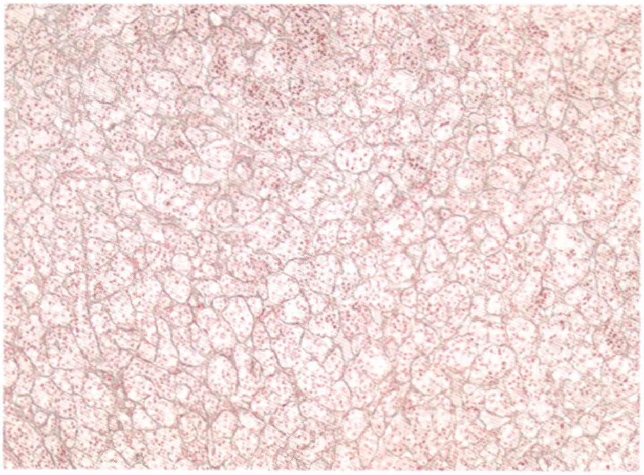

Figure 6-10. Anterior pituitary parenchyma: The orderly nesting pattern is highlighted (Reticulin; original magnification: 100×).

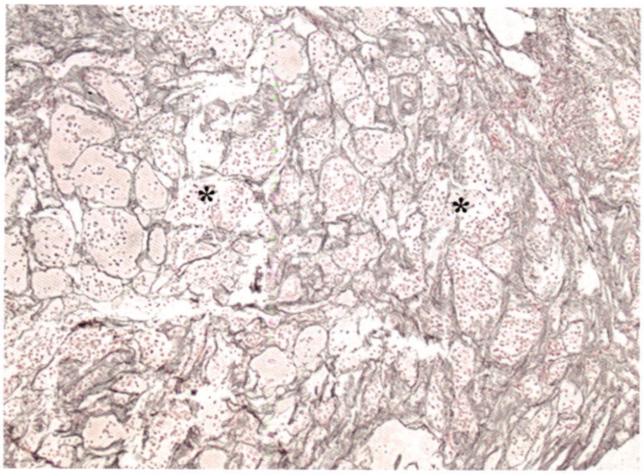

Figure 6-11. Hyperplastic anterior pituitary parenchyma: The usual orderly nesting pattern is effaced with irregular expansions and distortions. Several acini with increased cellularity, as indicated by expansion of the surrounding reticulin network, appear to be merging (*asterisk*) due to disruption of the intervening reticulin (Reticulin; original magnification: 100×).

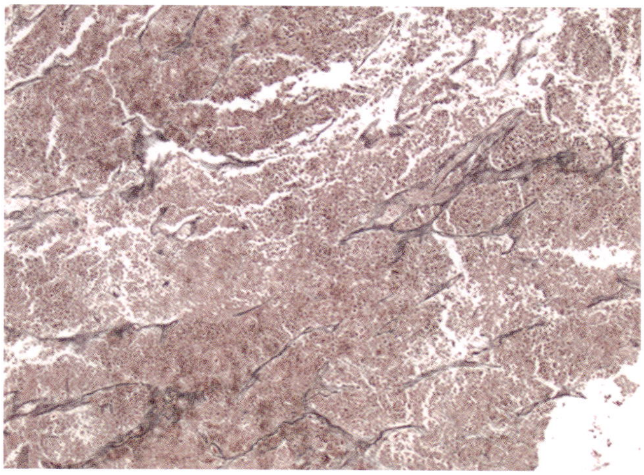

Figure 6-12. Pituitary adenoma: The usual reticulin network of the anterior pituitary parenchyma is essentially entirely wiped out, with reticulin remaining only around blood vessels scattered in sheets of cells. This particular case showed extensive infarct of the adenoma, and reticulin stain was used to highlight the adenomatous nature of the lesion (Reticulin; original magnification: 100×).

hyperplasia **(Fig. 6-11)** and completely lost in adenoma. In adenoma, reticulin remains essentially limited to perivascular areas. In small tissues sent for intraoperative consultation, the distinction of adenomatous from nonadenomatous tissue may be extremely difficult. Although not a widely used method, a rapid reticulin staining method is available for frozen sections.[45] In pituitary tissue with infarcts, a reticulin stain can still highlight the tissue architecture in the background of the infarct and allow one to confirm the presence of an adenoma **(Fig. 6-12)**. Likewise, reticulin stain can be used to evaluate the background tissue architecture as needed in other infarcts or necrotic tissue samples. Typically in *lymphoma*, which typically has an angiocentric pattern, the lymphoma cells are seen to infiltrate among the concentric layers of perivascular reticulin.[46] This is not a specific feature of lymphoma, however, and can be seen with inflammatory infiltrates also.

Reticulin stain is also useful similar to trichrome stain in highlighting the collagen in *abscess* wall. This contrasts with the reticulin pattern restricted to perivascular areas in *glioblastoma multiforme*, helping with the differential diagnosis of rich vascular tissue **(Fig. 6-13)**. In addition, the reticulin fibers are aligned circumferentially in the outer fibrous layer of the abscess wall, while irregular in inner granulation tissue layer. *Gummas* in meningovascular syphilis may be very similar to the necrotizing granulomas of tuberculosis. In gummas, reticulin stain shows the preservation of

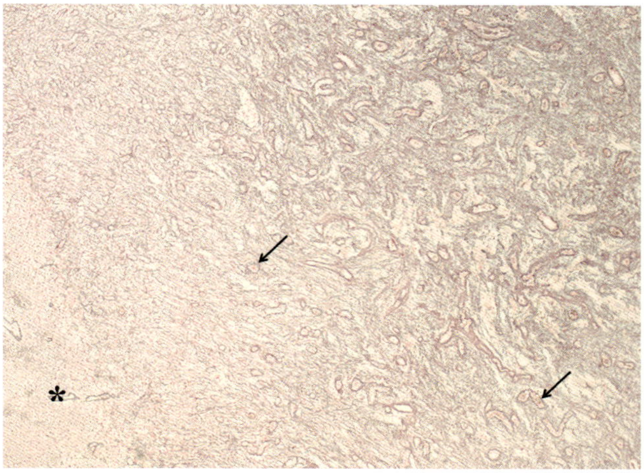

Figure 6-13. Abscess: The entire abscess wall shows rich, confluent reticulin, in which the lumens of thin-walled vessels are seen as mostly round, well-defined holes (*arrows*), in contrast to glioblastoma multiforme where the parenchyma is typically devoid of reticulin and the proliferating multichannel vessels can be highlighted by reticulin stain. Abscess lumen (*asterisk*) is in the bottom left and is devoid of reticulin fibers (Reticulin; original magnification: 40×).

central reticulin, whereas it is lost in the necrotic center of *tuberculous granulomas*.[7]

Collagen Stains

Collagen is ubiquitous in tissues.[35] Of the six major types, types I and III are more widespread in general in fibrovascular soft tissues, while collagen type II is present in elastic cartilage and type IV in basement membranes. Among several collagen stains termed trichrome stains, the most commonly used collagen stain is Masson's trichrome, which stains the collagen blue, while other tissues and especially muscle stain dark red. Van Gieson stain is another method that stains collagen red in the background of other tissues that stain yellow. Masson's trichrome is a method that is more commonly used and is more familiar to most pathologists. It can also provide additional information (see below) that appears to be easier to interpret. The identification of mainly collagen types I and III this way correlates with reticulin pattern, although reticulin provides a more delicate staining pattern, allowing more detailed evaluation of the network. Therefore, Masson's trichrome stain also highlights the collagenous balloons seen in *myxopapillary ependymoma*, as well as the collagen-rich spindle cell component of *desmoplastic infantile ganglioglioma/astrocytoma* and *pleomorphic xanthoastrocytoma*. The delicate pericellular pattern is better evaluated by reticulin stains, however. Likewise, identification of collagen pattern in the differentiation of *abscess* wall from *glioblastoma multiforme* is also similar to that seen with reticulin stain in principle.

List of Findings/Checklist for Collagen Stains

• AT A GLANCE

- Myxopapillary ependymoma
- Desmoplastic infantile ganglioglioma/astrocytoma
- Pleomorphic xanthoastrocytoma
- Abscess
- Glioblastoma multiforme
- Vascular malformations
- Fibrin/vascular injury
- Amyloid

In the evaluation of *vascular malformations*, collagen stains are useful to highlight the vessel walls, which are mostly collagenized, in a background of hemorrhage. Especially in cavernous angiomas, a thick hyalinized change in the vessel walls is present almost uniformly in the lesion. Trichrome stain in this context also highlights smooth muscle rich walls of the venous malformations. The distinction between cavernous angioma and arteriovenous malformation is more characteristic using elastic tissue stains (see elastic tissue stains). In the evaluation of vascular injury, especially in aneurysms, Masson's trichrome stain can help identify the microscopic rupture/hemorrhage sites by highlighting the *fibrin* as bright red. It is also useful due to its same property in highlighting Charcot-Bouchard microaneurysms in a background of hematoma, along with fibrin in the rupture site (see Fig. 2-128). Also in vasculitis cases, it can help highlight the fibrinoid necrosis of the vessel walls as bright red areas.

In vessel walls that show an eosinophilic, hyalinized-appearing thickening, the consideration is the presence of *amyloid*, in addition to collagen. Masson's trichrome may show a somewhat "dirty" brown staining in cases of amyloid accumulation and allows one to suspect amyloid. This is observed mainly in the modification of Masson's trichrome where light green is used instead of methyl blue **(Fig. 6-14)**. In such situations, further evaluation for amyloid should be performed.

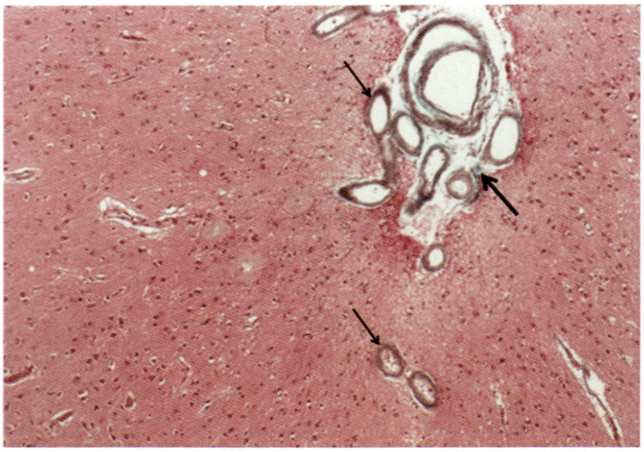

Figure 6-14. Cerebral amyloid angiopathy: The affected thickened vessel walls show a brown discoloration (*thin arrows*) instead of the bright green color of collagen, which is still focally visible (*thick arrow*) in this modification of Masson's trichrome stain (Masson's trichrome; original magnification: 100×).

Elastic Tissue Stain

Verhoeff-van Gieson is the classical elastic tissue stain. It stains the elastic tissue as black lines and is combined with van Gieson as a counter stain. Van Gieson stains collagen red. It is used mainly to highlight internal elastic laminae of arteries to aid in the distinction of arterial versus venous vessels, as well as evaluating the abnormalities of internal elastic lamina, such as duplications and disruptions.

In cases of *giant cell arteritis*, the abnormalities of the internal elastic lamina in the form of fragmentation and reduplication can be identified with this stain,[47] although it may not contribute significantly to the number of cases that would have been otherwise diagnosed without this stain and the abnormalities seen with this stain may not be specific for giant cell arteritis.[48] Fragments of internal elastic lamina can be identified within the cytoplasm of multinucleated giant cells with this stain to aid in the diagnosis. Similar findings can be seen in the intracranial giant cell arteritis/primary angiitis of the central nervous system cases. Likewise, it is also useful in the evaluation of *aneurysms* to identify microscopic defects. It is useful in the evaluation of saccular aneurysms,[49] especially if their histologic features are obscured within the hemorrhage. Even though van Gieson component allows evaluation of vessel wall as well, depending on the preference, Masson's trichrome may be separately performed to aid in this evaluation. This combination may be useful in the evaluation of *hemorrhagic or necrotic material* to highlight any vascular or collagenous tissue hidden in the background.

In *vascular malformations*, the identification of hybrid arteriovenous vessels seen as partial presence of internal elastic lamina is characteristic of arteriovenous malformation[50] **(Fig. 6-15)**, while cavernous angiomas do not have internal elastic lamina in their vessels. It stains the polyvinyl alcohol (PVA) embolization material as black also[51] **(Fig. 6-15)**.

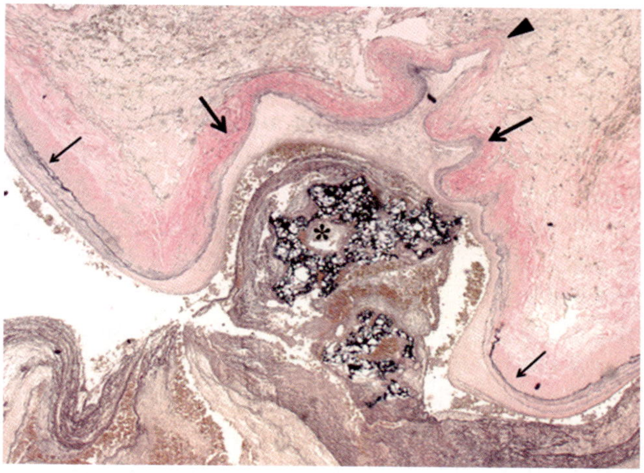

Figure 6-15. Arteriovenous malformation: A large malformed hybrid vessel has both arterial and venous features. A thick internal elastic membrane (*thin arrows*), which is reduplicated, with the underlying thick smooth muscle layer represents arterial features. They both gradually become thin in other areas, with smooth muscle mostly replaced by bright pink collagen (*thick arrows*). The segment with venous features (*arrow head*) has a thin wall and no internal elastic membrane. The black-staining amorphous material in the lumen (*asterisk*) is PVA used for preoperative embolization (Verhoeff-van Gieson; original magnification: 40×).

List of Findings/Checklist for Elastic Tissue Stain

AT A GLANCE

- Giant cell arteritis
- Aneurysms
- Hemorrhagic/necrotic material
- Vascular malformations

Microorganisms

Although a variety of serologic tests and immunologic staining methods are available for various microorganisms, traditional histochemical methods remain as the standard and most practical first step in routine diagnostic practice for the most commonly encountered microorganisms.[52]

List of Findings/Checklist for Microorganisms

AT A GLANCE

- Gram stain and bacteria
- Acid-fast stains and acid-fast microorganisms
- Grocott's methenamine silver stain and fungal microorganisms
- Warthin-Starry stain and spirochetes

Many infections can be suspected based on the histologic and cytologic changes identified by light microscopy, such as granulomas, the type of inflammatory infiltrate, and viral cytopathic effect (see "Inflammation and Bone Marrow-derived Cells" in Chapter 2).

Gram stain is the standard staining method for *bacteria*. It can be performed on air-dried cytologic preparations obtained from fresh specimens to provide a rapid impression, and a modification, Gram-Twort, is more suitable for formalin-fixed, paraffin-embedded tissue sections. Whenever there is an acute inflammation, abscess, or cerebritis with a predominance of polymorphonuclear (PMN) leukocytes, stains for microorganisms should be performed. In most cases, it is preferable to also perform special stains for fungal microorganisms in this setting. Obvious cases will commonly show small groups of bacteria, mostly cocci, upon diligent search. Depending on the situation, many of these cases have already been cultured in the operating room. In such cases, additional staining may not be necessary and does not add much to what is already known. However, in many other situations, it is the responsibility of the pathologist evaluating the sections to include infectious etiology in the differential diagnosis and show an effort to identify any microorganisms, as needed, even though these efforts may be fruitless in a large subpopulation of such cases. With Gram stain, gram-positive bacteria stain blue-black and gram-negative bacteria stain pink-red. A diligent search for bacteria, especially those that are intracytoplasmic, should be done on high-power magnification. Care should be taken not to mistake various artifacts for bacteria, since these inflammatory specimens contain large amount of cellular debris. Especially, eosinophil PMN leukocyte granules and nuclear fragments, which tend to stain red with this stain, can be notorious pitfalls. Elastic fibers may stain black and if fragmented, may lead to confusion. It may not work optimally in some situations, for example, with *Tropheryma whipplei* in Whipple disease as the bacteria may be degenerated; therefore, PAS and/or GMS stains may be more useful, necessitating a panel approach in such suspected cases.[7]

Ziehl-Neelsen is the main staining method for *acid-fast microorganisms* and is especially used for the identification of mycobacteria. Ziehl-Neelsen and GMS (see below) stains are indicated when any type of granuloma is seen, especially in necrotizing granulomas but also in nonnecrotizing granulomas and in the workup of suspected sarcoidosis cases. These stains should not be scanned at low power and concluded as negative within seconds, as especially acid-fast bacilli are notorious for being rare in the tissue. Therefore, an average high-power search, which may last many minutes, should be carried out before concluding them as being negative. Mycobacteria stain red with Ziehl-Neelsen. While *Mycobacterium tuberculosis* is typically very rare and identifying a few of them will be gratifying in many situations, *M. avium intracellulare* tends to be abundant, packing the macrophage cytoplasm. A modified acid-fast stain, *Fite* method, is preferred for *Mycobacterium leprae* due to technical aspects in regard to its capsular characteristics. This is important in the evaluation of granulomatous disease in peripheral nerve specimens. Acid-fast staining is also useful in the identification of mycobacterial pseudotumor and its differential diagnosis from other neoplastic lesions. Some fungi and Russell bodies can stain with Ziehl-Neelsen stain. Other acid-fast microorganisms, especially Nocardia[53] and Cryptosporidium,[54] should also be kept in mind during interpretation.

GMS is the standard staining method for *fungal microorganisms* and is sufficient in routine practice to at least suggest the diagnosis of most common fungi, which can be further sorted out depending on the presence of hyphae, yeast forms, septation, and branching, together with the clinical information and pathologic lesion **(Fig. 6-16)**. Fungal elements stain black. One drawback of GMS stain is that it is very prone to artifacts. Nonspecific staining of nonfungal elements, such as melanin pigment, cellular debris, PMN leukocyte granules, as well as stain residue may render the interpretation difficult. Fortunately, fungal elements, even the smallest of the yeast forms, such as Histoplasma, stain very crisply and can be detected among artifacts. It may stain cocci resulting in a picture somewhat reminiscent of Histoplasma **(Fig. 6-17)**. It may also show mycobacteria if they are dead, and routine stain does not work due to loss of their capsule, for example, after treatment. PAS stain is an alternative stain for fungal microorganisms but is also fraud with nonspecific staining of many cell components and artifacts.

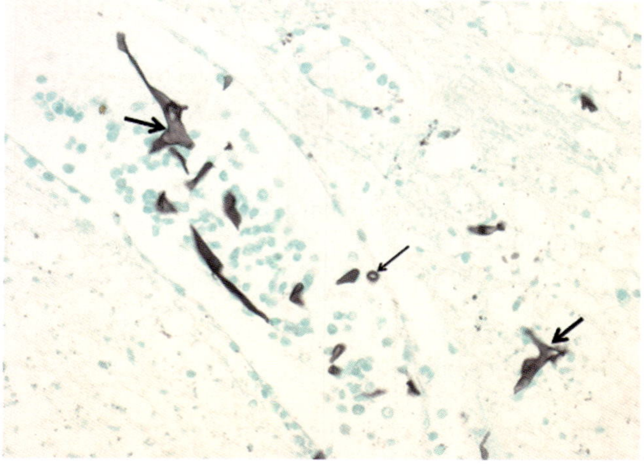

Figure 6-16. Mucormycosis: Many fungal hyphae are seen in a necrotic background in association with a vessel. They show approximately right-angle branching (*thick arrows*), have irregular walls, and show no septations in contrast to Aspergillus hyphae, which tend to be thinner and show acute-angle branching, have almost perfectly parallel walls and septations. Cross sections of some hyphae may mimic yeast forms (*thin arrow*) (Grocott's methenamine silver; original magnification: 400×).

In the rare case of *spirochete infections*, *Warthin-Starry* stain is used to identify spirochetes such as *Borrelia burgdorferi* in Lyme disease and *Treponema pallidum* in syphilis.

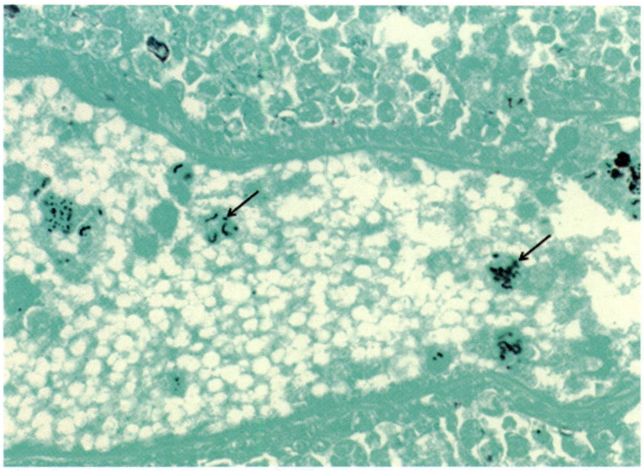

Figure 6-17. Cocci: The cocci in this septic embolus stain with GMS to mimic small yeast forms such as *Histoplasma* spp., especially when they form small colonies, further mimicking intracytoplasmic yeast forms (*arrows*). They are, however, much smaller than Histoplasma and do not have a cell wall or pallor in the center (Grocott's methenamine silver; original magnification: 400x).

Pigment Stains

In the great majority of situations, the pigments are self-evident and do not require further workup. If needed, however, special stains are available for identifying many pigments.[55] Fontana-Masson stain stains *melanin* pigment black. Its use is limited, however, as many melanocytic lesions may not necessarily have melanin pigment, and IHC plays a crucial role in specifically identifying melanocytic cells as well as in their differential diagnosis. In heavily pigmented lesions, melanin bleaching technique can both confirm the presence of melanin and also allow better evaluation of cells that may have been obscured by melanin. In addition, this technique can be performed after IHC using diaminobenzidine (DAB) as chromogen, which is not affected by bleaching.[1] This way, the pigment can be dealt with and the IHC evaluation of the cells can be carried out on the same slide, as needed.

Perls' Prussian blue stains *ferric iron* dark blue. Again, the recognition of obvious hemosiderin pigment usually does not require a special stain, and the identification of melanin forming cells can be done by IHC. However, rarely iron stain may be useful to identify the presence of tissue iron. For instance, *ferritinopathy*[56] (neuroferritinopathy, neurodegeneration with brain iron accumulation type II), neurodegeneration with brain iron accumulation type I (pantothenate kinase-associated neurodegeneration; Hallervorden-Spatz disease), and superficial siderosis[57] are characterized by iron accumulation in the involved areas.

Lipofuscin gives autofluorescence **(Fig. 6-18)** and also stains weakly with acid-fast stains, such as Ziehl-Neelsen. It does not stain as strongly as melanin with Fontana-Masson stain. Instead, the periphery of the granules stain.[3] It can be stained

List of Findings/Checklist

AT A GLANCE

- Melanin
- Iron
  - Ferritinopathy
- Lipofuscin
- Bile
- Copper

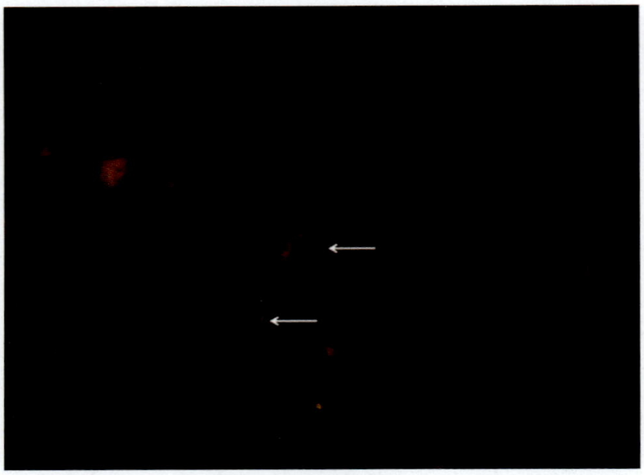

Figure 6-18. Lipofuscin autofluorescence: The cell bodies of several neurons are visible due to the autofluorescence of cytoplasmic lipofuscin pigment (*arrows*), while the nuclear contours are also seen as negative images (Unstained section; fluorescence microscopy; original magnification: 400×).

by PAS and Sudan stains, but a stain that is more specific for lipofuscin is Schmorl's method, which stains lipofuscin dark blue and melanin lighter blue. Lipofuscin also accumulates in a variety of disorders, mainly metabolic and inherited in nature (see Chapter 2).

Identification of *bile* and *copper* is rarely, if any at all, needed as conditions such as kernicterus and Wilson's disease are diagnosed by their typical gross and histologic findings in the right clinicopathologic context.

Other Methods

Congo red is the standard stain for amyloid in formalin-fixed, paraffin-embedded tissue sections and stains the *amyloid* pink-red.[58] It also creates an "apple green" birefringence in the areas of amyloid accumulation when examined under polarized light **(Fig. 6-19)**. The pink-red color is not always easy to identify, especially in small amount of accumulation. Elastic fibers can also yield a pink-red color. Specifically in the CNS, it is useful in amyloidoma; pituitary adenomas associated with amyloid accumulation; cerebral amyloid angiopathy (CAA), which is also referred to as congophilic angiopathy due to Congo red positivity; and the evaluation of plaque pathology in Alzheimer's disease. While it is a general screening stain for amyloid, in CAA and Alzheimer pathology, IHC for beta-amyloid is used more commonly and is more sensitive in identifying even minuscule amounts of accumulation without the difficulties associated with polarization of Congo red stain and subjectivity of the evaluator for the diagnostic color. Several pitfalls should be considered in the evaluation of Congo red stain in the CNS or in the skeletal muscle and peripheral

List of Findings/Checklist for Other Methods

AT A GLANCE

- Congo red
  - Amyloid
  - Pitfalls and technical aspects
- Birefringence
  - Apple green
  - Others
- Mucin stains
  - Glandular cells
  - Cryptococcus
- Phosphotungstic acid hematoxylin
  - Glial fibers
  - Striations
  - Amebae

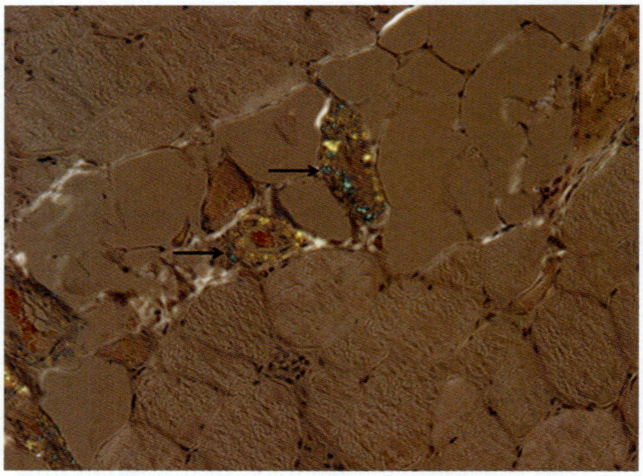

Figure 6-19. Amyloid: Polarized light examination of Congo red–stained paraffin section of skeletal muscle shows the "apple green" birefringence in the vessel walls (*arrows*) that is characteristic for amyloid (Congo red; original magnification: 200×).

nerve specimens. Birefringence of collagen can especially become confusing, and it too can have a green color in some cases; however, the characteristic fibrillarity of collagen is still obvious and should be taken into account to avoid false-positive results in such cases. The microscope used for polarized light can also have a technical effect on the evaluation. Same slide may appear brightly "apple green" in some microscopes, while it is negative in some others. This appears to be related to the intensity of light source of the microscope, more intense light resulting in brighter and easier identification of diagnostic birefringence. Prolonged formalin fixation and long-term archiving of blocks may result in reduced intensity of staining. Likewise, larger amount of amyloid in the tissue, probably due to its long-standing nature in the tissue, may have a weaker staining compared to smaller amounts of recently formed accumulations. Sections should be 8 to 10 μm in thickness for optimal results. Fluorescence microscopic examination of Congo red–stained sections shows fluorescence, though it is not as specific as the "apple green" birefringence. It should also be kept in mind, especially in the evaluation of muscle and nerve specimens, that amyloid accumulation is usually patchy and can be very focal. In addition, electron microscopic examination may reveal very small accumulations that may not have been identified by routine light microscopic techniques. Another amyloid structure that can be highlighted by Congo red is Biondi bodies in choroid plexus cells and ependymal cells.

Birefringence, in addition to that with amyloid on Congo red–stained paraffin sections, can be seen in some other situations, though not with such diagnostic implications as in amyloid. Accumulations in Niemann-Pick disease, which can show a Maltese cross birefringence (as in talc granules) in its early stages,[59] Fabry disease, and Farber disease can be birefringent. Calcium oxalate crystals in ethylene glycol ingestion can be highlighted by polarized light with their typical morphology.[60] Likewise, talc powder contamination of tissues and many foreign materials are also birefringent. Therefore, polarized light can be used in search of foreign material in tissues to support penetrating trauma, previous surgical changes, and in the evaluation of granulomas, especially when foreign body giant cells are present.

Mucin stains consist mainly of mucicarmine and Alcian blue for routine diagnostic purposes. Mucin is also PAS positive and diastase resistant, but these other stains are more specific for mucin. Alcian blue has the added advantage of distinguishing mesenchymal and epithelial mucins if pH is adjusted accordingly; however, this is not a crucial property again due to the involvement and accuracy of IHC in many differential diagnoses. Mucin stains are mainly used to identify *glandular cells*, be it looking for glandular cells to suggest Rathke cleft cyst origin of a stratified squamous epithelium–lined suprasellar cyst or further classifying a metastatic poorly differentiated non–small cell carcinoma of lung origin as adenocarcinoma for more specific chemotherapeutic protocols. They can also be used in cerebrospinal fluid cytology to identify metastatic carcinoma, although cytokeratin IHC has broader coverage and accuracy. While it is useful in further identifying a fungal yeast form as *Cryptococcus*, this feature can be more useful in cases where cryptococci degenerated and fragmented to look like smaller yeast forms, such as Histoplasma spp. Even though their capsules are also degenerated, mucicarmine may still highlight the remnants of their capsules even in the macrophage cytoplasm **(Fig. 6-20)**.

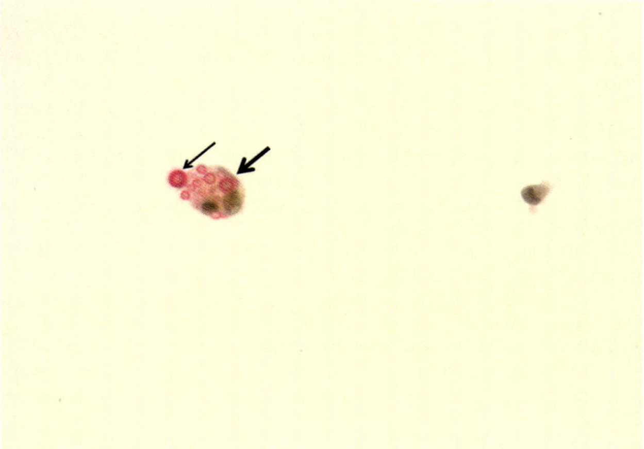

Figure 6-20. Cryptococcosis: Degenerated yeast forms (*thick arrow*) in the cytoplasm of a macrophage are seen in this cytologic preparation of cerebrospinal fluid. They could otherwise mimic intracytoplasmic small yeast forms of Histoplasma without the mucin stain confirming the presence of a mucinous capsule around them. An intact yeast is apparently about to be ingested (*thin arrow*) (Mucicarmine; original magnification: 400×).

Phosphotungstic acid hematoxylin (PTAH),[1] though rarely used in diagnostic practice after the introduction of GFAP IHC, not to mention the disadvantages such as time-consuming preparation and performance, stains the *glial fibers* dark blue and can be used in highlighting these processes in gliomas and reactive gliosis. It highlights the *striations of skeletal muscle* and can be useful in the search for skeletal muscle differentiation in neoplasms such as medulloblastoma with myoblastic differentiation, or in sarcomas. *Ameba* can also be highlighted as dark blue structures. Collagen stains deep brown–red.

References

1. Dawson TP, Neal JW, Llewellyn L, et al. *Neuropathology Techniques*. London: Arnold; 2003.

2. Bancforft JD, Gamble M. *Theory and Practice of Histological Techniques*. 6th ed. Philadelphia, PA: Churchill Livingstone; 2008.

3. Nestor SL. Techniques in neuropathology. In: Bancforft JD, Gamble M, et al. *Theory and Practice of Histological Techniques*. 6th ed. Philadelphia, PA: Churchill Livingstone; 2008: 365–403.

4. Mirra SS, Heyman A, McKeel D, et al. The Consortium to Establish a Registry for Alzheimer's Disease (CERAD). Part II. Standardization of the neuropathologic assessment of Alzheimer's disease. *Neurology*. 1991;41:479–486.

5. Braak H, Braak E. Neuropathological staging of Alzheimer-related changes. *Acta Neuropathol*. 1991;82:239–259.

6. Feany MB, Dickson DW. Widespread cytoskeletal pathology characterizes corticobasal degeneration. *Am J Pathol*. 1995;146: 1388–1396.

7. Ellison D, Love S, Chimelli L, et al. Neuropathology. *A Reference Text of CNS Pathology*. Philadelphia, PA: Elsevier; 2004.

8. Brat DJ. Neuronal and glioneuronal neoplasms. In: Perry A, Brat DJ, et al. *Practical Surgical Neuropathology: A Diagnostic Approach*. Philadelphia, PA: Churchill Livingstone; 2010: 125–150.

9. Reznik M, Schoenen J. Lhermitte-Duclos disease. *Acta Neuropathol*. 1983;59:88–94.

10. Friede RL, Schachenmayr W. Early stages of status marmoratus. *Acta Neuropathol*. 1977;38:123–127.

11. Ortiz-Hidalgo C, Weller RO. Peripheral nervous system. In: Mills SE, et al. *Histology for Pathologists*. 3rd ed. Philadelphia, PA: Lippincott Williams & Wilkins; 2007:243–271.

12. American Oil Chemists' Society (AOCS): http://lipidlibrary.aocs.org/lipids/ Editor in-chief: Dr. William W. Christie, Dec. 2011.

13. Jones LM. Lipids. In: Bancforft JD, Gamble M, et al. *Theory and Practice of Histological Techniques*. 6th ed. Philadelphia, PA: Churchill Livingstone; 2008:187–215.

14. Ho KL. Ultrastructure of cerebellar capillary hemangioblastoma. VI. Concentric lamellar bodies of endoplasmic reticulum in stromal cells. *Acta Neuropathol*. 1987;74: 345–353.

15. Lazzaro B, Gonick P, Katz SM. Renal cell carcinoma vs. renal oncocytoma. Report of a case with overlap features and review of the literature. *Urology*. 1991;37:52–56.

16. Burger PC, Scheithauer BW, Vogel FS. *Surgical Pathology of the Nervous System and its Coverings*. Philadelphia, PA: Churchill Livingstone; 2002.

17. Minauf M. The so-called amaurotic idiocies. Clinical, morphological and biochemical findings as a basis for modern classification. *Veroffentlichungen aus der Pathologie*. 1975;96:1–89.

18. Narita T, Nakazawa H, Hizawa Y, et al. Glycogen storage disease associated with Niemann-Pick disease: histochemical, enzymatic, and lipid analyses. *Mod Pathol*. 1994;7:416–421.

19. Pizzoni C, Sarandria C, Pierangeli E. Clear-cell meningioma of the anterior cranial fossa. Case report and review of the literature. *J Neurosurg Sci*. 2009;53:113–117.

20. Markesbery WR, Brooks WH, Milsow L, et al. Ultrastructural study of the pineal germinoma in vivo and in vitro. *Cancer*. 1976;37:327–337.

21. Siami-Namini K, Shuey-Drake R, Wilson D, et al. A 15-year-old female with progressive myelopathy. *Brain Pathol*. 2005;15:265–267.

22. Matyja E, Naganska E, Zabek M, et al. Meningioma with the unique coexistence of secretory and lipomatous components: a case report with immunohistochemical and ultrastructural study. *Clin Neuropathol*. 2005;24:257–261.

23. Yoshiki T, Itoh T, Shirai T, et al. Primary intracranial yolk sac tumor: immunofluorescent demonstration of alphafetoprotein synthesis. *Cancer*. 1976;37:2343–2348.

24. Fuller GN, Perry A. Epithelial, neuroendocrine, and metastatic lesions. In: Perry A, Brat DJ, ed. *Practical Surgical Neuropathology: A Diagnostic Approach*. Philadelphia, PA: Churchill Livingstone; 2010;287–313.

25. Arima K, Yanagawa S, Ito N, et al. Cerebral arterial pathology of CADASIL and CARASIL (Maeda syndrome). *Neuropathology*. 2003;23:327–334.

26. Ben Romdhane K, Lacombe MJ, Boddaert A, et al. Alveolar soft part sarcomas. Apropos of 6 cases and review of the literature. *Annales de Pathologie*. 1985;5:159–166.

27. Scheithauer BW, Kovacs K, Horvath E, et al. Pathology of the pituitary and sellar region. In: Perry A, Brat DJ, ed. *Practical Surgical Neuropathology: A Diagnostic Approach*. Philadelphia, PA: Churchill Livingstone; 2010;371–416.

28. Striano P, Ackerley CA, Cervasio M, et al. 22-year-old girl with status epilepticus and progressive neurological symptoms. *Brain Pathol*. 2009;19:727–730.

29. Stoltenburg-Didinger G, Punder I, Peters B, et al. Glial fibrillary acidic protein and RNA expression in adult rat hippocampus following low-level lead exposure during development. *Histochem Cell Biol*. 1996;105:431–442.

30. Lomas DA. Molecular mousetraps, alpha1-antitrypsin deficiency and the serpinopathies. *Clin Med*. 2005;5:249–257.

31. Baisden BL, Lepidi H, Raoult D, et al. Diagnosis of Whipple disease by immunohistochemical analysis: a sensitive and specific method for the detection of *Tropheryma whipplei* (the Whipple bacillus) in paraffin-embedded tissue. *Am J Clin Pathol*. 2002;118:742–748.

32. Adachi Y, Kobayashi Y, Ida H, et al. An autopsy case of fetal Gaucher disease. *Acta Paediatr Jpn*. 1998;40:374–377.

33. Jesionek-Kupnicka D, Majchrowska A, Krawczyk J, et al. Krabbe disease: an ultrastructural study of globoid cells and reactive astrocytes at the brain and optic nerves. *Folia Neuropathol*. 1997;35:155–162.

34. Alroy J, Castagnaro M, Skutelsky E, et al. Lectin histochemistry of infantile lysosomal storage disease associated with osteopetrosis. *Acta Neuropathol*. 1994;87:594–597.

35. Jones ML, Bancroft JD, Gamble M. Connective tissues and stains. In: Bancforft JD, Gamble M, et al. *Theory and Practice of Histological Techniques*. 6th ed. Philadelphia, PA: Churchill Livingstone; 2008:135–160.

36. Khaddage A, Chambonniere ML, Morrison AL, et al. Desmoplastic infantile ganglioglioma: a rare tumor with an unusual presentation. *Ann Diagn Pathol*. 2004;8:280–283.

37. Martinez-Diaz H, Kleinschmidt-DeMasters BK, Powell SZ, et al. Giant cell glioblastoma and pleomorphic xanthoastrocytoma show different immunohistochemical profiles for neuronal antigens and p53 but share reactivity for class III betatubulin. *Arch Pathol Lab Med*. 2003;127:1187–1191.

38. Katsetos CD, Herman MM, Frankfurter A, et al. Cerebellar desmoplastic medulloblastomas. A further immunohistochemical characterization of the reticulin-free pale islands. *Arch Pathol Lab Med*. 1989;113:1019–1029.

39. Pasquier B, Gasnier F, Pasquier D, et al. Papillary meningioma. Clinicopathologic study of seven cases and review of the literature. *Cancer*. 1986;58:299–305.

40. Burger PC, Scheithauer BW. *Tumors of the Central Nervous System, AFIP Atlas of Tumor Pathology*. Washington, DC: American Registry of Pathology; 2007.

41. Perry A, Louis DN, Scheithauer BW, et al. Meningiomas. In: Louis DN, Ohgaki H, Wiestler OD, et al., eds. *WHO Classification of Tumours of the Central Nervous System*. Lyon, France: IARC Press; 2007:164–172.

42. Shidoh S, Yoshida K, Takahashi S, et al. Parasagittal solitary fibrous tumor resembling hemangiopericytoma. *Brain Tumor Pathol*. 2010;27:35–38.

43. Hasselblatt M, Jeibmann A, Ger J, et al. Cellular and reticular variants of hemangioblastoma revisited: a clinicopathologic study of 88 cases. *Neuropathol Appl Neurobiol*. 2005;31:618–622.

44. Horvath E. Pituitary hyperplasia. *Pathol Res Pract*. 1988;183:623–625.

45. Velasco ME, Sindely SO, Roessmann U. Reticulum stain for frozen section diagnosis of pituitary adenomas. Technical note. *J Neurosurg*. 1977;46:548–550.

46. Guinto G, Felix I, Arechiga N, et al. Primary central nervous system lymphomas in immunocompetent patients. *Histol Histopathol*. 2004;19:963–972.

47. Ly KH, Regent A, Tamby MC, et al. Pathogenesis of giant cell arteritis: more than just an inflammatory condition? *Autoimmun Rev*. 2010;9:635–645.

48. Foss F, Brown L. An elastic Van Gieson stain is unnecessary for the histological diagnosis of giant cell temporal arteritis. *J Clin Pathol*. 2010;63:1077–1079.

49. Yong-Zhong G, van Alphen HA. Pathogenesis and histopathology of saccular aneurysms: review of the literature. *Neurol Res*. 1990;12:249–255.

50. Meng JS, Okeda R. Histopathological structure of the pial arteriovenous malformation in adults: observation by reconstruction of serial sections of four surgical specimens. *Acta Neuropathol*. 2001;102:63–68.

51. Kepes JJ, Yarde WL. Visualization of injected embolic material (polyvinyl alcohol) in paraffin sections with Verhoeff-van Gieson elastic stain. *Am J Surg Pathol*. 1995;19:709–711.

52. Bartlett JH. Microorganisms. In: Bancforft JD, Gamble M, et al., eds. *Theory and Practice of Histological Techniques*. 6th ed. Philadelphia, PA: Churchill Livingstone; 2008:309–331.

53. Ambrosioni J, Lew D, Garbino J. Nocardiosis: updated clinical review and experience at a tertiary center. *Infection*. 2010;38:89–97.

54. Cordero E, Lara C, Canas E, et al. Usefulness of cerebral biopsy in focal cerebral lesions in patients with human immunodeficiency virus infection. *Medicina Clinica*. 1996;107:738–741.

55. Churukian CJ. Pigments and Minerals. In: Bancforft JD, Gamble M, et al., eds. *Theory and Practice of Histological Techniques*. 6th ed. Philadelphia, PA: Churchill Livingstone; 2008:233–259.

56. Burn J, Chinnery PF. Neuroferritinopathy. *Semin Pediatr Neurol*. 2006;13:176–181.

57. Koeppen AH, Michael SC, Li D, et al. The pathology of superficial siderosis of the central nervous system. *Acta Neuropathol*. 2008;116:371–382.

58. Vowles GH. Amyloid. In: Bancforft JD, Gamble M, et al., eds. *Theory and Practice of Histological Techniques*. 6th ed. Philadelphia, PA: Churchill Livingstone; 2008:261–281.

59. Elleder M, Hrodek J, Cihula J. Niemann-Pick disease: lipid storage in bone marrow macrophages. *Histochem J*. 1983;15:1065–1077.

60. Froberg K, Dorion RP, McMartin KE. The role of calcium oxalate crystal deposition in cerebral vessels during ethylene glycol poisoning. *Clin Toxicol*. 2006;44:315–318.

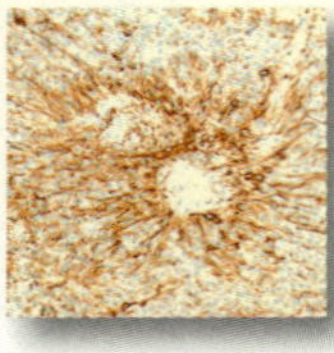
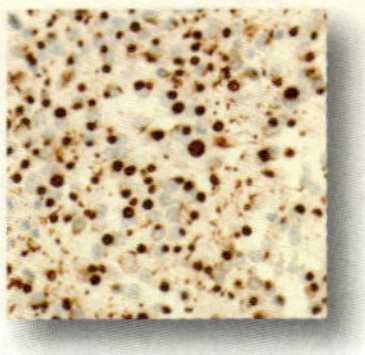
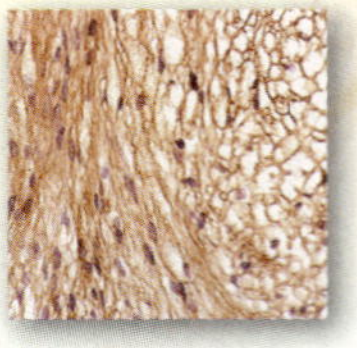

CHAPTER 7

Immunohistochemical Features

Introduction

This chapter is not intended as a comprehensive text on immunohistochemistry (IHC). It is not even a review of the immunohistochemical markers and their technical aspects, including control tissues, which are the subjects of other texts written specifically on IHC. Rather, it focuses on how they are used in diagnostic neuropathology, the evaluation of staining results, and how they apply to particular lesions. As is the case in other subspecialties of pathology, new antibodies are constantly added to the list, and many of them also apply to some lesions that can be seen in the nervous system. Therefore, awareness of not only nervous system–related markers but also those utilized commonly in other organ systems is important. Further complicating the subject is the fact that over time, the initial use and value of a given marker may change. It is not unusual for one antibody to be described as specific and diagnostic for one particular neoplasm and subsequent studies to show it to also apply to several other neoplasms. Changes in the specifications of the same antibody produced by different companies may also become important. In addition, not just positivity but also the pattern of staining, and which cells are staining, becomes very important in differential diagnosis[1] **(Table 7.1)**. Furthermore, immunophenotypical identification also takes into account various combinations of positivity, as well as negativity, and the correlation of the results with the cytohistomorphologic features, rendering IHC a lot more complicated than simply being brown (or another color depending on the chromogen used) or not. It should be remembered that the sections on which the IHC is performed are additional deeper sections obtained from the same block the initial H&E sections came from, that is, they are deeper sections for all practical purposes. As such, new findings aside from the IHC results may emerge on these new sections and may significantly influence the interpretation. For instance, the appearance of necrosis in an astrocytoma or brain invasion in meningioma should not be overlooked while quickly scanning for the "brown color" at low power magnification.

Glial Fibrillary Acidic Protein

Glial fibrillary acidic protein (GFAP) is an intermediate filament protein that is expressed mainly in glial cells. In spite of its name, implying that it is a glial marker, in practice, it is most useful for the identification of astrocytic and ependymal lineages and not so much for the oligodendroglial cells.[2] The *astrocytic processes* are highlighted, as well as any *cytoplasm* when it becomes prominent, as in the case of *gemistocytes* and *reactive astrocytes*. GFAP can be used to highlight the astrocytic population in cases with low cellularity and with a differential diagnosis of reactive gliosis versus low-grade astrocytoma, to evaluate the distribution of astrocytes,

TABLE 7.1 Typical or predominant staining patterns, other than cytoplasmic,[a] according to antibodies and neoplasms

Pattern	Antibody	Neoplasm
Membranous	Synaptophysin	Neurons in resting state
	EMA	Meningioma Carcinoma
	E-cadherin	Carcinoma Choroid plexus and its neoplasms
	ACTH	Crook's hyaline change (peripheral cytoplasmic rim)
	CD117 (c-kit)	Germinoma
	Podoplanin (D2-40)	Germinoma Embryonal carcinoma Epithelioid MPNST
	Beta-catenin	Anterior pituitary parenchyma Pituitary adenoma Adamantinomatous craniopharyngioma Carcinoma
	GLUT-1	Renal cell carcinoma
	Collagen type IV	Schwannoma
	CD99	PNET/EWS (p-PNET) Ependymoma
Nuclear	Neu-N	Relatively differentiated neuronal cells and neoplasms
	Hu	Neuronal cells and neoplasms
	Ki-67	Proliferating cells
	PCNA	Proliferating cells
	PHH3	Mitotic cells
	P53	Cells with *TP53* mutation
	ER and PR	Meningioma
	Ubiquitin (various nuclear inclusions)	FTLD-U FTLD-MND Kennedy's disease Huntington's disease
	TDP-43	FTLD-U FTLD-MND Motor neuron disease Amyotrophic lateral sclerosis
	FUS	FTLD-FUS NIFID BIBD
	OCT3/4	Germinoma
	MiTF	Melanocytic cells and neoplasms
	Viral inclusions	CMV HSV JC Virus (PML) EBV (EBNA)
	TTF-1	Lung and thyroid carcinomas Others (see text)
	Beta-catenin	Pituitary adenoma Adamantinomatous craniopharyngioma Medulloblastoma
	Brachyury	Chordoma
	Myogenin and Myo-D1	Skeletal muscle differentiation
Nuclear absence of staining	INI1	ATRT Others (see text)

TABLE 7.1 Typical or predominant staining patterns, other than cytoplasmic,[a] according to antibodies and neoplasms *(Continued)*

Pattern	Antibody	Neoplasm
Paranuclear dot (Golgi pattern)	Synaptophysin	Large cell medulloblastoma Oligodendroglioma
	Cytokeratin	Neuroendocrine carcinoma
	Prolactin	Sparsely granulated prolactinoma
	Growth hormone	Sparsely granulated somatotroph adenoma
	CAM 5.2	Sparsely granulated somatotroph adenoma (fibrous bodies) Acidophil stem cell adenoma (fibrous bodies)
Perinuclear rim	GFAP	Alzheimer type II glia
	CAM 5.2	Crook's hyaline change Densely granulated somatotroph adenoma
Nuclear and Cytoplasmic	S-100 protein	PNST Gliomas Melanocytic cells and neoplasms

[a]Any positivity with any antibody is considered cytoplasmic by default, unless a specific pattern is mentioned as in this table.
EMA, epithelial membrane antigen; PNET/EWS, primitive neuroectodermal tumor/Ewing sarcoma; p-PNET, peripheral primitive neuroectodermal tumor; PCNA, proliferating cell nuclear antigen; PHH3, phosphohistone H3 protein; ER, estrogen receptor; PR, progesterone receptor; FTLD-U, frontotemporal lobar degeneration with ubiquitin-positive inclusions; FTLD-MND, frontotemporal lobar degeneration with motor neuron disease; FUS, fused in sarcoma protein; FTLD-FUS, frontotemporal lobar degeneration with FUS accumulation; NIFID, neurofilament intermediate filament inclusion disease; BIBD, basophilic inclusion body disease; MiTF, microphthalmia transcription factor; CMV, cytomegalovirus; HSV, Herpes simplex virus; PML, progressive multifocal leukoencephalopathy; EBV, Epstein-Barr virus; EBNA, Epstein-Barr nuclear antigen; TTF-1, thyroid transcription factor-1; ATRT, atypical teratoid rhabdoid tumor; GFAP, glial fibrillary acidic protein; PNST, peripheral nerve sheath tumor.

List of Findings/Checklist for Glial Fibrillary Acidic Protein

AT A GLANCE

- Astrocytes
  - Reactive
  - Neoplastic
  - Background
- Gemistocytes
- Oligodendroglioma
  - Minigemistocytes
  - Gliofibrillary oligodendrocytes
- Oligoastrocytoma
- Glioblastoma multiforme and variants
- Gliosarcoma
- Desmoplastic infantile ganglioglioma/astrocytoma
- Granular cell astrocytoma
- Pleomorphic xanthoastrocytoma
- Others
  - Pilocytic astrocytoma
  - Subependymal giant cell astrocytoma
  - Angiocentric glioma
  - Astroblastoma
  - Chordoid glioma
  - Pituicytoma
- Ependymoma
- Central neurocytoma
- Meningioma and brain invasion
- Non-glial neoplasms
  - Fibroblastic meningioma
  - Schwannoma
  - Choroid plexus neoplasms
  - Primitive neuroectodermal tumor/Medulloblastoma
  - Atypical teratoid/rhabdoid tumor
  - Papillary tumor of the pineal region
- Folliculostellate cells
- Paraganglioma
- Malignant peripheral nerve sheath tumors
- Chondroid neoplasms
- Chordoma
- Carcinoma

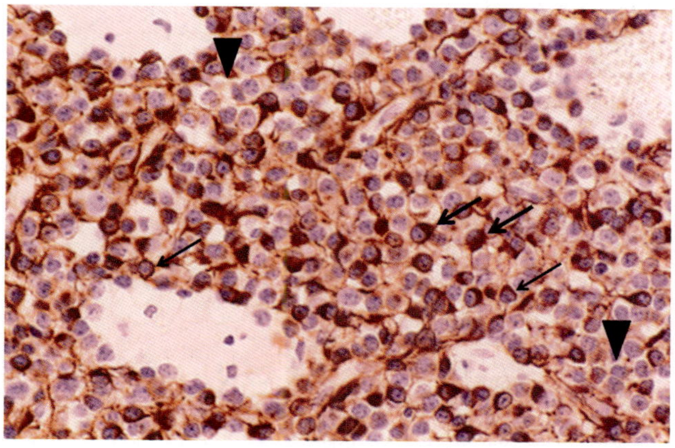

Figure 7-1. GFAP in oligodendroglioma: A subpopulation of cells shows variable cytoplasmic GFAP positivity. Some tend to have a plumper, eccentric and dense cytoplasm (*thick arrows*) and represent minigemistocytes, while others show a thin, perinuclear rim of staining, representing gliofibrillary oligodendrocytes (*thin arrows*). Many cells show no staining and are better identified when they are side-by-side in small groups (*arrowheads*) (GFAP IHC; original magnification: 400×).

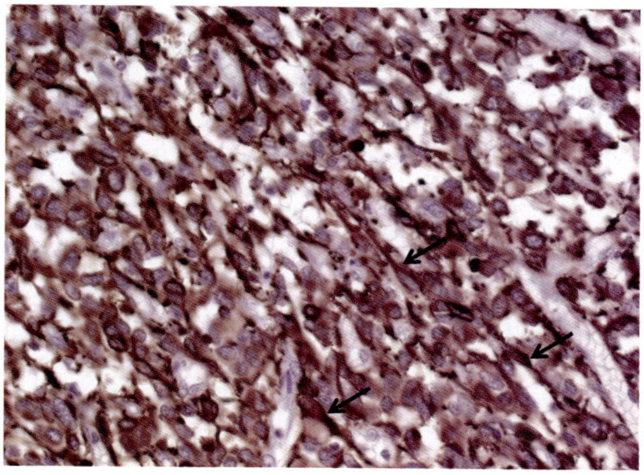

Figure 7-2. GFAP in small cell astrocytoma: In spite of its resemblance to oligodendroglioma due to small, round nuclei, small cell astrocytoma has a different staining pattern by GFAP, which highlights many elongated, delicate processes that can be traced to emanate from the bipolar cells (*arrows*), creating a roughly parallel, streaming fibrillarity (GFAP IHC; original magnification: 400×).

since an orderly distribution favors a reactive process, while irregular groupings favors a neoplastic process. Alzheimer type II glia do not have a prominent cytoplasm but may have a thin perinuclear rim of GFAP positivity. Some ghost NFT that are left in the neuropil after the death of the neuron can appear as GFAP positive due to the astrocytic reaction toward them.[3]

In a mixed *oligoastrocytoma* or in a case in which astrocytic or oligodendroglial origin is not clear, GFAP aids in identifying a GFAP-negative oligodendroglial population, keeping in mind that not every GFAP-negative population is oligodendroglial. In *oligodendrogliomas*, GFAP highlights the *minigemistocytes*. In contrast, in *gliofibrillary oligodendrocytes*, the other cell that can be positive for GFAP in oligodendroglioma, has only a thin perinuclear rim of cytoplasm that is positive for GFAP, whereas the typical round cells of the oligodendroglioma are negative[4] **(Fig. 7-1)**. These, however, should not be taken as a finding to support a diagnosis of mixed oligoastrocytoma, as minigemistocytes are part of the oligodendroglioma. As in any neoplastic process, entrapped reactive astrocytes can also be seen. Therefore, the interpretation of GFAP, just as the interpretation of any stain in general, should take into consideration the location, strength, and shape of the positivity, as well as the morphologic features of the positive cells, rather than simply equating brown color with positivity. In a *glioblastoma multiforme (GBM)*, GFAP will not be diffusely and strongly positive in most cases. As with many other poorly differentiated neoplasms in general, as the degree of differentiation is decreased, the cells lose their ability to recapitulate their cell of origin, not only in appearance but also in functionality, in this case, with less and less production of GFAP. Therefore, patchy and weak positivity for GFAP should not be a surprise in GBM. This should be taken into account in the evaluation of the stain, especially in small specimens. In *small cell astrocytoma/GBM*, GFAP highlights the delicate astrocytic processes of the bipolar cells[5] **(Fig. 7-2)**. In *gliosarcoma*, it can be used to show the glial component to complement the other stains, such as reticulin stain, by creating a negative image of it since sarcomatous areas are stained densely with reticulin stain. Likewise, in *GBM with oligodendroglioma component*, or with *primitive neuroectodermal tumor (PNET)-like foci*, GFAP also serves a similar purpose by highlighting the GBM component and separating it from the other elements. In contrast to the spindle cell or "sarcomatous" areas of gliosarcomas, *desmoplastic infantile ganglioglioma/astrocytoma (DIG/DIA)* show prominent GFAP positivity in its spindle cell, mesenchymal-appearing component,[6] as there are numerous glial cells present in this component creating a collagenous reaction by infiltrating the meninges. GFAP can be used as part of a panel of stains in the evaluation of the *granular cell component* in an astrocytic neoplasm to distinguish them from macrophages.[7] It also helps confirm the astrocytic nature of the xanthomatous cells in *pleomorphic xanthoastrocytoma (PXA)*[8] which may become a problem in small tissue samples. GFAP may help highlight the cytoplasmic xanthomatous vacuoles in the large cells of PXA that may not be otherwise as obvious, by creating a negative image of the vacuoles in the GFAP-positive cytoplasm. GFAP can also be used to highlight the long piloid processes of *pilocytic astrocytoma*. Although the diagnosis of pilocytic astrocytoma does not depend on the GFAP findings, some pilocytic astrocytomas can have a prominent oligodendroglial-like population with round nuclei and even with clear cytoplasms, that is, fried egg appearance, which may cause confusion, especially in small biopsies when other typical features of pilocytic astrocytoma are not present. In such cases, identification of the piloid GFAP-positive processes, which tend to be present even in the oligodendroglial-like areas, helps support the diagnosis of pilocytic astrocytoma. The large cells of *subependymal giant cell astrocytoma (SEGA)* may resemble gemistocytes, although their cytoplasm is pale compared to the bright eosinophilic cytoplasm of gemistocytes. GFAP is positive only in a subpopulation of these cells in SEGA,[9] sometimes as a weak blush, while a more uniform and strong GFAP positivity is expected in gemistocytic astrocytomas. GFAP is diffusely positive in *angiocentric glioma*, highlighting elongated processes of bipolar neoplastic cells. Most cells and their processes are arranged parallel to vessel walls, a peculiar feature better highlighted by GFAP. *Astroblastoma* is positive for GFAP with its elongated and thick processes becoming more prominent when stained. GFAP is useful in discriminating *chordoid glioma* from its mimickers,[10] such as chordoma and chordoid meningioma, keeping in mind, however, the occasional chordoma that can be positive for GFAP,[11] although this appears to be a sporadic finding in the literature, and in most cases, this distinction is not a problem due to the peculiar anterior third ventricular location of the chordoid glioma. *Pituicytoma* is a glial neoplasm that arises from the pituicytes in the posterior pituitary and can be variably positive for epithelial membrane antigen (EMA), along with variable GFAP positivity.[12] GFAP positivity is especially useful in its differential diagnosis from meningioma, as it may histologically resemble meningioma. While the diagnosis of *ependymoma* with its typical histology is a relatively easy diagnosis with ample amount of specimen having at least the pseudorosettes, these features may be obscured in anaplastic or highly cellular ependymomas. In such cases, GFAP can also be used together with other stains to confirm the ependymal nature of the neoplasm, as opposed to PNET or oligodendroglial origin. GFAP positivity of the pseudorosettes of the ependymoma **(Fig. 7-3)** and negative synaptophysin staining contrasts with the opposite immunophenotype of the perivascular fibrillary areas of central neurocytoma, even though GFAP positive apparently reactive entrapped astrocytes can be present in central neurocytoma. In addition, variable GFAP positivity has been reported in *central neurocytoma*,[13] and it has been suggested that increased GFAP may be associated with an aggressive course.[14]

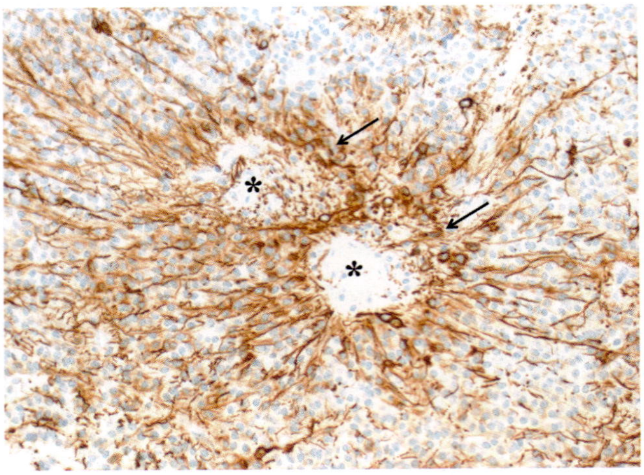

Figure 7-3. GFAP in ependymoma: Many ependymoma cells do not stain with GFAP. Instead, pseudorosettes are highlighted due to the positivity of cell processes in a radial arrangement (*arrows*) around blood vessels (*asterisk*). (GFAP IHC; original magnification: 200×).

By highlighting the neuroglial parenchyma, GFAP helps identify the invasive nature of the meningioma. *Brain invasion in meningioma* may not be obvious or may be questionable in tissues with surgical or other artifacts, in cases with overwhelming invasion where the brain tissue is essentially entirely overrun by meningioma, or in cases where the brain–meningioma border is irregular. It can also be combined with a stain that highlights endothelial cells, such as CD31 or CD34, to evaluate if some meningioma cell groups in the brain parenchyma are actually invasive or are perivascular in the Virchow-Robin spaces, as the latter should not be overinterpreted as brain invasion.

While GFAP is helpful in the identification of glial nature of a lesion in general, certain pitfalls should be kept in mind during its interpretation in certain settings. For instance, in an apparently spindle cell neoplasm of the spinal cord, where the differential diagnosis is *tanycytic ependymoma, fibroblastic meningioma, and schwannoma*, it should also be remembered that focal GFAP positivity can be seen in schwannoma[15] and rarely in meningioma,[16] which can be especially useful in the workup of meningiomas in extracranial locations. In the evaluation of nonastrocytic neoplasms and various nonneoplastic lesions, GFAP may still highlight the *background glial processes* in the parenchyma. This may sometimes cause confusion by creating an "astrocytic" impression for the lesion. Scattered cells can be positive in *choroid plexus neoplasms*,[17] but the diffuse positivity is more consistent with papillary ependymoma. Central nervous system *(CNS) PNET and medulloblastoma* may show areas of glial differentiation, identified by GFAP, and may be associated with more aggressive behavior.[18] It is less frequent than neuronal differentiation, especially in medulloblastomas and usually is in the form of small foci or scattered cells. Some scattered GFAP-positive cells may also represent entrapped reactive astrocytes. In addition, the thin rim of cytoplasm of some neoplastic cells can also be GFAP positive. *Atypical teratoid rhabdoid tumor (ATRT)* is known for its heterogeneous immunophenotype. It is positive at least focally for EMA and smooth muscle actin (SMA), commonly for vimentin, and often for GFAP, cytokeratin, synaptophysin, and neurofilament, with the diagnostic feature being the loss of immunohistochemical expression of INI1.[19] Focal GFAP positivity in *papillary tumor of the pineal region (PTPR)* is useful in its differential diagnosis from metastatic carcinomas, as both are positive for pancytokeratin.[20] *Folliculostellate cells* of the anterior pituitary gland are mainly S-100 protein positive, and occasional cells may be GFAP positive[21]; however, the spindle cell oncocytoma of the anterior pituitary that was suggested to be possibly of folliculostellate cell origin is not GFAP positive.[22] Among several other neoplasms that have been reported to show rare, variable, and typically focal GFAP positivity, those that can be commonly seen in neuropathology practice include the sustentacular cells of *paraganglioma*,[23] *malignant peripheral nerve sheath tumors (MPNSTs)*,[24] *chondroid neoplasms*, and *chordomas*.[25] Rare *carcinomas* with potential myoepithelial features can also show focal GFAP positivity.[26,27]

S-100 Protein

S-100 protein is a calcium binding protein[28] typically used as a general *glial* marker and a marker for neural crest–derived cells, aside from its usual and well-known role as a screening marker for *melanocytic* neoplasms and *peripheral nerve sheath tumors*.[29,30] In fact, it was first identified in the glial cells. Although it has alpha and beta subunits with

List of Findings/Checklist for S-100 Protein

AT A GLANCE

- Glial cells/gliomas
  - Oligodendroglioma
  - Subependymal giant cell astrocytoma
- Melanocytes/melanocytic neoplasms
- Hemangioblastoma
- Paraganglioma
- Others
  - Choroid plexus neoplasms
  - Fibroblastic meningioma
  - Synovial sarcoma
  - Leiomyosarcoma
  - Lipomatous neoplasms
  - Chondroid neoplasms
  - Langerhans cell and non-Langerhans cell histiocytoses
- Peripheral nerve sheath tumors
  - Schwannoma
  - Neurofibroma
  - Malignant peripheral nerve sheath tumor
  - Perineurioma
  - Nerve sheath myxoma
  - Granular cell tumor

their specific antibodies and a differential and preferential expression in various cell types,[31] S-100 protein antibody used in general routine practice covers both subunits and their combinations. The positivity is typically both nuclear and cytoplasmic. Even though S-100 protein as a calcium binding protein is located in the nucleus, it also results in a simultaneous nuclear and cytoplasmic, and sometimes even more prominent cytoplasmic staining, possibly due to diffusion of molecules into the cytoplasm or partially cytoplasmic location of the molecules.[1] Since essentially all gliomas are positive for this marker, it can be used in conjunction with GFAP to supplement its findings. Especially in cases of *oligodendroglioma* with no significant minigemistocyte or gliofibrillary oligodendrocyte population to stain with GFAP, S-100 protein positivity can be useful to support the glial and, therefore, oligodendroglial nature of the neoplasm.

Just like GBM, melanoma can have variable microscopic appearances, each one creating a different set of differential diagnostic possibilities, and may catch one by surprise even if there is a previous history. S-100 protein is useful as a screening marker for melanoma as part of an initial panel; however, due to its low specificity relative to its high sensitivity for melanocytic lesions, the diagnosis should be supported by more specific markers (see "Melanocytic Markers").

SEGA is positive for S-100 protein, and due to the intermediate features of its cells between neurons and astrocytes, it may have variable subpopulations of cells that are variably positive for GFAP, and for neuronal markers such as synaptophysin, chromogranin, and neurofilament.[9] Variable degrees of, but usually partial, positivity is seen in *choroid plexus neoplasms* and is useful in their differential diagnosis from metastatic carcinomas.[17] It is important to remember that S-100 protein can be focally positive in *fibroblastic meningioma,*[15] a feature that may be important to note in the differential diagnosis of fibroblastic meningiomas from schwannomas. S-100 protein positivity is diffuse and strong in *schwannoma*, which also shows pericellular collagen type IV positivity due to basement membrane production by Schwann cells, and negative for EMA, in contrast to meningiomas. Basement membrane is also present in meningioma, but it is focal, discontinuous, and irregular **(Table 7.2)**. In addition, S-100 protein is useful in distinguishing *melanocytoma* from fibroblastic meningioma together with other distinguishing features. Melanocytoma is diffusely and strongly positive for S-100 protein. *Hemangioblastoma* can show focal S-100 protein positivity,[32] which can be useful along with other markers in the rare challenging case that is difficult to distinguish from metastatic renal cell carcinoma.

TABLE 7.2 Characteristic immunophenotypical differential diagnosis of meningioma and schwannoma

Antibody	Meningioma	Schwannoma
S-100 protein	–; focally +	+; diffuse, strong
EMA	+; variable	–
Collagen type IV	+; focal irregular weak	+; pericellular, strong
PR	+ in most	–
GFAP	–; rarely +	+; focal

(–), negative; (+), positive; EMA, epithelial membrane antigen; PR, progesterone receptor; GFAP, glial fibrillary acidic protein.

S-100 protein highlights the sustentacular cells of *paraganglioma*, also referred to as type II cells, surrounding the zellballen formed by the chief cells.[23] Some studies found the latter can also show a weak cytoplasmic positivity for S-100 protein[33]; however, this does not appear to be a consistent and well-recognized finding, and sustentacular cells stand out due to their stronger positivity. In cases where sustentacular cells are not prominent, this S-100 protein positivity in chief cells, together with the organoid pattern, may result in confusion with melanoma. In addition, the paucity or absence of sustentacular cells as identified by S-100 protein has been linked to poor prognosis in adrenal and extra-adrenal paragangliomas.[34] This association with prognosis has not been reported in spinal paragangliomas, which are by definition indolent neoplasms that correspond to WHO grade I.[35] Salt and pepper chromatin pattern and diffuse synaptophysin and chromogranin positivity should be useful in favoring paraganglioma in this context. *Folliculostellate cells* of the anterior pituitary gland,[21] and a recently recognized neoplasm, *spindle cell oncocytoma of the anterior pituitary* that possibly arises from them, are positive for S-100 protein[22] **(Table 7.3)**.

TABLE 7.3 Characteristic immunophenotypical differential diagnosis of sellar region neoplasms

Antibody	PA	SCOAH	GCT	Pituicytoma	Meningioma
S-100 protein	–	+	+	+	±
GFAP	–	–	–	±	
TTF-1	–	+	+	+	–
Synaptophysin	+	–	–	–	–
CAM 5.2	±[a]	–	–	–	–
Pituitary hormones	+	–	–	–	–
Vimentin	–	+	+	+	+
EMA	±[b]	+	–	±	+

[a]Predominantly positive in some types (somatotroph and corticotroph).
[b]Predominantly positive in some types (corticotroph).
+, positive; –, negative; ±, mostly negative.
PA, pituitary adenoma; SCOAH, spindle cell oncocytoma of the adenohypophysis; GCT, granular cell tumor; GFAP, glial fibrillary acidic protein; TTF-1, thyroid transcription factor-1; EMA, epithelial membrane antigen.

In cases that are of hematolymphoid, more specifically histiocytic in nature, S-100 protein is used as a marker for the histiocytic cells of *Langerhans cell histiocytosis*,[36] with variable positivity in *non-Langerhans cell histiocytoses* such as Rosai-Dorfman disease,[37] juvenile xanthogranuloma,[38] and Erdheim-Chester disease,[39] although it can be negative in juvenile xanthogranuloma[38] and Erdheim-Chester disease.[40] It can be positive or negative in *histiocytic sarcoma*.[41]

Even though schwannoma and neurofibroma are strongly positive, the latter in a subpopulation of cells, diffuse and strong positivity is inconsistent with a diagnosis of *malignant peripheral nerve sheath tumor (MPNST)*. S-100 protein positivity in MPNST is focal at best, but can be more prominent in *epithelioid MPNST*,[42] potentially resulting in confusion with melanoma. S-100 protein may be focally positive in *monophasic synovial sarcoma*, a common differential diagnostic possibility with MPNST,[43] while *lipomatous and chondroid neoplasms* are generally strongly and diffusely positive. *Intraneural perineurioma*, also sometimes referred to as *localized hypertrophic neuropathy*,[44] creates a pseudo-onion bulb histology due to perineurial cell proliferation, mimicking *hereditary sensory motor neuropathy (HSMN)*, which also has onion bulb histology due to Schwann cell proliferation. Perineurial cells are S-100 protein–negative and EMA positive, in contrast to Schwann cells, which help distinguish these two lesions, although the diffuse nature of HSMN is also helpful in the differential diagnosis. *Soft tissue perineurioma* is a spindle cell neoplasm composed of fascicles and whorls and can be distinguished from schwannoma and neurofibroma with EMA-positive and S-100 protein–negative immunophenotype. This feature is more useful in the sclerosing variant of perineurioma with increased collagen.[45] A mixture of S-100 protein–positive and EMA-positive cells are present in *nerve sheath myxoma*,[46] while *neurothekeoma* is typically negative for S-100 protein,[47] although there appears to be a continuum of S-100 protein positivity in myxoid neurothekeomas to gradual disappearance of this positivity toward the cellular end of the spectrum.[48] *Granular cell tumors* are typically S-100 protein positive, including those seen usually as incidental findings in posterior pituitary.

Neuronal Markers

Synaptophysin is a presynaptic vesicle-associated protein.[49] It is positive in the *axons* and also stains the *neuron cell body* in a membranous pattern. It typically shows a granular staining pattern. In *abnormal neurons*, neoplastic or otherwise, the neuron cell bodies stain in a diffuse cytoplasmic pattern. This feature helps identify the neoplastic ganglion cells and other abnormal cells with neuronal features. Otherwise, *normal neurons* in tissues infiltrated by neoplasms or in tissues

List of Findings/Checklist for Neuronal Markers

AT A GLANCE

Synaptophysin
- Normal neurons
- Ganglion cell neoplasms
- Central neurocytoma
- Pineal parenchymal neoplasms
- PNET/Medulloblastoma and variants
- Paraganglioma
- Non-neuronal neoplasms
  - Pilocytic astrocytoma
  - Subependymal giant cell astrocytoma
  - Pleomorphic xanthoastrocytoma
  - Oligodendroglioma
  - Choroid plexus neoplasms
  - Atypical teratoid rhabdoid tumor
  - Papillary tumor of the pineal region
- Pituitary adenoma
- Brain-invasive meningioma

Chromogranin
- Central neurocytoma
- Pituitary adenoma
- Subeendymal giant cell astrocytoma
- Neurodegenerative diseases (see below)

Neuron-Specific Enolase
Neurofilament
- Neuronal differentiation
- Evaluation of glioma borders (infiltrative vs. well-circumscribed)
- Subependymal giant cell astrocytoma
- Focal cortical dysplasia
- Dysmorphic ganglion cells
- Pineocyte and pineocytoma cell processes
- Pineocytomatous rosettes
- Grading of pineal parenchymal tumors
- Medulloblastoma
- Atypical teratoid rhabdoid tumor
- Pleomorphic xanthoastrocytoma
- Axonal spheroids
- Dystrophic axons
- Demyelination versus destructive lesion
- Swollen neurons
  - Chromatolytic
  - Neurodegenerative disease
- Amyotrophic lateral sclerosis
- Spinal muscular atrophy
- Pick disease
- Neurofilament inclusion disease

Neu-N
- Nonneoplastic neurons
- Malformations of cortical development/cortical dysplasias
- Ganglioglioma
- Desmoplastic/nodular medulloblastoma
- Embryonal tumor with abundant neuropil and true rosettes
- Pineal parenchymal tumors

Others
- CD56 (NCAM)
- CD57 (Leu-7)
- PGP 9.5
- Nestin
- Microtubule-associated proteins (MAP 1 and 2)
- Peripherin
- Hu
- Alpha-internexin
- Beta-tubulin

adjacent to a pathologic process can also show cytoplasmic synaptophysin positivity as a result of interruption of their axonal transport and should not be misinterpreted as pathologic cells.[50] In practice, it is often used to identify neuronal differentiation or neuronal component in various neoplasms.

Ganglion cell component of *ganglion cell neoplasms* is positive and is useful in the identification of neuronal differentiation in cells in which ganglion cell features are not obvious.[50] In addition, dysmorphic or binucleated ganglion cells can be easily identified when the cytoplasm is highlighted by synaptophysin staining. In some glioneuronal tumors that cannot be further classified, the large cell population with abundant cytoplasm may be difficult to identify as astrocytic or neuronal. In such cases, synaptophysin clarifies the issue easily by highlighting any population with ganglion cell differentiation.[51] In the differential diagnosis of ependymoma and *central neurocytoma*, the perivascular fibrillary pseudorosette-like areas of the central neurocytoma are synaptophysin positive[52] since they are formed by neurites, and are negative for GFAP, which contrasts with the GFAP-positive and synaptophysin-negative pseudorosettes of ependymoma. Synaptophysin helps highlight the pineocytomatous rosettes of *pineocytoma* and *atypical pineocytoma*. While synaptophysin is predominantly positive in the fibrillary areas within the rosettes and less so in the perinuclear cytoplasm, neurofilament is positive in both. Their expressions are decreased to scattered cells in *pineal parenchymal tumors of intermediate differentiation (PPTID)*, especially the high-grade ones. Chromogranin in this context is more prominent in the pseudolobulated variant of PPTID.[53] Neurocytic rosettes in other neoplasms, namely, the rosette-forming glioneuronal tumor of the fourth ventricle, can be highlighted.

Medulloblastoma tends to have more synaptophysin-positive cells in contrast to the CNS PNET. In fact, medulloblastoma is commonly diffusely positive for synaptophysin in contrast to other small blue cell tumors of neuroectodermal origin. In *desmoplastic/nodular medulloblastoma*, the neuropil-like background composed of the processes of cells with neurocytic differentiation can be stained with synaptophysin, making the nodules more prominent. Paranuclear dot-like staining is typically seen in *large cell medulloblastoma*[54] **(Fig. 7-4)**. Diffuse and strong positivity is seen in the chief cells of *paraganglioma*. In the setting of primitive neoplasms, *metastatic small cell carcinoma* and other neuroendocrine carcinomas may present a challenge. While the neuroendocrine differentiation can be easily identified with synaptophysin positivity, cytokeratin is also needed to confirm their carcinomatous nature. *Primitive neuroectodermal tumors (PNETs)* are by definition composed of undifferentiated cells and are negative for neuronal and glial markers; however, it is not unusual for them to show variable degrees of neuronal and/or glial differentiation, which can be identified by neuronal markers, such as synaptophysin, and GFAP, respectively. These differentiations are only rarely overwhelming to obscure the true nature of the neoplasm and result in differential diagnostic problems. Medulloblastomas, on the other hand, are more commonly positive for neuronal markers, especially synaptophysin.

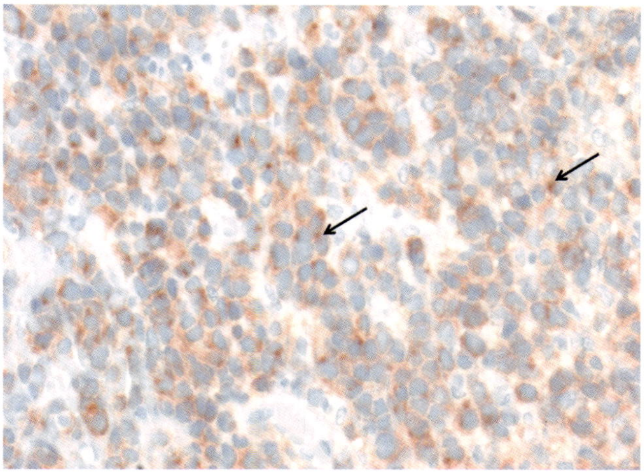

Figure 7-4. Synaptophysin in large cell medulloblastoma: Although synaptophysin positivity is common in medulloblastomas, a peculiar paranuclear dot-like Golgi pattern of positivity (*arrows*) is commonly seen in large cell medulloblastoma (Synaptophysin IHC; original magnification: 400×).

Many other CNS neoplasms may have variable synaptophysin positivity, even though they are not clearly neuronal neoplasms. *Pilocytic astrocytoma* may have synaptophysin positivity, although other neuronal markers are negative.[55] Occasional cells may be positive for synaptophysin in *SEGA*, similar to GFAP.[56] Synaptophysin positivity is not unusual in *PXA* and can be useful in distinguishing it from giant cell glioblastoma.[57] Its positivity should not prompt a diagnosis of a ganglion cell neoplasm, although a rare composite tumor of PXA and ganglioglioma can occur.[58] Neuronal features have been consistently identified in *oligodendroglioma*,[59] where a paranuclear dot-like positivity for synaptophysin may be seen. Variable degree of and typically focal positivity is seen in *choroid plexus neoplasms*, which can be useful if used as part of a panel, in their differential diagnosis from metastatic carcinomas.[60] *ATRT* is known for its heterogeneous immunophenotype. It is positive at least focally for EMA and SMA, commonly for vimentin, and often for GFAP, cytokeratin, synaptophysin, neurofilament, with the diagnostic feature being the loss of immunohistochemical expression of INI1.[19] *PTPR* can show variable, usually focal positivity for synaptophysin[20] and CD56.[61]

Pituitary adenomas are positive for both synaptophysin and chromogranin, although prolactin and adrenocorticotropic hormone (ACTH) producing adenomas tend to be negative for chromogranin.[62] Nonetheless, synaptophysin positivity may sometimes be needed to confirm the neuroendocrine nature of the adenoma cells, as pituitary adenoma may mimic a variety of other neoplasms such as plasma cell lesions and ependymoma due to its variable microscopical appearances. In *meningioma*, just like GFAP, synaptophysin can help with evaluation of brain invasion by highlighting the neuroglial parenchyma.

Synaptophysin quantitation can be used for evaluation of synaptic loss, mainly in research setting.[63] Axonal spheroids may be highlighted,[64] though neurofilament IHC or Bielschowsky silver stain can provide a better view of these structures.

Chromogranins A, B, and C are proteins associated with the *neuroendocrine granules*[65] and yield results similar to synaptophysin, with some exceptions that need to be kept in mind. Chromogranin A, against which the antibody is directed, is expressed most abundantly.[65] It can be variably positive in various *neuronal cells*, such as the neoplastic ganglion cells in ganglioglioma and chief cells of paraganglioma; however, *neurocytoma* and *SEGA* tend to be negative for chromogranin, while they are positive for other neuronal markers such as synaptophysin and Neu-N.[56] Pituitary adenomas are positive for both synaptophysin and chromogranin, although *prolactin and ACTH-producing adenomas* tend to be negative for chromogranin.[62] In general, while the results can be variable, synaptophysin appears to be more consistent and provide more reliable results in practice. For instance, some cases of small cell carcinoma may show more cells with stronger staining with one or the other marker, rendering them advisable to be used together in a panel. It can be identified in association with some swollen neurons and some plaque pathology in *neurodegenerative diseases*.[3]

Neuron-specific enolase (NSE) is an enolase that is present in higher concentrations in neuronal and neuroendocrine cells. For this reason, it is not highly specific for these cells and can be positive in many other cell type and their neoplasms.[66] This realization has earned it the infamous nickname of nonspecific enolase over time and took away its competitive edge with synaptophysin and chromogranin.

Neurofilament, the neuronal intermediate filament protein, is used as a *neuronal differentiation* marker.[67] Three different molecular weight subtypes and their phosphorylated and nonphosphorylated forms are present in different components of the neurons.[68] Therefore, the knowledge of the specific antibody used and caution with the interpretation of the results are required. Most antibodies in routine diagnostic practice are in the form of a cocktail. Even though it is expressed in cells with neuronal features, such as neuroblastic and ganglion cell neoplasms, paragangliomas, and even neuroendocrine carcinomas, synaptophysin is used more commonly for this purpose. However, neurofilament has its uses that are superior to other markers.

Especially in cases of astrocytic neoplasms, identification of their invasive nature, that is, well-circumscribed versus infiltrative (diffuse) glioma, is important for the purposes of intraoperative and postoperative management, as well as prognostic information. The *infiltrative nature of a glial neoplasm* is typically readily obvious along with its diagnosis, and performing neurofilament IHC is not necessary for practical purposes. However, it can be performed in difficult cases in which a definitive distinction between a pilocytic astrocytoma and a WHO grade II (low-grade) infiltrating astrocytoma cannot be made, such as cases where the specimen does not include the periphery of the lesion to allow assessment of a gradual fading of cellular density as one moves away from the neoplasm, or in small specimens where definitive features are not adequately represented. Neurofilament highlights the axons and allows one to evaluate the presence of *entrapped axons within the infiltrating neoplasm* **(Fig. 7-5)**, as opposed to well-circumscribed gliomas, in which at most a small number of entrapped axons can be seen at the peripheral areas of the neoplasm. The latter also implies that even in the well-circumscribed gliomas, some degree of "infiltration" is present, though limited to the periphery of the neoplasm, and they are considered well-circumscribed for practical purposes compared to the truly infiltrative gliomas. Some pilocytic astrocytomas may show a diffuse pattern similar to an infiltrative astrocytoma. As long as they have the typical features of a pilocytic astrocytoma, they are diagnosed as pilocytic astrocytoma and are not necessarily associated with any worse prognosis because of this pattern.[69] Neurofilament IHC can be useful in supporting the well-circumscribed nature of such lesions. Likewise, the evaluation of infiltrative borders by neurofilament may be useful in distinguishing some unusually well-circumscribed glial neoplasms from *metastatic*

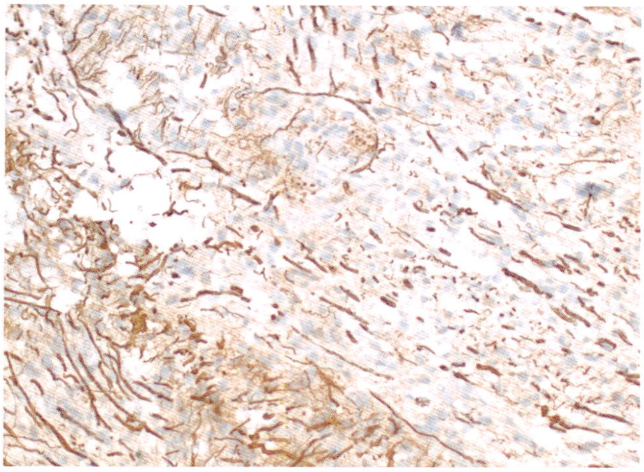

Figure 7-5. Neurofilament in infiltrating glial neoplasm: The neurofilament-positive axons are separated by and entrapped within the infiltrating neoplasm, a useful feature in distinguishing infiltrating glial neoplasms from well-circumscribed ones in small tissue samples (Neurofilament IHC; original magnification: 200×).

carcinomas. For instance, some glioblastomas and anaplastic oligodendrogliomas can have abundant, epithelioid cytoplasms, mimicking a metastatic carcinoma. In such cases, evaluation of the borders of the neoplasm, no matter how well circumscribed it may appear radiologically, intraoperatively, and even histologically, reveals its infiltrative nature among axons, supporting its glial nature.

The cell bodies of large neurons in some *SEGA* stain for neurofilament.[9] It also stains the dysplastic cells with neuronal and glial features found in *cortical dysplasias* in tuberous sclerosis, along with synaptophysin, Neu-N, and GFAP.[70] *Dysmorphic ganglion cell* processes and cell bodies are positive, a useful finding in the identification of a ganglion cell or other neuronal population, such as the dysmorphic neurons of cortical dysplasia,[71] when their typical features are not prominent. The *club-shaped terminal processes* of *pineocytes and pineocytoma cells* that are highlighted by Bielschowsky silver stain[72] are more difficult to appreciate by neurofilament. They can also occasionally be found in atypical pineocytomas. Neurofilament helps highlighting the *pineocytomatous rosettes* of pineocytoma and atypical pineocytoma. While synaptophysin is predominantly positive in the fibrillary areas in the rosettes, and less so in the perinuclear cytoplasm, neurofilament is positive in both. In addition, neurofilament immunohistochemistry has been proposed to be used formally in the *grading of pineal parenchymal tumors*,[53] suggesting that the degree of positivity provides insight to the neuronal differentiation and helps grading. This type of interpretation calls for caution not to interpret the strong positivity in the surrounding nonneoplastic parenchyma as true positivity in the neoplasm to avoid undergrading. *Medulloblastoma* tends to show a tendency for positivity for markers of neuronal differentiation, such as synaptophysin and Neu-N, more prominently in the more mature neurocytic areas of the pale islands. Neurofilament positivity is less pronounced.[73] *ATRT* is known for its heterogeneous immunophenotype. Neurofilament is among several markers that can show variable positivity in ATRT.[19] Neurofilament positivity can be seen in scattered neoplastic cells in *PXA*, similar to other neuronal markers.[57,58]

Neurofilament is useful in the *evaluation of axons*. In this setting, it is more informative by providing information on the cytoskeletal properties of the neurons compared to synaptophysin. It can help identify *axonal spheroids* in cases of *diffuse axonal injury*, *chemotherapy-induced leukoencephalopathy* and in the evaluation of *focal white matter lesions* to distinguish *demyelination*, where axons are expected to be relatively spared, from *infarct*, where axonal spheroids are expected at the periphery of the lesion. In that sense, the utility of neurofilament is similar to Bielschowsky silver stain and technically more practical to perform with more consistent results compared to Bielschowsky silver stain in surgical neuropathology setting. On the other hand, Bielschowsky silver stain provides a somewhat more delicate and consistent staining of the axons for this type of evaluation. Likewise, neurofilament can also help with the identification and evaluation of *dystrophic neurites*, which are irregular swellings and distortions rather than actual axonal spheroids and are associated with a variety of neurodegenerative diseases such as Alzheimer's disease. Neurofilament can help highlight some features of toxic-metabolic disorders that affect axons. Axonal spheroids of variable sizes and shapes seen in association with *vitamin E deficiency* and *neuroaxonal dystrophy* have peripheral staining with neurofilament.[3] *Carbon disulfide poisoning*, resulting in swelling of distal spinocerebellar tracts are highlighted due to prominent neurofilament accumulation based mainly on animal studies.[74] *Toxic oil syndrome* is a toxic cooking oil–related illness with chromatolysis, vacuolation, and neurofilament accumulation in large neurons of spinal cord.[3] Perikaryal neurofilament accumulation is seen in *cytosine arabinoside toxicity*.[75] Neurofilament accumulation in dystrophic axonal alterations seen in association with *vincristine*[76,77] and *fludarabine*[3] treatments are highlighted by neurofilament IHC.

In *swollen neurons* of various types, such as *axonal reaction (chromatolysis)* and other disease states, phosphorylated neurofilament that is normally present in the axon accumulates in the cell body. Swollen anterior horn motor neurons in *amyotrophic lateral sclerosis* show neurofilament accumulation in the cell body.[3] Similar finding is seen in the residual swollen neurons of the *spinal muscular atrophy* (SMA)[78,79] and the swollen neurons of *Pick disease*. Cytoskeletal pathology can be evaluated by neurofilament in neurodegenerative diseases of Alzheimer[80] and non-Alzheimer[81] type. *Cortical Lewy bodies* also contain neurofilament.[81] Likewise, *cytoplasmic inclusions* in *neurofilament inclusion disease (NID)* are also neurofilament positive.[82]

Neu-N recognizes a neuronal nuclear antigen, resulting in nuclear positivity in neuronal cells and is expressed better in those neuronal cells that are advanced or better differentiated in their development.[83] It has been identified as a useful marker for neoplasms with a neuronal lineage.[84] A variable degree but usually weak staining can also be seen in the cytoplasm. In spite of its usefulness in many situations in identifying cells with neuronal differentiation, it tends to be negative in a significant subpopulation of the ganglion cell component of most *gangliogliomas*.[85] This is not a significant problem, as there are other markers for identification of ganglion cells with subtle features, such as synaptophysin and neurofilament. In fact, it can even be used as a feature to support the neoplastic nature of the ganglion cell component in cases where the differential is ganglioglioma versus infiltration of resident neuronal population by a glioma, as *nonneoplastic neuron nuclei* are strongly positive for Neu-N. Those ganglion cells that are positive for Neu-N in ganglioglioma also tend to be positive for CD34, an additional useful finding.[86] Neu-N can be used to highlight the neurons in the cortical ribbon to facilitate the evaluation for abnormalities with cortical layering in the context of *malformations of cortical development/cortical dysplasias*. This approach especially helps with the identification of subtle alterations. Balloon cells in focal cortical dysplasias are negative.[70]

As a marker of differentiated neuronal lineage, Neu-N brings out the nodules of differentiated neuronal areas in *desmoplastic/nodular medulloblastoma*,[87] in which the primitive cells among these nodules are largely negative and may show only scattered positive nuclei. This creates a negative image with the Ki-67 pattern, which shows prominent proliferative activity in the primitive cell population but is essentially absent within the nodules. Likewise, Neu-N highlights the differentiated neurocytic background of *embryonal tumor with abundant neuropil and true rosettes (ETANTR)*, while the primitive cells forming the rosettes are negative.[88] *Pineal parenchymal tumors* are usually negative for Neu-N.[89] This feature can be useful in the pineal parenchymal tumor of intermediate differentiation, which may resemble neurocytoma in its sheet-like growth pattern, as neurocytoma is usually positive for this marker.[90]

There are *other markers* that can be useful in the evaluation of neuronal features in cells; however, they have not been well established as the first line commonly used markers in routine diagnostic practice. *CD56 (Neural Cell Adhesion Molecule; NCAM)* is widely present in various neural and nonneural tissues. It can be used as a neuroendocrine/neural marker in the appropriate context as part of a panel of antibodies. Neuroblastoma,[91] medulloblastoma,[92] olfactory neuroblastoma,[93] as well as benign and MPNSTs[94,95] show variable positivity. *CD57 (Leu-7)* is a natural killer cell–associated antigen, but also recognizes a myelin-associated protein in central and peripheral nervous systems.[96] As such, it can show patchy positivity in schwannomas and also can be used in the workup of MPNSTs. Because it has low sensitivity and specificity for neural tissues, it is best used as part of a panel and the results interpreted in that given context. Although originally isolated from brain and thought to be specific for neural tissues, *protein gene product 9.5 (PGP 9.5)* has later been shown to be less specific for neuroectodermal tissues than it was originally thought. It is positive in neurons and neuronal processes, as well as benign and MPNSTs. In addition, it is used to identify small nerve fibers in the epidermis in the evaluation of skin biopsies for small fiber neuropathy.[97] On the other hand, it has been identified in a wide variety of mesenchymal neoplasms.[98] Originally identified as a marker of neural stem and neural progenitor cells, *nestin* is positive in a wide range of neural and nonneural tissues and is thought to be a marker of embryonal stem cell–derived tissue-specific progenitor cells.[99] As such, neuronal precursor cells, radial glia, neural crest cells, Schwann cells, and oligodendrocyte precursors are positive.[100] It has been found in primitive neural cells with primitive neuroectodermal, as well as glial features.[99,101] *Microtubule-associated proteins (MAP 1 and 2)* are expressed in neuronal cells.[91,102,103] Although they have not been widely studied in the diagnostic IHC setting, they have been shown to be useful in the diagnosis and differential diagnosis of neuroblastomas in children. *Peripherin* is a neuron-associated intermediate protein that is involved in the development of peripheral nervous system. Melanocytic lesions of the skin,[104] peripheral nerve sheath tumors,[105] and, to some extent, CNS neoplasms can express peripherin.[106] It appears to have a high specificity for peripheral nervous system and neural crest–derived tissues, with extraskeletal myxoid chondrosarcoma being an exception.[107] *Hu family of proteins* has been shown to reliably identify neuronal neoplasms, neuroblastoma, medulloblastoma, and small cell carcinoma with a nuclear staining pattern.[108] *Alpha-internexin* is another neuronal intermediate filament protein expressed in most neuronal cells.[109] It has been identified in neuroblastomas[103] and medulloblastomas.[110] *Class III beta-tubulin* is a member of tubulins, the major component of microtubules[111] in the neurons and therefore can be identified in neoplasms with neuronal features, such as olfactory neuroblastoma,[112] pineal parenchymal tumors,[113] ganglioglioma, and dysembryoplastic neuroepithelial tumor.[114]

Epithelial Markers

The utility of epithelial markers in the practice of diagnostic neuropathology is largely limited to the workup of metastatic carcinomas. Primary epithelial lesions of the CNS are mainly limited to various cysts, the nature of which is readily obvious in most cases. Low molecular weight keratin can yield peculiar and helpful findings in the workup of pituitary adenomas. On the other hand, cytokeratins comprise a large group of antibodies consisting of numerous subtypes based on molecular weight with their various uses that are subject of general pathology practice.[115] For these reasons, the discussion here will be brief and will emphasize those areas that are relevant for the surgical neuropathology practice, including any pitfalls. It should be kept in mind, however, that due to the fact that brain is the recipient of many metastatic neoplasms and especially carcinomas, many times the pathologic evaluation of the cerebral metastatic neoplasm provides the first and only information about the malignancy, and that continuous changes in the classification of malignancies of various organs obligates the neuropathologist to be in touch with the updates in the classification systems and the information needed by the oncologists. One such example is the recent emphasis put on distinguishing squamous cell carcinomas and adenocarcinomas of the lung from each other, a diagnosis which used to be conveniently lumped under non–small cell lung carcinoma, as more specific treatments become available for them.[116,117]

Cytokeratin is an epithelial marker used in the identification of epithelial nature of cells, most notably *metastatic carcinoma* in neuropathology. Usually, a pancytokeratin marker such as AE1/AE3 is a good antibody for general purposes; however, it can show some degree of positivity, although weak, in *astrocytes*, due to what is generally thought to be an apparent cross reactivity with GFAP **(Fig. 7-6)**. In fact, it is sometimes referred to as "poor man's GFAP" due to this feature, implying that it could even be used instead of GFAP if one did not have GFAP antibody in the lab. Therefore, especially reactive astrocytes, gemistocytes, and the epithelioid cells of glioblastoma can be positive, as well as astrocytic processes, creating a pitfall in the interpretation of this stain. In most cases, with the incorporation of other features, the overall nature of the lesion becomes clear and this cross reactivity does not pose a significant problem. If this becomes an issue, another cytokeratin, such as CAM 5.2, or another epithelial marker, such as EMA, that is known to not result in this cross reactivity can be used. On the other hand, demonstration of cytokeratins in glioma cells by molecular techniques indicates that this staining

List of Findings/Checklist for Epithelial Markers

• AT A GLANCE

Cytokeratins and Subtypes (AE1/AE3, CK7, CK20, CK18, CAM 5.2)

- Epithelial cysts
- Metastatic carcinoma
- Positivity in astrocytes
- Epithelial metaplasia
- Neuroendocrine carcinoma
- Choroid plexus neoplasms
- Papillary tumor of the pineal region
- Atypical teratoid rhabdoid tumor
- Meningioma
- Paraganglioma
- Epithelioid malignant peripheral nerve sheath tumor
- Leiomyosarcoma
- Primitive neuroectodermal tumor/Ewing sarcoma
- Epithelioid angiosarcoma
- Germ cell neoplasms
- Endolymphatic sac tumor
- Pituitary adenoma

Epithelial Membrane Antigen

- Ependymoma
- Angiocentric glioma
- Papillary tumor of the pineal region
- Chordoid glioma
- Choroid plexus neoplasms
- Atypical teratoid rhabdoid tumor
- Pituicytoma
- Meningioma
- Metastatic adenocarcinoma
- Perineurium and perineurioma
- Nerve sheath myxoma
- Epithelioid malignant peripheral nerve sheath tumor
- Leiomyosarcoma
- Hematopoietic neoplasms

Carcinoembryonic Antigen

- Metastatic adenocarcinoma
- Secretory meningioma
- Chordoma
- Germ cell neoplasms

E-cadherin

- Metastatic carcinoma
- Choroid plexus neoplasms
- Chordoma
- Meningioma

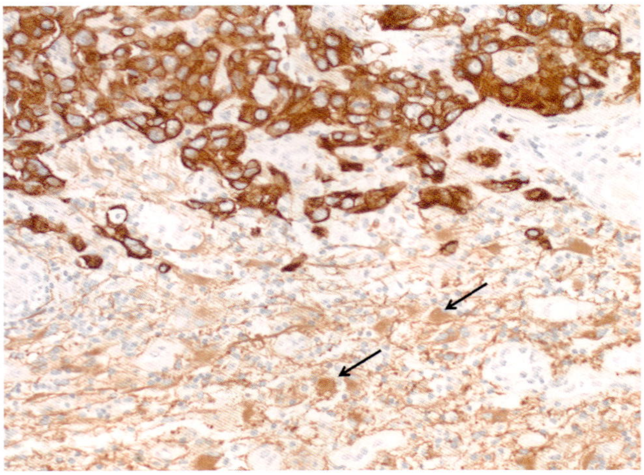

Figure 7-6. Cytokeratin in reactive astrocytes: Although relatively weak, a distinct cytokeratin positivity is seen in the cell bodies and processes of reactive astrocytes (*arrows*) surrounding the well-circumscribed metastatic carcinoma (**top**) (AE1/AE3 IHC; original magnification: 100×).

may represent true positivity.[118] At any rate, the fact that especially astrocytic cells may stain with cytokeratins should be considered in the differential diagnostic workup of high-grade neoplasms. In the context of glioblastoma, and with the use of any kind of epithelial marker, the possibility of *epithelial metaplasia* should be remembered.[119,120] Those foci are strongly and distinctly positive, however, and usually stand out in the general background of the main neoplasm and are relatively easy to recognize as long as they are kept in mind. Carcinomas with neuroendocrine features tend to show a paranuclear Golgi pattern of staining with cytokeratin, alerting one to the possibility of *neuroendocrine differentiation* especially in non–small cell carcinomas.

In the primary CNS neoplasms, cytokeratin positivity is also useful in the differential diagnosis of *choroid plexus neoplasms* from other papillary neoplasms, such as papillary ependymoma, which are more diffusely GFAP positive. Choroid plexus neoplasms, relative to metastatic carcinomas, tend to be more diffusely and strongly positive for CAM 5.2 compared to AE1/AE3 and for CK7 than for CK20.[17,121] Pancytokeratin can be focally expressed in *papillary tumor of the pineal region (PTPR)* and can be helpful in its differentiation from pineal parenchymal tumors. Cytokeratin positivity can be useful in distinguishing it from ependymoma. On the other hand, it may result in difficulty in distinguishing it from metastatic carcinoma; however, PTPR is typically only focally positive for EMA and in a cytoplasmic dot-like pattern, in contrast to the diffuse and strong positivity of many carcinomas. PTPR is also diffusely and strongly positive for vimentin, in contrast to many carcinomas.[122] *ATRT* is known for its heterogeneous immunophenotype. Along with other markers, it is positive at least focally for EMA and cytokeratin, adding to the typical mix and match immunophenotype.[19] *Meningioma* can show a focal cytokeratin positivity,[123] but this feature is especially prominent in secretory meningioma in the cells surrounding the secretory material (i.e., the so-called pseudopsammoma bodies).[124] Similar positivity in malignant meningiomas can be more confusing together with their cytohistologically malignant appearance, but diffuse and strong vimentin positivity as well as the presence of areas of more obvious and lower-grade meningioma along with the commonly present history of multiple recurrences and resections make this differential a relatively easy one. The chief cells of *paraganglioma* can be positive for cytokeratin,[23] resulting in confusion with metastatic carcinoma, especially in cases where nuclear atypia is prominent. Diffuse and strong synaptophysin and chromogranin positivity and S-100–positive sustentacular cells should alert one to the possibility of paraganglioma.

Cytokeratin can be used to highlight *epithelial metaplastic areas* that can be found in various primary neoplasms of the CNS, such as glioblastoma, gliosarcoma, and malignant meningioma. Many *sarcomas*, namely, leiomyosarcoma, MPNST and synovial sarcoma,[125] *PNET/EWS*,[126] and *angiosarcoma*[127] can show positivity for keratins. All of these neoplasms have other more typical microscopical and immunophenotypic features to help avoid confusing them with an epithelial malignancy. See below for cytokeratin expression in germ cell neoplasms.

Among many cytokeratin types, *cytokeratin 7 and 20* (CK7/CK20) profiles provide a typical immunophenotype that are associated with particular neoplasms; however, it should be kept in mind that they only provide a most common pattern, as various combinations are possible in subpopulations of various types of carcinomas.[128]

In the CNS, *choroid plexus neoplasms* are typically CK7+/CK20–.[17] This is similar to several other carcinomas that can metastasize to brain and may be in the differential of choroid plexus carcinoma. Although the latter is predominantly seen in young children, a rare case seen in adults may create significant problems in diagnosis. Other carcinomas that are typically CK7+/CK20– are breast, lung, ovarian, and biliary origin[128] and are positive with a variety of other markers that are negative in choroid plexus carcinoma. *Endolymphatic sac tumors* are also typically CK7+/CK20–.[129] *PTPR* can be confused with choroid plexus neoplasms due to its epithelioid appearance and papillary component.[122] In addition to its positivity for pancytokeratin, CK7 negativity also becomes a useful feature in this differential. *CK18* is diffusely positive in PTPR and can be helpful in its differential from pineal parenchymal tumors and choroid plexus neoplasms. In addition to pancytokeratin, *CAM 5.2* is also positive in *PTPR* and is useful in distinguishing this intraventricular neoplasm from choroid plexus neoplasms, although it can show a dot or ball-like staining in some *choroid plexus neoplasms*.

CAM 5.2 identifies simple epithelia such as secretory epithelial cells over squamous epithelial cells. More specifically, it identifies CK7 and 8, although it has been commonly and inappropriately used interchangeably to mean CK8 and 18.[130] Therefore, it may not always be clear what types of cytokeratins are in fact included in a particular study; however, whether CK7 and 8 or CK8 and 18 are used, there does not appear to be a significant difference in their target cells and staining results in practice. At any rate, CAM 5.2 provides an alternative cytokeratin antibody in cases where the positivity of AE1/AE3 in *astrocyte cytoplasm* may pose a problem. Usually, this situation is self-evident and does not pose a significant diagnostic problem. It highlights the *fibrous bodies of sparsely granulated growth hormone cell adenomas* of the pituitary gland[131] **(Fig. 7-7)** and can be seen in acidophil stem cell adenoma also.[132] ACTH cell adenomas are particularly strongly and diffusely positive for

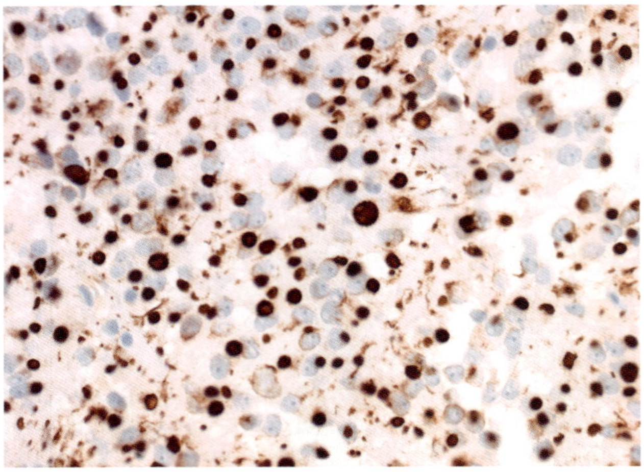

Figure 7-7. CAM 5.2 in sparsely granulated somatotroph adenoma: Fibrous bodies are abundant and are highlighted as round paranuclear cytoplasmic structures of variable sizes (CAM 5.2 IHC; original magnification: 400×).

cytokeratins. In addition, perinuclear circular accumulation of cytokeratin (*Crooke's hyaline change*) is highlighted as stronger positivity in such cells. In the evaluation of pituitary adenomas, CAM 5.2 provides a more widespread and stronger staining compared to AE1/AE3. Both AE1/AE3 and CAM 5.2 positivity is present in *chordoma*,[133] which may potentially add to the confusion with metastatic carcinoma; however, with the typical midline location along with vimentin, S-100 protein, and EMA coexpression, this should not be a significant problem. In addition, expression of cytokeratins in chordoma is useful in distinguishing it from chondrosarcoma,[134] a common differential diagnostic challenge in skull base **(Table 7.4)**.

Epithelial membrane antigen (EMA) highlights the luminal surfaces of the *true rosettes in ependymoma*. In addition, *intracytoplasmic lumens* are also highlighted by EMA as minute circles or even smaller dots **(Fig. 7-8)**, even though they may not be visible on H&E preparations. While the typical histologic appearance of ependymoma is quite diagnostic, EMA positivity is especially helpful in small tissue samples and in cases where the diagnostic features are not readily identified, such as clear cell ependymoma. On the other hand, *myxopapillary ependymomas* do not show EMA positivity, a feature that should be kept in mind in the differential diagnosis of neoplasms with myxoid background.[135] A *dot-like cytoplasmic positivity*, among other patterns of positivity, may be present in *angiocentric glioma*, suggesting an ependymal origin.[136] A similar pattern is also seen in *PTPR*. *Chordoid glioma* is also thought to have a histogenesis related to specialized ependyma associated with subventricular organs and, as such, has variable focal EMA positivity.[10] Since it is also GFAP positive, it is unlikely to be confused with chordoma and chordoid meningioma, especially when its specific location in the anterior third ventricle is taken into account. Some *choroid plexus neoplasms* are also positive.[17] *ATRT* is known for its heterogeneous immunophenotype, and EMA is one of the markers that is commonly positive in this peculiar

TABLE 7.4 Characteristic immunophenotypical differential diagnosis of myxoid/mucinous neoplasms

Antibody	Chordoma	CS	Carcinoma[a]	ME	PG
Cytokeratins	+	–	+	–	–
EMA	+	–	+	–	–
S-100 protein	+	+	–	+	+ (sustentacular cells)
Vimentin	+	+	–/+	–/+	+
GFAP	+	–	–	+	–
Brachyury	+	–	–	–	–
E-cadherin	+	–	+	–	–
CEA	–/+	–	+	–	–
Synaptophysin	–	–	+ (neuroendocrine differentiation)	–	+

[a]Carcinomas are also positive for other more specific markers depending on their origin.
+, positive; –, negative; –/+, predominantly negative.
CS, chondrosarcoma; ME, myxopapillary ependymoma; PG, paraganglioma; EMA, epithelial membrane antigen; GFAP, glial fibrillary acidic protein; CEA, carcinoembryonic antigen.

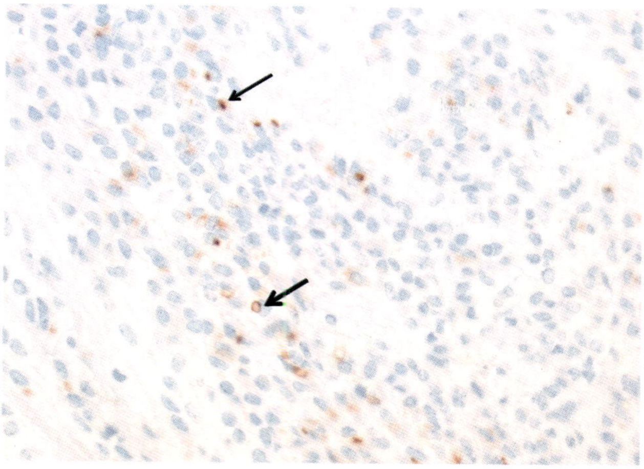

Figure 7-8. EMA in ependymoma: Subtle clues to ependymal differentiation can be obtained by the identification of cytoplasmic microlumens seen as small circles (*thick arrow*), as well as dots (*thin arrow*). They may be discarded as stain artifact at low magnification, especially focal and few, and require careful evaluation (EMA IHC; original magnification: 400×).

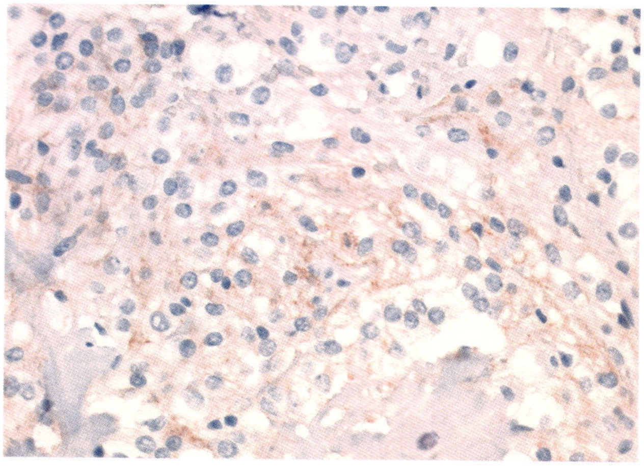

Figure 7-9. EMA in meningioma: A weak blush may be all there is by EMA in some meningiomas, a finding that can be discarded as a stain artifact since it is not as crisp and strong as would be the case in carcinomas. Threshold for positivity or the antibody concentration need to be adjusted for accurate evaluation (EMA IHC; original magnification: 400×).

neoplasm.[19] *Pituicytoma*, a glial neoplasm that arises from the pituicytes in the posterior pituitary, can be variably positive for EMA, along with variable GFAP positivity.[137]

Meningioma is positive for EMA as a rule; however, its positivity is variable, weak, and focal **(Fig. 7-9)**. This pattern contrasts sharply with the staining pattern of a *metastatic adenocarcinoma*. In the evaluation of EMA staining in a meningioma, the threshold for positivity should be lowered. Obtaining staining results in meningioma comparable to carcinoma is possible by making technical adjustments, such as using a higher concentration of the antibody; however, this is not practical for the laboratories in many practice settings that do not have meningioma cases frequent enough to justify such an adjustment. It is more practical to be aware of this pitfall with meningioma and to adjust interpretation threshold to accept this type of focal and weak staining as positive in a neoplasm that appear to be meningothelial in origin. Similar remarks are in order for EMA staining in *perineurioma*. While perineurial cells and its neoplasms are positive for EMA, they tend to stain weakly, requiring extra care in the interpretation. It highlights the pseudo-onion bulbs in intraneural perineurioma, as well as the spindle cells of the soft tissue perineurioma, and is useful in its diagnosis especially in the sclerotic variant in which the bland neoplastic cells may be obscured.[45] Perineurioma component of composite peripheral nerve sheath tumors is also identified by EMA. In the setting of peripheral nerve sheath tumors, EMA can be used to highlight the *perineurium* in some cases,[138] such as the palisaded encapsulated neuroma of the skin and superficial soft tissues or intraneural neurofibroma and plexiform neurofibroma or schwannoma. Identification of perineurium with EMA is especially useful in those plexiform neoplasms where the perineurium has been breached and the neoplasm has spread into the surrounding tissues, obscuring its plexiform nature. Perineurium is present around small nerve fascicles in amputation neuromas and in mucosal neuromas. Usually those in association with multiple endocrine neoplasia IIb (MEN-IIb) may have multiple small fascicles surrounded by perineurium, resembling an amputation neuroma.[139] *Nerve sheath myxoma* contains scattered EMA-positive spindle cells along with many S-100 protein–positive cells in a myxoid background. *Epithelioid malignant peripheral nerve sheath tumor* can be focally or widely cytokeratin and EMA positive in an occasional case, creating confusion with metastatic carcinoma. It is also more prominently positive for S-100 protein than the conventional MPNST, causing additional confusion with melanoma.[140] Focal EMA staining can be seen in *leiomyosarcoma*.[141]

Of the hematopoietic cells and their neoplasms, EMA positivity can be identified in plasma cells and plasma cell myeloma,[142] some types of Hodgkin lymphoma,[143] and non-Hodgkin lymphoma.[144]

Carcinoembryonic antigen (CEA) is a glycoprotein with several subtypes and is useful in the workup of *metastatic carcinomas*. Typically, adenocarcinomas of the lung, gastrointestinal tract including pancreatobiliary tract, upper respiratory tract, and breast are positive, while renal, prostatic, adrenal endometrial, and ovarian serous carcinomas are negative. Polyclonal CEA is particularly useful in highlighting the bile canalicular pattern in hepatocellular carcinomas. In the CNS, CEA is useful in highlighting the secretory material (pseudopsammoma bodies) and the surrounding cells in *secretory meningioma*. It has been suggested that secretory meningioma may cause an elevation of serum CEA,[124] potentially interfering with the follow-up of patients with colorectal carcinoma. Some *chordomas* can have CEA positivity, which may add to the potential confusion with metastatic carcinoma[145] (see above). It may, however, help in distinguishing chordoma from chondrosarcoma by being negative in the latter.[25] CEA may be useful in identifying some *germ cell neoplasm* components as it can be positive in yolk sac tumor, germinoma and choriocarcinoma, but negative in embryonal carcinoma.[146]

Present in a membranous staining pattern normally in epithelial cells except for the luminal surfaces and in carcinoma, *E-cadherin* can be positive in *choroid plexus neoplasms*, which may be important to note as a pitfall in distinguishing these neoplasms from metastatic carcinomas. In the context of their differential diagnosis from papillary ependymoma, however, e-cadherin positivity is useful as ependymomas are negative. It has also been identified in *chordomas*,[147,148] but not in chondrosarcomas,[147,149] as well as in *meningiomas*.[150]

Pituitary Hormones

IHC is important in accurately *classifying an adenoma*, by identifying densely or sparsely granulated, plurihormonal, silent (lacking clinical and biochemical evidence for hormone secretion but

List of Findings/Checklist for Pituitary Hormones

AT A GLANCE

Pituitary Hormones

- Prolactin
- Growth hormone
- Adrenocorticotropic hormone
- Thyroid-stimulating hormone
- Follicle-stimulating hormone
- Luteinizing hormone
- GATA-2
- Pit-1
- SF-1
- Alpha-subunit

Pituitary Adenomas

- Prolactinoma
    - Densely granulated
    - Sparsely granulated
- Somatotroph adenoma
    - Densely granulated
    - Sparsely granulated
- Mixed somatotroph and lactotroph adenoma
- Somatomammotroph adenoma
- Acidophil stem cell adenoma
- Corticotroph adenoma
- Silent corticotroph adenoma
    - Densely granulated (silent subtype I)
    - Sparsely granulated (silent subtype II)
- Crooke's cell change
- Crooke's cell adenoma
- Thyrotroph adenoma
- Gonadotroph adenomas
- Plurihormonal adenoma
- Silent subtype III adenoma
- Null cell adenoma
- Ganglion cell differentiation

Nonneoplastic Conditions

- Pituitary hyperplasia
- Resting pituitary parenchyma
- Normal cell distribution
- Basophil invasion of posterior pituitary

positive by IHC), or null cell adenomas. Some adenomas may have various combinations of hormone secretion with variable clinical and immunohistochemical features and may not fit into any of the defined categories **(Table 7.5)**. If *nonneoplastic parenchymal fragments* are present in the specimen, they provide a good internal control for hormone IHC, both for adenoma and for hyperplasia, by being positive for essentially all hormones and by providing an idea about the normal distribution of

TABLE 7.5 Characteristic immunophenotypes of pituitary adenoma subtypes

Antibody Positivity	Adenoma	Other Features
Growth hormone Pit-1 Alpha-subunit	Densely granulated somatotroph Sparsely granulated somatotroph	CAM 5.2 + (cytoplasmic) CAM 5.2 + (fibrous bodies)
Growth hormone Prolactin Pit-1 Alpha-subunit	Mixed somatotroph–lactotroph Somatomammotroph	
Growth hormone Prolactin TSH Pit-1 Alpha-subunit	Plurihormonal	
Growth hormone Prolactin Pit-1	Acidophil stem cell	CAM 5.2 + (fibrous bodies)
Prolactin Pit-1	Densely granulated lactotroph Sparsely granulated lactotroph	Prolactin (diffuse cytoplasmic) Prolactin (Golgi pattern)
TSH Pit-1 Alpha-subunit	Thyrotroph	PAS + (scattered cytoplasmic granules)
ACTH Tpit	Densely granulated corticotroph Sparsely granulated corticotroph Crooke cell Silent corticotroph (no clinical and biochemical ACTH excess) Densely granulated (silent subtype I) Sparsely granulated (silent subtype II)	 CAM 5.2 + (perinuclear, dense, Crooke's hyaline change); ACTH (peripheral cytoplasmic rim)
FSH and/or LH SF-1 Alpha-subunit	Gonadotroph	
Various combinations of hormones except as mentioned above	Plurihormonal	
Growth hormone Prolactin TSH	Silent subtype III (no clinical and biochemical hormone excess)	
No hormone positivity by IHC Alpha-subunit only	Null cell	

+, positive; TSH, thyroid-stimulating hormone; ACTH, adrenocorticotropic hormone; FSH, follicle-stimulating hormone; LH, luteinizing hormone; SF-1, steroidogenic factor-1.

various types of hormone-producing cells to compare with hyperplastic tissue and a reference point for the reticulin network of the resting pituitary parenchyma in cases of nodular hyperplasia. In general, performance and evaluation of IHC is not advisable in *necrotic or hemorrhagic tissue* as the results are usually misleading. The details of pituitary adenoma histogenesis, practical pathologic pints, and classification based on IHC and other factors are well-detailed elsewhere.[151–153] This discussion only reiterates the various staining patterns that can be encountered in association with particular situations. Such hormonal classification is not only important to shed light to clinical findings but also has prognostic implications in some cases.[154] For instance, highest invasion rates have been identified in treated PRL cell adenomas, ACTH adenomas of Nelson's syndrome, silent ACTH adenomas of subtype II, and silent subtype III adenomas.

Prolactin positivity in *densely granulated prolactinoma (lactotroph adenoma)* is strong and *diffuse cytoplasmic*, while it shows a *paranuclear dot-like staining*, that is, Golgi pattern, in *sparsely granulated prolactinoma*. As in prolactinoma, depending on the extent and strength of *growth hormone* positivity, *growth hormone–secreting adenomas (somatotroph adenoma)* are divided into densely or sparsely granulated adenomas. *Densely granulated adenoma* shows *diffuse cytoplasmic positivity*, while *sparsely granulated adenoma* show a *paranuclear dot-like Golgi pattern* of positivity in a subpopulation of cells. Sparsely granulated adenoma also shows *fibrous bodies*, which can be highlighted by cytokeratin, especially CAM 5.2. *Combined prolactin and growth hormone positivity* is also variably present in *acidophil stem cell adenoma*, in which prolactin positivity is typically stronger than growth hormone positivity, which may sometimes be negative. Acidophil stem cell adenoma can be distinguished from others by its characteristic acidophil cells, vacuolated cytoplasms, and nuclear atypia. Fibrous bodies may be present. *Mixed somatotroph and lactotroph adenoma* shows growth hormone and prolactin positivity in different populations of cells in the same adenoma, while *somatomammotroph adenoma* shows positivity for both in the same population of cells. Some of these adenomas can also secrete thyroid-stimulating hormone (TSH), alpha-subunit, and even gonadotropins.

Adrenocorticotropic hormone (ACTH) identifies the *ACTH-producing (corticotroph) adenomas*. *Silent ACTH-producing adenomas* are characterized by immunohistochemical ACTH positivity in the absence of biochemical ACTH elevation or clinical findings of ACTH excess. ACTH staining may be strong or weak, corresponding to *densely or sparsely granulated nature of the silent adenoma*, which may also be called *silent subtype I and II*, respectively. In cells with well-developed *Crooke's hyaline change*, ACTH provides a negative image of cytokeratin stain, by being positive as a *peripheral rim*, similar to cytoplasmic membranous staining pattern. *Crooke's cell adenoma* is composed predominantly of such cells. Production of alpha-subunit and prolactin can be seen in occasional ACTH cell adenomas.

Thyroid-stimulating hormone (TSH) cell (thyrotroph) adenomas are variably positive. Many may show a *weak staining* and may appear like a cytoplasmic blush. *Gonadotroph cell adenomas* producing luteinizing hormone (LH) and/or follicle-stimulating hormone (FSH) are positive for their respective hormones in a *variable pattern* and usually in the form of *scattered cells*. They are typically of sparsely granulated type. TSH and/or gonadotropin secretion can be seen together with growth hormone and prolactin secretion. Some pituitary adenomas can produce more than one type of hormone, that is, they are *plurihormonal adenomas*. They exclude, by definition, the aforementioned combinations of growth hormone, prolactin and TSH; or LH and FSH. They more commonly combine TSH, FSH, and growth hormone; or prolactin and TSH. *Silent subtype III adenomas* often show focal and weak positivity for a variety of combinations of hormones, usually only with immunohistochemical evidence of growth hormone, prolactin, and TSH. They may sometimes be classified as null cell adenomas; however, electron microscopically, they are relatively differentiated compared to the truly *null cell adenoma*, which is typically an indolent neoplasm, while silent subtype III adenoma is an aggressive neoplasm. Null cell adenoma is also clinically and biochemically silent and, in addition, immunohistochemically negative for pituitary hormones. Occasionally, a focal and weak staining for gonadotropins, TSH, or alpha subunit may be seen.

Pit-1 is a transcription factor that is needed for the differentiation of somatotrophs, lactotrophs, mammosomatotrophs, and thyrotrophs, and its positivity places an adenoma in this category, excluding gonadotroph and corticotroph adenomas. It also, at least in part, explains the common combinations of these hormones in some adenomas. *Tpit* is involved in corticotroph differentiation, while *GATA-2* and *steroidogenic factor-1 (SF-1)* are involved in gonadotroph differentiation. GATA-2 is also involved in thyrotroph differentiation. *Alpha-subunit* is a component of glycoprotein hormones, that is, the gonadotropins and TSH and is associated with the adenomas secreting these hormones, including those adenomas where they accompany as a minor component other primary hormone secretion, such as mixed somatomammotroph adenoma with TSH secretion. It can be present in densely (but not sparsely) granulated somatotroph adenoma, as well as in somatomammotroph adenoma. *Ganglion cell differentiation* can be seen in an otherwise ordinary adenoma. These ganglion cells are also positive for the *pituitary hormones* that the adenoma is secreting, as well as for *cytokeratin*, supporting a metaplastic origin from the adenoma.

Predominance of one or more types of hormone positivity is seen in *hyperplasia* and may be mistaken for adenoma in small tissue samples. To avoid such confusion, IHC evaluation should be correlated with reticulin stain. This will also help avoid the pitfall of mistaking *topographical differences* in the frequency of cell types in resting pituitary parenchyma with hyperplasia or adenoma. Prominent examples include the predominance of growth hormone–secreting cells in the lateral, and ACTH-secreting cells in the middle sections of the gland. Another pitfall is the common uniform ACTH positivity of the basophilic cells spilling into the posterior pituitary parenchyma, that is, the so-called *basophil infiltration of the posterior pituitary*, which should not be taken as evidence of an invasive corticotroph adenoma.

List of Findings/Checklist for Prognostic and Predictive Markers

AT A GLANCE

Ki-67 Proliferation Index

- Meningioma
- Pituitary adenoma
- Pineal parenchymal neoplasms
- Reactive versus neoplastic astrocytic proliferations
- Recurrent/residual astrocytic neoplasm versus radiation change/reactive astrocytosis
- Ganglion cell neoplasms
- PXA versus glioblastoma
- Choroid plexus neoplasms
- Neurocytoma
- Astroblastoma
- Adamantinomatous craniopharyngioma

Proliferating Cell Nuclear Antigen
Phosphohistone H3
P53

- Pituitary adenoma
- Reactive versus neoplastic astrocytic proliferations
- Astrocytes versus other cell types
- Oligoastrocytoma
- Pilocytic astrocytoma versus infiltrating astrocytoma
- Ependymoma
- Peripheral nerve sheath neoplasms
  - Malignant peripheral nerve sheath tumor versus neurofibroma
- Li-Fraumeni syndrome

Sex Steroid Hormone Receptors

- Progesterone receptor
- Estrogen receptor
- Androgen receptor
- HER2
- Breast carcinoma
- Meningioma
- Craniopharyngioma

Isocitrate Dehydrogenase 1 and 2

- Reactive versus neoplastic astrocytic proliferations
- Pilocytic astrocytoma versus infiltrating astrocytoma
- Primary versus secondary glioblastoma

O^6-Methylguanin-DNA Methyltransferase

- Glioblastoma
- Anaplastic astrocytoma
- Low-grade astrocytoma, oligodendroglioma and oligoastrocytoma

Cyclooxygenase 2
CD133

Prognostic and Predictive Markers

Ki-67 represents an antigen that is associated with the nuclei of the cells in the G_1, S, G_2, and M phases of the cell cycle and is absent in the quiescent G_0 phase,[155] providing a marker for proliferative activity.[156] It identifies the cells in the entire proliferative phase, in contrast to mitotic count, which identifies the cells only in the M phase. Therefore, it is not surprising that the results of the mitotic counts and Ki-67 proliferation indices may or may not correlate, that is, a high proliferation index does not necessarily translate into a high mitotic count. The first antibody that works on formalin-fixed, paraffin-embedded tissue sections was MIB-1.[157] For this reason, even though there are different clone names by different companies, MIB-1 has been traditionally and somewhat inaccurately used interchangeably with any Ki-67 immunohistochemical antibody regardless of its source and is sometimes referred to in combination as Ki-67/MIB-1.

In general, Ki-67 *proliferation index* tends to increase with increasing grade of the neoplasm[158]; however, there are no definitive cutoff values for individual neoplasms or grades.[159] Rather, variable and overlapping ranges of indices are available, making it necessary to be used with caution and in specific contexts. No definitive grading or diagnosis should be based solely on Ki-67 staining. Similar to the obstacles and pitfalls associated with mitotic counts (see Chapter 2 "Mitotic Activity"), there are issues with the evaluation of Ki-67 proliferation index. Differences in the antibody source[160] and evaluation methods can affect the results. The well-known histologic heterogeneity of the nervous system neoplasms and especially glial neoplasms is also reflected in the proliferation indices. It is not unusual to see a high variability in the frequency of positive nuclei, with very active foci alternating with quite low proliferative activity. While it is tempting and intuitive to concentrate on the more active areas, it may not always provide the best information applicable to the entire neoplasm. For instance, based on the comparison of two methods for counting the positive nuclei in meningiomas, the results obtained by counting random areas appeared to correlate better with recurrence and tumor growth compared to those results obtained by counting the areas of highest activity, although the results of either method correlated with the WHO grading.[161] In addition, there may be differences in the intensity of staining, creating subjectivity as to what is really positive. Using different intensity levels as cutoff for counting, a wide overlap was identified in meningiomas across all three WHO grades[162] **(Fig. 7-10)**. Even if interobserver and intraobserver subjectivity and variability may be overcome by using image analysis systems, the decision of a particular intensity cutoff point will still be subjective. This method, however, will likely provide consistency within the same institution, although reaching a consensus across institutions would still remain a problem. Most likely at least in part due to such issues with interpretation, some neuropathologists tend to indicate the results as "low" or "high" depending on the situation. Nonetheless, this issue is far from the strict criteria that are being implemented for the interpretation and reporting of the results of other prognostic studies in breast lesions.[163,164] Evaluation in general should take into account the positivity in the atypical and obviously neoplastic cells because there may be many other cell types, such as inflammatory cells, macrophages/microglia, and vascular cells, especially in the reactive or proliferating vessels, that can result in falsely

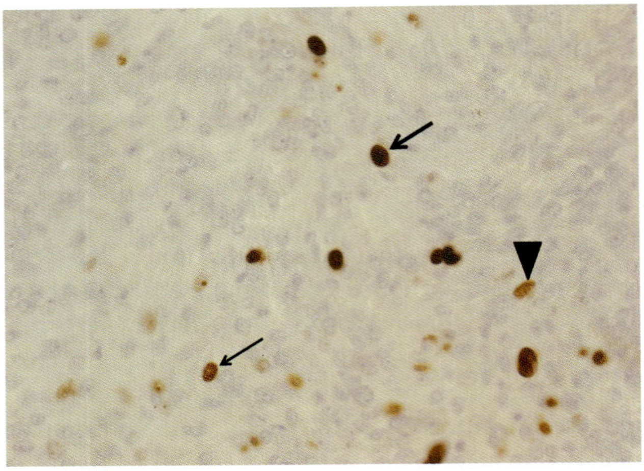

Figure 7-10. Proliferation index: Roughly three different staining intensities are highlighted as intense (*thick arrow*), intermediate (*thin arrow*), and weak (*arrowhead*). Although all are technically positive, counting of each will clearly result in widely variable and overlapping results in this meningioma (Ki-67 IHC; original magnification: 400×).

high proliferative indices. Aside from these practical issues, no definitive numerical cutoff values have been identified for any given neoplasm and the meaning of any given number in any given case remains open for speculation. On the other hand, useful information can be obtained from proliferation index in some cases.

According to WHO classification, *meningiomas* with a high proliferation index have a greater likelihood of recurrence and/or aggressive behavior grade by grade, although proliferation index does not affect grading.[165] Although there is broad overlap, proliferation indices increase from a mean of 3.8% in benign meningiomas to a mean of 7.2% in atypical and 14.7% in anaplastic/malignant meningiomas,[166] with the suggestion that proliferation indices greater than 4% indicate a behavior similar to atypical meningioma while values greater than 20% indicate a behavior similar to anaplastic meningioma.[167] It may also add one more piece of information in cases with borderline features, that is, those that may be difficult to grade between WHO grades I and II and between II and III. Proliferation index, similar to mitotic activity, may be higher around necrotic areas as a reaction, especially around the large areas of necrosis in embolized meningiomas,[168] requiring caution in interpretation. *Pituitary adenomas* are further evaluated by Ki-67 and p53, as well as mitotic counts in an attempt to subclassify some as atypical adenomas to indicate a more aggressive biologic behavior and likelihood of recurrence. A Ki-67 proliferation index greater than 3%, p53 positivity, and increased mitotic activity appear to indicate a more aggressive behavior, though the correlation is less than optimal in some cases.[169,170] As in meningiomas, Ki-67 proliferation index has been proposed as a formal component in the grading of *pineal parenchymal neoplasms* as a correlation was identified between proliferation indices and grades of these neoplasms.[53]

Proliferation index can provide supportive information in confusing situations and help with difficult differential diagnoses; however, it should not be used as the sole determinant of a diagnosis or grading. For instance, in the differential diagnosis of *reactive gliosis versus low-grade glioma*, identification of even low proliferative activity is a useful feature to favor glioma (see also Chapter 2, "Hypercellularity"). Again, one should make sure that the positive nuclei belong to the cell type of interest, that is, the astrocytes, and not to inflammatory cells, vascular cells, especially endothelial cells, macrophages, or activated microglia. In *recurrent neoplasms*, subsequent resections do not necessarily show an increase in the grade of the neoplasm; however, comparison with the histology of previous specimens may show a gradually increasing cytologic atypia and/or mitotic count. Likewise, Ki-67 staining can also provide a means of comparison in regard to the proliferative activity of subsequent neoplasms. Again, an increased Ki-67 index favors *recurrent/residual neoplasm versus radiation change or reactive gliosis* (see Chapter 2, "Hypercellularity"). Under circumstances when *small size of the tissue and/or various artifacts*, especially crush artifact, preclude optimal evaluation of mitotic activity, Ki-67 can provide a tool to assess proliferative activity, keeping in mind that mitotic count and proliferation index do not always mirror each other.

Similar to the situation with reactive gliosis versus low-grade infiltrating glioma, Ki-67 can be used to gauge the proliferative activity of the background of *ganglion cell neoplasms* in subtle cases to decide on the presence of a glioma component, with similar caveats. In addition, a proliferation index of 5% or more may be associated with atypical ganglioglioma.[86]

In the face of a *highly pleomorphic neoplasm* such as *PXA*, and when working with a small amount of tissue in which definitive diagnostic features are not obvious, distinguishing it from a high-grade glial neoplasm may become a challenge. In such a situation, high proliferation index is useful to favor the latter as a typical PXA has a proliferation index of about 3% or less.[171] The possibility of PXA with anaplastic features should be remembered in this situation, however, as they can have proliferation indices of about 20%.[171] In distinguishing *choroid plexus papilloma* from nonneoplastic choroid plexus, essentially any Ki-67 positivity in the epithelial cells favors papilloma.[172] Some *neurocytomas*, central or extraventricular, can have more than an occasional mitotic figure, are associated with vascular proliferation and necrosis, and have been designated as atypical neurocytomas, without a WHO grade. They also tend to have a Ki-67 proliferation index of more than 2%.[173] An anaplastic version of neurocytoma, however, has not yet been designated and is debatable. A difference in proliferation index is useful in subclassifying *astroblastoma* into well-differentiated and anaplastic (malignant), with the well-differentiated astroblastoma having a proliferation index of about 3% and anaplastic versions usually more than 10%.[174] Usefulness of proliferative index as a significant prognostic indicator in *adamantinomatous craniopharyngioma* is debated based on the higher proliferation indices found in recurrent neoplasms.[175]

In some *biphasic neoplasms*, Ki-67 highlights the high- and low-proliferating areas, such as the small cell, PNET-like foci of DIG with high proliferative index relative to spindle cell, glial component, as well as the PNET component versus the more differentiated ganglion cell areas for a ganglioneuroblastoma. Ki-67 brings out the nodules of differentiated neuronal areas in *desmoplastic medulloblastoma* by being essentially negative in these areas and highlighting the prominent proliferative activity in the primitive cells among these nodules. This creates a negative image with the Neu-N pattern, which is positive in the differentiated cells within the nodules but is negative in the primitive cell population among them.

Proliferating cell nuclear antigen (PCNA) is a nonhistone nuclear protein that is necessary in DNA synthesis and appears in the late G1 phase and remains throughout the rest of the proliferative cycle.[176] It has been reported to be a less sensitive marker for proliferating cells compared to Ki-67 but to be relatively more specific for the S-phase of the proliferation cycle.[177] Although a correlation with PCNA labeling index and the grade of various CNS neoplasms has been identified, it was not found to be reliable for predicting the prognosis of the disease in individual cases.[178] Since it also tends to remain even after the cell division, inaccurately high results are not unusual.[156]

Phosphohistone H3 (PHH3) is a histone protein that is associated with mitosis[179] and antibodies against it has been shown to identify the nuclei in mitosis in meningiomas[180] and astrocytomas.[181] It has been found to be a more sensitive marker for mitotic index than counting mitotic figures on routine sections in meningiomas and, apparently for this reason, a higher mitotic index can be obtained in a given case,[182,183] resulting in an upgrading of some cases unless new cutoff values are identified. Nonetheless, it can be used with caution to highlight the mitotic figures and the mitotically active areas, as well as helping distinguishing mitotic figures from apoptotic cells. In addition, in cases where simply the presence of mitotic figures, but not necessarily their accurate counting, are critical, this antibody can help easily identify their presence.

P53 is the protein product of tumor suppressor gene, *TP53*. When activated, p53 functions as a checkpoint by stopping the cell cycle or sending the cell to apoptosis,[184] preventing the multiplication of damaged cells, thereby reducing the chances of mutations and neoplastic growth.[185] This tumor suppressor function suffers if there are mutations of *TP53*, resulting in defective p53 protein, which accumulates in the nucleus, in contrast to the normal protein, which has a short half-life.[186] This accumulation can then be detected by IHC as a nuclear stain. Sometimes, p53 accumulation and its immunohistochemical detection may occur without the presence of mutations through epigenetic mechanisms,[187] that is, false-positive results. *Pituitary adenomas* are further evaluated by Ki-67 and p53, as well as mitotic counts in an attempt to identify atypical adenomas to indicate a more aggressive biologic behavior and likelihood of recurrence. Atypical adenoma shows p53 overexpression[169,170] (see Ki-67). Nuclear p53 protein overexpression is identified in a significant subpopulation of neoplastic processes, although only in those with astrocytic features, and essentially in none of the nonneoplastic lesions.[188] While similar results have been reproduced for neoplastic processes, some *nonneoplastic lesions*, such as progressive multifocal leukoencephalopathy (PML), have been found to be overexpressing p53.[189] It has subsequently been shown that p53 overexpression is not limited to *astrocytic neoplasms* but is also seen in a wide variety of *reactive processes* and *other cell types*, likely due to binding to MDM-2 resulting in extended half-life without associated mutations.[190] Other studies on *oligoastrocytomas* suggested that p53 overexpression was present in the astrocytic-appearing cells in the subpopulation of the neoplasms that showed overexpression.[191] P53 overexpression has been associated with a worse prognosis in *ependymomas*.[192] Only a small subpopulation of *pilocytic astrocytomas* show p53 overexpression,[193] providing an immunohistochemical tool that can potentially be used to differentiate pilocytic astrocytomas, especially in small tissue samples, from *infiltrating astrocytomas*, which tend to more commonly overexpress p53, keeping in mind the small overlapping population in each group.

In *peripheral nerve sheath tumors*, p53 overexpression can be used to identify malignant transformation in subtle cases, along with identification of mitotic figures and increased Ki-67 proliferation index.[194] P53 tends to be overexpressed in a high percentage of *malignant peripheral nerve sheath tumors* in contrast to *neurofibromas*. In addition, the overexpression tends to be more prominent in MPNST than in neurofibromas.[195] P53 staining is weak in *cellular schwannoma* and shows no correlation with recurrence.[196]

Multiple organ cancers, including various brain neoplasms are seen in *Li-Fraumeni syndrome*, which is associated with germline mutations of *TP53*.[197] Astrocytomas predominate among the CNS neoplasms and peripheral nerve sheath neoplasms can also be seen.[198] No histologic differences to allow the distinction of syndromic neoplasms from their sporadic counterparts are identified, including p53 IHC.[197]

Evaluation of *sex steroid hormone receptors* by IHC, in addition to their routine use in *breast carcinoma* in general surgical pathology and in cases metastatic to the brain, is also utilized in *meningiomas*. Their identification may contribute to the explanation of accelerated meningioma growth in high hormone level states, such as pregnancy.[199] *Progesterone receptor (PR)* is present in nonneoplastic arachnoid cells[200] and has been identified in meningiomas.[201] As in the case of Ki-67 proliferation index, since no definitive guidelines exist, when cases were considered to be "positive" for PR with more than 1% of neoplastic nuclei are staining, immunohistochemical positivity for PR gradually decreased with increasing WHO grades of meningiomas.[202] Although only 51% of WHO grade I meningiomas were positive for PR, no significant differences were identified between recurrent and nonrecurrent WHO grade I meningiomas by PR status. Any such differences became more significant with increasing grade, in spite of a wide overlap among different grades.[202] PR positivity is typically patchy, not uniform, with alternating groups of positive and negative nuclei, superficially resembling a checkerboard pattern.[203] It appears that the prognostic significance of PR status is closely associated with other parameters and not as an independent marker.[165] Nonetheless, when needed in borderline clinical situations, it may provide useful information. *Estrogen receptor (ER)*, on the other hand, has not generated as much interest. It is not present in nonneoplastic meningothelial cells[204] but can be identified in a subpopulation of meningiomas, and in combination with PR, additional information may be generated. It has been suggested that ER- and PR-negative and ER-positive meningiomas are associated with more aggressive behavior.[205] Despite these findings, no clinically significant progress has been made in the treatment of meningiomas with antihormonal agents. No difference in hormone receptor expression was found among histologic types of meningiomas, and ER expression was noted to parallel *androgen receptor (AR)* status.[206] AR has not been utilized in diagnostic clinical practice. Meningiomas with *HER2* overexpression and gene amplification were found to have higher recurrence rates,[150] although its value as an independent prognostic factor may need further investigation, as HER2-positive meningiomas were also found to have a tendency toward being PR-negative and having higher proliferation indices.[207] The incidence of postoperative tumor regrowth was found to be significantly higher in patients whose *craniopharyngiomas* were negative for ER and PR than in those positive for both receptors.[175]

Isocitrate dehydrogenase 1 and 2 (IDH1 & 2) are involved in the conversion of isocitrate to alpha-ketoglutarate and reduce nicotinamide adenine dinucleotide phosphate (NADP+). IDH1 is located in peroxisomes, and IDH2 is present in mitochondria.[208] The great majority of IDH1 mutations are R132H, while others, as well as IDH2 mutations, also occur.[209] They have been identified in *low-grade and anaplastic astrocytoma*, *oligodendroglioma*, and *oligoastrocytoma*, as well as in *secondary glioblastoma*, while they are rare in *primary glioblastoma* and *pleomorphic xanthoastrocytoma* and absent in *ependymoma*, *pilocytic astrocytoma*, *pediatric glioblastoma*, *medulloblastoma*, and *non-CNS neoplasms*.[210] *Reactive conditions* were also devoid of these mutations.[211] These findings suggest that IDH1 & 2 status can be potentially used to distinguish reactive gliosis from low-grade astrocytoma, primary from secondary glioblastoma, glioblastoma from pleomorphic xanthoastrocytoma, and pilocytic astrocytoma from infiltrating astrocytoma. It is also useful in the identification of well-circumscribed versus infiltrative nature of the borders of the neoplasms by highlighting any infiltrating neoplastic cells.[212] It has been suggested that IHC for R132H, the most common type of IDH1 mutation, may be a more sensitive method than sequencing.[213] However, since it leaves out the other types of mutations and IDH2 mutations, molecular techniques may be preferred for a more comprehensive approach to identify all mutations. While the functions of the enzymes and the effects of the mutations are not exactly clear, identification of these mutations may provide prognostic information since the presence of IDH1 mutation has been associated with a better prognosis in gliomas as an independent marker,[214] even though they are also closely associated with 1p/19q deletions and O^6-methylguanine-DNA methyltransferase (MGMT) methylation status.[214,215] IDH1 positivity in oligodendrogliomas was also found to be a good marker to distinguish them from their mimics, including those neoplasms with oligodendroglial-like components, as well as pediatric oligodendrogliomas, which are all negative.[216]

O^6-methylguanine-DNA methyltransferase (MGMT), sometimes also referred to as O^6-alkylguanine-DNA-alkyltransferase, is a DNA repair protein that counteracts the effect of alkylating agents in gliomas by repairing the DNA damage caused by these agents.[217] *MGMT* promoter methylation is associated with the disruption of this repair mechanism, resulting in increased efficacy of the alkylating agent and better response by *anaplastic astrocytoma*[218] and *glioblastoma,*[218,219] as well as *low-grade astrocytomas*, *oligodendrogliomas*, and *oligoastrocytomas*.[220] Unfortunately, molecular techniques such as semiquantitative methyl-specific polymerase chain reaction (SQ-MSP) and pyrosequencing, significantly correlated with overall survival, while no correlation was identified between the immunohistochemical values and survival,[221] indicating that IHC is not a useful method for this purpose.

Cyclooxygenase-2 (COX-2), an enzyme involved in the metabolism of arachidonic acid, has been identified by IHC in myxopapillary ependymomas and a subpopulation of other types of ependymomas,[222] as well as in a variety of other, preferably high-grade gliomas,[223] suggesting that COX-2 inhibitors may potentially have a role in their treatment.

CD133 identifies stem cells with the capacity to self-renew and have been identified in neoplasms as cancer stem cells.[224] CD133-positive stem cells have been identified in the subventricular zone and other locations of the brain in autopsy studies of patients with neoplastic and nonneoplastic conditions.[225,226] Their presence in gliomas has been correlated with chemoresistance and poor prognosis.[227,228] Whether this will lead to a systematical routine evaluation of these neoplasms by CD133 as a prognostic marker remains to be seen. CD133-positive stem cells are not restricted to nervous system and its tumors and have been identified in a diverse group of neoplasms.

Immunohistochemistry in Neurodegenerative Diseases

Various abnormal accumulations associated with well-defined nuclear or cytoplasmic inclusions, or simply as accumulations without an inclusion formation, are seen in many neurodegenerative diseases. These can be highlighted by immunohistochemical stains and based on their positivity, inclusion types and distribution, neurodegenerative diseases are further characterized.[229,230] (See also Chapter 2 "Cytoplasmic Inclusions"). Here, the major immunohistochemical stains used for this purpose will be reviewed and the main findings they help identify will be discussed.

Tau is a microtubule-associated protein that becomes hyperphosphorylated and accumulates as paired helical filament-tau (PHF-tau) in *tauopathies*,[231] such as Alzheimer's disease (AD),[232] where the pathologic hallmarks are typically negative for alpha-synuclein. Depending on its chemical

List of Findings/Checklist for Immunohistochemistry in Neurodegenerative Diseases

AT A GLANCE

- Tau
- Alpha-synuclein
- Ubiquitin
- Alpha-beta-crystalline
- TDP-43
- FUS
- Ataxin
- Huntingtin
- Neuroserpin
- Neurofilament (see Neuronal Markers)
- Prion protein

structure and whether it has three or four microtubule binding sites, it can be 3-repeat (3R) tau as in Pick disease, or 4-repeat (4R) tau as in corticobasal degeneration (CBD), progressive supranuclear palsy (PSP), and argyrophilic grain disease, while all isoforms are abnormally phosphorylated and aggregate into paired helical filaments in AD.[233] In practical use, unless specifically designated, tau antibodies recognize both types of accumulation. Its staining results mirror those of Bielschowsky silver stain. Therefore, *neurofibrillary tangles (NFTs)* associated with AD, PSP, and others are highlighted. *Dystrophic neurites* are highlighted as in the neuritic plaques in AD and in neuropil in other tauopathies. In addition, *neuropil threads* can be seen in the background neuropil **(Fig. 7-11)**. Neurofibrillary tangles are not necessarily only associated with neurodegenerative diseases per se (see Chapter 2, "Cytoplasmic Inclusions") and can be seen in other conditions such as the neurons of malformative lesions[234] or in Niemann-Pick disease,[235] extending into the dendrites resulting in thickenings around the cell body in the latter. Tau can be positive in neurons without the formation of typical neurofibrillary tangles, indicating the presence of abnormal tau within the cell. Tau may not always stain the *extracellular NFT* that are left behind and are degenerating after the death of the neuron, but those are better seen with Bielschowsky stain. Some neuritic plaques in AD may be *tau-negative*, but may be ubiquitin positive only, sometimes with some degree of *chromogranin* positivity. This situation has a tendency to occur in sparse plaques in elderly patients without cognitive impairment.[3] *Swollen neurons* seen in Pick disease and CBD are tau positive, although they can be identified on routine sections due to their size. They, as well as several other neurodegenerative diseases, can be associated with chromogranin positivity.[236]

Tau-positive accumulations are seen in *glial cells* in various diseases. For instance, thorn-like and especially tufted astrocytes are seen in *PSP*. Tau-positive glial cells are present in the affected areas in *postencephalitic parkinsonism. Astrocytic plaques* are typically seen in CBD and are identified by tau IHC.[233]

Alpha-synuclein is the marker for those diseases associated with its accumulation, called *synucleinopathies*, where the pathologic hallmarks are typically negative for tau. Alpha-synuclein–positive inclusions are seen mainly in *Lewy body disorders*, that is, *Parkinson disease*[237] *(classical Lewy bodies)* and *dementia with Lewy bodies (*in this case, *cortical Lewy bodies)* **(Fig. 7-12)**,[238] and

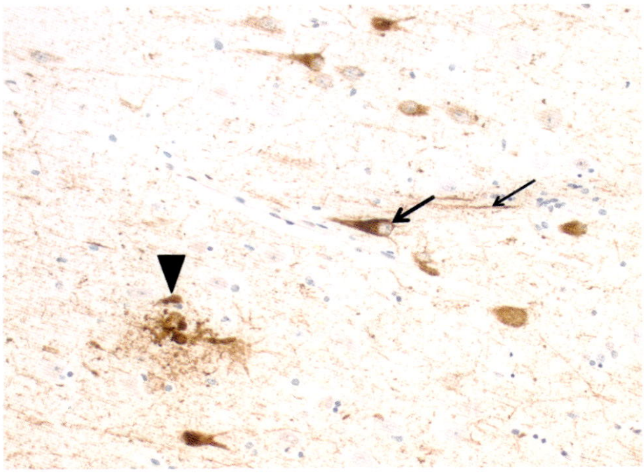

Figure 7-11. PHF-Tau in Alzheimer's disease: Various components of tau pathology are shown. Dystrophic axons in a neuritic plaque (*arrowhead*) are seen as irregular distorted thickenings. Neuropil threads (*thin arrow*) are abundant in the background, creating a tau-positive fibrillarity. While many neuron cell bodies are positive mainly in a finely granular pattern, some have a thicker and denser staining, corresponding to neurofibrillary tangles (*thick arrow*) (PHF-Tau IHC; original magnification: 200×).

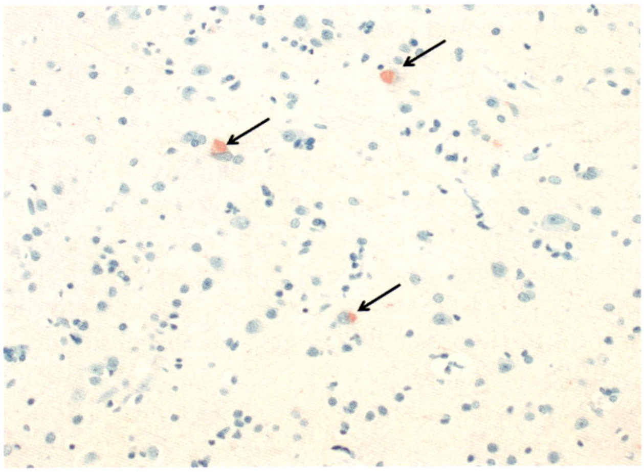

Figure 7-12. Alpha-synuclein in dementia with Lewy bodies: Three cortical Lewy bodies (*arrows*) are present in the cytoplasm of neurons. They are about the size of the nucleus, filling the cytoplasm almost entirely (Alpha-synuclein IHC; original magnification: 200×).

multiple system atrophy (MSA, not to be confused with muscle specific actin below). It is also positive in the *pale bodies*, which are presumably the precursors of Lewy bodies.[239] The dystrophic neurites in the background neuropil in these diseases stain with alpha-synuclein and are referred to as *Lewy neurites*.[240] The inclusions of MSA *(Papp-Lantos inclusions)* are also positive for this antibody.[241]

Alpha-synuclein accumulation is seen in amygdala in *Guam-parkinsonism dementia complex* and coexists with tau pathology, even in the same inclusion.[242] In *diffuse NFTs with calcification*, in addition to tau-positive NFTs and tau neurites, there are alpha synuclein–positive neuronal and astrocytic inclusions.[243]

Ubiquitin is a normal component of ubiquitin–proteasome system in the cell and can be immunohistochemically identified when *conjugated with various abnormal accumulations*, providing an indirect means for their detection.[244] Essentially all inclusions and accumulations that are seen by tau, such as *NFTs* and *neuritic plaques, Pick bodies*, frontotemporal lobar degeneration (*FTLD*), or by alpha-synuclein, such as *Lewy bodies*, are variably ubiquitin positive. Therefore, ubiquitin IHC is a practical screening method for such abnormalities, in spite of its inability to further characterize them.[229,245] *FTLD with ubiquitin-positive inclusions (FTLD-U)* and *FTLD with motor neuron disease (FTLD-MND)* have rod-shaped nuclear and dot-like cytoplasmic inclusions that are positive only for ubiquitin and negative for tau.[246]

Globose NFTs in small neurons may be compact and may look like cortical Lewy bodies by ubiquitin. Many other normal and abnormal accumulations are highlighted by ubiquitin. *Marinesco bodies*, age-related *cytoplasmic inclusions in inferior olive neurons*[247] that may be shadowed by lipofuscin pigment, *granulovacuolar degeneration* are ubiquitin positive.[248] Granular ubiquitin positivity can be seen in the axons with aging.[249] Nuclear ubiquitin–positive inclusions in neurons of affected regions, as well as in other tissues such as skin, heart, kidney and testis are seen in *spinobulbar muscular atrophy* (Kennedy's disease; X-linked bulbospinal neuronopathy).[250] Similar nuclear inclusions are present in the affected neurons in *spinal cerebellar atrophy*.[3] Remaining, somewhat swollen neurons in *spinal muscular atrophies* tend to show a peripheral granular ubiquitin positivity in their cell bodies without distinct inclusions.[251] Neuronal nuclei, nuclear inclusions, and axons are ubiquitin positive in *Huntington disease*.[252] The axonal swellings in *neuroaxonal dystrophy* can be ubiquitin positive.[253]

Alpha–beta crystalline is a small heat shock protein that interferes with apoptotic pathways, playing an inhibitory role in some of its steps.[254,255] It tends to accumulate in the cell body of *swollen neurons* in various disease states, such as CBD and Pick disease, with the exception of those swollen neurons in pellagra.[3]

Trans-active response (TAR) DNA-binding protein 43 (TDP-43) acts as a transcriptional repressor.[256] It is widely present in normal neurons and glial cells in the cytoplasm, but abnormal accumulation results in cytoplasmic and nuclear inclusions, as well as localization into the nucleus. It has been identified as the disease protein in cases of *sporadic and familial FTLD-U without or with motor neuron disease (FTLD-MND)*, and in *sporadic motor neuron disease (MND)* or *amyotrophic lateral sclerosis*.[257–259] FTLD-U is also known as FTLD-TDP due to the positivity for only TDP-43 and ubiquitin, but not for tau or alpha-synuclein (see above). The repertoire of diseases associated with TDP-43, that is, TDP-43 proteinopathies, is expanding.

Fused in sarcoma (FUS) protein is also widely expressed in neurons and glia, resulting in nuclear inclusions in some neurodegenerative diseases such as FTLD-U with FUS accumulation (FTLD-FUS), neurofilament intermediate filament inclusion disease (NIFID), and basophilic inclusion body disease (BIBD), potentially creating a new category of diseases, which may be termed FUS proteinopathies.[260]

In addition, there are highly specialized antibodies for the detection and confirmation of specific diseases. They are directed against the protein product of the genes involved and are positive in the inclusions containing them. Some examples are *ataxin* in spinocerebellar ataxia (SCA),[261] *huntingtin* in Huntington disease,[262] and *neuroserpin* in dementia with neuroserpin accumulation.[263] In addition to these main findings associated with the major neurodegenerative diseases, various other patterns of protein accumulations, overlapping expressions, and accumulations in other settings have been described.[230] *Prion protein* can be identified by IHC and is more reliable than increased 14-3-3 protein levels in cerebrospinal fluid[264,265]; however, it is best limited to specialized laboratories that can perform more definitive molecular testing and that are well equipped to handle such specimens in a safe manner, as contamination of the laboratory equipment and personnel is a major concern. IHC for 14-3-3 protein and its isoforms is also available, although its role in practice needs to be evaluated.[266]

Markers for Germ Cell Neoplasms

Although germinoma, the prototypical neoplasm that is histomorphologically similar to seminoma, is the main type seen in the CNS, practically all types of germ cell neoplasms can be seen in isolation or in various combinations as in the gonads. Therefore, their accurate diagnosis and differential diagnosis come into play especially in pineal region and suprasellar region lesions and are similar to their counterparts seen in other parts of the body and encountered in surgical pathology practice **(Table 7.6)**. In addition, compared to the studies on extracranial germ cell neoplasms, studies on intracranial germ cell neoplasms are relatively limited, and therefore, many of the generalizations are based on the results obtained from extracranial germ cell neoplasms.

Placental-like alkaline phosphatase (PLAP) is a sensitive marker for seminomatous and nonseminomatous germ cell neoplasms[267]; however, it can also be positive in a subpopulation of carcinomas, such as pulmonary adenocarcinomas.[268] It is useful especially as a screening marker for germ cell neoplasms as part of a panel in the workup of a neoplastic process in the right context. *SALL-4* is also a recently investigated general germ cell marker with similar results in the germ cell neoplasms of the CNS,[269] which can also be positive in some carcinomas.[270] *OCT3/4* (also known commonly as OCT3 or OCT4, among others) is a transcription factor that shows nuclear positivity. It is a highly sensitive

List of Findings/Checklist for Markers for Germ Cell Neoplasms

AT A GLANCE

- Placental-like alkaline phosphatase
- SALL-4
- OCT3/4
- CD117
- CD30
- D2-40
- Beta-human chorionic gonadotropin
- Alpha-fetoprotein
- CD34
- Germinoma/seminoma
- Embryonal carcinoma
- Choriocarcinoma
- Yolk sac tumor
- Teratoma
- Metastatic carcinoma
- Glioma

TABLE 7.6 Characteristic immunophenotypical differential diagnosis of germ cell neoplasms

Antibody	Germinoma	Embryonal Carcinoma	Yolk Sac Tumor	Choriocarcinoma
PLAP	+	+	+	+
OCT3/4	+	+	−	−
CD117	+	−/+	−/+	−
CD30	−	+	−	−
Cytokeratin	−/+	+	+	+
HCG	−	−	−	+
AFP	−	−/+	+	−
Podoplanin (D2-40)	+	−/+	−	−

+, positive; −, negative; −/+, mostly negative.
PLAP, placental-like alkaline phosphatase; HCG, beta-human chorionic gonadotropin; AFP, alpha-fetoprotein.

marker for germinomas that is comparable and even better than that of PLAP.[271] It is also commonly positive in embryonal carcinoma, but not in other types of germ cell neoplasms.[272] Interestingly, it has been identified in gliomas, including oligodendrogliomas[273] (see Chapter 2 for clear cells), and in colorectal[274] and more importantly in a subset of ovarian clear cell carcinomas,[275] adding a word of caution to its interpretation. The absence or only weak and focal cytokeratin staining in intracranial germinomas should be useful in such cases. To more specifically identify germ cell components that are not readily apparent, other more specific markers should be used.

CD117 (c-kit) identifies a cell-surface transmembrane tyrosine kinase receptor (CD117) encoded by *c-kit*.[276] It has been popularized both as a diagnostic marker as well as an indicator of favorable response to treatment by tyrosine kinase inhibitors in gastrointestinal stromal tumor (GIST).[277] Though attempt has been made to recapitulate that role in glial neoplasms[278] and it may prove useful in the rare case of a GIST metastatic to the brain,[279] its current utility in surgical neuropathology practice is mainly limited to the immunohistochemical workup of germ cell neoplasms. In this context, CD117 positivity typically in a membranous pattern supports the diagnosis of germinoma,[280] as other germ cell neoplasms are largely negative for this marker. In contrast, and to complement this finding, *CD30* is positive in the great majority of embryonal carcinomas with a high specificity for this neoplasm among other germ cell neoplasms.[281,282] Confusion with anaplastic large cell lymphoma is unlikely in the face of other more specific lymphoid and epithelial markers for lymphomas and embryonal carcinoma, respectively. *Podoplanin (D2-40)* is positive in seminomas in a membranous pattern and focally in an apical pattern in embryonal carcinomas, but not in other types of germ cell neoplasms.[282] It has been identified in pineal germinomas, although the number of cases studied was small.[283]

Beta-human chorionic gonadotropin (β-HCG) is strongly positive in the syncytiotrophoblasts and weak or negative in cytotrophoblasts and therefore is a very sensitive and specific marker for choriocarcinoma. β-HCG can highlight the syncytiotrophoblasts even in necrotic areas, a feature that is especially useful in practice since choriocarcinoma usually presents as an extensively necrotic and hemorrhagic lesion. Scattered syncytiotrophoblastic cells can be present in germinomas[284] and may result in elevated serum β-HCG levels, mimicking the presence of a choriocarcinoma component. These cells are also immunohistochemically positive for β-HCG, resulting in a pitfall for mistaking this occurrence for the presence of a choriocarcinoma component. *Alpha-fetoprotein (AFP)* is predominantly positive in yolk sac tumor,[285] but it can be seen in embryonal carcinoma and glands in a mature teratoma, especially in the endodermal component. At least a focal *CD34* positivity has been reported in a subpopulation of yolk sac tumors, but not in other types of germ cell neoplasms,[286] a feature that can be used with caution in the context of germ cell neoplasms.

Hematolymphoid and Macrophage Markers

Involvement of CNS by leukemia and lymphoma is not uncommon. In addition, many inflammatory processes occur and may need to be proven to be nonneoplastic, as discussed in Chapter 2. Therefore, IHC for hematolymphoid markers is frequently utilized. With many types of lymphomas, Hodgkin and non-Hodgkin, and a lot more IHC markers, all leading to the separate subspecialty practice of hematopathology, it can be overwhelming to cover all there is to be covered in practice.[287] Therefore, the neuropathologist should not hesitate to obtain hematopathology consultation when faced with unusual lesions and situations. On the other hand, not all hematopathologists may be familiar with the patterns of involvement in the CNS, such as lymphomatosis cerebri **(Fig. 7-13)**. The good news for the neuropathologist is that CNS has a limited repertoire of hematolymphoid malignancies and many, especially leukemic infiltrates have a previous history to provide some direction. Unfortunately, due to the entrapment of cells in the rich fibrillarity of neuroglial parenchyma, tissues submitted for flow cytometric evaluation almost always result in inadequate cell recovery, with the exception of bulky cellular lesions. This problem is compounded by the small tissue amount that is

List of Findings/Checklist for Hematolymphoid and Macrophage Markers

AT A GLANCE

- CD45 (LCA)
- CD20
- CD79a
- MUM-1
- CD10
- BCL-6
- BCL-2
- Light chains
- CD3 and other T-cell antigens
- ALK
- CD30
- EMA
- CD1a
- CD207
- CD117
- CD43
- CD68
- CD163
- Inflammatory/reactive
- Malignant
  - Diffuse large B-cell
  - Mature B-cell neoplasms
  - Lymphomatosis cerebri
  - Plasma cell myeloma
  - Malignant large cells in a small cell reactive background
    - T-cell rich B-cell lymphoma
    - Hodgkin lymphoma
    - Lymphomatoid granulomatosis
    - Anaplastic large cell lymphoma
- Solitary fibrous tumor
- Langerhans cell histiocytosis
- Non-Langerhans cell histiocytosis
- Histiocytic sarcoma
- Myeloid sarcoma
- Microglia/macrophages
- Epitheliod histiocytes/multinucleated giant cells
- Granular cell astrocytoma
- Aberrant expressions
- Neurothekeoma/plexiform fibrohistiocytic tumor

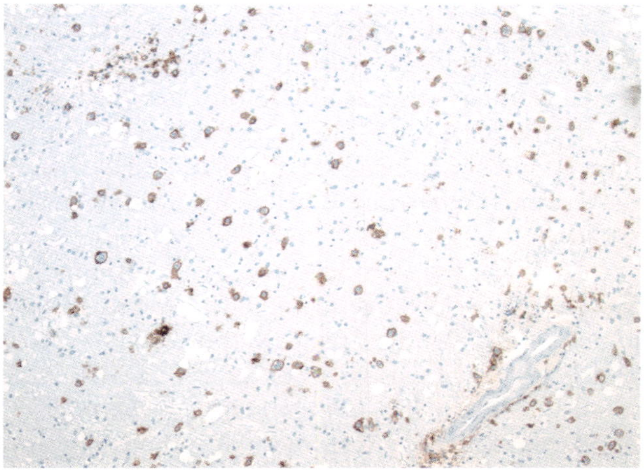

Figure 7-13. CD20 in lymphomatosis cerebri: What appeared to be a mildly hypercellular tissue with a differential diagnosis of gliomatosis versus gliosis on routine sections is identified as lymphomatosis cerebri due to the presence of many, diffusely infiltrating CD20-positive large cells (CD20 IHC; original magnification: 200×).

characteristic for the biopsy specimens. All these emphasize prioritizing the use of IHC in the workup of lymphoid lesions of CNS. At any rate, a basic knowledge of hematopathology is needed for an appropriate approach, while details have been outlined elsewhere.[288,289] The following discussion is a limited one to emphasize the main practical issues and any pitfalls, without turning it into a text on hematopathology or IHC.

Inflammatory/reactive lymphoid infiltrate is typically composed of a predominance of small T lymphocytes, while most *lymphoid malignancies* involving the CNS are of B-cell type, and the overwhelming majority of those are of diffuse large B-cell lymphoma. Therefore, the simple panel of *CD3* and *CD20 (L26)*, together with cytohistomorphologic features, should provide good baseline information, with the inflammatory/reactive infiltrates being CD3-positive T-cell predominant, while malignant infiltrates are predominantly composed of CD20 positive B cells; however, exceptions to this general rule have been reported.[290] As a general rule, a general antibody that is known to be positive for the suspected cell type should be included to confirm the preservation of antigenicity in the sample, in this case *CD45RB (leukocyte common antigen; LCA)* for lymphoid cells. It should be kept in mind that in cases that have been previously diagnosed and have undergone anti-CD20 antibody treatment,[291] the tissue expression of CD20 may be weak or it may be negative. Therefore, an additional antibody to identify B-cell lineage, such as *CD79a* should also be considered in such cases.[292] Although plasma cells are typically negative, a subset of *plasma cell myelomas* can be CD20 positive.[293] A subset of *microglia* can be *LCA*-positive[294] and LCA expression may apparently be upregulated in activated microglia in various processes[295,296] (see below for microglia). *Lymphomatosis cerebri*[297] may masquerade as gliosis or infiltrating glioma, can be suspected by the nuclear features and confirmed by IHC workup.

In general, even if a reactive-appearing lymphoid infiltrates is identified after immunohistochemical workup, it is necessary to pay attention to the cytologic features of the population with particular emphasis on scattered admixed cells that do not fit into the general population. Although relatively infrequent in the brain, *T-cell rich B-cell lymphoma* and *Hodgkin lymphoma* can be deceiving due to their malignant cells scattered in a reactive small lymphoid population. *Lymphomatoid granulomatosis* also is a malignant angiocentric process with large B cells that are CD20 positive as well as variably CD30 positive, distributed in a reactive lymphoid population. Therefore, not only the positivity and the number of positive cells but the cytologic features of cells that are positive for B-cell markers should be evaluated. Usually, in a mixed population, if there are malignant cells as in these examples, they tend to be the larger cells. *Clonality* can be studied by using IHC for lambda and kappa light chains; however, the results may not be easy to interpret and the technique may suffer from high background staining, with the exception of plasma cell lesions, where there are abundant intracytoplasmic light chains. Likewise, in situ hybridization for light chain mRNA can be very useful in the evaluation of clonality in plasma cell lesions, as well as in non-Hodgkin lymphomas.[298] Nodal and extranodal diffuse large B-cell lymphomas have been divided into subgroups with prognostic implications,[299] resulting in germinal center and nongerminal center subtypes based on *CD10, BCL-6, and MUM-1* expression. Most primary CNS diffuse large B-cell lymphomas have been found to be of nongerminal center type[300]; however, this classification was not shown to have a significant prognostic implication in the CNS according to some,[301] but not according to other studies.[302] In cases with extensive necrosis, IHC for at least some of the lymphoid markers such as LCA, CD20, CD79a, and CD3 still yield satisfactory results[303] and may be tried in suspected cases and interpreted with caution and with the understanding that accurate classification may not be possible.

Further characterization and classification of *mature B-cell neoplasms* can be more complicated and requires a broader panel approach and interpretation.[288] These are low-grade, small B-cell lymphomas such as mucosa-associated lymphoid tissue (MALT) type, mantle cell lymphoma, small lymphocytic lymphoma, and lymphoplasmacytic lymphoma that rarely involve the CNS. When they do, they tend to be superficial and associated with meninges, clinically and radiologically mimicking meningioma. *T-cell lymphomas* are rare, and although they may be suspected by the loss of one or more *T-cell antigens*, they may be essentially impossible to diagnose and at least accurately classify without the help of T-cell receptor gene rearrangement studies. Therefore, a high degree of suspicion is important in their initial identification. To further complicate the issue, some of them may express aberrant B-cell antigens, especially CD20.

ALK, the protein of anaplastic lymphoma kinase gene, is positive in *anaplastic large cell lymphoma*, which is also typically positive for CD30 and EMA. They can be T-cell or B-cell type. ALK has been identified in *inflammatory myofibroblastic tumor* and separates it from the histologically similar inflammatory pseudotumor.[304] *BCL-2*, other than its use in the classification of lymphomas, is positive in *solitary fibrous tumor* and hemangiopericytoma, allowing their distinction from histologically similar lesions, such as fibroblastic meningioma.[305] *CD1a* is a transmembrane protein present in Langerhans cells, providing a marker for

TABLE 7.7 Characteristic immunophenotypical differential diagnosis of Langerhans cell and major non-Langerhans cell histiocytic proliferations

Antibody	LCH	RDD	JXG	ECD	Granuloma
CD1a	+	−	−	−	−
Langerin (CD207)	+	−	−	−	−
S-100 protein	+	+	−	−	−
Factor XIIIa	−	+/−	+	+	+
CD68	−/+	+	+	+	+
CD163	−	+	+	+	−

+, positive; −, negative; +/−, mostly positive; −/+, mostly negative. LCH, Langerhans cell histiocytosis; RDD, Rosai-Dorfman disease; JXG, (Juvenile) xanthogranuloma; ECD, Erdheim-Chester disease.

Langerhans cell histiocytosis **(Table 7.7).** A subset of T-lymphoblastic leukemia/lymphoma can also be positive. *CD207 (Langerin)* is a membrane protein associated with Birbeck granules and is therefore present in Langerhans cells, although langerin was found to be expressed in some *histiocytic sarcomas* in the same study.[306] Both CD1a and CD207 are useful in the diagnosis of Langerhans cell histiocytosis while in ruling out the non-Langerhans cell histiocytoses. Some *myeloid sarcomas* (a.k.a., granulocytic sarcoma, chloroma, extramedullary myeloid tumor) may present as a mass lesion mimicking any other mass lesion and may be the first presentation of a myeloproliferative process without any history of myeloid leukemia. They appear as poorly differentiated or undifferentiated neoplasms. Their hematologic origin may be suspected upon careful evaluation, identification of some cytoplasmic granularity and nuclear irregularities. *CD117 (c-kit)* can be very useful in the workup of such cases as part of a panel. They also are positive for CD68 and *CD43*, but not with CD3 or other lymphoid markers. These features should prompt further evaluation.

Identification of *microglia and macrophages* is extremely important especially in diagnostic surgical neuropathology to avoid overinterpretation of cellularity as a neoplasm and to avoid pitfalls associated with *pseudoneoplastic conditions*. In addition to CD45 mentioned above, microglia are positive for *CD68 and CD163*.[307] The latter two markers also are positive in macrophages. CD68 is a lysosome-phagosome–associated protein, which is naturally expressed prominently in macrophages,[308] but has low specificity for the same reason. CD163 is a scavenger receptor superfamily[309] and therefore has a higher specificity for macrophages. While both identify nonneoplastic or neoplastic cells with scavenger function, for example, chronic myeloid leukemias, CD68 positivity can be seen in some carcinomas, Langerhans cell histiocytosis, melanoma, and granular cell tumors.[310] It has to be remembered that *epithelioid histiocytes and multinucleated giant cells* are negative for CD163,[307] even though they are positive for CD68. This may become important in the evaluation of granulomatous diseases, such as sarcoidosis. Other histiocytic lesions such as Rosai-Dorfman disease can also be positive for macrophage markers.[311] *Histiocytic sarcoma* is difficult to diagnose as it appears like a poorly differentiated or undifferentiated neoplasm with no obvious clues, and CD68 and CD163 may be useful as part of a panel in the workup of such neoplasms. These markers can also be useful in the workup of granular cell astrocytomas by distinguishing the granular cells of astrocytic origin from actual macrophages. In this case, CD163 is more reliable as CD68 may be positive in those cells. An interesting observation is the expression of macrophage markers by the cells of some carcinomas.[312] In addition, macrophages that are associated with neoplasms may absorb or ingest proteins from degenerating neoplastic cells to stain for them resulting in false-positive results, potentially creating a pitfall in small tissue samples. The identification of CD68 positivity in some neurothekeoma variants, as well as in plexiform fibrohistiocytic tumor, may support a continuum between these neoplasms, which likely represent the two extremes of a spectrum.[48]

Melanocytic Markers

Primary melanomas of the CNS are uncommon, but *metastatic melanomas* are frequently seen. In addition, there are primary neoplasms with melanocytic differentiation, such as medulloblastoma with melanocytic differentiation and psammomatous

List of Findings/Checklist for Melanocytic Markers

AT A GLANCE

- S-100 protein
- HMB-45
- MART-1
- MiTF-1
- Tyrosinase
- Melanoma
  - Metastatic
  - Primary
- Melanocytoma
- Others with melanocytic/melanotic features

melanotic schwannoma. Melanin pigment can be present in variable amounts in some other neoplasms that are otherwise typical for their respective types, such as in choroid plexus neoplasms and ependymomas (see below). As discussed in Chapter 2, many melanocytic neoplasms do not necessarily have melanin pigment to alert one to this possibility. Therefore, a high index of suspicion and including markers to address this possibility in the immunohistochemical panel should avoid such problems.

The fact that melanoma can have many cytohistomorphologic appearances and can mimic any type of neoplasm necessarily brings it into the differential diagnosis of many metastatic neoplasms. For the general initial screening purposes of a neoplasm of unknown origin, *S-100 protein* serves as a good screening marker for melanoma due to its high sensitivity. On the other hand, due to its low specificity, especially in the context of CNS neoplasms where there are many others that can show variable positivity for S-100 protein, any positivity needs to be corroborated with other markers that are more specific for melanocytic neoplasms. *HMB-45* identifies a premelanosome protein, which also explains its positivity in some other lesions such as angiomyolipoma and lymphangioleimyomatosis[313] and clear cell sarcoma (melanoma of soft tissues).[314] Interestingly, some oligodendrogliomas have been reported to have HMB-45 positivity.[315] Some variants of renal cell carcinoma can be HMB-45 positive.[316] In the peripheral nervous system, especially in the evaluation of skin and subcutaneous tissue lesions, neurothekeoma[47] and pigmented schwannoma[317] should be kept in mind as potentially HMB-45–positive neoplasms. *Melan-A* and *melanoma antigen recognized by T-cells-1 (MART-1)* are antibodies against melanocyte-specific glycoproteins, with the exception of their positivity in adrenocortical carcinoma, which should be kept in mind in the workup of malignancy of unknown origin. Both HMB-45 and MART-1/Melan-A are antibodies related to PMel17/gp100 associated with melanocytic lineage, which interestingly has also been identified in the normal retina and substantia nigra.[318]

Microphthalmia transcription factor-1 (MiTF-1) is a protein that is involved in the melanocyte development and regulation of melanogenesis, and is present in the melanocytes of neural crest and brain origin, such as retinal pigment epithelium.[319] It results in a nuclear staining pattern with high sensitivity and specificity for melanocytes and melanomas.[320] *Tyrosinase* is an enzyme involved in the production of melanin pigment,[321] providing a specific marker for melanocytic cells and lesions.

It is important to note in skin and subcutaneous soft tissue lesions that spindle cell/desmoplastic melanoma, while positive for S-100 protein, tends to be negative for other melanocytic markers,[322] potentially resulting in a pitfall to mistake it for peripheral nerve sheath neoplasm. Many otherwise typical lesions can occasionally have *melanocytic differentiation* and melanotic variations. Melanotic schwannoma,[323] psammomatous melanotic schwannoma,[324] subependymoma and ependymoma with melanin formation,[325] medulloblastoma with melanotic differentiation,[54] melanotic neuroectodermal tumor of infancy (a.k.a. progonoma or retinal anlage tumor),[326] pineal anlage tumor,[327] medulloepithelioma,[328] pilocytic astrocytoma,[329] ganglioglioma,[330] and choroid plexus papilloma[331] can have melanocytic features, but this usually does not cause significant diagnostic problems, as the true nature of the neoplasm is readily obvious.

Microorganisms

Of the many techniques available for the identification of microorganisms, only those immunohistochemical stains widely available for the most

List of Findings/Checklist for Microorganisms

AT A GLANCE

- Herpes simplex virus
- Cytomegalovirus
- JC Virus
- Epstein-Barr virus
- Toxoplasma gondii

commonly encountered ones in routine diagnostic neuropathology practice will be discussed here. They are mainly viral markers. In many cases, there is some clinical and/or radiologic indication to consider an infectious process. In those cases for which an intraoperative consultation is performed, additional support for that view may be provided by the neuropathologist, prompting submitting tissue for microbiologic evaluation directly from the operating room. As a result, only those cases with an unexpected need for a search for microorganisms remain to be evaluated by IHC. For the histochemical stains such as Grocott's methenamine silver for fungal microorganisms, see Chapter 6.

Although involvement patterns, typical lesions and cytopathic changes that they produce are highly characteristic, *herpes simplex virus (HSV)* and *cytomegalovirus (CMV)* may need to be confirmed. IHC for these viruses stain the viral particles and highlight the inclusions in subtle cases or in those cases where they cannot be identified in the necroinflammatory background, especially in HSV. CMV can be especially subtle in the setting of human immunodeficiency virus (HIV) infection and may need to be specifically searched for. A common opportunistic viral infection in the setting of HIV and less commonly these days in other immunocompromised states is *JC virus* infection, a papovavirus resulting in *progressive multifocal leukoencephalopathy (PML)*. The characteristic nuclear inclusions may not be present in the small biopsy sample, although clinical, radiologic, and other histologic features such as atypical reactive astrocytes may be highly suspicious. IHC and in situ hybridization are available for its identification and show positivity for viral antigens not only in the obvious inclusions but also in the relatively unremarkable oligodendroglial nuclei, but IHC not necessarily in the astrocytes with atypical changes. The antibody is not specific for JC virus but reacts with an antigen common to JC, BK, and SV40 viruses[332]; however, in the appropriate setting, its identification is considered diagnostic for PML in neuropathology practice. In situ hybridization identifies the viral genome in both oligodendroglial and astrocytic cells. Therefore, if PML is suspected in a small tissue sample, it can be identified even without the presence of typical inclusions in that sample. *Epstein-Barr virus (EBV)* is associated with several lymphoid and nonlymphoid malignancies[333] and is seen in neuropathology practice mainly due to its involvement in the immunodeficiency-associated neoplasms, most notably diffuse large B-cell lymphoma and lymphomatoid granulomatosis. Other types of lymphomas such as Burkitt lymphoma and Hodgkin lymphoma can also be associated with EBV. CNS diffuse large B-cell lymphoma associated with immunocompromised states tends to be more multifocal and largely necrotic compared to its counterpart seen in immunocompetent hosts.[302,334] It is almost always associated with EBV,[335] in contrast to its counterparts in immunocompetent hosts.[334]

A peculiar neoplasm is EBV-associated leiomyosarcoma that is seen in immunodeficiency states and is relatively commonly seen in the CNS.[336,337] In general, Epstein-Barr virus encoded RNA (EBER) in situ hybridization is commonly used to identify the presence of EBV genome. In addition, IHC to identify latency-related proteins such as Epstein-Barr nuclear antigen (EBNA) and latent membrane protein (LMP), are available and can be used in the workup of neoplasms in the appropriate setting.[334,335] EBER in situ hybridization is the preferred method for the identification of EBV in the formalin-fixed, paraffin-embedded tissue sections.[334] The diagnosis of *toxoplasmosis* may turn into a nightmare when one is stuck with a small and mostly necrotic biopsy sample in a context that is highly suspicious for toxoplasmosis.[338] When cyst forms are absent, tachyzoites can be impossible to distinguish from nuclear debris in the necrotic background and IHC is especially useful under such circumstances **(Fig. 7-14)**. Still, extra caution is needed due to background staining. IHC is available for many other microorganisms such as ameba and their subtyping,[339] West Nile virus,[340] HIV,[341] and many viruses that cause encephalitides. In suspected cases, central and specialized laboratories may be consulted for further workup of such cases.

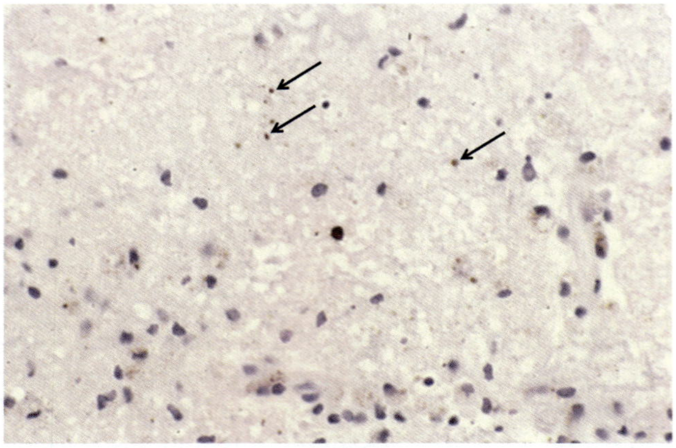

Figure 7-14. Toxoplasma cerebritis: Tachyzoites may be impossible to distinguish from nuclear debris in the necrotic background on routine sections. IHC can help identify the tachyzoites (*arrows*) and is especially helpful in the absence of cyst forms in small tissue samples. The results should be interpreted in the right clinical, radiologic, and pathologic context, as necrotic debris may also show nonspecific staining, especially if there is high background staining (Toxoplasma IHC; original magnification: 400×).

Other Markers

Amyloid in the CNS is mainly limited to β-amyloid with the exceptions of light chain amyloid (AL) mainly associated with lambda light chain and amyloid accumulation associated with chronic inflammation (AA). *β-amyloid* is found in association with *Alzheimer pathology,* and its accumulation is considered to be the fundamental abnormality in Alzheimer's disease.[342] IHC highlights any areas of accumulation in the neuropil as geographical patches of staining, as well as the more distinct plaque pathology, including those mature plaques with a central dense core of staining **(Fig. 7-15)**. Some ghost NFTs left behind after the death of the neuron can appear as amyloid positive when admixed with the amyloid in the neuropil. In the context of AD, *cerebral amyloid angiopathy* (Congophilic angiopathy)[343] can easily be highlighted by β-amyloid IHC. This way, even very small amount of partial accumulations in vessel walls can be identified. β-amyloid IHC is

List of Findings/Checklist for Other Markers

AT A GLANCE

β-Amyloid
- Alzheimer's disease
- Cerebral amyloid angiopathy
- Spongiform encephalopathies
- Biondi bodies

β-Amyloid Precursor Protein
- Axonal injury
  - Traumatic
  - Nontraumatic

Collagen Type IV and Laminin
- Schwannoma
- Neurofibroma
- Perineurioma
- Malignant peripheral nerve sheath tumor (MPNST)
- Smooth muscle neoplasms
- Endothelial neoplasms
- Choroid plexus neoplasms
- Hemangiopericytoma
- Chordoma

INI1 (Loss of Nuclear Positivity)
- Atypical teratoid rhabdoid tumor (ATRT)
- Renal and extrarenal rhabdoid tumors
- Clear cell sarcoma
- NF2-associated schwannoma (mosaic pattern)
- Choroid plexus neoplasms
- Cribriform neuroepithelial tumor
- Poorly differentiated chordoma

WT1
- Neoplastic astrocytes (vs. reactive astrocytes)
- Vascular neoplasms
- Sarcomas and carcinomas

CD34
- Ganglion cell neoplasms
- Anaplastic ganglioglioma
- Epilepsy-associated lesions
- Dysplastic/malformed neurons
- Pleomorphic xanthoastrocytoma (PXA)
- Vascular neoplasms
- Hemangiopericytoma/solitary fibrous tumor (HPC/SFT)
- Peripheral nerve sheath tumors

List of Findings/Checklist for Other Markers *(Continued)*

AT A GLANCE

CD99
- Hematolymphoid neoplasms
- Neuroblastoma
- Primitive neuroectodermal tumor (PNET)/Ewing sarcoma
- Ependymoma
- HPC/SFT
- Synovial sarcoma (vs. MPNST)
- Neurothekeoma

TTF-1 (Nuclear Positivity)
- Lung carcinoma
- Thyroid carcinoma of follicular origin
- Neuroendocrine carcinoma
- Pituicytoma
- Granular cell tumor of neurohypophysis
- Spindle cell oncocytoma of the adenohypophysis

β-Catenin
- Membranous–cytoplasmic
  - Anterior pituitary and adenoma
- Nuclear
  - Pituitary adenoma
  - Adamantinomatous craniopharyngioma
  - Medulloblastoma

Brachyury (Nuclear Positivity)
- Chordoma/chondroid chordoma (vs. chondrosarcoma and other mesenchymal neoplasms)
- Hemangioblastoma (vs. clear cell renal cell carcinoma)

D2-40 (Podoplanin)
- Germ cell neoplasms
- Hemangioblastoma
- Chondrosarcoma
- Peripheral nerve sheath tumors

Inhibin
- Hemangioblastoma
- Adrenal cortical carcinoma

Retinal S-Antigen (Arrestin, S-Ag)
- Pineal gland
- Pineal parenchymal neoplasms
- Medulloblastoma

Transthyretin (TTR, Prealbumin)
- Choroid plexus neoplasms
- Pineal parenchymal neoplasms
- Papillary tumor of the pineal region
- Carcinomas

Factor XIIIa
- Juvenile xanthogranuloma
- Erdheim-Chester disease

GLUT-1
- Perineurioma
- Hemangioblastoma (endothelial)
- Renal cell carcinoma (membranous in carcinoma cells)

Claudin-1
- Meningioma
- Perineurioma

Myelin Basic Protein
- Myelin

Olig-2
- Oligodendroglioma
- Dysembryoplastic neuroepithelial tumor (DNT)
- Astrocytic neoplasms
- Central neurocytoma
- Clear cell ependymoma

Nestin
- Stem cells
- Gliomas
- PNET
- Medulloblastoma
- Germ cell neoplasms
- Mesenchymal and epithelial neoplasms

Markers of Myogenic Differentiation
- Smooth muscle neoplasms
- Skeletal muscle neoplasms
- Myogenic differentiation
  - Medulloblastoma
  - Triton tumor
  - Gliosarcoma
- Rhabdoid cells
  - Rhabdoid meningioma
  - ATRT
- Myofibroblastic lesions
- HPC/SFT
- Meningeal fibrosarcoma
- Hirano body
- Thalamic inclusions

(Continued)

List of Findings/Checklist for Other Markers *(Continued)*

AT A GLANCE

Vimentin
- Glial neoplasms
- Medulloblastoma (vs. metastatic small cell carcinoma)
- Malignant meningioma (vs. metastatic carcinoma)
- Coexpression with cytokeratin
  - Chordoma
  - ATRT
  - Papillary tumor of the pineal region
- Metastatic neoplasms
- Mesenchymal neoplasms

very useful in the workup of vasculopathies and hemorrhages **(Fig. 7-15)**. β-amyloid accumulation is also seen in *spongiform encephalopathies*[344] (see Chapter 2, "Neuropil Features, Background and Accumulations"). *Biondi bodies* in ependymal and choroid plexus cells are β-amyloid positive.[345]

β-Amyloid precursor protein (β-APP) IHC is useful mainly in the identification of early *axonal injury*, before the axonal spheroids form, in cases of *diffuse axonal injury*. This way, pathology can be highlighted as early as 2 to 4 hours, before

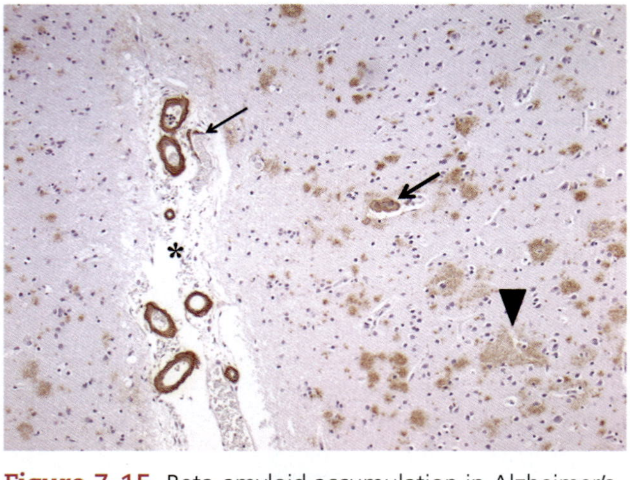

Figure 7-15. Beta-amyloid accumulation in Alzheimer's disease: Numerous foci of beta-amyloid accumulation are present in the cerebral cortex. Some are denser and more compact (*thick arrow*) corresponding to neuritic plaques, while others are in the form of weakly staining irregular patches (*arrowhead*) representing early stages of accumulation. The walls of leptomeningeal vessel in a sulcus (*asterisk*) are also strongly positive, while one vessel shows partial positivity (*thin arrow*), a common occurrence (Beta-amyloid IHC; original magnification: 100×).

other histologic findings, including axonal distortions and varicosities, appear. On the other hand, β-APP positivity is not specific for traumatic injury and can be seen in association with *nontraumatic axonal injury* such as intoxications[346] and hypoxic–ischemic damage,[347] as well. The patterns of different lesions and their staining characteristics by β-APP IHC may help distinguish some of these lesions.[348] Multifocal/diffuse positivity where axonal spheroids are scattered throughout the white matter was seen in a variety of conditions, including traumatic brain injury, hypoglycemia, carbon-monoxide poisoning, cardiac arrest, and status epilepticus. A "Z"-shaped or geographical linear pattern with a suggestion of the borders of an infarct was not identified in isolation but was seen as part of what is described as a mixed pattern admixed with the diffuse pattern in cases of increased intracranial pressure with subsequent vascular compromise due to internal herniation.

Basement membrane components laminin and collagen type IV can be used in the differential diagnosis of particular neoplasms whose cells produce basement membrane. In diagnostic surgical neuropathology practice, their main use is in the diagnosis of *schwannoma*, which can create problems especially in the cerebellopontine angle in differentiation from fibroblastic meningioma. Schwannoma typically has a distinct and orderly pericellular staining **(Fig. 7-16)**, while the basement membrane material in meningioma is scattered about with no particular pattern. *Perineurioma*[349] and *neurofibroma*[350] also have variable staining for basement membrane components. In cases of *MPNST* where the differential diagnosis is another especially high-grade neoplasm, immunohistochemical identification of basement membrane components favors

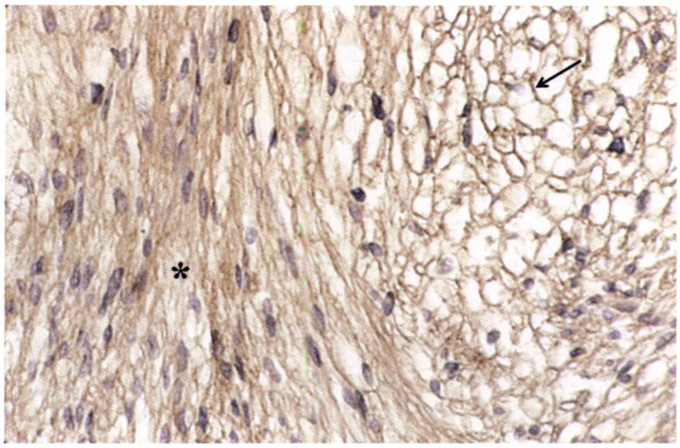

Figure 7-16. Collagen type IV in schwannoma: a pericellular pattern of positivity (*arrow*) is easier to appreciate in the cross sections of fascicles and appears as fibrillary positivity in areas with longitudinal orientation of cells (*asterisk*) (Collagen type IV IHC; original magnification: 400×).

MPNST over its mimics, such as fibrosarcoma. On the other hand, one of its greatest mimics, synovial sarcoma, is also commonly positive.[351] It should be remembered that *smooth muscle cells* and *endothelial cells*, as well as their respective neoplasms, also produce basement membrane. A pericellular staining pattern is identified in the cellular nodules of neurothekeoma,[47] as well as in its myxoid variant nerve sheath myxoma.[46] Likewise, *choroid plexus neoplasms* also have prominent basement membrane production, which helps distinguish them from papillary ependymoma and papillary meningioma. Carcinomas and other epithelial cells also produce basement membrane; however, the need for basement membrane antibodies practically never arises in their workup in neuropathology, in contrast to those situations where invasive versus in situ nature should be evaluated in other organs. Therefore, these antibodies are most useful in the limited context of a few primary CNS neoplasms. *Hemangiopericytoma* can also show a pericellular collagen type IV positivity; however, this is a focal finding. A subpopulation of *chordomas* is positive.[352]

INI1 is the protein product of the tumor suppressor gene *INI1 (SMARCB1/hSNF5/BAF47)* that plays a role in transcriptional regulation.[353] Mutations of this gene results in the *loss of immunohistochemical staining in the nuclei* for its protein INI1. The prototypical neoplasm with distinctive loss of nuclear INI1 positivity is *ATRT*.[354] In addition, some ATRTs can have a prominent and predominant small blue cell component that may obscure the characteristic rhabdoid elements and lead to a misdiagnosis of medulloblastoma in a young child with a cerebellar mass, although ATRT is not typically a midline mass. INI1 should be utilized in such small blue cell tumors since it will be lost in such cases and help identify such ATRTs obscured by a PNET-like component.[355] Loss of nuclear staining has subsequently been identified in neoplasms other than ATRT. These include *renal and extrarenal malignant rhabdoid tumors* and *epithelioid sarcomas*.[356] INI1 is retained in schwannomas, but a peculiar patchy loss described as a *mosaic pattern* is seen in those *schwannomas associated with NF2* and schwannomatosis, potentially providing a tool to differentiate syndromic schwannomas from sporadic ones.[357] Since rhabdoid change can be seen in other neoplasms, for example, rhabdoid meningioma and choroid plexus neoplasms, accurate identification of ATRT is supported by the absence of nuclear INI1 staining. However, examples of *choroid plexus neoplasms* of all grades with inactivation of *INI1* have been reported.[358] Another example of the INI1–negative neoplasms is a rare nonrhabdoid neoplasm called *cribriform neuroepithelial tumor (CRINET)*.[359] Since at least the initial examples of this neoplasm have been described in the third and fourth ventricles in young. It potential confusion with unusual histologic variations of ATRT should be avoided, as CRINET appears to have a relatively favorable prognosis. A recent addition to this group of neoplasms is *poorly differentiated chordoma* that is typically seen in childhood. It presents with a highly malignant, sarcoma-like morphology and rhabdoid features, and is difficult to recognize as a chordoma.[360] In general, endothelial cells are used as an internal positive control in the interpretation of immunohistochemical stain in these widely INI1–negative neoplasms.

WT1 is a zinc-finger transcription factor encoded by Wilms tumor suppressor gene and is associated with genitourinary malformations.[361] WT1 has two major antibodies: Polyclonal (C19, against the carboxy terminus) and monoclonal (6F-H2, against the amino terminal). They identify preferentially some malignancies better than the others,[362] and their positivity may be variably cytoplasmic and/or nuclear.[363] In a large survey of malignancies of various types and origins, nuclear staining was identified only occasionally, while the great majority of positive cases were cytoplasmic. In addition, a large number of *sarcomas and carcinomas* were positive for WT1. Of interest for the neuropathologist is the cytoplasmic positivity identified in various glial neoplasms.[363] More importantly, WT1 positivity has been proposed as an additional tool in the armamentarium to distinguish nonneoplastic/reactive astrocytic proliferations from *astrocytic neoplasms* by being positive in the latter.[364] In some situations in a glial neoplasm, where GFAP may be negative due to high-grade and poorly differentiated nature of the neoplasm, WT1 may provide a potential marker for glial origin in this limited context. *Endothelial cells* provide internal positive control, and WT1 can also be a marker for *vascular neoplasms* in the appropriate setting as part of a panel.[365]

CD34 is a hematopoietic progenitor cell antigen and is also expressed by the *endothelial cells*. As such, it provides a marker for *vascular neoplasms*, although it suffers from low specificity by being positive variably in many other neoplasms. The main use of CD34 in the CNS is in the evaluation of *ganglion cell neoplasms*. In the great majority of ganglion cell neoplasms, ganglion cells are positive for CD34. This way, CD34 provides an additional tool in the differential diagnosis of resident neurons infiltrated by a glioma versus the neoplastic ganglion cells of ganglioglioma. CD34 appears to be positive predominantly in gangliogliomas, and rarely in other glial and glioneuronal neoplasms, suggesting additional potential use for this antibody. The number of CD34-positive cells decrease in *anaplastic ganglioglioma*. In these high-grade gangliogliomas, the presence of CD34 staining of neoplastic cell processes correlated with shorter overall survival.[366] An extensive survey of *epilepsy-associated neoplastic and malformative lesions*, including infiltrating gliomas, identified CD34 positivity more commonly in the lesions associated with epilepsy in contrast to their non–epilepsy-associated counterparts.[367] Likewise, dysplastic neurons in *focal cortical dysplasias* were also found to be CD34 positive.[368] Positivity is seen in variable numbers of neoplastic cells in *PXA*, but not in diffuse astrocytomas, providing an additional tool for this differential diagnosis.[369]

Solitary fibrous tumor/hemangiopericytoma is variably positive for CD34,[370] though more commonly in those neoplasms with typical solitary fibrous tumor histology, a feature useful in the differential diagnosis of a spindle cell neoplasm with areas of keloid-like collagen and hemangiopericytomatous vascular pattern from fibroblastic meningioma, even though typical hemangiopericytomas[371] and fibroblastic meningiomas[15] can also have some degree of CD34 positivity. *Peripheral nerve sheath tumors* such as neurofibroma,[372] including plexiform neurofibroma,[373] perineurioma,[45] MPNST,[373] dermatofibrosarcoma protuberans,[374] as it may come into the differential diagnosis of peripheral nerve sheath tumors, can also be positive for CD34, as well as many other soft tissue neoplasms. In the skin, it is useful in distinguishing neurofibroma from desmoplastic melanoma by being frequently positive in the former.[375]

CD99 is the protein product of *MIC-2* gene that is involved in intercellular interactions and is expressed in a variety of *hematolymphoid malignancies,*[376] *neuroblastoma*, PNET/EWS, and other mesenchymal neoplasms, such as MPNST, synovial sarcoma,[377] and mesenchymal chondrosarcoma.[378] In the setting of nervous system neoplasms, *peripheral PNET/EWS* is diffusely and strongly positive for CD99 in contrast to CNS counterparts, that is, central PNET, and other high-grade neoplasms such as glioblastoma.[379] *Ependymomas* show membranous positivity, as well as a cytoplasmic dot-like positivity with this marker.[380] *Solitary fibrous tumor/hemangiopericytoma* is another neoplasm where CD99 can be useful in differentiating from those neoplasms with similar presentation and overlapping microscopical features.[381] It can be useful as part of a panel to distinguish *synovial sarcoma* from *MPNST* by being more diffusely and strongly positive in synovial sarcoma.[377] *Neurothekeoma* is the peripheral nervous system neoplasm with a high rate of positivity for CD99.[47]

Thyroid transcription factor-1 (TTF-1) is a member of NKx2 family of homeodomain transcription factors[382] identified in thyroid, in respiratory epithelial cells, and in developing brain.[383,384] Its main use is in the workup of metastatic carcinomas, as it is typically positive in *lung and thyroid carcinomas,*[385] as well as *neuroendocrine carcinomas*.[386] In the CNS, in the occasional situation when the papillary configuration of endolymphatic sac tumor mimics papillary thyroid carcinoma, TTF-1 positivity supports metastatic papillary thyroid carcinoma. Fetal and adult pituicytes, *pituicytoma, granular cell tumor of the neurohypophysis,* and *spindle cell oncocytoma of the adenohypophysis* have been found to be TTF-1 positive, providing a useful tool for the differential diagnosis of these neoplasms from their mimickers.[387]

β-Catenin, along with other catenins and cadherins, is involved in cell adhesion,[388] as well as in the Wnt signaling pathway.[389] Its translocation into the nucleus is thought to be an important mechanism in the progression of malignancy.[390] Therefore, it is normally seen immunohistochemically as *membranous and weak cytoplasmic positivity*. Conflicting information has been reported on its specificity, some suggesting that *nuclear positivity* is restricted to *adamantinomatous craniopharyngioma*,[391] while others reported nuclear positivity in *pituitary adenomas* also[392] **(Fig. 7-17)**. It has been suggested that nuclear positivity of β-Catenin in *medulloblastomas* may indicate a favorable prognosis in general, including large cell/anaplastic medulloblastoma as well as those medulloblastomas presenting with metastatic disease.[393]

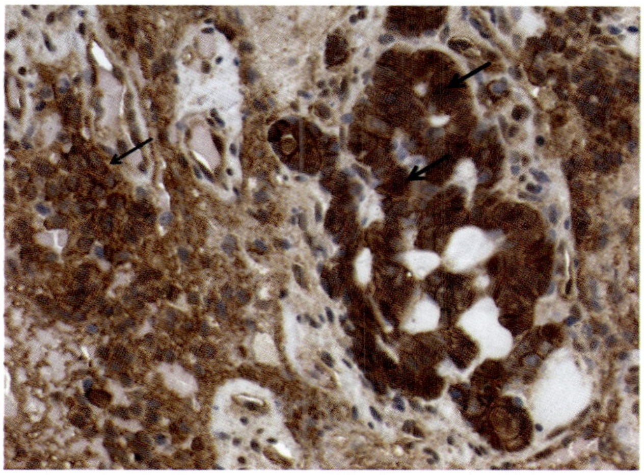

Figure 7-17. Beta-catenin in craniopharyngioma and pituitary adenoma: While variable results have been reported (see text) in these neoplasms, in this example of composite pituitary adenoma and craniopharyngioma, beta-catenin shows both cytoplasmic and membranous positivity in pituitary adenoma (*thin arrow*), as well as in craniopharyngioma component, where nuclear positivity is also present (*thick arrows*). (Beta-catenin IHC; original magnification: 400×).

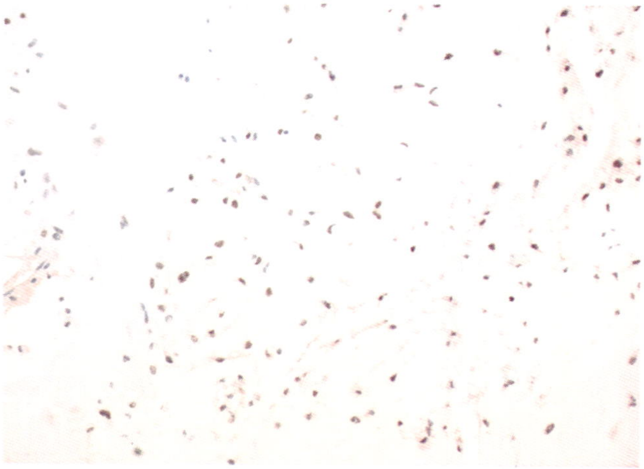

Figure 7-18. Brachyury in chondroid chordoma: Many nuclei are positive in this chondroid neoplasm, supporting the diagnosis chondroid chordoma over chondrosarcoma (Brachyury IHC; original magnification: 200×).

Brachyury is a transcription factor involved in mesenchymal differentiation, including notochord development and has been identified as a highly specific marker for *chordoma*, including *chondroid chordoma*, with a nuclear staining pattern **(Fig. 7-18)**. It is especially useful in the setting of a chordoid/chondroid neoplasm with the differential diagnosis of chordoma versus *chondrosarcoma* by supporting the diagnosis of chordoma. In addition, it has also been found to be negative in many other *mesenchymal neoplasms*.[394] It has been subsequently shown to also have a high specificity for *hemangioblastoma*,[395] which adds to the armamentarium for the differential diagnosis of this neoplasm from its clear cell mimics, especially metastatic clear cell *renal cell carcinoma*. Rare *testicular germ cell neoplasms* may also show focal positivity.[395]

D2-40 (podoplanin),[396,397] in addition to its role in germ cell neoplasms (see "Markers for Germ Cell Neoplasms"), has been identified in *hemangioblastoma* along with *inhibin* and in *chondrosarcoma*,[135,398] especially in low-grade chondrosarcoma. Inhibin, in the work-up of metastatic carcinomas, can be included as a marker for *adrenal cortical carcinoma*. Benign and malignant *peripheral nerve sheath neoplasms*, as well as epithelioid MPNST, are found to coexpress podoplanin along with S-100 protein, in contrast to melanomas, in which podoplanin was negative. Schwannomas showed a cytoplasmic pattern, while epithelioid MPNST had a membranous pattern of positivity.[42]

Transthyretin (TTR, prealbumin) is a transport protein identified in the human choroid plexus.[399] *Choroid plexus neoplasms*[400] are variably positive for transthyretin. On the other hand, its positivity in some carcinomas[401] makes it necessary to include it as part of a panel and interpret the results carefully. Since it is positive in nonneoplastic choroid plexus, its positivity is not an indication of a neoplastic process.[402] It is also identified in pineal gland and *pineal parenchymal tumors*[403] and *PTPR*.[20]

Retinal S-antigen (arrestin, S-Ag) is a marker of neurosensory differentiation and has been used as a marker of *pineal gland* and its *parenchymal neoplasms*, that is, pineocytoma, pineal parenchymal tumor of intermediate differentiation, and pineoblastoma.[404,405] It can also be focally expressed in the primitive cells of *medulloblastoma*.[406] It has not become a widely used antibody in daily practice as the typical clinical and pathologic features, as well as the availability of other common glial neuronal markers, leave little room for the differential diagnoses of these neoplasms.

Factor XIIIa is a dendritic cell marker, and in the nervous system, it can be used as part of a panel in the workup of some histiocytic proliferations, such as *juvenile xanthogranuloma*[407] and sometimes in *Erdheim-Chester disease*.[408] It is also variably present in hemangiopericytoma/solitary fibrous tumor and fibroblastic meningioma.[409]

Glucose transporter (GLUT-1) protein is normally expressed in erythrocytes, perineurial cells, renal tubules, germinal centers of lymphoid tissue, and some carcinomas.[410] While schwannoma and neurofibroma are negative, *perineurioma* is strongly positive.[411] It has also been identified as a useful marker in distinguishing *hemangioblastoma* from *renal cell carcinoma*, as the stromal cells of hemangioblastoma are negative, but its endothelia are positive, while the reverse is true for renal cell carcinoma, which shows membranous positivity in the carcinoma cells.[412]

Claudin-1 is a tight junction–associated protein that has been identified in *meningiomas* and *perineuriomas* and can be useful in the differential diagnosis of meningiomas from their mimics such as schwannoma and hemangiopericytoma/solitary fibrous tumor,[15,413,414] and though it has a low sensitivity, it has a high specificity and may be useful as part of a panel.[15]

IHC for *myelin basic protein (MBP)* has been available for a long time.[415] It has been demonstrated only in the oligodendroglia of infants in either fixed or frozen tissues, but not in older children or adults; however, it has not been successfully applied to the study of oligodendrogliomas.[416,417] Interestingly, it has not been identified in Schwann cells[418] and could not replace S-100 protein as a Schwann cell marker in this setting. It is used by some to evaluate *myelination* in place of Luxol fast blue or other myelin stains (see Chapter 6),[419] but IHC for MBP or other myelin components has not enjoyed any significant popularity in the diagnostic surgical neuropathology practice.

Olig-2 is a transcription factor that regulates oligodendroglial development.[420] As such, it has been positive in the nuclei of oligodendroglial cells and *oligodendrogliomas*.[421] It is also positive in a subpopulation of cells in *astrocytic neoplasms*, including glioblastoma and pilocytic astrocytoma, but is negative in central neurocytoma and schwannoma.[421] Although it was found to be useful in distinguishing oligodendroglioma and *DNT* with their widespread staining from clear cell ependymoma, central neurocytoma, and clear cell meningioma, which were all negative or showed only focal staining,[422] considerable overlap between the positivity of oligodendroglial and astrocytic neoplasms has been found in other studies,[423] destroying once again the high hopes for a specific oligodendroglial marker to finally put an end to the agony of going through the oligodendroglioma versus astrocytoma versus oligoastrocytoma differential diagnosis that neuropathologists commonly face.

Nestin is an intermediate filament protein expressed in neural precursor cells.[424] During the early stages of development, the precursor cells express both nestin and GFAP,[425] while nestin is limited to *neural precursors* in later stages.[426] It is a stem cell marker like CD133.[427] In *gliomas*, it has been associated with higher histologic grade and worse prognosis.[428] It has been identified in a variety of glial neoplasms, including pilocytic astrocytoma, ependymoma, and *PNET*, but not in metastatic carcinomas.[429] *Medulloblastomas* are also positive for nestin.[99] Germ cell tumors in the CNS, except for mature teratomas, were found to be nestin positive, especially those that showed dissemination, suggesting that it may be used to identify the subset of *germ cell neoplasms* that is more likely to disseminate.[430] It was subsequently identified in a wide variety of *mesenchymal and epithelial neoplasms* in other sites and has not found a useful, specific application in diagnostic surgical neuropathology.

Many *markers of myogenic differentiation* are available, both for skeletal and for smooth muscle differentiation and only a few used more commonly will be mentioned here. *Actin* is directed against the contractile protein family of actins and has multiple isoforms. Although sometimes confused with each other or used interchangeably, *smooth muscle actin (SMA)* and *muscle specific actin (MSA, not to be confused with multiple system atrophy above)* are different antibodies, with MSA having somewhat more specificity for myogenic differentiation, but both can also be positive in other cells such as myofibroblasts, myoepithelial cells, and pericytes.[431,432] *Desmin* is an intermediate filament protein expressed in *skeletal muscle* and its neoplasms.[431] Desmin and MSA have been identified in occasional cases of *MPNST* and *GBM*, [432] but this typically should not result in any confusion in these neoplasms together with their overall phenotype. Certainly, any of the muscle markers can be seen as part of a myogenic differentiation in either of these neoplasms, more specifically *triton tumor* and *gliosarcoma*. *Myogenin* and *Myo-D1* are nuclear antigens that are expressed in the developing, immature skeletal muscle cells. The well-developed, mature skeletal muscle nuclei are negative. As such, *embryonal and alveolar rhabdomyosarcomas* are positive for these markers,[433] along with cytoplasmic desmin and actin. *Leiomyosarcomas*, therefore, are diffusely and strongly positive for desmin and actin, but not for myogenin or Myo-D1. In contrast, *myoglobin* is the iron-binding protein in skeletal muscle and is expressed in mature skeletal muscle and is therefore present in tissues and neoplasms with features of *mature skeletal muscle*,[434] in contrast to more primitive neoplasms.

Aside from the general soft tissue–related use of these markers, in the nervous system, a few specific uses are present, such as the identification or confirmation of *medulloblastoma with myogenic differentiation*.[54] Rhabdoid cells of *rhabdoid meningioma* may show, in addition to strong vimentin positivity, occasional GFAP and desmin positivity, which may overlap with *ATRT* in some situations in pediatric population.[435] ATRT is known for its heterogeneous immunophenotype. It is positive at least focally for EMA and SMA, commonly for vimentin, and often for GFAP, cytokeratin, synaptophysin, neurofilament, with the diagnostic feature being the loss of immunohistochemical expression of INI1.[19] In the context of meningeal spindle cell neoplasms, *inflammatory myofibroblastic tumor*[436] and *hemangiopericytoma/solitary fibrous tumor*[437] show focal positivity for SMA. *Hirano bodies* are actin positive.[438]

Historically recognized as a mesenchymal marker in its earlier days, *vimentin* is an intermediate filament protein that is now considered quite nonspecific, as it can be variably positive in many neoplasms. On the other hand, although it has been labeled as "a marker of mammalian cell" by some of our surgical pathologist colleagues who are frustrated with its nonspecificity, it may still be useful in certain differential diagnostic situations in a given neuropathologic context. In general, a tendency to become vimentin positive is seen in *glial neoplasms*,[439,440] and the positivity becomes stronger and more widespread as the histologic grade increases.[439] In the presence of other more specific markers, however, vimentin has not been widely used for this purpose. Normal neuroglial cells are negative for vimentin. Even in the workup of *metastatic neoplasms*, it has lost its importance in the presence of more specific markers for specific types of carcinomas. In some ways and as part of a panel, it can still provide some insight in some cases, for example, cytokeratin and vimentin coexpression in renal cell carcinoma and vimentin-positive/cytokeratin-negative adrenal cortical carcinoma. In the differential diagnosis of a small cell neoplasm in the cerebellum of an adult, *medulloblastoma* is typically diffusely vimentin positive, while its positivity will be limited to scattered cells in *metastatic small cell carcinoma* (high-grade neuroendocrine carcinoma), although positivity of the latter for cytokeratin and TTF-1 will obviate the need for the use of vimentin. Another similar feature is seen in *malignant (WHO grade III; anaplastic) meningioma*. One of the definitions of such a meningioma is a microscopic appearance that is similar to a carcinoma, sarcoma, or melanoma, that is, obviously malignant. When diffuse, such cases may create considerable difficulty in the identification of their meningothelial nature, although fortunately, there are lower grade, relatively easily recognizable meningioma areas in many cases, as well as a history of previous diagnoses with multiple resections, hinting to the malignant transformation in a meningioma. Such meningiomas can have focal cytokeratin positivity but are also diffusely and strongly positive for vimentin, helping their separation from metastatic carcinoma. In *chordoma*, vimentin is diffusely and strongly positive, in contrast to a metastatic carcinoma, one of its histologic mimics. *ATRT* is another neoplasm known for its heterogeneous immunophenotype, typically with coexpression of a variety of markers such as at least focally for EMA and SMA, commonly for vimentin, and often for GFAP, cytokeratin, synaptophysin, and neurofilament, with the diagnostic feature being the loss of immunohistochemical expression of INI1.[19] *PTPR* is also diffusely and strongly positive for vimentin, variably along with other markers such as GFAP and S-100 protein, and this feature is useful in distinguishing it from metastatic carcinomas, as PTPR is also positive for cytokeratin.[20]

References

1. Cheuk W, Chan JK. Subcellular localization of immunohistochemical signals: knowledge of the ultrastructural or biologic features of the antigens helps predict the signal localization and proper interpretation of immunostains. *Int J Surg Pathol*. 2004;12:185–206.

2. Reifenberger G, Szymas J, Wechsler W. Differential expression of glial- and neuronal-associated antigens in human tumors of the central and peripheral nervous system. *Acta Neuropathol*. 1987;74:105–123.

3. Ellison D, Love S, Chimelli L, et al. *Neuropathology. A Reference Text of CNS Pathology*. Philadelphia, PA: Elsevier. 2004.

4. Kros JM, Schouten WC, Janssen PJ, et al. Proliferation of gemistocytic cells and glial fibrillary acidic protein (GFAP)-positive oligodendroglial cells in gliomas: a MIB-1/GFAP double labeling study. *Acta Neuropathol*. 1996;91:99–103.

5. Perry A, Aldape KD, George DH, et al. Small cell astrocytoma: an aggressive variant that is clinicopathologically and genetically distinct from anaplastic oligodendroglioma. *Cancer*. 2004;101:2318–2326.

6. Komori T, Scheithauer BW, Parisi JE, et al. Mixed conventional and desmoplastic infantile ganglioglioma: an autopsied case with 6-year follow-up. *Mod Pathol*. 2001;14: 720–726.

7. Brat DJ, Scheithauer BW, Medina-Flores R, et al. Infiltrative astrocytomas with granular cell features (granular cell astrocytomas): a study of histopathologic features, grading, and outcome. *Am J Surg Pathol*. 2002;26:750–757.

8. Grant JW, Gallagher PJ. Pleomorphic xanthoastrocytoma. Immunohistochemical methods for differentiation from fibrous histiocytomas with similar morphology. *Am J Surg Pathol*. 1986;10:336–341.

9. Buccoliero AM, Franchi A, Castiglione F, et al. Subependymal giant cell astrocytoma (SEGA): Is it an astrocytoma? Morphological, immunohistochemical and ultrastructural study. *Neuropathology*. 2009;29:25–30.

10. Brat DJ, Scheithauer BW, Staugaitis SM, et al. Third ventricular chordoid glioma: a distinct clinicopathologic entity. *J Neuropathol Exp Neurol*. 1998;57:283–290.

11. Kasantikul V, Shuangshoti S. Positivity to glial fibrillary acidic protein in bone, cartilage, and chordoma. *J Surg Oncol*. 1989;41:22–26.

12. Brat DJ, Scheithauer BW, Staugaitis SM, et al. Pituicytoma: a distinctive low-grade glioma of the neurohypophysis. *Am J Surg Pathol*. 2000;24:362–368.

13. Schmidt MH, Gottfried ON, von Koch CS, et al. Central neurocytoma: a review. *J Neurooncol*. 2004;66:377–384.

14. Elek G, Slowik F, Eross L, et al. Central neurocytoma with malignant course. *Pathol Oncol Res*. 1999;5:155–159.

15. Hahn HP, Bundock EA, Hornick JL. Immunohistochemical staining for claudin-1 can help distinguish meningiomas from histologic mimics. *Am J Clin Pathol*. 2006;125:203–208.

16. Rushing EJ, Bouffard JP, McCall S, et al. Primary extracranial meningiomas: an analysis of 146 cases. *Head Neck Pathol*. 2009;3:116–130.

17. Gyure KA, Morrison AL. Cytokeratin 7 and 20 expression in choroid plexus tumors: utility in differentiating these neoplasms from metastatic carcinomas. *Mod Pathol*. 2000;13:638–643.

18. Janss AJ, Yachnis AT, Silber JH, et al. Glial differentiation predicts poor clinical outcome in primitive neuroectodermal brain tumors. *Ann Neurol*. 1996;39:481–489.

19. Mohapatra I, Santosh V, Chickabasaviah YT, et al. Histological and immunohistochemical characterization of AT/RT: a report of 15 cases from India. *Neuropathology*. 2010;30:251–259.

20. Fevre-Montange M, Hasselblatt M, Figarella-Branger D, et al. Prognosis and histopathologic features in papillary tumors of the pineal region: a retrospective multicenter study of 31 cases. *J Neuropathol Exp Neurol*. 2006;65:1004–1011.

21. Acosta M, Filippa V, Mohamed F. Folliculostellate cells in pituitary pars distalis of male viscacha: immunohistochemical, morphometric and ultrastructural study. *Eur J Histochem*. 2010;54:e1.

22. Vajtai I, Beck J, Kappeler A, et al. Spindle cell oncocytoma of the pituitary gland with follicle-like component: organotypic differentiation to support its origin from folliculo-stellate cells. *Acta Neuropathol*. 2011;122:253–258.

23. Moran CA, Rush W, Mena H. Primary spinal paragangliomas: a clinicopathological and immunohistochemical study of 30 cases. *Histopathology*. 1997;31:167–173.

24. Giangaspero F, Fratamico FC, Ceccarelli C, et al. Malignant peripheral nerve sheath tumors and spindle cell sarcomas: an immunohistochemical analysis of multiple markers. *Appl Pathol*. 1989;7:134–144.

25. Oakley GJ, Fuhrer K, Seethala RR. Brachyury, SOX-9, and podoplanin, new markers in the skull base chordoma vs. chondrosarcoma differential: a tissue microarray-based comparative analysis. *Mod Pathol*. 2008;21:1461–1469.

26. Leibl S, Gogg-Kammerer M, Sommersacher A, et al. Metaplastic breast carcinomas: are they of myoepithelial differentiation?: immunohistochemical profile of the sarcomatoid subtype using novel myoepithelial markers. *Am J Surg Pathol*. 2005;29:347–353.

27. Shah SS, Chandan VS, Wilbur DC, et al. Glial fibrillary acidic protein and CD57 immunolocalization in cell block preparations is a useful adjunct in the diagnosis of pleomorphic adenoma. *Arch Pathol Lab Med*. 2007;131:1373–1377.

28. Baudier J, Briving C, Deinum J, et al. Effect of S-100 proteins and calmodulin on Ca2+-induced disassembly of brain microtubule proteins in vitro. *FEBS Lett*. 1982;147:165–168.

29. Nakajima T, Watanabe S, Sato Y, et al. An immunoperoxidase study of S-100 protein distribution in normal and neoplastic tissues. *Am J Surg Pathol*. 1982;6:715–727.

30. Perentes E, Rubinstein LJ. Recent applications of immunoperoxidase histochemistry in human neuro-oncology. An update. *Arch Pathol Lab Med*. 1987;111:796–812.

31. Takahashi K, Isobe T, Ohtsuki Y, et al. Immunohistochemical study on the distribution of alpha and beta subunits of S-100 protein in human neoplasm and normal tissues. *Virchows Arch B Cell Pathol* 1984;45:385–396.

32. Ishizawa K, Komori T, Hirose T. Stromal cells in hemangioblastoma: neuroectodermal differentiation and morphological similarities to ependymoma. *Pathol Int*. 2005;55:377–385.

33. Rumana M, Santosh V, Khursheed N, et al. Primary spinal paragangliomas: a clinicopathological and immunohistochemical study of six cases. *Ind J Pathol Microbiol*. 2007;50:528–532.

34. Achilles E, Padberg BC, Holl K, et al. Immunocytochemistry of paragangliomas—value of staining for S-100 protein and glial fibrillary acid protein in diagnosis and prognosis. *Histopathology*. 1991;18:453–458.

35. Scheithauer BW, Brandner S, Soffer D. Spinal paraganglioma. In: *WHO Classification of Tumours of the Central Nervous System*. Louis DN, Ohgaki H, Wiestler OD, et al., eds. Lyon, France: IARC Press; 2007;117–120.

36. Bergmann M. Yuan Y. Bruck W, et al. Solitary Langerhans cell histiocytosis lesion of the parieto-occipital lobe: a case report and review of the literature. *Clin Neurol Neurosurg*. 1997;99:50–55.

37. Z'Graggen WJ, Sturzenegger M, Mariani L, et al. Isolated Rosai-Dorfman disease of intracranial meninges. *Pathol Res Pract*. 2006;202:165–170.

38. Yamamoto Y, Kadota M, Nishimura Y. A case of S-100-positive juvenile xanthogranuloma: a longitudinal observation. *Pediatr Dermatol*. 2009;26:475–476.

39. Kenn W, Eck M, Allolio B, et al. Erdheim-Chester disease: evidence for a disease entity different from Langerhans cell histiocytosis? Three cases with detailed radiological and immunohistochemical analysis. *Hum Pathol*. 2000;31:734–739.

40. Ivan D, Neto A, Lemos L, et al. Erdheim-Chester disease: a unique presentation with liver involvement and vertebral osteolytic lesions. *Arch Pathol Lab Med*. 2003;127:e337–e339.

41. Hornick JL, Jaffe ES, Fletcher CD. Extranodal histiocytic sarcoma: clinicopathologic analysis of 14 cases of a rare epithelioid malignancy. *Am J Surg Pathol*. 2004;28:1133–1144.

42. Jokinen CH, Dadras SS, Goldblum JR, et al. Diagnostic implications of podoplanin expression in peripheral nerve sheath neoplasms. *Am J Clin Pathol*. 2008;129:886–893.

43. Smith TA, Machen SK, Fisher C, et al. Usefulness of cytokeratin subsets for distinguishing monophasic synovial sarcoma from malignant peripheral nerve sheath tumor. *Am J Clin Pathol*. 1999;112:641–648.

44. Boyanton BL Jr, Jones JK, Shenaq SM, et al. Intraneural perineurioma: a systematic review with illustrative cases. *Arch Pathol Lab Med*. 2007;131:1382–1392.

45. Hornick JL, Fletcher CD. Soft tissue perineurioma: clinicopathologic analysis of 81 cases including those with atypical histologic features. *Am J Surg Pathol*. 2005;29:845–858.

46. Fetsch JF, Laskin WB, Miettinen M. Nerve sheath myxoma: a clinicopathologic and immunohistochemical analysis of 57 morphologically distinctive, S-100 protein- and GFAP-positive, myxoid peripheral nerve sheath tumors with a predilection for the extremities and a high local recurrence rate. *Am J Surg Pathol*. 2005;29:1615–1624.

47. Fetsch JF, Laskin WB, Hallman JR, et al. Neurothekeoma: an analysis of 178 tumors with detailed immunohistochemical data and long-term patient follow-up information. *Am J Surg Pathol*. 2007;31:1103–1114.

48. Jaffer S, Ambrosini-Spaltro A, Mancini AM, et al. Neurothekeoma and plexiform fibrohistiocytic tumor: mere histologic resemblance or histogenetic relationship? *Am J Surg Pathol*. 2009;33:905–913.

49. Thomas L, Hartung K, Langosch D, et al. Identification of synaptophysin as a hexameric channel protein of the synaptic vesicle membrane. *Science*. 1988;242:1050–1053.

50. Quinn B. Synaptophysin staining in normal brain: importance for diagnosis of ganglioglioma. *Am J Surg Pathol*. 1998;22:550–556.

51. Rodriguez FJ, Scheithauer BW, Port JD. Unusual malignant glioneuronal tumors of the cerebrum of adults: a clinicopathologic study of three cases. *Acta Neuropathol*. 2006;112:727–737.

52. Chen CL, Shen CC, Wang J, et al. Central neurocytoma: a clinical, radiological and pathological study of nine cases. *Clin Neurol Neurosurg*. 2008;110:129–136.

53. Jouvet A, Saint-Pierre G, Fauchon F, et al. Pineal parenchymal tumors: a correlation of histological features with prognosis in 66 cases. *Brain Pathol*. 2000;10:49–60.

54. Giangaspero F, Eberhart CG, Haapasalo H, et al. Medulloblastoma. In: *WHO Classification of Tumours of the Central Nervous System*. Louis DN, Ohgaki H, Wiestler OD, et al., eds. Lyon, France: IARC Press; 2007:132–140.

55. Tihan T, Ersen A, Qaddoumi I, et al. Pathologic characteristics of pediatric intracranial pilocytic astrocytomas and their impact on outcome in 3 countries: a multi-institutional study. *Am J Surg Pathol*. 2012;36:43–55.

56. You H, Kim YI, Im SY, et al. Immunohistochemical study of central neurocytoma, subependymoma, and subependymal giant cell astrocytoma. *J Neurooncol*. 2005;74:1–8.

57. Martinez-Diaz H, Kleinschmidt-DeMasters BK, Powell SZ, et al. Giant cell glioblastoma and pleomorphic xanthoastrocytoma show different immunohistochemical profiles for neuronal antigens and p53 but share reactivity for class III beta-tubulin. *Arch Pathol Lab Med*. 2003;127:1187–1191.

58. Giannini C, Scheithauer BW, Lopes MB, et al. Immunophenotype of pleomorphic xanthoastrocytoma. *Am J Surg Pathol*. 2002;26:479–485.

59. Vyberg M, Ulhoi BP, Teglbjaerg PS. Neuronal features of oligodendrogliomas—an ultrastructural and immunohistochemical study. *Histopathology*. 2007;50:887–896.

60. Kepes JJ, Collins J. Choroid plexus epithelium (normal and neoplastic) expresses synaptophysin. A potentially useful aid in differentiating carcinoma of the choroid plexus from metastatic papillary carcinomas. *J Neuropathol Exp Neurol*. 1999;58:398–401.

61. Shibahara J, Todo T, Morita A, et al. Papillary neuroepithelial tumor of the pineal region. A case report. *Acta Neuropathol*. 2004;108:337–340.

62. Scheithauer BW, Kovacs K, Horvath E, et al. Pathology of the pituitary and sellar region. In: *Practical Surgical Neuropathology*. Perry A, Brat DJ, eds. Philadelphia, PA: Churchill Livingstone; 2010:371–416.

63. Lippa CF. Synaptophysin immunoreactivity in Pick's disease: comparison with Alzheimer's disease and dementia with Lewy bodies. *Am J Alzheimers Dis Other Demen*. 2004;19:341–344.

64. Jortner BS, Dyer K, Walton A, et al. Synaptophysin immunoreactive axonal swelling in p-bromophenylacetylurea-induced neuropathy. *Neurotoxicology*. 1997;18:161–168.

65. Lloyd RV, Wilson BS. Specific endocrine tissue marker defined by a monoclonal antibody. *Science*. 1983;222:628–630.

66. Vinores SA, Bonnin JM, Rubinstein LJ, et al. Immunohistochemical demonstration of neuron-specific enolase in neoplasms of the CNS and other tissues. *Arch Pathol Lab Med*. 1984;108:536–540.

67. Trojanowski JQ, Lee VM, Schlaepfer WW. An immunohistochemical study of human central and peripheral nervous system tumors, using monoclonal antibodies against neurofilaments and glial filaments. *Hum Pathol*. 1984;15:248–257.

68. Nixon RA. The regulation of neurofilament protein dynamics by phosphorylation: clues to neurofibrillary pathobiology. *Brain Pathol*. 1993;3:9–38.

69. Burger PC, Scheithauer BW. Tumors of the central nervous system. In: *Armed Forces Institute of Pathology Atlas of Tumor Pathology*, Series 4, Fascicle 7. Washington, DC: AFIP Press; 2007.

70. Han CW, Min BW, Kim Y, et al. Immunohistochemical analysis of developmental neural antigen expression in the balloon cells of focal cortical dysplasia. *J Clin Neurosci*. 2011;18:114–118.

71. Tassi L, Colombo N, Garbelli R, et al. Focal cortical dysplasia: neuropathological subtypes, EEG, neuroimaging and surgical outcome. *Brain*. 2002;125:1719–1732.

72. Rubinstein LJ. Tumors of the central nervous system. In: *Armed Forces Institute of Pathology Atlas of Tumor Pathology*, Series 2, Fascicle 6. Washington, DC: AFIP Press; 1972.

73. Maraziotis T, Perentes E, Karamitopoulou E, et al. Neuron-associated class III beta-tubulin isotype, retinal S-antigen, synaptophysin, and glial fibrillary acidic protein in human medulloblastomas: a clinicopathological analysis of 36 cases. *Acta Neuropathol*. 1992;84:355–363.

74. Song F, Zhao X, Zhou G, et al. Carbon disulfide-induced alterations of neurofilaments and calpains content in rat spinal cord. *Neurochem Res*. 2006;31:1491–1499.

75. Vogel H, Horoupian DS. Filamentous degeneration of neurons. A possible feature of cytosine arabinoside neurotoxicity. *Cancer*. 1993;71:1303–1308.

76. Dahl D, Bignami A, Bich NT, et al. Immunohistochemical characterization of neurofibrillary tangles induced by mitotic spindle inhibitors. *Acta Neuropathol*. 1980;51:165–168.

77. Dettmeyer R, Driever F, Becker A, et al. Fatal myeloencephalopathy due to accidental intrathecal vincristine administration: a report of two cases. *Forensic Sci Int*. 2001; 122:60–64.

78. Chou SM, Wang HS. Aberrant glycosylation/phosphorylation in chromatolytic motoneurons of Werdnig-Hoffmann disease. *J Neurol Sci*. 1997;152:198–209.

79. Sasaki S, Toi S, Shirata A, et al. Immunohistochemical and ultrastructural study of basophilic inclusions in adult-onset motor neuron disease.[Erratum appears in *Acta Neuropathol* (*Berl*) 2002 Jan;103:88] *Acta Neuropathol*. 2001;102:200–206.

80. Hof PR, Cox K, Morrison JH. Quantitative analysis of a vulnerable subset of pyramidal neurons in Alzheimer's disease: I. Superior frontal and inferior temporal cortex. *J Comp Neurol*. 1990;301:44–54.

81. Dickson DW, Feany MB, Yen SH, et al. Cytoskeletal pathology in non-Alzheimer degenerative dementia: new lesions in diffuse Lewy body disease, Pick's disease, and corticobasal degeneration. *J Neural Trans*. 1996;47:31–46.

82. Cairns NJ, Armstrong RA. Quantification of the pathological changes in the temporal lobe of patients with a novel neurofilamentopathy: neurofilament inclusion disease (NID). *Clin Neuropathol*. 2004;23:107–112.

83. Mullen RJ, Buck CR, Smith AM. NeuN, a neuronal specific nuclear protein in vertebrates. *Development*. 1992;116:201–211.

84. Preusser M, Laggner U, Haberler C, et al. Comparative analysis of NeuN immunoreactivity in primary brain tumours: conclusions for rational use in diagnostic histopathology. *Histopathology*. 2006;48:438–444.

85. Wolf HK, Buslei R, Schmidt-Kastner R, et al. NeuN: a useful neuronal marker for diagnostic histopathology. *J Histochem Cytochem*. 1996;44:1167–1171.

86. Blumcke I, Wiestler OD. Gangliogliomas: an intriguing tumor entity associated with focal epilepsies. *J Neuropathol Exp Neurol*. 2002;61:575–584.

87. Eberhart CG, Kaufman WE, Tihan T, et al. Apoptosis, neuronal maturation, and neurotrophin expression within medulloblastoma nodules. *J Neuropathol Exp Neurol*. 2001;60:462–469.

88. Dunham C, Sugo E, Tobias V, et al. Embryonal tumor with abundant neuropil and true rosettes (ETANTR): report of a case with prominent neurocytic differentiation. *J Neurooncol*. 2007;84:91–98.

89. Vasiljevic A, Fevre-Montagne M, Jouvet A. Pineal parenchymal tumors. In: *Practical Surgical Neuropathology*. Perry A, Brat DJ, eds. Philadelphia, PA: Churchill Livingstone; 2010:151–164.

90. Soylemezoglu F, Onder S, Tezel GG, et al. Neuronal nuclear antigen (NeuN): a new tool in the diagnosis of central neurocytoma. *Pathol Res Pract*. 2003;199:463–468.

91. Krishnan C, Higgins JP, West RB, et al. Microtubule-associated protein-2 is a sensitive marker of primary and metastatic neuroblastoma. *Am J Surg Pathol*. 2009;33:1695–1704.

92. Son EI, Kim IM, Kim DW, et al. Immunohistochemical analysis for histopathological subtypes in pediatric medulloblastomas. *Pathol Int*. 2003;53:67–73.

93. Cordes B, Williams MD, Tirado Y, et al. Molecular and phenotypic analysis of poorly differentiated sinonasal neoplasms: an integrated approach for early diagnosis and classification. *Hum Pathol*. 2009;40:283–292.

94. Miettinen M, Cupo W. Neural cell adhesion molecule distribution in soft tissue tumors. *Hum Pathol*. 1993;24: 62–66.

95. Shimada S, Tsuzuki T, Kuroda M, et al. Nestin expression as a new marker in malignant peripheral nerve sheath tumors. *Pathol Int*. 2007;57:60–67.

96. Mechtersheimer G, Staudter M, Moller P. Expression of the natural killer cell-associated antigens CD56 and CD57 in human neural and striated muscle cells and in their tumors. *Cancer Res*. 1991;51:1300–1307.

97. Lauria G, Lombardi R, Camozzi F, et al. Skin biopsy for the diagnosis of peripheral neuropathy. *Histopathology*. 2009;54:273–285.

98. Campbell LK, Thomas JR, Lamps LW, et al. Protein gene product 9.5 (PGP 9.5) is not a specific marker of neural and nerve sheath tumors: an immunohistochemical study of 95 mesenchymal neoplasms. *Mod Pathol*. 2003;16:963–969.

99. Tohyama T, Lee VM, Rorke LB, et al. Nestin expression in embryonic human neuroepithelium and in human neuroepithelial tumor cells. *Lab Invest*. 1992;66:303–313.

100. Wiese C, Rolletscheka A, Kaniaa G, et al. Nestin expression—a property of multi-lineage progenitor cells? *Cell Mol Life Sci*. 2004;61:2510–2522.

101. Tohyama T, Lee VM, Rorke LB, et al. Monoclonal antibodies to a rat nestin fusion protein recognize a 220-kDa polypeptide in subsets of fetal and adult human central nervous system neurons and in primitive neuroectodermal tumor cells. *Am J Pathol*. 1993;143:258–268.

102. Artlieb U, Krepler R, Wiche G. Expression of microtubule-associated proteins, MAP-1 and MAP-2, in human neuroblastomas and differential diagnosis of immature neuroblasts. *Lab Invest*. 1985;53:684–691.

103. Willoughby V, Sonawala A, Werlang-Perurena A, et al. A comparative immunohistochemical analysis of small round cell tumors of childhood: utility of peripherin and alpha-internexin as markers for neuroblastomas. *Appl Immunohistochem Mol Morphol*. 2008;16:344–348.

104. Prieto VG, McNutt NS, Lugo J, et al. The intermediate filament peripherin is expressed in cutaneous melanocytic lesions. *J Cutan Pathol*. 1997;24:145–150.

105. Prieto VG, McNutt NS, Lugo J, et al. Differential expression of the intermediate filament peripherin in cutaneous neural lesions and neurotized melanocytic nevi. *Am J Surg Pathol*. 1997;21:1450–1454.

106. Gokden M, Fuller GN: Peripherin expression in central and peripheral nervous systems: an immunohistochemical study. *J Neuropathol Exp Neurol*. 2000;59:453.

107. Okamoto S, Hisaoka M, Ishida T, et al. Extraskeletal myxoid chondrosarcoma: a clinicopathologic, immunohistochemical, and molecular analysis of 18 cases. *Hum Pathol*. 2001;32:1116–1124.

108. Gultekin SH, Dalmau J, Graus Y, et al. Anti-Hu immunolabeling as an index of neuronal differentiation in human brain tumors: a study of 112 central neuroepithelial neoplasms. *Am J Surg Pathol*. 1998;22:195–200.

109. Kaplan MP, Chin SS, Fliegner KH, et al. α-internexin, a novel neuronal intermediate filament protein, precedes the low molecular weight neurofilament protein (NF-L) in the developing brain. *J Neurosci*. 1990;10:2735–2748.

110. Kaya B, Mena H, Miettinen M, et al. Alpha-internexin expression in medulloblastomas and atypical teratoid-rhabdoid tumors. *Clin Neuropathol*. 2003;22:215–221.

111. Goldman JE, Yen S-H. Cytoskeletal protein abnormalities in neurodegenerative diseases. *Ann Neurol*. 1986;19:209–223.

112. Hirose T, Scheithauer BW, Lopes MB, et al. Olfactory neuroblastoma. An immunohistochemical, ultrastructural, and flow cytometric study. *Cancer*. 1995;76:4–19.

113. Sato K, Kubota T. Pathology of pineal parenchymal tumors. *Prog Neurol Surg*. 2009;23:12–25.

114. Hirose T, Scheithauer BW. Mixed dysembryoplastic neuroepithelial tumor and ganglioglioma. *Acta Neuropathol*. 1998;95:649–654.

115. Chu PG, Weiss LM. Keratin expression in human tissues and neoplasms. *Histopathology*. 2002;40:403–439.

116. Langer CJ, Besse B, Gualberto A, et al. The evolving role of histology in the management of advanced non-small-cell lung cancer. *J Clin Oncol*. 2010;28:5311–5320.

117. Scagliotti G, Brodowicz T, Shepherd FA, et al. Treatment-by-histology interaction analyses in three phase III trials show superiority of pemetrexed in nonsquamous non-small cell lung cancer. *J Thorac Oncol*. 2011;6:64–70.

118. Cosgrove MM, Rich KA, Kunin SA, et al. Keratin intermediate filament expression in astrocytic neoplasms: analysis by immunocytochemistry, western blot, and northern hybridization. *Mod Pathol*. 1993;6:342–347.

119. Mork SJ, Rubinstein LJ, Kepes JJ. Patterns of epithelial metaplasia in malignant gliomas. I. Papillary formations mimicking medulloepithelioma. *J Neuropathol Exp Neurol*. 1988;47:93–100.

120. Mork SJ, Rubinstein LJ, Kepes JJ, et al. Patterns of epithelial metaplasia in malignant gliomas. II. Squamous differentiation of epithelial-like formations in gliosarcomas and glioblastomas. *J Neuropathol Exp Neurol*. 1988;47:101–118.

121. Miettinen M, Clark R, Virtanen I. Intermediate filament proteins in choroid plexus and ependyma and their tumors. *Am J Pathol*. 1986;123:231–240.

122. Dahiya S, Perry A. Pineal tumors. *Adv Anat Pathol*. 2010;17:419–427.

123. Miettinen M, Paetau A. Mapping of the keratin polypeptides in meningiomas of different types: an immunohistochemical analysis of 463 cases. *Hum Pathol*. 2002;33: 590–598.

124. Tsunoda S, Takeshima T, Sakaki T, et al. Secretory meningioma with elevated serum carcinoembryonic antigen level. *Surg Neurol*. 1992;37:415–418.

125. Miettinen M. Keratin subsets in spindle cell sarcomas. Keratins are widespread but synovial sarcoma contains a distinctive keratin polypeptide pattern and desmoplakins. *Am J Pathol*. 1991;138:505–513.

126. Srivastava A, Rosenberg AE, Selig M, et al. Keratin-positive Ewing's sarcoma: an ultrastructural study of 12 cases. *Int J Surg Pathol*. 2005;13:43–50.

127. Kurian KM, Tagkalakis P, Erridge SC, et al. Primary intracranial angiosarcoma of the Pineal gland: an unusual cause of recurrent intraventricular haemorrhage and superficial haemosiderosis. *Neuropathol Appl Neurobiol*. 2006;32: 557–561.

128. Wang PN, Zee S, Zarbo RJ, et al. Coordinate expression of cytokeratins 7 and 20 defines unique subsets of carcinomas. *Appl Immunohistochem*. 1995;3:99–107.

129. Perry A. Familial tumor syndromes. In: *Practical Surgical Neuropathology*. Perry A, Brat DJ, eds. Philadelphia, PA: Churchill Livingstone; 2010:427–454.

130. Lin WL, Chen FL, Kuo JF, et al. Cytokeratin 8/18 monoclonal antibody was dissimilar to anti-cytokeratin CAM 5.2. *Exp Mol Pathol*. 2011;91:323–324.

131. Sano T, Ohshima T, Yamada S. Expression of glycoprotein hormones and intracytoplasmic distribution of cytokeratin in growth hormone-producing pituitary adenomas. *Pathol Res Pract*. 1991;187:530–533.

132. Horvath E, Kovacs K, Singer W, et al. Acidophil stem cell adenoma of the human pituitary. *Arch Pathol Lab Med*. 1977;101:594–599.

133. O'Hara BJ, Paetau A, Miettinen M. Keratin subsets and monoclonal antibody HBME-1 in chordoma: immunohistochemical differential diagnosis between tumors simulating chordoma. *Hum Pathol*. 1998;29:119–126.

134. Huse JT, Pasha TL, Zhang PJ. D2-40 functions as an effective chondroid marker distinguishing true chondroid tumors from chordoma. *Acta Neuropathol*. 2007;113:87–94.

135. Cho HY, Lee M, Takei H, et al. Immunohistochemical comparison of chordoma with chondrosarcoma, myxopapillary ependymoma, and chordoid meningioma. *Appl Immunohistochem Mol Morphol*. 2009;17:131–138.

136. Wang M, Tihan T, Rojiani AM, et al. Monomorphous angiocentric glioma: a distinctive epileptogenic neoplasm with features of infiltrating astrocytoma and ependymoma. *J Neuropathol Exp Neurol*. 2005;64:875–881.

137. Cenacchi G, Giovenali P, Castrioto C, et al. Pituicytoma: ultrastructural evidence of a possible origin from folliculo-stellate cells of the adenohypophysis. *Ultrastruct Pathol*. 2001;25:309–312.

138. Argenyi ZB. Immunohistochemical characterization of palisaded, encapsulated neuroma. *J Cutan Pathol*. 1990;17:329–335.

139. Scheithauer BW, Woodruff JM, Spinner RJ. Peripheral nerve sheath tumors. In: *Practical Surgical Neuropathology*. Perry A, Brat DJ, eds. Philadelphia, PA: Churchill Livingstone; 2010:235–286.

140. Laskin WB, Weiss SW, Bratthauer GL. Epithelioid variant of malignant peripheral nerve sheath tumor (malignant epithelioid schwannoma). *Am J Surg Pathol*. 1991;15:1136–1145.

141. Iwata J, Fletcher CD. Immunohistochemical detection of cytokeratin and epithelial membrane antigen in leiomyosarcoma: a systematic study of 100 cases. *Pathol Int*. 2000;50:7–14.

142. Ngo NT, Brodie C, Giles C, et al. The significance of tumour cell immunophenotype in myeloma and its impact on clinical outcome. *J Clin Pathol*. 2009;62:1009–1015.

143. Nguyen PL, Ferry JA, Harris NL. Progressive transformation of germinal centers and nodular lymphocyte predominance Hodgkin's disease: a comparative immunohistochemical study. *Am J Surg Pathol*. 1999;23:27–33.

144. Fraga M, Sánchez-Verde L, Forteza J, et al. T-cell/histiocyte-rich large B-cell lymphoma is a disseminated aggressive neoplasm: differential diagnosis from Hodgkin's lymphoma. *Histopathology*. 2002;41:216–229.

145. Hoch BL, Gunnlaugur P, Nielsen GP, et al. Base of skull chordomas in children and adolescents: a clinicopathologic study of 73 cases. *Am J Surg Pathol*. 2006;30:811–818.

146. Pan CC, Chen PC, Tsay SH, et al. Differential immunoprofiles of hepatocellular carcinoma, renal cell carcinoma, and adrenocortical carcinoma: a systemic immunohistochemical survey using tissue array technique. *Appl Immunohistochem Mol Morphol*. 2005;13:347–352.

147. Naka T, Oda Y, Iwamoto Y, et al. Immunohistochemical analysis of E-cadherin, alpha-catenin, beta-catenin, gamma-catenin, and neural cell adhesion molecule (NCAM) in chordoma. *J Clin Pathol*. 2001;54:945–950.

148. Mori K, Chano T, Kushima R, et al. Expression of E-cadherin in chordomas: diagnostic marker and possible role of tumor cell affinity. *Virchows Arch*. 2002:440:123–127.

149. Sato H, Hasegawa T, Abe Y, et al. Expression of E-cadherin in bone and soft tissue sarcomas: a possible role in epithelial differentiation. *Hum Pathol*. 1999;30:1344–1349.

150. Loussouarn D, Brunon J, Avet-Loiseau H, et al. Prognostic value of HER2 expression in meningiomas: an immunohistochemical and fluorescence in situ hybridization study. *Hum Pathol*. 2006;37:415–421.

151. DeLallis RA, Lloyd RV, Heitz PU, et al. Pathology and genetics: Tumours of the endocrine organs. In: *World Health Organization Classification of Tumours*. 3rd ed. Lyon, France: International Agency for Research on Cancer (IARC) Press; 2004.

152. Asa SL. Practical pituitary pathology: what does the pathologist need to know? *Arch Pathol Lab Med*. 2008;132:1231–1240.

153. Asa SL, Ezzat S. The pathogenesis of pituitary tumors. *Annu Rev Pathol* 2009;4:97–126.

154. Scheithauer BW, Gaffey TA, Lloyd RV, et al. Pathobiology of pituitary adenomas and carcinomas. *Neurosurgery*. 2006; 59:341–353.

155. Scholzen T, Gerdes J. The Ki-67 protein: From the known and the unknown. *J Cell Physiol*. 2000;182:311–322.

156. Prayson RA. Cell proliferation and tumors of the central nervous system, part II: radiolabeling, cytometric, and immunohistochemical techniques. *J Neuropathol Exp Neurol*. 2002;61:663–672.

157. Cattoretti G, Becker MHG, Kay G, et al. Monoclonal antibodies against recombinant parts of the Ki-67 antigen (MIB1 and MIB3) detect proliferating cells in microwave processed formalin-fixed paraffin sections. *J Pathol*. 1992;168:357–364.

158. Burger PC, Shibata T, Kleihues P. The use of the monoclonal antibody Ki-67 in the identification of proliferating cells: application to surgical neuropathology. *Am J Surg Pathol*. 1986;10:611–617.

159. Karamitopoulou E, Perentes E, Diamantis I, et al. Ki-67 immunoreactivity in human central nervous system tumors: a study with MIB 1 monoclonal antibody on archival material. *Acta Neuropathol*. 1994;87:47–54.

160. Torp SH. Proliferative activity in human glioblastomas: Evaluation of different Ki-67 equivalent antibodies. *J Clin Pathol*. 1997;50:198–200.

161. Nakasu S, Li DH, Okabe H, et al. Significance of MIB-1 staining indices in meningiomas: comparison of two counting methods. *Am J Surg Pathol*. 2001;25:472–478.

162. Gokden M. Staining intensity in the evaluation of proliferation index. *J Neuropathol Exp Neurol*. 2009;68:586.

163. Wolff AC, Hammond ME, Schwartz JN, et al. American Society of Clinical Oncology/College of American Pathologists guideline recommendations for human epidermal growth factor receptor 2 testing in breast cancer. Oncology/College of American Pathologists. *Arch Pathol Lab Med*. 2007;131:18–143.

164. Hammond ME, Hayes DF, Dowsett M, et al. American Society of Clinical Oncology/College of American Pathologists guideline recommendations for immunohistochemical testing of estrogen and progesterone receptors in breast cancer (unabridged version). American Society of Clinical Oncology. College of American Pathologists. *Arch Pathol Lab Med*. 2010;134:e48–e72.

165. Perry A, Louis DN, Scheithauer BW, et al. Meningiomas. In: *WHO Classification of Tumours of the Central Nervous System*. Louis DN, Ohgaki H, Wiestler OD, et al., eds. Lyon, France: IARC Press; 2007:164–172.

166. Maier H, Wanschitz J, Sedivy R, et al. Proliferation and DNA fragmentation in meningioma subtypes. *Neuropathol Appl Neurobiol*. 1997;23:496–506.

167. Perry A, Stafford SL, Scheithauer BW, et al. The prognostic significance of MIB-1, p53, and DNA flow cytometry in completely resected primary meningiomas. *Cancer*. 1998;82:2262–2269.

168. Ng HK, Poon WS, Goh K, et al. Histopathology of post-embolized meningiomas. *Am J Surg Pathol*. 1996;20:1224–1230.

169. Lloyd RV, Kovacs K, Young WF Jr, et al. Pituitary tumors: introduction. In: *World Health Organization Classification of Tumours. Pathology and Genetics: Tumours of Endocrine Organs*. DeLellis RA, Lloyd RV, Heitz PU, et al., eds. Lyon, France: IARC Press; 2004:10–13.

170. Salehi F, Agur A, Scheithauer BW, et al. Ki-67 in pituitary neoplasms: a review—part I. *Neurosurgery*. 2009;65:429–437.

171. Hirose T, Ishizawa K, Sugiyama K, et al. Pleomorphic xanthoastrocytoma: a comparative pathological study between conventional and anaplastic types. *Histopathology*. 2008;52:183–193.

172. Carlotti CG Jr, Salhia B, Weitzman S, et al. Evaluation of proliferative index and cell cycle protein expression in choroid plexus tumors in children. *Acta Neuropathol*. 2002;103:1–10.

173. Sharma MC, Deb P, Sharma S, et al. Neurocytoma: a comprehensive review. *Neurosurg Rev*. 2006;29:270–285.

174. Brat DJ, Hirose Y, Cohen KJ, et al. Astroblastoma: clinicopathologic features and chromosomal abnormalities defined by comparative genomic hybridization. *Brain Pathol*. 2000;10:342–352.

175. Izumoto S, Suzuki T, Kinoshita M, et al. Immunohistochemical detection of female sex hormone receptors in craniopharyngiomas: correlation with clinical and histologic features. *Surg Neurol*. 2005;63:520–525.

176. Bravo R, Frank R, Blundell PA, et al. Cyclin/PCNA is the auxiliary protein of DNA polymerase. *Nature*. 1987;326:515–517.

177. Louis DN, Edgerton S, Thor AD, et al. Proliferating cell nuclear antigen and Ki-67 immunohistochemistry in brain tumors: a comparative study. *Acta Neuropathol*. 1991;81:675–679.

178. Karamitopoulou E, Perentes E, Melachrinou M, et al. Proliferating cell nuclear antigen immunoreactivity in human central nervous system neoplasm. *Acta Neuropathol*. 1993;85:316–322.

179. Shibata K, Inagaki M, Ajiro K. Mitosis-specific histone H3 phosphorylation in vitro in nucleosome structure. *Eur J Biochem*. 1990;192:87–93.

180. Fukushima S, Terasaki M, Sakata K, et al. Sensitivity and usefulness of anti-phosphohistone-H3 antibody immunostaining for counting mitotic figures in meningioma cases. *Brain Tumor Pathol*. 2009;26:51–57.

181. Habberstad AH, Gulati S, Torp SH. Evaluation of the proliferation markers Ki-67/MIB-1, mitosin, survivin, pHH3, and DNA topoisomerase II alpha in human anaplastic astrocytomas—an immunohistochemical study. *Diagn Pathol*. 2011;6:43.

182. Ribalta T, McCutcheon IE, Aldape KD, et al. The mitosis-specific antibody anti-phosphohistone-H3 (PHH3) facilitates rapid reliable grading of meningiomas according to WHO 2000 criteria. *Am J Surg Pathol*. 2004;28:1532–1536.

183. Kim YJ, Ketter R, Steudel WI, et al. Prognostic significance of the mitotic index using the mitosis marker anti-phosphohistone H3 in meningiomas. *Am J Clin Pathol*. 2007;128:118–125.

184. Benchimol S. p53-dependent pathways of apoptosis. *Cell Death Differ*. 2001;8:1049–1051.

185. Bourdon JC, Laurenzi VD, Melino G, et al. p53: 25 years of research and more questions to answer. *Cell Death Differ*. 2003;10:397–399.

186. Linden MD, Nathanson SD, Zarbo RJ. Evaluation of anti-p53 antibody staining immunoreactivity in benign tumors and nonneoplastic tissues. *Appl Immunohistochem*. 1995;3:232–238.

187. Kuerbitz SJ, Plunkett BS, Walsh WV, et al. Wild-type p53 is a cell cycle checkpoint determinant following irradiation. *Proc Natl Acad Sci U S A*. 1992;89:7491–7495.

188. Bruner JM, Saya H, Moser RP. Immunocytochemical detection of p53 in human gliomas. *Mod Pathol*. 1991;4:671–674.

189. Yaziji H, Massarani-Wafai R, Gujrati M, et al. Role of p53 immunohistochemistry in differentiating reactive gliosis from malignant astrocytic lesions. *Am J Surg Pathol*. 1996;20:1086–1090.

190. Kurtkaya-Yapicier O, Scheithauer BW, Hebrink D, et al. p53 in nonneoplastic central nervous system lesions: an immunohistochemical and genetic sequencing study. *Neurosurgery*. 2002;51:1246–1254.

191. Beckmann MJ, Prayson RA. A clinicopathologic study of 30 cases of oligoastrocytoma including p53 immunohistochemistry. *Pathology*. 1997;29:159–164.

192. Verstegen MJ, Leenstra DT, Ijlst-Keizers H, et al. Proliferation- and apoptosis-related proteins in intracranial ependymomas: an immunohistochemical analysis. *J Neurooncol*. 2002;56:21–28.

193. Horbinski C, Hamilton RL, Lovell C, et al. Impact of morphology, MIB-1, p53 and MGMT on outcome in pilocytic astrocytomas. *Brain Pathol*. 2010;20:581–588.

194. Kindblom LG, Ahlden M, Meis-Kindblom JM, et al. Immunohistochemical and molecular analysis of p53, MDM2, proliferating cell nuclear antigen and Ki67 in benign and malignant peripheral nerve sheath tumours. *Virchows Arch.* 1995;427:19–26.

195. Halling KC, Scheithauer BW, Halling AC, et al. p53 expression in neurofibroma and malignant peripheral nerve sheath tumor. An immunohistochemical study of sporadic and NF1-associated tumors. *Am J Clin Pathol.* 1996;106:282–288.

196. Casadei GP, Scheithauer BW, Hirose T, et al. Cellular schwannoma. A clinicopathologic, DNA flow cytometric, and proliferation marker study of 70 patients. *Cancer.* 1995;75:1109–1119.

197. Ohgaki H, Olivier M, Hainaut P. Li-Fraumeni syndrome and TP53 germline mutations. In: *WHO Classification of Tumours of the Central Nervous System.* Louis DN, Ohgaki H, Wiestler OD, et al., eds. Lyon, France: IARC Press; 2007:222–225.

198. Varley JM, McGown G, Thorncroft M, et al. Germ-line mutations of TP53 in Li-Fraumeni families: an extended study of 39 families. *Cancer Res.* 1997;57:3245–3252.

199. Bickerstaff ER, Small JM, Guest IA. The relapsing course of certain meningiomas in relation to pregnancy and menstruation. *J Neurol Neurosurg Psychiatry.* 1958;21:89–91.

200. Verhagen A, Go KG, Visser GM, et al. The presence of progesterone receptors in arachnoid granulations and in the lining of arachnoid cysts: its relevance to expression of progesterone receptors in meningiomas. *Br J Neurosurg.* 1995;9:47–50.

201. Carroll RS, Glowacka D, Dashner K, et al. Progesterone receptor expression in meningiomas. *Cancer Res.* 1993;53:1312–1316.

202. Perry A, Cai DX, Scheithauer BW, et al. Merlin, DAL-1, and progesterone receptor expression in clinicopathologic subsets of meningioma: a correlative immunohistochemical study of 175 cases. *J Neuropathol Exp Neurol.* 2000;59:872–879.

203. Perry A. Meningiomas. *Practical Surgical Neuropathology: A Diagnostic Approach.* Perry A, Brat DJ, eds. Philadelphia, PA: Churchill Livingstone; 2010:185–218.

204. Koehorst SGA, Jacobs HM, Thijssen JHH, et al. Wild type and alternatively spliced estrogen receptor messenger RNA in human meningioma tissue and MCF7 breast cancer cells. *J Steroid Biochem Mol Biol.* 1993;45:227–233.

205. Pravdenkova S, Al-Mefty O, Sawyer J, et al. Progesterone and estrogen receptors: opposing prognostic indicators in meningiomas. *J Neurosurg.* 2006;105:163–173.

206. Leães CGS, Meurer RT, Coutinho LB, et al. Immunohistochemical expression of aromatase and estrogen, androgen and progesterone receptors in normal and neoplastic human meningeal cells. *Neuropathology.* 2010;30:44–49.

207. Abdelzaher E, El-Gendi SM, Yehya A, et al. Recurrence of benign meningiomas: predictive value of proliferative index, BCL2, p53, hormonal receptors and HER2 expression. *Br J Neurosurg.* 2011;25:707–713.

208. Thompson CB. Metabolic enzymes as oncogenes or tumor suppressors. *N Engl J Med.* 2009;360:813–815.

209. Horbinski C, Kofler J, Kelly LM, et al. Diagnostic use of IDH1/2 mutation analysis in routine clinical testing of formalin-fixed, paraffin-embedded glioma tissues. *J Neuropathol Exp Neurol.* 2009;68:1319–1325.

210. Yan H, Parsons DW, Jin G, et al. IDH1 and IDH2 mutations in gliomas. *N Engl J Med.* 2009;360:765–773.

211. Camelo-Piragua S, Jansen M, Ganguly A, et al. Mutant IDH1-specific immunohistochemistry distinguishes diffuse astrocytoma from astrocytosis. *Acta Neuropathol.* 2010;119:509–511.

212. Capper D, Weissert S, Balss J, et al. Characterization of R132H mutation-specific IDH1 antibody binding in brain tumors. *Brain Pathol.* 2010;20:245–254.

213. Capper D, Zentgraf H, Balss J, et al. Monoclonal antibody specific for IDH1 R132H mutation. *Acta Neuropathol.* 2009;118:599–601.

214. Sanson M, Marie Y, Paris S, et al. Isocitrate dehydrogenase 1 codon 132 mutation is an important prognostic biomarker in gliomas. *J Clin Oncol.* 2009;27:4150–4154.

215. Labussiere M, Idbaih A, Wang XW, et al. All the 1p19q codeleted gliomas are mutated on IDH1 or IDH2. *Neurology.* 2010;74:1886–1890.

216. Capper D, Reuss D, Schittenhelm J, et al. Mutation-specific IDH1 antibody differentiates oligodendrogliomas and oligoastrocytomas from other brain tumors with oligodendroglioma-like morphology. *Acta Neuropathol.* 2011;121:241–252.

217. Drablos F, Feyzi E, Aas PA, et al. Alkylation damage in DNA and RNA—repair mechanisms and medical significance. *DNA Repair.* 2004;3:1389–1407.

218. Esteller M, Garcia-Foncillas J, Andion E, et al. Inactivation of the DNA-repair gene MGMT and the clinical response of gliomas to alkylating agents. *N Engl J Med.* 2000;343:1350–1354.

219. Hegi ME, Diserens AC, Gorlia T, et al. MGMT gene silencing and benefit from temozolomide in glioblastoma. *N Engl J Med.* 2005;352:997–1003.

220. Everhard S, Kaloshi G, Criniere E, et al. MGMT methylation: A marker of response to temozolomide in low-grade gliomas. *Ann Neurol.* 2006;60:740–743.

221. Karayan-Tapon L, Quillien V, Guilhot J, et al. Prognostic value of O6-methylguanine-DNA methyltransferase status in glioblastoma patients, assessed by five different methods. *J Neurooncol.* 2010;97:311–322.

222. Roma AA, Prayson RA. Expression of cyclo-oxygenase-2 in ependymal tumors. *Neuropathology.* 2006;26:422–428.

223. Deininger MH, Weller M, Streffer J, et al. Patterns of cyclo-oxygenase-1 and -2 expression in human gliomas in vivo. *Acta Neuropathol.* 1999;98:240–244.

224. Martin-Villalba A, Okuducu AF, von Deimling A. The Evolution of Our Understanding on Glioma. *Brain Pathol.* 2008;18:455–463.

225. Zhai X, Goodacre JA, Hassan HT. A very small population of Cells expressing the CD133 haematopoietic stem cell antigen in Normal Adult Substantia Nigra and Striatum Brain Tissues. *Haematologica.* 2006;91 (Suppl. 1):515–516.

226. Schrot RJ, Ma JH, Greco CM, et al. Organotypic distribution of stem cell markers in formalin-fixed brain harboring glioblastoma multiforme. *J Neurooncol.* 2007;85:149–157.

227. Liu G, Yuan X, Zeng Z, et al. Analysis of gene expression and chemoresistance of CD133+ cancer stem cells in glioblastoma. *Mol Cancer.* 2006;5:67–78.

228. Zeppernick F, Ahmadi R, Campos B, et al. Stem cell marker CD133 affects clinical outcome in glioma patients. *Clin Cancer Res.* 2008;14:123–129.

229. Lowe J. Establishing a pathological diagnosis in degenerative dementias. *Brain Pathol.* 1998;8:403–406.

230. Kovacs GG, Botond G, Budka H. Protein coding of neurodegenerative dementias: the neuropathological basis of biomarker diagnostics. *Acta Neuropathol.* 2010;119:389–408.

231. Feany MB, Dickson DW. Neurodegenerative disorders with extensive tau pathology: a comparative study and review. *Ann Neurol.* 1996;40:139–148.

232. Reddy PH. Abnormal tau, mitochondrial dysfunction, impaired axonal transport of mitochondria, and synaptic deprivation in Alzheimer's disease. *Brain Res.* 2011;1415:136–148.

233. Yoshida M. Cellular tau pathology and immunohistochemical study of tau isoforms in sporadic tauopathies. *Neuropathology.* 2006;26:457–470.

234. Kakita A, Kameyama S, Hayashi S, et al. Pathologic features of dysplasia and accompanying alterations observed in surgical specimens from patients with intractable epilepsy. *J Child Neurol.* 2005;20:341–350.

235. Saito Y, Suzuki K, Nanba E, et al. Niemann-Pick type C disease: accelerated neurofibrillary tangle formation and amyloid beta deposition associated with apolipoprotein E epsilon 4 homozygosity. *Ann Neurol.* 2002;52:351–355.

236. Yasuhara O, Kawamata T, Aimi Y, et al. Expression of chromogranin A in lesions in the central nervous system from patients with neurological diseases. *Neurosci Lett.* 1994;170:13–16.

237. Forno LS. Neuropathology of Parkinson's disease. *J Neuropathol Exp Neurol*. 1996;55:259–272.

238. McKeith IG, Galasko D, Kosaka K, et al. Consensus guidelines for the clinical and pathologic diagnosis of dementia with Lewy bodies (DLB): report of the consortium on DLB international workshop. *Neurology*. 1996;47:1113–1124.

239. Wakabayashi K, Tanji K, Mori F, et al. The Lewy body in Parkinson's disease: molecules implicated in the formation and degradation of alpha-synuclein aggregates. *Neuropathology*. 2007;27:494–506.

240. Spillantini MG, Schmidt ML, Lee VM, et al. Alpha-synuclein in Lewy bodies. *Nature*. 1997;388:839–840.

241. Papp MI, Kahn JE, Lantos PL. Glial cytoplasmic inclusions in the CNS of patients with multiple system atrophy (striatonigral degeneration, olivopontocerebellar atrophy and Shy-Drager syndrome). *J Neurol Sci*. 1989;94:79–100.

242. Yamazaki M, Arai Y, Baba M, et al. Alpha-synuclein inclusions in amygdala in the brains of patients with the parkinsonism-dementia complex of Guam. *J Neuropathol Exp Neurol*. 2000;59:585–591.

243. Habuchi C, Iritani S, Sekiguchi H, et al. Clinicopathological study of diffuse neurofibrillary tangles with calcification. With special reference to TDP-43 proteinopathy and alpha-synucleinopathy. *J Neurol Sci*. 2011;301: 77–85.

244. Mayer RJ, Lowe J, Landon M, et al. Ubiquitin and the lysosome system: molecular immunopathology reveals the connection. *Biomed Biochim Acta*. 1991;50:333–341.

245. Lowe J, Mayer J, Landon M, et al. Ubiquitin and the molecular pathology of neurodegenerative diseases. *Adv Exp Med Biol*. 2001;487:169–186.

246. Rohn TT. Cytoplasmic inclusions of TDP-43 in neurodegenerative diseases: a potential role for caspases. *Histol Histopathol*. 2009;24:1081–1086.

247. Dickson DW, Wertkin A, Kress Y, et al. Ubiquitin immunoreactive structures in normal human brains. Distribution and developmental aspects. *Lab Invest*. 1990;63:87–99.

248. Okamoto K, Hirai S, Iizuka T, et al. Reexamination of granulovacuolar degeneration. *Acta Neuropathol*. 1991;82: 340–345.

249. Iseki E, Odawara T, Li F, et al. Age-related ubiquitin-positive granular structures in non-demented subjects and neurodegenerative disorders. *J Neurol Sci*. 1996;142:25–29.

250. Gallo JM. Kennedy's disease: a triplet repeat disorder or a motor neuron disease? *Brain Res Bull*. 2001;56:209–214.

251. Hiraga T, Leipold HW, Cash WC, et al. Reduced numbers and intense anti-ubiquitin immunostaining of bovine motor neurons affected with spinal muscular atrophy. *J Neurol Sci*. 1993;118:43–47.

252. Schwab C, Arai T, Hasegawa M, et al. Colocalization of transactivation-responsive DNA-binding protein 43 and huntingtin in inclusions of Huntington disease. *J Neuropathol Exp Neurol*. 2008;67:1159–1165.

253. Bacci B, Cochran E, Nunzi MG, et al. Amyloid beta precursor protein and ubiquitin epitopes in human and experimental dystrophic axons. Ultrastructural localization. *Am J Pathol*. 1994;144:702–710.

254. Mao YW, Liu JP, Xiang H, et al. Human alphaA- and alphaB-crystallins bind to Bax and Bcl-X(S) to sequester their translocation during staurosporine-induced apoptosis. *Cell Death Differ*. 2004;11:512–526.

255. Li DW, Liu JP, Mao YW, et al. Calcium-activated RAF/MEK/ERK signaling pathway mediates p53-dependent apoptosis and is abrogated by alpha B-crystallin through inhibition of RAS activation. *Mol Biol Cell*. 2005;16:4437–4453.

256. Buratti E, Baralle FE. Characterization and functional implications of the RNA binding properties of nuclear factor TDP-43, a novel splicing regulator of CFTR exon 9. *J Biol Chem*. 2001;276:36337–36343.

257. Neumann M, Sampathu DM, Kwong LK, et al. Ubiquitinated TDP-43 in frontotemporal lobar degeneration and amyotrophic lateral sclerosis. *Science*. 2006;314:130–133.

258. Kwong LK, Neumann M, Sampathu DM, et al. TDP-43 proteinopathy: the neuropathology underlying major forms of sporadic and familial frontotemporal lobar degeneration and motor neuron disease. *Acta Neuropathol*. 2007;114:63–70.

259. Geser F, Lee VM-Y, Trojanowski JQ. Amyotrophic lateral sclerosis and frontotemporal lobar degeneration: A spectrum of TDP-43 proteinopathies. *Neuropathology*. 2010;30:103–112.

260. Frank S, Tolnay M. Frontotemporal lobar degeneration: toward the end of conFUSion. *Acta Neuropathol*. 2009;118:629–631.

261. Uchihara T, Fujigasaki H, Koyano S, et al. Non-expanded polyglutamine proteins in intranuclear inclusions of hereditary ataxias—triple-labeling immunofluorescence study. *Acta Neuropathol*. 2001;102:149–152.

262. Maat-Schieman M, Roos R, Losekoot M, et al. Neuronal intranuclear and neuropil inclusions for pathological assessment of Huntington's disease. *Brain Pathol*. 2007;17:31–37.

263. Davis RL, Holohan PD, Shrimpton AE, et al. Familial encephalopathy with neuroserpin inclusion bodies. *Am J Pathol*. 1999;155:1901–1913.

264. Kubler E, Oesch B, Raeber AJ. Diagnosis of prion diseases. *Br Med Bull*. 2003;66:267–279.

265. Kovacs GG, Voigtlander T, Gelpi E, et al. Rationale for diagnosing human prion disease. *World J Biol Psychiatry*. 2004;5:83–91.

266. Umahara T, Uchihara T, Yagishita S, et al. Intranuclear immunolocalization of 14-3-3 protein isoforms in brains with spinocerebellar ataxia type 1. *Neurosci Lett*. 2007;414: 130–135.

267. Manivel JC, Jessurun J, Wick MR, et al. Placental alkaline phosphatase immunoreactivity in testicular germ-cell neoplasms. *Am J Surg Pathol*. 1987;11:21–29.

268. Saad RS, Landreneau RJ, Liu Y, et al. Utility of immunohistochemistry in separating thymic neoplasms from germ cell tumors and metastatic lung cancer involving the anterior mediastinum. *Appl Immunohistochem Mol Morphol*. 2003;11:107–112.

269. Mei K, Liu A, Allan RW, et al. Diagnostic utility of SALL4 in primary germ cell tumors of the central nervous system: a study of 77 cases. *Mod Pathol*. 2009;22:1628–1636.

270. Cao D, Li J, Guo CC, et al. SALL4 is a novel diagnostic marker for testicular germ cell tumors. *Am J Surg Pathol*. 2009;33:1065–1077.

271. Hattab EM, Tu PH, Wilson JD, et al. OCT4 immunohistochemistry is superior to placental alkaline phosphatase (PLAP) in the diagnosis of central nervous system germinoma. *Am J Surg Pathol*. 2005;29:368–371.

272. Jones TD, Ulbright TM, Eble JN, et al. OCT4 staining in testicular tumors: a sensitive and specific marker for seminoma and embryonal carcinoma. *Am J Surg Pathol*. 2004;28: 935–940.

273. Guo Y, Liu S, Wang P, et al. Expression profile of embryonic stem cell-associated genes Oct4, Sox2 and Nanog in human gliomas. *Histopathology*. 2011;59:763–775.

274. Ong CW, Kim LG, Kong HH, et al. CD133 expression predicts for non-response to chemotherapy in colorectal cancer. *Mod Pathol*. 2010;23:450–457.

275. Howell NR, Zheng W, Cheng L, et al. Carcinomas of ovary and lung with clear cell features: can immunohistochemistry help in differential diagnosis? *Int J Gynecol Pathol*. 2007;26:134–140.

276. Yarden Y, Kuang WJ, Yang-Feng T, et al. Human proto-oncogene c-kit: a new cell surface receptor tyrosine kinase for an unidentified ligand. *EMBO J*. 1987;6:3341–3351.

277. Dagher R, Cohen M, Williams G, et al. Approval summary: imatinib mesylate in the treatment of metastatic and/or unresectable malignant gastrointestinal stromal tumors. *Clin Cancer Res*. 2002;8:3034–3038.

278. Cetin N, Dienel D, Gokden M. CD117 expression in glial tumors. *J Neurooncol*. 2005;75:195–202.

279. Janku F, Kidney D, Coyne J. Unusual presentation of gastrointestinal stromal tumor with early cerebral involvement. *Ir J Med Sci*. 2011;180:765–766.

280. Leroy X, Augusto D, Leteurtre E, et al. CD30 and CD117 (c-kit) used in combination are useful for distinguishing embryonal carcinoma from seminoma. *J Histochem Cytochem*. 2002;50:283–285.

281. Ferreiro JA. Ber-H2 expression in testicular germ cell tumors. *Hum Pathol*. 1994;25:522–524.

282. Lau SK, Weiss LM, Chu PG. D2-40 immunohistochemistry in the differential diagnosis of seminoma and embryonal carcinoma: a comparative immunohistochemical study with KIT (CD117) and CD30. *Mod Pathol*. 2007;20:320–325.

283. Nakamura Y, Kanemura Y, Yamada T, et al. D2-40 antibody immunoreactivity in developing human brain, brain tumors and cultured neural cells. *Mod Pathol*. 2006;19:974–985.

284. Yonezawa H, Shinsato Y, Obara S, et al. Germinoma with syncytiotrophoblastic giant cells arising in the corpus callosum. *Neurol Med Chir*. 2010;50:588–591.

285. Wang F, Liu A, Peng Y, et al. Diagnostic utility of SALL4 in extragonadal yolk sac tumors: an immunohistochemical study of 59 cases with comparison to placental-like alkaline phosphatase, alpha-fetoprotein, and glypican-3. *Am J Surg Pathol*. 2009;33:1529–1539.

286. Hamazaki S, Okada S. Expression of CD34 antigen in testicular mixed germ cell tumor. *Pathol Int*. 2003;53:853–857.

287. Swerdlow SH, Campo E, Harris NL, et al. *WHO Classification of Tumours of Haematopoietic and Lymphoid Tissues*. 4th ed. Lyon, France: IARC Press; 2008.

288. Higgins RA, Blankenship JE, Kinney MC. Application of immunohistochemistry in the diagnosis of non-Hodgkin and Hodgkin lymphoma. *Arch Pathol Lab Med*. 2008;132:441–461.

289. Garcia CF, Swerdlow SH. Best practices in contemporary diagnostic immunohistochemistry panel approach to hematolymphoid proliferations. *Arch Pathol Lab Med*. 2009;133:756–765.

290. Myung J, Kim B, Yoon B-W, et al. B-cell dominant lymphocytic primary angiitis of the central nervous system: Four biopsy-proven cases. *Neuropathology*. 2010;30:123–130.

291. Boyle EM, Morschhauser F. Ongoing development of monoclonal antibodies and antibody drug-conjugates in lymphoma. *Curr Oncol Rep*. 2011;13:386–397.

292. Chu PG, Arber DA. CD79a: a review. *Appl Immunohistochem Mol Morphol*. 2001;9:97–106.

293. Robillard N, Avet-Loiseau H, Garand R, et al. CD20 is associated with a small mature plasma cell morphology and t(11;14) in multiple myeloma. *Blood*. 2003;102:1070–1071.

294. Mittelbronn M, Dietz K, Schluesener HJ, et al. Local distribution of microglia in the normal adult human central nervous system differs by up to one order of magnitude. *Acta Neuropathol*. 2001;101:249–255.

295. Masliah E, Mallory M, Hansen L, et al. Immunoreactivity of CD45, a protein phosphotyrosine phosphatase, in Alzheimer's disease. *Acta Neuropathol*. 1991;83:12–20.

296. Sasaki A, Hirato J, Nakazato Y. Immunohistochemical study of microglia in the Creutzfeldt-Jakob diseased brain. *Acta Neuropathol*. 1993;86:337–344.

297. Rollins KE, Kleinschmidt-DeMasters BK, Corboy JR, et al. Lymphomatosis cerebri as a cause of white matter dementia. *Hum Pathol*. 2005;36:282–290.

298. Beck RC, Tubbs RR, Hussein M, et al. Automated colorimetric in situ hybridization (CISH) detection of immunoglobulin (Ig) light chain mRNA expression in plasma cell (PC) dyscrasias and non-Hodgkin lymphoma. *Diagn Mol Pathol*. 2003;12:14–20.

299. Hans CP, Weisenburger DD, Greiner TC, et al. Confirmation of the molecular classification of diffuse large B-cell lymphoma by immunohistochemistry using a tissue microarray. *Blood*. 2004;103:275–282.

300. Hattab EM, Martin SE, Al-Khatib SM, et al. Most primary central nervous system diffuse large B-cell lymphomas occurring in immunocompetent individuals belong to the nongerminal center subtype: a retrospective analysis of 31 cases. *Mod Pathol*. 2010;23:235–243.

301. Raoux D, Duband S, Forest F, et al. Primary central nervous system lymphoma: Immunohistochemical profile and prognostic significance. *Neuropathology*. 2010;30:232–240.

302. Gualco G, Weiss LM, Barber GN, et al. Diffuse large B-cell lymphoma involving the central nervous system. *Int J Surg Pathol*. 2011;19:44–50.

303. Strauchen JA, Miller LK. Lymph Node Infarction An Immunohistochemical Study of 11 Cases. *Arch Pathol Lab Med*. 2003;127:60–63.

304. Swain RS, Tihan T, Horvai AE, et al. Inflammatory myofibroblastic tumor of the central nervous system and its relationship to inflammatory pseudotumor. *Hum Pathol*. 2008;39:410–419.

305. Tihan T, Viglione M, Rosenblum MK, et al. Solitary fibrous tumors in the central nervous system: a clinicopathologic review of 18 cases and comparison to meningeal hemangiopericytomas. *Arch Pathol Lab Med*. 2003;127:432–439.

306. Lau SK, Chu PG, Weiss LM. Immunohistochemical expression of Langerin in Langerhans cell histiocytosis and non-Langerhans cell histiocytic disorders. *Am J Surg Pathol*. 2008;32:615–619.

307. Backe E, Schwarting R, Gerdes J, et al. Ber-MAC3: new monoclonal antibody that defines human monocyte/macrophage differentiation antigen. *J Clin Pathol*. 1991;44:936–945.

308. Saito N, Pulford KA, Breton-Gorius J, et al. Ultrastructural localization of the CD68 macrophage-associated antigen in human blood neutrophils and monocytes. *Am J Pathol*. 1991;139:1053–1059.

309. Law SK, Micklem KJ, Shaw JM, et al. A new macrophage differentiation antigen which is a member of the scavenger receptor superfamily. *Eur J Immunol*. 1993;23:2320–2325.

310. Lau SK, Chu PG, Weiss LM. CD163: a specific marker of macrophages in paraffin-embedded tissue samples. *Am J Clin Pathol*. 2004;122:794–801.

311. Nguyen TT, Schwartz EJ, West RB, et al. Expression of CD163 (hemoglobin scavenger receptor) in normal tissues, lymphomas, carcinomas, and sarcomas is largely restricted to the monocyte/macrophage lineage. *Am J Surg Pathol*. 2005;29:617–624.

312. Shabo I, Svanvik J. Expression of macrophage antigens by tumor cells. *Adv Exp Med Biol*. 2011;714:141–150.

313. Hoon V, Thung SN, Kaneko M, et al. HMB-45 reactivity in renal angiomyolipoma and lymphangioleiomyomatosis. *Arch Pathol Lab Med*. 1994;118:732–734.

314. Hisaoka M, Ishida T, Kuo TT, et al. Clear cell sarcoma of soft tissue: a clinicopathologic, immunohistochemical, and molecular analysis of 33 cases. *Am J Surg Pathol*. 2008;32:452–460.

315. Taddei GL, Arganini L, Raspollini MR, et al. Oligodendroglioma: HMB-45 positivity using catalyzed signal amplification method: an immunohistochemical (HMB-45, CD31, p53, Mib-1) and ultrastructural study. *Appl Immunohistochem Mol Morphol*. 2001;9:35–41.

316. Wu A, Kunju LP, Cheng L, et al. Renal cell carcinoma in children and young adults: analysis of clinicopathological, immunohistochemical and molecular characteristics with an emphasis on the spectrum of Xp11.2 translocation-associated and unusual clear cell subtypes. *Histopathology*. 2008;53:533–544.

317. Boyle JL, Haupt HM, Stern JB, et al. Tyrosinase expression in malignant melanoma, desmoplastic melanoma, and peripheral nerve tumors. *Arch Pathol Lab Med*. 2002;126:816–822.

318. Wagner SN, Wagner C, Schultewolter T, et al. Analysis of Pmel17/gp100 expression in primary human tissue specimens: implications for melanoma immuno- and gene-therapy. *Cancer Immunol Immunother*. 1997;44:239–247.

319. Hodgkinson CA, Moore KJ, Nakayama A, et al. Mutations at the mouse microphthalmia locus are associated with defects in a gene encoding a novel basic helix-loop-helix zipper protein. *Cell*. 1993;74:395–404.

320. King R, Weilbaecher KN, McGill G, et al. Microphthalmia transcription factor. A sensitive and specific melanocyte marker for Melanoma Diagnosis. *Am J Pathol*. 1999;155:731–738.

321. Lerner AB, Fitzpatrick TB. Biochemistry of melanin formation. *Physiol Rev*. 1950;30:91–126.

322. Ohsie SJ, Sarantopoulos GP, Cochran AJ, et al. Immunohistochemical characteristics of melanoma. *J Cutan Pathol*. 2008;35:433–444.

323. Smith AB, Rushing EJ, Smirniotopoulos JG. Pigmented lesions of the central nervous system: radiologic-pathologic correlation. *Radiographics*. 2009;29:1503–1524.

324. Kurtkaya-Yapicier O, Scheithauer B, Woodruff JM. The pathobiologic spectrum of Schwannomas. *Histol Histopathol*. 2003;18:925–934.

325. Rosenblum MK, Erlandson RA, Aleksic SN, et al. Melanotic ependymoma and subependymoma. *Am J Surg Pathol*. 1990;14:729–736.

326. Kapadia SB, Frisman DM, Hitchcock CL, et al. Melanotic neuroectodermal tumor of infancy. Clinicopathological, immunohistochemical, and flow cytometric study. *Am J Surg Pathol*. 1993;17:566–573.

327. Schmidbauer M, Budka H, Pilz P. Neuroepithelial and ectomesenchymal differentiation in a primitive pineal tumor ("pineal anlage tumor"). *Clin Neuropathol*. 1989;8:7–10.

328. Sharma MC, Mahapatra AK, Gaikwad S, et al. Pigmented medulloepithelioma: report of a case and review of the literature. *Childs Nerv Syst*. 1998;14:74–78.

329. Vajtai I, Yonekawa Y, Schauble B, et al. Melanotic astrocytoma. *Acta Neuropathol*. 1996;91:549–553.

330. Soffer D, Lach B, Constantini S. Melanotic cerebral ganglioglioma: evidence for melanogenesis in neoplastic astrocytes. *Acta Neuropathol*. 1992;83:315–323.

331. Watanabe K, Ando Y, Iwanaga H, et al. Choroid plexus papilloma containing melanin pigment. *Clin Neuropathol*. 1995;14:159–161.

332. Sunden Y, Suzuki T, Orba Y, et al. Characterization and application of polyclonal antibodies that specifically recognize JC virus large T antigen. *Acta Neuropathol*. 2006;111:379–387.

333. Hsu JL, Glaser SL. Epstein-Barr virus-associated malignancies: epidemiologic patterns and etiologic implications. *Critic Rev Oncol Hematol*. 2000;34:27–53.

334. Bergmann M, Blasius S, Bankfalvi A, et al. Primary non-Hodgkin lymphomas of the CNS-proliferation, oncoproteins and Epstein-Barr-virus. *Gen Diagn Pathol*. 1996;141:235–242.

335. Guterman KS, Hair LS, Morgello S. Epstein-Barr virus and AIDS-related primary central nervous system lymphoma. Viral detection by immunohistochemistry, RNA in situ hybridization, and polymerase chain reaction. *Clin Neuropathol*. 1996;15:79–86.

336. Gupta S, Havens PL, Southern JF, et al. Epstein-Barr virus-associated intracranial leiomyosarcoma in an HIV-positive adolescent. *J Pediatr Hematol Oncol*. 2010;32:e144–e147.

337. Sivendran S, Vidal CI, Barginear MF. Primary intracranial leiomyosarcoma in an HIV-infected patient. *Int J Clin Oncol*. 2011;16:63–66.

338. Khoury H, Adkins D, Brown R, et al. Successful treatment of cerebral toxoplasmosis in a marrow transplant recipient: contribution of a PCR test in diagnosis and early detection. *Bone Marrow Transplant*. 1999;23:409–411.

339. Guarner J, Bartlett J, Shieh WJ, et al. Histopathologic spectrum and immunohistochemical diagnosis of amebic meningoencephalitis. *Mod Pathol*. 2007;20:1230–1237.

340. Armah HB, Wang G, Omalu BI, et al. Systemic distribution of West Nile virus infection: postmortem immunohistochemical study of six cases. *Brain Pathol*. 2007;17:354–362.

341. Rhodes RH, Ward JM. Immunohistochemistry of human immunodeficiency virus in the central nervous system and an hypothesis concerning the pathogenesis of AIDS meningoencephalomyelitis. *Prog AIDS Pathol*. 1989;1:167–179.

342. O'Brien RJ, Wong PC. Amyloid precursor protein processing and Alzheimer's disease. *Annu Rev Neurosci*. 2011;34:185–204.

343. Grinberg LT, Thal DR. Vascular pathology in the aged human brain. *Acta Neuropathol*. 2010;119:277–290.

344. Mikol J. Neuropathology of prion diseases. *Biomed Pharmacother*. 1999;53:19–26.

345. Wen GY, Wisniewski HM, Kascsak RJ. Biondi ring tangles in the choroid plexus of Alzheimer's disease and normal aging brains: a quantitative study. *Brain Res*. 1999;832: 40–46.

346. Niess C, Grauel U, Toennes SW, et al. Incidence of axonal injury in human brain tissue. *Acta Neuropathol*. 2002;104:79–84.

347. Oehmichen M, Meissner C, Schmidt V, et al. Pontine axonal injury after brain trauma and nontraumatic hypoxic-ischemic brain damage. *Int J Legal Med*. 1999;112:261–267.

348. Graham DI, Smith C, Reichard R, et al. Trials and tribulations of using beta-amyloid precursor protein immunohistochemistry to evaluate traumatic brain injury in adults. *Forensic Sci Int*. 2004;146:89–96.

349. Rankine AJ, Filion PR, Platten MA, et al. Perineurioma: a clinicopathological study of eight cases. *Pathology*. 2004;36:309–315.

350. Haraida S, Nerlich AG, Bise K, et al. Comparison of various basement membrane components in benign and malignant peripheral nerve tumours. *Virchows Arch A Pathol Anat Histopathol*. 1992;421:331–338.

351. O'Sullivan MJ, Kyriakos M, Zhu X, et al. Malignant peripheral nerve sheath tumors with t(X;18). A pathologic and molecular genetic study. *Mod Pathol*. 2000;13:1336–1346.

352. Folpe AL, Agoff SN, Willis J, et al. Parachordoma is immunohistochemically and cytogenetically distinct from axial chordoma and extraskeletal myxoid chondrosarcoma. *Am J Surg Pathol*. 1999;23:1059–1067.

353. Biggar SR, Crabtree GR. Continuous and widespread roles for the Swi-Snf complex in transcription. *EMBO J*. 1999;18:2254–2264.

354. Biegel JA, Zhou JY, Rorke LB, et al. Germ-line and acquired mutations of INI1 in atypical teratoid and rhabdoid tumors. *Cancer Res*. 1999;59:74–79.

355. Haberler C, Laggner U, Slavc I, et al. Immunohistochemical analysis of INI1 protein in malignant pediatric CNS tumors: Lack of INI1 in atypical teratoid/rhabdoid tumors and in a fraction of primitive neuroectodermal tumors without rhabdoid phenotype. *Am J Surg Pathol*. 2006;30:1462–1468.

356. Sigauke E, Rakheja D, Maddox DL, et al. Absence of expression of SMARCB1/INI1 in malignant rhabdoid tumors of the central nervous system, kidneys and soft tissue: an immunohistochemical study with implications for diagnosis. *Mod Pathol*. 2006;19:717–725.

357. Patil S, Perry A, Maccollin M, et al. Immunohistochemical analysis supports a role for INI1/SMARCB1 in hereditary forms of schwannomas, but not in solitary, sporadic schwannomas. *Brain Pathol*. 2008;18:517–519.

358. Gessi M, Giangaspero F, Pietsch T. Atypical teratoid/rhabdoid tumors and choroid plexus tumors: when genetics "surprise" pathology. *Brain Pathol*. 2003;13:409–414.

359. Hasselblatt M, Oyen F, Gesk S, et al. Cribriform neuroepithelial tumor (CRINET): a nonrhabdoid ventricular tumor with INI1 loss and relatively favorable prognosis. *J Neuropathol Exp Neurol*. 2009;68:1249–1255.

360. Mobley BC, McKenney JK, Bangs CD, et al. Loss of SMARCB1/INI1 expression in poorly differentiated chordomas. *Acta Neuropathol*. 2010;120:745–753.

361. Buckler AJ, Pelletier J, Haber DA, et al. Isolation, characterization, and expression of the murine Wilms' tumor gene (WT1) during kidney development. *Mol Cell Biol*. 1991;11:1707–1712.

362. Hill DA, Pfeifer JD, Marley EF, et al. WT1 staining reliably differentiates desmoplastic small round cell tumor from Ewing sarcoma/primitive neuroectodermal tumor. An immunohistochemical and molecular diagnostic study. *Am J Clin Pathol*. 2000;114:345–353.

363. Nakatsuka S, Oji Y, Horiuchi T, et al. Immunohistochemical detection of WT1 protein in a variety of cancer cells. *Mod Pathol*. 2006;19:804–814.

364. Schittenhelm J, Mittelbronn M, Nguyen T-D, et al. WT1 expression distinguishes astrocytic tumor cells from normal and reactive astrocytes. *Brain Pathol*. 2008;18:344–353.

365. Timár J, Mészáros L, Orosz Z, et al. WT1 expression in angiogenic tumours of the skin. *Histopathology*. 2005;47:67–73.

366. Majores M, von Lehe M, Fassunke J, et al. Tumor Recurrence and Malignant Progression of Gangliogliomas. *Cancer*. 2008;113:3355–3363.

367. Blumcke I, Giencke K, Wardelmann E, et al. The CD34 epitope is expressed in neoplastic and malformative lesions associated with chronic, focal epilepsies. *Acta Neuropathol*. 1999;97:481–490.

368. Deb P, Sharma MC, Tripathi M, et al. Expression of CD34 as a novel marker for glioneuronal lesions associated with chronic intractable epilepsy. *Neuropathol Appl Neurobiol*. 2006;32:461–468.

369. Reifenberger G, Kaulich K, Wiestler OD, et al. Expression of the CD34 antigen in pleomorphic xanthoastrocytomas. *Acta Neuropathol*. 2003;105:358–364.

370. Brunnemann RB, Ro JY, Ordonez NG, et al. Extrapleural solitary fibrous tumor: a clinicopathologic study of 24 cases. *Mod Pathol*. 1999;12:1034–1042.

371. Sundaram C, Uppin SG, Uppin MS, et al. A clinicopathological and immunohistochemical study of central nervous system hemangiopericytomas. *J Clin Neurosci*. 2010;17:469–472.

372. Hasegawa T, Matsuno Y, Shimoda T, et al. Frequent expression of bcl-2 protein in solitary fibrous tumors. *Jpn J Clin Oncol*. 1998;28:86–91.

373. Zhou H, Coffin CM, Perkins SL, et al. Malignant peripheral nerve sheath tumor: a comparison of grade, immunophenotype, and cell cycle/growth activation marker expression in sporadic and neurofibromatosis 1-related lesions. *Am J Surg Pathol*. 2003;27:1337–1345.

374. Sachdev R, Sundram U. Expression of CD163 in dermatofibroma, cellular fibrous histiocytoma, and dermatofibrosarcoma protuberans: comparison with CD68, CD34, and Factor XIIIa. *J Cutan Pathol*. 2006;33:353–360.

375. Yeh I, McCalmont TH. Distinguishing neurofibroma from desmoplastic melanoma: the value of the CD34 fingerprint. *J Cutan Pathol*. 2011;38:625–630.

376. Riopel M, Dickman PS, Link MP, et al. MIC2 analysis in pediatric lymphomas and leukemias. *Hum Pathol*. 1994;25:396–399.

377. Folpe AL, Schmidt RA, Chapman D, et al. Poorly differentiated synovial sarcoma: immunohistochemical distinction from primitive neuroectodermal tumors and high-grade malignant peripheral nerve sheath tumors. *Am J Surg Pathol*. 1998;22:673–682.

378. Granter SR, Renshaw AA, Fletcher CD, et al. CD99 reactivity in mesenchymal chondrosarcoma. *Hum Pathol*. 1996;27:1273–1276.

379. Ishii N, Hiraga H, Sawamura Y, et al. Alternative EWS-FLI1 fusion gene and MIC2 expression in peripheral and central primitive neuroectodermal tumors. *Neuropathology*. 2001;21:40–44.

380. Choi YL, Chi JG, Suh YL. CD99 immunoreactivity in ependymoma. *Appl Immunohistochem Mol Morphol*. 2001;9:125–129.

381. Bisceglia M, Galliani C, Giannatempo G, et al. Solitary Fibrous Tumor of the Central Nervous System: A 15-year Literature Survey of 220 Cases (August 1996–July 2011). *Adv Anat Pathol*. 2011;18:356–392.

382. Guazzi S, Price M, De Felice M, et al. Thyroid nuclear factor 1 (TTF-1) contains a homeodomain and displays a novel DNA binding specificity. *EMBO J*. 1990;9:3631–3639.

383. Lazzaro D, Price M, De Felice M, et al. The transcription factor TTF-1 is expressed at the onset of thyroid and lung morphogenesis and in restricted regions of the fetal brain. *Development*. 1991;113:1093–1104.

384. Kimura S, Hara Y, Pineau T, et al. The T/ebp null mouse: thyroid-specific enhancer-binding protein is essential for the organogenesis of the thyroid, lung, ventral forebrain, and pituitary. *Genes Dev*. 1996;10:60–69.

385. Ordonez NG. Thyroid transcription factor-1 is a marker of lung and thyroid carcinomas. *Adv Anat Pathol*. 2000;7:123–127.

386. Kaufmann O, Dietel M. Expression of thyroid transcription factor-1 in pulmonary and extrapulmonary small cell carcinomas and other neuroendocrine carcinomas of various primary sites. *Histopathology*. 2000;36:415–420.

387. Lee EB, Tihan T, Scheithauer BW, et al. Thyroid transcription factor 1 expression in sellar tumors: a histogenetic marker? *J Neuropathol Exp Neurol*. 2009;68:482–488.

388. Takeichi M. Cadherin cell adhesion receptors as a morphogenetic regulator. *Science*. 1991;251:1451–1455.

389. Behrens J, Lustig B. The Wnt connection to tumorigenesis. *Int J Dev Biol*. 2004;48:477–487.

390. Polakis P. Wnt signaling and cancer. *Genes Dev*. 2000;14:1837–1851.

391. Buslei R, Nolde M, Hofmann B, et al. Common mutations of beta-catenin in adamantinomatous craniopharyngiomas but not in other tumours originating from the sellar region. *Acta Neuropathol*. 2005;109:589–597.

392. Semba S, Han S-Y, Ikeda H, et al. Frequent nuclear accumulation of beta-Catenin in pituitary adenoma. *Cancer*. 2001;91:42–48.

393. Ellison DW, Onilude OE, Lindsey JC, et al. beta-Catenin status predicts a favorable outcome in childhood medulloblastoma. *J Clin Oncol*. 2005;23:7951–7957.

394. Vujovic S, Henderson S, Presneau N, et al. Brachyury, a crucial regulator of notochordal development, is a novel biomarker for chordomas. *J Pathol*. 2006;209:157–165.

395. Tirabosco R, Mangham DC, Rosenberg AE, et al. Brachyury expression in extra-axial skeletal and soft tissue chordomas: a marker that distinguishes chordoma from mixed tumor/myoepithelioma/parachordoma in soft tissue. *Am J Surg Pathol*. 2008;32:572–580.

396. Kalof AN, Cooper K. D2-40 immunohistochemistry—so far! *Adv Anat Pathol*. 2009;16:62–64.

397. Rivera AL, Takei H, Zhai J, et al. Useful immunohistochemical markers in differentiating hemangioblastoma versus metastatic renal cell carcinoma. *Neuropathology*. 2010;30:580–585.

398. Sangoi AR, Dulai MS, Beck AH, et al. Distinguishing chordoid meningiomas from their histologic mimics: an immunohistochemical evaluation. *Am J Surg Pathol*. 2009;33:669–681.

399. Herbert J, Wilcox JN, Pham KC, et al. Transthyretin: a choroid plexus-specific transport protein in human brain. The 1986 S. Weir Mitchell Award. *Neurology*. 1986;36:900–911.

400. Hasselblatt M, Bohm C, Tatenhorst L, et al. Identification of novel diagnostic markers for choroid plexus tumors: a microarray-based approach. *Am J Surg Pathol*. 2006;30:66–74.

401. Ang LC, Taylor AR, Bergin D, et al. An immunohistochemical study of papillary tumors in the central nervous system. *Cancer*. 1990;65:2712–2719.

402. Herbert J, Cavallaro T, Dwork AJ. A marker for primary choroid plexus neoplasms. *Am J Pathol*. 1990;136:1317–1325.

403. Raisanen J, Vogel H, Horoupian DS. Primitive pineal tumor with retinoblastomatous and retinal/ciliary epithelial differentiation: an immunohistochemical study. *J Neurooncol*. 1990;9:165–170.

404. Perentes E, Rubenstein LJ, Herman MM, et al. S-Antigen immunoreactivity in human pineal glands and pineal parenchymal tumors. A monoclonal antibody study. *Acta Neuropathol*. 1986;71:224–227.

405. Lopes MB, Gonzalez-Fernandez F, Scheithauer BW, et al. Differential expression of retinal proteins in a pineal parenchymal tumor. *J Neuropathol Exp Neurol*. 1993;52:516–524.

406. Bonnin JM, Perentes E. Retinal S-antigen immunoreactivity in medulloblastomas. *Acta Neuropathol*. 1988;76:204–207.

407. Kraus MD, Haley JC, Ruiz R, et al. "Juvenile" xanthogranuloma: an immunophenotypic study with a reappraisal of histogenesis. *Am J Dermatopathol*. 2001;23:104–111.

408. Rushing EJ, Bouffard JP, Neal CJ, et al. Erdheim-Chester disease mimicking a primary brain tumor. Case report. *J Neurosurg*. 2004;100:1115–1118.

409. Perry A, Scheithauer BW, Nascimento AG. The immunophenotypic spectrum of meningeal hemangiopericytoma: a comparison with fibrous meningioma and solitary fibrous tumor of meninges. *Am J Surg Pathol*. 1997;21:1354–1360.

410. Younes M, Lechago LV, Somoano JR, et al. Wide expression of the human erythrocyte glucose transporter Glut 1 in human cancers. *Cancer Res*. 1996;56:1164–1167.

411. Yamaguchi U, Hasegawa T, Hirose T, et al. Sclerosing perineurioma: a clinicopathological study of five cases and diagnostic utility of immunohistochemical staining for glut-1. *Virchows Arch*. 2003;443:159–163.

412. North PE, Mizeracki A, Mihm MC Jr, et al. GLUT1 immunoreaction patterns reliably distinguish hemangioblastoma from metastatic renal cell carcinoma. *Clin Neuropathol*. 2000;19:131–137.

413. Folpe AL, Billings SD, McKenney JK, et al. Expression of claudin-1, a recently described tight junction-associated protein, distinguishes soft tissue perineurioma from potential mimics. *Am J Surg Pathol*. 2002;26:1620–1626.

414. Rajaram V, Brat DJ, Perry A. Anaplastic meningioma versus meningeal hemangiopericytoma: immunohistochemical and genetic markers. *Hum Pathol*. 2004;35:1413–1418.

415. Sternberger N, Tabira T, Kies MW, et al. Immunohistochemical staining of basic protein in CNS myelin. *Trans Am Soc Neurochem*. 1977;8:157.

416. Itoyama Y, Sternberger NH, Kies MW, et al: Immunocytochemical method to identify myelin basic protein in oligodendroglia and myelin sheaths of the human nervous system. *Ann Neurol*. 1980;7:157–166.

417. Bonnin JM, Rubinstein LJ. Immunohistochemistry of central nervous system tumors. Its contributions to neurosurgical diagnosis. *J Neurosurg*. 1984;60:1121–1133.

418. Clark HB, Minesky JJ, Agrawal D, et al. Myelin basic protein and P2 protein are not immunohistochemical markers for Schwann cell neoplasms. A comparative study using antisera to S-100, P2, and myelin basic proteins. *Am J Pathol*. 1985;121:96–101.

419. Oehmichen M, Auer RN, Konig HG. *Forensic Neuropathology and Associated Neurology*. Berlin, Germany: Springer-Verlag; 2009.

420. Lu QR, Yuk D, Alberta JA, et al. Sonic hedgehog-regulated oligodendrocyte lineage genes encoding bHLH proteins in the mammalian central nervous system. *Neuron*. 2000;25:317–329.

421. Yokoo H, Nobusawa S, Takebayashi H, et al. Anti-human Olig2 antibody as a useful immunohistochemical marker of normal oligodendrocytes and gliomas. *Am J Pathol*. 2004;164:1717–1725.

422. Preusser M, Budka H, Rossler K, et al. OLIG2 is a useful immunohistochemical marker in differential diagnosis of clear cell primary CNS neoplasms. *Histopathology*. 2007;50:365–370.

423. Jung TY, Jung S, Lee KH, et al. Nogo-A expression in oligodendroglial tumors. *Neuropathology*. 2011;31:11–19.

424. Lendahl U, Zimmerman LB, McKay RD. CNS stem cells express a new class of intermediate filament protein. *Cell*. 1990;60:585–595.

425. Fukuda S, Kato F, Tozuka Y, et al. Two distinct subpopulations of nestin-positive cells in adult mouse dentate gyrus. *J Neurosci*. 2003;23:9357–9366.

426. Kronenberg G, Reuter K, Steiner B, et al. Subpopulations of proliferating cells of the adult hippocampus respond differently to physiologic neurogenic stimuli. *J Comp Neurol*. 2003;467:455–463.

427. Dell'Albani P. Stem cell markers in gliomas. *Neurochem Res*. 2008;33:2407–2415.

428. Strojnik T, Rosland GV, Sakariassen PO, et al. Neural stem cell markers, nestin and musashi proteins, in the progression of human glioma: correlation of nestin with prognosis of patient survival. *Surg Neurol*. 2007;68:133–143.

429. Almqvist PM, Mah R, Lendahl U, et al. Immunohistochemical detection of nestin in pediatric brain tumors. *J Histochem Cytochem*. 2002;50:147–158.

430. Sakurada K, Saino M, Mouri W, et al. Nestin expression in central nervous system germ cell tumors. *Neurosurg Rev*. 2008;31:173–176.

431. Jones H, Steart PV, Du Boulay CE, et al. Alpha-smooth muscle actin as a marker for soft tissue tumours: a comparison with desmin. *J Pathol*. 1990;162:29–33.

432. Rangdaeng S, Truong LD. Comparative immunohistochemical staining for desmin and muscle-specific actin. A study of 576 cases. *Am J Clin Pathol*. 1991;96:32–45.

433. Wang NP, Marx J, McNutt MA, et al. Expression of myogenic regulatory proteins (myogenin and MyoD1) in small blue round cell tumors of childhood. *Am J Pathol*. 1995;147:1799–1810.

434. Furlong MA, Mentzel T, Fanburg-Smith JC. Pleomorphic rhabdomyosarcoma in adults: a clinicopathologic study of 38 cases with emphasis on morphologic variants and recent skeletal muscle-specific markers. *Mod Pathol*. 2001;14:595–603.

435. Nozza P, Raso A, Rossi A, et al. Rhabdoid meningioma of the tentorium with expression of desmin in a 12-year-old Turner syndrome patient. *Acta Neuropathol*. 2005;110:205–206.

436. Qiu X, Montgomery E, Sun B. Inflammatory myofibroblastic tumor and low-grade myofibroblastic sarcoma: a comparative study of clinicopathologic features and further observations on the immunohistochemical profile of myofibroblasts. *Hum Pathol*. 2008;39:846–856.

437. Knosel T, Schulz B, Katenkamp K, et al. Solitary fibrous tumor and haemangiopericytoma: what is new? *Pathologe*. 2010;31:123–128.

438. Hirano A. Hirano bodies and related neuronal inclusions. *Neuropathol Appl Neurobiol*. 1994;20:3–11.

439. Yoshimine T, Maruno M, Ushio Y, et al. Intermediate filaments and anaplastic change of ENU-induced gliomass: immunohistochemical study with vimentin and astroprotein (GFAP). *J Neurooncol*. 1987;5:377–385.

440. Paetau A. Glial fibrillary acidic protein, vimentin and fibronectin in primary cultures of human glioma and fetal brain. *Acta Neuropathol*. 1988;75:448–455.

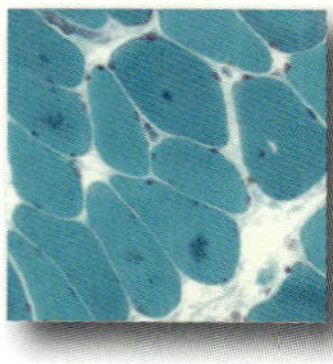 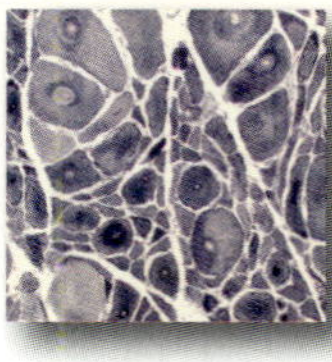 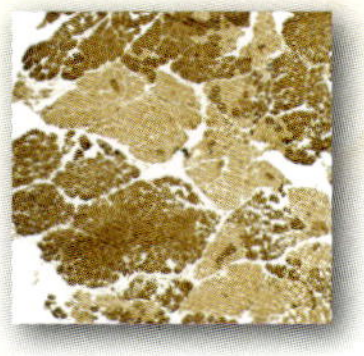

CHAPTER 8

Nonneoplastic Diseases of Skeletal Muscle

Introduction

Although the general idea of approach to the evaluation of skeletal muscle biopsy specimens remains the same, consistent with the theme of this book, the discussion in this chapter is tailored to the different tissue types and their disorders. This discussion is limited to the nonneoplastic diseases that are seen in neuropathology practice. Routine evaluation of skeletal muscle tissue involves multiple modalities, stains, and reactions. Frozen sections and enzyme reactions performed on frozen sections are a routine part of tissue processing. The type of special studies included in the routine evaluation is a matter of personal and institutional preference, suggestions ranging from a few[1] to all inclusive. Regardless, additional immunohistochemical and immunofluorescence stains can be added depending on the special situation. Tissue saved routinely for electron microscopic evaluation can be processed for semi-thin plastic sections, and further electron microscopical evaluation can be performed as needed. Securing additional frozen tissue for possible further studies such as for mitochondrial disorders and biochemical testing for metabolic disorders may also be necessary. In addition, a close correlation exists between the pathologic findings and the clinical and other laboratory findings, such as clinical laboratory tests and electromyography, influencing the interpretation. Since a relatively limited repertoire of elementary findings is present, their interpretation should be done in the specific clinicopathologic context. Technical aspects of tissue processing, the details of clinical features, and some ancillary techniques, as well ultrastructural features, are beyond the scope of this text and are discussed in detail elsewhere.[2–4] Given all the involvement of diverse techniques and information from different sources, the discussion in this chapter is limited to the findings that are most likely to be identified during the initial routine evaluation to remain consistent with the general theme of this book.

Fiber Size Variation

Fiber size variation results from myofiber atrophy, hypertrophy or both, but is usually due to variable degrees and extents of *atrophy* that can be present in many diseases. Only a few scattered atrophic fibers may be present in subtle forms, or it can be extensive and be associated with other findings to provide clues to its etiology. Acute denervation can be subtle and in the form of a few scattered *angulated atrophic fibers*. Due to loss of their innervation, the fibers that are otherwise normal simply become atrophic and assume concave contours with pointy corners **(Fig. 8-1)**. Some of them may be extremely small and linear, making it difficult to identify if not searched for specifically or highlighted by special stains. Due to the shrinkage of the volume as a result of denervation atrophy, the internal structure of the myofiber is condensed, creating *dark*

List of Findings/Checklist for Nonneoplastic Diseases of Skeletal Muscle

• AT A GLANCE

Fiber Size Variation
- Atrophy
  - Angulated atrophic fibers
  - Small group atrophy
  - Large group atrophy
  - Rounded atrophic fibers
  - Perifascicular atrophy
  - Type 1 fiber atrophy
  - Type 2 fiber atrophy
- Hypertrophy
- Artifacts

Nuclear Features
- Syncytial nuclear clumps
- Multinucleation
- Internal nuclei
- Regenerative changes

Vacuoles
- Rimmed vacuoles
- Autophagic vacuoles
- Storage diseases
- Ice crystal artifact

Accumulations and Inclusions
- Cytoplasmic body
- Reducing body
- Hyaline body
- Nemaline (rod) body
- Lafora body
- Basophilic body
- Tubular aggregates
- Ragged red fibers
- Ragged blue fibers
- Protein accumulations
- Calcifications
- Glycogen storage
- Lipid storage

Fibers with Structural Changes
- Splitting fibers
- Ring fibers
- Coil (whorled) fibers
- Target fibers
- Targetoid fibers
- Central cores
- Mini-/multi-cores
- Moth-eaten fibers
- Trabecular (lobulated) fibers
- Necrotic fibers
  - Degenerating fibers
  - Segmental necrosis
  - Rhabdomyolysis

Inflammation
- Inflammatory myopathies
  - Polymyositis
  - Dermatomyositis
  - Inclusion body myositis
- Lymphorrhages
- Plasma cells
- Macrophages
- Polymorphonuclear leukocytes
- Infections

Connective Tissue
- Endomysial fibrosis
- Amyloidosis

Vascular Changes
- Vasculitis
- Perivascular inflammation

Others
- Peripheral nerve fibers
- Muscle spindles

Mixed Patterns

Histochemistry
- Gomori's trichrome
- ATPase
- NADH-TR
- Oil red O
- Succinic dehydrogenase
- Cytochrome oxidase
- Phosphorylase
- Phosphofructokinase
- Acid phosphatase
- Nonspecific esterase

Immunohistochemistry
- Lymphoid markers
- Markers for protein accumulations
- Markers for deficient proteins
- Myosins

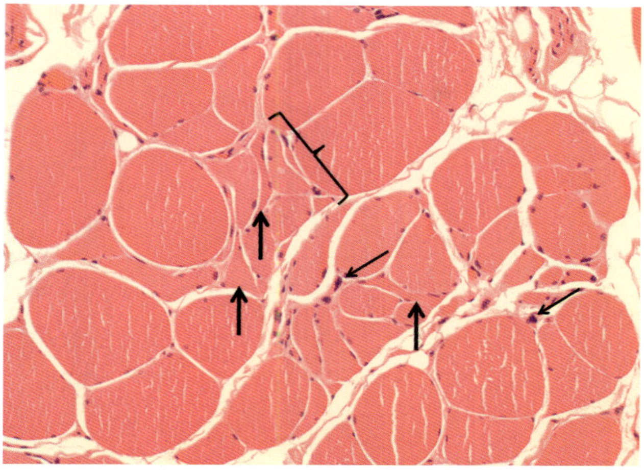

Figure 8-1. Denervation atrophy: Many angulated atrophic fibers (*thick arrows*) are present with concave contours and pointy corners, squeezed among other fibers. Atrophic fibers form small groups (*bracket*) within the fascicle. Several syncytial nuclear clumps (*thin arrows*) are also seen (H&E; original magnification: 200×).

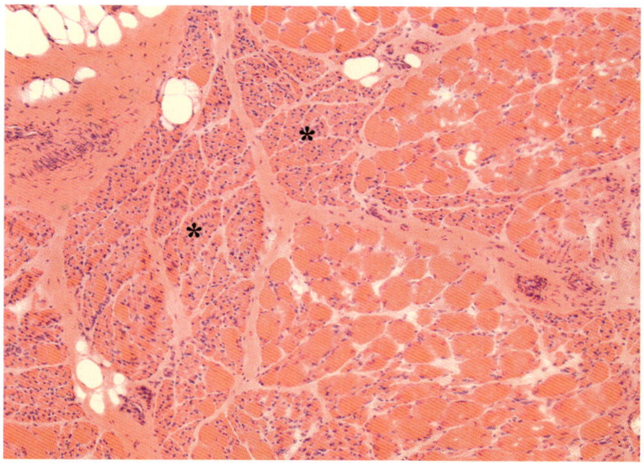

Figure 8-3. Large group atrophy: Entire fascicles (*asterisk*) are uniformly composed of atrophic fibers. They alternate with relatively normal fascicles, and their component fibers are likely of the same fiber type as a result of previous reinnervation (see Fig. 8-28) in this case of Werdnig-Hoffmann disease (spinal muscular atrophy type 1) (H&E; original magnification: 100×).

fibers on reduced nicotinamide adenine dinucleotide-tetrazolium reductase (NADH-TR) **(Fig. 8-2)** and esterase reactions. These darkly reacting fibers provide further support for the denervation nature of the atrophy. Type 1 fibers are normally darker than the type 2 fibers by NADH-TR reactions; however, the angulated atrophic dark fibers should not be used for typing and should not be taken as type 1 fibers because they are dark. Several adjacent angulated atrophic fibers can form *small group atrophy* **(Fig. 8-1)**. There may be one or more groups within the fascicles. Angulated atrophic fibers can be seen in some other conditions, including myopathic processes, such as facioscapulohumeral muscular dystrophy.[5] Type 2 myofiber atrophy and age-related changes also have fibers with angular contours. In contrast, *large group atrophy* tends to involve all or the great majority of a fascicle **(Fig. 8-3)**. It is formed as a result of denervation of large groups or fascicles that are being reinnervated to form fiber type grouping (see below) after initial denervation[6] and therefore indicate an ongoing denervation process. As such, it is typically associated with progressive neurodegenerative disorders such as spinal muscular atrophy or repeated bouts of neural injury. In contrast to angulated atrophic fibers, *rounded atrophic fibers* have also lost their usual polygonal appearance and assumed rounded contours **(Fig. 8-4)**. They are commonly associated with variably increased fibrous connective tissue in which they are entrapped. They are typically seen in the later stages of myopathic disorders that are

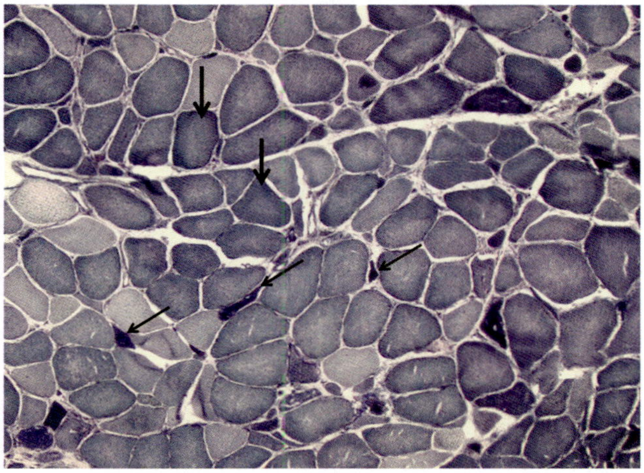

Figure 8-2. Dark fibers: Several angulated atrophic fibers appear dark (*thin arrows*) due to condensation of their otherwise normal sarcoplasm in a smaller volume in this patient with acute denervation. They are darker than the type 1 fibers (*thick arrows*) and their fiber type cannot be ascertained without ATPase reactions or myosin immunohistochemistry (see text for details) (NADH-TR; original magnification: 200×).

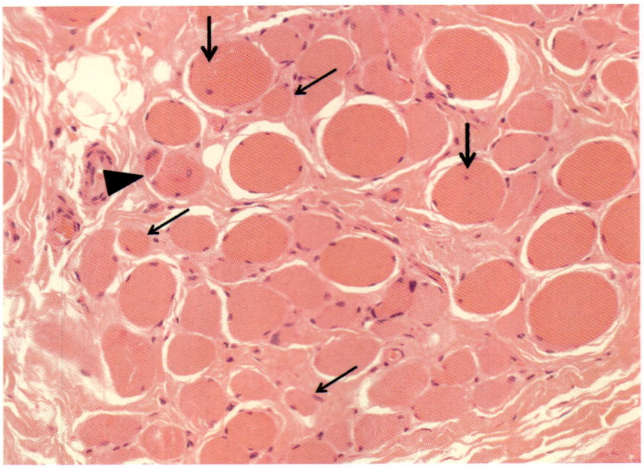

Figure 8-4. Rounded atrophic fibers and endomysial fibrosis: Prominent fiber size variation is present due to many atrophic fibers with round contours (*thin arrows*). The fibers are separated from each other by and are entrapped within increased amount of endomysial connective tissue. Some fibers also have internal nuclei (*thick arrows*). One fiber appears to be split (*arrowhead*) in this myopathic process (H&E; original magnification: 200×).

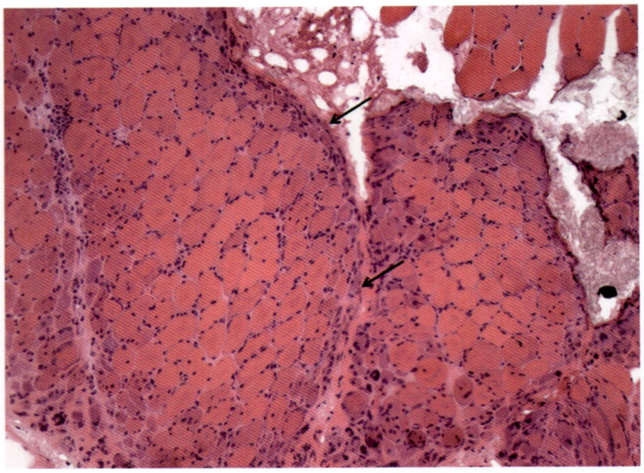

Figure 8-5. Perifascicular atrophy: Predominantly, those fibers at the periphery of the fascicles are atrophic (*arrows*) in this case of dermatomyositis. Many of the atrophic fibers are also basophilic due to regenerative activity (H&E; original magnification: 100×).

characterized by ongoing myofiber degeneration and scarring, such as muscular dystrophies and chronic or healing stages of inflammatory myopathies. Although they tend to be randomly scattered throughout the fascicles, they too can be seen in groups but are typically of variable sizes and are usually separated by increased endomysial fibrous connective tissue, in contrast to the back-to-back arrangement of angulated atrophic fibers in small group atrophy. Rarely, split fibers can result in a group of a few atrophic fibers that mimic small group atrophy. Fiber splitting is a finding that is associated with myopathic rather than neurogenic processes; the presence of other myopathic changes and absence of typical angulated atrophic fibers should facilitate this distinction. Intrafusal fibers of the muscle spindle form a small group of fibers with smaller caliber and may mimic small group atrophy. It should be kept in mind that fibers are uniformly small and round in pediatric population. For this reason, age-matched controls may provide a reference for evaluation. *Perifascicular atrophy* refers to a peculiar distribution of atrophic fibers to involve the periphery of the fascicles **(Fig. 8-5)**. It is considered an ischemic change as a result of vascular pathology and is particularly associated with dermatomyositis.[7] The fibers are not only atrophic but many are also regenerating. *Selective type 1 myofiber atrophy* involves the type 1 myofibers and requires fiber typing techniques such as ATPase reactions (see below) to evaluate **(Table 8.1)**. It can be associated with some congenital myopathies and myotonic dystrophy, especially of type 1.[8,9] Selective *type 2 myofiber atrophy* is the uniform atrophy of type 2 fibers and also requires fiber typing techniques such as ATPase reaction to evaluate. It is more common than type 1 fiber atrophy and

TABLE 8.1 Histochemical differences between fiber types

Feature	Type 1	Type 2
ATPase low pH	Dark	Light
ATPase high pH	Light	Dark
Gomori's trichrome	More mitochondria (red dots)	Fewer mitochondria
NADH-TR	Dark	Light
COX	Dark	Light
SDH	Dark	Light
Oil red O	More lipid droplets	Fewer lipid droplets
PAS	Light	Dark
Phosphorylase	Light	Dark
PFK	Light	Dark

COX, cytochrome oxidase; SDH, succinic dehydrogenase; PAS, periodic acid-Schiff; PFK, phosphofructokinase.

is typically a secondary change in the muscle due to problems that are outside the muscle. Common causes are corticosteroid excess, either exogenous or endogenous as in ectopic production or endocrine abnormalities, and disuse such as prolonged bed rest and other conditions that restrict mobility. A relatively smaller type 2 fiber population is also seen in association with aging. Atrophic type 2 fibers appear somewhat angulated and may create an acute denervation picture.[10] Toxic effect of alcohol, especially in chronic alcoholism, can also result in type 2 myofiber atrophy. Cachexia associated with malignancy and the so-called chronic carcinomatous myopathy also typically result in the atrophy of type 2 fibers. Chronic hyperthyroid myopathy can sometimes show type 2 myofiber atrophy, or variable atrophy of both types. Lambert-Eaton myasthenic syndrome, myasthenia gravis, polymyalgia rheumatica, acute quadriplegic myopathy (a.k.a., intensive care myopathy), and osteomalacia myopathy can have variable degrees of type 2 fiber atrophy.[3,11,12] By ATPase reactions, angulated atrophy of denervation involves both fiber types in contrast to selective involvement of type 2 myofibers. *Hypertrophic fibers* also contribute to fiber size variation. Although atrophy and hypertrophy usually occur together, rare cases where fibers are exclusively or predominantly hypertrophic may create a false atrophic picture. This situation may be seen in some congenital myopathies. Typically, hypertrophic fibers scattered or in groups are seen as a compensatory change in any case that is characterized by atrophic fibers. The evaluation of both atrophy and hypertrophy may be difficult in subtle cases with minimal pathologic changes. Utilization of automated and computerized evaluation of fiber types and diameters, and comparisons with age- and sex-matched controls may be a way of overcoming this subjectivity; however, this approach may not prove practical in a daily practice setting. Hypertrophy of type 2 fibers without atrophy of type 1 fibers can be a feature of proximal myotonic dystrophy. Common *artifacts* may contribute to the fiber size variation. Scattered hypereosinophilic larger fibers can be seen in some cases. They commonly represent fibers that show hypercontraction as a result of artifact during biopsy procedure if appropriate techniques to keep the muscle in its original stretched position are not used. They appear as having alternating hyper- and

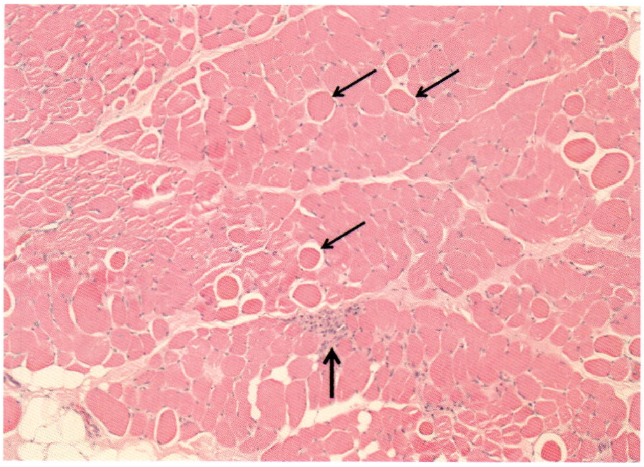

Figure 8-6. Hypercontracted fibers: Larger, round, and darker eosinophilic fibers (*thin arrows*) are scattered in a background of a myopathic process with fiber size variation, focal degenerating and regenerating fibers (*thick arrow*), and adjacent areas of increased amount of endomysial connective tissue in this case of Duchenne muscular dystrophy (H&E; original magnification: 100×).

hypoeosinophilic bands along its length on longitudinal sections. In most cases, they are easily recognized, are only few, and do not interfere with the evaluation. Although a few hypereosinophilic fibers can be seen in an otherwise unremarkable tissue, frequent hypereosinophilic/hypercontracted fibers are a common finding especially in Duchenne muscular dystrophy[13] **(Fig. 8-6)**. They may show a thin radial tear on cross section, called delta lesion,[14] which may be difficult to distinguish from artifact. If a perfect cross section cannot be obtained due to malorientation or distortion of the tissue, some fibers are cut longitudinally or obliquely in various planes, contributing to fiber size variation. Focal fiber size variation with some increase in the amount of endomysial connective tissue is seen at the myotendinous junction, along with internal nuclei in some fibers, mimicking a myopathic process. Adjacent dense regular fibrous connective tissue representing the tendon, the focal nature of these changes, and an awareness of this pitfall help distinguish it from truly pathologic processes.

Nuclear Features

The *changes in the nuclei* are somewhat limited compared to those described in Chapter 2. In a

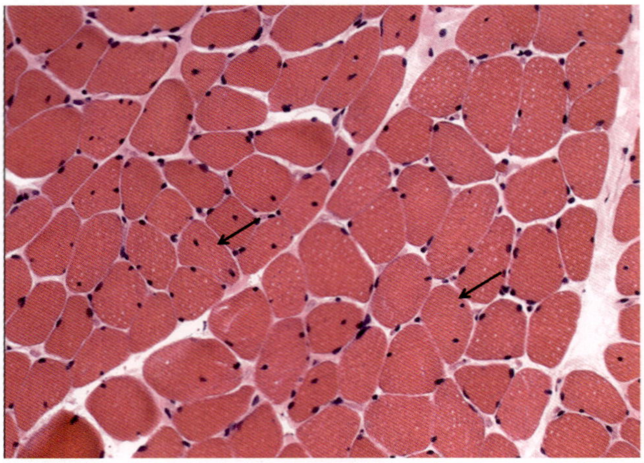

Figure 8-7. Internal nuclei: Increased number of fibers with one or more internal nuclei (*arrows*) are present. There is also a mild fiber size variation. There appears to be a mild and focal increase in the amount of endomysial connective tissue in the upper left corner of the picture, resulting in a slight separation of the fibers from each other (H&E; original magnification: 200×).

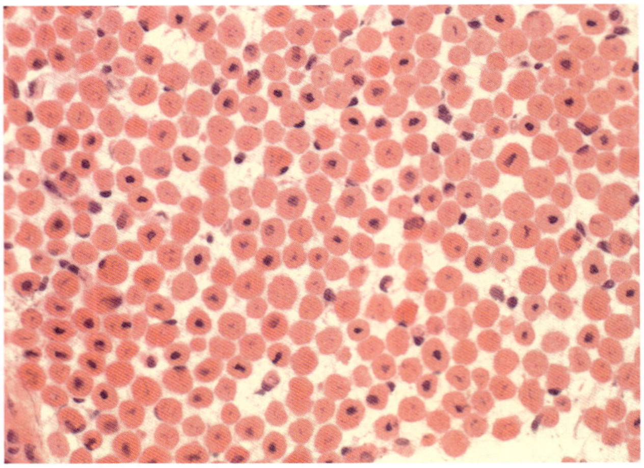

Figure 8-8. Centronuclear myopathy: Many fibers have a perfectly centrally placed internal nucleus. Others appear without a nucleus due to the plane of section. The fibers are small and round with central nuclei similar to the myotube stage of muscle development (H&E; original magnification: 400×).

given section, only a few of the many normally subsarcolemmal nuclei are seen in a myofiber. The resting nuclei normally appear pyknotic, round-to-oval, and somewhat angulated. As in the case of dark fibers described above in the context of acute denervation, when the denervated myofiber becomes atrophic, its nuclei accumulate in the sarcoplasm of the collapsed myofiber to form a multinucleated cell, variably referred to as *syncytial nuclear clumps*, knots, or bags **(Fig. 8-1)**. It is not unusual to find scattered fibers with internal nuclei, and to be more technical, it is generally considered by many that up to 3% of myofibers may have *internal nuclei*, although their significance should be interpreted in the given context. An increase in the number of fibers with internal nuclei is typically associated with myopathic processes **(Fig. 8-7)**, although they may also be seen in chronic neuropathies. In myotonic dystrophy, the fibers predominantly have internal nuclei. There is some increase in proximal myotonic myopathy, which is considered a variant of myotonic dystrophy[15] and does not contain ring fibers.[16] Schwartz-Jampel syndrome is also associated with increased internal nuclei as well as a fiber size variation due to the presence of atrophic and hypertrophic fibers.[3] In centronuclear myopathy,[17] a congenital myopathy also known as myotubular myopathy, myofibers uniformly have centrally placed nuclei **(Fig. 8-8)**. Sometimes, myotubular myopathy is used to refer to the X-linked form of the disease.[18] Internal nuclei in general may form longitudinal chains arranged in a line at the center of the fiber, as seen on longitudinal sections. The central nuclei of the centronuclear myopathy on longitudinal sections are not back to back but are lined with some distance from each other. The interpretation of internal nuclei may be deceiving on longitudinal sections as tangential sections or superimposed sarcoplasm over normally placed nuclei may create the appearance of internal nuclei. Central nuclei have been described in a syndrome associated with congenital hypothyroidism (Kocher-Debré-Semelaigne syndrome) along with ring fibers and type 2 fiber atrophy.[19] Internal nuclei may be seen as part of the changes seen at the myotendinous junction. Some internal nuclei may be associated with the early stages of fiber splitting, and close evaluation may reveal the splitting of the sarcoplasm along the internal nuclei. Fetal muscle normally contains central nuclei, reminiscent of a picture seen in centronuclear myopathy. The *nuclei of regenerating fibers*, internal or not, are enlarged and are very active with open chromatin pattern and prominent nucleoli, creating an "atypical" appearance. They are easy to identify as reactive/regenerative due to their association with basophilic/regenerating fibers and can be distinguished from syncytial nuclear clumps based on the quality of their nuclei and cytoplasm.

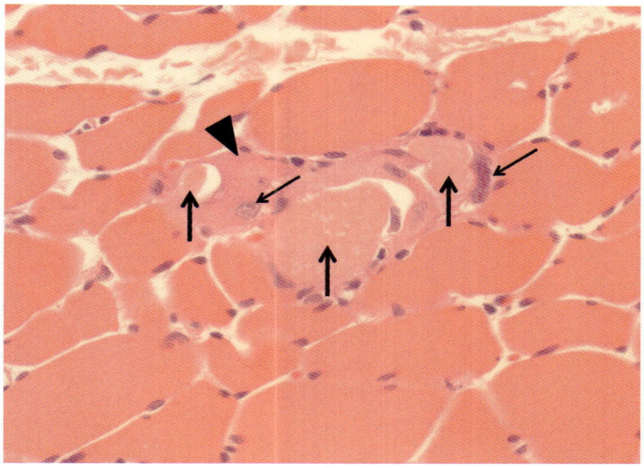

Figure 8-9. Regenerating fibers: Residual sarcoplasms of several degenerating fibers (*thick arrows*) are surrounded by the regenerating portions of the fiber. The latter has enlarged nuclei with prominent nucleoli (*thin arrows*) and a relatively basophilic cytoplasm (*arrowhead*), both indicating regenerative activity (H&E; original magnification: 400×).

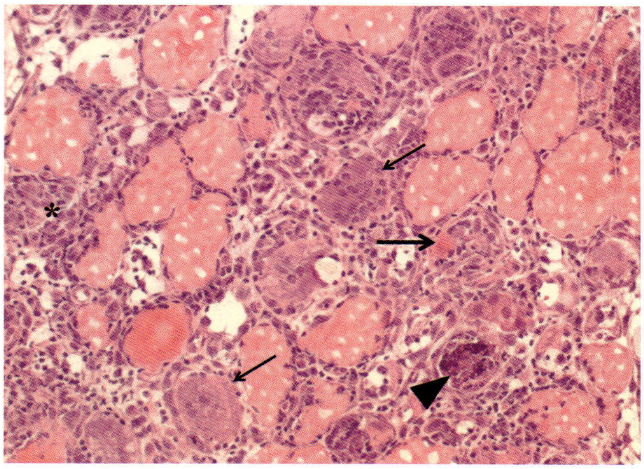

Figure 8-10. Giant cells and granulomas: Large numbers of histiocytes are present among the myofibers. Some appear to form granulomas (*asterisk*). Multinucleated giant cells (*thin arrows*) are also present. Some appear to occur within or invade the muscle fibers, associated with residual sarcoplasmic fragments (*thick arrow*) in this patient with thymoma. One degenerated fiber has microcalcifications (*arrowhead*) (H&E; original magnification: 200×).

Their cytoplasm is amphophilic due to the presence of abundant ribosomes and associated RNA in the cytoplasm, all part of the extensive protein synthesis to facilitate regeneration **(Fig. 8-9)**. *Multinucleation* is commonly present at the myotendinous junction and in areas of previous injury, such as previous surgical intervention sites or ischemic injury. These are commonly seen at the surgical margins of the amputation specimens in surgical pathology. Multinucleated giant cells representing macrophages can be a part of various processes, most notably granulomatous inflammations as discussed in detail in Chapter 2. A peculiar multinucleation is seen in giant cell myositis **(Fig. 8-10)**, where the giant cells are mainly associated with granulomas, but some are also of myogenic in origin and can be seen together with thymoma.[3,20,21]

Vacuoles, Accumulations, and Inclusions

Sarcoplasmic vacuoles can have different appearances associated with different types of processes. The most notable vacuole is the *rimmed vacuole* that is seen in association with inclusion body myositis. It is best seen on H&E- and Gomori's trichrome–stained frozen sections due to peripheral basophilic stippling **(Fig. 8-11)**. Granular debris may be present in within the vacuole, but in spite of the name of the disease, it is not associated with viral diseases, any peculiar accumulations, or

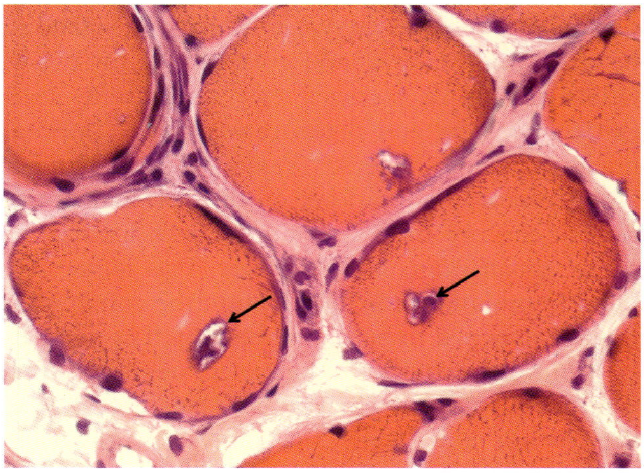

Figure 8-11. Rimmed vacuoles: Peculiar irregular vacuoles with peripheral basophilic stippling and granular debris within the lumen (*arrows*) are seen in this case of inclusion body myositis. There is also a mild increase in the amount of endomysial connective tissue, resulting in the separation of fibers from each other (H&E; original magnification: 400×).

true inclusions. They can be positive for ubiquitin, beta-amyloid, and TDP-43.[22] Vacuoles similar to rimmed vacuoles can be seen in oculopharyngeal muscular dystrophy, the so-called distal myopathies, which may be considered familial inclusion body myopathies, as well as in other myopathic conditions such as X-linked vacuolar myopathy. A number of disorders with rimmed vacuoles have been described, indicating that rimmed vacuoles are not diagnostic of inclusion body myositis.[23] Rimmed vacuoles can be seen in Marinesco-Sjögren syndrome, along with fiber size variation, degenerating and regenerating fibers, and eventually increased endomysial fibrosis, mimicking inclusion body myositis.[24] Chloroquine[25] and colchicine[26] myopathies are also characterized by vacuoles. A group of diseases associated with *autophagic vacuoles* have genetic basis, and although the vacuoles may look similar to rimmed vacuoles, they are mainly seen in pediatric population. A variety of diseases including some metabolic/storage disorders are also included in this group. They are further classified according to the characteristics of their vacuoles.[23,27] *Freeze artifact* occurs as a result of slow freezing and/or repeated thawing and refreezing and creates variably sized clear vacuoles that frequently distort the fibers to interfere with evaluation. *Glycogen and lipid storage diseases* also create vacuoles and can be further investigated by special studies. The vacuoles of *periodic paralysis* are typically clear. They tend to be large, one or more, and present in many fibers. Other myopathic changes may be present, such as degenerating and regenerating fibers, internal nuclei, and split fibers.[28] Various accumulations and structural alterations of the internal structure of the myofiber may appear as vacuoles on some *special stains and reactions*. This is because the accumulation may not contain the component that is supposed to be highlighted by that particular stain or reaction. For instance, nemaline rods (see below) do not react in ATPase reactions as they do not contain myosin. Many different vacuolations can occur as a result of dilatation of cellular organelles, such as lysosomes, T tubules, and peroxisomes.

Sarcoplasmic accumulations and inclusions, excluding those seen in storage diseases mentioned above, can be specific to indicate particular diseases or can be nonspecific findings. *Cytoplasmic bodies* are round-to-oval, erythrocyte-like eosinophilic cytoplasmic structures that are dark blue to bright red on Gomori's trichrome stain **(Fig. 8-12)**. They are quite nonspecific, seen in a wide variety of disorders, including denervation, and represent a structural change in the fiber.[29] They can be seen in human immunodeficiency virus (HIV)-associated myopathy and zidovudine treatment. *Reducing bodies* are blue-green accumulations seen in reducing body myopathy. Their nature is not clear. Although they resemble cytoplasmic bodies, they are positive with menadione-nitro-blue tetrazolium reaction.[30] *Hyaline accumulations* have been described as hyaline body myopathy,[31,32] where they appear as homogeneous areas only within type 1 myofibers, pale eosinophilic on H&E, and pale green on Gomori's trichrome stain. *Rod (nemaline) bodies* are elongated spindled structures best seen on Gomori's trichrome stain as dark blue-purple accumulations. They may appear as patchy discolorations eccentrically located in the fiber when they are abundant. They are most typical for nemaline myopathy (rod myopathy)[33] but can also be present in other myopathies. A myopathy without inflammation but with nemaline bodies can be seen in association with HIV infection.[34] *Tubular aggregates* are eccentric patches of accumulations within the fiber that appear basophilic on H&E and red on

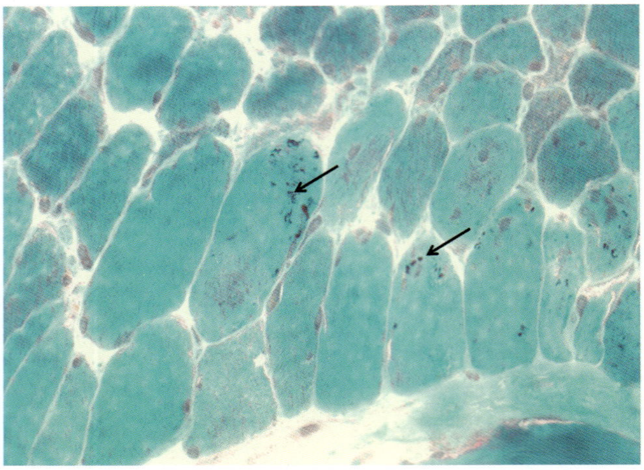

Figure 8-12. Cytoplasmic bodies: Many fibers have round to oval or spindled structures scattered within their sarcoplasm individually or in groups. Some are larger and eosinophilic (*arrows*). Others may mimic nemaline bodies; however, nemaline bodies are darker green or blue and tend to be more uniform (Gomori's trichrome; original magnification: 400×).

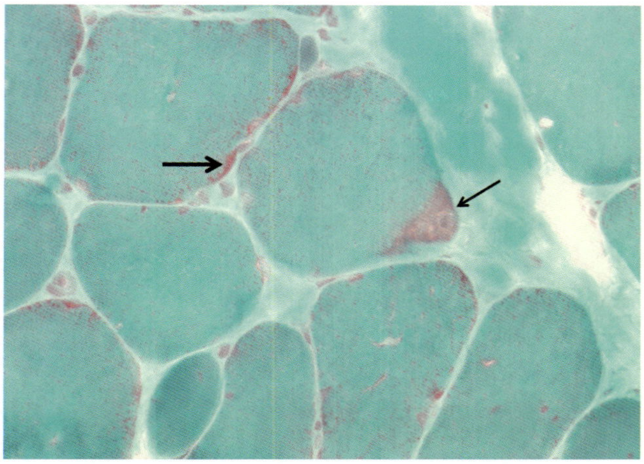

Figure 8-13. Tubular aggregates: Typically eccentric within the fiber is an aggregate (*thin arrow*). It has a dull red and globular quality relative to the bright red and fine granules representing somewhat increased mitochondria (*thick arrow*) (Gomori's trichrome; original magnification: 400×).

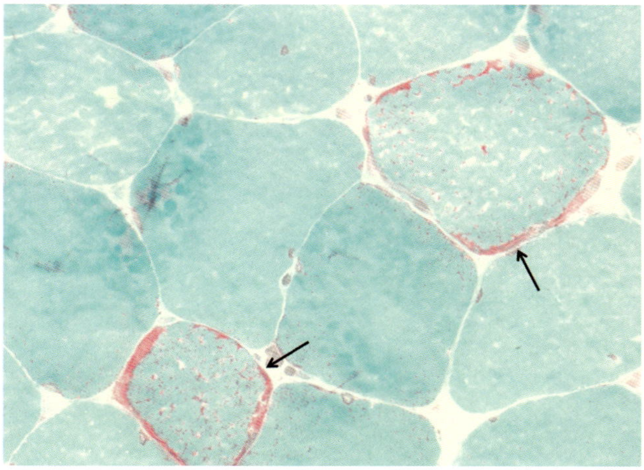

Figure 8-14. Ragged red fibers: Two fibers with irregular granular peripheral zones are seen (*arrows*). The red dots within the fibers correspond to mitochondria, and the red peripheral granular areas indicate mitochondrial proliferation (Gomori's trichrome; original magnification: 400×).

Gomori's trichrome stain **(Fig. 8-13)**. They are also prominent on NADH-TR reactions. For this reason, they may mimic ragged red fibers with increased mitochondria (see below). In contrast to ragged red fibers, these areas react with cytochrome oxidase (COX) and do not react with succinic dehydrogenase (SDH). They can be seen in a wide variety of conditions[35] and are not particularly a significant finding for any group of disorders, as well as in scattered fibers in otherwise unremarkable muscle tissue. They are more commonly seen in periodic paralysis and less commonly in familial tubular aggregate myopathies. *Ragged red fibers* form as a result of increased mitochondria typically at the periphery of the myofiber. The zones of mitochondrial proliferation and accumulation at the periphery of the fiber appear basophilic on H&E and red on Gomori's trichrome stains **(Fig. 8-14)**. These fibers also become prominent as *ragged blue fibers* on SDH reactions **(Fig. 8-15)** and are COX-negative **(Fig. 8-16)**; however, both the Gomori's trichrome and H&E stains can identify only the fully developed ragged red fibers, while the so-called ragged red equivalents, that is, those fibers with abnormally increased mitochondria are not enough to be identified on routine stains, can still be identified by SDH. These changes are characteristic for mitochondrial myopathies but are not diagnostic for them without further confirmation. Mitochondrial myopathies can be part of many syndromes. Mitochondrial encephalomyopathy lactic acidosis and stroke like episodes (MELAS), myoclonic epilepsy with ragged red fibers (MERRF), and Kearns-Sayre syndrome are some of the better-known examples.[36] On the other hand, the absence of these changes does not

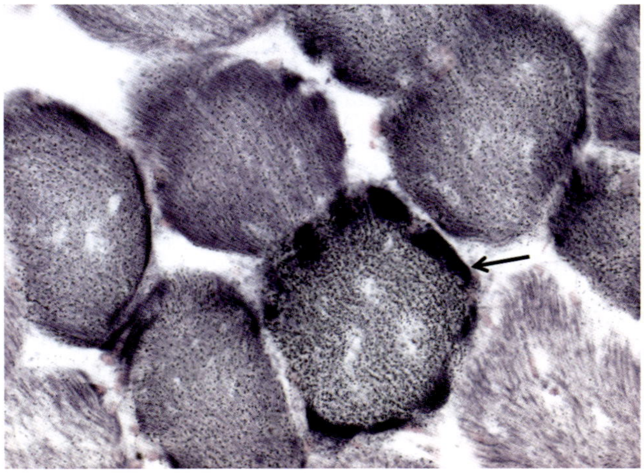

Figure 8-15. Ragged blue fiber: A fiber with darker blue irregular and granular peripheral zone (*arrow*) is seen. The blue dots correspond to mitochondria. The ragged red fibers on Gomori's trichrome stain and the so-called ragged red equivalents are then seen as ragged blue fibers on this reaction (Succinic dehydrogenase [SDH]; original magnification: 400×).

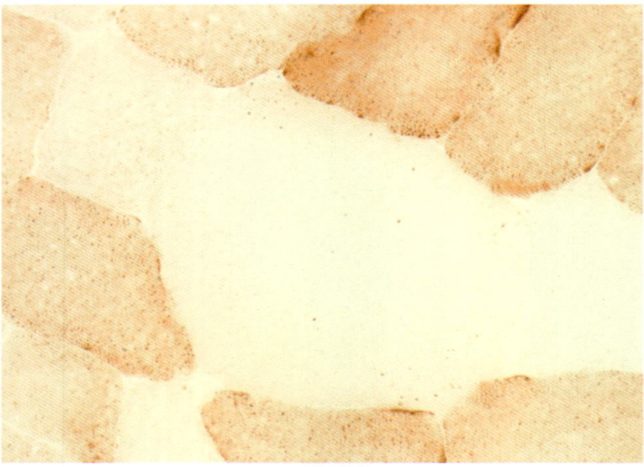

Figure 8-16. Cytochrome oxidase (COX)-negative fibers: Three fibers in the center are essentially entirely negative for COX activity. These fibers correspond to ragged red and ragged blue fibers. Type 1 fibers are normally darker (**right upper corner**), while type 2 fibers are lighter (**left upper and lower corners**); however, the light reaction of type 2 fibers should not be mistaken for reduced COX activity (COX; original magnification: 400×).

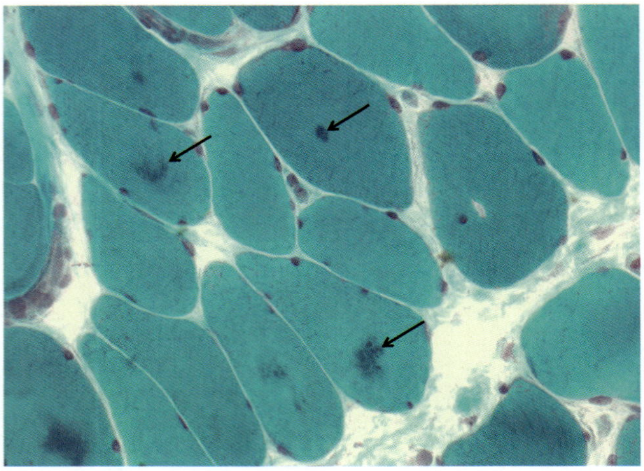

Figure 8-17. Myofibrillary accumulations: several fibers have dark blue-green granular to globular irregular densities (*arrows*) randomly distributed in their sarcoplasm in this protein accumulation myopathy in which the accumulations were positive for desmin by immunohistochemistry (Gomori's trichrome; original magnification: 200×).

rule out mitochondrial disease, while in some mitochondrial disorders such as Leber's optic atrophy[37] and Leigh's disease in which COX reaction can be generally decreased, and neuropathy ataxia retinitis pigmentosa (NARP), ragged red fibers are few or absent.[38] Mitochondrial disorders under the age of five tend not to have ragged red fibers. Scattered ragged red fibers can be seen as an incidental finding in an otherwise unremarkable muscle, especially in older individuals. Mitochondria may be increased in regenerative states as well as in athletes.[39] A group of cases that otherwise appear to have features of polymyositis or inclusion body myositis also have ragged red fibers and have been described as inflammatory myopathies with COX-negative fibers.[40,41] Ragged red fibers can be seen in some cases of myotonic dystrophy. Therefore, diagnostic criteria have been developed for respiratory chain disorders both for adults and children.[42] HIV-associated myopathies, polymyositis, and zidovudine treatment have been associated with ragged red fibers. *Myofibrillary myopathies (protein accumulation myopathies)* can show subtle or prominent accumulations in the myofibers that are better appreciated by Gomori's trichrome stain as dark green-blue irregular patches of compact areas with decreased or absent mitochondria[43–45] **(Fig. 8-17)**. They can be further characterized by immunohistochemistry as to what type of protein is accumulating, such as desmin in desminopathy or myotilin in myotilinopathy. The accumulations may be amorphous or variable oval to spherical inclusion-like, and negative for oxidative enzyme reactions. Irregular areas of dense staining on Gomori's trichrome stain can be seen in Schwartz-Jampel syndrome and may mimic nemaline rods or other accumulations.[3,46] *Lafora bodies* seen in Lafora disease appear as rounded sarcoplasmic inclusions that are basophilic on H&E and dark blue to purple on Gomori's trichrome stain.[47] They react strongly on NADH-TR reaction and are periodic acid-Schiff (PAS)-positive and diastase-resistant. Some cases of phosphofructokinase (PFK) deficiency can show polyglucosan-like accumulations with sharp outlines and are PAS-positive and diastase-resistant. *Calcification* within the myofiber can be demonstrated in many conditions with special stains. Dystrophic calcium accumulation may occur in necrotic, degenerating fibers **(Fig. 8-10)**. Dead parasites may become calcified. Focal disorders such as myositis ossificans show prominent calcification. Calcium accumulation has been described in association with juvenile dermatomyositis and other rheumatic diseases.[48] Childhood HIV infection may be associated with vascular calcifications.[49] Its accumulation may generate a foreign body giant cell reaction. Accumulations in *glycogen*[50–52] *and lipid*[53,54] *storage disorders* can appear like irregular vacuolations but can be highlighted as PAS-positive, diastase-sensitive, and oil red O positive material, respectively. The features of various types of storage disorders are in general similar to their overall features elsewhere. Glycogen accumulation is not very prominent in myophosphorylase deficiency (McArdle's disease; glycogenosis type V), but myophosphorylase reaction shows the absence of its activity. It should be noted that phosphorylase reaction rapidly fades if not kept in the dark and needs to be evaluated as soon as possible, ideally the same day that it is performed. If that is not possible, the faded slide can be retreated with iodine solution and restained. Likewise, tissue phosphorylase is depleted rapidly, rendering autopsy tissues and tissues that are not frozen immediately after biopsy less than optimal for this evaluation. PFK deficiency can be diagnosed by the absence of PFK activity, but some glycogen accumulation can be seen by PAS or as vacuoles on H&E in subsarcolemmal location. Large amount of subsarcolemmal glycogen accumulation is present in myxedema. These patients can also have basophilic irregular accumulations in myofibers close to the myotendinous junction, referred to as *basophilic bodies*.[55] Their diagnoses require multimodal approach and biochemical and genetic testing.

Structural Changes in Myofibers

Fibers with structural abnormalities come in several varieties. *Split or splitting fibers*[56] may be seen as a group of small fibers grouped together within the confines of an apparent fiber, mimicking small group atrophy or rounded atrophic fibers. It is more commonly seen as a larger fiber partially or completely divided into two, one usually smaller than the other **(Fig. 8-18)**. In its early stages, the impending splitting may be highlighted by the lining up of internal nuclei along the future splitting line. Fiber splitting is apparently a regenerative or adaptation change that is typically seen in hypertrophic fibers. While it is more commonly seen in myopathic processes, some chronic neurogenic disorders can also show fiber splitting. *Ring fibers* are seen best on cross sections of frozen tissue by H&E, PAS, and NADH-TR reaction and are characterized by a peripheral ring of longitudinally arranged layer of myofibrils **(Fig. 8-19)**. They are not diagnostic of any particular disorder but are common in myotonic dystrophy[57] and limb-girdle muscular dystrophy. Scattered ring fibers can be seen in many other conditions as well as in otherwise unremarkable muscle tissue as an incidental finding. Sometimes, they occur as an artifact on

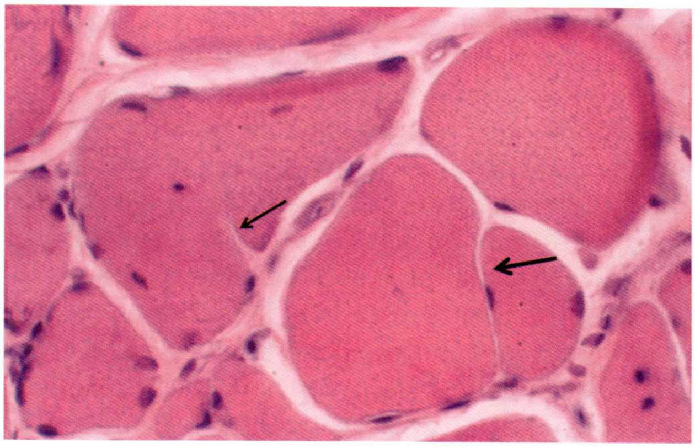

Figure 8-18. Splitting or split fibers: The fiber shown in center left, which also has an internal nucleus, is developing a groove (*thin arrow*), that is, splitting, while the one on the right appears to have recently split with two fibers. Their contours are matching each other (*thick arrow*) and the general boundaries of a larger, original fiber (H&E; original magnification: 400×).

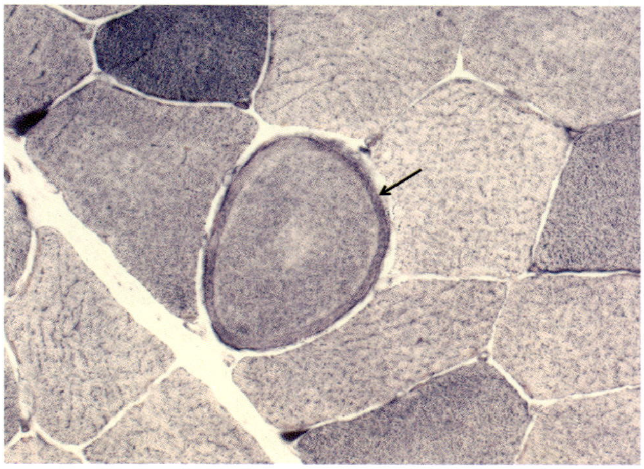

Figure 8-19. Ring fiber: one fiber has a peculiar peripheral "ring" (*arrow*) in which its striations can be seen by focusing up and down due to the longitudinal orientation of the myofibrils (NADH-TR; original magnification: 400×).

frozen sections if cut by a dull knife. They are then seen above the surface of the rest of the section. Probably a variation of ring fibers is the *coil fibers or whorled fibers*, which have irregularly whorled internal myofibrillary network, seen as swirling of the internal structure of the myofiber especially on NADH-TR reaction. These fibers tend to be larger and form small groups of a few. They can be associated with many disorders including muscular dystrophies and chronic denervation. *Target/targetoid fibers* are best seen on NADH-TR reactions and consist of a central pale area surrounded by alternating rings of stronger and weaker oxidative enzyme activity **(Fig. 8-20)**. They are referred to as target or targetoid depending on how closely they mimic the target sign based on the presence of well-formed rings. Though the diagnostic differences may not be significant, targetoid fibers may be considered less specific and can also be seen in myopathic disorders. Target fibers are typically associated with chronic denervation and tend to involve type 1 fibers predominantly; however, they tend to be rare in amyotrophic lateral sclerosis. *Central cores* may resemble targetoid fibers due to a thin rim of peripherally increased oxidative activity and are also best appreciated on NADH-TR reactions. Their periphery is also accentuated on PAS stain. Both target/targetoid fibers and central cores have a predilection to involve type 1 fibers. Central cores are most prominent and widespread in central core myopathy,[17] but occasional cores can be seen in other myopathic conditions. Their smaller and less well-developed versions are called *mini-cores*,[58] which occur as multiple pale areas in the fiber, also seen better by NADH-TR reactions. They are also identified in myopathic processes, including central core myopathy and other dystrophies. *Moth-eaten fibers*, also commonly seen in type 1 fibers and best with NADH-TR reaction, consist of patchy irregular small areas of reduced or absent oxidative enzyme reaction within the fiber. It may be difficult to tell them apart from fibers with mini-cores, except that they are more irregular than mini-cores. They are also nonspecific, but at least in some situations, they may represent partially reinnervated fibers. *Trabecular* fibers also known as *lobulated fibers* have peculiar internal architecture by NADH-TR reaction. They have alternating patches of decreased and increased oxidative enzyme activity, creating a trabecular or lobulated appearance to the fibers **(Fig. 8-21)**. They tend to be type 1 fibers, are usually smaller than other fibers, and have somewhat irregular contours. They are nonspecific findings but can be especially

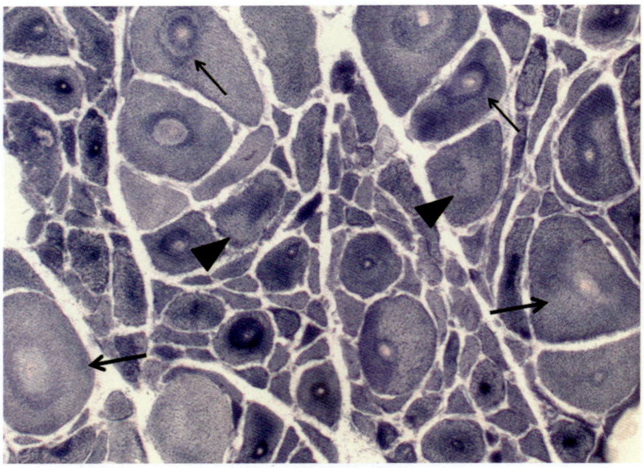

Figure 8-20. Target and targetoid fibers: Though they represent a similar process, target fibers have multiple light and dark rings (*thin arrows*), while targetoid fibers are less well-developed (*thick arrows*). Poorly developed changes are seen as pale areas and may be difficult to distinguish in isolation from central cores (*arrowheads*). Group atrophy and a few darkly reacting angulated atrophic fibers are also seen among the larger fibers in this case of neurogenic atrophy (NADH-TR; original magnification: 200×).

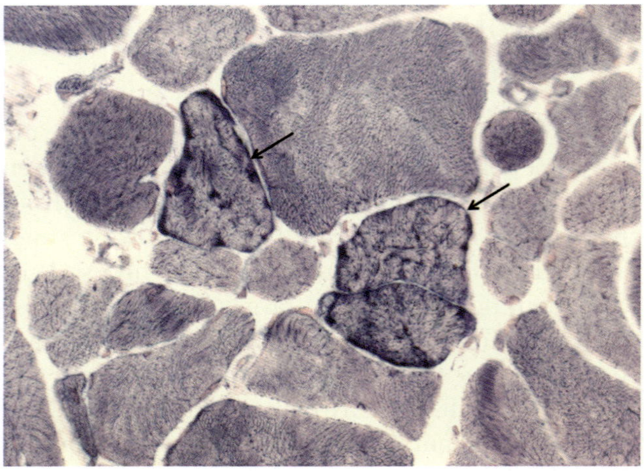

Figure 8-21. Trabecular fibers: The internal structures of several fibers appear to be divided into pale compartments by denser and darker trabeculae, resulting in trabecular or lobulated fibers (*arrows*) (NADH-TR; original magnification: 400×).

prominent in trabecular fiber myopathy[59] and some limb-girdle muscular dystrophies,[60] and occasionally in other conditions[61] such as inclusion body myositis, facioscapulohumeral dystrophy, and some congenital myopathies. Fibers with increased subsarcolemmal reaction on NADH-TR are different than the trabecular/lobulated fibers. Though nonspecific, they have been identified in Schwartz-Jampel syndrome.[3]

Processes associated with myofiber degeneration/rhabdomyolysis are also associated with variable numbers of regenerating fibers. *Degenerating fibers* are those fibers that appear partially or entirely pale depending on the stage of degeneration. They may be fragmented and the details of their internal architecture cannot be identified. They may be infiltrated by macrophages in an effort to clean up the debris **(Fig. 8-22)**. Lymphocytes may be present, especially if the process is an inflammatory one in nature. The degenerating fibers represent segmental necrosis, and the segmental nature of this process is better seen on longitudinal sections as a degenerating segment of otherwise unremarkable myofiber. They simply indicate a process with myofiber damage and are associated with a wide variety of myopathic processes, including inflammatory myopathies such as polymyositis, dystrophies such as Duchenne muscular dystrophy, and drug-induced myopathies such as myopathies of statin group of medications (hydroxymethylglutaryl coenzyme-A reductase inhibitors). Carnitine palmitoyltransferase (CPT) deficiency can show scattered degenerating and regenerating fibers, especially after episodes of myoglobinuria. Chloride channel myotonias can have scattered degenerating and regenerating fibers with increased caliber in type 2 fibers. *Rhabdomyolysis*[62] is also necrosis of the myofibers but implies a more widespread, severe, and acute condition **(Fig. 8-23)**. It also typically results in myoglobinuria. Malignant hyperthermia; extensive muscle damage due to trauma; toxic myopathies associated with drugs, especially drugs of abuse, or poisoning for instance by organophosphates; and severe inflammatory myopathies tend to be associated with rhabdomyolysis with resultant extremely elevated plasma creatine kinase myoglobin levels and the danger of renal failure. Diabetes mellitus can be associated with a focal myonecrosis **(Fig. 8-23)** that typically involves the quadriceps muscle and presents as a painful mass, mimicking a surgical condition and therefore resulting in the performance of a surgical biopsy.[63] Hemorrhage can be present in these lesions. Extensive rhabdomyolysis is seen in malignant hyperthermia if the biopsy is performed during or immediately

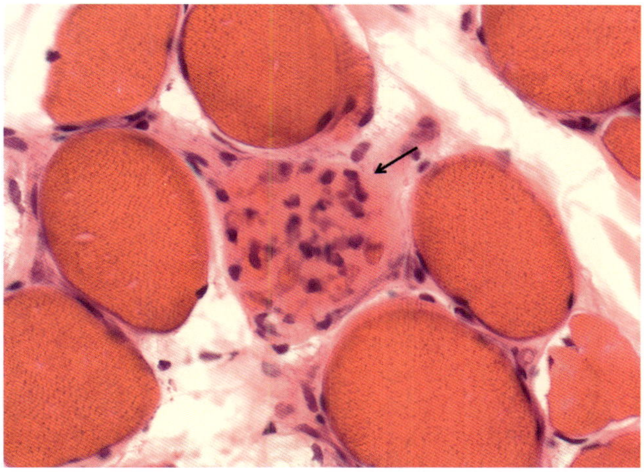

Figure 8-22. Degenerating fiber: The fiber in the center has essentially entirely degenerated (*arrow*) and has been infiltrated by histiocytes. These areas are seen as segments of degeneration on longitudinal sections, representing segmental necrosis (H&E; original magnification: 400×).

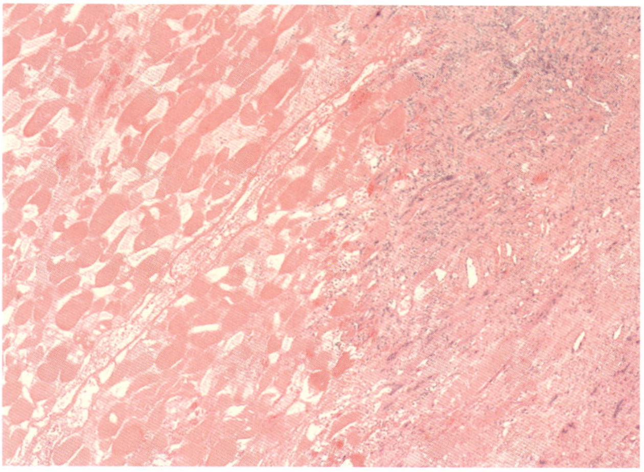

Figure 8-23. Rhabdomyolysis: A large zone of myofibers in the left side of the picture can only be recognized based on their ghost outlines, while the right side of the picture shows regenerating fibers in this case of diabetic myonecrosis which presented as a mass lesion in the quadriceps muscle (H&E; original magnification: 40×).

after the acute episode, but only mild myopathic changes can be identified afterward. A necrotizing myopathy can be associated with malignancies as a paraneoplastic syndrome.[64] Necrotizing autoimmune myopathy is histologically characterized by myocyte necrosis without inflammation.[65]

Hematolymphoid cells

Inflammation can be present in the muscle in a variety of conditions, including infections, and can be composed of different cell types similar to inflammations in other tissues; however, inflammation in the muscle specifically brings mind *inflammatory myopathies* unless further specified. Most inflammatory infiltrates in the muscle are predominantly or exclusively *lymphocytic*. These are mainly polymyositis, dermatomyositis, and inclusion body myositis.[7,66] In polymyositis, the inflammatory infiltrate is lymphocytic and is predominantly present within the fascicles, in the endomysium, circling and infiltrating myofibers, and is referred to as endomysium heavy. Scattered degenerating fibers are also present as well as regenerating fibers. In the later stages of the disease, variable increase in the endomysial connective tissue can be seen **(Fig. 8-24)**. Dermatomyositis, in contrast, is associated with a perimysium-heavy inflammation, which tends to be perivascular in this location **(Fig. 8-25)**. There is typically a perifascicular atrophy admixed with basophilic regenerating fibers **(Fig. 8-5)**. There are also additional differences in the composition of lymphocytic infiltrates as well as in some immunohistochemical markers between the two diseases.[67] In polymyositis, lymphocytes are essentially exclusively T cells with a predominance of CD8-positive lymphocytes over CD4-positive lymphocytes. In contrast, dermatomyositis has a more prominent CD4-positive cell population over CD8-positive cell population. In addition, B cells, as identified by CD20, are also more prominent. Major histocompatibility antigen class I (MHC-I) is normally present only in the blood vessels, but sarcolemma and sarcoplasms become positive in many pathologic states, including inflammatory myopathies and muscular

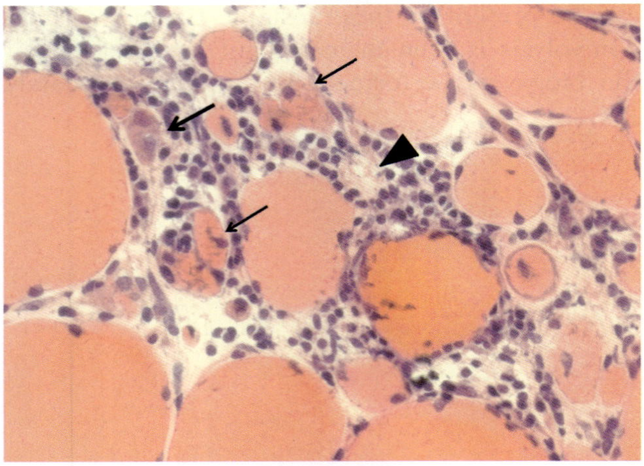

Figure 8-24. Inflammatory myopathy: Prominent lymphocytic inflammation is present in the endomysium. Some fibers have degenerated with sarcoplasmic remnants (*arrowhead*) seen in the inflammatory background. Others have basophilic sarcoplasms and enlarged nuclei, representing regenerating fibers (*thick arrow*). Some are irregular, fragmented, and infiltrated by lymphocytes (*thin arrows*), probably degenerating, but also show some regenerative activity as evidenced by a somewhat basophilic sarcoplasm and enlarged nuclei. These features favor polymyositis (H&E; original magnification: 400×).

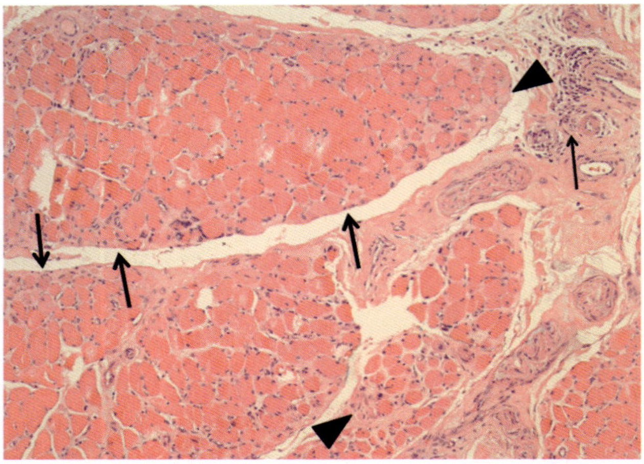

Figure 8-25. Inflammatory myopathy: In this case, inflammation is more prominent in the perimysium around the vessels (*thin arrow*). The fascicles have a suggestion of perifascicular atrophy (*thick arrows*) with the fibers at the periphery of the fascicle being somewhat smaller than those in the central areas. In some areas of the fascicles, increased perimysial connective tissue also extends into the endomysium to result in the rounded atrophy and separation of fibers from each other (*arrowheads*). These features favor dermatomyositis (H&E; original magnification: 40×).

dystrophies. While it tends to be uniformly positive in a sarcolemmal pattern in polymyositis, its positivity is limited to the damaged fibers in dermatomyositis, where it highlights the perifascicular fibers. Likewise in inclusion body myositis, it tends to be positive only in the damaged fibers, while the remaining fibers are negative. It tends to label those fibers infiltrated by lymphocytes in inclusion body myositis. Regenerating fibers are also positive. Polymyositis associated with HIV infection and myopathies with or without the features of polymyositis seen in HTLV-1–associated myositis[68] also show MHC-I positivity on all fibers. Fibers in X-linked vacuolar myopathies and the boundaries of their vacuoles are also MHC-I–positive. C5b-9 (membrane attack complex; MAC) is positive in the vessel walls in dermatomyositis.[69] Partial infiltration of intact, that is, nondegenerating/nonnecrotic, myofibers by lymphocytes can be seen in polymyositis and inclusion body myositis **(Fig. 8-26)**. Inclusion body myositis is associated with a variable amount and distribution of inflammation consisting predominantly of CD8-positive lymphocytes similar to polymyositis. Its characteristic feature is the presence of rimmed vacuoles (see above) **(Fig. 8-11)**. Inflammation in inflammatory myopathies can be extremely focal. Therefore, if it is not readily identified in a suspicious case, multiple levels should be evaluated before concluding the absence of inflammation in that sample. Likewise, paying attention to various findings on special stains/reactions other than their colors is advisable as new findings such as focal inflammation may emerge on those sections. A typical polymyositis picture can be associated with HIV infection.[70] Alternatively, interstitial lymphocytic aggregates can be found in association with HIV infection, without definitive features of an inflammatory myopathy. An inflammatory myopathy picture can be seen as a toxic effect of *D*-penicillamine.[71] Lymphorrhages are focal endomysial collections of lymphocytes typically seen in myasthenia gravis[72] or in connective tissues in collagen vascular diseases. Dermatomyositis can commonly be seen as a paraneoplastic presentation associated with adenocarcinomas of various internal organs and lymphomas, while polymyositis can be associated with lymphomas.[73] *Plasma cells* may be seen as a minor component in some inflammatory myopathies. Involvement of muscle by hematolymphoid malignancies, including plasma cell myeloma, may be difficult to distinguish from inflammatory infiltrates without a high degree of suspicion to initiate appropriate workup (see Chapter 2). *Macrophages* can be present within and around degenerating fibers to remove the debris; however, this should not be interpreted as a primary inflammatory process, even though it technically represents a reaction to tissue injury. Truly inflammatory processes usually have other inflammatory cells also and reveal their true nature in other areas of the tissue. A focal inflammatory process composed predominantly of macrophages with an admixture of lymphocytes has been termed macrophagic myofasciitis and has been associated with vaccinations. The inclusions seen ultrastructurally in the macrophage cytoplasms were identified as aluminum hydroxide, a vaccine adjuvant.[74] *Polymorphonuclear (PMN) leukocytes* can be seen in areas of previous injury, such as electromyography needle sites, physical trauma, or at the biopsy site, especially if the procedure lasted unusually long. They can be abundant in bacterial infections and abscess. Parasitic infections are also associated with an abundance of eosinophil PMN leukocytes.[75] Trichinella infection can be associated with abundant leukocytes, including eosinophil PMN leukocytes.[76] Eosinophil PMN leukocytes

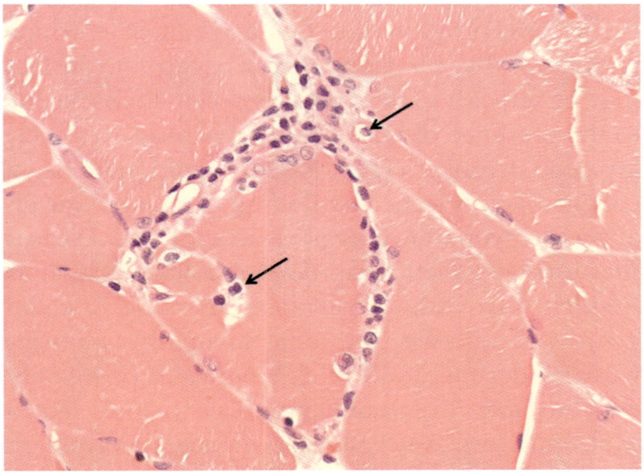

Figure 8-26. Lymphocytes infiltrating myofibers: A mild lymphocytic infiltrate is present in the endomysium, surrounding the fiber in the center as well as infiltrating two fibers (*arrows*), which appear otherwise unremarkable in this case of polymyositis (H&E; original magnification: 400×).

are abundant and accompany histiocytes, plasma cells, and lymphocytes in the endomysium and perimysium in eosinophilic polymyositis. Variable myopathic changes, including myofiber necrosis, are also seen. Abundant eosinophil PMN leukocyte infiltrates preferentially involve the subcutaneous soft tissues in Shulman's syndrome,[77] while the inflammatory infiltrate is present within the perimysium and fascia, together with myofiber damage and prominent myopathic changes in eosinophilia-myalgia syndrome.[78] A focal inflammatory mass-forming lesion that can present more commonly as a surgical process similar to diabetic muscle infarction has been appropriately termed *focal myositis* and consists of a mixed inflammatory infiltrate, fibrosis, predominantly myopathic, and many times focal neurogenic changes. Predominantly, CD4-positive T cells and an admixture of B cells and plasma cells are present. IgG4 and MHC-I are focally positive.[79] Various *infections*, including bacterial, fungal, viral, and parasitic, can cause suppurative or granulomatous inflammations, and their specific features are similar to those elsewhere. Various inflammatory, vasculitic-vasculopathic, and myopathic features are seen in cases of lupus erythematosus, mixed connective tissue disease, rheumatoid arthritis, scleroderma, and Sjögren syndrome. Plasma cells may be prominent in the latter. Aside from the typical granulomatous infections, granulomas in the muscle can be seen in giant cell myositis (see above), sarcoidosis,[21] and Crohn's disease.[80]

Connective Tissues, Vessels, and Nerves

Increased connective tissue is usually a secondary change in response to ongoing myofiber damage. In long-standing and progressive diseases such as muscular dystrophies or in chronic stages of inflammatory myopathies, a gradual scar formation occurs especially in the endomysial connective tissue in the form of fibrosis, in which entrapped rounded atrophic fibers are seen **(Fig. 8-4)**. Normally, myofibers are seen as barely touching their neighboring myofibers with only an inconspicuous endomysial connective tissue that is visible at the points where capillaries are located. At the initial stages of endomysial fibrosis, a thin band of connective tissue becomes easily visible and gradually and heterogeneously increases to widely separate the myofibers. In the advanced stages of this process, mature adipose tissue also contributes to the increase in the amount of endomysial connective tissue. In some cases, scattered adipocytes appear as vacuoles in the endomysium. Eventually, the process progresses to end-stage muscle, which is not suitable for diagnostic workup and in fact may be difficult to recognize as skeletal muscle due to the presence of only a few remaining extremely atrophic myofibers **(Fig. 8-27)**. A mild increase in collagen is a nonspecific finding associated generally with myopathic processes. In addition, diseases that involve genetic disorders of collagen, such as Bethlem myopathy, show some increase in collagen, with otherwise minimal myopathic changes with no degeneration or regeneration of myofibers, but may eventually progress to look like a dystrophic process.[81] Skeletal muscle involvement in nephrogenic fibrosing dermopathy (dialysis-associated systemic fibrosis), which is thought to be associated with contrast-enhancing material use for radiologic evaluation in patients with renal disease,[82] results in prominent endomysial and perimysial fibrosis. It can be associated with calcifications. Subcutaneous tissues are also involved.[83]

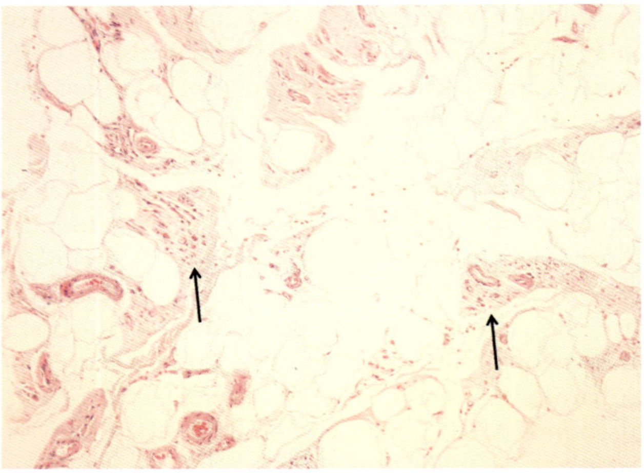

Figure 8-27. End-stage muscle: The tissue looks like mature adipose tissue. Several extremely atrophic fibers can be identified entrapped within fibrosis (*arrows*) upon closer evaluation. No further comments can be made regarding the pathologic process based on such end-stage muscle (H&E; original magnification: 100×).

Some cases of amyloidosis show extensive involvement of endomysium and perimysium, resulting in firm fibrotic pseudohypertrophic appearance of the muscles,[84] similar to nephrogenic fibrosing dermopathy. Amyloid accumulation can occur as a result of various processes and involve the muscle to various extents,[85] sometimes associated with or mimicking other specific muscle diseases.[86] Many amyloidogenic substances have also been identified and may be associated with specific pathologic processes. Therefore, identification of amyloid should initiate further clinical and pathologic investigation, potentially including spectrophotometric evaluation to identify the exact nature of this accumulation.[87]

Vascular changes can be seen and may be prominent in some conditions. Various *vasculitides* may involve the blood vessels in the muscle[88] and are in general similar to those discussed in Chapters 2 and 9. Perivascular lymphocytic cuffs without evidence of vasculitis can be seen commonly, sometimes without a definitive explanation and sometimes in association with inflammatory myopathies and collagen vascular diseases.[89] The number of capillaries per myofiber is increased especially in endurance athletes. There are differences based on age and fiber size, as well. Dermatomyositis may be associated with a decrease in the number of capillaries due to destruction of vessels before the typical histologic changes ensue.[90] These types of evaluations require morphometric studies and are not practical in daily routine. Highlighting the vessels by immunohistochemical stains such as CD31 or CD34 is useful for this purpose. A concentric collagenous thickening of vessels is common in diabetes mellitus and is due to reduplicated basement laminae.[91,92] In some mitochondrial disorders, for instance, MELAS, mitochondria are increased in vascular smooth muscle cells, which can be seen while evaluating SDH for ragged blue fibers.[93]

Other components of the tissue may occasionally show some changes. For instance, small *peripheral nerve twigs* within the muscle may show changes relevant to nerve disorders, such as demyelination; however, these changes are difficult, if not impossible, to appropriately evaluate for a definitive diagnosis. *Muscle spindles* can be abnormal in many conditions.[3,94] In some dystrophies and neurologic diseases, muscle spindles may have abnormally increased numbers of intrafusal fibers, capsular thickening, and other changes.[95,96] Intrafusal fibers can be involved by the pathologic process affecting the muscle. For instance, they can show glycogen storage in acid maltase deficiency myopathy.[97]

Mixed patterns mainly consisting of overlapping neurogenic and myopathic features are common and can be confusing and difficult to sort through based solely on pathologic evaluation. Long-standing and severe neurogenic atrophy eventually develops secondary myopathic features, and in addition to the typical neurogenic findings, changes such as degenerating fibers and increase in the amount of endomysial connective tissue can be seen. In some cases, a pathologic process may affect both the skeletal muscle and motor nerve, resulting in a mixed pattern. These are usually diseases with systemic involvement, such as various vasculitides, collagen vascular diseases, infections, and toxins or drugs that can cause myopathy and neuropathy. Another scenario is the presence of more than one pathologic process, such as the development of an unrelated myopathic process in a patient with herniated nucleus pulposus or motor neuron disease. The interpretation of the biopsy findings requires close correlation with the history and clinical and other laboratory findings. It should also be remembered that, while many findings indicate toward a primary muscle or nerve related problem **(Table 8.2)**, not every individual finding is definitely either myopathic or neurogenic. For instance, angulated atrophic fibers, while typical for acute denervation, can be seen in some other conditions. Targetoid fibers can also be seen in both categories of diseases (see above for discussions of individual features). A source of confusion for the unwary is the presence of clear cut and severe neurogenic atrophy in the muscle biopsy with an accompanying largely unremarkable sural nerve biopsy. This discrepancy is due to the completely sensory nature of the sural nerve, while the neurogenic changes in the muscle are the result of motor nerve involvement. Nonetheless, if not only motor nerve involvement but a generalized neurogenic problem is present, sural nerve can yield important information. This way, both the motor and sensory nervous system can be evaluated (see Chapter 9).

TABLE 8.2 Typical features of predominantly myopathic or neurogenic processes

Myopathic	Neurogenic
Fiber size variation	Fiber size variation
Rounded atrophic fibers	Angulated atrophic fibers
Increased endomysial connective tissue	Small group atrophy
Degenerating fibers	Large group atrophy
Regenerating fibers	Fiber type grouping (ATPase)
Splitting fibers	Target/targetoid fibers
Internal nuclei	Dark fibers (NADH-TR, esterase)
Inflammation	Syncytial nuclear clumps
Vacuoles	
Inclusions	
Accumulations	
Ragged red fibers	
Ragged blue fibers	
Ring fibers	
COX-negative fibers	
Type 2 fiber atrophy	
Perifascicular atrophy	

COX, cytochrome oxidase.

Histochemistry

In addition to those features mentioned in various discussions above, some of the additional features that can be seen by special stains and reactions are mentioned here.[4,98–100] Also see Table 8.1 for the normal staining of fiber types. *Gomori's trichrome stain* is one of the most important stains for the evaluation of muscle tissue. It provides information about the internal architecture of the myofiber and highlights many accumulations and inclusions. Mitochondria are stained as red dots. Myelin stains red and the intramuscular peripheral nerve twigs become prominent. *Adenosine triphosphatase (ATPase)* reaction is used to differentiate fiber types with a normal checkerboard pattern. Depending on the pH the reaction is performed, type 1 and 2 fibers and sometimes subtypes of type 2 fibers can be identified. Differentiation of fiber types starts in the fetus. In cases where there is extensive degeneration and fiber injury, chronic myopathic and neurogenic processes, fiber types may lose their differentiation. Normally, at low pH, typically at 4.4, type 1 fibers are dark and type 2 fibers are light, while the reverse is true at high pH, typically at 9.4. At intermediate pH such as 4.6, it is possible to identify type 2A and 2B fibers as having intermediate activity. This way, type 1 and type 2 fiber atrophy or involvement of both can be identified. Selective atrophy of a particular type of fiber tends to be associated with particular processes (see above Fiber Size Variation). ATPase reactions tend to fade after several months. In general, approximately 1/3 of fibers are type 1, 1/3 is type 2A, and 1/3 is 2B. When more than about 55% of fibers are of type 1, type 1 fiber predominance is identified, while when more than 80% of fibers are of type 2, type 2 fiber predominance is identified. Type 1 fiber predominance is usually associated with myopathic conditions, including some rare syndromes such as Marinesco-Sjögren syndrome,[101] while type 2 fiber predominance is usually associated with neurogenic conditions. Fiber type grouping is also an important finding seen by ATPase reactions. It indicates reinnervation of the denervated fibers by adjacent nerves, switching their types, resulting in large groups of fibers of similar type **(Fig. 8-28)**. While this situation is obvious in most cases, subtle forms can be diagnosed when there are at least 16 fibers of similar type in the same group.[3] Fiber type grouping may be difficult to distinguish from fiber type predominance in small tissues and especially when the typed groups are extremely large. The small groups of fibers that appear like small group atrophy due to forking and splitting of one fiber into multiple fibers as a regenerative attempt also are of similar types of fibers, mimicking fiber type grouping. They are sometimes referred to as myopathic fiber type grouping as they are associated with myopathic processes such as Duchenne muscular dystrophy. Fiber type disproportion can be a congenital abnormality.[102] Fiber types are also variable depending on the location. Weight-bearing muscles that need to endure for long periods of time, such as those in the lower extremity, may have more type 1 fibers than upper extremity, where type 2 fibers may be prominent due to their strength-related activities. Other factors such as training, innervation, and aging also affect the fiber type composition of the muscle. In general, ATPase reactions highlight the presence of myofibrillary ATPase activity and can show the absence of such activity in areas of various accumulations. In

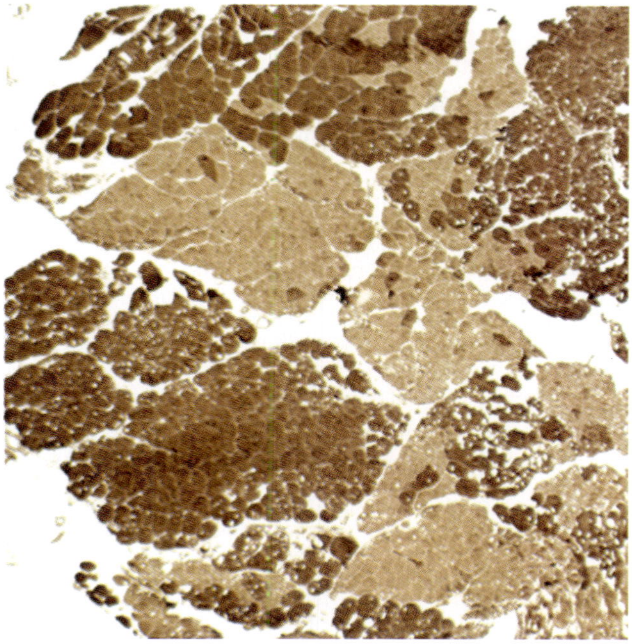

Figure 8-28. Fiber type grouping: The usual checkerboard pattern of fiber types is lost. Entire fascicles are composed of one type of fiber, while others are entirely composed of the other type of fiber as a result of reinnervation in this neurogenic process. Small biopsy tissues consisting entirely of one large fascicle may mimic fiber type predominance in such cases (ATPase at pH 9.4; light-colored fibers are type 1, dark-colored fibers are type 2; original magnification: 40×).

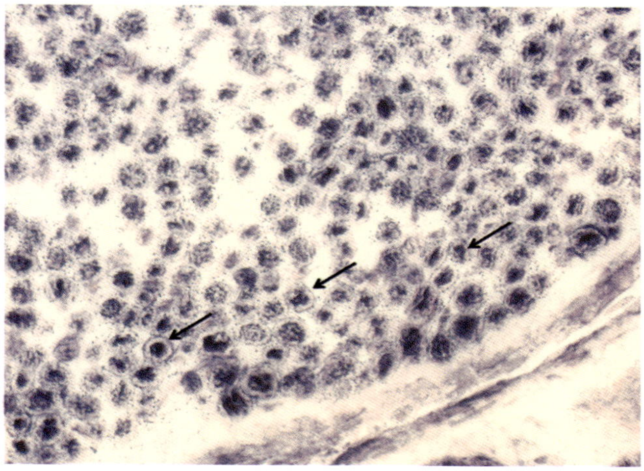

Figure 8-29. Centronuclear myopathy: Oxidative activity has a tendency to be prominent toward the center of the fibers, leaving a pale halo at their periphery (*arrows*) (NADH-TR; original magnification: 400×).

addition, some pathologic processes tend to involve preferentially one type of fiber over the other. For instance, central cores tend to occur more frequently in type 1 fibers, while tubular aggregates are seen more frequently in type 2 fibers. Fiber typing can be relatively easily and more accurately done by using *immunohistochemistry for myosin types* (see below, "Immunohistochemistry"). *NADH-TR reactions* provide information on internal structure of the fiber through evaluation of the intermyofibrillary network and by highlighting the mitochondria through oxidative activity. As such, any accumulations or disturbances that interfere with the internal structure of the myofiber can be relatively easily seen. Common findings are moth-eaten appearance, central cores, minicores, trabecular and target/targetoid fibers, and darkly reacting atrophic fibers. It shows the condensation of mitochondria toward the center of the fiber in myotubular myopathy with peripheral pale halos **(Fig. 8-29)**. Although it highlights the mitochondria through oxidative enzyme activity, it is not a good tool to evaluate mitochondrial disorders, as it tends to show only normal mitochondria and not necessarily the abnormal ones seen in mitochondrial disorders. *Oil red O* stains the lipids as orange-red droplets. Increased lipid is identified especially in type 1 fibers in lipid storage myopathies and mainly in CPT deficiency. Fasting, through increased plasma lipids, results in increased lipid content in the fibers. At least a focal excess in lipid content can be seen in dermatomyositis. Many other conditions can show a high lipid content, making the interpretation of this stain difficult. In addition, the stained lipid droplets can float on the slide under the coverslip and become displaced for instance from adjacent adipose tissues, resulting in potential misinterpretations. *SDH* and *COX* reactions are explained above in the discussion of ragged red fibers and mitochondrial disorders, which are their main uses. *Phosphorylase* and *PFK* reactions are explained above in the discussion of accumulations. *Acid phosphatase* activity can be present in the connective tissue and macrophages but should not be present within the myofibers, although some staining in scattered fibers may be associated with lipofuscin accumulation and aging. In both cases, the reaction tends to be subsarcolemmal and around the nuclei. Otherwise, it is abnormal and may indicate degenerating fibers. Many vacuolar changes and lysosomal disorders are also positive. There may be many positive foci in many fibers in congenital myotonic dystrophy. Vitamin E deficiency can also result in increased acid phosphatase reactivity in the myofibers.[4] Although *nonspecific esterase* reaction can also show lysosomal activity and therefore is especially useful for macrophages, its main use is to highlight motor end plates. Angulated atrophic fibers of acute denervation tend to show a dark reaction, similar to the darkly reacting fibers on NADH-TR.

Immunohistochemistry

Immunohistochemistry[67,100] can be used to further characterize an *inflammatory infiltrate* as discussed above under inflammation. Plasma cells and macrophages can be highlighted. Clonality of a lymphoid population can be studied as in other tissues. MHC-I and C5b-9 help further characterize inflammatory myopathies, as also discussed above under "Inflammation". *Accumulations* can be characterized by immunohistochemistry.[43,45] Desmin normally stains the myofibers weakly but shows strong staining of accumulations in desminopathy. Likewise, other protein accumulation disorders, such as ZASPopathy, myotilinopathy, etc., can also be studied. The *absence of a protein* that is normally present on sarcolemma and that becomes deficient due to a genetic defect can be confirmed by immunohistochemistry or immunofluorescence microscopy.[67,100] Most notable example is dystrophin in Duchenne and Becker muscular dystrophies. Sarcoglycans, dystroglycans, dysferlin, and caveolin are other examples, among many others. The pattern of absence of staining can also provide some information. For instance, a reduced intensity of staining or uneven/patchy staining for dystrophin may suggest Becker's muscular dystrophy. Immunohistochemistry for *myosin heavy chain isoforms* can be used to distinguish type 1 and type 2 fibers based on their slow or fast isoform content, respectively.[103] Neonatal form gradually disappears and should not be present after about 1 year of age. Its identification indicates immature and regenerating fibers.[104] Myosin immunohistochemistry may be more useful in autopsy tissue where enzymatic activity may be reduced or lost for proper ATPase reaction.

References

1. Cohen ML. Skeletal muscle and peripheral nerve disorders. In: *Neuropathology*. Prayson RA, ed. Philadelphia, PA: Elsevier; 2005:537–581.
2. Pearl GS, Ghatak NR. Muscle biopsy. *Arch Pathol Lab Med*. 1995;119:303–306.
3. Carpenter S, Karpati G. *Pathology of Skeletal Muscle*. 2nd ed. New York: Oxford University press; 2001.
4. Dubowitz V, Sewry AC. *Muscle Biopsy: A Practical Approach*. Philadelphia, PA: Elsevier; 2007.
5. Lin MY, Nonaka I. Facioscapulohumeral muscular dystrophy: muscle fiber type analysis with particular reference to small angular fibers. *Brain Dev*. 1991;13:331–338.
6. Anthony DC, Frosch MP, Girolamu UD. Peripheral nerve and skeletal muscle. In: *Robbins and Cotran Pathologic Basis of Disease*. Kumar V, Abbas AK, Fausto N, et al., eds. 8th ed. Philadelphia, PA: Saunders; 2010:1257–1278.
7. Dalakas MC. Review: an update on inflammatory and autoimmune myopathies. *Neuropathol Appl Neurobiol*. 2011;37: 226–242.
8. Bassez G, Chapoy E, Bastuji-Garin S, et al. Type 2 myotonic dystrophy can be predicted by the combination of type 2 muscle fiber central nucleation and scattered atrophy. *J Neuropathol Exp Neurol*. 2008;67:319–325.
9. Pisani V, Panico MB, Terracciano C, et al. Preferential central nucleation of type 2 myofibers is an invariable feature of myotonic dystrophy type 2. *Muscle Nerve*. 2008;38:1405–1411.
10. Lexell J. Human aging, muscle mass, and fiber type composition. *J Gerontol A Biol Sci Med Sci*. 1995;50:11–16.
11. Kojima S, Takagi A, Ida M, et al. Muscle pathology in polymyalgia rheumatica: histochemical and immunohistochemical study. *Jpn J Med*. 1991;30:516–523.
12. Squier M, Chalk C, Hilton-Jones D, et al. Type 2 fiber predominance in Lambert-Eaton myasthenic syndrome. *Muscle Nerve*. 1991;14:625–632.
13. Lotz BP, Engel AG. Are hypercontracted muscle fibers artifacts and do they cause rupture of the plasma membrane? *Neurology*. 1987;37:1466–1475.
14. Boxler K, Jerusalem F. Hyperreactive (hyaline, opaque, dark) muscle fibers in Duchenne dystrophy. A biopsy study of 16 dystrophy and 205 other neuromuscular disease cases and controls. *J Neurol*. 1978;219:63–72.
15. Kurihara T. New classification and treatment for myotonic disorders. *Intern Med*. 2005;44:1027–1032.
16. Eisenschenk S, Triggs WJ, Pearl GS, et al. Proximal myotonic myopathy: clinical, neuropathologic, and molecular genetic features. *Ann Clin Lab Sci*. 2001;31:140–146.
17. Fujimura-Kiyono C, Racz GZ, Nishino I. Myotubular/centronuclear myopathy and central core disease. *Neurol India*. 2008;56:325–332.
18. Pierson CR, Tomczak K, Agrawal P, et al. X-linked myotubular and centronuclear myopathies. *J Neuropathol Exp Neurol*. 2005;64:555–564.
19. Afifi AK, Najjar SS, Mire-Salman J, et al. The myopathology of the Kocher-Debre-Semelaigne syndrome. Electromyography, light- and electron-microscopic study. *J Neurol Sci*. 1974;22: 445–470.
20. Pascuzzi RM, Roos KL, Phillips LH. Granulomatous inflammatory myopathy associated with myasthenia gravis. A case report and review of the literature. *Arch Neurol*. 1986;43:621–623.
21. Prayson RA. Granulomatous myositis: clinicopathologic study of 12 cases. *Am J Clin Pathol*. 1999;112:63–68.
22. Dubourg O, Wanschitz J, Maisonobe T, et al. Diagnostic value of markers of muscle degeneration in sporadic inclusion body myositis. *Acta Myologica*. 2011;30:103–108.
23. Nishino I. Autophagic vacuolar myopathies. *Curr Neurol Neurosci Rep*. 2003;3:64–69.
24. Sasaki K, Suga K, Tsugawa S, et al. Muscle pathology in Marinesco-Sjögren syndrome: a unique ultrastructural feature. *Brain Dev*. 1996;18:64–67.

25. Nucci A, Queiroz LS, Samara AM. Chloroquine neuromyopathy. *Clin Neuropathol*. 1996;15:256–258.

26. Fernandez C, Figarella-Branger D, Alla P, et al. Colchicine myopathy: a vacuolar myopathy with selective type I muscle fiber involvement. An immunohistochemical and electron microscopic study of two cases. *Acta Neuropathol*. 2002;103:100–106.

27. Nishino I. Autophagic vacuolar myopathy. *Semin Pediatr Neurol*. 2006;13:90–95.

28. Martin JJ, Ceuterick C, Mercelis R, et al. Familial periodic paralysis with hypokalemia. Study of a muscle biopsy in the myopathic stage of the disorder. *Acta Neurol Belg*. 1984;84:233–242.

29. Caron A, Gohel C, Mollaret K, et al. Study of some components of the cytoskeleton in muscular disorders with nonspecific cytoplasmic bodies. *Acta Neuropathol*. 1999;97:267–274.

30. Bertini E, Salviati G, Apollo F, et al. Reducing body myopathy and desmin storage in skeletal muscle: morphological and biochemical findings. *Acta Neuropathol*. 1994;87:106–112.

31. Rafay MF, Halliday W, Bril V. Hyaline body myopathy: adulthood manifestations. *Can J Neurol Sci*. 2005;32:253–256.

32. Shingde MV, Spring PJ, Maxwell A, et al. Myosin storage (hyaline body) myopathy: a case report. *Neuromuscul Disord*. 2006;16:882–886.

33. Gyure KA, Prayson RA, Estes ML. Adult-onset nemaline myopathy: a case report and review of the literature. *Arch Pathol Lab Med*. 1997;121:1210–1213.

34. Rowland LP. HIV-related neuromuscular diseases: nemaline myopathy, amyotrophic lateral sclerosis and bibrachial amyotrophic diplegia. *Acta Myol*. 2011;30:29–31.

35. Morgan-Hughes JA. Tubular aggregates in skeletal muscle: their functional significance and mechanisms of pathogenesis. *Curr Opin Neurol*. 1998;11:439–442.

36. Filosto M, Tomelleri G, Tonin P, et al. Neuropathology of mitochondrial diseases. *Biosci Rep*. 2007;27:23–30.

37. DiMauro S, Schon E. Mitochondrial mutations in human disease. *Am J Med Genet*. 2001;106:18–26.

38. Yis U, Seneca S, Dirik E, et al. Unusual findings in Leigh syndrome caused by T8993C mutation. *Eur J Paediatr Neurol*. 2009;13:550–552.

39. Walker UA, Schon EA. Neurotrophin-4 is up-regulated in ragged-red fibers associated with pathogenic mitochondrial DNA mutations. *Ann Neurol*. 1998;43:536–540.

40. Blume G, Pestronk A, Frank B, et al. Polymyositis with cytochrome oxidase negative muscle fibres. Early quadriceps weakness and poor response to immunosuppressive therapy. *Brain*. 1997;120:39–45.

41. Temiz P, Weihl CC, Pestronk A. Inflammatory myopathies with mitochondrial pathology and protein aggregates. *J Neurol Sci*. 2009;278:25–29.

42. Bernier FP, Boneh A, Dennett X, et al. Diagnostic criteria for respiratory chain disorders in adults and children. *Neurology*. 2002;59:1406–1411.

43. Selcen D. Myofibrillar myopathies. *Curr Opin Neurol*. 2008;21:585–589.

44. Vattemi G, Neri M, Piffer S, et al. Clinical, morphological and genetic studies in a cohort of 21 patients with myofibrillar myopathy. *Acta Myol*. 2011;30:121–126.

45. Selcen D. Myofibrillar myopathies. *Neuromuscul Disord*. 2011;21:161–171.

46. Cao A, Cianchetti C, Calisti L, et al. Schwartz-Jampel syndrome. Clinical, electrophysiological and histopathological study of a severe variant. *J Neurol Sci*. 1978;35:175–187.

47. Iannaccone S, Zucconi M, Quattrini A, et al. Early detection of skin and muscular involvement in Lafora disease. *J Neurol*. 1991;238:217–220.

48. Boulman N, Slobodin G. Rozenbaum M, et al. Calcinosis in rheumatic diseases. *Semin Arthritis Rheum*. 2005;34:805–812.

49. Liu J, Sulh MA, Zagzag D, et al. Disseminated calcification with predominant muscle and cerebral involvement in a child with acquired immunodeficiency syndrome: a case report. *Pediatr Pathol Lab Med*. 1997;17:593–600.

50. Dimaur S, Andreu AL, Bruno C, et al. Myophosphorylase deficiency (glycogenosis type V: McArdle disease). *Curr Mol Med*. 2002;2:189–196.

51. Ozen H. Glycogen storage diseases: new perspectives. *World J Gastroenterol*. 2007;13:2541–2553.

52. Bembi B, Cerini E, Danesino C, et al. Diagnosis of glycogenosis type II. *Neurology*. 2008;71:4–11.

53. Liang WC, Nishino I. State of the art in muscle lipid diseases. *Acta Myol*. 2010;29:351–356.

54. Liang WC, Nishino I. Lipid storage myopathy. *Curr Neurol Neurosci Rep*. 2011;11:97–103.

55. Ho KL. Basophilic degeneration of skeletal muscle in hypothyroid myopathy. Histochemical and ultrastructural studies. *Arch Pathol Lab Med*. 1984;108:239–245.

56. Chou SM, Nonaka I. Satellite cells and muscle regeneration in diseased human skeletal muscles. *J Neurol Sci*. 1977;34:131–145.

57. Pongratz D, Schultz D, Koppenwallner C, et al. Diagnostic value of muscle biopsy findings in myotonic dystrophy (Curschmann-Steinert). *Klin Wochenschr*. 1979;57:215–224.

58. Jungbluth H. Multi-minicore disease. *Orphanet J Rare Dis*. 2007;2:31.

59. Weller B, Carpenter S, Lochmuller H, et al. Myopathy with trabecular muscle fibers. *Neuromuscul Disord*. 1999;9:208–214.

60. Gallardo E, Saenz A, Illa I. Limb-girdle muscular dystrophy 2A. *Handb Clin Neurol*. 2011;101:97–110.

61. Figarella-Branger D, El-Dassouki M, Saenz A, et al. Myopathy with lobulated muscle fibers: evidence for heterogeneous etiology and clinical presentation. *Neuromuscul Disord*. 2002;12:4–12.

62. Cervellin G, Comelli I, Lippi G. Rhabdomyolysis: historical background, clinical, diagnostic and therapeutic features. *Clin Chem Lab Med*. 2010;48:749–756.

63. Trujillo-Santos AJ. Diabetic muscle infarction: an underdiagnosed complication of long-standing diabetes. *Diabetes Care*. 2003;26:211–215.

64. Hocar O, Poszepczynska-Guigne E, Faye O, et al. Severe necrotizing myopathy subsequent to Merkel cell carcinoma. *Ann Dermatol Venereol*. 2011;138:130–134.

65. Liang C, Needham M. Necrotizing autoimmune myopathy. *Curr Opin Rheumatol*. 2011;23:612–619.

66. Dalakas MC. Polymyositis, dermatomyositis, and inclusion-body myositis. *N Engl J Med*. 1991;325:1487–1498.

67. Bornemann A, Anderson LV. Diagnostic protein expression in human muscle biopsies. *Brain Pathol*. 2000;10:193–214.

68. Inose M, Higuchi I, Yoshimine K, et al. Pathological changes in skeletal muscle in HTLV-I-associated myelopathy. *J Neurol Sci*. 1992;110:73–78.

69. Jain A, Sharma MC, Sarkar C, et al. Detection of the membrane attack complex as a diagnostic tool in dermatomyositis. *Acta Neurol Scand*. 2011;123:122–129.

70. Gabbai AA, Schmidt B, Castelo A, et al. Muscle biopsy in AIDS and ARC: analysis of 50 patients. *Muscle Nerve*. 1990;13:541–544.

71. Chappel R, Willems J. D-penicillamine-induced myositis in rheumatoid arthritis. *Clin Rheumatol*. 1996:15:86–87.

72. Pascuzzi RM, Campa JF. Lymphorrhage localized to the muscle end-plate in myasthenia gravis. *Arch Pathol Lab Med*. 1988;112:934–937.

73. Aggarwal R, Oddis CV. Paraneoplastic myalgias and myositis. *Rheum Dis Clin North Am*. 2011;37:607–621.

74. Gherardi RK, Coquet M, Cherin P, et al. Macrophagic myofasciitis lesions assess long-term persistence of vaccine-derived aluminium hydroxide in muscle. *Brain*. 2001;124:1821–1831.

75. Arness MK, Brown JD, Dubey JP, et al. An outbreak of acute eosinophilic myositis attributed to human Sarcocystis parasitism. *Am J Trop Med Hyg*. 1999;61:548–553.

76. Taratuto AL, Venturiello SM. Trichinosis. *Brain Pathol.* 1997;7:663–672.

77. Pellissier JF, Figarella-Branger D, Serratrice G. Neuromuscular diseases with eosinophilia. *Med Trop*. 1998;58: 471–476.

78. Philen RM, Eidson M, Kilbourne EM, et al. Eosinophilia-myalgia syndrome. A clinical case series of 21 patients. New Mexico Eosinophilia-Myalgia Syndrome Study Group. *Arch Intern Med*. 1991;151:533–537.

79. Auerbach A, Fanburg-Smith JC, Wang G, et al. Focal Myositis. A Clinicopathologic Study of 115 Cases of an Intramuscular Mass-like Reactive Process. *Am J Surg Pathol.* 2009;33:1016–1024.

80. Christopoulos C, Savva S, Pylarinou S, et al. Localised gastrocnemius myositis in Crohn's disease. *Clin Rheumatol.* 2003;22:143–145.

81. Bonnemann CG. The collagen VI-related myopathies: muscle meets its matrix. *Nat Rev Neurosci*. 2011;7:379–390.

82. Penfield JG, Reilly RF. Gadolinium and nephrogenic systemic fibrosis: have we overreacted? *Semin Dial.* 2011;24:480–486.

83. Levine JM, Taylor RA, Elman LB, et al. Involvement of skeletal muscle in dialysis-associated systemic fibrosis (nephrogenic fibrosing dermopathy). *Muscle Nerve*. 2004;30: 569–577.

84. Whitaker JN, Hashimoto K, Quinones M. Skeletal muscle pseudohypertrophy in primary amyloidosis. *Neurology*. 1977;27:47–54.

85. Prayson RA. Amyloid myopathy: clinicopathologic study of 16 cases. *Hum Pathol*. 1998;29:463–468.

86. Kazmi SAJ, McComb RD, Gokden M, et al. Amyloid myopathy associated with dysferlinopathy: comparison with light chain amyloidosis. *J Neuropathol Exp Neurol*. 2011;70:524.

87. Vrana JA, Gamez JD, Madden BJ, et al. Classification of amyloidosis by laser microdissection and mass spectrometry-based proteomic analysis in clinical biopsy specimens. *Blood*. 2009;114:4957–4959.

88. Prayson RA. Skeletal muscle vasculitis exclusive of inflammatory myopathic conditions: a clinicopathologic study of 40 patients. *Hum Pathol*. 2002;33:989–995.

89. Engel AG, Arahata K. Mononuclear cells in myopathies: quantitation of functionally distinct subsets, recognition of antigen-specific cell-mediated cytotoxicity in some diseases, and implications for the pathogenesis of the different inflammatory myopathies. *Hum Pathol*. 1986;17:704–721.

90. Pestronk A, Schmidt RE, Choksi R. Vascular pathology in dermatomyositis and anatomic relations to myopathology. *Muscle Nerve*. 2010;42:53–61.

91. Tilton RG, Hoffmann PL, Kilo C, et al. Pericyte degeneration and basement membrane thickening in skeletal muscle capillaries of human diabetics. *Diabetes*. 1981;30:326–334.

92. Feingold KR, Browner WS, Siperstein MD. Prospective studies of muscle capillary basement membrane width in prediabetics. *J Clin Endocrinol Metab*. 1989;69:784–789.

93. Hasegawa H, Matsuoka T, Goto Y et al. Strongly succinate dehydrogenase-reactive blood vessels in muscles from patients with mitochondrial myopathy, encephalopathy, lactic acidosis, and strokelike episodes. *Ann Neurol*. 1991;29: 601–605.

94. Cazzato G, Walton JN. The pathology of the muscle spindle. A study of biopsy material in various muscular and neuromuscular diseases. *J Neurol Sci*. 1968;7:15-70.

95. Kararizou E, Manta P, Kalfakis N, et al. Morphological and morphometrical study of human muscle spindles in Werdnig-Hoffmann disease (infantile spinal muscular atrophy type I). *Acta Histochem*. 2006;108:265–269.

96. Kararizou EG, Manta P, Kalfakis N, et al. Morphologic and morphometrical study of the muscle spindle in muscular dystrophy. *Anal Quant Cytol Histol*. 2007;29:148–152.

97. van der Walt JD, Swash M, Leake J, et al. The pattern of involvement of adult-onset acid maltase deficiency at autopsy. *Muscle Nerve*. 1987;10:272–281.

98. Dawson TP, Neal JW, Llewellyn L, et al. *Neuropathology Techniques*. London, UK: Arnold; 2003.

99. Nestor SL, Bancroft JD. Enzyme histochemistry and its diagnostic applications. *Theory and Practice of Histological Techniques*. Bancforft JD, Gamble M, eds. 6th ed. Philadelphia, PA: Churchill Livingstone; 2008:405–432.

100. Paciello O, Papparella S. Histochemical and immunohistological approach to comparative neuromuscular diseases. *Folia Histochem Cytobiol*. 2009;47:143–152.

101. Komiyama A, Nonaka I, Hirayama K. Muscle pathology in Marinesco-Sjögren syndrome. *J Neurol Sci.* 1989;89:103–113.

102. Clarke NF, North KN. Congenital fiber type disproportion—30 years on. *J Neuropathol Exp Neurol*. 2003;62: 977–989.

103. Raheem O, Huovinen S, Suominen T, et al. Novel myosin heavy chain immunohistochemical double staining developed for the routine diagnostic separation of I, IIA and IIX fibers. *Acta Neuropathol*. 2010;119:495–500.

104. Fanin M, Pegoraro E, Angelini C. Absence of dystrophin and spectrin in regenerating muscle fibers from Becker dystrophy patients. *J Neurol Sci*. 1994;123:88–94.

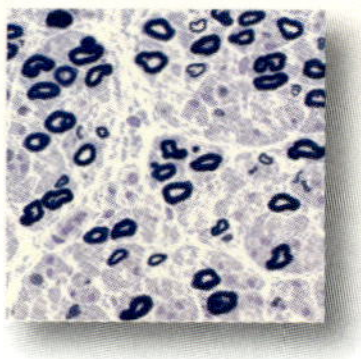
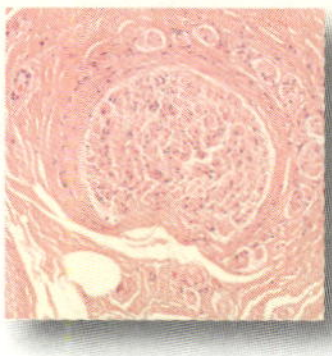
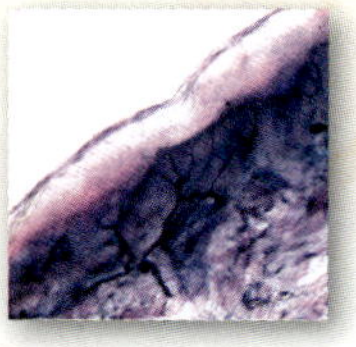

CHAPTER 9

Nonneoplastic Diseases of Peripheral Nerve

Introduction

In practice, many peripheral nerve neoplasms are seen in surgical pathology, soft tissue, and dermatopathology setting since they present as deep or subcutaneous soft tissue masses. While some of those are seen by neuropathologists in consultation, neuropathologists' exposure to the neoplasms of peripheral nerve is mainly limited to those lesions originating from neurosurgery. Nonetheless, many features that characterize the neoplastic proliferations of the peripheral nerve components are discussed in Chapters 1 and 2. In this chapter, the discussion focuses on the features of nonneoplastic lesions seen in the context of peripheral nerve biopsy performed for the evaluation of neurologic disorders. These specimens are essentially limited to sural nerve biopsy specimens, with rare exceptions. This discussion is limited to light microscopic features and aims to provide an initial guidance for the diagnostic approach **(Fig. 9-1)**. It should be kept in mind, however, that the so-called thick sections or semi-thin sections of the epoxy-resin–embedded nerve obtained after glutaraldehyde fixation and special processing are necessary **(Figs. 9-2 and 9-3)**, as is electron microscopy in many cases for appropriate evaluation of the nerve biopsy specimen.[1] Evaluation of semi-thin sections under immersion oil is helpful in providing sufficient detail and electron microscopy, while essential in some situations, is mainly used to confirm the findings identified on semi-thin sections for the most part. Teased fiber preparations[1] are also useful in the evaluation of individual fibers on longitudinal view throughout long segments; however, they are difficult to prepare and require skill, experience, patience, and time, and this method is unfortunately becoming condemned to extinction from routine diagnostic practice. Unfortunately, the information that can be obtained from the evaluation of peripheral nerve biopsy is not high in specificity, with sural nerve biopsy resulting in a specific diagnosis in about 29% of cases and about 14% showing mild or no abnormalities.[2] On the other hand, a previously unsuspected or nonpreferred diagnosis can be made in 14% of patients,[3] and it was found to be essential for correct management in 21% of patients and helpful in an additional 22%.[4] In many situations, a general categorization such as axonopathy or demyelination, providing an additional idea on the activity and the severity of the process, is also very useful, with Guillain-Barré syndrome, vasculitis, hereditary motor and sensory neuropathy (HMSN), leprosy, diabetic neuropathy, and amyloidosis being among the more commonly diagnosed disorders.[2] Many genetic and metabolic diseases of the nerve are now diagnosed using special genetic and biochemical testing with decreasing need for nerve biopsy.[5] As with any other specimens in pathology, but especially as with skeletal muscle biopsy specimens, highly specific and diagnostic findings are rare, and in most cases, a constellation of several features, identified by various modalities, should be interpreted together with clinical and other laboratory data. The purpose of this discussion is to provide guidelines on various abnormal features and on how to identify and interpret them.

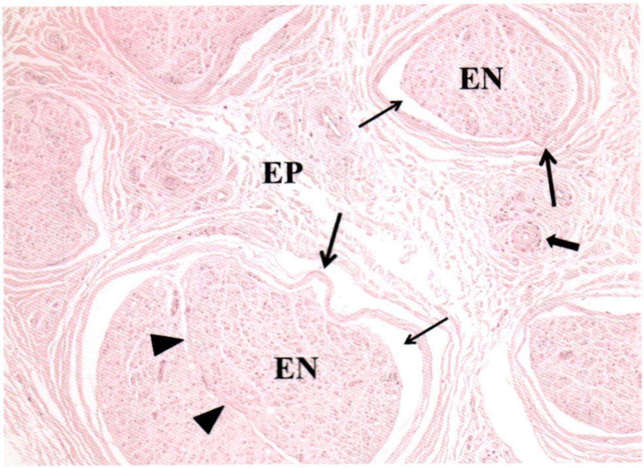

Figure 9-1. Normal compartments of peripheral nerve and fixation artifact: Epineurium (EP) is a loose connective tissue that contains the vessels (*block arrow*) of arteriolar, capillary, and venular types. Endoneurium (EN) is the compartment where the axons are located and is ensheathed by perineurium (*thick arrows*) to form altogether the nerve fascicle. Multiple but variable numbers of fascicles are present within the EN on cross section depending on the particular nerve and the particular site the tissue is obtained. Perineurium can be wrinkled and irregular (*thick arrows*) as an artifact of formalin fixation, which may result in differential shrinkage of tissues to cause separation (*thin arrows*) of EN from perineurium. One of the fascicles appears to be divided into two by a thin connective tissue band (*arrowheads*), possibly close to a branching point (H&E; original magnification: 100×).

Epineurium

Epineurium (EP) is the outermost supportive layer, which consists of loose fibroadipose connective tissue and which is usually not distinguishable as a separate "layer" especially in the more distal nerves, as it merges and is continuous with the surrounding connective tissue **(Fig. 9-1)**. As such, it can be affected by any other pathologic process in the adjacent connective tissues. Systemic diseases, for instance, granulomatous processes and hematolymphoid neoplasms, can be seen in the EP. Specifically for nerve pathology, it can participate in the inflammatory/infectious processes of the nerve. Many of the vasculitides of the nerve are centered in the arterioles, capillaries, and venules located in the EP. Other vasculopathies, for example, amyloidosis, can be identified in the

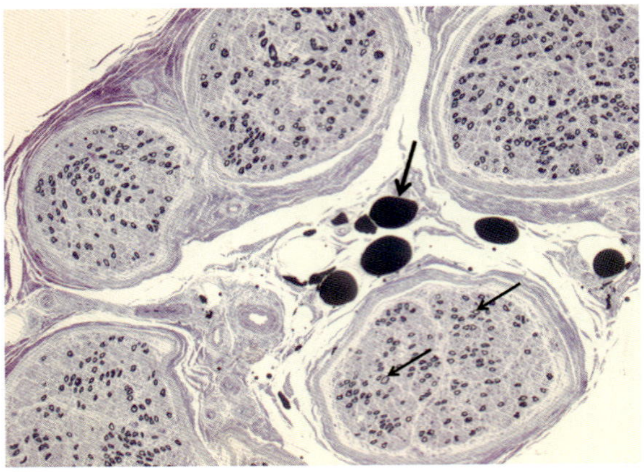

Figure 9-2. Semi-thin section: Although the general structural features are the same as with H&E, their appearances are different. Dark, round, or oval globules in the epineurium (*thick arrow*) represent lipid in the adipocytes. Myelinated nerve fibers (*thin arrows*) in the endoneurium are more prominent due to dark blue staining of their myelin sheaths (Toluidine blue–stained semi-thin epoxy-resin section; original magnification: 100×).

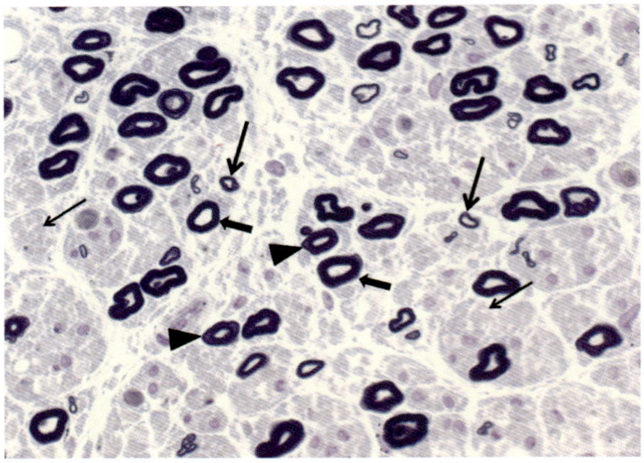

Figure 9-3. Axons and myelin on semi-thin section: *Dark blue* myelin sheaths surround the central pale or clear-appearing area, representing the axon. While large myelinated (*block arrows*) and small myelinated (*thick arrows*) fibers can be easily identified, unmyelinated fibers, which are also the smallest in diameter, are difficult to identify and can be seen as tiny vacuoles (*thin arrows*) embedded in the cytoplasm of Schwann cells associated with them (Remak cells). The myelin sheaths of an occasional large myelinated fiber seem to have a circular pale zone (*arrowheads*), which likely corresponds to Schmidt-Lanterman incisures. Note that the thickness of the myelin sheaths is proportional to the axon caliber. Many fibers are artifactually distorted, when they are supposed to be almost perfectly round (Toluidine blue–stained semi-thin epoxy-resin section; original magnification: 600×).

List of Findings/Checklist for Nonneoplastic Diseases of Peripheral Nerve

AT A GLANCE

Epineurium
- Vascular disorders
- Inflammations/infections
- Acute panautonomic neuropathy (pandysautonomia)
- Various systemic or neighboring processes
- Minifascicles

Perineurium
- Contours of fascicles
- Thickening/fibrosis
    - Chronic neuropathies
    - Morton's neuroma
- Inflammation
    - Idiopathic perineuritis
- Infection
    - Leprosy
- Increased cellularity
    - Regeneration
- Accumulations
    - Calcium
    - Lipid

Subperineurial region
- Shrinkage artifact
- Edema
- Renaut bodies
- Accumulations
    - Mucopolysaccharides
    - Amyloid
    - Cryoglobulin

Endoneurium
- Edema
- Fibrosis/collagenous expansion
- Increased fibrous bands/compartmentalization
- Accumulations
    - Amyloid
    - Immunoglobulins
    - Light chain deposition disease
- Increased cellularity
    - Schwann cells
- Proliferation/regeneration (nuclear changes)
- Nuclear atypia (ataxia-telangiectasia)
    - Onion bulbs (hypertrophic neuropathies)
- Chronic inflammatory demyelinating polyneuropathy (CIDP)
- Genetic diseases (Charcot-Marie-Tooth, Dejerine-Sottas, Refsum)
- POEMS (Crow-Fukase) syndrome
- Toxic neuropathy (tacrolimus, lead)
- Metabolic (diabetes mellitus)
- Paraneoplastic neuropathy
- Storage diseases (Niemann-Pick)
- Mitochondrial disease (mitochondrial neurogastrointestinal encephalomyopathy)
- Leukodystrophy (adrenoleukodystrophy)
- Recurrent compressive neuropathy
    - Pseudo-onion bulbs
- Perineurial cells (intraneural perineurioma)
- Schwann cell basal lamina duplication
- Congenital hypomyelinating neuropathy
- Charcot-Marie-Tooth type 4
- Schwann cells with unmyelinated fibers
- Immature/developing onion bulbs
    - Burnt-out onion bulbs

Hematolymphoid cells
- Lymphocytes
    - Demyelination
    - Infection
- Macrophages
    - Demyelination
    - Axonal degeneration
    - Infection
    - Sarcoidosis
    - Xanthomatous neuropathy
- Polymorphonuclear leukocytes
- Plasma cells
- Mast cells
- Vasculitis (Table 9.1)
- Hematolymphoid malignancies

Vacuolations, inclusions, and accumulations
- Schwann cells
    - Myelin breakdown (digestion chambers)
    - Lipid (Tangier disease, Krabbe disease, Fabry disease)
    - Glycogen (hypothyroidism)
    - Pi granules
    - Pigment (metachromatic leukodystrophy)
    - Chediak-Higashi syndrome
- Fibroblasts
- Perineurial cells
- Endothelial cells
- Foamy macrophages
    - Xanthomatous change
    - Leprosy
- Holes in place of axons

(Continued)

List of Findings/Checklist for Nonneoplastic Diseases of Peripheral Nerve *(Continued)*

AT A GLANCE

Vessels
- Collagenous thickening
- Cellular thickening
- Amyloid accumulation
- Vasculitis (Table 9.1)
- Perivascular lymphocytes
  - Lymphocytic vasculitis/perivasculitis (Table 9.1)
  - Diabetes mellitus
  - Collagen vascular diseases
  - CIDP
  - Acute inflammatory demyelinating polyneuropathy
  - Diabetic neuropathy
  - HIV infection
  - Lyme disease
  - Toxic oil syndrome
  - Lymphoma
  - Paraneoplastic neuropathy
- Petechial hemorrhages
- Endothelial cells
  - Swelling
  - Cytomegalovirus inclusions
  - Lipid accumulation (Fabry disease)
- Subintimal fibrosis (Degos-Kohlmeier syndrome)
- Cerebral autosomal dominant arteriopathy with subcortical infarcts and leukoencephalopathy (CADASIL)

Axons
- Axonal degeneration
- Wallerian degeneration
- Regenerating clusters
- Mixed degeneration–regeneration pattern
- Persistent Schwann cell basal lamina
- Enlargement
  - Giant axonal dystrophy
  - Neuroaxonal dystrophy
  - Polyglucosan bodies
  - Swollen axons
- Atrophy
- Axonal density
- Preferential involvement of fiber types
  - Large myelinated fibers
  - Small myelinated fibers
  - Unmyelinated fibers
- Small fiber neuropathy
  - Skin biopsy

Myelin sheaths
- Myelin loss
  - Primary demyelination
  - Secondary demyelination
  - Myelin debris
- Thin myelin sheaths
- Mixed demyelination–remyelination pattern
- Hypomyelination
- Thick myelin sheaths/hypermyelination
- Shape and appearance of myelin sheaths
  - Curved/irregular shapes
  - Jelly roll appearance
  - Tomaculae
  - Folded myelin sheaths
  - Collapsed/wrinkled myelin sheaths
  - Double-barrel appearance
  - Pale myelin sheaths

Ongoing demyelination and active axonal degeneration

Others
- Ischemic changes
- Heterogeneous involvement of fascicles
- End-stage nerve
- Developing nerve

Special stains and techniques
- Histochemistry
  - Myelin
  - Axons
  - Trichrome
  - Elastic tissue
  - Amyloid
- Immunohistochemistry
  - Neurofilament
  - Epithelial membrane antigen
  - S-100 protein
  - Collagen type IV
  - Lymphoid markers
  - Amyloid markers
- Immunofluorescence microscopy
  - Immunoglobulins (light and heavy chains)
- Epoxy-resin semi-thin sections
  - Toluidine blue
- Electron microscopy

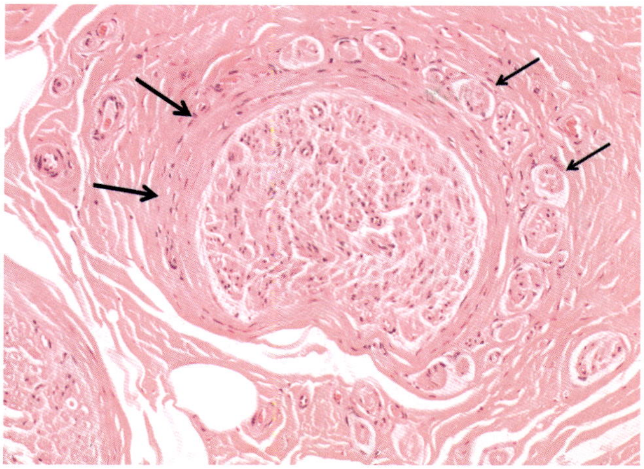

Figure 9-4. Minifascicles: Multiple small fascicles (*thin arrows*) are seen in the EP immediately outside and surrounding the perineurium of the fascicle in the center. Perineurium (*thick arrows*) is thickened and appears fibrotic, possibly due to previous injury or an injury at a different level (H&E; original magnification: 200×).

vessels in this compartment. Many *minifascicles* in the EP immediately outside the perineurium suggest that at some point during the pathologic process, the perineurium may have been involved and damaged,[6] and the sprouting axons grew through the perineurium to proliferate around it **(Fig. 9-4)**. In general, minifascicle formation is a regenerative response in the injured nerve.[7] Similar but more exaggerated versions of this type of proliferation are seen in amputation neuroma **(Fig. 9-5)**.

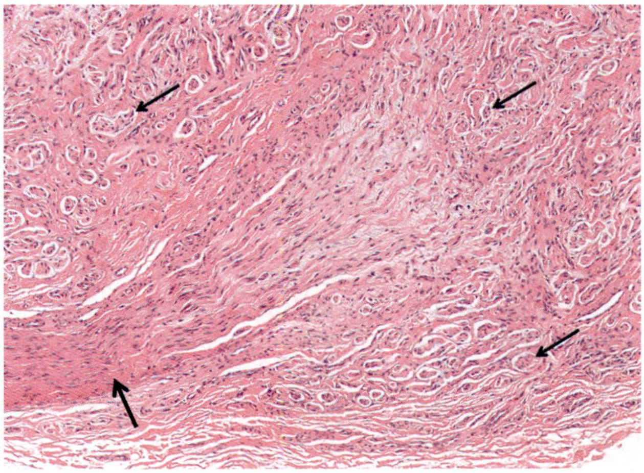

Figure 9-5. Amputation neuroma: A nerve fascicle (*thick arrow*) is proliferating to form numerous minifascicles (*thin arrows*) into which it blends and disappears. This is a desperate attempt of the proximal stump to connect to the distal segment, if any, as part of the regenerative process. Since, however, the distal segment of the nerve has either completely degenerated or is not there anymore as a result of amputation or resection of an organ, such as gallbladder, the disorganized proliferation ends up forming a nodule (H&E; original magnification: 100×).

Perineurium

Wrinkling of the outlines of the fascicles **(Fig. 9-1)** is commonly seen as a result of shrinkage of the tissues due to formalin fixation. This can create a zigzag appearance on longitudinal sections. *Perineurial thickening* **(Fig. 9-4)** may occur as a result of perineuritis, such as seen in leprous neuritis[8] or sensory perineuritis,[9] but can also be seen in association with a wide variety of conditions, such as diabetic neuropathy and rheumatoid arthritis,[10,11] and in idiopathic perineuritis after the exclusion of any other specific etiologies.[4] Increased concentric fibrosis in perineuritis may constrict the nerve, resulting in axonal degeneration. In addition to the presence of any inflammatory cells where applicable, perineurium is thickened and assumes a collagenous appearance. Macrophages, when present, may create a vague granulomatous appearance. Epithelial membrane antigen (EMA) immunohistochemistry may be helpful by highlighting the loss of orderly concentric arrangement of normal perineurium, its thickening and irregularities.[12] In other situations, variable degrees of perineurial fibrosis can be seen together with increased endoneurial collagenization in chronic axonal degenerations. Perineurial cell basement membrane thickening is an electron microscopic finding and is especially prominent in diabetes mellitus.[13] In some cases of nerve damage, perineurial cells show reactive changes and proliferation as part of the regenerative process, for example, in response to regeneration after ischemic damage. In such cases, perineurium may appear thick and cellular, sometimes in an asymmetrical pattern. Extensive fibrous thickening of perineurium, along with degeneration of nerve fibers and endoneurial fibrosis, resulting in prominent atrophy of the nerve fascicles is typical of the biopsy specimens seen in Morton's neuroma[14] **(Fig. 9-6)**, which represents a chronic repeated traumatic injury of the nerve most commonly seen in the interdigital

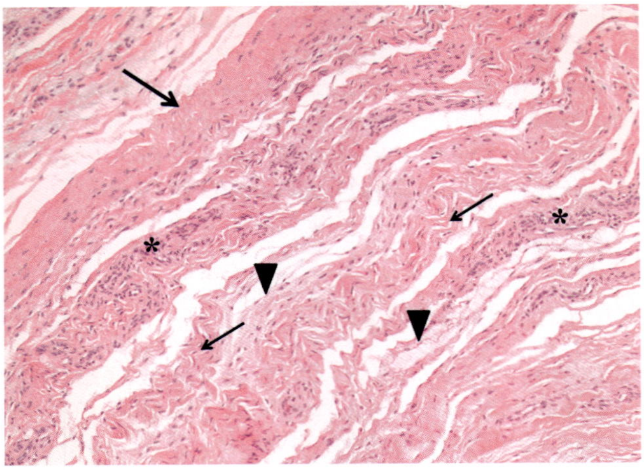

Figure 9-6. Morton's neuroma: This longitudinal section shows atrophic nerve fascicles (*thin arrows*) admixed with fibrotic and edematous endoneurial connective tissue (*arrowheads*). There may be some inflammation and increased vascularity (asterisk). The perineurium (*thick arrow*) and surrounding epineurium and connective tissues are usually fibrotic, and the entire nerve can sometimes be palpated as a thick cord (H&E; original magnification: 100×).

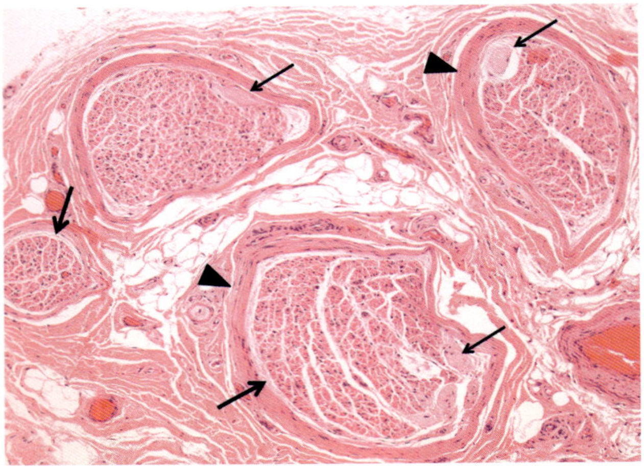

Figure 9-7. Subperineurial edema and Renaut bodies: Subperineurial areas appear concentrically loosely textured and lightly basophilic (*thick arrows*) in subperineurial edema, a nonspecific finding simply indicating injury to the fascicle. There are also basophilic, also loosely textured subperineurial nodules (*thin arrows*) in three larger fascicles. These are Renaut bodies. The perineuria of especially these three larger fascicles show collagenous thickening (*arrowheads*), supporting a chronic traumatic injury or healed inflammatory process (H&E; original magnification: 100×).

nerve between the third and fourth metatarsal bones and less commonly in the prepatellar nerve. Morton's neuroma is different than the amputation neuroma, which represents a haphazard nonneoplastic proliferation of regenerating nerve, forming a nodule **(Fig. 9-5)**, typically seen after transections such as accidents or surgeries. As such, the term traumatic neuroma is sometimes used more comprehensively to cover both of these situations. *Calcium accumulation* selectively in the perineurium has been described as a nonspecific finding in diabetes mellitus and other chronic neuropathies.[15] *Lipid accumulation* in the perineurial cells are seen in Fabry disease.[16,17]

Subperineurial expansion may result from subperineurial edema. Shrinkage artifact associated with formalin fixation can also result in the separation of endoneurium (EN) from perineurium. Subperineurial edema is seen as an expansion of the subperineurial area as a thin and loosely textured connective tissue without dense collagen, although collagen bands can be seen in it **(Fig. 9-7)**. It may push the perineurium outward, resulting in bowing of any septae that traverses subperineurial space. Edema is a nonspecific finding that is commonly associated with many neuropathies but tends to be especially associated with chronic demyelination.[18] *Renaut bodies* **(Fig. 9-7)** are large nodular pools of loosely textured edematous appearing subperineurial structures that are of no known significance, although they apparently increase in number in various pathologic states.[19] Actual Renaut bodies or somewhat similar apparently mucopolysaccharide accumulations can be seen in the EN of fascicles that suffer from chronic repetitive traumatic injury,[20] such as seen in Morton's neuroma (see above). An amorphous material that is not amyloid can accumulate in the subperineurium in chronic inflammatory demyelinating polyneuropathy (CIDP).[21] Amyloid accumulations can also be seen in the subperineurial location, resulting in expansion of this compartment. In an appropriately processed normal nerve tissue, no subperineurial space or expansion should be seen. Carcinoma cells infiltrating the nerve tend to localize subperineurially. Although this is a rare and incidental occurrence in a peripheral nerve biopsy for neurologic problems, it is commonly seen in surgical pathology practice during the evaluation of resection margins and extent of malignancies, especially of the head and neck.

Endoneurium

Endoneurial expansion refers to the increase in the acellular compartment of the EN with an accompanying decrease in the number of axons and is typically due to prominent axon loss and resultant collagenization, such as seen in diabetes mellitus among many others, or an accumulation, such as amyloid,[22] immunoglobulin deposition as seen in dysproteinemic neuropathy and light chain deposition disease.[23] Otherwise, the nerve is not actually thickened or enlarged, but the relative contributions of various components have changed. *Endoneurial edema* is also seen as an expansion of this compartment but with edema, seen as a loose, hypocellular change. It typically accompanies inflammatory processes, such as demyelination and vasculitis **(Fig. 9-8)**. *Fibrous bands* in the EN dividing the fascicle into a few compartments and containing the endoneurial capillaries are normal. Sometimes, they may indicate the branching site of the fascicle **(Fig. 9-1)**. These bands contain perineurial cells. In a fascicle recuperating from an injury, this septation may be exaggerated, resulting in a busy compartmentalization of the EN. The cells in such septae have features of fibroblasts that have not yet developed into perineurial cells, and this can be shown by their lack of positivity for EMA.

Increased endoneurial cellularity can be due to inflammation, but more specifically, a proliferation of Schwann cells as a result of a demyelinating process as well as some degree of endoneurial collapse is also common. This is a subjective finding; however, as with every other feature, a familiarity with "normal" is helpful. A better overall idea about cellularity can be obtained by the evaluation of longitudinal sections, but section thickness variability may become an issue. The nuclei of active *Schwann cells* may appear reactive and enlarged with nucleolar prominence. Extremely large Schwann cell nuclei have been identified in ataxia-telangiectasia.[24] A peculiar concentric Schwann cell proliferation can present with a pattern of *onion bulb formation* **(Fig. 9-9)**. It is described as at least two layers of Schwann cells completely surrounding an axon.[12] Onion bulbing is present around the thinly myelinated axons and indicates a process with repeated

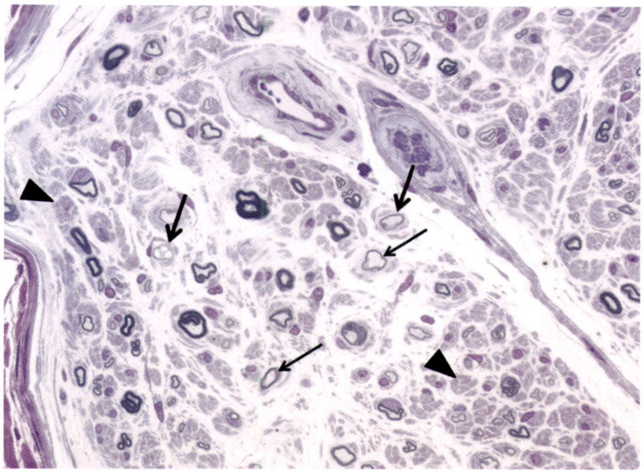

Figure 9-8. Endoneurial edema, thinly myelinated fibers, and immature onion bulbs: There is a prominent loss of small and large myelinated fibers. Endoneurium appears rarified, hypocellular, and loose due to edema, which is also seen in the subperineurium (**upper left**). Many axons are thinly myelinated (*thin arrows*), indicating remyelination. There has apparently been recurrent demyelination and remyelination, as there are some onion bulb–like formations (*thick arrows*), although they are not fully developed and represent immature onion bulbs or a version of pseudo-onion bulbs. Unmyelinated fibers can be seen as tiny vacuoles in groups (*arrowheads*) (Toluidine blue–stained semi-thin epoxy-resin section; original magnification: 400×).

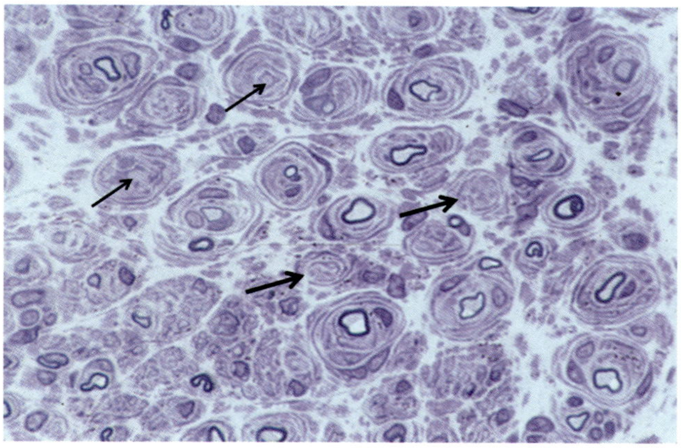

Figure 9-9. Onion bulb formation: Many nerve fibers are surrounded by concentric proliferations of Schwann cells, resulting in a multilayered structure. Many of them contain a central axon with a myelin sheath that is thin relative to the axon caliber. Some onion bulbs have a central axon that is difficult to see due to the absence of myelin (*thin arrows*), while some other onion bulbs contain no axons (*thick arrows*), that is, burnt-out onion bulbs, in this hypertrophic neuropathic process (Toluidine blue–stained semi-thin epoxy-resin section; original magnification: 400×).

demyelination and remyelination; hence, the central axon typically has a thin myelin sheath as part of remyelination process or is devoid of myelin. CIDP, also considered as chronic Guillain-Barré syndrome, is characterized by onion bulbing, with or without a residual inflammatory component, although onion bulbs are seen in a subpopulation of cases and their absence should not exclude this diagnosis.[21] The myelinated fiber population is also decreased and variable degrees of endoneurial edema can be seen.[25] Other diseases associated with onion bulb formation can be genetic, Charcot-Marie-Tooth (CMT), Dejerine-Sottas (CMT type 3), and Refsum disease,[26,27] where the onion bulb formation is uniformly prominent, in contrast to CIDP, where it appears heterogeneous with onion bulbs at different stages of development, with or without inflammation and variable endoneurial edema. A CIDP-like picture can be associated with POEMS (polyneuropathy, organomegaly, endocrinopathy, M-protein, and skin changes) syndrome, diabetic neuropathy, as part of a paraneoplastic neuropathy in association with malignancy,[28] sarcoidosis and vasculitis,[29] and tacrolimus toxicity.[30] Onion bulbs are most prominent in CMT type 1 (formerly known as HMSN type 1) and are essentially absent in CMT type 2 (formerly known as HMSN type 2; axonal form of CMT disease), while CMT type X appears to have some onion bulbs and pseudo-onion bulbs (see pseudo-onion bulbs below).[27] Lead neuropathy,[31] compressive neuropathy,[32] adrenoleukodystrophy,[33] mitochondrial neurogastrointestinal encephalomyopathy, and Niemann-Pick disease can also have onion bulb formation.[21] Some onion bulb structures are formed by concentric basal lamina reduplication, rather than actual Schwann cell cytoplasms, and require electron microscopy for identification. They have been described in congenital hypomyelinating neuropathy[34] and CMT type 4.[21] The central axon in some onion bulbs may eventually degenerate, leaving the concentric Schwann cell proliferation behind, which is called *burnt-out onion bulb* **(Fig. 9-9)**. The group of diseases associated with onion-bulb formation is descriptively referred to as *hypertrophic neuropathies* due to the thickening of the nerve, sometimes including the following disorders. Intraneural perineurioma is characterized by perineurial cell proliferations around axons, resulting in onion bulb appearance, and is referred to as *pseudo-onion bulb*.[35] Since they are perineurial cells and not Schwann cells, they are positive for EMA and negative for S-100 protein and lack the pericellular collagen type IV staining by immunohistochemistry. Intraneural perineurioma causes focal thickening of the nerve. Though the terms may sometimes be used interchangeably, localized hypertrophic neuropathy is another lesion that, as the name implies, causes a focal hypertrophy of the nerve and is characterized by onion bulbs formed by Schwann cells. It is thought to be a focal, nonneoplastic, and reactive process.[36] To add to the possible confusion caused by this sophisticated terminology on onion bulbs, it should be noted that the term pseudo-onion bulb can sometimes also be used to describe an onion bulb structure that is formed by a central myelinated fiber surrounded by the Schwann cells associated with unmyelinated fibers, representing a sprouting axon, that is, a regenerative cluster. This particular arrangement has been described in CMT type X.[21] Rarely, pseudo-onion bulb may be used to refer to early, immature, or false onion bulb–like structures that have not yet fully developed to fulfill the rule of two concentric layers of Schwann cells **(Fig. 9-8)**.

Hematolymphoid Cells

Lymphocytes can be present around the endoneurial vessels and are usually associated with a demyelinating process. The perivascular distribution of the lymphocytic infiltrate may be difficult to appreciate in the EN, especially on longitudinal sections. Perineuritis shows a lymphocytic infiltration centered in the perineurium. Lymphocytes in the EP are quite nonspecific but may be seen in inflammatory/infectious disorders involving other compartments of the nerve, in vasculitis, and also in cases of acute panautonomic neuropathy (pandysautonomia),[37,38] the latter along with a relative loss of small myelinated and unmyelinated fibers. Lymphocyte subsets may provide additional supportive information for the diagnosis. For instance, CD4-positive T cells are predominant in Guillain-Barré syndrome (acute inflammatory demyelinating polyneuropathy; AIDP), while CD8-positive T cells are predominant in the AIDP seen in the context of HIV infection and can be otherwise identical to the typical (AIDP).[39] Same is true for the CIDP[40] in which T-cell subsets are variable and HIV-associated CIDP,[41] in which CD8-positive T-cells predominate. *Macrophages* should alert one to the

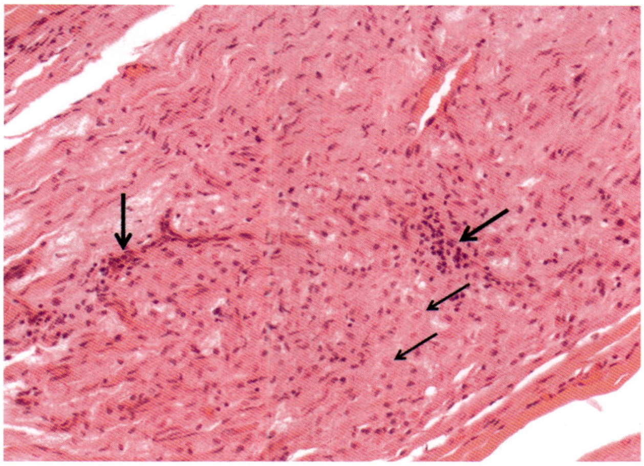

Figure 9-10. Endoneurial inflammation: There is a predominantly lymphocytic infiltrate in the endoneurium on this longitudinal section of the nerve. This infiltrate is more prominent around the endoneurial capillaries (*thick arrows*). Scattered macrophages (*thin arrows*) are also suspected based on their nuclear features. The foamy or granular appearance in the background likely represents degenerating myelin, although some may be associated with foamy macrophages. While the findings on H&E are nonspecific, they are suspicious for AIDP (Guillain-Barré syndrome) in the correct clinicopathologic setting and should be further evaluated by semi-thin sections (H&E; original magnification: 200×).

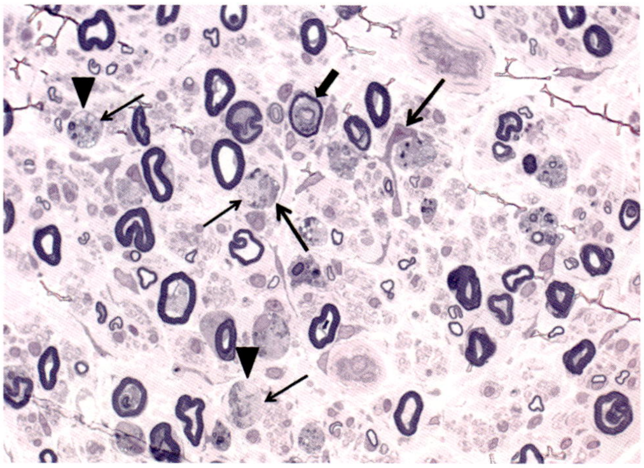

Figure 9-11. Macrophage-mediated demyelination: A prominent loss of myelinated fibers is seen. The myelin sheaths of several fibers are degenerating and appear as granular blue debris (*thin arrows*). Although this may be difficult to distinguish from a degenerating axon (see Fig. 9-14), the axons can still be identified in this picture along with some of the debris as a round-to-oval structure (*arrowheads*). In addition, the macrophages, which can also be seen in axonal degeneration, are in very close association with the degenerating myelin in this case, essentially "hugging" the degenerating myelin (*thick arrows*). Some myelin sheaths are in the early stages of degeneration (*block arrow*) and may show by electron microscopic evaluation the macrophages actively stripping the myelin from the axon (Toluidine blue–stained semi-thin epoxy-resin section; original magnification: 600×).

possibility of demyelination, and myelin breakdown products should be sought in their cytoplasm. They are also present in association with axonal degeneration, as they need to clean up the debris from axons and myelin, as well. The distinction of Guillain-Barré syndrome from other types of demyelination may be difficult or even impossible solely based on histologic evaluation. In Guillain-Barré syndrome,[42] a lymphocytic inflammation is also commonly present, especially in the most commonly recognized clinicopathologic form, AIDP **(Fig. 9-10)**, but may not be so obvious in other forms, for example, axonal forms, which presents predominantly with axonal degeneration (acute motor axonal neuropathy), where macrophages tend to be underneath the myelin sheaths but leaving them intact.[43] Regardless, the main and diagnostic finding in AIDP form of Guillain-Barré syndrome is the identification of macrophages in close association with myelin sheaths **(Fig. 9-11)**, seen as stripping the myelin sheaths by electron microscopy, or at least their identification immunohistochemically by macrophage markers in close association with the myelin sheaths. Otherwise, it may be difficult to distinguish active axonal degeneration from demyelination and to decide whether the thinly myelinated axons are remyelinating after demyelination or as part of regeneration of axons. In such situations, the identification of degenerating axons and regenerative clusters favors axonal degeneration as the primary process. AIDP-like picture has been seen in association with suramin toxicity[44] and as part of a paraneoplastic neuropathy associated with Hodgkin[45] and non-Hodgkin lymphoma[46] as well as leukemia[47] and in association with chemotherapy.[48] Granulomas associated with a variety of etiologies, including leprosy, can be identified and are in general similar to those seen in other sites. Endoneurial microgranulomas can be seen in pure neuritic leprosy, the diagnosis of which is mainly by peripheral nerve biopsy.[49] Lipid-laden foamy macrophages (also see Vacuolations below) may infiltrate

TABLE 9.1 Typical features of vasculitides commonly seen in peripheral nerve

Predominantly Involved Vessel	Inflammatory Cells	Vasculitis Type	Other Features
Medium and small arteries, epineurial arterioles	Fibrinoid necrosis n-PMNL, e-PMNL, lymphocytes, histiocytes, granulomas	Polyarteritis nodosa	
Epineurial arterioles, capillaries, and venules	Fibrinoid necrosis n-PMNL, e-PMNL, lymphocytes, histiocytes, granulomas	Churg-Strauss syndrome	PR3-ANCA +
Epineurial arterioles, capillaries, and venules	Fibrinoid necrosis Necrotizing granulomas Lymphocytes, n-PMNL	Wegener's granulomatosis	MPO-ANCA +
Endoneurial capillaries	Fibrinoid necrosis n-PMNL, leukocytoclasia	Microscopic polyangiitis	MPO-ANCA +
Epineurial arterioles, capillaries, venules, and endoneurial capillaries	Variable, like any of the above (Intimal proliferation in rheumatoid arthritis)	Collagen vascular diseases	Immune complex deposition in vessels, cryoglobulins in cryoglobulinemic vasculitis
Epineurial arterioles, capillaries, venules, and endoneurial capillaries	Mostly T cells, No B cells, Perivascular No vascular damage	Lymphocytic vasculitis (perivasculitis)	

n-PMNL, neutrophil polymorphonuclear leukocytes; e-PMNL, eosinophil polymorphonuclear leukocytes; PR3-ANCA, cytoplasmic antineutrophil cytoplasmic antibody (cANCA); MPO-ANCA, perinuclear antineutrophil cytoplasmic antibody (pANCA).

the perineurium in the so-called xanthomatous neuropathy, which has been described in association with primary biliary cirrhosis,[50] hyperlipidemia,[51] and Fabry disease.[52] A vague granulomatous appearance can occur in cases of severe idiopathic perineuritis and should not be misinterpreted as sarcoidosis or an infectious process. Inflammation around the vessels should be evaluated for the presence of an actual *vasculitis* **(Table 9.1)**. The general features of vasculitis are similar to those seen in other sites,[53–56] although detailed diagnostic criteria have been outlined for vasculitic neuropathy.[57,58] It is typically identified in the EP, but this may require the examination of multiple additional sections due its focal nature **(Fig. 9-12)**, so much so that combined muscle and nerve biopsy has been found to increase the diagnostic yield.[59] Perivascular lymphocytes and vasculitis features can be seen in association with sarcoidosis and may result in ischemic changes and axonal degeneration. *Polymorphonuclear (PMN) leukocytes* are seen in cases of vasculitis and infections. Some degree of PMN leukocyte extravasation may raise suspicion for vasculitis in the right context, but the possibility that this may be related to procedure lasting longer than usual should be ruled out. *Plasma cells* also participate in many inflammatory conditions, including vasculitis and CIDP. A few *mast cells* are normally found in the EN and EP. They show variable and nonspecific increase in number in various pathologic states. Rarely, mast cells with extremely enlarged granules have been observed in association with Chediak-Higashi syndrome.[60] Involvement of peripheral nerve by *lymphomas and plasma cell myeloma* is also possible, with features

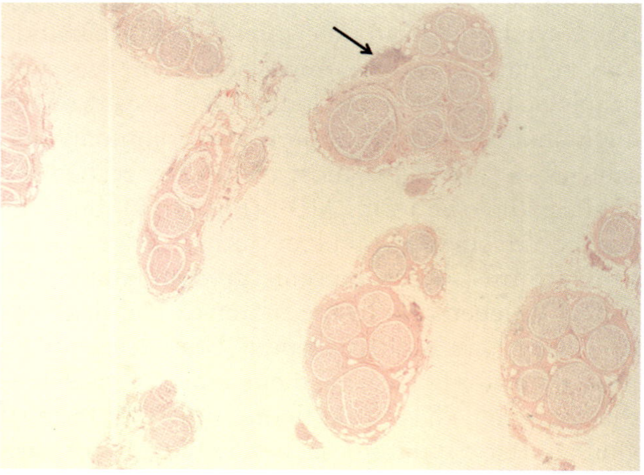

Figure 9-12. Vasculitis: Of multiple cross sections in this picture and many levels, only one epineurial focus (*arrow*) shows the vascular lesion, attesting to the notoriously focal nature of these lesions (H&E; original magnification: 40×).

similar to general features of these neoplasms. This may be secondary to a systemic malignancy or in the form of a primary involvement, that is, neurolymphomatosis, although the term can be used for any involvement of peripheral nervous system by lymphoma.[61] These may masquerade as inflammation and may mimic inflammatory diseases such Guillain-Barré syndrome.

Vacuolations, Accumulations, and Inclusions

Various *vacuolations and accumulations* can be seen in various cells. Vacuoles seen on longitudinal sections may be *digestion chambers* in the Schwann cells with granular debris representing myelin breakdown **(Fig. 9-13)**. They represent ongoing axonal and/or myelin degeneration and can be seen on paraffin sections. Some of the granular material represent myelin breakdown products and can be highlighted by myelin stains. Cytoplasmic vacuolations in Schwann cells may be seen in Tangier disease,[62] a lipid metabolism disorder, and represent dissolved lipid droplets during paraffin processing. They can be seen in endothelial cells and pericytes, also.[63] Accumulation of glycogen in Schwann cells may appear as vacuolations and can be seen in the neuropathy associated with hypothyroidism. Similar glycogen accumulation is also present in perineurial cells, in endothelial cells, and in the axons.[64] *Fibroblast vacuolation* has been seen in cases of hereditary sensory neuropathies and in hypertrophic neuropathies.[65] *Foam cells* are vacuolated macrophages and can be present in the EN in leprosy, called lepra cells,[66] as well as in other conditions where various lipid substances can accumulate in their cytoplasm, such as leukodystrophies. *Mycobacterium leprae* may be seen as blue dots within the vacuoles on semi-thin sections and can be confirmed by acid-fast stains. Although technically there should not be any *holes in the tissue*, sometimes there may be a hole in place of an axon. These likely are artifacts, may represent retraction of the axon during processing, and very rarely, may be related to a degenerating axon[12] **(Fig. 9-14)**. *Inclusions* in Schwann cell cytoplasm can be seen. Some Schwann cells can have granular material in

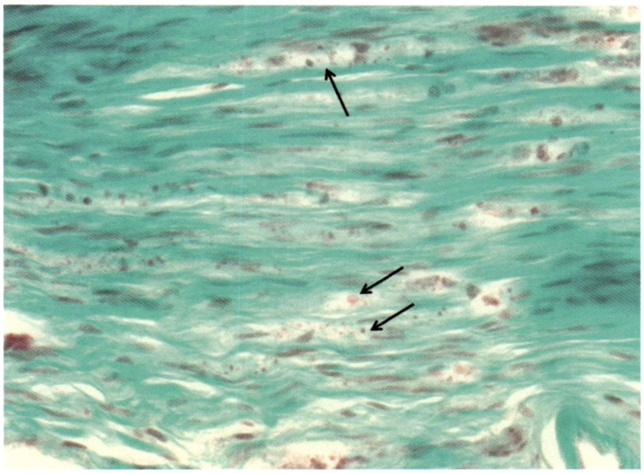

Figure 9-13. Degenerating myelin: On this longitudinal section, the nerve fascicle is essentially entirely devoid of myelin, although this trichrome stain is not ideal for this type of evaluation. Many granules and vacuoles (*arrows*) are seen with red fragments representing degenerating myelin. This does not, however, indicate whether the primary process is demyelination or axonal degeneration with secondary myelin degeneration. The observation that the fascicle appears somewhat cellular may suggest that there is a component of axon loss (Gomori's trichrome; original magnification: 400×).

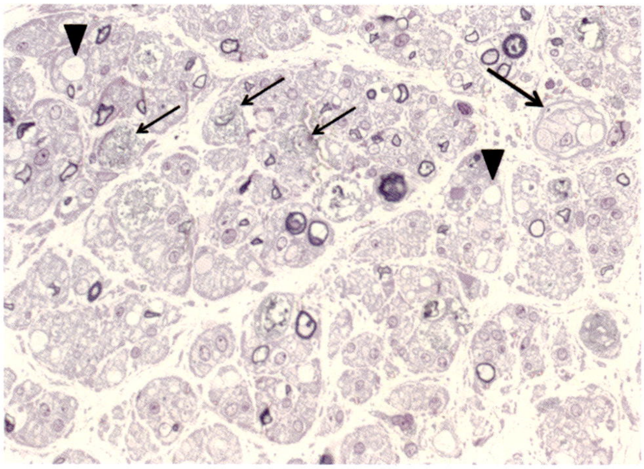

Figure 9-14. Axonal degeneration: Many fibers, both axons and myelin, are degenerating and are seen as round structures with granular debris (*thin arrows*). The fascicle shows prominent fiber loss. Several vacuoles (*arrowheads*) likely represent spaces left from recently degenerated axons in this context, although some of them may be artifact. An endoneurial capillary has reactive changes with swollen endothelial cells (*thick arrow*) (Toluidine blue–stained semithin epoxy-resin section; original magnification: 400×).

their cytoplasm, accumulating typically in the perinuclear location. These are called *Pi (π) granules (of Reich)*. They have no known significance and seem to increase with age. When present, they are in the cytoplasm of Schwann cells associated with myelinated fibers or demyelinated fibers, but not in Remak cells, which are the Schwann cells associated with unmyelinated fibers. They may resemble lipofuscin pigment and are metachromatic with toluidine blue[12] on paraffin sections and are seen as clear, somewhat rectangular holes on epoxy-resin sections. Metachromatic accumulations in Schwann cells and macrophages, together with myelin loss, are also seen in metachromatic leukodystrophy.[67] Peripheral nerve biopsy in this and other leukodystrophies is typically not performed as their diagnoses can now be made by biochemical and genetic testing. Other rare inclusions in Schwann cells may be seen in Chediak-Higashi syndrome.[68]

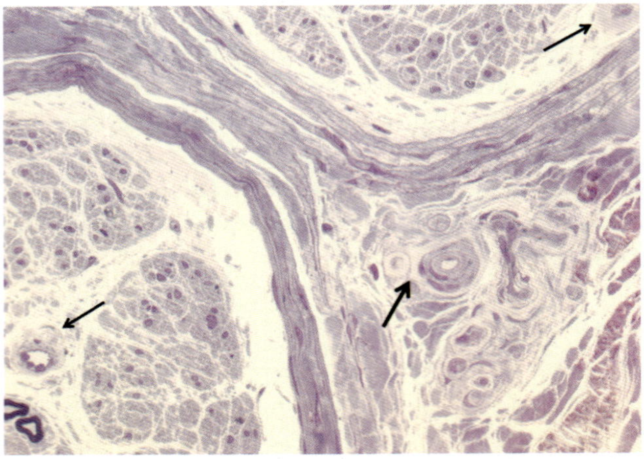

Figure 9-16. Amyloid neuropathy: Both endoneurial (*thin arrows*) and epineurial (*thick arrow*) vessels are thickened with homogeneous amorphous accumulations. The fascicles show severe fiber loss with only a rare myelinated fiber remaining (**lower left**). Special stains and electron microscopic evaluation are needed for confirmation of amyloid (Toluidine blue–stained semi-thin epoxy-resin section; original magnification: 400×).

Vascular Features

Vascular changes can be seen in different compartments. *Collagenous thickening of endoneurial vessels* **(Fig. 9-15)** is a change associated with chronic conditions but is also seen with increasing age.[69] It is also commonly associated with diabetic neuropathy. This vascular change appears in parallel with the endoneurial collagen increase in chronic conditions associated with axonal degeneration and gradual loss of axons. It consists of multiple layers of reduplicated basement membrane and can be seen by electron microscopy or highlighted by collagen type IV immunohistochemistry. A similar thickening can be seen due to amyloid accumulation.[22] As in elsewhere, it results in a bright eosinophilic thickening of the vessel wall and is seen as pale blue amorphous thickening of the vessel wall on semi-thin sections **(Fig. 9-16)**, which may have irregular borders spreading into the EN. A *cellular or hyalinized thickening of vessels* can be associated with diabetes mellitus and can result in ischemic changes.[70] *Thickening of basal laminae*, especially relatively easily seen in Schwann cells, is an electron microscopic finding. In general by light microscopy, variable loss of the involved fiber types, thickening of endoneurial vessel walls due to basement membrane reduplication and collagen accumulation,[71] and collagenous expansion of the EN are seen. Various types of *vasculitides* can commonly involve the peripheral nerves[53–58] **(Table 9.1)**. The changes may be of active vasculitis with

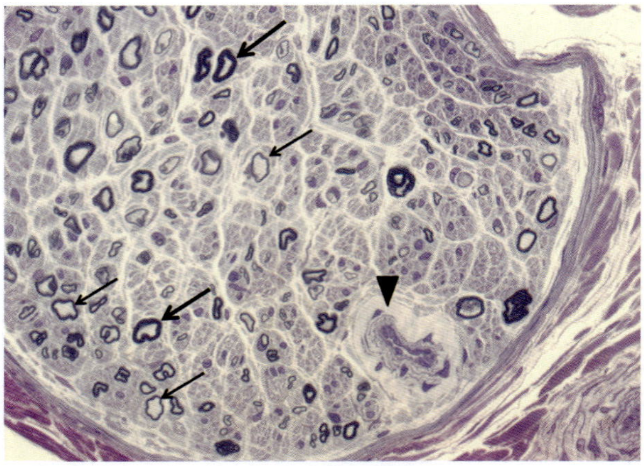

Figure 9-15. Thick endoneurial capillary: An endoneurial capillary is concentrically thickened with a collagenous wall (*arrowhead*), a common nonspecific finding that can be seen more commonly with aging and diabetes mellitus. There is prominent loss of myelinated fibers with scattered thinly myelinated fibers (*thin arrows*) as well as unremarkable fibers with apparently normal myelin thickness (*thick arrows*) (Toluidine blue–stained semi-thin epoxy-resin section; original magnification: 400×).

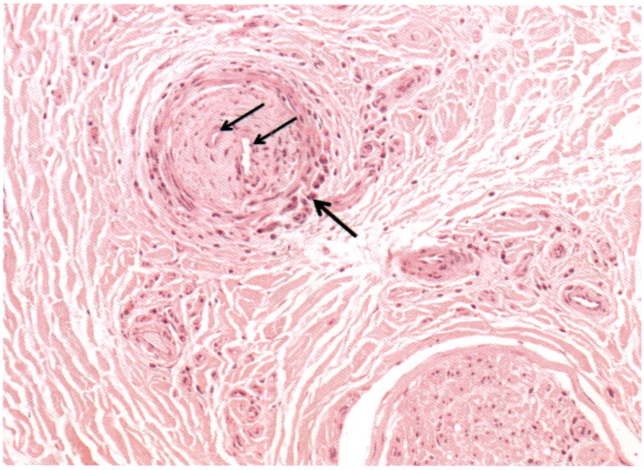

Figure 9-17. Vasculitis: The lumen is obliterated apparently by a recanalized thrombus, resulting in multiple channels (*thin arrows*). A few residual inflammatory cells are still seen around the vessel (*thick arrow*) in this burnt-out or healed lesion (H&E; original magnification: 100×).

features characteristic of the type of vasculitis, or only thrombosed, recanalized, fibrotic vessels with some perivascular lymphocytes and hemosiderin pigment can be left as a residual lesion from a healed or burnt-out lesion **(Figs. 9-17 and 9-18)**. The presence of perivascular lymphocytes without infiltration of vessel walls and without vascular damage has been termed *lymphocytic vasculitis or perivasculitis*.[72] It is quite nonspecific with associations from actual vasculitis to collagen vascular diseases, infections and neoplastic processes, CIDP, and Guillain-Barré syndrome.[73,74] The lymphocytes are typically essentially all T-cells. A vasculitis-like microscopic picture with epineurial perivascular lymphocytes but with no vascular damage, together with perineurial thickening and variable axon loss in different fascicles, has been described in a form of diabetic neuropathy called diabetic lumbosacral radiculoplexus neuropathy.[75] A perivascular lymphocytic infiltrate around endoneurial vessels can be seen as part of the vasculitis seen in the setting of HIV infection, although microscopic findings can show any changes seen in various vasculitides.[76] Diffuse infiltrative lymphocytosis syndrome seen in the setting of HIV infection is also characterized by endoneurial and epineurial perivascular lymphocytic infiltrates.[77] A similar picture may also be identified in Lyme disease,[78] which can also involve perineurium.[79] Perivascular inflammation in all compartments of the nerve with or without vasculitis and sometimes together with eosinophil PMN leukocytes can be associated with toxic oil syndrome.[80–82] *Pacinian corpuscle*, the end organ responsible for detection of vibration, consists of concentric and loosely arranged layers of perineurial-like cells around a central axon. It can be seen in the EP, and may sometimes be next to nerve fascicles and should not be confused with a concentrically thickened, thrombosed, or organized vessel **(Fig. 9-19)**. Pacinian corpuscles may be involved in inflammatory processes affecting the nerve, which may make their recognition difficult. They may lose their central axon if associated with diseased nerves, together with the axon loss seen in their parent nerve.[26] *Petechial or larger hemorrhages* can be seen as a result of systemic hemorrhagic diatheses and can be difficult clinically to distinguish from vasculitis. *Swelling of endothelial cells*, indicating possible damage to the blood–nerve barrier at least in some situations, is a nonspecific finding but can be seen in those situations associated with endoneurial edema. Such changes have been described in POEMS syndrome.[83]

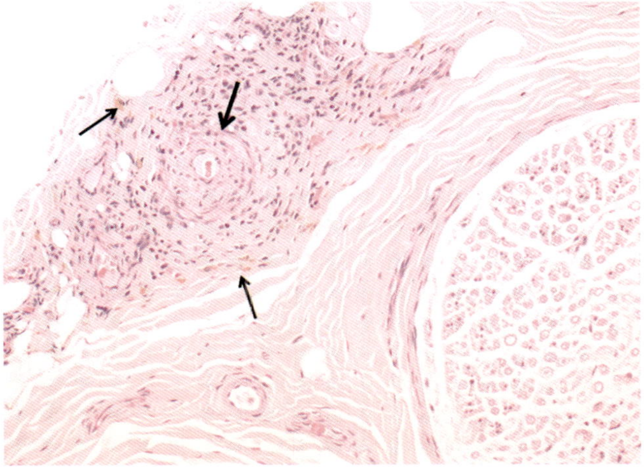

Figure 9-18. Vasculitis: An epineurial arteriole is thickened (*thick arrow*) and considerable perivascular inflammatory infiltrate still present. Although no infiltration of the vessel wall, or definitive features of vascular damage, such as fibrinoid necrosis, thrombosis in the lumen, or endothelial changes are seen, there is perivascular hemosiderin pigment (*thin arrows*), indicating previous vascular damage and leakage (H&E; original magnification: 100×).

Cytomegalovirus (CMV) inclusions can be present in the endothelial cells in CMV infection, with secondary inflammatory and/or ischemic damage

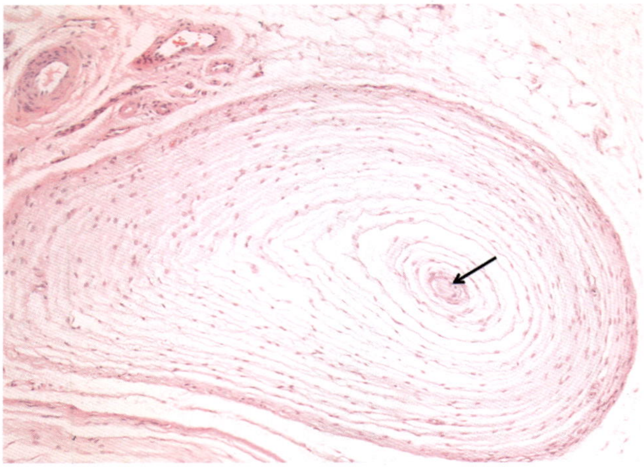

Figure 9-19. Pacinian corpuscle: Concentric loose layers of perineurial-like cells surround a central axon (*arrow*), which may be lost if affected by the axonal degenerating process that involves the nerve (H&E; original magnification: 100×).

in the nerve fascicles.[84] Rare and peculiar conditions involving the vessels can result in distinct syndromes. *Degos-Kohlmeier syndrome (malignant atrophic papulosis)* results in prominent subintimal fibrosis in the arterioles, with gradual obliteration of the lumen. Although it typically involves gastrointestinal tract, skin, and central nervous system,[85] involvement of peripheral nerve vessels can rarely be seen.[86] *Lipid accumulation* can be seen in the cytoplasm of endothelial and smooth muscle cells of the vessels in Fabry disease.[87] Cerebral autosomal dominant arteriopathy with subcortical infarcts and leukoencephalopathy (CADASIL) involves the arterioles in the peripheral nerve, where granular periodic acid-Schiff (PAS)-positive accumulations corresponding electron microscopically to granular osmiophilic material associated with smooth muscle and basement membranes are seen, requiring electron microscopic evaluation for definitive diagnosis.[88]

Axons

The main and most dramatic finding seen in *axons* is *axonal degeneration*. Any pathologic process that involves the axons can be associated with axonal degeneration. The number of degenerating axons may vary from rare to many. They may or may not be accompanied by other features to help further characterize this axonal degeneration. Axonal degeneration is difficult to identify on paraffin sections and is better seen on semi-thin sections as granular debris in place of an axon **(Fig. 9-14)**. While the identification of axon loss is relatively easy, its cause is usually not obvious in the tissue sample. Many disorders that are associated with axonal degeneration and subsequent loss, for example, vasculitis at another level of the nerve, or axonopathies related to toxic and neurodegenerative diseases; diseases involving the neuron cell body, that is, neuronopathy such as involvement of dorsal root ganglia; and some forms of paraneoplastic neuropathies associated with solid neoplasms present in a similar manner in the nerve biopsy specimen. To further complicate the interpretation, some disorders are typically focal, notable examples being vasculitis **(Fig. 9-12)** and amyloidosis, and the actual diagnostic changes may not be present in the tissue examined. Macrophages are present to clear up the debris from degenerating axons and myelin (see "Macrophages" above); however, in contrast to demyelination, they are not identified in close association with myelin sheaths stripping them off the axons. Metabolic disorders associated with vitamin deficiencies, diabetes mellitus, toxins and medications, paraneoplastic conditions, and endocrine disorders may result in a nonspecific neuropathic process characterized by axonal degeneration. In such cases, the clinical investigation sheds light to the potential cause, and a nerve biopsy is typically not needed. The presence of *regenerating clusters*, which are clusters of several thinly myelinated fibers, indicates axonal sprouting, with associated remyelination **(Fig. 9-20)**. In other words, they indicate the regeneration of previously damaged axons and suggest a primarily axonal process. *Persistent Schwann cell basal lamina* represents the remaining basal lamina of the Schwann cell that used to surround a myelinated fiber before that fiber degenerated. The basal lamina is seen as a circular structure and may contain a regenerating cluster in its center as a result of sprouting of that axon. This finding strongly suggests diabetic neuropathy as it is commonly seen in that condition.[89]

A distinct form of axonal degeneration is *Wallerian degeneration*. It refers to a series of quite constant chronologic events involving sequential degeneration and subsequent regeneration of the

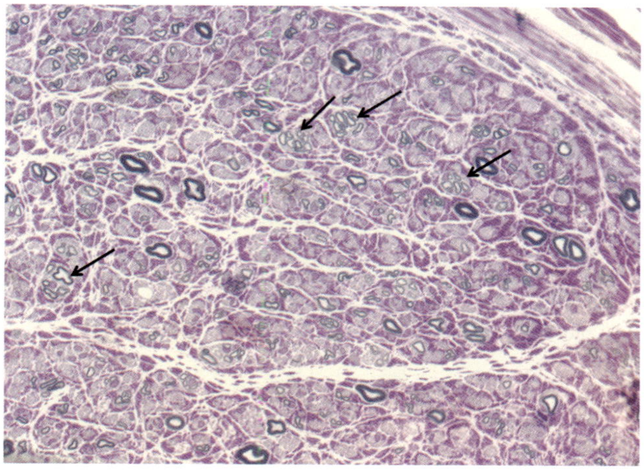

Figure 9-20. Regenerating clusters: In this fascicle with prominent fiber loss, there are groups of smaller and thinly myelinated fibers (*arrows*). They represent sprouting axons after axonal degeneration, which are also remyelinating as part of this regenerative process. No active axonal degeneration is seen in this picture, however (H&E; original magnification: 400×).

axon distal to a specific injury site, such as crush injury, transection, or vasculitic damage. As such, when a nerve biopsied from a site distal to the injury site is examined, fairly uniform and homogeneous changes are seen in fascicles, the degeneration being uniformly at the same stage of development. In other types of axonal degeneration, especially in chronic neuropathies where the multiple and metachronous insults cause axonal degeneration, it is possible to find coexisting degeneration and regeneration, that is, regenerating clusters, and the axonal degeneration tends to be in different stages of progression.[21] Nonetheless, some cases may be difficult to definitively distinguish, and the terms Wallerian degeneration and axonal degeneration are sometimes used interchangeably, though inaccurately. Wallerian degeneration has been identified, for unknown reasons, in porphyric neuropathy.[90,91]

Enlargement of axons by basophilic or amphophilic round accumulations is seen in *giant axonal dystrophy (or neuropathy)*.[92,93] It is characterized by scattered extremely enlarged axons due to neurofilament accumulation, which are seen as fusiform axonal expansions on longitudinal sections. Usually, the giant axons are scattered in a background of unremarkable axons. They have thin myelin sheaths or no myelin. Similar giant axons may be seen in disulfiram toxicity.[94] *Neuroaxonal dystrophy*[21,95] is characterized by round expansions of axons similar to axonal spheroids. Only a rare axonal spheroid is seen in any given fascicle. They are PAS positive, but in contrast to polyglucosan bodies, they are also positive by silver stains (such as Bielschowsky) and by neurofilament immunohistochemistry. Dystrophic axons may be identical to giant axons by light microscopy but are different electron microscopically.[92] They are also seen in Niemann-Pick disease type C.[96] What appears to be giant axons may represent *polyglucosan bodies* in polyglucosan body disease[97] **(Fig. 9-21)**, where round, amorphous, lightly basophilic structures are found within the axons of myelinated fibers. They have ill-defined concentric laminations reminiscent of corpora amylacea and are PAS positive. They are not diagnostic of polyglucosan body disease and can also be seen in Andersen disease (glycogen storage disease type IV)[98] and other conditions, including, normally, aging.[99] *Swollen axons* can be seen in glycogen storage disease type 3 (Cori-Forbes disease) as a result of glycogen accumulation in the axon in addition to in the cytoplasm of Schwann cells and in the EN.[100] Scattered swollen axons are seen in glue-sniffing neuropathy.[101,102]

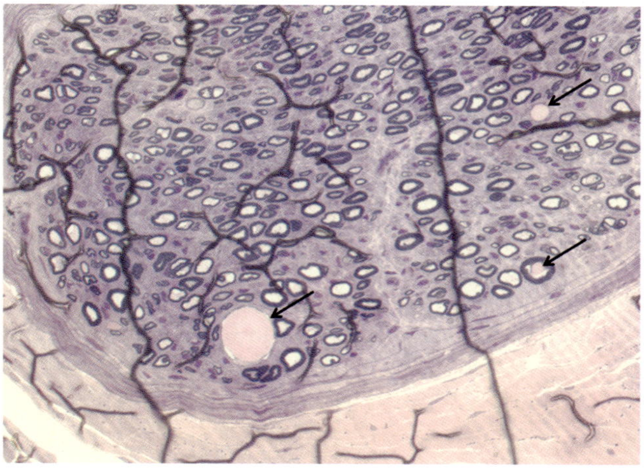

Figure 9-21. Polyglucosan bodies: Pale, round structures are present (*arrows*) in three fibers, which have very thin myelin sheaths, except for the fiber that contains the smallest polyglucosan body. The largest polyglucosan body shows a faint concentric lamination, reminiscent of the corpora amylacea in the central nervous system (Toluidine blue–stained semi-thin epoxy-resin section; original magnification: 400×).

They are larger than the general population of axons due to neurofilament accumulation and have relatively thin myelin sheaths. In contrast, *atrophy of the axons* can be seen and may mimic thick myelin sheaths. While it may be difficult to assess the axon and myelin thickness and their ratios, and morphometric studies may be required, in general, axonal atrophy has been described in HMSNs,[103] hereditary sensory and autonomic neuropathies (HSANs),[104] Friedreich's ataxia,[105] some toxic and metabolic conditions and uremia,[106] and HIV neuropathy.[107] Atrophic axons collapse and the myelin sheaths assume an irregularly wrinkled appearance, which may mimic artifact.

Although morphometric evaluation is available, a semiquantitative evaluation of axon loss can be performed **(Fig. 9-3)**, which requires familiarity with the "normal" *density of small and large myelinated axons and unmyelinated axons*, which in turn are dependent on age[69] and location.[108] The latter does not become an issue as sural nerve is the nerve that is biopsied almost exclusively. Sural nerve is exclusively a sensory nerve. In some cases where both muscle and sural nerve are biopsied, muscle may show prominent neurogenic atrophy, and sural nerve may appear entirely unremarkable if the pathologic process is limited to motor nerves. This situation may cause confusion for and questioning of the diagnosis by the unwary. Though they are readily identifiable on semi-thin sections, axons can be made more prominent on paraffin sections by special stains for myelin, which helps provide an indirect idea only about myelinated fibers, and by stains for axons, such as neurofilament immunohistochemistry. Myelinated axons have larger calibers on cross sections and are distributed individually throughout the EN, while unmyelinated axons are seen as small vacuoles grouped together **(Figs. 9-3 and 9-8)**.

In spite of the presence of many *fiber types* with detailed features,[21] recognition of three major types of fibers is important for practical diagnostic purposes[108] **(Fig. 9-3)**. Various disorders tend to preferentially affect different types of fibers **(Fig. 9-22)**. For instance, diabetes mellitus, in its different clinicopathologic presentations, can be associated with the involvement of unmyelinated fibers, a mixture of small and large myelinated fibers or large myelinated fibers.[109] Tangier disease and autonomic disorders tend to show a preferential loss of small myelinated fibers and unmyelinated fibers,[110] while predominantly large myelinated fibers are lost in CMT type X,[111] mitochondrial disorders affecting the peripheral nervous system,[112] Friedreich ataxia,[113] thalidomide toxicity,[114] vitamin E deficiency,[115] and abetalipoproteinemia (Bassen-Kornzweig disease).[116] Small myelinated fibers are preferentially lost in HSAN.[117] Small myelinated fibers tend to be relatively preserved, while large myelinated fibers and unmyelinated fiber loss are more prominent in Chediak-Higashi syndrome.[60] Antiretroviral medications may result in a preferential loss of unmyelinated fibers.[118] The evaluation of small myelinated fibers and unmyelinated fibers has been facilitated by the introduction of *skin biopsy*, which allows for the evaluation of unmyelinated fibers innervating the epidermis, large myelinated fibers of the corpuscles, and the autonomic fibers of the sweat glands, blood vessels, and arrectores pilorum muscles. The more common *small fiber neuropathies* that can be investigated this way are diabetic neuropathy, amyloid neuropathy, idiopathic distal sensory neuropathy, inherited neuropathies, HIV-associated neuropathy, and immune-mediated neuropathies. The technique involves immunohistochemical staining of frozen sections of the skin sample with PGP9.5 and quantitative and qualitative evaluation of the nerve

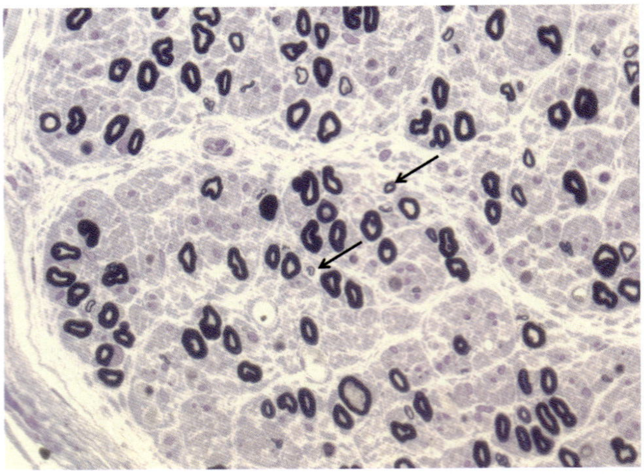

Figure 9-22. Preferential loss of small myelinated fibers: Almost all remaining myelinated fibers are large myelinated fibers, and only a rare residual small myelinated fiber (*arrows*) can be identified. There appear to be many unmyelinated fibers in the background, but this is difficult to evaluate without electron microscopy (Toluidine blue–stained semi-thin epoxy-resin section; original magnification: 400×).

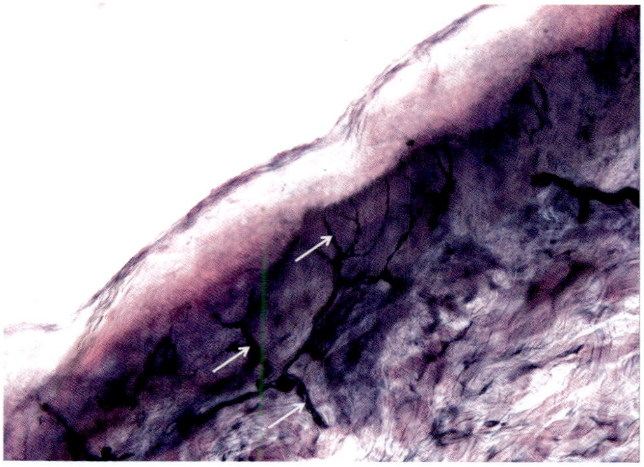

Figure 9-23. Intraepidermal nerve fibers: This frozen section of skin biopsy specimen shows the intraepidermal nerve fibers (*arrows*), which are unremarkable in this case. Their quantitative and qualitative changes can provide valuable information about many diseases, especially small fiber neuropathies (PGP 9.5 immunohistochemistry; original magnification: 200×). (Courtesy of Sakir Humayun Gultekin, M.D., Oregon Health & Science University, Portland, OR.)

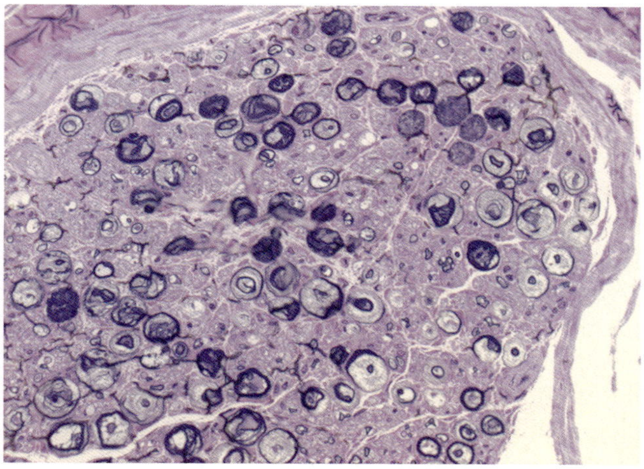

Figure 9-24. Myelin artifact: Delayed or improper fixation and mechanical factors such as poor tissue handling with stretching and crushing of nerve fibers result in this type of smudgy and disintegrated myelin sheaths, which may be difficult at times to distinguish from actual pathologic change (Toluidine blue–stained semi-thin epoxy-resin section; original magnification: 400×).

fibers **(Fig. 9-23)**.[119,120] Evaluation of nerve fibers in skin biopsy specimens can also be utilized in the diagnosis of many other disorders of the central and peripheral nervous systems as a relatively simple and convenient method.[5,121–124]

Myelin

Myelin sheaths are very prone to artifacts. They can be easily crushed and stretched during handling of the tissue **(Fig. 9-24)**. Herringbone appearance to the myelin can occur as an artifact of fixation. Some myelinated axons may appear to have myelin sheaths undulated in a clover leaf arrangement on semi-thin sections. These represent sections corresponding to the paranodal regions. In contrast to myelin sheath irregularities seen in axonal atrophy (see above), the undulations are very orderly and the axon is not atrophic. *Curved or irregular shapes* to both axons and myelin sheaths are common artifacts, but they may also be deformed by external compressions of individual fibers. In Krabbe disease (globoid cell leukodystrophy), accumulations in Schwann cell cytoplasms result in distortions of fiber contours.[125] Similar accumulations and distortions can be seen with other accumulations, such as in Farber disease, though the accumulations tend to have rounder borders in those cases.[126] Myelin sheaths are generally about the one-third of the thickness of their axon's thickness, expressed as the *g* ratio.[127] Fibers with thin myelin sheaths relative to their axon caliber **(Figs. 9-8, 9-9, and 9-15)** indicate remyelinating axons after an injury. Axons, which are large enough to be myelinated but are without a myelin sheath, indicate myelin loss. They can be difficult to identify due to their pale appearance. Some myelin debris may be present in their Schwann cell cytoplasm. Whether the myelin damage is due to primary demyelination or is secondary to axonal degeneration can be difficult to assess. Many thinly myelinated fibers without axonal degeneration and without significant axon loss favor a primary demyelinating process, also referred to as segmental demyelination. The patchy nature of myelin loss is better appreciated on longitudinal sections with a myelin stain such as Luxol fast blue (LFB), which also highlights the myelin debris in these areas. The axons are relatively preserved, while the myelin sheaths are degenerating or completely lost, as in the demyelinating diseases of the central nervous system (see Chapter 2). Variable numbers of macrophages can be present, containing intracytoplasmic myelin debris. Some axons have thin myelin sheaths relative to their axon caliber, indicating remyelination. Among many diverse causes in addition to the typical demyelinating diseases mentioned above (see macrophages), some toxins, such as diphtheria toxin[128] and hexachlorophene,[129] and hypothyroidism result in demyelination.[130] Longer periods of sustained compression can result in demyelination through ischemia (see "Ischemic Changes" below). *Hypomyelination* refers to the absence of or uniformly thin myelin in axons with a diameter that is large enough to suggest that they should be myelinated. Its uniform appearance throughout the fascicle helps distinguish it from thin myelin sheaths of remyelination, which tends to be heterogeneous within the fascicle. Congenital hypomyelinating neuropathy[131] and Dejerine-Sottas disease are examples where hypomyelinated axons are prominent.[132] Farber disease, a sphingolipidosis, also shows hypomyelination with a preserved fiber density.[21] *Thickening of myelin sheaths or hypermyelination* is a relatively rare occurrence and is seen as a result of increase in the number of myelin lamellae. Hereditary neuropathy with liability to pressure palsies is a hereditary recurrent focal neuropathy. It shows on semi-thin sections a peculiar thickening of myelin sheaths in scattered fibers, characterized by an interwoven appearance to the myelin, described as *"jelly roll"* where myelin layers forming layers on themselves in a spiral fashion. They are seen as sausage-like expansions on longitudinal sections and are called *"tomaculae"* **(Fig. 9-25)**, hence tomaculous neuropathy. Onion bulbs and evidence of demyelination–remyelination are also present (see above). Tomaculae can also be present in other conditions such as CIDP and some cases of CMT, and therefore, specific names should be used to refer to these diseases rather than the descriptive term tomaculous neuropathy.[133,134] Thick myelin can also be seen in association with paraproteinemic neuropathy[135] and in some HMSN.[136] Another descriptive terminology is hereditary neuropathy with focally folded myelin, where irregular folds and undulations of myelin sheaths are present.[137] Myelin folding can also be seen in some types of CMT disease.[138,139] Myelin sheaths may have a *collapsed and wrinkled appearance* when their axon becomes atrophic (see above Axonal Atrophy). The myelin sheaths of occasional axons can show a *double-barrel appearance*, as though there are two concentric layers of myelin. This may be an artifact, but it likely also represents the Schmidt-Lanterman incisures **(Fig. 9-3)**, a normal structure that provides connection between the inner and outer Schwann cell compartments through the myelin sheath. *Pale-staining myelin sheaths* on semi-thin sections may be due to abnormal myelin periodicity, described as widely spaced myelin by electron microscopy, which is required for definitive identification. While it is most commonly known to be associated with Waldenstrom's macroglobulinemia,[140] where IgM can be shown in the myelin sheaths by immunostains, it can also be associated with IgG,[141] Guillain-Barré syndrome, and CIDP.[142]

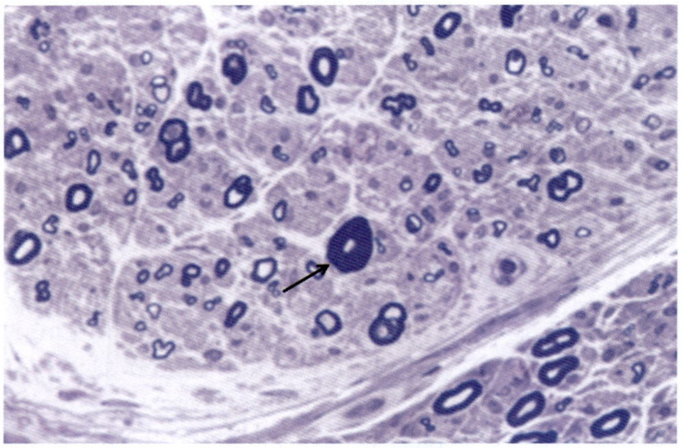

Figure 9-25. Tomaculous neuropathy: A hypermyelinated fiber (*arrow*) with a myelin sheath that is very thick for its axon caliber (tomaculum) is seen (Toluidine blue–stained semi-thin epoxy-resin section; original magnification: 400×).

Mixed Patterns and Other Features

In many situations, especially those that have a progressive or chronic course, both *demyelination and remyelination*, or both *axonal degeneration and regeneration*, can be seen. Especially in axonopathies, in addition to axonal degeneration, remyelination of the regenerating axons can result in a confusing picture. The identification of the primary process may be very difficult in such cases. In long-standing demyelinating conditions, some degree of axon loss will eventually occur in axons that are devoid of their myelin sheaths for long periods of time. *Ongoing demyelination and active axonal degeneration* can coexist in some diverse disorders such as cerebrotendinous xanthomatosis;[143] HTLV-1 infection;[144] dysproteinemic neuropathy;[21] toxicity of gold,[145] disulfiram,[146] metronidazole,[147] and perhexiline;[148] and mitochondrial neurogastrointestinal encephalomyopathy.[149]

Unmyelinated axons can be identified but are relatively difficult to evaluate by light microscopy **(Figs. 9-3 and 9-8)** and commonly require electron microscopy for appropriate evaluation. Their loss is commonly seen in autonomic neuropathies,[150] and the structures termed collagen pockets, an electron microscopic finding referring to Schwann cell cytoplasmic processes encircling collagen instead of unmyelinated fibers in cases of significant unmyelinated axon loss, can be mistaken for unremarkable population of unmyelinated fibers on semi-thin sections even when using immersion oil.

Ischemic changes in the nerve result from vascular insufficiency due to partial or complete blockage of blood supply, the latter resulting in frank infarcts. Notable causes are diabetic vascular changes and vasculitic (including sarcoidosis—see above) **(Fig. 9-26)** or occlusive, for example, embolic or cryoglobulinemic.[151] Focal ischemia can occur as a result of compression, such as the brief episodes of limbs falling asleep, and do not result in clinical problems and biopsy procedures. Longer and sustained compression and ischemia can cause a myelin loss, which can heal over time. Even longer exposure to such compressive ischemia can result in the infarct of the nerve. An *asymmetrical, uneven, or heterogeneous involvement of adjacent fascicles* by fiber loss at a given level is typically due to focal lesions at that level or at a higher level. The most notable process that can result in this type of heterogeneous involvement is vasculitis. This is best appreciated on semi-thin sections that show multiple adjacent fascicles. It is even possible to see the partial involvement of single fascicles in some cases **(Fig. 9-27)**. Some degree of fiber density variation can be seen among fascicles with increasing age[26] as well as in association with compression neuropathies.[152] It is also seen in vasculopathies with associated hypoxic–ischemic injury to the nerve as well as with dysproteinemic neuropathies.[21] *End-stage nerve* is an entirely devastated nerve with essentially no residual axons, or any clues to the pathologic process are left to diagnose **(Fig. 9-28)**. *Developing nerve*[12,21] from fetal autopsies is essentially completely devoid of any myelin sheaths and may appear like end-stage nerve to the unwary.

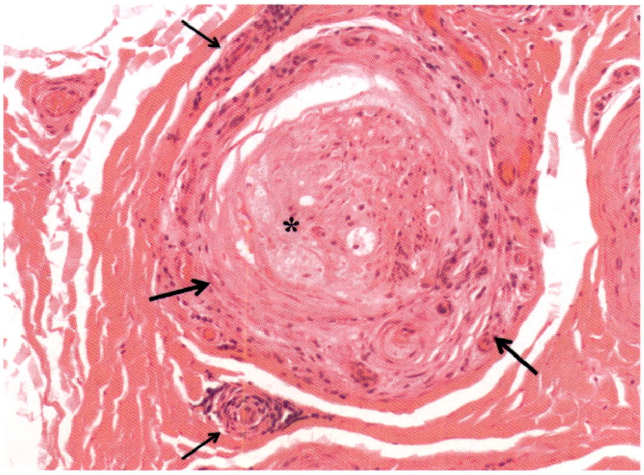

Figure 9-26. Ischemic changes: Almost one-half of this fascicle shows infarct (*asterisk*). Epineurial vessels (*thin arrows*) have perivascular inflammation that infiltrates the vessel wall, with a fibrin thrombus in the lumen of the bottom one. Perineurium (*thick arrows*) is thick (H&E; original magnification: 200×).

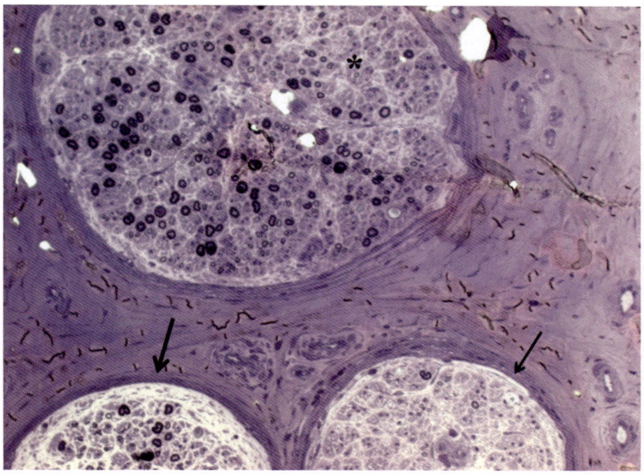

Figure 9-27. Uneven involvement of fascicles: Of the three fascicles in this picture, the large one at the top has the least fiber loss, while another one (*thin arrow*) is completely wiped-out of myelinated fibers and yet another (*thick arrow*) is moderately involved. In addition, a part of the larger fascicle at the top (*asterisk*) is involved more than the rest of that fascicle (Toluidine blue–stained semi-thin epoxy-resin section; original magnification: 400×).

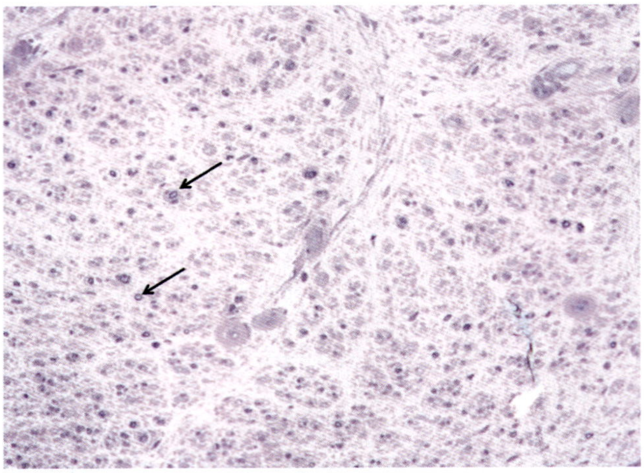

Figure 9-28. End-stage nerve: The entire fascicle is devastated with only a rare small myelinated fiber remaining (*arrows*), and no clues to the pathologic process can be obtained (Toluidine blue–stained semi-thin epoxy-resin section; original magnification: 400x).

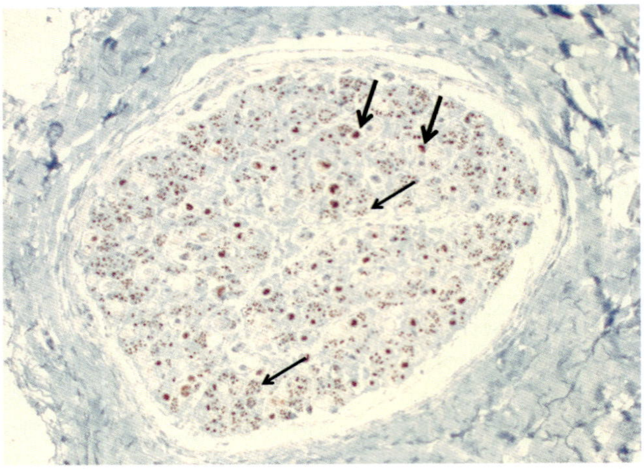

Figure 9-29. Evaluation of axons by special stains: It is possible to have an idea about the axons and myelin if semi-thin sections are not available or will be delayed. By neurofilament immunohistochemistry, individually placed large caliber axons (*thick arrows*) represent myelinated fibers, although further characterization of their size is difficult. Smaller ones arranged in groups (*thin arrows*) are unmyelinated fibers. Based on this picture, there appears to be a prominent loss of myelinated fibers (Neurofilament immunohistochemistry; original magnification: 200×).

Special Studies

A variety of *techniques and special stains* are used to obtain the most information;[1] some are standard general pathology techniques and some are special to peripheral nerve specimens. *Histochemical stains* are mainly done to evaluate myelin loss and myelin debris most commonly with LFB/PAS/cresyl violet (CV), while an axon stain such as Bielschowsky silver stain helps with the evaluation of axonal loss, irregularities, or relative preservation of axons. The same can also be done by neurofilament immunohistochemistry **(Fig. 9-29)**. Unless a cocktail antibody is utilized, high molecular weight (200 kDa) neurofilament should be used since this type of neurofilament is the most prominent in the axons (see Chapter 6). Trichrome stain and especially Goldner or Gomori trichrome stains can help highlight myelin sheaths on paraffin sections, in addition to evaluation of collagen. An elastic tissue stain such as Verhoeff-van Gieson is useful in the evaluation of vessels. Congo red stain for amyloid and its evaluation using polarized light are useful for the initial screening for amyloid. Stains for microorganisms are utilized as needed. *Immunohistochemical stains* to further characterize amyloid types, identify inflammatory cells and their subpopulations, as well as to work up potentially neoplastic populations are used as in other areas of diagnostic neuropathology. Although resorting to special stains is usually not needed to identify endoneurial lymphocytes as they are prominent when they are in numbers that are of clinical significance, in a rare case, CD45RB (LCA; leukocyte common antigen) can be utilized. The identification of more than three to four LCA-positive endoneurial cells per fascicle on cross section should be considered abnormal.[2] S-100 protein, collagen type IV, and EMA are useful for the Schwann cells and perineurial cells. *Immunofluorescence microscopy* or immunohistochemistry[153] for immunoglobulin heavy and light chains is useful in the evaluation of dysproteinemic neuropathy. Toluidine blue and lipid stains can be utilized on frozen sections as needed in search for various metachromatic or lipid accumulations, respectively. Toluidine blue is also the stain of choice for the epoxy-resin semithin sections. *Electron microscopic techniques* and findings, as important, valuable, and standard as they are in the evaluation of peripheral nerve tissue, are not included in this discussion, which is limited to light microscopic findings consistent with the scope of this text.

References

1. Dawson TP, Neal JW, Llewellyn L, et al. *Neuropathology Techniques*. London: Arnold; 2003.

2. Bilbao JM. Peripheral nerves. In: Rosai J, ed. *Rosai and Ackerman's Surgical Pathology*. 9th. ed. Vol. 2, Edinburgh, UK: Mosby; 2004:2623–2662.

3. Gabriel C, Howard R, Kinsella N, et al. Prospective study of the usefulness of sural nerve biopsy. *J Neurol Neurosurg Psychiatry*. 2000;69:442–446.

4. Midroni G, Bilbao J. *Biopsy Diagnosis of Peripheral Neuropathy*. Boston, MA: Butterworth-Heinemann; 1995.

5. Goebel HH. Extracerebral biopsies in neurodegenerative diseases of childhood. *Brain Dev*. 1999;21:435–443.

6. Sommer C, Galbraith JA, Heckman HM, et al. Pathology of experimental compression neuropathy producing hyperesthesia. *J Neuropathol Exp Neurol*. 1993;52:223–233.

7. Hall SM. Regeneration in the peripheral nervous system. *Neuropathol Appl Neurobiol*. 1989;15:513–529.

8. Tzourio C, Said G, Millan J. Asymptomatic nerve hypertrophy in lepromatous leprosy: a clinical, electrophysiological and morphological study. *J Neurol*. 1992;239:367–374.

9. Bourque CN, Anderson BA, Martin del Campo C, et al. Sensorimotor perineuritis—an autoimmune disease? *Can J Neurol Sci*. 1985;12:129–133.

10. Hill RE, Williams PE. Perineurial cell basement membrane thickening and myelinated nerve fibre loss in diabetic and nondiabetic peripheral nerve. *J Neurol Sci*. 2004;217:157–163.

11. Agarwal V, Singh R, Wiclaf, et al. A clinical, electrophysiological, and pathological study of neuropathy in rheumatoid arthritis. *Clin Rheumatol*. 2008;27:841–844.

12. King RH. *Atlas of Peripheral Nerve Pathology*. London, UK: Arnold; 1999.

13. Peltonen JT, Kalliomaki MA, Muona PK. Extracellular matrix of peripheral nerves in diabetes. *J Peripher Nerv Syst*. 1997;2:213–226.

14. Lassmann G, Lassmann H, Stockinger L. Morton's metatarsalgia. Light and electron microscopic observations and their relation to entrapment neuropathies. *Virchows Arch A Pathol Anat Histol*. 1976;370:307–321.

15. King RH, Llewelyn JG, Thomas PK, et al. Perineurial calcification. *Neuropathol Appl Neurobiol*. 1988;14:105–123.

16. Sima AA, Robertson DM. Involvement of peripheral nerve and muscle in Fabry's disease. Histologic, ultrastructural, and morphometric studies. *Arch Neurol*. 1978;35:291–301.

17. Van Lis JM, Jennekens FG, Veldman H. Calcium deposits in the perineurium and their relation to lipid accumulation. *J Neurol Sci*. 1979;43:367–375.

18. Kulkarni GB, Mahadevan A, Taly AB, et al. Sural nerve biopsy in chronic inflammatory demyelinating polyneuropathy: are supportive pathologic criteria useful in diagnosis?. *Neurol India*. 2010;58:542–548.

19. Asbury AK. Renaut bodies. A forgotten endoneurial structure. *J Neuropathol Exp Neurol*. 1973;32:334–343.

20. Jefferson D, Neary D, Eames RA. Renaut body distribution at sites of human peripheral nerve entrapment. *J Neurol Sci*. 1981;49:19–29.

21. Bilbao JM, Schmidt R, Hawkins C. Diseases of peripheral nerve. In: Love S, Louis DN, Ellison DW, eds. *Greenfield's Neuropathology*. 8th ed. Vol. 2, London, UK: Hodder Arnold; 2008:1609–1724.

22. Simmons Z, Specht CS. The neuromuscular manifestations of amyloidosis. *J Clin Neuromuscul Dis*. 2010;11:145–157.

23. Grassi F, Clerici C, Perin M, et al. Light chain deposition disease neuropathy resembling amyloid neuropathy in a multiple myeloma patient. *Ital J Neurol Sci*. 1998;19:229–233.

24. Malandrini A, Guazzi GC, Alessandrini C, et al. Peripheral nerve involvement in ataxia telangiectasia: histological and ultrastructural studies of peroneal nerve biopsy in two cases. *Clin Neuropathol*. 1990;9:109–114.

25. Prineas JW, McLeod JG. Chronic relapsing polyneuritis. *J Neurol Sci*. 1976;27:427–458.

26. Johnson PC. Peripheral nerve. In: Davis RD, Robertson DM, eds. *Textbook of Neuropathology*. Baltimore, MD: Williams & Wilkins; 1997:1233–1323.

27. Keller MP, Chance PF. Inherited peripheral neuropathy. *Semin Neurol*. 1999;19:353–362.

28. Wadwekar V, Kalita J, Misra UK. Does the chronic inflammatory demyelinating polyradiculoneuropathy due to secondary cause differ from primary? *Neurol India*. 2011;59: 664–668.

29. Vital A, Lagueny A, Ferrer X, et al. Sarcoid neuropathy: clinico-pathological study of 4 new cases and review of the literature. *Clin Neuropathol*. 2008;27:96–105.

30. Wilson JR, Conwit RA, Eidelman BH, et al. Sensorimotor neuropathy resembling CIDP in patients receiving FK506. *Muscle Nerve*. 1994;17:528–532.

31. Ohnishi A, Dyck PJ. Retardation of Schwann cell division and axonal regrowth following nerve crush in experimental lead neuropathy. *Ann Neurol*. 1981;10:469–477.

32. Said G. Fusiform enlargement of mechanic origin of a peripheral nerve. *Acta Neuropathol*. 1976;35:47–54.

33. Ohori N, Yamashita Y, Ohnishi A. A case of adult cerebral X-linked adrenoleukodystrophy (X-ALD) accompanying typical hypertrophic neuropathy with marked onion-bulb formation. *Rinsho Shinkeigaku Clin Neurol*. 1999;39:1144–1146.

34. Fidzianska A, Drac H, Rafalowska J. Phenomenon of Schwann cell apoptosis in a case of congenital hypomyelinating neuropathy with basal lamina onion bulb formation. *Brain Dev*. 2002;24:727–731.

35. Boyanton BL Jr, Jones JK, Shenaq SM, et al. Intraneural perineurioma: a systematic review with illustrative cases. *Arch Pathol Lab Med*. 2007;131:1382–1392.

36. Tsang WY, Chan JK, Chow LT, et al. Perineurioma: an uncommon soft tissue neoplasm distinct from localized hypertrophic neuropathy and neurofibroma. *Am J Surg Pathol*. 1992;16:756–763.

37. Young RR, Asbury AK, Adams RD, et al. Pure pan-dysautonomia with recovery. *Trans Am Neurol Assoc*. 1969;94:355–357.

38. Young RR, Asbury AK, Corbett JL, et al. Pure pan-dysautonomia with recovery. Description and discussion of diagnostic criteria. *Brain*. 1975;98:613–636.

39. Cornblath DR, McArthur JC, Kennedy PG, et al. Inflammatory demyelinating peripheral neuropathies associated with human T-cell lymphotropic virus type III infection. *Ann Neurol*. 1987;21:32–40.

40. Hughes RA, Allen D, Makowska A, et al. Pathogenesis of chronic inflammatory demyelinating polyradiculoneuropathy. *J Peripher Nerv Syst*. 2006;11:30–46.

41. de la Monte SM, Gabuzda DH, Ho DD, et al. Peripheral neuropathy in the acquired immunodeficiency syndrome. *Ann Neurol*. 1988;23:485–492.

42. Winer JB. Guillain-Barré syndrome. *Mol Pathol*. 2001;54:381–385.

43. Vucic S, Kiernan MC, Cornblath DR. Guillain-Barré syndrome: an update. *J Clin Neurosci*. 2009;16:733–741.

44. Peltier AC, Russell JW. Recent advances in drug-induced neuropathies. *Curr Opin Neurol*. 2002;15:633–638.

45. Correale J, Monteverde DA, Bueri JA, et al. Peripheral nervous system and spinal cord involvement in lymphoma. *Acta Neurol Scand*. 1991;83:45–51.

46. Seffo F, Daw HA. Non-Hodgkin lymphoma and Guillain-Barré syndrome: a rare association. *Clin Advan Hematol Oncol*. 2010;8:201–203.

47. D'Arena G, Vigliotti ML, Pizza V, et al. Guillain-Barré syndrome complicating mobilization therapy in a case of B-cell chronic lymphocytic leukemia. *Leuk Lymph*. 2004;45: 1489–1490.

48. Melguizo I, Gilbert M, Tummala S. Guillain-Barré syndrome and glioblastoma. *J Neurooncol*. 2011;104:371–373.

49. Suneetha S, Arunthathi S, Kurian N, et al. Histological changes in the nerve, skin and nasal mucosa of patients with primary neuritic leprosy. *Acta Leprol*. 2000–2001;12:11–18.

50. Thomas PK, Walker JG. Xanthomatous neuropathy in primary biliary cirrhosis. *Brain*. 1965;88:1079–1088.

51. Ludwig J. Xanthomatous neuropathy associated with hyperlipidemia. (Letter) *Hum Pathol*. 1994;25:215.

52. Thomas PK. Inherited neuropathies related to disorders of lipid metabolism. *Advan Neurol*. 1988;48:133–144.

53. Jennette JC, Thomas DB, Falk RJ. Microscopic polyangiitis (microscopic polyarteritis). *Semin Diag Pathol*. 2001;18:3–13.

54. Lacroix C, Lozeron P, Ferreira A, et al. Peripheral neuropathy due to necrotizing arteritis (NA) in non-connective tissue disorders (NCTD): a clinicopathological study. *J Neurol*. 2003;250(suppl 2):25.

55. Said G, Lacroix C. Primary and secondary vasculitic neuropathy. *J Neurol*. 2005;252:633–641.

56. Mitchell RN, Schoen FJ. Blood vessels. In: Kumar V, Abbas AK, FaustoN, Aster JC, eds. *Robbins and Cotran Pathologic basis of Disease*. 8th ed. Philadelphia, PA: Saunders; 2010:487–528.

57. Collins MP, Dyck PJ, Gronseth GS, et al. Peripheral Nerve Society. Peripheral Nerve Society Guideline on the classification, diagnosis, investigation, and immunosuppressive therapy of non-systemic vasculitic neuropathy: executive summary. *J Peripher Nerv Syst*. 2010;15:176–184.

58. Vrancken AF, Gathier CS, Cats EA, et al. The additional yield of combined nerve/muscle biopsy in vasculitic neuropathy. *Eur J Neurol*. 2011;18:49–58.

59. Said G, Lacroix-Ciaudo C, Fujimura H, et al. The peripheral neuropathy of necrotizing arteritis: a clinicopathological study. *Ann Neurol*. 1988;23:461–465.

60. Misra VP, King RHM, Harding AE, et al. Peripheral neuropathy in the Chediak-Higashi syndrome. *Acta Neuropathol (Berlin)*. 1991;81:354–358.

61. Baehring JM, Damek D, Martin EC, et al. Neurolymphomatosis. *Neuro-Oncol*. 2003;5:104–115.

62. Sinha S, Mahadevan A, Lokesh L, et al. Tangier disease—a diagnostic challenge in countries endemic for leprosy. *J Neurol Neurosurg Psych*. 2004;75:301–304.

63. Fazio R, Nemni R, Quattrini A, et al. Acute presentation of Tangier polyneuropathy: a clinical and morphological study. *Acta Neuropathol*. 1993;86:90–94.

64. Pollard JD, McLeod JG, Honnibal TG, et al. Hypothyroid polyneuropathy. Clinical, electrophysiological and nerve biopsy findings in two cases. *J Neurol Sci*. 1982;53:461–471.

65. Asbury AK, Cox SC, Baringer JR. The significance of giant vacuolation of endoneurial fibroblasts. *Acta Neuropathol*. 1971;18:123–131.

66. Ohkawa S. Activation of human monocytes in leprosy. *Microbiol Immunol*. 1985;29:265–274.

67. Meier C, Bischoff A. Sequence of morphological alterations in the nervous system of metachromatic leukodystrophy. Light- and electron microscopic observations in the central and peripheral nervous system in a prenatally diagnosed foetus of 22 weeks. *Acta Neuropathol*. 1976;36:369–379.

68. Sung JH, Meyers JP, Stadlan EM, et al. Neuropathological changes in Chediak-Higashi disease. *J Neuropathol Exp Neurol*. 1969;28:86–118.

69. Jacobs JM, Love S. Qualitative and quantitative morphology of human sural nerve at different ages. *Brain*. 1985;108:897–924.

70. Powell HC, Rosoff J, Myers RR. Microangiopathy in human diabetic neuropathy. *Acta Neuropathol*. 1985;68:295–305.

71. Bradley J, Thomas PK, King RH, et al. Morphometry of endoneurial capillaries in diabetic sensory and autonomic neuropathy. *Diabetologia*. 1990;33:611–618.

72. Prayson RA, Sedlock DJ. Clinicopathologic study of 43 patients with sural nerve vasculitis. *Hum Pathol*. 2003;34:484–490.

73. Schmidt B, Toyka KV, Kiefer R, et al. Inflammatory infiltrates in sural nerve biopsies in Guillain-Barré syndrome and chronic inflammatory demyelinating neuropathy. *Muscle Nerve*. 1996;19:474–487.

74. Terrier B, Lacroix C, Guillevin L, et al. Diagnostic and prognostic relevance of neuromuscular biopsy in primary Sjogren's syndrome-related neuropathy. *Club Rhumatismes et Inflammation Arthritis Rheum*. 2007;57:1520–1529.

75. Kelkar P, Masood M, Parry GJ. Distinctive pathologic findings in proximal diabetic neuropathy (diabetic amyotrophy). *Neurology*. 2000;55:83–88.

76. Gherardi R, Belec L, Mhiri C, et al. The spectrum of vasculitis in human immunodeficiency virus-infected patients. A clinicopathologic evaluation. *Arthritis Rheum*. 1993;36:1164–1174.

77. Chahin N, Temesgen Z, Kurtin PJ, et al. HIV lumbosacral radiculoplexus neuropathy mimicking lymphoma: diffuse infiltrative lymphocytosis syndrome (DILS) restricted to nerve?. *Muscle Nerve*. 2010;41:276–282.

78. Meier C, Grahmann F, Engelhardt A, et al. Peripheral nerve disorders in Lyme-Borreliosis. Nerve biopsy studies from eight cases. *Acta Neuropathol*. 1989;79:271–278.

79. Elamin M, Alderazi Y, Mullins G, et al. Perineuritis in acute lyme neuroborreliosis. *Muscle Nerve*. 2009;39:851–854.

80. Ricoy JR, Cabello A, Rodriguez J, et al. Neuropathological studies on the toxic syndrome related to adulterated rapeseed oil in Spain. *Brain*. 1983;106:817–835.

81. Mateo IM, Izquierdo M, Fernandez-Dapica MP, et al. Toxic epidemic syndrome: musculoskeletal manifestations. *J Rheumatol*. 1984;11:333–338.

82. Altenkirch H, Stoltenburg-Didinger G, Koeppel C. The neurotoxicological aspects of the toxic oil syndrome (TOS) in Spain. *Toxicology*. 1988;49:25–34.

83. Kanda T. Usefulness of sural nerve biopsy in the genomic era. *Neuropathology*. 2009;29:502–508.

84. Cornford ME, Ho HW, Vinters HV. Correlation of neuromuscular pathology in acquired immune deficiency syndrome patients with cytomegalovirus infection and zidovudine treatment. *Acta Neuropathol*. 1992;84:516–529.

85. Strole WE Jr, Clark WH Jr, Isselbacher KJ. Progressive arterial occlusive disease (Kohlmeier-Degos). A frequently fatal cutaneosystemic disorder. *New Engl J Med*. 1967;276: 195–201.

86. Asbury AK, Johnson PC. Pathology of peripheral nerve. In: Bennington JL, Series ed. *Major Problems in Pathology*. Vol. 9, Philadelphia, PA: W.B. Saunders; 1978.

87. Pellissier JF, Van Hoof F, Bourdet-Bonerandi D, et al. Morphological and biochemical changes in muscle and peripheral nerve in Fabry's disease. *Muscle Nerve*. 1981;4:381–387.

88. Schroder JM, Zuchner S, Dichgans M, et al. Peripheral nerve and skeletal muscle involvement in CADASIL. *Acta Neuropathol*. 2005;110:587–599.

89. King RH, Llewelyn JG, Thomas PK, et al. Diabetic neuropathy: abnormalities of Schwann cell and perineurial basal laminae. Implications for diabetic vasculopathy. *Neuropathol Appl Neurobiol*. 1989;15:339–355.

90. Albers JW, Fink JK. Porphyric neuropathy. *Muscle Nerve*. 2004;30:410–422.

91. Lin CS, Lee MJ, Park SB, et al. Purple pigments: the pathophysiology of acute porphyric neuropathy. *Clin Neurophysiol*. 2011;122:2336–2344.

92. Mahadevan A, Santosh V, Gayatri N, et al. Infantile neuroaxonal dystrophy and giant axonal neuropathy—overlap diseases of neuronal cytoskeletal elements in childhood? *Clin Neuropathol*. 2000;19:221–229.

93. Nafe R, Trollmann R, Schlote W. The giant axonal neuropathy—clinical and histological aspects, differential diagnosis and a new case. *Clin Neuropathol*. 2001;20:200–211.

94. Bergouignan FX, Vital C, Henry P, et al. Disulfiram neuropathy. *J Neurol*. 1988;235:382–338.

95. Duncan C, Strub R, McGarry P, et al. Peripheral nerve biopsy as an aid to diagnosis in infantile neuroaxonal dystrophy. *Neurology*. 1970;20:1024–1032.

96. Hahn AF, Gilbert JJ, Kwarciak C, et al. Nerve biopsy findings in Niemann-Pick type II (NPC). *Acta Neuropathol*. 1994;87:149–154.

97. Milde P, Guccion JG, Kelly J, et al. Adult polyglucosan body disease. *Arch Pathol Lab Med*. 2001;125:519–522.

98. Tay SK, Akman HO, Chung WK, et al. Fatal infantile neuromuscular presentation of glycogen storage disease type IV. *Neuromuscul Disord*. 2004;14:253–260.

99. Cavanagh JB. Corpora amylacea and the family of polyglucosan diseases. *Brain Res Rev*. 1999;29:265–295.

100. Ugawa Y, Inoue K, Takemura T, et al. Accumulation of glycogen in sural nerve axons in adult-onset type III glycogenosis. *Ann Neurol*. 1986;19:294–297.

101. Altenkirch H, Mager J, Stoltenburg G, et al. Toxic polyneuropathies after sniffing a glue thinner. *J Neurol*. 1977;214:137–152.

102. Escobar A, Aruffo C. Chronic thinner intoxication: clinico-pathologic report of a human case. *J Neurol Neurosurg Psych*. 1980;43:986–994.

103. Hahn AF. Hereditary motor and sensory neuropathy: HMSN type II (neuronal type) and X-linked HMSN. *Brain Pathol*. 1993;3:147–155.

104. Rotthier A, Baets J, De Vriendt E, et al. Genes for hereditary sensory and autonomic neuropathies: a genotype-phenotype correlation. *Brain*. 2009;132:2699–2711.

105. Koeppen AH, Morral JA, Davis AN, et al. The dorsal root ganglion in Friedreich's ataxia. *Acta Neuropathol*. 2009;118:763–776.

106. Ahonen RE. Peripheral neuropathy in uremic patients and in renal transplant recipients. *Acta Neuropathol*. 1981;54:43–53.

107. Fuller GN, Jacobs JM, Guiloff RJ. Nature and incidence of peripheral nerve syndromes in HIV infection. *J Neurol Neurosurg Psych*. 1993;56:372–381.

108. Cohen ML. Skeletal muscle and peripheral nerve disorders. In: Prayson RA, ed. *Neuropathology*. Philadelphia, PA: Elsevier; 2005:537–581.

109. Zochodne DW. Diabetic neuropathies: features and mechanisms. *Brain Pathol*. 1999;9:369–391.

110. Gibbels E, Schaefer HE, Runne U, et al. Severe polyneuropathy in Tangier disease mimicking syringomyelia or leprosy. Clinical, biochemical, electrophysiological, and morphological evaluation, including electron microscopy of nerve, muscle, and skin biopsies. *J Neurol*. 1985;232:283–294.

111. Capasso M, Di Muzio A, Ferrarini M, et al. Internerves and intra-nerve conduction heterogeneity in CMTX with Arg(15)Gln mutation. *Clin Neurophysiol*. 2004;115:64–70.

112. Chu CC, Huang CC, Fang W, et al. Peripheral neuropathy in mitochondrial encephalomyopathies. *Eur Neurol*. 1997;37:110–115.

113. Zouari M, Feki M, Ben Hamida C, et al. Electrophysiology and nerve biopsy: comparative study in Friedreich's ataxia and Friedreich's ataxia phenotype with vitamin E deficiency. *Neuromus Disord*. 1998;8:416–425.

114. Chaudhry V, Cornblath DR, Corse A, et al. Thalidomide-induced neuropathy. *Neurology*. 2002;59:1872–1875.

115. Puri V, Chaudhry N, Tatke M, et al. Isolated vitamin E deficiency with demyelinating neuropathy. *Muscle Nerve*. 2005;32:230–235.

116. Hirsch E, Simon M, Villemin B, et al. Role of the electrophysiologic examination in the diagnosis of Bassen-Kornzweig syndrome. *Neurophysiol Clin*. 1988;18:469–475.

117. Esteban-Garcia A, Salinero-Paniagua E, Traba A, et al. Hereditary sensory and autonomic neuropaties. The neurophysiological and pathological aspects of two cases with congenital insensitivity to pain. *Revista de Neurologia*. 2004;39:525–529.

118. Pardo CA, McArthur JC, Griffin JW. HIV neuropathy: insights in the pathology of HIV peripheral nerve disease. *J Peripher Nerv Syst*. 2001;6:21–27.

119. Devigili G, Tugnoli V, Penza P, et al. The diagnostic criteria for small fibre neuropathy: from symptoms to neuropathology. *Brain*. 2008;131:1912–1925.

120. Lauria G, Lombardi R, Camozzi F, et al. Skin biopsy for the diagnosis of peripheral neuropathy. *Histopathology*. 2009;54: 273–285.

121. Arsenio-Nunes ML, Goutieres F, Aicardi J. An ultramicroscopic study of skin and conjunctival biopsies in chronic neurological disorders of childhood. *Ann Neurol*. 1981;9:163–173.

122. Kimura S. Sasaki Y. Warlo I, et al. Axonal pathology of the skin in infantile neuroaxonal dystrophy. *Acta Neuropathol*. 1987;75:212–215.

123. Malandrini A, Gaudiano C, Gambelli S, et al. Diagnostic value of ultrastructural skin biopsy studies in CADASIL. *Neurology*. 2007;68:1430–1432.

124. Ikemura M, Saito Y, Sengoku R, et al. Lewy body pathology involves cutaneous nerves. *J Neuropathol Exp Neurol*. 2008;67:945–953.

125. Thomas PK, Halpern JP, King RHM, et al. Galactosylceramide lipidosis: novel presentation as a slowly progressive spinocerebellar degeneration. *Ann Neurol*. 1984;16: 618–620.

126. Vital C, Battin J, Rivel J, et al. Aspects ultrastructuraux des lesions du nerf peripherique dans un cas de maladie de Farber. *Revue Neurologique (Paris)*. 1976;132: 419–423.

127. Schmitt F, Bear R. The optical properties of vertebrate nerve axons as related to fiber size. *J Cell Comp Physiol*. 1937;9:261–273.

128. Solders G, Nennesmo I, Persson A. Diphtheritic neuropathy, an analysis based on muscle and nerve biopsy and repeated neurophysiological and autonomic function tests. *J Neurol Neurosurg Psych*. 1989;52:876–880.

129. Pleasure D, Towfighi J, Silberberg D, et al. The pathogenesis of hexachlorophene neuropathy: in vivo and in vitro studies. *Neurology*. 1974;24:1068–1075.

130. Shirabe T, Tawara S, Terao A, et al. Myxoedematous polyneuropathy: a light and electron microscopic study of the peripheral nerve and muscle. *J Neurol Neurosurg Psych*. 1975;38:241–247.

131. Kochanski A, Drac H, Kabzinska D, et al. A novel MPZ gene mutation in congenital neuropathy with hypomyelination. *Neurology*. 2004;62:2122–2123.

132. Guzzetta F, Ferriere G, Lyon G. Congenital hypomyelination polyneuropathy. Pathological findings compared with polyneuropathies starting later in life. *Brain*. 1982;105: 395–416.

133. Adlkofer K, Martini R, Aguzzi A, et al. Hypermyelination and demyelinating peripheral neuropathy in Pmp22-deficient mice. *Nat Genet*. 1995;11:274–280.

134. Adlkofer K, Frei R, Neuberg DH, et al. Heterozygous peripheral myelin protein 22-deficient mice are affected by a progressive demyelinating tomaculous neuropathy. *J Neurosci*. 1997;17:4662–4671.

135. Nardelli E, Pizzighella S, Tridente G, et al. Peripheral neuropathy associated with immunoglobulin disorders an immunological and ultrastructural study. *Acta Neuropathol Suppl*. 1981;7:258–261.

136. Lutschg J, Vassella F, Boltshauser E, et al. Heterogeneity of congenital motor and sensory neuropathies. *Neuropediatrics*. 1985;16:33–38.

137. Houlden H, King RH, Wood NW, et al. Mutations in the 5′ region of the myotubularin-related protein 2 (MTMR2) gene in autosomal recessive hereditary neuropathy with focally folded myelin. *Brain*. 2001;124:907–915.

138. Salih MA, Maisonobe T, Kabiraj M, et al. Autosomal recessive hereditary neuropathy with focally folded myelin sheaths and linked to chromosome 11q23: a distinct and homogeneous entity. *Neuromus Disord*. 2000;10:10–15.

139. Vallat JM, Magy L, Lagrange E, et al. Diagnostic value of ultrastructural nerve examination in Charcot-Marie-Tooth disease: two CMT 1B cases with pseudo-recessive inheritance. *Acta Neuropathol (Berl)*. 2007;113:443–449.

140. Vital C, Vital A, Deminiere C, et al. Myelin modifications in 8 cases of peripheral neuropathy with Waldenstrom's macroglobulinemia and anti-MAG activity. *Ultrastruct Pathol*. 1997;21:509–516.

141. Vallat JM, Magy L, Sindou P, et al. IgG neuropathy: an immunoelectron microscopic study. *J Neuropathol Exp Neurol*. 2005;64:386–390.

142. Vital C, Dumas P, Latinville D, et al. Relapsing inflammatory demyelinating polyneuropathy in a diabetic patient. *Acta Neuropathol*. 1986;71:94–99.

143. Donaghy M, King RH, McKeran RO, et al. Cerebrotendinous xanthomatosis: clinical, electrophysiological and nerve biopsy findings, and response to treatment with chenodeoxycholic acid. *J Neurol*. 1990;237:216–219.

144. Kiwaki T, Umehara F, Arimura Y, et al. The clinical and pathological features of peripheral neuropathy accompanied with HTLV-I associated myelopathy. *J Neurol Sci*. 2003;206:17–21.

145. Katrak SM, Pollock M, O'Brien CP, et al. Clinical and morphological features of gold neuropathy. *Brain*. 1980;103:671–693.

146. Nukada H, Pollock M. Disulfiram neuropathy. A morphometric study of sural nerve. *J Neurol Sci*. 1981;51:51–67.

147. Bradley WG, Karlsson IJ, Rassol CG. Metronidazole neuropathy. *Br Med J*. 1977;2:610–611.

148. Said G. Perhexiline neuropathy: a clinicopathological study. *Ann Neurol*. 1978;3:259–266.

149. Said G, Lacroix C, Plante-Bordeneuve V, et al. Clinicopathological aspects of the neuropathy of neurogastrointestinal encephalomyopathy (MNGIE) in four patients including two with a Charcot-Marie-Tooth presentation. *J Neurol*. 2005;252:655–662.

150. Freeman R. Autonomic peripheral neuropathy. *Neurol Clin*. 2007;25:277–301.

151. Tredici G, Petruccioli MG, Cavaletti G, et al. Sural nerve bioptic findings in essential cryoglobulinemic patients with and without peripheral neuropathy. *Clin Neuropathol*. 1992;11:121–127.

152. MacKinnon SE, Dellon AL, Hudson AR, et al. Chronic human nerve compression. *Neuropathol Appl Neurobiol*. 1986;12: 547–565.

153. Liebert UG, Seitz RJ, Weber T, et al. Immunocytochemical studies of serum proteins and immunoglobulins in human sural nerve biopsies. *Acta Neuropathol*. 1985;68:39–47.

Index

Note: Page numbers in *italics* denote figures; those followed by a t denote tables.

C

D

E

F

G

H

N

R

S

T